Healthcare Documentation:

Fundamentals & Practice
Fourth Edition

Health Professions Institute

Ellen A. Drake, CMT, B.A.

Sally Crenshaw Pitman, M.A.

John H. Dirckx, M.D.

PEARSON

Boston   Columbus   Indianapolis   New York   San Francisco   Upper Saddle River
Amsterdam   Cape Town   Dubai   London   Madrid   Milan   Munich   Paris   Montreal   Toronto
Delhi   Mexico City   Sao Paulo   Sydney   Hong Kong   Seoul   Singapore   Taipei   Tokyo

Publisher: Julie Levin Alexander
Publisher's Assistant: Regina Bruno
Editor-in-Chief: Marlene McHugh Pratt
Executive Editor: Joan Gill
Associate Editor: Bronwen Glowacki
Editorial Assistant: Stephanie Kiel
Director of Marketing: David Gesell
Marketing Manager: Katrin Beacom
Senior Marketing Coordinator: Alicia Wozniak
Marketing Specialist: Michael Sirinides
Marketing Assistant: Crystal Gonzalez
Managing Production Editor: Patrick Walsh

Production Editor: Julie Boddorf
Senior Media Editor: Matt Norris
Media Project Manager: Lorena Cerisano
Manufacturing Manager: Lisa McDowell
Creative Director: Andrea Nix
Senior Art Director: Chris Weigand
Cover Designer: Kevin Kall
Cover Image: YanLev/Shutterstock
Composition: Sally C. Pitman, Health Professions Institute
Printing and Binding: R.R. Donnelley/Willard
Cover Printer: Lehigh-Phoenix Color/Hagerstown

Credits and acknowledgments borrowed from other sources and reproduced, with permission, in this textbook appear on appropriate page within text.

Every effort has been made to provide accurate and current Internet information in this book. However, the Internet and information posted on it are constantly changing, so it is inevitable that some of the Internet addresses listed in this textbook will change.

10 9 8 7 6 5 4 3 2 1

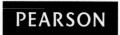

ISBN 13: 978-0-13-298814-8
ISBN 10: 0-13-298814-3

Brief Contents

Contents

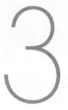

Healthcare Documentation Technology 59

Medical Transcription Practices 78

Perspectives on Style 109

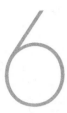

6 Psychiatry 137

7 Dermatology 169

Family Medicine 205

Internal Medicine 247

10 Pulmonary Medicine 301

15

Gastroenterology 511

18 Diagnostic Imaging 621

Preface

Of all the people on the healthcare team, the well-trained, experienced medical transcriptionist (MT) is quite possibly the one nonclinician whose medical knowledge is on par with some of those on the clinical team. That's not to say, of course, that an MT could treat a patient, prescribe medicines, or perform surgery.

We're merely saying that the depth and breadth of medical knowledge acquired by MTs through training and experience allow them to anticipate the diagnostic tests and medications that the physician may order, to readily spot inconsistencies or incongruities in a report, and to use that knowledge to construct a complete and accurate document that is commensurate with the finest patient care.

Indeed, clinical healthcare workers who have transitioned into medical transcription for a variety of reasons almost always exclaim that they had no idea medical transcription was so intense. As technology changes healthcare, the MT's role has evolved and will continue to evolve to keep pace with those changes. In fact, the new title of *healthcare documentation specialist*, established by the Association for Healthcare Documentation Integrity (AHDI), is designed to reflect these changes.

At the heart of all future projected roles for the MT is a solid core of medical knowledge and the critical thinking and problem-solving skills that accompany it. Attaining this level of knowledge as you continue your studies and your career will ensure that there will always be a place for you in the healthcare arena.

Healthcare Documentation: Fundamentals and Practice, 4th edition, is the most comprehensive transcription learning system available in a single package. We've designed this course for learners with no prior experience as well as those looking for refresher training. This course is ideal as a module within programs of medical assisting, medical or legal transcription, and business technology. This course includes a textbook, 10 hours of authentic physician dictation, and additional online study materials. It was written to provide a reasonably priced, comprehensive, authentic training course at a basic or introductory level. It provides a broad overview of medical transcription as a career yet is short and compact enough to be used a stand-alone course or incorporated into other programs as noted above.

Healthcare Documentation: Fundamentals and Practice does not teach medical language, anatomy and physiology, or pathophysiology. Rather, it reviews key knowledge in anatomy, medical vocabulary, clinical medicine, common diseases, diagnostic and surgical procedures, laboratory procedures, and pharmacology. In addition, students will read real-world contributions from experienced medical transcriptionists and physicians who have played important roles in the medical transcription profession. Students will transcribe reports and complete other activities using authentic physician dictation. No other book or course provides such a succinct yet thorough introduction to medical transcription.

Coordinating medical readings with transcription practice in the related specialty or body system is a sound teaching methodology unequaled by other products at this level. This approach was pioneered by Health Professions Institute and has been refined over time to provide medical transcription training that enables students who successfully complete this program to transcribe for physicians and clinics. In addition, it provides a strong foundation for students who want to continue with advanced training in order to qualify to work in acute care and sit for credentialing exams offered by the professional association for medical transcription.

Organization

The textbook is divided informally into three sections. The first part consists of five chapters that present the fundamentals of medical transcription. Chapter 1, Healthcare Documentation Profession, lists prerequisite skills and describes the role of the medical transcriptionist and healthcare documentation specialist as well as provides self-assessment tools for those interested in this career. It discusses the state of the industry from the perspective of leaders in the profession and also reviews medicolegal and ethics considerations and professional and regulatory organizations.

Chapter 2, The Healthcare Record, starts students on their journey to understanding the importance and structure of the medical documents they transcribe. Chapter 3, Healthcare Documentation Technology, provides an overview of digital dictation and transcription, speech recognition technology, the electronic health record, and security and encryption. Chapter 4, Medical Transcription Practices, gets into the nitty gritty of everyday transcription practices including the nuances of interpreting medical dictation, developing research skills, techniques and practices that distinguish editing straight transcription and speech-recognized drafts, and productivity and quality issues. Chapter 5, Perspectives on Style, is a quick-reference style guide that students will be able to use throughout the course to ensure that their transcripts conform to the standards recommended in the AHDI *Book of Style for Medical Transcription*.

The second part of the book consists of 14 chapters, each addressing a medical specialty or body system. The specialty/body system approach for transcription training is a proven effective strategy that incorporates coordinated reading and learning activities with hands-on transcription practice of progressive difficulty. These chapters have been organized in a graduated fashion from the less difficult to the more difficult, both within each individual chapter and so far as possible from chapter to chapter.

Each medical chapter follows a standard outline. Much of the content is specific to the dictations that the student will transcribe after reading the chapter and completing the exercises. Each chapter begins with a brief introduction, an overview of anatomy, a medical vocabulary list with brief definitions, and a feature box that compares lay terms to their medical counterparts.

Medical readings follow; these include an overview of the content of the history and physical examination pertaining to the body system or specialty and common diseases. At the end of each of the medical readings, Pause for Reflection questions enable the student to review and summarize what they have read before going on. The chapters conclude with an overview of diagnostic and surgical procedures, laboratory procedures, and pharmacology, again with an emphasis on content that will be encountered in transcription practice.

Each chapter concludes with transcription tips that specifically relate to typical problems encountered in transcribing the specialty. A special feature of each chapter is the Spotlight that provides students with real-world insights from experienced medical transcriptionists and others in the healthcare documentation field. End-of-chapter exercises and sample reports follow. Finally, the student is directed to the online site for additional audio exercises and transcription practice on authentic physician dictation.

The final chapter, Professional Issues, provides the student with information related to work environments and staying healthy while working. It also includes guidance on job searching, resumé writing, self-assessment and employment tests, and job interviews. It encourages students to become involved in professional associations and to network as well as to consider lifelong learning and becoming credentialed. Additionally, it provides helpful information on various professional pathways for graduates.

Physician Dictations

Perhaps the most important component of this course is the unique combination of authentic physician dictation and coordinated readings and exercises by medical specialty, with supplementary information vital to every medical transcription student. This instructional technique provides a distinct learning advantage over programs using professional readers as dictators. It is only by transcribing actual medical dictation that a student develops the selective auditory skills and experience necessary to gain competency as a medical transcriptionist.

While the authenticity of the dictation will be immediately apparent, the dictations have been edited to remove protected health information (PHI), demographics, and long sections of silence, hemming and hawing, and background noise. Students will be able to add demographics to their transcripts using a patient census and physician roster for which the names, medical record numbers, and dates have been generated using online name, number, and date-generating applications.

The dictation is sequenced from simple to complex, encompassing a broad spectrum of terminology for each medical specialty. Within the general framework for this course, students are exposed to many dictating variables in style and punctuation as well as genuine distractions such as hospital noises and voices in the background. Male and female physicians and regional and foreign accents have been included.

The dictated reports include chart notes, initial office evaluations, consultations, history and physical examinations, discharge summaries, operative reports, emergency department reports, procedure notes, and diagnostic studies from each of the medical specialties.

The dictations and accompanying transcripts have been carefully reviewed by certified medical transcriptionists, educators, and a medical doctor to ensure that the reports reflect an accurate and representative sample of each medical specialty.

Special Features of the Textbook

Transcription Tips offer handy suggestions to improve accuracy and avoid the error traps that students and new MTs often encounter. Exercises reinforce vocabulary and medical content and prepare the student for transcription practice. Comic Relief provides a light touch and points out humorous yet common errors made in transcription.

Sample Reports offer model transcribed reports prepared according to the recommendations of the AHDI *Book of Style for Medical Transcription*, 3rd ed. (Modesto, CA: Association for Healthcare Documentation Integrity, 2008). Online Audio Exercises and Transcription Practice provide students opportunities to apply the concepts they've learned in their readings and study.

Highlights of the 4th Edition

- Ten hours of new dictation covering major medical specialties, with footnoted transcript keys consistent with the current edition of the AHDI *Book of Style* and explanatory notes.
- New content and exercises on all topics in the nonmedical chapters (Chapters 1-5 and 20), with Pause for Reflection questions interspersed throughout the text.
- In the 14 medical chapters (Chapters 6-19), updated and revised content and exercises specifically related to the dictations, including diseases, diagnoses, medications, lab tests and other diagnostics, and surgical procedures.
- Online dictated vocabulary research and sound-alike exercises related to the dictations which should be completed prior to transcription practice.
- Online proofreading and editing practice using transcripts and audio for each specialty chapter, focusing on the types of errors common in speech recognition editing and traditional editing.

- Appendices including laboratory tests with reference values organized by test panel or profile and also alphabetical and common abbreviations.
- Fifty audio clips with a 100-item multiple choice online practice exam for the Registered Healthcare Documentation Specialist credential.

Online resources include additional sample reports with audio of some of the same voices, report types, or surgical procedures that students will encounter in transcription practice.

The goal of *Healthcare Documentation: Fundamentals & Practice*, 4th edition, is to familiarize students with the transcription of dictation in the basic medical and surgical specialties. Students seeking employment as medical transcriptionists will find that this course prepares them for entry-level positions in physician offices or medical group practices, clinics, and specialty departments.

An online practice exam is provided for students wishing to become a Registered Healthcare Documentation Specialist (RHDS). Those wanting to become a Certified Healthcare Documentation Specialist (CHDS) and expand their employment options to hospitals and transcription services will want to continue their education through advanced training.

As comprehensive as this course is, the authors assume that students will have had a medical terminology and anatomy course prior to embarking on this course of study. The medical terminology and anatomy content of this program is intended for review and not in-depth study. Students should be required to have a medical and an English dictionary. Pharmacology and other references are optional but would be helpful.

This fourth edition of *Healthcare Documentation: Fundamentals & Practice* represents a major revision of the entire course—text, supplemental materials, and dictation—and reflects the feedback and recommendations of many current users as well as selected reviewers. We appreciate the feedback and have endeavored to incorporate most of the suggestions. Those familiar with the course will be happily surprised at the new and updated content and the new look. Those using the course for the first time will be impressed with its usefulness and comprehensiveness.

Sally Crenshaw Pitman, M.A.
Ellen A. Drake, CMT, B.A.
Health Professions Institute

A Note to Students

Most students have probably taken courses where they "learned" the material just long enough to do well on a test and make an acceptable grade for the course. This isn't one of those types of courses. It's unfortunate when an education system teaches students that memorization and regurgitation of facts is learning, for it is not.

Learning is understanding. Learning is the ability to relate new knowledge to that data bank of knowledge and experience in your brain. Learning is being able to act on knowledge, to apply knowledge to new situations and circumstances. Learning is being able to extrapolate and make those intellectual leaps that are pictured in cartoons as light bulbs over the head. Learning is being able to think critically and reason clearly so as to solve problems.

The ability to solve problems and use critical thinking is of primary importance in medical transcription. Please keep these thoughts in mind as you pursue your new career in healthcare documentation.

If you are unsure of your reading, note-taking, and study skills, be aware that there are numerous online resources that will help you improve in these areas. Suggested search phrases are "become a better learner," "study skills," and "using critical thinking as a student" (omit the quotation marks). You may also want to read "The Science of Studying Science," by Georgia Green, CMT, which can be found on the free Downloads page of the Health Professions Institute website (**www.hpisum.com**).

To make the most of this course of study, it is important that you understand the features of this course and how best to maximize your training. Please read the Preface to familiarize yourself with the content and features of the course. Take the time to page through the book, looking at the different features. Read the objectives for each chapter, note the outline, and observe the hierarchy of headings. Become familiar with the appendiceal material following Chapter 20 (Resources, Glossary, Normal Laboratory Test Values, and Index).

The first three chapters introduce you to medical transcription as a career choice and to the medicolegal and technological aspects of healthcare documentation. Chapter 4, Medical Transcription Practices, provides a number of tools to enhance your studies as you proceed through the course. It is one of the most important chapters in the book. You will want to review its content frequently as you proceed through the course. Chapter 5 is an abbreviated style reference. It should be sufficient to complete this course, but as noted elsewhere, we follow and recommend the AHDI *Book of Style for Medical Transcription* as an arbiter of healthcare documentation style.

Chapters 6 through 19 are the medical specialty chapters. Check the Anatomy Review at the beginning of each chapter. Although general in nature, many of these terms will be encountered in your readings as well as later in transcription practice. The Vocabulary Review offers abbreviated definitions or explanations of terms that you will also encounter in reading the chapter or in transcription practice. The intent of the Medical Readings in the specialty chapters is to give you a context in which to place the diseases, diagnostic procedures, and therapeutic maneuvers that follow, and yes, again, the readings will inform your transcription practice.

Throughout each chapter, you will find Pause for Reflection questions. These questions are designed to ensure that you are capturing the most important points in your reading and that you understand what you have read. Many of the questions are open-ended, so answers can vary, but your instructor will have sample responses of appropriate answers that we have prepared.

The Exercises at the end of each chapter, while covering the content of the chapter, also prepare you for transcription practice, as do the Online Audio Exercises, all of which should be completed prior to transcribing the authentic medical dictations provided for transcription practice. In addition, you will find online audio samples of reports similar to those you will be transcribing, some of which are by the same dictators.

Are you getting the idea that everything is leading up to **transcription practice**? It most assuredly is! The important point is this: You cannot skip steps and jump to transcription practice because you think that is where all the learning takes place. Trying to transcribe without proper preparation is like falling off a boat in the middle of the ocean and not knowing how to swim. If you survive, it won't be easy or pretty.

When first introduced to dictation and medical transcription, you have myriad things to remember. You're learning intellectual and physical coordination skills you've never had to use before. You're struggling with format and style and punctuating occasionally nonstandard syntax "on the fly." And, of course, you're developing auditory discrimination and trying to recognize what you hear as vocabulary you've actually studied in medical terminology. With all these things to do, it's easy to develop a kind of "remote control" habit of just typing sounds and failing to connect with the meaning of the words coming into your ears and brain.

It's important that you take time to understand the medical content of the reports you're transcribing. By doing so, you begin to make connections between symptoms and diseases, diseases and diagnostic procedures, diseases and treatments, drugs and interactions, diagnoses and outcomes. These are the connections that enable the experienced transcriptionist to decipher difficult or garbled dictation and to spot and report inconsistencies, omissions, and risk management issues.

After you have transcribed the practice dictations, your instructor may assign additional exercises called Engaging the Content. The questions will be similar to the Transcript Forensics questions at the end of each specialty chapter, only on a deeper level because they will relate to entire reports selected from your transcription practice dictations. Some of the questions do nothing more than encourage you to translate the medical content into lay language. Others focus on auditory discrimination skills. Some require you to see relationships and corollaries. Almost all require you to justify your answers using information contained in the medical content of the report. All the questions will help develop your problem-solving and critical thinking skills and make you a better transcriptionist or healthcare documentation specialist.

I hope you find these exercises of benefit. These are techniques I have been developing throughout my years of teaching. I've found that my students have become better and better thinkers as I find more ways for them to engage the content.

Ellen A. Drake, CMT
Development Editor
Health Professions Institute

Healthcare Documentation: Fundamentals & Practice, fourth edition, was written and developed by the editorial staff and associates of Health Professions Institute (HPI), Salt Lake City, Utah.

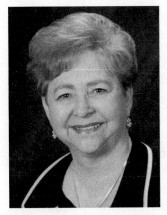

Sally Crenshaw Pitman is editor, publisher, and CEO of Health Professions Institute. Since 1985 she has published 11 editions of *Vera Pyle's Current Medical Terminology* and numerous periodicals, primarily the quarterly *Perspectives on the Medical Transcription Profession* since 1990. She edited and published *The SUM Program for Medical Transcription Training*, the *Career Development Series*, numerous textbooks and quick-reference books as well as other educational materials for medical transcriptionists, teachers, supervisors, and business owners. She owned a medical transcription service for 10 years (until 1982), having previously taught English in a community college for five years. She has B.S. and M.A. degrees in English.

Sally Pitman was a founding director of AAMT (1978-1984), now AHDI, editor and publisher of AAMT publications for eight years (until September 1986). She was also the founder and executive director of the Medical Transcription Industry Alliance (MTIA) in the early 1990s. In 1985 she received the Distinguished Member Award from AAMT, in 2006 the Lifetime Achievement Award from MTIA, and in 2011 AHDI's Distinguished Service Award, recognizing her service in the medical transcription profession over the past 30 years. She and her husband Leon have two children and six grandchildren.

Ellen A. Drake, CMT, B.A., is the development editor for Health Professions Institute (HPI) where she helped develop *The SUM Program for Medical Transcription Training*, the *Career Development Series* for continuing education for MT practitioners, and other HPI books and training materials. She is coauthor with her husband Randy of the *Saunders Pharmaceutical Word Book* and author of the *Sloane Medical Word Book*. She is also an editorial consultant and contributor to the *Dorland's Medical Speller* and *Taber's*

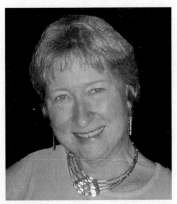

Medical Dictionary. She has contributed to several textbooks and written dozens of articles for medical transcription and HIM publications.

Ellen Drake has worked as an onsite and remote MT, QA specialist, and MT/QA manager in diverse settings. She has owned an MT service and taught medical transcription at a community college and online. She has a B.A. in Education and taught high school English for five years. In her leisure time, Ellen enjoys reading and writing. She also loves to travel, having made a recent solo 9000-mile road trip from Florida to Washington state to southern California and back to Florida. She has four "children"—rescue kitties Aristotle, Nefertiti, Chat Noir, and Soft Kitty.

John H. Dirckx, M.D., retired in 2003 after 35 years as director of the student health center at the University of Dayton (Ohio). His longstanding interest in classical and modern languages has led to the writing of numerous books and articles on the language, literature, and history of medicine. He is the author of *The Language of Medicine: Its Evolution, Structure, and Dynamics*, 2nd ed. (New York: Praeger Publishers, 1983), *H&P: A Nonphysician's Guide to the Medical History and Physical Examination*, 4th ed. (HPI, 2009), *Human Diseases*, 2nd ed. (HPI, 2003), and *Laboratory Tests and Diagnostic Procedures in Medicine* (HPI, 2004).

He has been medical consultant for *The SUM Program for Medical Transcription Training* and all HPI products for 27 years. He has edited medical journals as well as Lippincott Williams & Wilkins' line of Stedman's medical reference works. He and his wife Joyce have five daughters and ten grandchildren.

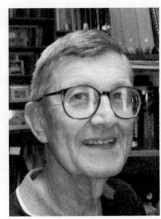

Acknowledgments

Healthcare Documentation: Fundamentals & Practice, fourth edition, has been greatly expanded to meet the needs of medical transcription students of the 21st century. The new arrangement of material is designed to enhance learning in each medical specialty, and extensive material has been added in every chapter.

What makes this transcription course unique is not only the inclusion of ten hours of new authentic dictation but also the pertinent medical readings by physicians, the interesting articles by medical transcriptionists and other healthcare colleagues about the profession, and the challenging exercises and learning tools.

Ellen A. Drake, an educator par excellence, has been the lead author on this fourth edition, having developed the new outline, assembled the most interesting essays about the profession and the industry, developed quizzes on readings throughout the textbook and end-of-chapter exercises to test knowledge and application of the material. In addition, she reviewed hundreds of authentic physician dictations in order to select the best ten hours for student practice; she spent many hours editing the transcripts for medical content accuracy and style, removing personal health information, and developing explanatory footnotes to contribute to student understanding of the dictations. Not stopping with the textbook and dictations, she has developed numerous online audio exercises to enhance understanding of the medical specialties.

Notable contributions to this edition came from Linda C. Campbell, longtime educator, author, and researcher for Health Professions Institute. Many of her writings appear in introductory material in several chapters, along with feature boxes containing anecdotes, fast facts, and other interesting contributions, particularly in cardiology, gastroenterology, orthopedic, and pediatric chapters. They add humor, wit, fresh insights, and knowledge to the text.

A large body of material from other HPI publications provides the bulk of the text, and we have John H. Dirckx, M.D., to thank for so many contributions: his scholarly and astute editing of the medical transcripts as well as numerous excerpts from his writings, including *H&P: A Nonphysician's Guide to the Medical History and Physical Examination*; *Laboratory Tests and Diagnostic Procedures in Medicine*; *Human Diseases*; and timeless articles published in HPI's quarterly magazine, *Perspectives on the Medical Transcription Profession* (1990-2010). Working on this edition went on a little longer than he had expected, but he always leapt to the task of writing new material as we identified the need for it in the medical specialty chapters.

The healthcare documentation profession and industry is a moving target in today's fast-paced society, and we could not have portrayed it as comprehensively in this moment in time without the help of leaders in the field. Brenda Hurley and Georgia Green contributed many articles on electronic healthcare records, healthcare documentation technology, and health information management to help us portray an industry in a constant state of change. In addition, Brenda Hurley and Randy Drake proofread the entire text for accuracy and consistency in style and format.

We are most grateful to Joan Gill, executive editor of health professions at Pearson Health, for her enthusiastic support of the editorial staff at Health Professions Institute in its valiant effort to produce the best edition of HDFP for tomorrow's healthcare documentation specialists and medical transcriptionists. Her encouragement of our efforts to provide quality education for medical transcription students has contributed greatly to the success of this book.

Thanks are also due the staff and associates of Pearson Health for the dynamic graphic design and layout and for the colorful medical illustrations that make this textbook a great visual learning tool. I am especially grateful to the staff of Pearson Health for their patience and graciousness in working with me in my multiple roles of writer, editor, and compositor.

Sally Crenshaw Pitman, M.A.
Editor & Publisher
Health Professions Institute
Salt Lake City, Utah

Healthcare Documentation Profession

Learning Objectives

▶ Describe the attributes that distinguish the professional medical transcriptionist.

▶ Given abbreviations related to health record privacy, identify the correct expanded form.

▶ Define vocabulary related to health record privacy.

▶ Identify appropriate examples of PHI and/or disclosure of PHI under the HIPAA privacy rule.

▶ Identify the individuals and/or organizations that are defined as accountable parties or business associates under the HIPAA rule.

▶ Describe the processes involved in creating a healthcare record for an individual patient.

▶ Explain the role of the healthcare documentation specialist in creating a healthcare record and in the revenue cycle.

▶ Demonstrate knowledge of the healthcare documentation profession by accurately completing the exercises in this chapter.

Healthcare Documentation Profession

Every time you see a doctor, are admitted to a hospital, go to an emergency department, get a lab test done, or have an x-ray or other procedure, one or more reports must be created to document the event. These reports may include office chart notes, history and physical examinations (H&Ps), consultations, letters, memos, admission notes, emergency department notes, operative reports, discharge summaries, and many specialized laboratory, imaging, and other diagnostic studies.

The results of some diagnostic studies, such as those that come from a clinical laboratory (blood and chemistry studies), are machine-generated. Other diagnostic studies, such as electrodiagnostic studies on the heart and brain, may be documented with both electronic results and narrative summaries. The content and format of these reports will be discussed in more detail in Chapter 2.

Transcription of the narrative portion of medical reports has long belonged to the **medical transcriptionist (MT)**. These reports encompass a variety of medical specialties, and each day's work presents a unique challenge and opportunity for learning, as you will discover in the readings and transcription practice in chapters 6 through 19. By the time you complete this course, you will have developed the knowledge and skills of a medical transcriptionist.

A strong MT skill set prepares you to transcribe medical dictation in a variety of settings. It also serves as the basis for building skills as a **speech recognition editor (SRE)** and **quality assurance (QA) specialist** as well as roles that are still emerging in healthcare documentation such as auditing provider **electronic medical record (EMR)** entries, **electronic health record (EHR)** system trainers, implementers of EHR systems, data abstractors, and more that are still to be determined—all of which fall under the umbrella of the **healthcare documentation specialist (HDS)**. It is the medical transcription skill set that really sets an HDS apart from

---

THE MIND BEHIND THE MACHINE

If there is one thing that medical transcriptionists are known for, it is our love for words. This is the common thread in our profession. It is what makes us professionals. If I were cast away on a desert island, the book I would probably want to take with me is an unabridged English dictionary, and I could be happy for years.

Transcriptionists can get lost in a dictionary. We look up a word and we see something else that looks interesting, and then we look up another word, and so on. Words are truly exciting. I would much rather have a dozen new medical words all researched and defined than a five-pound box of candy. I hope that you too will come to share this feeling.

Some years ago I was transcribing the manuscript of a textbook by a physician for whom I had worked in the past. He is a well-educated, extremely literate person. He is a published poet, a musician, a composer, a teacher—a real Renaissance man. So it was with some trepidation that I presumed to suggest changes. I transcribed the page the way he dic-

tated it, and then I gave him my version as well. He read it and beamed. "This is a tremendous improvement," he said. "You know, Vera, together we could rule the world."

It was a charming proposition. However, it is not my ambition to rule the world. All I want is recognition for what I know and how accurately and intelligently I can convey that information—my contribution to the delivery of the best possible healthcare for a patient.

Some 30 years ago, our hospital got the prototype of one of the first word processing machines. Our medical record director brought in a group of interns and residents to see this marvel. Pointing to the machine proudly, she said, "And this is the machine that transcribes your reports."

Not so, I thought then, and now. The machines we use are simply tools. Without the knowledge contained in the mind of the transcriptionist, the machines are impotent. **The transcriptionist is the mind behind the machine.**

Vera Pyle

others who work with healthcare records because, more than anyone else in the healthcare documentation arena, MTs really get into the actual thought processes of providers as they compose.

Whether you call yourself a medical transcriptionist, speech editor, or healthc are documentation specialist, you are a vital member of the professional healthcare team. The medical transcriptionist provides an important service to both physician and patient by transcribing, or editing if speech recognition is used for the first draft, dictated medical reports that document a patient's medical care and condition. Because each dictated report represents a part of a patient's healthcare record, the MT transcribes it with care, demonstrating an extensive knowledge of medical terminology, anatomy, pharmacology, human diseases, surgical procedures, diagnostic studies, and laboratory tests, in order to produce an accurate and complete permanent medical record.

While not as visible to the general public as those members of the team providing hands-on care, such as physicians, nurses, therapists, technicians, dietitians, and other healthcare support staff, the healthcare documentation specialists play an important role in documenting the quality of patient care and the continuity and accuracy of the healthcare record through their commitment to excellence.

Vocabulary Review

account number A number assigned by a healthcare facility for each patient visit or encounter. Also called billing number, or visit number.

ADT (admission, discharge, transfer) information Demographic data about the patient that includes name, patient number, and dates of admission and discharge or transfer and can include age, sex, and other information. This data is electronic and can often be incorporated directly into a medical report.

back-end speech recognition technology (BE-SRT) The use of editors to proofread and correct text drafts generated by a speech recognition engine, a process that also contributes to further training of the recognition engine.

biometric identifier Biological characteristics that identify an individual. The most commonly used identifiers are fingerprints, handprints, and eye iris and/or retina scans.

SELF-ASSESSMENT SURVEY OF "SOFT" TRAITS
Do you have what it takes to become a successful medical transcriptionist? Rate yourself from 1 to 5 (with 1 being "doesn't describe me at all" and 5 being "yes, that's me!") on these important personal and professional characteristics of a successful medical transcriptionist. Be honest.

You do not have to be a 5 for every one of these characteristics, but if you can't choose 4 or 5 for a good number of them, you may have some work to do.

___ I am interested in medical science.
___ I enjoy learning something new every day.
___ I see challenges as opportunities for learning and growing.
___ I see myself as a problem-solver; I think things through.
___ I am very detail-oriented.
___ I enjoy reading for fun and information.
___ I enjoy solving puzzles, crossword puzzles, jigsaw puzzles.
___ I am self-motivated and work well independently.
___ I usually meet required deadlines and deliver on what I promise.
___ I adapt well to change.
___ I care about quality and excellence.
___ I am an honest and ethical person.
___ I desire a professional career in healthcare.

clinicians Healthcare professionals who treat patients or provide direct patient care of any type. These include physicians, nurses, and allied health professionals (technologists and therapists).

electronic health record (EHR) A longitudinal electronic record of patient health information generated by one or more encounters in any care delivery setting able to be shared among different systems and healthcare providers.

electronic medical record (EMR) The electronic version of a patient's chart. It is not the same as the electronic health record. See *electronic health record*.

face sheet The first page of a patient's printed healthcare record; it contains demographic data, the reason for admission and the final diagnosis, as well as a list of any procedures performed.

SELF-ASSESSMENT SURVEY
OF "HARD" SKILLS AND ABILITIES
This survey of skills and abilities may seem incomplete compared to the survey of personal and professional characteristics. That's because, while you can probably always improve on your personal and professional characteristics, those are the defining traits that will help you determine whether medical transcription is right for you.

On the other hand, most of the knowledge and technical skills and abilities needed for this career can be acquired through diligent study. For example, you have probably already had or are taking concurrently several medical science courses including medical terminology, anatomy and physiology, and perhaps others. You may have taken a computer skills course.

If you do not have at least some foundation in the skills outlined below, your course of study will likely be longer than it would be coming in with a solid foundation in these areas. Rate yourself from 1 to 5 (with 1 being "doesn't describe me at all" and 5 being "yes, that's me!") on these important "hard" skills.

__ I have excellent English language skills (spelling, grammar, and punctuation).
__ I have a strong English language vocabulary and enjoy learning new words.
__ I am comfortable using a computer and word processing software.
__ I can type at least 50 corrected words per minute.
__ I am comfortable using an Internet browser and email.
__ I understand English fractions and decimals.
__ I have good hearing acuity.

flags, flagging Marking or electronically tagging blanks or discrepancies in a healthcare document for the originator to resolve.

front-end speech recognition technology (FE-SRT) Editing of speech-recognized draft text by the originator of the text in real time while dictating.

healthcare documentation specialist (HDS) An umbrella designation for numerous positions related to healthcare documentation including medical transcriptionist, speech recognition editor, quality assurance specialist, auditor of provider EMR entries, EHR system trainers, implementers of EHR systems, data abstractors, and others that are to be determined.

Joint Commission, The An independent, not-for-profit organization that accredits and certifies more than 19,000 healthcare organizations and programs in the U.S.

meaningful text Accurate and complete healthcare documentation that represents what the originator meant. Documentation that contributes to quality patient care.

medical record number (MRN) A permanent patient identifier assigned by a healthcare facility that identifies the patient on each subsequent visit.

medical transcriptionist (MT) One who transcribes medical reports from dictation, a role that has expanded to include the speech recognition editor (SRE). See *speech recognition editor* and *healthcare documentation specialist*.

medication reconciliation The process of comparing a patient's medication orders to all of the medications that the patient has been taking to avoid medication errors such as omissions, duplications, dosing errors, or drug interactions.

quality assurance specialist One who ensures that healthcare documentation is accurate and complete and who provides feedback to MTs and SREs regarding errors and blanks. Often, the quality assurance specialist serves as a mentor and on-the-job trainer.

speech recognition editor (SRE or SE) One who edits drafts of text generated by a speech recognition engine.

speech recognition technology (SRT) A technology by which speech is converted to text.

structured-text system The use of templates, outlines, or check boxes to document patient care.

T-form system A means of creating structured text using predesigned templates, each created with language specific to the chief complaint of the patient whereby healthcare providers simply choose which T-form to use, check the boxes, and a report is generated.

third-party payer An insurance company, Medicare, Medicaid, etc. that will pay all or a portion of a patient's covered medical expenses.

Meaningful Text

Healthcare documentation requires a skill that few people—many of those who hire MTs and even some HDSs—truly understand. Many people think it is basically a physical skill—typing or keyboarding. And that's part of it, a very small part. However, even the physical aspects encompass much more than hitting the correct keys on a keyboard because properly equipped MTs are also operating a foot pedal or hand control, which has a forward, fast forward, and reverse. Because they sit for long hours, MTs must be cognizant of their posture and their physical environment. But none of this comes close to describing what an MT actually does with his or her brain!

The medical transcriptionist listens to the spoken word, which can be marked by poor grammar and usage, disorganization, back-tracks, nonlanguage vocalizations, misspeaks, corrections, variable voice volume, and variable speed sometimes approaching Mach 2. In addition, MTs must overcome obstacles that other listeners don't have. No face to look at, no body language, no gestures. Some experts estimate that 80% of communication is through body language! Yet, the MT must interpret and translate these disembodied sounds, which pretty much correspond to a foreign language, into **meaningful text** (while continuing to control the fingers on the keyboard and the foot or finger on the pedal and keep the body in an ergonomic position).

While interpreting the spoken word into meaningful text, the MT is also organizing, formatting and paragraphing the text; applying grammar, punctuation, spelling, and style rules; correcting usage; and making sure that the finished report meets the specifications of the dictator or client. In addition, the MT is proofreading on-screen what has just been transcribed, while transcribing what was just heard and listening to the next set of sounds.

Essentially, the brain is performing multiple intellectual functions along with several physical functions. We can think of no other activity or skill that requires the intense mental processing, physical involvement, and concentrated focus of the medical transcriptionist.

Learning medical language is akin to learning a foreign language. Indeed, it contains many foreign words and phrases, primarily but not limited to expressions of Latin or Greek origin. Medical dictation also contains many abbreviations, brief forms, shortcuts, jargon, medical vernacular, and word coinages that are an integral part of the language of medicine. Because medical

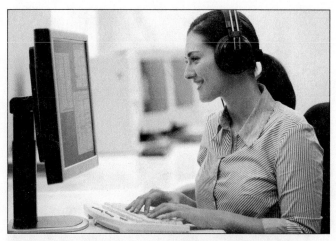

Source: Monkey Business Images, Shutterstock

reports are dictated, their tone and style are often informal, even conversational.

A mastery of English grammar, structure, and style, a knowledge of transcription practices, skill in typing, spelling, and proofreading, and the highest professional standards contribute to the medical transcriptionist's ability to interpret, translate, and edit medical dictation for content and clarity.

With the advent of the electronic health record (EHR), it is anticipated that the medical transcriptionist's role will evolve into a more technological-based position which will require advanced clinical knowledge, greater problem-solving skills, and mastery of a variety of computer software programs such as database management and spreadsheet programs.

For all these reasons, medical transcriptionists must be critical thinkers—that is, they must be able to use their interpretive medical language skills and the context clues in the report to detect and correct errors, to make decisions about leaving blanks and flagging, and to spot potential risk management issues. These topics and more will be covered in chapters 4 and 5.

Professional Readings
Evolution of the Medical Transcription Role

by Brenda J. Hurley

Throughout my career as a medical transcriptionist, I have been repeatedly told that medical transcription will "go away" and that we will become extinct, much like the PBX operators and the dinosaurs. In my 40 years in the industry, I have heard versions of this tale repeated and predicted now for over 30 years.

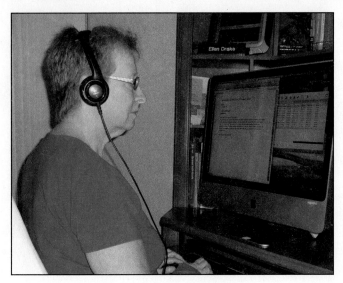

Source: Bella Modella Studio

First it was speech recognition that would be the answer. Just imagine healthcare providers everywhere stepping up to their PCs, talking into them, and bingo, out pop their words—eliminating the need for MTs. While we are closer to this scenario today than we were 10 years ago, mostly due to faster PC processors, larger capacity hard drives, noise-canceling microphones, and improved telephony, it is still not the reality in every setting for every healthcare provider. In fact, **front-end** speech recognition technology (SRT) is actually moving quickly to the use of **back-end** speech recognition systems, and MTs are transitioning now to **SRT editors** at a rapid pace in many healthcare environments.

Next it was the **T-forms** that would eliminate MTs. With hundreds of predesigned T-forms to choose from, each created with language specific to the chief complaint of the patient, healthcare providers simply needed to choose which T-form to use, check the boxes, and bingo, the report was done! Later this system evolved to scanning the completed paper-based T-forms to electronically capture the information provided by the checked boxes. Then "canned" structured text would be generated for each item.

For example, if the practitioner checked the boxes for Ambulance, 83, Caucasian, Female, Chest Pain, the scanned version would read something like: This 83-year-old Caucasian female arrived by ambulance complaining of chest pain. Sounds perfect, right? Not quite. It seems that the healthcare providers constantly changed their minds by trying to unmark boxes, marked too many boxes, skipped important boxes, or did not clearly place their mark within the boxes provided. Scanning difficulties consistently caused

errors in reports generated by this process which resulted in report completion delays, billing discrepancies, and incomplete or inaccurate healthcare documentation.

The T-form system has evolved again. Today, healthcare providers have electronic templates to point and click on their desktop PC, tablet, or pad. Many similarities exist. Templates are often designed around chief complaints, allowing for structured text to be inserted with a mouse click and/or a touch on a screen.

This system has advantages over its paper-based origin. The fact that it is electronic is critical for its integration within today's healthcare record. It has the capability to overcome input errors by not allowing the report to be closed until the critical information has been entered, alerts when inconsistent information has been entered (i.e., right vs. left), and reminders that entries have been skipped. Sounds perfect, right? Well, not quite. It does have some limitations.

The safeguards do not entirely eliminate all input errors. Additionally, there are many different systems on the market today, and more in development. They all operate a little differently. Perhaps in time, these conflicts can be resolved as manufacturers realize that healthcare providers have their own office needs, and many have staff privileges at multiple different hospitals. Standardizing data input processes will assure a wider acceptance by users of these systems.

As an example, consider automobiles. If Chevy, Ford, and other car makers all made cars that operate differently, it would be very cumbersome to learn how to drive each of them when you are required to drive more than one type. Instead cars have a standard way they operate with the steering wheel, the gas pedal, and brake so each user does not need to be trained on these basic operations for each vehicle type.

Another important limitation of the **structured-text system** is the lack of content flexibility. Despite the predesigned templates for hundreds of ailments, there are times when one just does not cover what needs to be said. The option to type in those comments seems less appealing to healthcare providers than the option of speaking it. Some astute programmers have listened to their customers and now offer the option for "insert dictation," allowing the healthcare provider to dictate portions of the report content. In fact, many healthcare providers today are enjoying the benefits of their handheld PCs, tablets, and pads, and are now utilizing software on them for dictation.

Perhaps the reason that medical transcription has endured over the years is because the process, although not perfect, provides a service to healthcare that has not been replicated by other modalities. Is that a bold or self-serving statement? Perhaps. As noted before, few truly understand the dictation/transcription process and the factors related to it. It is very easy to simplify it to "the doctor speaks, it is recorded, the HDS transcribes it, and bingo, the report appears!" Well, it is not quite that easy.

Frequently MTs are provided dictations that are cluttered with background noises, side conversations between the dictator and others, cell phone or portable phone static, beepers going off, sounds that require deciphering from whispers and mumbles, in speeds that would make auctioneers jealous. Also, there are problems with the English language that challenge many healthcare providers in today's medical settings.

Dictation is not a perfect process. I remember as a hospital supervisor explaining to a physician how difficult his dictation was for our staff to transcribe; he replied simply, "I hate to dictate." A few years ago some felt that saving the recorded dictation without transcribing it would be the solution and save many healthcare dollars by eliminating the need for MTs. That sounded like a great idea until it became apparent that it was not an efficient way for healthcare providers to get the information they needed.

One can read much faster than one can listen, and listening to the dictation is not easy (due to the reasons listed above). For the first time, many heard "real" dictation recorded by other healthcare professionals. They found it amazing that they could not understand the dictation performed by their own colleagues, although they had frequent conversations with them and felt they could understand them perfectly during those times. It is the dictation phenomenon that takes over, the hurry up, get it over with, too busy to slow down, the "I hate to dictate" mode.

If I sound like a whiny MT complaining about doctors, let me assure you that I, and my fellow HDSs, have profound respect for physicians. We hear in their voices their compassion, their concern, and even at times their frustration as they work long hours to treat and care for patients in many different settings. Through the years, we have been participants, albeit behind the scenes, when we shared the joy of the miracle of birth and when we joined in the grief over the loss of a life. MTs want to provide perfect reports in a timely fashion; however, we are often handicapped by the dictation provided by healthcare providers.

Congratulations to those who do understand and dictate clearly in a conversational tone and speed, to assure that their dictation is the foundation of a quality report that will become a permanent component of the patient's legal health record.

With all that has changed, some things have not. The interpretation of the spoken medical language to text is a craft that is difficult to learn and takes time to perfect. Technology can assist, and does in many ways, but it still comes down to people. Even with the transition of MTs to SREs to HDSs, medical language interpretation skills are still imperative for a quality report.

Every day errors are made in dictation. MTs "fix" or edit them, or flag them when appropriate for the dictator's review. MTs have always served as the "safety net" for dictators. This has always been an essential element of the healthcare documentation process. Consider that in a conversation we often make small errors when speaking (i.e., wrong subject-verb use, mispronunciation, etc.); however, the listener automatically interprets what is said and the meaning is understood. Dictation, however, is recorded, so you hear exactly what is said, not always what was meant.

It is the skill of the MT that adds clarity to the communication without altering the intent of its meaning or the style of the dictator. This is why when asked about speech recognition, I have often responded that the best you will get is exactly what you said, not what you really meant to say.

While many of the new technologies provide greater efficiencies in the documentation process, it is the interpretation of the medical language that skilled HDSs bring to healthcare communication that cannot be replicated by technology alone. Our skills have transitioned for decades as we moved from typewriters to computers, then as editors of SRT draft documents, and continue to transition as we work within EHR systems to assure quality reports that are complete and accurate. We have repeatedly proven our adaptability, and we are here to stay.

Evolution of the Healthcare Documentation Specialist
by April Martin

Many of us were not even aware transcription existed as a profession until we fell into it. Some were medical assistants or doctor's office secretaries who were pushed into transcription as part of their duties. Some went to

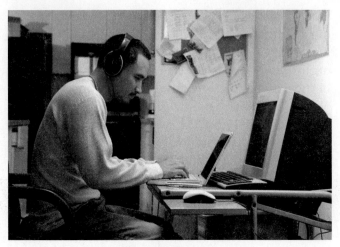

Source: iofoto, Shutterstock.

school and earned degrees or certificates. Whatever the circumstances, we all found ourselves in a profession we are passionate about.

Not all of us share the same roles. We are transcriptionists, editors, trainers, educators, consultants, supervisors, managers, and service operators; however, we are ALL healthcare documentation specialists.

Just as the profession of transcription continues to evolve, so must the skills and knowledge base of the transcriptionists. The once very green and inexperienced MT continues to learn, grow, and evolve into an experienced MT and then possibly moves on to become lead MT, trainer, QA editor, or even a supervisor or manager. It takes years of experience to fine-tune the skills necessary, and continuing education is necessary to remain relevant.

Experienced MTs, when they were just starting in this field, will remember listening over and over to the same phrase in a dictation and not having a clue what Dr. Speedracer was trying to say. When they asked for help, they wondered how on earth their experienced coworker could very confidently tell them exactly what the doctor just dictated. However, on listening again and now knowing what it was, it would be as clear as day. Six months later, they were the ones telling the new MT exactly what was dictated and seeing the same look of astonishment on the new MT's face.

Many MTs work from home; however, one of the greatest challenges for a new home MT is that you do not have the advantage of having that "second ear." A good transcription company will have a system set up for every new person to be assigned to a trainer or editor—that second ear. This allows work done by a student to be sent to an experienced person for proofing prior to delivery and also for a relatively new but learning MT to have a trouble spot in a dictation filled in.

This allows for continuing education for the new MT. It is critical that feedback be provided and is timely to assist in their training. This evolution in technology and in the profession has created a need for qualified MTs to serve as healthcare documentation specialists.

The skills needed to be a great transcriptionist are the very foundation of a healthcare documentation specialist: excellent proofreading skills, at least two years of acute-care experience, a good ear, proficient research abilities, and strong communication skills.

One of the great benefits of being a transcriptionist or an editor is that we all learn something new every day, but even more so as an editor. As you listen to dictation and review transcribed documents done by a student or new person, proofreading skills are enhanced, and you have the ability to learn from others' mistakes. There are skill-building exercises available to help hone these skills.

Editing medical reports is where superb communication skills come into play. Corrected reports and constructive feedback are critical to the success of new MTs. The first reports are strewn with blanks and incorrect terms. As time progresses and the communication cycle continues, you will see fewer and fewer blanks and incorrect terms. You will see perfect reports eventually, and the gratitude of the new MTs is immeasurable. You share in their accomplishments.

An often-overlooked role of the MT of today and the future is that of editor. The increased use of offshore transcription has created a demand for experienced MTs to serve as editors who understand the idiosyncrasies of the English language, ones who understand the difference between a veteran who was "deployed to Iraq" versus one who was "decoyed to a rack."

As speech recognition technology continues to improve, so will the demand for experienced MTs to serve as medical editors. There will always be the clinician who is unable to use speech recognition for a myriad of reasons, so there will always be the need for the essential MT skill set; however, the MT of the future needs to transform into much more—a hybrid MT. That MT must develop editing skills.

How the HDS Fits into Healthcare Documentation
by Georgia Green

The creation and maintenance of individual healthcare records is a fundamental requirement for licensure and accreditation of today's healthcare facilities, but the practice of healthcare documentation is more than 2000 years old. In the 5th century BC, Hippocrates, the Father of Medicine, recommended that physicians record the causes and course of various diseases so that these records could be passed down and used by other physicians. The most extensive surviving set of medical records dates back to the 17th century, with the case-books of Forman and Napier, British astrologers, who were regarded as physicians of their day.

By the 20th century, healthcare documentation began to be seen as a tool that could improve health-care quality, assist in the management and prevention of communicable disease, standardize medical educa-tion, and aid in research that would yield advances in treatments and improve patient outcomes.

Modern healthcare documentation serves as a method of communication among health professionals to ensure continuity of a patient's care. Healthcare records are the basis for reimbursement, which is essen-tial to the livelihood of the healthcare facility. Health-care records are used to evaluate quality assurance procedures, conduct performance reviews, facilitate accreditation processes and required inspections, and ensure thorough analysis of a critical incident. The healthcare record is a legal record that protects a health-care facility and helps it to manage and mitigate risk.

Healthcare documentation includes all forms of documentation by doctors, nurses, laboratory and imag-ing technologists, physical and occupational therapists, social workers, dietitians, and others, recorded in a pro-fessional capacity in relation to the provision of patient care. Healthcare documentation is seen as an essential part of clinical practice. It demonstrates a clinician's accountability and documents his or her professional judgment and critical thinking in the provision of patient care.

The **healthcare documentation specialist (HDS)** is a facilitator of healthcare documentation. Whether transcribing provider dictation, editing text generated from speech recognition technology, auditing direct provider input, or participating as a historian or scribe, the healthcare documentation specialist is a partner with clinicians in the documentation process.

The healthcare documentation process typically begins before the patient arrives at a facility. The moment an encounter is scheduled, a computer record is created, assigning a unique and permanent patient identifier that will be used for that patient at every sub-sequent encounter at that facility. In addition to the permanent patient identifier or medical record number (MRN), a number is assigned to identify that particular encounter. Each encounter will have its own number and may be referred to as an account number, billing number, or visit number.

Prior to a scheduled hospital visit, a patient is con-tacted to obtain insurance information for the purpose of establishing coverage and obtaining authorization from a third-party payer in advance of performing non-emergent services. Demographic information is col-lected from the patient and becomes part of the healthcare record.

If a facility maintains healthcare records on paper, often referred to as a patient's **"chart,"** the demographic information appears on the first page of the record and is referred to as a **face sheet**. The face sheet typically includes space to record the reason for admission and the final diagnosis, as well as a list of any procedures performed. The same information is contained in an **electronic medical record** but can be accessed and pre-sented on a viewing screen in a variety of ways, depend-ing upon who is accessing information and how it will be used.

At the time a patient arrives at the facility, whether for a scheduled visit or unexpectedly to receive emer-gency care, demographic information is confirmed by the registration department, photocopies or scans are made of photo ID and insurance cards, and signatures are requested to acknowledge the conditions of admis-sion, authorize treatment, and release information as necessary to third-party payers. The patient will be advised of his or her rights under HIPAA and any required notices associated with participation in gov-ernment-sponsored insurance, such as Medicare or Medicaid. This documentation becomes part of the patient's healthcare record.

In addition, any records brought by the patient from a primary care provider, e.g., an order for an x-ray or a lab test, or any records from another facility in the case of a transferring patient, are incorporated into the med-ical chart or electronic medical record. The registration department generates an identification bracelet that contains the patient's name, age, gender, MRN and account numbers, name of attending physician, and critical information such as allergies.

As the patient moves to a clinical area to receive care, either as an inpatient on a nursing floor or in an outpatient area like the emergency department or clin-ical laboratory, additional records are generated. In the outpatient setting, a clerk will record the arrival of the patient in the record, confirm the test to be performed, and communicate information to the patient about what to expect. When the technologist or other

THE JOINT COMMISSION

The Joint Commission (TJC), formerly known as the Joint Commission on Accreditation of Healthcare Organizations (JCAHO) is a nonprofit agency that accredits healthcare organizations in the U.S.

In many states, TJC accreditation is a prerequisite for licensure as a healthcare facility. TJC accreditation is also required for facilities seeking reimbursement from the Centers for Medicare and Medicaid services, the government agency that oversees these federal insurance programs.

Facilities undergoing accreditation are subject to on-site inspections by a team of TJC surveyors. There are different accreditation programs for different types of facilities, and each program has a specific set of standards it must meet.

The standards for hospitals are published annually in the *Comprehensive Accreditation Manual for Hospitals* (CAMH). Each standard consists of individual elements of performance, and a facility must be able to demonstrate strict compliance with every element of performance for every standard.

TJC standards and elements of performance that impact the work of the healthcare documentation specialist fall primarily under the category called Record of Care, Treatment, and Services (RC).

The first standard under this category is RC.01.01.01, "The hospital maintains complete and accurate medical records for each individual patient." Some examples of elements of performance that are measured under this standard include:

"The hospital defines the components of a complete medical record,"

"The medical record contains information unique to the patient, which is used for patient identification,"

"The medical record contains the information needed to support the patient's diagnosis and condition," and so on.

A hospital's director of health information management (HIM) is responsible for ensuring the facility's compliance with these standards.

provider interacts with the patient to record the service performed, entries are made to record each event. All entries are signed, dated, and timed if handwritten or electronically authenticated with the same information.

For patients admitted as inpatients, a unit secretary or ward clerk will begin making entries in the electronic record or, if relying on paper records, will compile a new patient chart containing various forms and templates ready for completion by the nursing staff who interact with the patient, e.g., a nursing admission assessment, a medication reconciliation record, medication administration records, physician order sheets, progress note pages, graphs for recording vital signs and the input and output of fluids, among others. The first clinical entry in the record for an inpatient is a physician's order for admission.

Within 24 hours of admission, the admitting physician must document an admission history and physical examination (H&P). For scheduled patients, an H&P performed within the prior 30 days can be supplied and will become part of the healthcare record for that admission. Often, an admission H&P is dictated, and this is where the **medical transcriptionist (MT)** becomes involved. The MT is responsible for transcribing the dictation promptly and ensuring demographic information is correct so that the transcribed document is associated both with the correct patient and the correct visit number.

Voluminous entries are made in the healthcare record of an inpatient, sometimes on an hourly basis, by everyone involved in the care of that patient. Over a 4-day hospital stay, as many as 50 staff members may interact with a patient, and every clinical interaction requires documentation in the healthcare record.

If a patient undergoes surgery or enters a critical care unit, the number of entries in the record increases dramatically as the level of care provided to the patient intensifies and a greater number of clinicians are involved. **The Joint Commission** requires surgeons to record essential details about surgical procedures as soon as surgery is complete and to provide a detailed record, typically dictated, within 24 hours. The medical transcriptionist is responsible for transcribing surgical dictations. A variety of dictated reports may be generated for critical care patients to ensure that details of the clinical decision-making process are documented.

At the conclusion of the inpatient stay, a narrative summary called a **discharge summary** is required to establish the final diagnosis, provide essential details about the care of the patient, and describe the plan for followup care after discharge. Discharge summaries are often dictated and transcribed.

In addition to the volume of entries in the healthcare record during a patient's inpatient stay or the more limited number of entries that record an outpatient visit, additional entries are recorded that are not part of the legal healthcare record but are a necessary part of the encounter. These entries represent the **charges for services** received. Many charges are calculated and entered automatically, e.g., the daily room rate. Other charges are entered as services are rendered, e.g., the charge associated with a laboratory test, an imaging study, or a medication administered. With an electronic medical record, the entering of charges may be associated with the clinical entry. Even in a paper healthcare record, charges are typically entered electronically into a system designed for that purpose. The healthcare documentation specialist who is transcribing, editing, or auditing a record may require access to patient charges for the purpose of resolving discrepancies in clinical documentation.

At the termination of a patient visit, the health information management (HIM) department assumes control of the record. Whether paper or electronic, healthcare records are scrutinized for accuracy and completeness. Any deficiencies in the record are noted, and clinicians are notified to complete their deficiencies. Deficiencies may include missing signatures, dates, or times on paper records, an omitted daily progress note, or an undictated H&P, surgical record, or discharge

DIAGNOSIS AND PROCEDURE CODING

Medical coding specialists typically perform diagnosis and procedure coding, and healthcare documentation specialists (HDSs) often encounter these codes in records they transcribe or edit.

The *International Classification of Diseases (ICD)* is a world-wide classification system that assigns numeric codes that classify diseases, symptoms, causes of injuries, and the names of operations. The 9th edition of ICD, called *ICD-9*, is the version currently in use in the U.S. and is based on 3-digit codes with the option to add 4th and 5th digits as decimals to provide additional information.

The medical term for a heart attack is *acute myocardial infarction*, but it could also be described as a cardiac arrest or coronary thrombosis, or the terms might be reversed (myocardial infarction, acute) or abbreviated as an MI, AMI, etc. No matter what words you use to describe a heart attack, it can be communicated clearly as an *ICD-9* code.

The *ICD-9* code for acute myocardial infarction is 410. This code includes cardiac infarction; coronary (artery) embolism, occlusion, rupture, or thrombosis; infarction of the heart, myocardium, or ventricle; rupture of the heart, myocardium, or ventricle; and ST elevation (STEMI) and non-ST elevation (NSTEMI) myocardial infarction. A myocardial infarction of the inferoposterior wall of the heart is assigned *ICD-9* code 410.3.

The 10th revision of the ICD is already in use in more than 25 countries. *ICD-10* contains more than 140,000 codes, compared to *ICD-9*'s 17,000, and utilizes alphanumeric coding with up to 7 digits. The need to upgrade computer software and database systems; provide training for physicians, coding specialists, and the myriad of professionals who currently use ICD coding; as well as manage the transition process from *ICD-9* to *ICD-10* has led to delays in its adoption in the U.S. It is currently scheduled to go live in October of 2014.

Diagnosis coding is utilized to document every patient encounter in a healthcare facility. In addition to diagnosis coding, a separate coding system called *Current Procedural Terminology*, or *CPT*, is used to document services performed. Insurers rely on CPT codes in determining reimbursement. CPT codes are 5 digits in length, with an optional 2-digit modifier appended with a hyphen. The CPT code for a chest x-ray, PA and lateral views, is 71020. The CPT code 71020-26 designates the professional fee for the radiologist's reading of that chest x-ray. A CPT manual is published annually by the American Medical Association.

Healthcare documentation specialists must be able to distinguish between diagnosis and procedure codes in order to format them correctly in the medical reports.

summary. Late dictations may be flagged as priority reports for the medical transcriptionist or speech recognition editor.

The **medical coder** then begins the process of reviewing the record to ensure that the documentation supports the discharging physician's final diagnosis and that all diagnoses and procedures are coded. Diagnosis and procedure coding for inpatients (**ICD-9** and/or **ICD-10**) is entered in a software program called a grouper that generates a **DRG code**, which stands for Diagnosis Related Grouping. The DRG code establishes the level of reimbursement a hospital will ultimately receive. Outpatient records are also subjected to diagnostic and procedure coding utilizing a combination of *ICD-9/ICD-10* and **CPT codes**, respectively.

Until medical coding is complete, a bill for services rendered cannot be generated. Most healthcare facilities are dependent upon rapid reimbursement in order to meet key financial obligations, like payroll. The number of days between the time the bill officially "drops" and a check arrives from a third-party payer is referred to as **A/R days** or accounts receivable days.

Many factors impacting the fluctuation of A/R days are outside the control of the healthcare facility, but those within the control of the healthcare facility include ensuring that there are no delays in the documentation process. Backlogs in transcription or coding can result in millions of dollars of unbilled accounts in a single facility. These delays cause A/R days to grow and cash reserves to shrink.

The healthcare documentation specialist plays a role in a healthcare facility's revenue cycle by ensuring timely and complete documentation. The individual HDS can impact the revenue cycle by ensuring demographic information is correct and complete and that discrepancies in a document that could interfere with accurate medical coding are resolved or flagged to the originating clinician's attention. Together with members of the registration department, HIM department, and billing departments, the healthcare documentation specialist is an essential part of the revenue cycle.

Pause for Reflection

1. List 4 common types of reports that could be used to document a patient's hospital stay.
2. Describe some of the important skills and traits for individuals who work in healthcare documentation.
3. List the purposes for healthcare documentation.
4. Outline the steps involved in the creation of a healthcare record prior to involvement by the medical transcriptionist.
5. What is the MT's role in the creation of the healthcare record?
6. What is the role of The Joint Commission?
7. For what reasons might an MT require access to a patient's billing information?
8. At what point does the HIM department assume control of the patient's healthcare record? What happens then?
9. Briefly define ICD-9, ICD-10, CPT, and DRG.
10. Explain how the healthcare documentation specialist is an essential part of the revenue cycle.

HIPAA—What Is It?

by Brenda J. Hurley

HIPAA is the **Health Insurance Portability and Accountability Act**, Public Law 104-191, enacted by Congress in 1996 as a broad attempt at healthcare reform. The Act had two major objectives. The first was to allow individuals to maintain their health insurance from one employer to another; this was relatively straightforward and was successfully implemented.

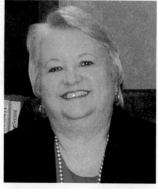

Brenda J. Hurley

The second objective was far more complex; it mandated the security and confidentiality of patient health information and the establishment of uniform standards for electronic data transmissions related to a patient's health information. HIPAA was the first federal legislation that protected the healthcare record; previously only state laws dealt with healthcare records, many of which had been outdated in respect to evolving technologies and the greater mobilization of individuals seeking healthcare services.

So why was HIPAA necessary? It was anticipated that with the establishment of new EHR systems and improved communication within the healthcare delivery system, a better and more efficient healthcare industry would yield enhanced quality in healthcare services but at the same time a need for improved security of the information in each patient's healthcare record and protection of the individual's privacy.

Individuals gained some important rights that are now protected by HIPAA. Healthcare providers and health plans must provide a Notice of Privacy Policies that describes how the individual's information will be used and identifies the individual's rights. In addition, providers must allow patients to

• Inspect and copy their protected health information.

• Request amendment or correction.

• Consent before information is released other than for use related to treatment, payment, and healthcare operations.

KEY HIPAA TERMS

biometric identifier: Biological characteristics that identify an individual. The most commonly used identifiers are fingerprints, handprints, and eye iris and/or retina scans.

breach: An "acquisition, access, use, or disclosure" of unsecured PHI that is not otherwise permitted under HIPAA "which compromises the security or privacy" of the PHI. Unsecured means unencrypted.

business associate (BA): A person who is not an employee of the covered entity or a company that assists in the performance of a function or activity for the covered entity involving the use or disclosure of individually identifiable health information.

covered entity (CE): (1) health plan, (2) healthcare clearinghouse, (3) healthcare provider, and (4) healthcare institutions (i.e., clinics, hospitals, imaging center, etc., places where patients go to seek healthcare services)

disclosure: The release, transfer, provision of access to, or divulging in any other manner of PHI outside the entity that holds the PHI.

encrypted: Secured through the use of a technology or methodology that renders the data unusable, unreadable, or undecipherable to unauthorized individuals.

HHS: Health and Human Services, the branch of the federal government that drafts the rules for implementing HIPAA. Within HHS, the Office of Civil Rights (OCR) is tasked with the responsibility for oversight and enforcement of HIPAA. See **www.hhs.gov/ocr/hipaa** for more information.

healthcare provider: A provider is any person or organization that furnishes medical or other healthcare services. This includes a long list, but some examples include hospitals, skilled nursing facilities, home health agencies, outpatient rehabilitation centers, clinics, physicians, clinical laboratories, pharmacies, nursing homes, and therapists.

individual: The person (patient) who is the subject of the protected health information.

individually identifiable health information: Information collected on an individual that is created or received by a healthcare provider, health plan, employer, or healthcare clearinghouse, that relates to the past, present, or future physical or mental health or condition or the provision of payment for healthcare services. It is determined to be individually identifiable health information if there is a reasonable basis to believe that the information can be used to identify the individual.

protected health information (PHI): Individually identifiable health information that is transmitted, maintained, or stored by any electronic media or in any other form of medium. PHI in its electronic form is referred to as ePHI, although PHI has become acceptable for either.

PROTECTED HEALTH INFORMATION (PHI)

PHI, by definition, contains individually identifiable elements that could lead to the patient's identity. Those identifying elements include:

Name
Geographic subdivisions
Dates, except year
Phone number
Fax number
E-mail address
Social Security number
Medical record number
Health plan number
Account number
Certificate/license number
Vehicle identifiers/license plate
Device identifiers
Web URLs
Internet protocol (IP)
Biometric identifiers
Full face photo
Other unique identifier

• Request restrictions on uses or disclosures.

• Complain about violations to health plan or healthcare provider and to HHS (Health and Human Services).

While the HIPAA Privacy Rule mandated responsibilities of the **covered entities (CEs)**, it recognizes that they often do not perform all the functions and activities themselves. Many times CEs require assistance from a variety of contractors and other businesses. A classification for the **business associate (BA)** was created in order for CEs to share **protected health information (PHI)** with these individuals and businesses enabling them to complete their designated tasks.

The obligations of both the CE and the BA are specified in a written document called a **business associate agreement** (or business associate contract). In general, business associates have to provide assurances that they will safeguard the PHI entrusted to them, use the PHI provided to them only to fulfill their contracted functions or services, notify the covered entity of any breach, make their internal practices and policies available to the covered entity to determine compliance,

and at the termination of the contract, the business associate will return or destroy all PHI in its possession.

Understanding the role of business associate is important for HDSs because businesses that perform medical transcription, called **medical transcription services**, are HIPAA business associates and often employ a large HDS workforce.

When it comes to HIPAA security of PHI, there are three categories: physical, technical, and administrative. The HIPAA Security Rule required the development and implementation of specific written **policies and procedures (P&Ps)** for all CEs and their business associates, some of which include the following:

1. Physical safeguards and technical security of access to computers, workstations, and/or networks.

2. Verification of individuals and entities before a connection to the network is allowed and an audit trail to track system access and failed access attempts.

3. Ensure that PHI is accessed only by properly authorized individuals.

4. Encryption for all health information transmitted outside of the organization.

5. Termination process for removal of access, passwords, security codes, etc.

6. Contingency plan for how data would be accessed when systems are down.

7. Ongoing internal audits for processing and monitoring all security procedures and appropriate access to PHI.

8. Formal HIPAA training program for all those who have access to PHI.

9. Proper disposal of all computer media, including diskettes, tapes, and other storage media that contains PHI.

10. Safeguards to prevent accidental or intentional breach of PHI.

11. Employee sanctions for violations of procedures.

Because HIPAA is so complex, portions of it have been presented and implemented in increments. The portion called the Privacy Rule was enacted in 2003, and the Security Rule in 2005. The HIPAA Privacy and Security Rules were then enhanced in 2010 with the modifications implemented within the American Recovery and Reinvestment Act (ARRA) and its Title XIII called the HITECH (Health Information Technology for Economic and Clinical Health) Act.

One of the significant changes made under the HITECH Act was the breach notification provision. Before this change, individuals had the right to request an accounting of their disclosures but if they did not request this, they likely were never notified of any wrongful disclosure of their PHI. The HITECH Act now requires the patient be notified if there is any breach of their PHI that could cause them significant risk of harm. Included within this scope of "harm" would be any potential significant physical, financial, or reputational loss resulting from that breach.

Guidelines address how to assess this potential significant risk of harm, and if it is determined that there is such a risk, the patient must be notified of the breach within 60 days under HIPAA; however, if state law requires less time for breach notification, the patient is notified in compliance with the state law. State law supersedes the federal law when it provides a higher level of protection to the individual or greater individual rights.

A major risk to healthcare institutions due to a lack of HIPAA compliance is not just from government fines, although they can be significant, but also from bad publicity that comes from major privacy violations. As consumers of healthcare services, when given a choice of providers to use, we would likely want to go to a facility that does the "right thing" in protecting our privacy, over the choice of a facility that has had a known breach of patient data.

The most common example of a breach of PHI in medical transcription is faxing a transcribed report to the wrong recipient. Physicians change practices and offices move, the transcription department or out-sourced transcription service is unfortunately seldom notified of this change; this is then discovered after a fax was sent. The most worrisome scenario is when a physician has closed an office and the phone number has been reassigned to the fax of another business or individual. When a business, such as a gas station, has received an operative report (which is PHI) on a patient, it can be difficult to mitigate potential significant risk of harm to the individual whose information has been breached, escalating the event to a reportable breach requiring patient notification.

An important way to prevent breaches is to use encryption to secure the PHI. HHS guidance for this is 128-bit or 256-bit encryption using the guidelines that are published by NIST (National Institute of Standards and Technology); this can be found at **www.nist.gov.** The encryption of PHI is critical because when PHI is "secured" through this encryption process, a breach is avoided. Even when unauthorized server access has

---

DOES HIPAA PROTECT PRIVACY?
A Gallup Poll taken before the implementation of HIPAA reported the following:

* 77% of Americans feel their health information privacy is very important.
* 84% said they were very concerned that their health information when computerized might be available to others without their consent.
* Only 7% said they are willing to store or transmit their personal information over the Internet, and only 8% said they felt a website could be trusted with this information.
* 90% said they trusted their doctor to keep their information private and secure, 66% trusted a hospital, 42% trusted an insurance company, and 35% trusted a managed care company to do the same.

---

occurred, if the PHI has been appropriately encrypted, no breach has taken place because the data has been rendered unusable, unreadable, and undecipherable.

A large breach is considered to be a breach when 500 or more individuals are affected. When a significant breach occurs, it is usually covered in the media, both locally and nationally. Also, HHS posts on their website the large breaches that have occurred; this is often called by the media the "wall of shame." This listing includes the healthcare institution, the number of individuals whose information was breached, date of the breach, a short description of what caused the breach, and if a business associate was involved the name of that business is listed. This is not a list that a healthcare institution or a business associate ever wants to be affiliated with!

When it comes to protecting health information, it is up to each one of us to do our part. By law, every individual who comes in contact with patient information, in any form, is responsible for protecting that information. Healthcare documentation specialists (HDSs) have access to dictation, faxed data, ADT (admission, discharge, transfer) information, and at times previously transcribed reports. Therefore, HDSs need to be HIPAA savvy in their daily procedures and processes to assure their compliance with the mandated regulations related to HIPAA.

Here are some tips for being HIPAA smart:

1. Protect your computer with password-required access, virus protection, and firewall. Your computer is at tremendous risk for enormous damage without these basic elements of protection to your computer system and for the files that reside in it. Limiting access to your computer helps to assure that files could not be viewed or altered by unauthorized individuals. Without the knowledge of or direction by the user, some viruses can send files from an infected computer to individuals listed in the e-mail address book. It is also possible for an unsuspecting user to transmit viruses while performing routine procedures.

2. When faxing any patient information, use a HIPAA notice of confidentiality on the coversheet. Also, double-check the fax number by using a test fax prior to sending any PHI in order to assure the fax number is accurate.

3. If electronically transferring any patient information, use encryption to secure it from any unauthorized access.

4. Shred all paper that contains any patient information. Do not put paper that contains any patient information in trash bins. If you do not own a shredder, buy one. It is a very small investment for compliance.

5. Do not leave any patient information in areas where unauthorized individuals may have access to it. An unauthorized individual is not just a person who may be a stranger, but also includes family members, friends, and visitors.

6. Locate printers and fax machines in a secured environment to avoid access by unauthorized individuals.

7. If you store PHI in your computer or portable media, encrypt it in order to assure the security of that data.

8. Do not participate in unsafe online practices or Internet activities that could compromise the security of the computer that you use for your work.

9. Analyze your workstation area for ways to be proactive in protecting your computer and the PHI you are entrusted with.

10. Do not disclose PHI beyond the scope of your responsibilities. You are provided PHI for a specific purpose and it can be used only for that purpose. For example, as a medical transcriptionist you will be provided PHI for the purpose of transcribing reports. You do not have authorization to use that PHI for other purposes, such as providing it to a pharmaceutical company for tracking of medication outcomes. That is beyond the scope of your responsibility, and would be considered a breach of PHI.

11. Report any breaches of PHI immediately. There will be times, despite your best efforts, when something slips and an inadvertent release of PHI happens. Do not ignore it. Often significant risk to the patient can be avoided through a quick response with appropriate mitigation processes following a breach.

As consumers of healthcare services, we should all welcome this high level of discretion and confidentiality of our personal health information and for our family's health information. HIPAA is not just one person's job. It is everyone's responsibility!

Pause for Reflection

1. What groups would be defined as HIPAA covered entities?
2. List 3 different types of technology used in the past or the present for capturing or creating healthcare documentation.
3. Describe some of the rights that patients have gained by the enactment of HIPAA.
4. What is the potential connection between HIPAA business associates and healthcare documentation specialists (HDSs)?
5. Briefly describe some of the potential risks to the security of PHI with the use of a remote workforce.
6. What type of information included in a report would cause it to be PHI?
7. Provide a common example of a breach of PHI in the HDS industry and how this can happen.
8. What technology can be used to protect PHI from a breach?

Patient Confidentiality

by Linda C. Campbell

Medical transcriptionists are pledged to protect the privacy and confidentiality of the individual health record (see Code of Ethics at **www.ahdionline.org**). They must never acknowledge or disclose that they are privy to personal, medical, or social patient information. Even if a patient is a relative, friend, or celebrity, the details of every report must remain absolutely confidential.

This is true in every work setting. A privately owned medical transcription company once ran an ad in several allied health publications picturing a home-based medical transcriptionist in her bathrobe, gossiping on the telephone to her friend, with a crying baby nearby in a playpen. The caption read, "Madge, you won't believe what I just found out about your neighbor!" The implication was that a medical transcriptionist working at home is more likely to breach confidentiality than one who is working in an office or within the confines of a hospital. Is this a valid conclusion?

In the past, medical transcriptionists who "came up through the ranks"—that is, those who were trained and then practiced medical transcription solely in the hospital or clinic environment—were often directly involved in some way with patients' medical records. This may have included accessing patient charts to find specific information or even "charting" transcribed reports (physically placing transcribed reports in patient charts). The need for confidentiality of the patient health record was well understood within this environment.

Today there are many practicing medical transcriptionists who have never set foot in a hospital health information or transcription department. Having learned their craft in a college setting or private company, they have gone on to work in transcription services or at home and have never worked directly with patient charts. These transcriptionists may have signed confidentiality agreements in which they commit to hold all patient information in the strictest confidence.

But merely signing a confidentiality agreement does not necessarily mean that they truly understand all that the term "breach" encompasses. Because breach of confidentiality is one of the few areas in health information management where the transcriptionist can be held liable, its importance cannot be overstated.

The following are true case histories that describe encounters with health information. Which are breaches of confidentiality?

1. A transcriptionist saw the name of a friend on a hospital inpatient roster. He phoned the patient's room and said, "I heard you're in the hospital. Would you like a visitor this evening?"

Case review. Unless the patient gave the hospital permission to release his name and room number, the transcriptionist was breaching confidential patient information by contacting his friend in the hospital. It doesn't matter that the transcriptionist avoided telling his friend where he got the information—the patient has the right to privacy. This incident indicates either inadequate education regarding the extent of confidentiality, or lack of professionalism on the part of the transcriptionist.

2. A transcriptionist overheard two lab technicians discussing a patient by name. Because she transcribed the patient's operative report earlier, the transcriptionist is familiar with the patient's history. As she listened to their conversation, she realized they have inaccurate information. "You've got it wrong," she interjected. "The woman in 413 had a therapeutic abortion, not just a D&C."

Case review. It's certainly possible that the transcriptionist felt it was all right to set the record straight with fellow workers; however, it was not her prerogative to do so under these circumstances. The information did not promote patient care and could even be construed as gossip. Knowledge obtained from transcribing a report should not be discussed with co-workers and must never be related to anyone other than those with a valid need to know.

3. Your mother has had quintuple bypass surgery. You are a medical transcriptionist working at home, and you want to help your mother better understand her medical condition. You call your friends in the health information department of the hospital where she is a patient and ask them to make photocopies for you of any report they transcribe on your mother.

Case review. The home worker was not utilizing proper channels to obtain report transcripts on her mother. The health information sought can be legally obtainable, but it must be procured in accordance with regulations. Even if the patient is a relative or friend, the details of every report must remain absolutely confidential; thus, the appropriate action on the part of hospital staff would be to deny the request.

4. A transcriptionist employed by a private company transcribed what she believed to be a sexual abuse case. The physician failed to report the case to the proper authorities. The transcriptionist contacted state authorities and related the incident.

Case review. This was a very serious breach of confidentiality. Even where state laws mandate the reporting of suspected child abuse, that reporting is the responsibility of the hospital or the examining physician, not the transcriptionist. (What actually transpired in this incident is that the transcriptionist was in error about the validity of the child abuse, and she was successfully sued for violation of confidentiality.)

5. A medical transcription service owner in a large metropolitan area interviewed job applicants. One applicant proudly showed the service owner samples of work she had transcribed at a different facility in the same city. The service owner observed that patient names appeared on the reports.

Case review. The applicant not only violated patient confidentiality by taking documents from a facility, but she left the patient names on the documents. The service owner who spoke with this applicant advised her that showing work samples was inappropriate since the sample documents could have been someone else's work. Furthermore, he would not hire the applicant under any circumstances because she had blatantly violated patient confidentiality by not removing or obscuring the names in the documents.

Protecting confidentiality. Make sure that your environment is secure from intruders. A hospital in California went to great expense to implement state-of-the-art computers networked to their satellite facilities, running sophisticated software programs, and then neglected to provide adequate locks and alarm systems. A resulting break-in resulted in the theft of millions of dollars' worth of computer equipment— and an untold amount of confidential patient information—when the thieves simply walked out of the hospital with computers in hand.

Finally, understand that the penalties for violation of confidential patient information will probably include immediate dismissal or termination of contract and legal liability for violations. In other words, **you can be fired and sued**.

Because confidentiality is a critical issue, your employer will inform you of the facility's policy about patient confidentiality. The employer may also require you to sign a confidentiality statement and will inform you of the penalties for violating patient confidentiality. In most facilities a breach of patient confidentiality is grounds for immediate dismissal from the job.

HEALTHCARE DOCUMENTATION SPECIALISTS

Healthcare documentation specialists have always done more than one thing. We have always been more than typists. We have always used our extensive knowledge of medical terminology, anatomy and physiology, laboratory values, diagnostic tests and other information in our positions. Professionals in our industry have known for a long time that their compensation and value to the industry were seen in relation to their manual dexterity and the ability to produce a certain number of lines of documentation per day. The term medical transcriptionist became synonymous with typist, and the knowledge base of these professionals often was overlooked.

Even coworkers thought that we sat at a desk all day and typed what we heard. They did not realize that we were also proofreading, analyzing, marking questionable text for clarification by the physician, flagging reports that seemed to have errors including medication and allergy conflicts, dosage amounts, and plans of care. All of these skills and talents are highlighted by the change to the healthcare documentation specialist title.

Recent changes in the industry are clearing away the fog that has kept healthcare documentation specialists out of view. At long last, physicians, nurses, and the industry as a whole, not to mention the federal government, are actually taking a long look at documentation issues within the industry.

Meaningful use initiatives are tied to accurate, timely, and clear documentation of patient encounters. Documentation improvement programs are springing up in every institution, with more and more of the focus being on developing methods to capture the true and accurate health story of each patient's care.

The seven criteria AHIMA has given for high-quality healthcare documentation are:
- legibility
- precision
- consistency
- timeliness.
- reliability
- completeness
- clarity

Those are the goals, and those are the areas where healthcare documentation specialists have historically been gatekeepers and protectors of the record.

Cynthia C. Alder

Spotlight On

How I Became a Medical Transcriptionist

by Bron Taylor

When I started my shift today, I turned on the computer, adjusted the ergonomic chair and keyboard tray from my desk partner's settings to mine, and changed the monitor to a fresh set of colors. Then I checked my electronic mailbox. I found a format for a new type of clinic note, which I downloaded, quickly read, and filed in my procedure manual. Next I looked at the statistics and saw that we were very caught up, so I relaxed a bit. I felt a little like an airline pilot, booting up and adjusting all this powerful equipment.

When I turned on my digital transcriber, my first piece of work was a stat discharge summary. During the dictation, the doctor mentioned the Kleihauer-Betke test. As it had been many months since I'd last heard this, I thought I'd better check it. Was it really Kleihauer or Kleihaure? I could have left my terminal and found it in a reference book, or asked a co-worker, but as I was working on a stat, I used our on-line "homemade dictionary" instead, confirming that I had all the vowels in the right places (yes; Kleihauer), and within seconds I was back in the report. When I was finished, I phoned from the off-site office where I work to the transcription unit at the medical center, to let them know a stat was being printed; it was already coming off the printer and was quickly sent to the floor.

I was 28 years old when I discovered there was such a thing as transcription. I was extremely fortunate in how I discovered it, and yet I don't think my story is that different from that of others who have been doing this work for more than 20 years. There were no formal training courses when we started. One way or another, we stumbled onto the existence of the job; usually someone in a position to give us a chance to learn, someone who always needed more MTs, became aware of us and made the connection for us. Some didn't have this kind of mentoring and had to gamble that they could learn on the job, promising skills they didn't have but quickly developed.

I'd gone to college straight out of high school and married straight out of college, so I was 28 and unskilled when I was finally looking for my first job in the early 1970s, after an amicable divorce. After a long search, I finally found an entry-level job in the file room at a university teaching hospital. As I'd always loved everything about medicine, and would have gone to medical school had my math skills been strong, I was pleased to be working in a medical center right in the midst of the real thing.

During the day there would be slow times when nobody wanted a record from my rows of files. I'd pull a thick chart and read it without looking at the name on it. One day a woman I knew only as "that nice lady who works in the back somewhere" caught me at it, but was smiling. Soon we were talking whenever she came looking for a chart, and she elicited from me that I'd been pre-med, loved to read, loved medicine, and, curiously, couldn't type. Why would she want to know that, I wondered. I had met Vera Pyle.

Soon I started working weekends, and part of my job was to change a broad band of tape when a bell rang. I didn't have the vaguest idea what I was doing, but carefully followed instructions. Vera Pyle was often in on weekends, and one day she asked if I'd like to be shown around the transcription department. "Yes," I said. So she showed me the cubicles, the correcting IBM Selectric typewriters, the reference material (at great length, as I was awed), and the "homemade dictionary." She told me how the dictionary had been developed in the transcription unit and how it was kept up-to-date. Any MT could make entries, but they had to be verified and not just "doctors' spelling." I wondered what that meant. She explained about the tape equipment and why I was changing belts. She asked me again if I could type, and I had to say no. It felt as if a door was closing.

The campus newspaper printed an article about transcriptionists, including Vera Pyle, and I read it again and again, not even realizing that I wanted to do this so badly I couldn't even admit it to myself. Vera could see that, though. In our talks she'd told me the ingredients for a good transcriptionist. One had to love medicine, love researching words, have a good feel for English grammar, and a good ear for accents. One had to

Spotlight On How I Became a Medical Transcriptionist, page 2

respect the patient behind the paper of the medical record and never ever guess what a physician was saying.

I can do that, I thought to myself, but couldn't type so I didn't even consider it. Sometimes I'd listen to the sound of fast typing from the transcription department in action, and it seemed hopeless. I didn't realize then that typing was the least of it. The university normally required an MT to have two years of acute care hospital experience before hiring, but Vera Pyle received permission to train me and a co-worker from the hospital laundry. She asked us if we'd commit to work on transcription for an hour each day if she agreed to teach us. We were speechless. We promised to read reports, read journals, and work as hard as we could to learn.

Over the years I learned transcription and then went on to learn transcription theory, editing, and editing theory, opening the door not only to a career I've enjoyed but to work as a writer and editor.

I was very tentative at first, in a room with such experts. The first documents I produced were thanks to a resident physician who was afraid of the phone, who handwrote all her consultations which then had to be copy-typed. None of the MTs wanted to do her work, which mystified me then, but now I understand. Happily for me, she was a pediatric endocrinologist with good handwriting, so my first documents were thick with complex lab work and gave me a sense of format. As Vera realized, of course, doing all of this copy-typing was good practice for my beginning typing skills. I typed as much as I could in the clerical part of the day.

During my "transcription hour," I'd work until I'd asked everyone in the room at least one question, like "Is there such a thing as Betadine?" After that I dared not bother anyone twice, so I'd retype the work. Of course, I quickly did learn how to type, and I'm now as irritable as anyone when someone walks into a room full of MTs, listens to rapid typing, and says, "Oooh, how fast do you type?"

Every piece of work I did was proofreaded by Vera Pyle. I think I had some of the most intensive proofreading anyone has ever had. I wanted to capture every nuance, every subtlety. I liked the

medical center's style, demanding full sentences in every part of the report with consistent tenses, with lab work written in narrative style and divided into the correct categories. BUN and creatinine were put in a separate sentence from electrolytes, never mind what the dictator said. We were expected to know that a differential was not part of a routine CBC and punctuate accordingly. Work coming out of our unit didn't look or read like something sent by Western Union. (It has taken me many years to lighten up and accept that in some cases a telegraphic or clipped style communicates just as well, and using it is not a moral failing.)

Now it's many years later. I've helped to write, edit, and proofread many books, and had many articles published by three publishers. I'm just as pleased with transcription and just as proud to be an MT and just as curious as to what the next dictation will reveal as I was at the beginning. Vera gave me a strong foundation, and when I later went to work as a proofreader for a large service, in pathology, in radiology, and at home for researchers. I was rarely challenged as I had been working for her at the university medical center.

Why do we have a rule "never guess"? Because a wrong guess, a soundalike but incorrect medication, will go into someone's permanent record and be picked up and repeated and could cause harm. The same rule that applies to everyone in the medical profession— Hippocrates' "First, do no harm"—applies to us too. Transcription decisions are made based on what in the end will best serve the patient.

Many of us were given a chance to learn transcription by a manager who needed more MTs and saw potential in someone with no experience. Very few of us knew that this niche in the medical field existed until one day we stumbled on it by accident. I don't think too many of us as children said, "I want to be a medical transcriptionist when I grow up." I'm glad that such good teaching materials exist now, and that transcription teachers are everywhere, with that field becoming a profession in itself. This raises the level of transcription and everyone benefits.

Exercises

Vocabulary Review

Instructions: Choose the best answer.

___ 1. Meaningful text is most likely to be captured by which of the following?
   A. Speech recognition technology.
   B. Structured text systems.
   C. Point-and-click templates.
   D. MTs with interpretive medical language skills.

___ 2. A major limitation of today's electronic healthcare record systems is their lack of
   _____
   A. standardization across different systems.
   B. alerts when inconsistent information has been entered.
   C. capability to overcome input errors by not allowing the report to be closed.
   D. reminders that entries have been skipped.

___ 3. According to author Hurley, the reason that medical transcription has endured over the years is because _____
   A. it is cheaper and faster than other modalities of healthcare documentation.
   B. other modalities of healthcare documentation have yet to be widely accepted.
   C. other methods of healthcare documentation are expensive, cumbersome and not user friendly.
   D. it deals with imperfect dictation/transcription process in a way that has not been replicated by other modalities.

___ 4. Which skill do the authors seem to believe is the trait that gives medical transcriptionists the advantage over technology?
   A. Knowledge of medical terminology, anatomy, and other clinical sciences.
   B. Interpretive skills that focus on intended meaning over what was said.
   C. Being able to apply grammar, punctuation, and style as one transcribes.
   D. Facility with computers and adaptability to changes in technology.

___ 5. The first federal legislation that protected the healthcare record was _____
   A. HIPAA.
   B. NIST.
   C. ARRA.
   D. HITECH.

___ 6. _____ is the acquisition, access, use, or disclosure of unsecured PHI that is not permitted under HIPAA.
   A. A disclosure
   B. A breach
   C. Encryption
   D. Protection

___ 7. Healthcare institutions (i.e., clinics, hospitals, imaging center, etc., places where patients go to seek healthcare services) are considered
   _____
   A. business associates.
   B. protected health information.
   C. covered entities.
   D. individually identifiable health information.

___ 8. Protected health information does NOT include _____
   A. a patient's marital status.
   B. the city and state in which a patient lives.
   C. phone number.
   D. date of birth.

___ 9. Which statement is NOT true?
   A. The HITECH Act requires the patient be notified if there is any breach of their PHI that could cause any potential significant physical, financial, or reputational loss resulting from that breach.
   B. State law supersedes the federal law when it provides a higher level of protection to the individual or greater individual rights.
   C. If it is determined that there has been a breach of patient privacy, the patient must be notified of the breach within 90 days after the breach occurred.
   D. The 2010 American Recovery and Reinvestment Act (ARRA) is an enhancement of HIPAA Privacy and Security Rules.

___ 10. Which incident constitutes a breach of patient privacy?
   A. Faxing a medical report to a fax number that has been changed and is not for a medical office involved in the treatment of the patient.
   B. Sending a copy of a medical report to the patient's insurance company for reimbursement purposes.
   C. Sharing individually identifiable health information in a letter to a physician requesting consultation services.
   D. Interpreting your mother-in-law's laboratory test results with her so that she can understand them.

Terms Review

Instructions: Match the following healthcare documentation terms to their descriptions or definitions. Some answers may be used more than once, some not at all.

___ 1. ADT (admission, discharge, transfer) information

___ 2. back-end speech recognition technology (BE-SRT)

___ 3. front-end speech recognition technology (FE-SRT)

___ 4. healthcare documentation specialist (HDS)

___ 5. meaningful text

___ 6. medical transcriptionist (MT)

___ 7. quality assurance (QA) specialist

___ 8. speech recognition editor (SRE or SE)

___ 9. speech recognition technology (SRT)

___ 10. structured-text system

A. Demographic data

B. A means of creating standardized text using predesigned templates

C. A method by which templates, outlines, or check boxes are used to document patient care

D. Accurate and complete healthcare documentation that contributes to quality patient care

E. Editing of speech-recognized draft text by the originator in real time while dictating

F. Editor or edits speech-recognized drafts.

G. Individual who produces medical reports from dictation

H. One who ensures that healthcare documentation is accurate and complete

I. Speech is converted to text by a computer using voice profile, language system, and dictionary

J. Umbrella designation for numerous positions related to healthcare documentation

K. Use of editors to proofread and correct speech-recognition drafts

Computer Skills Survey

Instructions: Complete this computer skills survey by matching the following computer concepts or terms to their descriptions or definitions. These are just some of the common concepts you should be familiar with at the beginning of the program, but it is not comprehensive. However, it should reveal any significant gaps and reflect your comfort level with computer technology. If you are unsure about your computer skills, you may want to investigate a basic computer skills course. Some answers may be used more than once, some not at all.

Computer Concept or Term

___ 1. Alt key

___ 2. caps lock

___ 3. CTRL key

___ 4. CTRL+W or CTRL+F4

___ 5. CTRL+BACKSPACE

___ 6. CTRL+C

___ 7. CTRL+DELETE

___ 8. CTRL+F

___ 9. CTRL+P

___ 10. CTRL+Q

___ 11. CTRL+S

___ 12. CTRL+V

___ 13. CTRL+X

___ 14. CTRL+Z

___ 15. email address (example)

___ 16. ESC

___ 17. hardware

___ 18. Internet Explorer

___ 19. Microsoft Excel

___ 20. Microsoft Windows

___ 21. Microsoft Word

___ 22. Microsoft Powerpoint

___ 23. monitor

___ 24. mouse

___ 25. Mozilla Firefox

___ 26. router

___ 27. shift key

___ 28. software

___ 29. tab key

___ 30. Web address (example)

Description or Definition

A. Indents text a predetermined amount of space

B. Delete an entire word to right of cursor.

C. A Web search engine

D. santaclaus@northpole.com

E. Exit out of a program

F. Cuts highlighted text from a document

G. Command to copy highlighted text

H. Widely used operating system for personal computers

I. A device used to point, click, select, or move information on the computer screen

J. Cancels an operation in progress

K. Software for creating presentations

L. Initiates a search inside a document or on a Web page

M. Device that allows networking of multiple computers and/or peripheral hardware

N. A key that changes the function when pressed in conjunction with another key

O. Changes letters to capitals and selects the symbols associated with the number keys

P. Popular word processing software

Q. www.myhealthprofessionskit.com

R. Toggles between open windows

S. Undoes a previous action

T. Display device for a computer

U. When this key is pressed, text will be in all capital letters.

V. The mechanical, magnetic, electronic, and electrical components making up a computer system

W. Delete an entire word to left of cursor.

X. Print command

Y. Command to close a window

Z. Spreadsheet software

AA. Saves a document or file

BB. Pastes previously copied text into a document

CC. This key, when pressed in conjunction with another key, will perform a special operation.

DD. Computer programs or written procedures for performing functions on a computer

English Vocabulary: Homophones

Instructions: Homophones, more commonly called "soundalikes," are very possibly the most common type of errors committed by both MTs and speech recondition engines. Both English and medicine abound with words and phrases that sound alike or very similar to other words and phrases. Being able to distinguish among these will give the novice transcriptionist or speech editor a leg up on more experienced practitioners. Take this little "soundalike" survey and see how well you do. Choose the correct word from the terms inside the parentheses. This is not a test. Look up any words about which you are uncertain. You may want to start a notebook in which you have a section for recording English and medical soundalike terms.

_____ 1. The patient was (councilled, counseled) to get psychiatric help.

_____ 2. The patient expressed strong (decent, descent, dissent) to the recommended bypass operation.

_____ 3. Venous (access, assess, axis, excess) was needed for IV administration of antibiotics, so a heparin lock was placed.

_____ 4. (Accept, Except) for a slight weakness in the left arm, the patient had no residual symptoms of stroke.

_____ 5. Because penicillin was not (affective, effective), the patient was put on another antibiotic.

_____ 6. The patient's wife made an (allusion, elusion, illusion) to possible alcoholism by stating that the patient drank a six-pack a day, but the patient denied a drinking problem.

_____ 7. My (advice, advise) to the patient was to drink plenty of liquids, get lots of sleep, and take aspirin for pain.

_____ 8. The patient complained of (a symptomatic, asymptomatic) cough for the last month, but it was nonproductive.

_____ 9. I would (access, assess, axis, excess) his chances of surviving the operation at 50:50.

_____ 10. The surgical (cite, sight, site) was dressed with a sterile bandage.

_____ 11. The patient was not (conscience, conscious) after the head injury.

_____ 12. Moderate exercise would certainly (complement, compliment) the patient's post-CABG therapy.

The Healthcare Record

2

Learning Objectives

▶ Explain the purpose of the healthcare record.

▶ Review the steps in the creation of an individual healthcare record and identify the individuals who participate in its creation.

▶ Expand selected abbreviations and define vocabulary related to healthcare and healthcare providers and facilities.

▶ Summarize the mission or role of the HIM department.

▶ Describe the components of a healthcare record, including those components that may not be dictated and transcribed.

▶ Describe the components of healthcare report types that are dictated, including chart notes, letters, initial office evaluations, emergency department reports, consultations, H&Ps, operative reports, and discharge summaries.

▶ Describe the two techniques used by the physician to gather data for a diagnosis.

▶ Explain the reasons physicians order laboratory tests.

▶ Distinguish among different drug dosage forms and delivery methods.

▶ Discuss the healthcare documentation specialist's role in preventing drug errors.

The Healthcare Record

Chapter 1 discusses healthcare documentation and the role of the healthcare documentation specialist in the creation of the healthcare record. In this chapter, we will go into detail about the components of the healthcare record and the types of reports that medical transcriptionists and speech recognition editors will most likely encounter in their work.

The healthcare record is a legal record detailing the healthcare services rendered to a patient. It may be paper, stored digitally in electronic format in a computer, or a combination of the two. The healthcare record is the property of the hospital or the medical facility or office in which it originates, and it cannot be removed from the premises without a subpoena or court order. In hospitals and usually in large multi-specialty clinics or health maintenance organizations (HMOs), the healthcare record is maintained in a **health information management (HIM)** department. The HIM department is usually headed by a **registered health information administrator (RHIA)**. Other duties in the HIM department are performed by a **registered health information technician (RHIT)**. RHIAs and RHITs are certified by **AHIMA (American Health Information Management Association)**.

Purpose of the Healthcare Record

The healthcare record is a measurement of care rendered in a medical facility. It is utilized to plan, communicate, and evaluate the quality of care given to each patient. It is "proof of work done," containing documentation to meet federal, state, and The Joint Commission standards and regulations, as well as requirements for reimbursement from third-party payers. The healthcare record is maintained for medicolegal protection for the patient, facility, staff, and physician. It is used for research, compiling statistics, and evaluation of healthcare delivery.

Origin of the Healthcare Record

Let's briefly review the creation of the healthcare record. In hospitals, the healthcare record begins in the admissions department, outpatient registration, or the emergency department (ED). Patients having surgery as outpatients check in at outpatient regis-tration, which registers elective surgery outpatients and clinic patients. These patients, after observation, may also be admitted. Patients may also enter the hospital after evaluation in the emergency department,

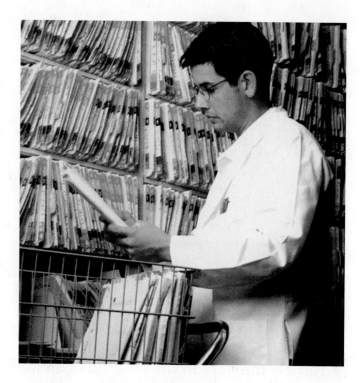

which collects patient identification and demographic information. The correct spelling of the patient's legal name and birthdate are critical elements to determine positive patient identification. The healthcare record number that is assigned is maintained for the lifetime of the patient when seeking services from that health-care facility and should be recorded on all transcribed reports.

Additional identification entries on patients are address, next of kin, birthplace, Social Security number, occupation, sex, marital status, ethnic origin, religious preference, and admitting diagnosis. Financial entries include the patient's employer, job title, address of company, insurance company, person responsible for emergency notification and payments, type of coverage, insurance identification number, and type of payment plan. All this information is recorded on an admission sheet or patient demographic face sheet.

Consents and Privacy Notice

The departments noted above also have responsibility for obtaining forms which include the patient's consent for treatment and outline of patient's responsibilities, including payment for services, and the assurance that confidentiality will be protected. Throughout a patient's care, additional informed consents for surgery, procedures, invasive diagnostic tests, transfer, etc., will be obtained as appropriate.

Admissions clerks will also often ask a patient about to be admitted if he or she has a "living will," a healthcare declaration that simply documents a person's wishes concerning treatment when those wishes can no longer be personally communicated. Some hospitals and physician offices provide a form for patients to complete if they do not already have a living will.

The **Health Insurance Portability and Accountability Act (HIPAA)** contains detailed directives regarding the confidentiality of all data contained in healthcare records (see Chapter 1). Under the terms of this legislation, a provider of healthcare must inform each patient of the extent of privacy protection, including exceptions (for example, sharing of historical or diagnostic information among physicians in a group practice), and must obtain the patient's signed authorization for any transfer of information to a third party, except as set forth in the regulations.

It is recommended that patients keep copies of their own medical reports in order to have a complete **personal health record (PHR)** available to emergency departments, hospitals, and their doctors. A PHR can help improve the quality of care a person receives by reducing or eliminating duplicate tests and allowing patients to receive faster, safer treatment and care in an emergency. In short, a PHR helps people play a more active role in their own healthcare. There are many websites that provide a way for individuals to safely store their PHR on the Internet. One such site that is free is MyPHR (**www.myphr.com**), hosted by AHIMA.

Pause for Reflection

1. What is the purpose of the healthcare record?
2. Where does the creation of the healthcare record begin?
3. What is a living will?
4. What is the purpose of HIPAA?
5. What is a PHR and how does it contribute to one's healthcare?

Vocabulary Review

admitting physician The doctor who admits the patient and generally oversees his/her care while an inpatient. Also called the *attending physician*.

American Health Information Management Association (AHIMA) The professional organization for health information administrators, technicians, coders, and health information technology (HIT) professionals.

assisted living facility (ALF) Although there is no nationally recognized definition of an assisted living facility, it is generally a residential facility in which patients with disabilities are provided assistance with **activities of daily living (ADLs)**.

Centers for Medicare and Medicaid Services (CMS) The government agency that sets regulations and manages reimbursement for those on Medicare and Medicaid.

CPT codes *Current Procedural Terminology* codes assigned to procedures for the purpose of reimbursement and other uses.

DRG codes Diagnosis-related group codes that determine the amount of reimbursement the hospital will receive.

extended care facility (ECF) A medical institution that provides prolonged care (as in cases of prolonged illness or rehabilitation from acute illness).

HCPS codes Codes similar to CPT codes that are required by the Centers for Medicare and Medicaid Services.

health information management (HIM) department The department that preserves and protects healthcare records.

Health Insurance Portability and Accountability Act (HIPAA) Federal legislation detailing the requirements for privacy and confidentiality of patient information.

hospitalist A physician who oversees the care of patients admitted to the hospital, works exclusively in a hospital, and does not have a private practice.

ICD codes *International Classification of Diseases* codes assigned to diagnoses and surgical procedures for purposes of reimbursement and other uses.

living will A healthcare declaration that documents a person's wishes concerning treatment when those wishes can no longer be personally communicated.

nurse practitioner (NP) An **advanced practice registered nurse (APRN)** or **advanced registered nurse practitioner (ARNP)**, depending on the state one is in, who has completed graduate-level education (either a Master of Nursing or Doctor of Nursing Practice degree). NPs assess patients, order and interpret diagnostic tests, make diagnoses, and initiate and manage treatment plans—including prescribing medications. NPs usually work closely with physicians but may also be the primary care provider in some clinic and community healthcare settings.

physician assistant (PA) A medical professional who works as part of a healthcare team under the supervision of a physician. PAs perform physical examinations, diagnose and treat illnesses, order and interpret lab tests, perform procedures, assist in surgery, provide patient education and counseling and make rounds in hospitals and nursing homes. All 50 states and the District of Columbia allow PAs to practice and prescribe medications.

primary care provider (PCP) The physician, usually a family practice or internal medicine specialist, who takes care of a patient's healthcare on a routine basis. The PCP may be an admitting or attending physician who has privileges at a hospital or other healthcare facility.

RAC audit Comparing of documentation to amount billed to Medicare or Medicaid, looking for discrepancies. See *Recovery Audit Contractor*.

Recovery Audit Contractor (RAC) A company designated by CMS to act as a bounty hunter looking for fraud and any indication of overcharging.

registered health information administrator (RHIA) A credentialed professional qualified by exam to oversee the creation and use of health information systems in healthcare settings and manage health information departments.

registered health information technician (RHIT) A technician who ensures and verifies medical record completeness, accuracy, and proper entry into computer systems.

Release of Information request A request for information by an entity outside the facility, especially insurance companies, attorneys, other healthcare providers, to the patients themselves, and to fulfill subpoenas. The requests are scrutinized to ensure they comply with all applicable regulations before copies of records are released.

skilled nursing facility (SNF) A residential nursing home, convalescent home, or skilled nursing unit in a larger healthcare facility that provides nursing care for patients on a short-term or long-term basis.

Professional Reading

A View from the HIM Director's Chair
by Georgia Green

You may never meet the Director of Health Information Management in the facility for which you transcribe, but that person is acutely aware of your performance. The HIM director is the legal guardian of the healthcare record and everything in it. Every document you transcribe is the responsibility of the HIM director.

In facilities with in-house transcription services, the HIM director may personally manage the medical transcription department or rely on a supervisor. When I entered the field of medical transcription 30 years ago, most MTs worked on-site, physically in or very nearby what was then called the medical record department. If our work ran low, we helped out in medical records with virtually every task, from filing charts to coding diagnoses.

The new generation of MTs works primarily off-site and few have seen the inside of a modern HIM department, and this puts them at a distinct disadvantage. A dictated document is very much impacted by the content of the healthcare record that the MT cannot see. In addition, the challenges faced by the HIM director guide decisions made about the transcription process—from the establishment of quality and productivity benchmarks to choosing software platforms to decisions made about employing speech recognition technology or outsourcing.

Last summer the HIM director in my hospital resigned, and I was asked to fill her role until a replacement could be recruited and hired. I lacked the necessary HIM credentialing, but as the on-site transcription supervisor for the previous four years, I knew the HIM staff and had a working knowledge of some of their processes. The rest I would have to learn quickly while I sat in the director's chair.

I looked first to the mission of the department:

• Guards the confidentiality of medical records and supervises their transmittal to those authorized to see them.

• Performs qualitative and quantitative analysis of each patient record to assure its consistency and completeness.

• Abstracts and codes all records and prepares them for billing and reimbursement.

- Facilitates record-keeping for the medical staff by providing transcription services and developing the most efficient procedures for record completion.
- Participates in quality assurance, utilization review, and risk management activities.
- Provides services and reports to various medical staff committees, and others as requested.

It helped that I regularly read HIM publications that are made available to MTs. I was also well versed on HIPAA and the laws pertaining to release of information. However, there were some areas for which I might be a little unprepared.

On my first day the chief financial officer, who had placed me in this role, told me my job was to keep things running smoothly, to keep people from bringing HIM problems to him, and to do something about the "unbilled" list. We had $8 million in outstanding billings that could not go out because coding was behind. I didn't know what that meant but it sounded bad.

My new team members were already known to me in the sense that we had mingled at department celebrations and had the occasional lunch or break together. Now I needed to know what they did when they were on the clock. They each explained their roles to me and took me through their process step by step. We were in the middle of transitioning to an electronic healthcare record, but we still had paper charts that contained both original records and copies of what was signed electronically.

Volunteers assembled skeletal healthcare records, commonly called "charts," at the direction of the HIM department and provided them to specific nursing floors. An OB chart contains different forms than a chart used on the medical floor. The unit secretary on each nursing floor was responsible for maintaining the chart until the patient was discharged. He or she would file test results and transcribed records in the appropriate sections and restock needed forms for doctor's orders, progress notes, intake and output records, medication administration records, and so on.

Every morning an HIM clerk would visit each of the nursing floors to pick up "discharged charts," the records of those patients who had been discharged the previous day. A designated assembler would go through each record and put the pages in the correct order. While a patient is in-house, most chart entries are on the top. When a patient is discharged, page order for individual types of documents, like lab tests or progress notes, needs to be chronological, with the most recent at the end. At that point the order of the documents

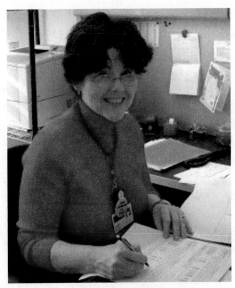

Georgia Green

also changed, with certain documents placed topmost and others at the back.

The assembler was responsible for knowing which documents were part of the legal healthcare record and which were not. Of those documents that didn't belong in the chart, some were returned where they belonged while others were safe to destroy. The assembler inserted the assembled record into the patient's existing chart, if any, as a new admission. If the folder grew too large, it was separated into volumes and older volumes remained on the shelves unless requested. An entry was made in the electronic tracking system indicating the chart was now physically located in the HIM department.

Next, the chart went to an analyst. If the assembler was also qualified as an analyst, he or she would do both jobs at once. The analyst scrutinized the record to ensure that every handwritten entry was signed, dated, and timed, as required by The Joint Commission. If any documents were missing, like a discharge summary, this would be noted as well. Missing documents or signatures were noted in the chart tracking program as "deficiencies." The chart then went to coding.

Each of the coders had a specialty area: outpatient services, physician office visits and procedures, emergency department visits, same-day surgery, inpatients with Medicare/Medicaid coverage, and inpatients with private insurance. One coder even specialized in "mommas and babies."

Coders would abstract a record, going through it page by page to determine if the diagnosis stated by the attending physician was supported by the documentation. They would then apply **ICD codes** to every diagnosis and surgical procedure, if an inpatient. Outpatient codes utilized **CPT codes** for every service as well as additional **HCPS codes** for Medicare/Medicaid patients, similar to CPT codes.

After the diagnostic codes were determined, they were entered into a software program called a grouper. A grouper assigns the **DRG**, or **diagnosis-related group. The DRG correlates the amount of reimbursement the hospital will receive.** Coders describe their legal and ethical responsibility with pride. They select only those codes justified by the documentation, and the coder's choice is final.

After coding, charts were released to the incomplete chart room for any needed signatures or missing documentation. When the record was complete, the appropriate entry would be made in the tracking system and the chart would be filed away. The filing process alone was not final as the shelves would quickly fill and it was necessary to constantly purge older charts and send them to off-site storage. Off-site storage was also limited, so the identification of records that could be designated for destruction was ongoing.

Charts seldom sat idle on the shelf waiting for the next admission. There were numerous audits for which charts needed to be pulled. Audits were conducted by nearly every department in the hospital, from the emergency department to the pharmacy to various medical staff subcommittees. Charts were pulled and the records scrutinized to assess compliance with current guidelines and review of outcomes to determine if guidelines should be changed. Audits were conducted by state and federal agencies, often without notice. Audits were also requested by insurance companies, sometimes on groups of records and other times a single record. Often the entire contents of a chart would be requested, requiring that every page be photocopied.

RAC (Recovery Audit Contractor) audits were especially challenging. RAC audits involved Medicare patients for which **CMS** (Centers for Medicare and Medicaid Services) designated a company to act as a bounty hunter looking for fraud and any indication of overcharging. As many as 200 records could be requested at a time. They would need to be scanned and transmitted electronically within a strict timeframe. The auditing agency would compare the documentation to the payment made by Medicare, and if it found a single discrepancy, the entire payment for that hospitalization would be immediately revoked. The hospital would have to appeal the finding to try to get

the money refunded. This process was so complex that it required hiring an additional HIM clerk to manage it.

The release of information specialists were involved any time information was to be provided to an outside entity, especially insurance companies, attorneys, other healthcare providers, to the patients themselves, and to fulfill subpoenas. The request would be scrutinized to ensure it complied with all applicable regulations before copies of records were released.

In addition to the numerous in-house departments and committees conducting audits of records, these same groups requested statistics. Through trial and error, I learned to use the abstracting program that would allow me to answer requests such as, "How many patients of Dr. X in the last two years had one of these three surgeries?" or "How many pediatric patients were inpatients for more than three days in the last year?" This abstracting software would prove useful in managing the transcription process when I returned to that role full time, as I would now have the ability to not just query how many operative reports were dictated by Dr. Z but how many laparoscopic cholecystectomies he did and quickly produce a list of the reports, should I need sample documents.

In addition to keeping track of the healthcare record from its creation until its resting place in the chart room, with all of its many side trips, the HIM director participates in numerous hospital committees and projects. They meet regularly with the representatives of the medical staff and with the medical staff's committee on quality and utilization review. Most members of the medical staff comply with record-keeping rules while others are "high maintenance" from the perspective of the HIM director. They have difficulty with compliance, refuse to comply, or insist on special treatment. It is in this role that the HIM director serves as a buffer between the dictators of transcribed records and the healthcare documentation specialists who transcribe them.

If a new type of form is needed anywhere in the hospital, it must be approved by the forms committee, which the HIM director chaired. There were regular meetings with business and accounts receivable people, with IT teams, and with ancillary departments, to identify and solve problems that prevented the billing and payment process from going smoothly. Invariably, documentation issues were implicated, and HIM's input was crucial in finding a solution.

The federal mandate to meet "meaningful use" with an electronic healthcare record was another source of ongoing meetings, as new software and processes were tested and discussed. The number of decisions that had already been made without consulting health information management was astounding. For example, an application that allowed doctors to enter their own progress notes electronically required the development of templates. These had been designed by people with nursing backgrounds without any input from healthcare documentation specialists. The resulting documents were hard to read and the medical staff, anxious for the convenience afforded by electronic charting, ultimately rejected this tool because dictated documents were easier to read and understand.

During the three months I spent in the director's chair, I learned a great deal about managing an HIM department, including the knowledge that managing health information management is not for me. I did, however, resolve the problem of the unbilled list, much to the delight of our CFO. Our turnaround times in the transcription area were stellar so that wasn't what was holding up coding. I learned that coders faced many of the same issues with productivity as did transcriptionists—awkward design of workflow processes, frequent interruptions, work assignments poorly matched to skill sets, and low morale.

While I had little power to fix big problems, minor tweaks were possible, and just having someone listen and genuinely care about challenges you have to overcome to do your work on a daily basis can lift morale. That $8 million backlog dwindled back down to normal levels. I returned to my crew with a new appreciation for what goes on in the HIM department.

Pause for Reflection

1. Why does working off-site put the remote medical transcriptionist at a disadvantage when it comes to working on the healthcare record?
2. Summarize the mission or duties of the health information management department as outlined by Georgia Green.
3. What is the unit clerk or ward clerk's role with respect to the healthcare record?
4. Briefly outline the path the patient's chart takes once the patient is discharged.
5. What happens to a chart after it is filed away?
6. What is the role of the release of information specialist?

Components of the Healthcare Record

Physician Orders

A patient is admitted and treated only on the order of an attending physician. The admission includes orders for diagnostic tests, medications, and treatments. Pharmacy orders may be entered electronically for safety reasons. Paper-based forms are usually multipart with a copy for the department.

From the physician's orders, the nurses generate a requisition for diagnostic tests. These are sent to the appropriate department, whose personnel perform the tests and document the results. Typical diagnostic results include the following.

Laboratory. Lab slips include the results of urinalyses, complete blood counts, electrolytes, chemistries, specimens, and blood transfusions. Pathology and autopsy results are also the responsibility of this department.

Radiology. Dictated reports include the clinical history, findings, and conclusions for any x-rays and diagnostic imaging performed.

Cardiology. Electrocardiograms, Holter monitor, and exercise stress test results are dictated, or reports are machine generated.

Neurophysiology. Electroencephalograms, electromyograms, and sleep disorder results are dictated or machine generated.

Nursing Entries

Nurses assess patients on admission by completing an admission history and physical, establish a patient care plan, and set up forms for documentation of graphic information such as vital signs (temperature, pulse, respiration, blood pressure, and weight). Intake and output of fluids, diet and hygiene records, medication records, as well as specialized forms for monitoring diabetes, operating room checklists, operating room record, recovery room record, and nurses' notes and observations become a part of every patient's healthcare record.

Therapist Entries

Physical, respiratory, occupational, speech, vocational, and recreational therapists, and social workers who might be requested to assist in the patient's care, write or dictate an initial evaluation and plans, ongoing progress notes, and a final summary with followup instructions.

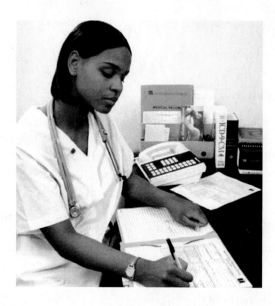

Ancillary Personnel Entries

Dietary personnel, discharge planners, utilization review managers, and others participating in the patient's care make a record of progress notes on each of their visits. Thus, the health information management department and medical transcription are vitally linked in the delivery of healthcare.

Physician Entries

Although any clinician involved in patient care may dictate narrative reports for the healthcare record, the majority of reports are dictated by the admitting physician, attending physician, hospitalist, or primary care provider (PCP). They, or occasionally their physician assistant (PA) or nurse practitioner (NP), dictate history and physical examinations upon the patient's admission and discharge summaries, also called clinical resumés, upon the patient's discharge. If the patient is discharged to a rehabilitation center, nursing home, assisted living facility (ALF), extended care facility (ECF), or skilled nursing facility (SNF), a transfer summary is dictated.

The physician may call in consultants as appropriate to assist in the patient's care. The consultant writes or dictates a consultation which includes a comprehensive review of the healthcare record and targeted physical examination and recommendations.

If the patient has a diagnostic procedure or a surgical procedure performed, the surgeon dictates preoperative and postoperative diagnoses, the name of the procedure, assistant, findings, technique, and outcome. The anesthesiologist completes a preanesthesia and postanesthesia evaluation.

All these physicians may write or dictate progress notes which include all pertinent plans and observations during the patient's care.

Demographics

Demographic data includes the patient's name, medical record number, and dates of admission and discharge or transfer and can include age, sex, and other information. This data is gathered on admission or at the time of an ED visit or outpatient procedure and kept electronically (the ADT data).

At the beginning of a dictation, the originator may be required to key in the patient's medical record number, along with other numeric codes that identify the dictator and the type of report. The dictation is then linked to the patient and on many if not most systems is pulled into the transcribed report or SR draft document electronically. Because physicians do not always key in the correct numbers, it is imperative that the MT or SRE compare the dictated patient's name and other data to the auto-populated electronic data.

A more accurate way to incorporate demographic data into a report is by means of a bar code which the dictator may swipe with a reader at the beginning of the dictation; however, the information should still be verified.

In some facilities, the MT may be required to look up the patient in the hospital's electronic master patient indexing system and manually enter the demographics into the report.

Demographics are displayed in many ways. It is important to note, however, that with the advent of the computerized patient record, demographic information may appear quite different, even foreign. Some EHRs use HL7 standards. An HL7 message looks like a combination of computer code, abbreviations, and text.

The name of each segment in the message is specified by the first field of the segment, which is always three characters long. Over 120 different segments are available for use in HL7 messages. A portion of an HL7 message might look like this (MSH identifies the message header; ADT is the beginning of the ADT feed: MSH | ^~ \& | EPIC | EPICADT | SMS | SMSADT | 199912271408 | CHARRIS | ADT^A04 | 1817457 | D | 2.5

It is not important for the medical transcriptionist to know HL7 codes or what they mean, just that an uncompleted field or error in the code would bounce the report back to someone who would correct the data before it could be uploaded into the patient's health record in the EHR. If the document needed to be printed, the codes would be stripped off, and only the pertinent data would appear on the printed document.

Time and Date Stamping

The Joint Commission (TJC) and Centers for Medicare and Medicaid Services (CMS) require time and date stamping on all entries in the health record. A draft entry, like a transcribed report, is still an entry. Electronic authentication would make this extra step unnecessary and most transcription applications automatically insert the time next to the date for both dictation and transcription (D&T). However, if you are working in a system that does not automatically insert the time with the D&T dates, then you must do so.

If a facility prints its reports, and the physician signs them manually, he or she is required to include the date and time with the signature. Some facilities include date and time labels with the signature line to remind the physician to do so. It is worth noting that compliance with the date/time rule is one of the most common causes of an RFI (requirement for improvement—the name for a negative finding on a TJC survey). TJC surveyors look at date and time of dictation and date and time of transcription specifically as evidence of compliance with other elements of performance, e.g., that an operative report be dictated within 24 hours of surgery or that an H&P is on the chart within 24 hours of admission.

CMS requirements for time and date stamping are as the follows:

All patient medical record entries must be legible, complete, dated, timed, and authenticated in written or electronic form by the person responsible for providing or evaluating the service provided, consistent with hospital policies and procedures.

The time and date of each entry (orders, reports, notes, etc.) must be accurately documented. Timing

---

AUTHENTICATION

The Book of Style for Medical Transcription, 3rd ed., states: "According to The Joint Commission, authentication must be done by the author of the record and cannot be delegated to anyone else, regardless of the process for inclusion of signature. The Joint Commission further defines authentication as: to prove authorship. Therefore, the legal responsibility for ensuring that all information in the record represents an accurate reflection of the patient encounter falls to the author of that record, not to the transcriptionist or any other ancillary personnel."

The BOS goes on to state further: "Automated or third-party inclusion of electronic signatures generates a critical risk management concern, where the assumption has been made that the transcribed report is without error or inconsistency, leaving the transcriptionist to unfairly shoulder the burden for the accuracy of the report—something the MT, who is clearly not the author of the record, is not legally qualified to do."

This means that MTs or SREs should not be asked or required, and should not agree, to electronically insert a provider's signature into a health record. Nor should MTs or SREs insert into the record the statement "dictated but not read," and should they be asked to do so, they should report this risk management concern to their supervisors.

---

establishes when an order was given, when an activity happened, or when an activity is to take place.

Timing and dating entries is necessary for patient safety and quality of care. Timing and dating of entries establishes a baseline for future actions or assessments and establishes a timeline of events.

Many patient interventions or assessments are based on time intervals or timelines of various signs, symptoms, or events.

The requirements for dating and timing do not apply to orders or prescriptions that are generated outside of the hospital until they are presented to the hospital at the time of service. Once the hospital begins processing such an order or prescription, it is responsible for ensuring that the implementation of the order or prescription by the hospital is promptly dated, and timed in the patient's medical record.

SAMPLE SIGNATURE BLOCK FOR A PAPER CHART

(Military time is used; OI stands for the originator's initials.)

_____   _____
Signature of Originator   Date/Time

OI:ead
D: 02/21/2013:1315
T: 02/21/2013:1804

The Medical Reports

A variety of medical reports are generated every day in physician offices, clinics, and hospitals. Medical transcriptionists should be familiar with those dictated in each work setting.

Physicians in private practice frequently dictate office chart notes, letters, initial office evaluations, and history and physical examinations. Medical reports dictated in hospitals and medical centers are numerous in category; however, they invariably include dictations from the "basic four" reports: History and Physical Examination, Consultation Report, Operative Report, and Discharge Summary. Emergency department reports, hospital progress notes, and diagnostic studies are often dictated as well. (See Sample Reports at the end of this chapter.) Every treatment, every diagnostic study, and every procedure must be documented in one way or another and placed in the patient's chart or permanent medical record.

Chart Note

The chart note (also called progress note or followup note) is dictated by a physician after talking with, meeting with, or examining a patient, usually in an outpatient setting, although progress notes may also be dictated on hospital inpatients. The chart note contains a concise description of the patient's presenting problem, physical findings, and the physician's plan of treatment, and may also include the results of laboratory tests.

Chart notes or progress notes become a permanent part of the patient's medical record. Chart notes can vary in length from one sentence to one or more pages, with the average note being two to four paragraphs long. Chart notes are sometimes dictated in an informal, staccato style using clipped sentences, abbreviations, and brief forms.

There are numerous formats for dictated chart notes. SOAP notes are those dictated in the SOAP format (an acronym for Subjective, Objective, Assessment, and Plan, which are headings within the note). Although formats vary from office to office, chart notes and progress notes should include the date of visit, patient's name, the patient's ID number, a signature line for the physician, and the transcriptionist's initials.

Letter

Physicians frequently dictate letters to communicate patient information to other physicians, insurance companies, patients' employers, and government offices. Medical transcriptionists need to be familiar with the various standard business letter formats. A dictator may express a preference for a specific letter format, although the full-block format (with the parts of the letter lined up on the left margin) is the one most commonly used. The patient's name and identification number are included in the Re (regarding) line.

Referral letters and consultation letters are not mere business letters; they are medical documents in letter form and as such should be transcribed with the same high degree of skill and accuracy as other medical reports. A copy of each letter must be kept and incorporated into the patient's medical record.

Initial Office Evaluation

Performed in the physician's office or clinic setting, the initial office evaluation is dictated after the physician sees a patient for the first time. It contains essentially the same information as the history and physical examination, although the physical examination in an initial office evaluation may be limited to specific areas of disease.

History and Physical Examination (H&P) Report

Shortly before or after a patient is admitted to the hospital, the physician obtains the patient's subjective history and conducts an objective physical examination.

These findings are then dictated by category and usually include the following.

Chief Complaint. This is the patient's main presenting problem and the reason for which the patient is seeking medical help. It can be a short sentence or a paragraph in length. Usually, the chief complaint is a rephrase of the patient's statement to the physician, but sometimes the dictator will quote the patient's exact words ("I fainted."). This is particularly true for psychiatric reports. When the patient's exact words are used, the statement is set off with quotation marks. The dictator may say "quote unquote" at the beginning of the sentence, and the MT must decide which dictation to put in quotation marks.

History of Present Illness. The history of present illness is a description of the events leading to the patient's presentation to the physician (or admission to the hospital). It can be a few lines to one or two paragraphs in length. Some of the material dictated under this heading may appear to be past history because it could have happened in the distant past, but if it relates to the admitting complaint or complaints, then it will likely be included in the history of the present illness.

Past Medical History. This category includes all medical and surgical problems from childhood to the present, including medications and allergies.

Family History. Family history is the medical condition of parents, other family members, and blood relatives. A complete family history (often not elicited) includes the age and state of health of all the immediate family members.

Social History contains a description of the patient's personal information—occupation, lifestyle, and habits. Asbestos and hazardous chemical exposure, for example, contain medical implications. The patient's use of caffeine, nicotine, alcohol, and prescription or illicit drugs is described here.

Review of Systems. The review of systems is subjective, that is, it reflects the patient's perception of symptoms as the physician asks questions about the major organ systems. Because this section reports on the patient's symptoms, physicians sometimes misspeak and say "review of symptoms" instead of "review of systems." The systems reviewed usually include Head, Eyes, Ears, Nose, Throat (HEENT); Cardiovascular (CV); Respiratory; Gastrointestinal (GI); Genitourinary (GU); Neuromuscular; Psychiatric; and occasionally Integumentary (Skin).

Physical Examination. The physical examination details the physician's objective findings on examina-

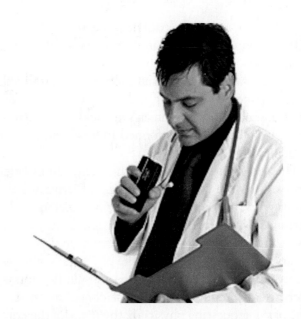

tion of the patient. The following subheadings are usually dictated: General Appearance, Vital Signs, Skin, HEENT (Head, Eyes, Ears, Nose, and Throat), Neck, Chest (Breasts, Heart, and Lungs), Abdomen, Back, Extremities, Genitalia or Pelvic, Rectal, Neurologic, and occasionally Mental Status Exam.

In addition, the History and Physical Examination often includes an Admitting Diagnosis or Impression, and often a proposed Treatment Plan. The H&P report is also known as the Admission History and Physical. More detailed information about the History and Physical Examination is covered later in this chapter.

Emergency Department Report

An emergency department report is much like an initial office evaluation, except that the patient is seen and treated in an emergency department of a hospital or acute care clinic. The Presenting Complaint, Present Illness, Physical Examination, and Course of Treatment are usually dictated. Sometimes the patient's condition is serious enough to warrant admission to the hospital, but more often the patient is seen, evaluated, treated, and then released to home with a recommended treatment plan.

Consultation

A consultation occurs when one physician requests the evaluation, opinion, and recommendations of another physician (almost always a board-certified specialist) in the care and treatment of a patient. The consultant bears no responsibility for patient care and, in fact, no doctor-patient relationship is established by the consultant until or unless the patient's care is either turned over to or shared with the consultant by the requesting physician. A consultation report must be generated by the consultant for each consultation service provided. The report becomes part of the consultant's records, part of the requesting physician's medical records, and, if the consultation was performed in a facility, part of the facility's medical records.

The report usually contains the subheadings Brief History of the Present Illness, Findings, Pertinent Laboratory Work, Working Diagnosis or Impression, and a Recommended Course of Treatment. The Consultation Report may be dictated in letter format and is to be transcribed on the stationery of the physician's office or the medical facility or on preprinted consultation forms, which usually require the date of consultation, the name of the requesting physician, the name of the consulting physician, and the reason for consultation.

Operative Report

After a surgical procedure is performed, a detailed description of the operation is dictated. Surgical procedures are carried out in hospitals, outpatient surgery centers, and occasionally in a physician's office.

The format used in dictating an operative report will depend to some extent on the surgeon's specialty and training, on the nature of the procedure, and on local conventions and institutional guidelines. The following discussion is based on an idealized format, some parts of which would be appropriate only for certain types of surgery. In addition, some pieces of information presented here under separate headings are regularly included by some dictators as part of the account of the operative procedure. Often a printed form or template is used for operative reports, containing a heading with spaces for entering the following information.

Identifying Data. The operative report must contain, as an absolute minimum, the name of the patient and any case or admission number assigned by the hospital for record-keeping purposes; the name of the surgeon; and the date on which the procedure was performed.

Name of Procedure. Generally, standard procedural terminology must be used, and in addition to the name of the operation, a code number, for insurance and statistical purposes, may be required to be entered by the surgeon or by a clerk.

Preoperative Diagnosis. The surgeon's provisional assessment of the patient's condition before beginning the operation, including the disease or condition that is the principal reason for the surgery. Again, standard terminology is required, followed by appropriate coding.

Postoperative Diagnosis. A more definitive and precise diagnosis established at or after operation, but often the same as the preoperative diagnosis.

Names of Surgeon(s) and Anesthesiologist(s). The surgeon, any surgical assistants, and the anesthesiologist(s) are ordinarily identified somewhere in the operative record. The name of the person dictating the operative report (who may not be the principal surgeon) will also appear at the end of the dictation. In some institutions, nurses or technicians assisting in the operating room are also identified.

Indications, History. Here the dictator elaborates on the preoperative diagnosis and explains the reasons that led to surgery on this patient and the choice of procedure and techniques used. This part of the operative report is not to be confused with the full clinical history of the patient contained elsewhere in the hospital record and perhaps dictated by someone other than the surgeon.

Clinical Status, Physical Examination. This information is a continuation of the preceding and may appear under the same heading. The surgeon describes the patient's physical condition (including results of pertinent laboratory tests or x-rays), particularly as it has a bearing on the need for surgery and the choice of procedure. Again, this is not to be confused with the complete physical examination report contained elsewhere in the patient's record.

Operative Report. The dictator's description of the actual surgical procedure may be given as a continuous narrative or may be presented under two or more of the following headings.

Anesthesia. A simple statement of the type of anesthetic used. The dictator may say simply "general" or "spinal," knowing that detailed information about the anesthetic will be recorded by the anesthesiologist.

Position. The position of the patient on the operating table is often passed over in silence unless some special positioning is required by the nature of the procedure.

Skin preparation. Scrubbing of the skin is usually a routine procedure carried out by an assistant or technician. The surgeon may record the name of the soap or disinfectant used and any special procedures used for sterile draping.

Incision. Under this heading the surgeon records the anatomic location and orientation of the incision by which access was gained to the operative site; for

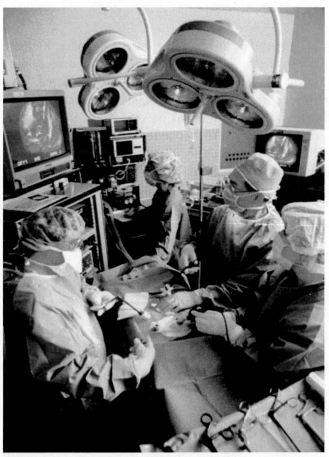

Endoscopy suite. Source: David Joel, Getty Images USA, Inc.

example, "right upper quadrant oblique" or "median sternotomy."

Procedure, Technique. A detailed, step-by-step narrative of the operation from beginning to end. Although parts of the operative report may be quite routine, each operation varies in some details from others, and a thorough and accurate report will reflect this uniqueness. The surgeon ordinarily includes in this narrative a record of the findings and some comment on their bearing on the choice of procedure and their implications for the future health of the patient.

Grafts, Implants. Any foreign objects or materials left in the patient, including grafts, artificial cardiac valves, stents, artificial joints, orthopedic fixation devices, pacemakers, shunts, mesh, screws, wire, and cement, must be fully identified. The brand names, chemical nature, origin, sizes, shapes, adjustments or settings, and exact anatomic location of such materials are all an essential part of the record. Serial numbers or other unique identifiers are included for devices such as pacemakers.

Closure. The repair of the incision and of any dissection or structural alterations performed during the surgery is described. Each layer of the body wall is closed

separately, often with a different type of stitch and a different suture material for each layer. The skin may be closed with metal clips or adhesive strips.

Drains, Packs, Dressings. These are devices or materials temporarily placed in or on the patient during or at the conclusion of the procedure. Since they must later be removed, recording their presence is of critical importance. Splints, casts, and other externally applied devices such as suction apparatus for evacuation of bleeding from the operative site may also be reported here.

Tourniquet Time. The number of minutes during which blood flow to an extremity was shut off by a tourniquet.

Specimens, cultures. Any materials removed from the patient during surgery and intended to be submitted for laboratory study.

Sponge and Needle Counts. In order that no foreign material or object may be inadvertently left inside the patient, it is standard practice for sponges, needles, and certain other articles to be counted before the commencement of surgery and again just before the surgeon begins to close the wound. Usually two persons perform the counts together for greater security. The surgeon does not begin closure of the wound until the sponge and needle counts are reported correct.

Estimated Blood Loss. Various measures are used during an operation to monitor blood loss, including close observation of blood absorbed by sponges and measurement of blood in the trap of the suction machine. The blood loss is measured in milliliters (mL), not cubic centimeters (cc).

Fluids Administered. Intravenous fluids, including whole blood, administered during the procedure are sometimes recorded in the operative report. This information is also part of the anesthesia record. The fluids are measured in milliliters (mL), not cubic centimeters (cc).

Condition of Patient at Conclusion of Operation. The surgeon reports that the patient left the operating room in satisfactory condition, or if this is not so, records any significant health problems occasioned by the surgery or anesthesia.

Complications. Under this heading the surgeon lists any unexpected and untoward consequences of the surgical procedure, such as accidental injury to healthy tissues or organs, extensive hemorrhage, or adverse reactions to anesthesia.

Postoperative Plan. The surgeon's intentions regarding postoperative care, including inhalation therapy, physical therapy, graded resumption of activities, followup examinations, and so on.

Discharge Summary

This report is sometimes referred to as a clinical resumé. By the time a patient is ready for discharge from the hospital, a variety of treatment modalities have been carried out. The Discharge Summary is the medical document that summarizes the patient's course in the hospital and may be short if the patient's stay in the hospital was brief and uncomplicated. (See Sample Reports at the end of this chapter.)

Most reports include a summary of the admission and discharge diagnoses, procedures or operations performed (if any), brief review of the patient's history, the physician's findings on physical examination, a report of laboratory work performed and pertinent findings, the patient's hospital course, discharge medications, and the discharge plan or disposition. This actual summary of the patient's hospital course becomes a part of the hospital's healthcare record for that patient but is also sent to and becomes a permanent part of the admitting physician's healthcare record for that patient. Discharge summaries can be extremely important in terms of followup care after the patient is discharged.

A transfer summary is a modified form of discharge summary that is prepared by the treating physician when a patient is discharged to a nursing home, a skilled nursing facility, or another hospital to ensure continuity of care.

Pause for Reflection

1. Which types of medical reports are primarily found in physician offices and clinics? Which types in hospitals and medical centers?
2. What are the primary components of a chart note? Describe a common format used for chart notes.
3. How do letters dictated in a medical setting differ from standard business letters?
4. How does an initial office evaluation differ from a history and physical examination?
5. List and briefly describe the main sections of a history and physical examination.
6. Describe an emergency department report and a consultation.
7. Briefly name the components of an operative report, and where it is not self-explanatory, describe the component.
8. Describe the content of a discharge summary or clinical resumé.

Laboratory Tests

In the past decade there has been a dramatic increase in both the number of new diagnostic laboratory tests as well as in the complexity of the tests offered. This explosive growth in the field of laboratory medicine has been due to the demand by physicians for new and improved diagnostic procedures, combined with the ever-expanding capacity of modern technology to meet the demand with increasingly sophisticated laboratory methods and equipment.

On a daily basis medical transcriptionists come in contact with dictation which details the results of laboratory tests performed on patients. In order to accurately transcribe this material, it is important to be familiar with the names and abbreviations of many laboratory tests, the reasons they are offered, and the meaning of the results.

Laboratory tests can be performed in many different settings: clinics, physicians' offices, health fairs, and sometimes even at home by patients themselves, though the greatest number of laboratory tests are performed within the hospital setting. Hospital laboratories are equipped with the most technologically advanced and automated equipment to handle hundreds of tests each day. The largest hospitals perform all standard laboratory tests as well as many uncommon ones which may be requested by smaller hospitals or clinics whose facilities are not equipped to handle unusual tests.

The laboratory of a hospital is divided into many smaller departments which perform specialized laboratory tests. This division of labor is also reflected to a great extent on the average laboratory slip which is used to report the results of laboratory tests. Various sections on the lab slip include hematology, blood bank, chemistry, coagulation, urinalysis, stool examination, microbiology, and cytology.

Hematology is concerned with the study of the formed components or cells of the blood. These cells include mature red blood cells, white blood cells, and platelets, as well as their immature forms. The function of the red blood cell is to carry oxygen from the lungs to the body tissues. The function of the white blood cell is to fight any foreign substances that enter the body, such as bacteria. Platelets function along with the coagulation factors in the blood to form a blood clot at the site of tissue injury. White blood cells are further differentiated into groups which have diagnostic value. These include lymphocytes, monocytes, neutrophils, eosinophils, basophils, and bands or immature neutrophils.

There are many brief forms, slang, and special terms associated with the blood. Brief forms are acceptable in medical reports, but transcriptionists should always spell out in full any slang words that are dictated. For example, *monos* is an acceptable brief form for monocytes, but *lytes* is a slang term that must be translated *electrolytes* in medical reports. (See Brief Forms and Medical Slang section in Chapter 5.)

A complete blood count (CBC) includes tests that measure red blood cell and white blood cell levels. A CBC with differential also measures the levels of all of the different types of white blood cells. Other common tests are the hemoglobin and hematocrit (which is often dictated as *H&H* but must be written out in full), which are indicative of the oxygen-carrying capacity of the blood as well as the percentage of red blood cells per blood sample. Normally the hematocrit is about three times greater than the hemoglobin level for the same patient, so that if the patient's hemoglobin level was reported as 15, you could expect that the hematocrit would be approximately 45.

The chemistry section of the laboratory performs tests on many different electrolytes, fats, and other substances found in the serum, or clear fluid which separates from a clotted blood sample. Blood chemistries include tests for electrolytes: sodium, potassium, calcium, and chloride. Lipids (fatty substances) include cholesterol and triglycerides. Other substances tested include bilirubin, ALT, AST, and LDH which are used to evaluate liver function. BUN and creatinine are useful indicators of kidney function. Uric acid levels are tested to diagnose the medical condition of gout.

Often the physician orders a combination of tests under one name. For example, by checking a box next to the entry "serum lipid profile" on the laboratory slip, the physician can order the tests for cholesterol, triglycerides, total lipids, and lipoproteins.

The microbiology department of the laboratory identifies infectious organisms through the use of microscopes and culture and sensitivity testing. Specimens for testing are obtained from urine, stool, blood, sputum, wound drainage, or other body fluids. A sample of the specimen is smeared onto a culture medium and incubated at 37°C for sufficient time to allow bacterial growth to occur. Antibiotic disks placed on the media of the culture plates permit evaluation of the sensitivity of the bacteria cultured to specific antibiotics. Antibiotic disks to which the bacteria are sensitive are surrounded by a ring or zone of inhibition of bacterial growth. Bacteria that are resistant to an antibiotic show no inhibition of growth around the disk.

A rapid method to tentatively identify a pathogenic bacterium is to smear a sample on a slide and then stain the slide with the Gram stain. This stain differentiates between organisms that are gram-positive and those that are gram-negative. The shape of the bacterium can provide further clues to the identity of the organism. The acid-fast stain is used to identify mycobacteria specifically.

Physicians order laboratory tests to be performed on patients for a variety of reasons:

1. To diagnose disease in a patient who is ill.
2. To screen for hidden diseases. Well-known examples include use of the Pap smear to identify cervical cancer, and the self-administered test for occult or hidden blood in the stool as an indicator of colon cancer.
3. To assess the extent of damage from disease processes.
4. To monitor the effectiveness of treatment prescribed by the physician.
5. To monitor blood levels of certain medications. Periodic blood samples can ensure that drug levels in the blood remain within the therapeutic range.
6. To monitor the course of a disease.
7. To confirm freedom from disease, or to detect recurrence, after a cure has apparently been achieved.

Laboratory test results are measured and reported most often in **SI** (Système International) **units**, including submultiples of the meter (centimeters, millimeters, cubic centimeters), the liter (milliliters), the gram (milligrams, micrograms), and the equivalent (milliequivalents).

If the reported value falls within the range observed in normal individuals, it is considered normal. If it falls outside of this range, it is considered abnormal. The age and sex of a patient cause variation in the normal range of laboratory values.

The accepted normal range for a particular laboratory test also varies from one laboratory to another, due to differences in equipment and methodology used in testing. Therefore, lab slips usually give the accepted normal range for that particular facility. The normal value is printed next to the blank space for the reported value for the individual patient. When transcribing, it is not unusual for the medical transcriptionist to hear the physician say, "Normal for our laboratory is . . . ," after dictating a patient's test result.

The transcription of laboratory test terminology presents certain challenges for the medical transcriptionist. Correctly transcribing the name of a laboratory test or its abbreviation is just the first step. Numerical results must be transcribed with absolute accuracy. Care must be taken to place decimal points accurately and to transcribe units of measure correctly.

It is also necessary to understand why a test was ordered and what the results indicate. Some dictations contain considerable detail concerning the test process, the use of special stains or dyes, as well as the significance of the results.

As a student, you will want to study this critical area of medical transcription diligently. As a practicing medical transcriptionist, you will always be increasing your knowledge of laboratory tests and procedures, as the technology of medicine increases daily.

Pause for Reflection

1. What might one be able to deduce from knowing the red blood cell count, the white blood cell count, and the platelet count based on knowing the function of these cells?
2. Which individual laboratory tests are included in a complete CBC with differential?
3. List the individual blood chemistry tests identified as electrolytes, tests included in a serum lipid profile, tests to evaluate liver function, tests to evaluate kidney function, and tests for gout and prostate cancer respectively.
4. What is culture and sensitivity testing?
5. Name two other laboratory methods used to identify bacteria.
6. What challenges confront the medical transcriptionist in transcribing laboratory test results?

Pharmacology

Pharmacology is the study of drugs and their interactions with living organisms. The term *pharmacology* comes from a Greek word meaning *medicine*. The term *drug* is derived from a Dutch word which means *dry* and refers to the use of dried herbs and plants as the first medicines. The Latin word for *drug* is *medicina*, from which we derive our term medicine. Pharmacology is concerned with the nature of drugs and medications, their actions in the body, drug dosages, side effects of drugs, and so on. Drugs are used to prevent, treat, and cure diseases, and in some instances to diagnose diseases.

Drug Forms

Different forms of a drug are appropriate for different routes of administration. Some common manufactured drug forms are tablets, capsules, transdermal patches, suppositories, creams, ointments, lotions, powders, oral suspensions, sprays, and foams. Some drugs are ineffective when administered in a certain form or by a certain route; other drugs may seriously injure the patient if administered in certain forms or by a certain route.

1. **Tablet**. This drug form contains dried, powdered, active drug as well as binders and fillers to provide bulk and ensure proper tablet size. A **scored** tablet has an indented line running across the middle. It can be easily broken into two pieces with a knife to produce two doses. **Enteric** tablets are covered with a special coating that resists stomach acid but dissolves in the alkaline environment of the small intestine to avoid irritating the stomach (e.g., Ecotrin). **Slow-release** tablets are manufactured to provide a continuous, sustained release of certain drugs. Often this is abbreviated as **XR (extended release)**, **SR (slow release)**, or **LA (long acting)** and included in the trade name of the drug (e.g., Dilacor XR, Dilatrate-SR, Cardizem LA, all used in the prophylaxis of angina pectoris). **Caplets** are coated tablets in the form of capsules. Tablets can also be designed to be dissolved in water before being taken orally (e.g., Alka-Seltzer effervescent tablets).

Some over-the-counter drugs come in the form of **lozenges**. These tablets are formed of a hardened base of sugar and water containing the drug and other flavorings. They are never swallowed, but are allowed to dissolve slowly in the mouth to release the drug topically to the tissues of the mouth and throat (e.g. Cepacol lozenges for sore throat). In prescriptions, *tablet* is sometimes abbreviated as *tab* or *tabs*.

2. **Capsule**. This drug form comes in two varieties. The first is a soft gelatin shell manufactured in one piece in which the drug is in a liquid form inside the shell (e.g., docusate [Colace, Surfak], a stool softener; fat-soluble vitamins such as A and E). The second type of capsule is a hard shell manufactured in two pieces which fit together and hold the drug, which is in a powdered or granular form. Many nonprescription cold remedies and pain medications were manufactured in this form until some Tylenol capsules were reported to be contaminated with cyanide in the early 1980s. Now, most pharmaceutical companies manufacture their nonprescription pain medications in a tablet or caplet form. Many prescription drugs, however, are still manu-

factured as hard-shell capsules. In written prescriptions, capsule is sometimes abbreviated as cap or caps.

3. **Cream**. A cream is a semisolid emulsion of oil (such as lanolin or petroleum) and water, the main ingredient being water. Emulsifying agents are added to keep the oil and water well mixed. Many topical drugs are manufactured in a cream base (e.g., hydrocortisone cream for skin inflammation).

4. **Ointment**. An ointment is a semisolid emulsion of drug, oil (such as lanolin or petroleum, and water, the main ingredient being oil. Many topical drugs are manufactured in an ointment base (e.g., Kenalog ointment for skin inflammation). Specially formulated ophthalmic ointments are made to be applied topically to the eye without causing irritation.

5. **Lotion**. A lotion is a semisolid suspension of drug dissolved in a thickened water base (e.g., calamine lotion for itching).

6. **Gel**. A gel is a semisolid suspension in which the drug particles are suspended in a thickened water base (e.g., MetroGel for acne rosacea).

7. **Powder**. A powder is a finely ground form of an active drug. Powdered drugs can be in capsules but also can be manufactured in glass vials where they must be reconstituted with sterile water before being injected (e.g., intravenous ampicillin, an antibiotic). Powders can also come in packets; the packet is opened and the powder is reconstituted for oral use (e.g., Metamucil, a laxative). Powders can also be sprinkled on topically or sprayed on (e.g., Tinactin, an antifungal drug for the skin). Powders can also be inhaled into the lungs with the help of a special inhalation device (e.g., Serevent Diskus, a bronchodilator).

8. **Liquid**. Liquids come in the form of either solutions or suspensions. Solutions contain the drug dissolved in a water base. Solutions never need to be mixed as the drug-to-water concentration is always the same in every part of the solution, even after prolonged standing. Solutions come in many forms: elixirs, syrups, tinctures, liquid sprays, and foams.

Elixirs are solutions that contain an alcohol and water base with added sugar and flavoring (e.g., Tylenol elixir for fever and pain). Elixirs are commonly used for pediatric or elderly patients who cannot swallow the tablet or capsule form of a drug.

Syrups are solutions that contain no alcohol and are a concentrated solution of sugar, water, and flavorings. Syrups are sweeter and more viscous (thicker) than elixirs. Most over-the-counter cough medications

---

ORPHAN DRUGS

An orphan drug is a drug or biological product for the diagnosis, treatment, or prevention of a rare disease or condition. A rare disease is one that affects less than 200,000 persons or for which there is no reasonable expectation that the cost of development and testing will be recovered through U.S. sales of the product.

Federal subsidies are provided to the manufacturer or sponsor for the development of orphan drugs. Applications for orphan status are made through the FDA, and may be made during drug development or after marketing approval.

Ellen Drake and Randy Drake
Saunders Pharmaceutical Word Book

---

have a syrup base which not only carries the drug but acts to soothe inflamed mucous membranes in the throat (e.g., guaifenesin [Robitussin] for coughs).

Liquid sprays contain a solution of drug combined with water or alcohol; they are sprayed by a pump or aerosol propellant. Spray liquid drugs are commonly used for topical application (e.g., Afrin nasal spray, a decongestant).

Foams contain a solution of drug that is expanded by tiny aerosol bubbles (e.g., Cortifoam, a hydrocortisone product used in the treatment of proctitis).

Suspensions contain fine, undissolved particles of drug suspended in a water base. With prolonged standing, these fine particles gradually settle to the bottom of the container. It is always important to shake suspensions well before using them, a fact that is noted on the label of these drugs (e.g., Maalox antacid). An **emulsion** is a suspension in which the drug is mixed with fat particles and water (e.g., Intralipid intravenous fat solution). Two general terms used to describe a liquid are *aqueous* (from the Latin word *aqua*, water), meaning of watery consistency, and viscous, which designates a nonwatery or thick liquid.

9. **Suppository**. A suppository is composed of a solid base of glycerin or cocoa butter that contains the drug. It is manufactured in appropriate sizes for rectal or vaginal insertion and in adult and pediatric sizes. Vaginal suppositories are most often used to treat vaginal infections. Rectal suppositories can deliver topical medicine to the rectal mucosa or can be used to admin-

ister drugs to patients who are vomiting and cannot take oral medication.

10. **Transdermal patches.** The transdermal form of a drug is a multilayered disk consisting of a drug reservoir, a porous membrane, and an adhesive layer to hold it to the skin. The porous membrane regulates the amount of drug released into the skin.

11. **Pellet/Bead.** A drug can be implanted in the body in the form of a pellet or bead that slowly releases the drug to the surrounding tissues (e.g., gentamicin beads [Septopal] on a surgical wire are inserted into the bone to treat chronic osteomyelitis).

Routes of Drug Administration

There are various routes of drug administration. These include oral, sublingual, nasogastric, gastrostomy or jejunostomy, rectal, vaginal, topical, transdermal, inhalation, parenteral, subcutaneous, intramuscular, intravenous, endotracheal, intra-arterial, intra-articular, intracardiac, intradermal, intrathecal, umbilical artery or vein.

1. **Oral.** The oral route is the most convenient route of administration and the most commonly used. Tablets, capsules, and liquids are all given orally. Even patients who have difficulty swallowing a tablet or capsule can usually take the liquid form of a drug without problems. Infants are given drugs in a liquid form mixed with a small amount of formula and administered through a nipple. Even unconscious patients can be given liquid medication through a nasogastric (NG) tube. The oral route is routinely abbreviated as *p.o.* (Latin for *per os*, meaning *through the mouth*).

Disadvantages of the oral route include the following: Some drugs (e.g., interferons, hormones such as insulin, and antibiotics such as gentamicin) are inactivated by stomach acid and cannot be given orally. After oral administration, some drugs (e.g., lidocaine [Xylocaine] for cardiac arrhythmias) are metabolized so quickly by the liver that a therapeutic blood level cannot be achieved. Some drugs (e.g., tetracycline) cannot be taken with certain foods and drinks because they combine chemically to form an insoluble complex. Other drugs (e.g., MAO inhibitors for depression) cannot be taken with certain foods or drinks because they produce adverse side effects.

2. **Sublingual.** Sublingual administration involves placing the drug (usually in a tablet form) under the tongue and allowing it to slowly dissolve. The tablet is not swallowed (because this would become oral admin-

istration). The drug is absorbed quickly through oral mucous membranes and into the large blood vessels under the tongue. The sublingual route provides a faster therapeutic effect than the oral route (e.g., nitroglycerin tablets for treating angina).

3. **Nasogastric** (abbreviated *NG*). This route is used to administer drugs to patients who cannot take oral medications. Nasogastric administration is accomplished with a nasogastric tube that passes from the nose through the esophagus and into the stomach. Only liquid drugs can be given by this route.

4. **Gastrostomy** or **jejunostomy**. These routes are used to administer drugs to patients who cannot take oral medications. These routes use a surgically implanted feeding tube to deliver liquid drugs directly into the stomach (gastrostomy) or jejunum (jejunostomy).

5. **Rectal.** This route is reserved for certain clinical situations, such as when the patient is vomiting and/or the medication cannot be given by injection (e.g., Tylenol suppositories). Absorption of a drug via the rectal route of administration is slow and often unpredictable, so this route is not used often. The rectal route is the preferred route, however, when drugs are administered locally to relieve constipation (e.g., Fleet enema) or treat hemorrhoids (e.g., Anusol) or ulcerative colitis (Proctofoam-HC).

6. **Vaginal.** The vaginal route is used to treat vaginal infections and vaginitis by means of creams and suppositories (e.g., Monistat 7 suppositories, Premarin vaginal cream). Contraceptive foams are inserted vaginally as well.

7. **Topical.** When a drug is applied directly to the skin or to the mucous membranes of the eyes, ears, nose, or mouth, it is administered via the topical route. The effects of the drug are generally local (e.g., bacitracin antibiotic ointment for skin abrasions, Sudafed nasal decongestant spray, Timoptic eye drops for glaucoma).

8. **Transdermal.** This route of administration differs from the topical route in that the drug is applied to the skin via physical delivery through a porous membrane, and the therapeutic effects are felt systemically, not just at the site of administration. Drugs delivered by the transdermal route are usually manufactured in the form of a patch. A transdermal patch is worn on the skin and releases the drug slowly over a 24-hour period, providing sustained therapeutic blood levels (e.g., Transderm-Nitro for prevention of angina pectoris).

9. **Inhalation.** This route of administration involves the inhaling of a drug that is in a gas, liquid, or powder

form. The drug is absorbed through the alveoli of the lungs (e.g., nitrous oxide, a general anesthetic; albuterol [Proventil], a bronchodilator).

10. **Parenteral.** Parenteral is a general term, taken from two Greek words, *para* and *enteron*, which literally mean *apart from the intestine*. Technically, parenteral administration means all routes of administration other than oral, but in clinical usage, parenteral commonly includes the following routes of administration: subcutaneous, intramuscular, and intravenous, and other less frequently used routes: endotracheal, intra-arterial, intra-articular, intracardiac, intradermal, intrathecal, and injection into the umbilical artery or vein.

Subcutaneous administration involves the injection of liquid into the subcutaneous tissue (the fatty layer of tissue just under the dermis of the skin but above the muscle layer) (e.g., insulin for diabetes mellitus, allergy shots). There are few blood vessels in this layer, so drugs are absorbed more slowly by this route than when given by intramuscular injection. Diabetics who inject insulin use approximately 10 to 12 different areas on the upper arms, thighs, and abdomen and rotate the site of each subcutaneous insulin injection. The term *subcutaneous* is abbreviated *subcu.*

Intramuscular (IM) administration involves the injection of a liquid into the belly (area of greatest mass) of a large muscle. The large muscles of the body are well supplied with blood vessels, and drugs are absorbed more quickly by this route than when given by subcutaneous injection. There are five intramuscular injection sites that can be used; injection at other sites invites damage to adjacent nerves and blood vessels.

> **deltoid**, located on the upper arm, lateral aspect.
> **vastus lateralis**, located on the midthigh, lateral aspect.
> **rectus femoris**, located on the midthigh, anterior aspect.
> **ventrogluteal**, located on the side of the hip .
> **dorsogluteal**, located in the upper outer quadrant of each buttock.

Examples of drugs given intramuscularly: Demerol for pain, vitamin B_{12} for pernicious anemia, Garamycin for bacterial infections. Some drugs cannot be given by intramuscular injection because they are not water soluble and would form precipitate particles in the tissue (e.g., Valium and Librium, antianxiety drugs).

Intravenous (IV) administration of a drug involves the injection of a liquid directly into a vein. The therapeutic effect of drugs given intravenously can often be

---

NEEDLE CLASSIFICATION

Needles are classified according to gauge and length. The gauge is the inside diameter of the needle. The lower the gauge number, the larger the inside diameter will be. For example, a 15-gauge needle is used for blood donation to allow the blood to flow freely through the needle and to decrease turbulence and damage to the red blood cells. An 18- to 22-gauge needle is used for intramuscular injections in adults. A 27-gauge needle is used for an intravenous line in a premature infant. The inside diameter of a needle is also known as the **bore**. The term *bore* is synonymous with *gauge,* but the bore is designated only as either small or large.

A **butterfly needle** is a specially designed needle of short length and high gauge with color-coded tabs of plastic on each side of the needle. These tabs facilitate control of the needle during insertion. This needle gets its name because the tabs on either side of the needle make it appear like the wings of a butterfly. Butterfly needles are most often used to start intravenous lines on premature infants or on elderly patients with poor veins.

Susan M. Turley
*Understanding Pharmacology
for Health Professionals*

---

seen immediately. This is because the drug does not need to be absorbed from tissue or muscle before it can exert an effect. IV administration can be done in one of three ways. The injection of a single dose of a drug (**bolus**) may be given through a **port** (rubber stopper) into an existing intravenous line. This is often referred to as **IV push** because the drug is manually pushed into the IV line in a short period of time. A drug may also be mixed with the fluid in an IV bag or bottle and administered continuously over several hours. This is known as **IV drip**. A drug may also be mixed in a very small IV bag or bottle and administered over an hour or less by IV drip. This small secondary IV bag or bottle is connected through tubing to a port in the existing primary IV line. This method is known as **IV piggyback** administration. Examples of drugs given intravenously include thiopental (Pentothal) for induction of general anesthesia, diazepam (Valium) to control continuous epileptic seizures, and most chemotherapy drugs.

Other parenteral routes that have specialized uses include the following:

- **endotracheal** This route is used during emergency resuscitation measures (e.g., epinephrine) and to deliver pulmonary drugs to intubated patients via the endotracheal tube.

- **intra-arterial** This route is used occasionally for direct injection of a chemotherapeutic agent to a tumor area. Generally, arterial lines are used for continuous monitoring of arterial blood pressure and are not used to administer drugs.

- **intra-articular** This route is used only to inject specific drugs, such as corticosteroids, into the joint to decrease severe inflammation and pain caused by a chronic disease such as arthritis. The Latin word *articulus* means *joint*.

- **intracardiac** This route is used only during emergency resuscitative measures (e.g., epinephrine is given directly through the chest wall into the heart to stimulate the heart muscle during cardiac arrest).

- **intradermal** This route involves the injection of a liquid into the dermis, the layer of skin just below the epidermis. The epidermis itself is only about 1 mm (less than 1/20 of an inch) thick; therefore, when an intradermal injection is correctly positioned, the tip of the needle is still plainly visible through the skin (e.g., Mantoux test for tuberculosis).

- **intrathecal** Intrathecal administration involves the injection of a liquid within the sheath or meninges of the spinal cord into the cerebrospinal fluid (e.g., spinal anesthesia). *Theka* is Greek for *sheath*.

- **umbilical artery** or **vein** This route is accessible only in newborn infants before the umbilical cord has dried. It is used to administer fluids and draw blood. It is generally not used to give drugs. Instead, an IV line is inserted peripherally in the hand, foot, or scalp for drug administration.

Drug Effects

Some drugs may be approved for use via more than one route and are manufactured in different forms appropriate for those different routes. Each route of administration has distinct advantages and disadvantages. A drug given by one route may be therapeutic, while given by another route it may be ineffective, harmful, or even fatal. Therefore, every drug prescription or drug order always includes the form of the drug as well as the route of administration.

Drugs exert their effects in a number of ways and at a number of sites within the body. Basically, drugs act in two ways: locally or systemically. A local effect is limited to the site of administration and those tissues immediately surrounding it. Drugs applied topically are an example of those that exert a local effect. A systemic drug effect is not limited to the site of application but can be felt throughout the body, particularly evident in certain organs and tissues. Drugs taken intravenously and intramuscularly always exert a systemic effect. Drugs taken orally and subcutaneously usually exert a systemic effect.

All drugs have an intended therapeutic effect and a side effect. The therapeutic effect is the drug's main action for which it was prescribed by the physician. The therapeutic effect will cure a disease, decrease disease symptoms, or prevent a disease. The perfect drug would have a complete therapeutic effect perfectly suited for its use with no side effects. Unfortunately, this perfect drug does not exist. Side effects vary widely with the type of drug administered. They may be mild or quite severe. Many drugs, for example, exert gastrointestinal side effects which include anorexia, nausea, vomiting, or diarrhea. Common side effects expressed in the central nervous system include drowsiness, excitement, or depression.

Drugs may react with other drugs in the system to cause side effects. Many patients are treated with more than one drug at a time. In particular, elderly patients with chronic medical problems may consume a number of medications several times a day. Some drugs react to each other in a particular way to either accentuate or diminish the action of each.

Pause for Reflection

1. List drug forms that are taken orally, applied topically, or injected, respectively. What forms do not fit into any of these categories?
2. List and briefly define each route of administration discussed in the text.
3. Define *bolus*, *IV push*, *IV drip*, *IV piggyback*, and *IV port*.
4. Distinguish between therapeutic effect and side effect of a drug.

Spotlight On

Our Health Story—Being a Patient Advocate

by Brenda J. Hurley

When medical transcriptionists apply what they have learned both through formal studies and from MT experience, they can use that knowledge to advantage when seeking healthcare services. For many years I helped my aging parents to compile their medical histories, medication lists, allergies, etc., and organize them in a typed document for their multiple physician office visits throughout the year. Even when I could not accompany them to all of their office visits, I provided them with updated health data sheets to take with them because accurate information is extremely important for healthcare providers.

As the health issues for my parents grew more serious, I attended doctor visits in order to ask questions on their behalf regarding diagnoses, treatment plans, and treatment options. Once home from the physician office, I would explain to my parents in easily understood language what was said by the doctor, the purpose for any scheduled studies, and the medications ordered.

In time my role as a healthcare advocate expanded beyond my parents to various family members who developed serious health issues and needed help in navigating the often confusing and occasionally scary world of healthcare. It was a natural progression in using my medical transcription skills as they needed an expert interpreter of the medical language. I explain it like this: There is nothing like having a doctor announce to you that you have cancer; your brain immediately turns to mush and you don't hear anything else that is said. That's when a healthcare advocate can help.

There are three key benefits for serving as a healthcare advocate. One is communication among healthcare providers regarding the patient's treatment and diagnoses. Some patients routinely seek care from three or more physicians, depending on their health needs. A cardiologist may prescribe a medication that the ophthalmologist may not know about that could cause a complication for the patient with a medication prescribed for an eye condition. Also, awareness of all allergies and drug sensitivities is critical to treatment decisions to optimize rather than jeopardize patient care. Providing healthcare professionals with updated and accurate information at the time the patient seeks healthcare services is an important way to improve communication.

The second benefit is to improve the delivery of healthcare services. Patients who do not "speak" or understand the language of medicine are often bewildered and confused when physicians talk in medicalese, often using a myriad of abbreviations that sound like alphabet soup to the untrained ear. Doctors and nurses communicate this way all the time, so for them there is nothing unusual about telling the patient things like "your BUN spiked so no p.o. fluids for the next 12 hours."

Elderly patients often feel inhibited in asking their doctor a question or comment about the difficulty of complying with the treatment plan because they do not know how to articulate this to their very busy and important doctor. All of these communications could be enhanced with a healthcare advocate who would keep both the healthcare provider and the patient on track for the delivery of quality healthcare services.

The third benefit is education for the patient. The healthcare advocate can explain the diagnosis made or suspected, why certain tests are ordered or medications prescribed in an easy-to-understand language in a conversational manner that allows the patient to absorb the information at their own pace. Often I provide literature from reputable websites that give more details so they can read and re-read it to formulate an understanding or generate new questions for me or for their healthcare provider. When patients are informed, it empowers and motivates them to follow treatment plans and seek resolution of their health issues—thus improving their opportunity for recovery.

When faced with health issues, yours or your family, use your professional skills as a healthcare advocate for improving communication as well as the efficiency and effectiveness of the healthcare services. You will be rewarded to know that your skills have made a difference in helping to make a patient's healthcare journey a little easier.

Exercises

Chapter Review

Instructions: Choose the best answer.

___ 1. The agency or organization that administers Medicare and Medicaid reimbursement is ____
   A. AHIMA.
   B. AHDI.
   C. CMS.
   D. RAC.

___ 2. Codes assigned to diagnoses and surgical procedures for purposes of reimbursement and other uses are _____
   A. DRG codes.
   B. CPT codes.
   C. HCPS codes.
   D. ICD codes.

___ 3. Federal legislation detailing the requirements for privacy and confidentiality of patient information is named _____
   A. ARRA.
   B. HIPAA.
   C. HITECH.
   D. RAC.

___ 4. Clinicians who may dictate healthcare documentation reports include all of the following EXCEPT _____
   A. RHIA.
   B. PCP.
   C. PA.
   D. RA.

___ 5. All of the following are codes that determine reimbursement EXCEPT _____
   A. ADT.
   B. CPT.
   C. HCPS.
   D. ICD.

___ 6. The individual responsible for knowing which documents were part of the legal healthcare record and which were not is the _____
   A. HIM volunteer.
   B. chart analyst.
   C. chart assembler.
   D. coder.

___ 7. The role of The Joint Commission is _____
   A. to ensure that patients' personal health information is protected.
   B. to ensure that every handwritten entry was signed, dated, and timed.
   C. to ensure that dangerous abbreviations be expanded to English words in medical reports to avoid confusion with similar abbreviations.
   D. to accredit hospitals and other healthcare institutions.

___ 8. Which of the following is often handwritten in the healthcare record?
   A. Daily progress notes by nurses and physicians.
   B. Requisitions for laboratory procedures.
   C. Orders for prescription medications.
   D. Admission H&P and discharge summary.

___ 9. Reports that are usually machine-generated include _____
   A. history and physical examinations.
   B. progress notes.
   C. initial office evaluations.
   D. clinical laboratory reports.

___ 10. The "basic four" reports in hospitals and larger healthcare facilities include all of the following EXCEPT _____
   A. history and physical examinations.
   B. consultations.
   C. emergency department reports.
   D. operative reports.

___ 11. Reports that are more commonly generated in physicians' offices rather than hospitals include _____
A. consultation reports.
B. SOAP notes.
C. operative reports.
D. x-ray reports.

___ 12. The laboratory study that includes hemoglobin and hematocrit is the _____
A. complete blood count.
B. blood chemistries.
C. lipid studies.
D. kidney function studies.

___ 13. Cholesterol and triglycerides are included on which laboratory panel?
A. Liver function study.
B. Kidney function study.
C. Lipid profile.
D. Electrolytes.

___ 14. Red and white blood cell counts are included in which laboratory study?
A. Blood chemistry profile or panel.
B. Complete blood count or CBC.
C. Electrolytes.
D. Kidney function tests.

___ 15. ALT, AST, and LDH are used to evaluate _____.
A. liver function.
B. kidney function.
C. lipids.
D. white and red blood cells.

___ 16. An electrolyte panel includes which of these studies?
A. Hemoglobin, hematocrit, and white blood cell count.
B. Cholesterol, triglycerides, total lipids, and lipoproteins.
C. Sodium, potassium, calcium, and chloride.
D. ALT, AST, and LDH.

___ 17. The microbiology department performs which of the following tests?
A. Complete blood count.
B. Platelet count.
C. White blood cell differential.
D. Culture and sensitivity.

___ 18. _____ are covered with a special coating that resists stomach acid but dissolves in the alkaline environment of the small intestine to avoid irritating the stomach.
A. Lozenges
B. Capsules
C. Enteric-coated tablets
D. Elixirs

___ 19. _____ contain fine, undissolved particles of drug suspended in a water base.
A. Elixirs
B. Suspensions
C. Foams
D. Suppositories

___ 20. Parenteral administration includes all of the following routes of administration EXCEPT _____
A. nasogastric.
B. endotracheal.
C. subcutaneous.
D. intramuscular.

Healthcare Industry Abbreviations

Instructions: Expand the following common healthcare industry abbreviations from Chapters 1 and 2. You may not need to transcribe these abbreviations, but you do need to know what they mean because they are essential to understanding healthcare industry communications.

Abbreviation   *Expansion*

1. ADT _____

2. AHDI _____

3. AHIMA _____

4. ARRA _____

5. BA _____

6. CE _____

7. CHDS _____

8. CMS _____

9. CPT _____

10. DRG _____

11. EHR _____

12. EMR _____

13. HDS _____

14. HHS _____

15. HIM _____

16. HIPAA _____

17. HITECH _____

18. ICD _____

19. ISMP _____

20. P&Ps _____

21. PHI _____

22. PHR _____

23. RAC _____

24. RHDS _____

25. RHIA _____

26. RHIT _____

27. SRT _____

28. TJC _____

Healthcare Documentation Abbreviations

Instructions: Expand the following common healthcare documentation abbreviations from Chapters 1 and 2. You may not need to transcribe these in reports but you need to know what they mean because they are essential to understanding terms and concepts related to healthcare documentation practice.

Abbreviation   *Expansion*

1. ALF _____

2. CBC _____

3. cc _____

4. H&H _____

5. H&P _____

6. HEENT _____

7. IM _____

8. IV _____

9. LA _____

10. mL _____

11. MRN _____

12. MT _____

13. NG _____

14. NP _____

15. PA _____

16. PCP _____

17. QA _____

18. SE or SRE _____

19. SOAP _____

20. SR _____

21. subcu _____

22. XR _____

Content of Reports

Instructions: For the headings or report content in column 1, identify the type of report in which it would appear in column 2. Answers may include more than one type of report.

Report Component   *Report Type*

1. Chief Complaint _____

2. History of Present Illness _____

3. Review of Systems _____

4. Social History _____

5. HEENT _____

6. Cardiovascular _____

7. Vital Signs _____

8. Genitalia _____

9. Preoperative Diagnosis _____

10. Findings _____

11. Estimated Blood Loss _____

12. Extremities _____

13. SOAP _____

14. General Appearance _____

15. Abdomen _____

Sample Reports

Sample medical reports appear on the following pages, illustrating a variety of reports. Fictional names are provided for illustration of proper format, and no resemblance to actual persons is intended. Sample transcripts were prepared according to *The Book of Style for Medical Transcription* (AHDI).

Letter

October 1, [add year]

Stanley Lessing, MD
1829 Apache Way
Cheyenne, CA 95555

Re: Laverne DeFazio

Dear Dr. Lessing:

I have seen the above-named patient for several visits since her colonoscopy, and I wanted to update you about what has transpired. After the colonoscopy, I increased the Azulfidine to 500 mg q.i.d. I also sent stool for *C. difficile*, which was negative, and ordered an upper GI with a small bowel series. This showed a small sliding-type hiatal hernia with rapid transit time through the small bowel. The remainder of the exam was normal.

I saw this patient again 3 months later, at which time she had a fever and sweats with temperature of 103 degrees. I referred her to your office to further assess whether the Azulfidine or Crohn's is the source of her fever. Also, when she took Lomotil for loose stools, she became obstipated. Metamucil may help avoid rebound constipation.

Thank you for allowing me to participate in this very lovely patient's care and management.

Very truly yours,

James Wood, MD

JW:hpi
D: 10/2/[add year]
T: 10/3/[add year]

Chart Note

BOKKER, JANICE
June 28, [add year]

The patient was seen today for skin testing, and all of her skin tests are negative. It is my impression, therefore, that she has intrinsic asthma.

She is to discontinue the Theo-24, as she has been experiencing episodes of tachycardia and anxiety. Switch to Proventil 2 mg tablets 4 times daily for wheezing. Return to see me again in 2 months.

ANTONIO FERRERIA, MD

AF:hpi
d: 6/28/[add year]
t: 6/29/[add year]

SOAP Note

FARR, LISA
#802741
October 1, [add year]

SUBJECTIVE
Patient is here for routine gynecologic examination. She is on Ortho-Novum and is having no difficulty with the pill. She forgets to take the pill occasionally.

OBJECTIVE
Breasts reveal no masses or tenderness. Abdomen negative. Pelvic exam was entirely negative. Pap smear taken.

ASSESSMENT
Normal gynecologic examination.

PLAN
Advised to use alternative forms of contraception when she misses a pill. Given a refill of Ortho-Novum 1/35. To return in 9 months.

LAURA NEUBURGER, MD

LN:hpi
d&t: 10/1/[add year]

History and Physical Examination

THOMAS, JEFFREY
April 8, [add year]

HISTORY
This 38-year-old male was admitted through the emergency department with a history of less than 1 day of acute ureteral colic on the left side. Patient had an intravenous pyelogram in the emergency department earlier today, which shows partial to complete obstruction of the left ureter at the ureterovesical junction with a large stone, approximately 8 x 5 mm, lodged at the ureterovesical junction. Patient has no other calcifications visible. Patient denies any previous history of urinary tract stones or other genitourinary problems except for prostatitis a couple of years ago. Patient has no other significant medical problems.

PAST MEDICAL HISTORY
Otherwise negative.

ALLERGIES
None.

REVIEW OF SYSTEMS:
HEENT on the system review is essentially unremarkable. He denies headache. He has a moderate hearing deficit.
Respiratory: No upper respiratory symptoms; no cough, congestion, or hemoptysis.
Cardiac: All symptoms are denied.
Gastrointestinal: There has been no history of hematemesis or melena. He denies significant fatty food intolerance.
Genitourinary: Ureteral colic as noted in the history.
Neuromuscular: Without complaint.
Musculoskeletal: Moderate arthritis.
Endocrine: No dysuria, polyuria, or polydipsia.
Hematologic: There is no history of anemia.
Integumentary: No significant skin problem.

MEDICATIONS
None. Follows usual diet.

FAMILY HISTORY
No familial history of kidney stones or other significant hereditary disease.

PHYSICAL EXAMINATION
GENERAL: Physical exam reveals a well-nourished, well-developed male in no acute distress.
HEENT: Eyes: Pupils equal, round, react to light. Ears, nose, and throat clear.
NECK: Neck supple. No jugular venous distention or bruit.

(continued)

History and Physical Examination *(continued)*

THOMAS, JEFFREY
April 8, [add year]
Page 2

LUNGS: Lungs clear to percussion and auscultation.
HEART: Regular rhythm, no murmur.
ABDOMEN: Abdomen soft. Slight left costovertebral angle tenderness, slight left lower quadrant tenderness. No rebound.
GENITALIA: Genitalia within normal limits. Penis: Normal male.
EXTREMITIES: No cyanosis, clubbing, or edema.
NEUROLOGIC: Neurologically oriented x3 with no gross deficits.

IMPRESSION
Left lower ureteral stone with obstruction.

RECOMMENDATION
Hydration, analgesia, observation, and if stone does not pass within 72 hours or less, will probably recommend patient for ureteroscopy and stone basketing and, if needed, ultrasonic lithotripsy. If the stone cannot be mobilized downward, push-back and extracorporeal shock wave lithotripsy might be considered.

ANNETTE MEHLHORN, MD

AM:hpi

d: 4/8/[add year]
t: 4/8/[add year]

Consultation

SKYLAR, SUNNY
#627582
Date: February 20, [add year]

HISTORY OF PRESENT ILLNESS

The patient is a 9-year-old student who allegedly was knocked down by kids playing a game, chasing each other in the gym. She apparently fell on her left knee and had immediate pain and swelling in the knee region. She quit playing the game immediately. Apparently initially she was unable to walk and had a lot of pain and her "complete left leg was swollen," according to her father. She denied any prior trouble with the left knee before the incident at school.

PAST MEDICAL HISTORY

The past medical history obtained was that she had had no major operations. She had had no serious illnesses other than presumably the usual childhood illnesses. She had no known food or drug allergies. She denied any serious accidents or injuries.

ORTHOPEDIC EXAMINATION

The orthopedic examination revealed a well-developed, well-nourished, alert 9-year-old Caucasian female child in apparent good general health and in no obvious severe pain but who did complain of discomfort as noted below. The skin in the left knee region was intact except there was a 1 to 2 mm dry scab at the left infrapatellar area said to be due to a mosquito bite. There was no obvious ecchymotic discoloration in the knee region. There was slight to moderate swelling at the medial left knee at the medial collateral ligament and medial joint line. There was rather marked tenderness at the medial left knee at the medial joint line and the entire length of the medial collateral ligament from the femoral attachment to the tibial attachment, and no tenderness at the left lateral knee either at the joint line or lateral collateral ligament or tenderness at the pre- or peripatellar area, except very slight tenderness with deep pressure at the medial border of the left patella. She extended the right knee fully to 180º and the left knee incompletely to 160º with complaint with maximal extension of the left knee. She flexed the right knee through a range of 150º without complaint and flexed the left knee only to a right angle with complaint. The circumferences of the thighs measured with the knees flexed to a right angle from the popliteal flexion crease to the suprapatellar area, right over left, were 11 inches over 11 inches. The circumferences of the legs at the level of maximum girth, right over left, were 10-1/2 inches over 10 inches in this right-handed person. Pinprick sensitivity in the lower extremities was normal and equal bilaterally, and peripheral circulation in the lower limbs was normal and equal bilaterally. The knee and ankle jerks were brisk and equal bilaterally. At 160º of extension of the left knee, the patient was noted to have good collateral stability medially and laterally, and at 90º of flexion there was a negative drawer sign. She did have some complaint of discomfort with stressing the ligaments of the left knee. One could not flex the left knee sufficiently to carry out a McMurray maneuver.

ROENTGENOGRAMS

AP and lateral x-rays of the patient's left knee were examined and felt to be negative or normal.

DIAGNOSIS

Medial collateral ligament strain, left knee. Rule out torn meniscus.

DONALD SCHAFFRAN, MD d: 02/20/[add year] t: 02/20/[add year]

Operative Report

CASSO, STEPHANIE
#718369
Date of surgery: 9/15/[add year]

PREOPERATIVE DIAGNOSIS
Cholelithiasis; recurrent biliary colic; chronic cholecystitis.

POSTOPERATIVE DIAGNOSIS
Cholelithiasis; recurrent biliary colic; chronic cholecystitis.

PROCEDURE PERFORMED
Laparoscopic cholecystectomy.

ANESTHESIA
General endotracheal anesthesia.

INDICATIONS
Presented for evaluation of recurrent, intermittent biliary colic. She needed a laparoscopic cholecystectomy in treatment for her symptoms.

PROCEDURE
After satisfactory general anesthesia was accomplished, a nasogastric tube and Foley catheter were placed for decompression of the stomach and urinary bladder. The anterior abdominal wall was sterilely prepped and draped. A curvilinear infraumbilical incision was made and the fascia grasped with two Kocher clamps. Two #1 PDS sutures were placed to assist with retraction of the fascia, and the Hasson trocar was placed in an incision in the fascia. The placement of the Hasson was preceded by digital examination of the peritoneal cavity to ensure that there were no periumbilical adhesions to the anterior abdominal wall. Pneumo-peritoneum was established, and the camera was placed through the Hasson retractor for placement of the other trocars under direct visualization. A 10 mm epigastric port was placed, and two lateral 5 mm ports were placed in the subcostal plane. Graspers were placed through the lateral ports and used to retract the fundus of the gallbladder over the edge of the liver and to retract the body to facilitate dissection of the hilar structures. Before this could be accomplished, some thin, filmy adhesions between the omentum and the gallbladder were taken down bluntly with the dissector. Then attention was directed to dissection of the hilar structures.

The cystic artery and cystic duct were isolated, doubly clipped proximally and doubly clipped distally, and then divided with the parrot scissors. Dissection was commenced with cautery, and the gallbladder was removed from the hilar structures to the fundus. The camera was moved to the epigastric port, and the gallbladder was removed through the Hasson umbilical port. The gallbladder was inspected and indeed found to have all the clips in the appropriate place. There was an approximately 2 cm stone in the gallbladder. The Hasson retractor was replaced in the umbilical port and the camera was replaced through

(continued)

Operative Report (continued)

CASSO, STEPHANIE
#718369
Date of surgery: 9/15/[add year]
Page 2

this. Inspection of the right upper quadrant revealed the hilar clips to be in good position. The right upper quadrant was copiously irrigated with saline and aspirated. Of note, there was no spillage of stones during the case; however, one of the graspers had disrupted the gallbladder wall early in the case, and there was some minimal spillage of clear yellow bile. All of this was irrigated and aspirated at the conclusion of the case.

The lateral ports were removed and revealed no bleeding. The epigastric port was removed and also revealed no bleeding. The Hasson retractor was withdrawn and pneumoperitoneum evacuated. The PDS sutures at the umbilical fascia were approximated to close the fascial defect, and an additional #1 PDS suture was placed to completely close this fascial defect. All skin incisions were closed with a running subcuticular 4-0 Vicryl suture. Steri-Strips were applied. The patient tolerated the procedure well and was returned to the recovery room in stable condition.

ANTHONY LOO, MD

AL:hpi

d: 9/15/[add year]
t: 9/16/[add year]

Discharge Summary

SCHONE, RANDALL
#558086
Admitted: 12/1/[add year]
Discharged: 12/3/[add year]

ADMITTING DIAGNOSIS
Fracture of right tibia, closed.

DISCHARGE DIAGNOSIS
Fracture of right tibia, closed.

OPERATION PERFORMED
Open reduction and internal fixation with Lottes nail, right tibia.

HISTORY
The patient was playing baseball on the day of admission. He was hit at second base and sustained an injury to his right leg with immediate pain and swelling. He was brought to the emergency department and diagnosed as having fractured his right tibia.

PHYSICAL EXAMINATION
The fracture site was tender to palpation. He had good sensation and circulation in the leg, but marked swelling was present.

X-RAYS
Multiple views of the tibia revealed there was a stairstep-type fracture at the distal portion of the middle one third of the tibia.

HOSPITAL COURSE
On the day of admission, the patient was taken to surgery and a Lottes nail inserted to fix the fracture. The patient's postoperative course was essentially benign. He was placed in a long leg cast and gradually ambulated on crutches.

DISCHARGE PLAN
The patient will remain on crutches for the next 6 weeks. At that time another set of x-rays will be carried out to assess the progress of healing. The patient is to call our office immediately if he notices increased pain, swelling, or duskiness of the toes.

DISCHARGE MEDICATIONS
Tylenol No. 3, one p.o. q.4h. p.r.n. pain.

KEITH BULLOCK, MD
KB:hpi   d: 12/1/[add year]   t: 12/3/[add year]

Comic Relief

Jest for the Health of It

by Richard Lederer, Ph.D.

It is ironic that the humor in hospitals, emergency departments, and doctors' offices—usually some of the scariest places—can be exceedingly hilarious. The giddy ghost of Mrs. Malaprop haunts medical halls and application forms, where we discover all manner of strange conditions, such as swollen asteroids, an erection nervosa, shudders (shingles!), and migrating headaches. All the malappropriate terms in this article were miscreated by anxious patients or hassled doctors and nurses.

An Austin, Texas, emergency medical technician answered a call at the home of an elderly woman whose sister had collapsed. As they were placing her into the ambulance, the lady wailed, "Oh, lawdy, lawdy. I know what's the matter with her. She done got the same thing what killed her brother. It's a heretical disease."

The technician asked what that would be, and the lady said, "The Smiling Mighty Jesus!" When the EMT got the sister to the county hospital, she looked up the brother's medical records to find he had died of spinal meningitis.

A woman rushed into the lobby of a hospital and exclaimed, "Where's the fraternity ward?" The receptionist calmly replied, "You must mean the maternity ward." The woman went on, "But I have to see the upturn." Patiently, the receptionist answered, "You must mean the intern." Exasperated, the woman continued, "Fraternity, maternity, upturn, intern—I don't care wherever or whoever. Even though I use an IOU, and my husband has had a bisectomy, I haven't demonstrated for two months and I think I may be fragrant!"

That same woman later became 3 cm diluted and, narrowly avoiding a mess carriage, she ultimately went into contraptions. Her baby was born with its biblical cord wrapped around its arm, and she asked if she could have the child circumscribed before leaving the hospital.

A man went to his eye doctor, who told him he had a case of myopera and would have to wear contract lenses. That was a lot better than his friend who had had a cadillac removed from his eye. Still, when he worked at his computer, he would have to watch out for harbor tunnel syndrome. He worried that his authoritis of the joints might be a signal of Old Timer's disease and fretted that a genital heart defect was causing a myocardial infraction and trouble with his duodemon.

Another man was in the hospital passing gullstones from his bladder while the doctor was treating a cracked dish from his spine. After the operation, his glands were completely prostrated. A hyannis hernia, hanging hammeroids, inflammation of the strocum, and a blockage of his large intesticle could have rendered him impudent.

We're not talking about just a deviant septum here. These symptoms were enough to give a body heart populations, high pretension, a peppery ulcer, and postmortem depression—even a cerebral hemorrhoid. But at least that's better than a case of headlights (head lice), sea roses of the liver, cereal palsy, or sick as hell anemia. Any of these could cause one to slip into a comma.

A woman experienced itching of the virginia during administration, which led to pulps all up her virginal area and they had to void her reproductions. This was followed by a tubular litigation and, ultimately, mental pause. Mental pause can cause one to become a maniac depressive and act like a cyclopath.

She didn't worry about her very close veins, but she thought that a mammy-o-gram and Pabst smear might show if she had swollen nymph glands and fireballs of the eucharist. That's "fibroids of the uterus," and it's something you can't cure with simple acnepuncture, Heineken maneuver, or a bare minimum enema. Apparently, evasive surgery would be required. Afterward, she would recuperate in expensive care.

Healthcare Documentation Technology

3

Learning Objectives

▶ Identify appropriate security measures for protecting PHI.

▶ Identify the recommended encryption standard of healthcare records under the HIPAA security rule.

▶ Identify documentation authentication practices considered dangerous by both The Joint Commission and DHHS.

▶ Given the abbreviation of a computer term, identify the correct expanded form.

▶ Given a computer technology term, identify the correct definition, or given a definition, identify the correct computer technology term.

▶ Given the abbreviation of a healthcare documentation technology term, identify the correct expanded form.

▶ Given a healthcare documentation technology term, identify the correct definition, or, given a definition, identify the correct healthcare documentation technology term.

▶ Given a term or abbreviation related to transcription technology or data exchange, identify the correct definition, or given a definition related to transcription technology or data exchange, identify the term or abbreviation.

Healthcare Documentation Technology

Introduction

The field of medical transcription has seen many changes in the area of dictation and transcription technologies that have dramatically altered how transcriptionists do what they do. Gone are the tape recorders and players and typewriters of yesterday. Today's transcriptionists use computers and keyboards to generate reports from narrative dictation that, for the most part, is digitally recorded and also delivered via computer. The technological innovation that has perhaps had the greatest impact so far on the dictation/transcription process is **speech recognition technology (SRT)**.

No one has a crystal ball and can predict with certainty what future technological changes will bring. SRT has changed *how* **medical transcriptionists (MTs)** do *what* they do, but the **electronic health record (EHR)** will dramatically change what transcriptionists do.

For this reason, it is important to emphasize again that it is medical transcriptionists' interpretive medical language skills, their reasoning and problem-solving abilities, their understanding of the context and content of clinical documentation, and their attention to quality and detail that will ensure their place in the future, regardless of what it brings.

Vocabulary Review

authentication (1) A system that keeps computer information safe by checking who the user is and checking that the information has not been changed. (2) Verification, usually by electronic signature or unique code, that an entry in the health record (like a medical report or physician order) is accurate and complete.

back-end speech recognition technology (BE-SRT) The use of editors to proofread and correct text drafts generated by a speech recognition engine, a process that also contributes to further training of the recognition engine.

Centers for Medicare & Medicaid Services (CMS) The government agency that sets regulations and manages reimbursement for those on Medicare and Medicaid.

clinical decision support (1) CMS definition: Health Information Technology (Health IT) functionality that "builds upon the foundation of an EHR to provide persons involved in care processes with general and person-specific information, intelligently filtered and organized, at appropriate times, to enhance health and healthcare." (2) The Health Information Management and Systems Society (HIMSS), definition: "…a process for enhancing health-related decisions and actions with pertinent, organized clinical knowledge and patient information to improve health and healthcare delivery." Whichever definition is used, the core intent for the practicing clinician is to actively assist in delivering optimal patient care.

clinical quality measures (CQMs) A set of standards designed to assess the quality of care and improve patient care by which CMS determines whether a provider using an EHR is eligible for financial incentives or must pay a penalty for failing to meet the standards.

computerized provider order entry (CPOE) The process of placing orders for pharmaceuticals, laboratory studies, and imaging studies in digital format in order to reduce errors and increase efficiency.

critical access hospitals (CAHs) A separate provider type recognized by CMS. These facilities are established under a State Medicare Rural Hospital Flexibility Program, operated 24/7, with no more than 25 inpatient beds (plus 10 more for a rehab or psychiatric unit), have an average annual length of stay of 96 hours or less per patient for acute care, and be located either more than a 35-mile drive from the nearest hospital or CAH or more than a 15-mile drive in areas with mountainous terrain or only secondary roads *or* designated as a "necessary provider" of healthcare services to residents in the area by the state prior to January 1, 2006.

EHR (electronic health record) A longitudinal electronic record of patient health information generated by one or more encounters in any care delivery setting. An EHR supports integration of a patient's health record across multiple health organizations and secure sharing of information with other providers, such as laboratories and specialists, providing clinical decision support and helping clinicians do a better job of managing patient care.

encryption A method of converting an original message of regular text into encoded text by means of an algorithm (i.e., type of procedure or formula). The receiving party who has the key to the code or access to another confidential process would be able to decrypt (i.e., translate) the text and convert it into plain, comprehensible text.. HHS guidance for this is 128-bit or 256-bit encryption using NIST guidelines. The goal of encryption is to protect electronic PHI from being accessed and viewed by unauthorized users.

front-end speech recognition technology (FE-SRT) Editing of speech-recognized draft text by the originator of the text in real time while dictating.

FTP (file transfer protocol) A standard network protocol used to transfer files from one host to another host over a TCP-based network, such as the Internet.

integrated transcription platform A multitasking application that includes dictation, transcription, ADT (admission, discharge, transfer) data, productivity tools, dictionaries, format tools, communication tools (instant messaging, flagging, or alerts), and other processes needed for the transcription process.

language model The probability distribution of words the speaker may use based on the speaker profile; the language model improves as the speech engine is "trained."

macros Key words or codes that are expanded to blocks of text by the text-generating software.

meaningful use A set of standards developed by the Centers for Medicare and Medicaid Services (CMS) that specifies clinical quality measures to improve patient care that must be met by users of certified EHR technology in order to qualify for financial incentives or avoid penalties for failure to meet the standards.

Office of the National Coordinator for Health Information Technology (ONC) The principal federal entity charged with coordination of nationwide efforts to implement and use the most advanced health information technology and the electronic exchange of health information. ONC is a division of the Department of Health and Human Services (HHS).

role-based limited access Users of a system are allowed access only to the systems that are needed for them to perform the tasks they are assigned to do.

secure web portal A secure Internet pipeline or entry point. Data passing through the web portal is encrypted in both directions.

speaker profile The stored data the speech engine has about a speaker that enables it to adapt to characteristics of the speaker. The profile includes the name of the speaker, speaker preferences, information about the vocabulary and word patterns of the speaker, pronunciation models, and acoustic data about the speaker's voice.

SRE (speech recognition editor) One who edits drafts of text generated by a speech recognition engine.

SRT (speech recognition technology) A technology by which speech is converted to text.

TAT (turnaround time), transcription The time elapsed between the completion of dictation and the delivery of the transcribed document either in printed medium or electronically to a repository.

templates Predetermined formats and content matched to specific report types, procedures, or diagnoses.

web portal A secured Internet pipeline or web site that brings information from diverse sources in a unified way.

Dictation and Transcription Systems

We still see some cassette tape dictation systems in place today, but most have been replaced with digital dictation systems. A digital dictation system works much the same as a compact disk (CD). The end result is digital dictation that is without any hiss or other extraneous sounds that are found on regular cassette tape.

In the digital dictation system, voice files are stored in "digital" (computer) format with file extensions like **.wav, .mp3, .mp4,** or **.wma** rather than "analog" (tape) format, and the dictation is usually free from mechanical noise. Digital dictation does not eliminate all background noise from the environment surrounding the dictator, however, nor does it correct poor dictation habits. The computer on which the digital voice files are stored may be in the same room as the dictator or in a room on the other side of the country and accessed via the Internet.

To dictate medical reports, doctors may use a hardwired dictation unit, an ordinary phone, a handheld pocket-sized digital recorder, or a headset with microphone attachment. With digital dictation, the physician is usually required to key in a personal ID number, a patient identification number, and a report type number, or the physician may swipe a bar code encoded with all the patient's **demographic data**. On some systems, this electronic information can be imported directly into a report without intervention by the transcriptionist. However, the MT still needs to verify that the information is correct.

The transcriptionist may access digital dictation by working on a proprietary platform that is local or on a personal computer in the next room or across the country. If the MT or **speech recognition editor (SRE)** works remotely, the dictation probably will be transferred via the Internet, either in encrypted form or via a secure **FTP (file transfer protocol)** site. Foot pedals may be connected to a computer via a USB connection or, less likely, a serial port. These pedals operate the audio player on the transcriptionist's computer or a proprietary player. A stereo headset is plugged into the speaker output. With these accessories, the computer completely replaces the transcriber equipment that is necessary for playing cassette tapes.

Once a report is transcribed using either proprietary software or widely available commercial software such as Microsoft Word, the MT will then "upload" the report, sending it securely to the employer, a quality assurance (QA) department, the client, or directly into an EHR system where it will be **authenticated** by the originator and become a permanent part of the patient's health record.

Pause for Reflection

1. List the common file formats or extensions for digital dictation files.
2. How is demographic information inserted into a dictation file?
3. How does the MT access the dictation in order to transcribe it or the SRE to edit the SR draft?
4. What happens to the transcribed reports?

Speech Recognition Technology

We are surrounded by speech recognition technology (SRT); few individuals in modern society can go a day without encountering its use in their lives. You encounter SRT every time you call your credit card company or use the phone to reserve a hotel room or make a flight reservation. When you tell your smart phone to "Call John Simmons" or your computer to "open MS Word," you are using SRT. When Raj on *Big Bang Theory* falls in love with Siri, iPhone's sultry-voiced voice-command computerized personal assistant, he is falling in love with SRT.

SRT has become ubiquitous and commonplace, and it has had a big impact on healthcare documentation. Originally predicted to make medical transcriptionists obsolete, SRT has become a tool by which MTs turned SREs (editors) have been able to increase production and improve **turnaround times (TAT)**.

SRT turns speech into text by means of a "voice recognition engine." We won't go into the math and science of how it operates, but basically, speech-recognition software applications consist of these components: a microphone, sound card, dictionary, **speaker profile**, **language model**, and recognition engine. The microphone and sound card convert speech into a digital waveform, just like the music you listen to on your MP3 player.

The initial training of the speech recognition engine is accomplished by matching a recording of the user's speech to a large file mapped to specific text (the speaker profile). This is what makes it possible for voice-recognition engines to recognize the speech of a Texan, a native of India, or a speaker from the West Indies. As the user continues to dictate (and the text is corrected as necessary), the engine continues to "learn."

Early SRT systems were referred to as **discrete speech** recognition systems; processing speeds were slow and the vocabulary databases (dictionaries) were limited. The dictator had to speak directly into a microphone attached to the computer and had to speak very slowly, enunciating each word, in order for the system to have a reasonable recognition rate. You can imagine how cumbersome this would have been for harried doctors who are always in a hurry.

Today's SRT systems, however, have much faster processors and very large dictionaries allowing for **continuous speech** recognition. Dictators can speak at a natural rate and rhythm and use a hard-wired microphone or dictate remotely using a telephone or mobile phone, just as they do with other dictation systems. To put this in perspective, early systems trained the dictators; today, it's the other way around.

Most speech recognition systems require continued training beyond the speaker profile to recognize the speech of different individuals. The amount of training required depends in large part on the amount of vocabulary that needs to be recognized. So you may be able to train your smart phone in a matter of minutes, but in order for a speech recognition system to accurately recognize dozens or even hundreds of dictators using very advanced and extensive medical vocabularies, more training is needed.

There are two methods of using SRT to generate medical reports. The first is referred to as **front-end speech recognition**. In front-end systems, text is generated as the physician dictates. The physician makes corrections as necessary while dictating. When the report is complete, it can be electronically authenticated or printed and signed, and immediately distributed to the patient's chart, other physicians, and from a reimbursement standpoint, to coding and billing. The benefit of this system is faster turnaround time. Presumably this enhances patient care and speeds reimbursement.

Speech recognition technology incorporates a number of other tools to save time and improve the quality of documentation. Dictation is often combined with **templates** (predetermined formats and content matched to specific report types, procedures, or diagnoses) which serve as the building blocks of a report. The dictator just adds new content unique to the patient or situation. Dictators may dictate **macros** (key words or codes) that are expanded to blocks of text by the text-generating software in much the same way that MTs use abbreviation expanders.

In combination with the electronic health record, stored text can be incorporated into or linked to a report, eliminating the need to repeat information already in the patient's medical record. For example, the results of a blood chemistry test do not have to be dictated for the History and Physical Examination, a consultation, and a discharge summary—they can simply be linked to electronically or, if a report needs to be printed, imported into a document prior to printing.

Some physicians have embraced front-end recognition but many, if not most, have not. The latter feel that their time would be better spent caring for their patients or seeing more patients. Unfortunately, in some settings, the decision to use front-end speech recognition is not made by the providers of healthcare.

While front-end speech recognition has its advantages, the disadvantages have led many to adopt **back-end speech recognition**, which is much more common in the industry. This is the behind-the-scenes editing (and training of the speech recognition engine) by MTs working as SR editors. Many times, dictators are not even aware that their dictation is being run through a speech recognition engine.

In this system, SR editors listen to the dictation while proofing and editing the speech-recognized draft. While turnaround is not as fast as when physicians edit their own dictation, this method often provides better quality and frees up the physician for the more important task of patient care. In Chapter 4, we will go into more detail about the do's and don'ts of speech editing and how it affects the "learning" of the speech engine.

There are still limitations to SRT. Background noise, disorganization of content dictated, and other poor dictation habits have a negative effect on the quality of recognition. SRT cannot correct misspeaks or other dictation errors, although some systems are programmed to catch some discrepancies like left-right. It won't query the dictator when something doesn't make sense or an important lab test result or diagnosis is missing.

Although speech recognition technology has improved dramatically in terms of recognition and tools that contribute to the quality of dictation, SRT is still not accurate enough for the reports that are generated to go straight to a patient's chart. This is why skilled SR editors are needed.

Pause for Reflection

1. Complete this sentence: Originally predicted to make medical transcriptionists obsolete, SRT has become a tool by which MTs turned SREs (editors) have been able to _____.
2. What are the components of a speech recognition system?
3. How are speech engines "trained"?
4. Distinguish between discrete speech and continuous speech.
5. Distinguish between front-end speech recognition and back-end speech recognition.
6. What tools to save time and improve the quality of documentation may be incorporated into healthcare documentation by SRT?
7. What are some of the limitations of SRT?

The Electronic Health Record

The **electronic health record (EHR)** is a longitudinal electronic record of patient health information generated by one or more encounters in any care delivery setting. Included in this information are patient demographics, progress notes, problems, medications, vital signs, past medical history, immunizations, laboratory data, and radiology reports. The EHR automates and streamlines the physician's workflow. The EHR has the ability to generate a complete record of a clinical patient encounter—as well as supporting other care-related activities directly or indirectly via interface—including evidence-based decision support, quality management, and outcomes reporting.

Some people use the terms *electronic health record* and *electronic medical record* (EMR) interchangeably. What's the difference? Electronic medical records are a digital version of the paper charts in the physician's office. An EMR contains the medical and treatment history of the patients in one practice. EMRs have advantages over paper records in that they allow physicians to track data over time, easily identify which patients are due for preventive screenings or checkups, check how their patients are doing on certain parameters—such as blood pressure readings or vaccinations—and monitor and improve overall quality of care within the practice.

However, the information in EMRs doesn't travel easily out of the practice. In fact, the patient's record might even have to be printed out and delivered by mail or electronically with special security to specialists and other members of the care team. In that regard, EMRs are not much better than a paper record.

Electronic health records (EHRs) do all those things—and more. EHRs focus on the total health of the patient. EHRs are designed to reach out beyond the health organization that originally collects and compiles the information and securely share that information with other providers, such as laboratories and specialists, and help providers do a better job of managing patient care. EHRs contain information from all the physicians involved in the patient's care, which, in turn, results in more open communication and more involvement on the patient's part.

Information moves electronically with the patient —to the specialist, the hospital, the nursing home, the next state or even across the country. By making it easier to use and share information, The National Alliance for Health Information Technology stated that EHR data "can be created, managed, and consulted by authorized physicians and staff across more than one healthcare organization."

When information is shared in a secure way, it becomes more powerful. Healthcare is a team effort, and shared information supports that effort. After all, much of the value derived from the healthcare delivery system results from the effective communication of information from one party to another and, ultimately, the ability of multiple parties to engage in interactive communication of information. In so doing, EHRs improve the accuracy of diagnoses and health outcomes, better coordinate patient care among multiple providers, and increase practice efficiencies and cost savings.

EHRs are designed to be accessed by all people involved in the patient's care—including the patients themselves. Indeed, that is an explicit expectation in the Stage 1 definition of "meaningful use" of EHRs.

With fully functional EHRs, all members of the team have ready access to the latest information allowing for more coordinated, patient-centered care. With EHRs:

• The information gathered by the primary care provider tells the emergency department physician about the patient's life-threatening allergy, so that care can be adjusted appropriately, even if the patient is unconscious.

• Patients can log on to their own records and see the trend of the lab results over the last year, which can help motivate them to take their medications and keep up with the lifestyle changes that have improved the numbers.

• The lab results run last week are already in the record to tell the specialists what they need to know without running duplicate tests.

• The physician's notes from the patient's hospital stay can help inform the discharge instructions and followup care and enable the patient to move from one care setting to another more smoothly.

Pause for Reflection

1. Distinguish between the EHR and the EMR.
2. Discuss advantages of an EHR.
3. How does an EHR benefit the patient?

Meaningful Use

Electronic health records can provide many benefits for providers and their patients, but the benefits depend on how they're used. **Meaningful use** is the set of standards defined by the **Centers for Medicare & Medicaid Services (CMS)** Incentive Programs that provide financial incentives for the "meaningful use" of certified EHR technology to improve patient care.

To receive an EHR incentive payment, providers have to show that they are "meaningfully using" their

EHRs by meeting thresholds for a number of objectives referred to as **clinical quality measures (CQMs)**. CMS has established the objectives for "meaningful use" that eligible professionals, eligible hospitals, and **critical access hospitals (CAHs)** must meet in order to receive an incentive payment.

There are 15 required core measures, and eligible providers (EPs) must choose an additional five measures from a list provided by CMS. Requirements include but are not limited to **computerized provider order entry (CPOE)** for prescriptions; maintenance of an active medication and allergy list; charting of changes in height, weight, blood pressure, and BMI, and for children, growth charts; providing patients with an electronic copy of their health information (diagnostic test results, problem list, medication lists, medication allergies, discharge summary, and procedures) upon request and an immediate clinical summary for each office visit; implementation of **clinical decision support**; the ability to exchange information with other providers; and securing of PHI and patient privacy.

In addition, the **Office of the National Coordinator for Health Information Technology** (ONC) has established standards and certification criteria for the certification of EHR technology, so eligible professionals and hospitals may be assured that the systems they adopt are capable of performing the required functions.

EHR adoption among physician offices and hospitals is increasing, primarily due to CMS incentives and penalties for failure to adopt, but the technical limitations, ease of use, interoperability, improved clinical decision support, and other hoped-for benefits of the EHR have yet to be fully realized.

EHR vendors who, like speech recognition technology vendors before them, thought that they could eliminate or reduce the need for healthcare documentation specialists are realizing that they were short-sighted. They have begun to work with other stakeholders in the healthcare documentation arena to integrate tools for the use of SRT and direct entry of narrative text from dictation or other sources.

Pause for Reflection

1. What is meaningful use?
2. List some of the CQMs by which CMS determines whether meaningful use is met.
3. What is the role of the ONC in certifying EHR technology?

Professional Readings

Technology, Security, and Beyond for the Remote Workforce

by Brenda J. Hurley

The medical transcription industry has used a remote workforce for nearly three decades. In the early years, the technologies allowed only for transcribing on typewriters from cassette tapes, and then printing and delivering reports to the clients (healthcare providers) via couriers. After years of this, dictation systems progressed to telephone call-in systems that recorded dictation so that the dictation could then be accessed with the use of a remote transcribe station via a telephone line.

More medical transcriptionists (MTs) ventured to work from their homes with the technology connecting to dictation via their telephone line. The workforce, however, was limited geographically to receiving dictation where they lived to avoid expensive long distance charges; there was no unlimited long distance service available then. Typewriters were then exchanged for word processor units and the improved efficiencies soon became a winner in the industry as productivity increased.

Before long the geographic limitation became a nonissue for the workforce when the dictation transitioned from analog (tape) to digital files (using computers), and then telephone access was replaced with Internet file transfers for both voice (dictation) and text (transcribed documents). The remote workforce exploded. In fact, today most MTs when hired by an MT service are given no opportunity to work on-site; they are expected to work off-site. Healthcare facilities that employ remote-based MTs do the same.

Through all of this time, a staggering number of healthcare documents and their companion dictation files have been exchanged between healthcare facilities to MT services, and then to the remote MT workforce, without major security breaches—truly, a testimony to the excellent job that the medical transcription industry has done in protecting confidential patient data.

Long before HIPAA, the HITECH Act, and state privacy laws were enacted, MT services built good security into their systems to protect the data entrusted to them by their clients. They were driven, not by laws, but by a desire to follow good business practices, high ethics, and excellent customer service. Hats off to those pioneers in the MT industry for setting their standards high!

But the compliance rules have changed, the risks are higher, the laws are more stringent, and what was good in the past is not considered good enough by today's standards. Because of this, it is important to evaluate the security and processes used by the MT remote workforce in order to raise the compliance bar even higher.

A risk analysis of the remote security and processes used is not an option; it is mandatory under HIPAA. Just as the technology has progressed over the decades in this industry, the risks, threats, and vulnerabilities have changed as well. For example, what was a risk with cassette tapes for dictation is not applicable to the organizations that no longer use tapes for recording dictation. But there are still a few facilities that use cassette tapes, so they would still need to establish and implement processes to protect those tapes and the PHI (protected health information) contained on them.

Few individuals outside of the MT industry understand the many technical complexities that are woven into the fabric of the 24/7/365 processes required in capturing dictation, instantaneous transmission to a data center, delivery to the right MT to do the work (that alone has another set of complex factors), report creation through transcription (or speech editing), transfer of completed report to the data center, sharing with a QA (quality assurance) specialist when required, delivering final report to the client, and fulfilling report distribution requirements—all within a handful of hours while maintaining flawless security and data integrity throughout the entire process. Because of the unique systems and processes used by each MT service, it is unlikely that there would be two organizations that do everything exactly the same. Given this, a security risk analysis will be different for each MT business.

There are many tools and articles published on security analysis, but as a very simple description, it is a process that is carried out by a team that represents several of the key steps in the path of the PHI throughout the organization. For example, you would want to

WHEN WORKING OFF-SITE OR FROM HOME

Here is a list of the items commonly expected to be furnished by either the MT who works remotely or by the employer. There may be variations to this list, depending on the employer.

- Hospitals will nearly always furnish a PC that will be used only for their work. Some MT services will furnish a PC; however, many will not. Often when a PC is provided, the MT needs to furnish the monitor, keyboard, and mouse. A 20-inch monitor or larger will ease eye strain, and a wireless mouse will allow greater flexibility in use.

- If you have to furnish your own PC, it is best to dedicate the PC only to work in order to avoid any inadvertent malware contamination or configuration changes unintentionally caused from your personal use.

- If you furnish the computer, you will need to maintain it with antivirus and firewall software.

- Ergonomic chair and desk.

- An office that is its own room with a door and key lock and with windows that lock.

- Appropriate lighting.

- Headset. A good quality headset that is comfortable will be worth every cent spent.

- Paper shredder. Although many remote MTs never need to print their transcripts, some do and they may need to shred confidential information as well. Some do not even have a printing option. Having a shredder is not a big expense and can be used for your personal papers to reduce your risk of identity theft.

- Phone with a messaging feature and caller ID. Avoid answering the phone while working; let it go to the messaging feature. If caller ID indicates your office is calling, then you can safely answer it.

- High-speed Internet access. Get the fastest speed you can; it will be worth the difference in productivity.

- Grounded electrical outlets with adequate circuit load. If your home is more than 40 years old, you may need to have your electrical outlets upgraded and your circuits evaluated by an electrician. If you overload a low-grade circuit with high-performance electrical equipment, you could be at risk for an electrical fire.

- Surge protector and uninterruptible power supply. Use these items for your computer and your cable or DSL modem box to avoid unwanted disruptions in function and connectivity.

- Reference materials—electronic and written.

- Digital pictures of your office space to provide to your employer, if required to do so.

include a representative from **information technology (IT)**, operations, transcription, and others as deemed needed. They would review a data flow document showing the PHI (dictation as well as the transcribed document) during all processes from the initial capture of dictation to the delivery of the final transcribed report back to the client, and all of those steps in between.

Once those processes and technologies are thoroughly analyzed for vulnerabilities, areas of risk, especially those of high risk, steps to mitigate those potential risks would be developed. As an example of this process, let's take a glimpse at a few of the typical vulnerabilities and consider solutions for minimizing the risks related to them.

Potential risks. We will assume for this exercise that the remote MT is working with encrypted voice and text files through a secure web portal on an integrated transcription platform that is designed with role-based limited system access with strong log-in authentication processes.

Let's break down those terms to understand what is included in this common MT work situation.

• An important way to prevent breaches is to use **encryption** to secure the PHI. HHS guidance for this is 128-bit or 256-bit encryption using the guidelines that are published by NIST (National Institute of Standards and Technology); this can be found at **www.nist.gov**. **Encryption** renders the files unusable, unreadable, or undecipherable to unauthorized individuals.

• **Secure web portal** indicates that the MT is working on-line through a secured Internet 'pipeline' referred to as a web portal. This also means that the actual application (or platform) that the MT is working on is not located on the MT's computer but is accessed remotely through the web portal. When established with **SSL technology** (secure socket layer), this type of access is very secure and utilizes a cryptographic system to encrypt the data being exchanged. If you do on-line banking, you are likely accessing your bank account via SSL technology.

• The phrase **integrated transcription platform** is used to indicate that this is a multitasking application that includes items needed for the transcription process. These would likely include dictation, transcription, ADT (admission, discharge, transfer) data, productivity tools, dictionaries, format tools, communication tool (instant messaging, flagging), and other items that would be needed in the transcription process.

In working on an integrated platform as an MT, when a new job (a new report to transcribe) is queued to an MT, a format for the report type will appear (this info is entered by the dictator at the time of dictation) on the screen with the appropriate report format section headings inserted, the ADT data will auto-populate the demographic section of the report, and the dictation readied is at that start position. During the transcription process, depending on the system, the MT will have available a word expander, an online dictionary (perhaps other on-line references), a line count tool, and a messaging tool for flagging a portion of the report for any discrepancy, inconsistency, or uncertainty.

• **Role-based limited access** allows users to access only the systems that are needed for them to perform the tasks they are assigned to do. For example, an MT would not have access to the client contract data because that would not be the role assigned to the MT to perform.

• Strong log-in authentication process will require signing on to the system with a complex **password** (more than 8 characters/numbers/symbols), and some systems may require a handheld device called a security token (other common names include key fob, cryptographic token, authentication token) that will generate a security code; this code will also be required to gain access to the system.

In a scenario like this, the ownership of the MT's computer is usually not an issue since the work is done on the organization's transcription platform; the MT's computer serves merely as an access device. Some MT platforms, however, may save the active document (the transcribed file) on the local PC (the MT's PC) to assure that a connectivity glitch does not lose or corrupt the report while being transcribed. That local save feature is generally programmed to be temporary and will delete that temp file within a specific time from when the report was completed.

The technical process has to be analyzed in a risk assessment to assure that if any file with PHI remains on the MT's computer, it is encrypted. This is where the ownership of the computer becomes an issue with the software licensing, compatible operating system versions, and updating of the software on a non-company-owned PC, all to assure that the required applications are fully functional. This can be fraught with many challenges. Also, it is hard to enforce limiting the use of social networking, personal emails, on-line games, and Internet website searching, or restrict who can use the PC when it is personally owned by the medical transcriptionist.

It is because of this that many organizations mitigate their potential risks and provide to their workforce a computer that is fully set up with administrator privileges locked from the remote user. These company-provided PCs usually do not allow local printing or connection with media storage devices, and load only the software that is needed for the performance of the tasks intended.

If the remote user changes his or her role within the organization, such as moves to a QA position, the applications needed for that role are remotely loaded on the PC by the company's IT staff. Also, routine remote security audits can be performed on this company-owned PC without individual privacy concerns. Given that some organizations have hundreds of MTs in their workforce, this investment in technology is costly.

Technology is not the only critical piece to security with a remote workforce. Training is mandatory under HIPAA and is paramount to good security practices. Even with the best technologies in place, if the people who use them handle situations inappropriately or fail to follow the established processes, security breaches can occur. Understanding is the first step to compliance, and this comes from education and training.

Let's take on the challenge of **report distribution**. Many organizations still use traditional faxing as their primary distribution tool for transcribed reports. Likely this is because it is the way it has been done for many years. Despite the fact that a traditional fax is not encrypted and is unprotected as defined by HIPAA, many organizations still insist on using unsecured faxing as their report distribution process for physician offices. Given this practice, making sure the fax number is accurate has taken on a whole new level of importance; in fact, it is critical.

What can and does sometimes happen is the physician dictates a note to send a copy of a report to Dr. Fred Flintstone, and then provides a fax number for Dr. Flintstone, a new physician in the area. The remote MT adds the name and number to the fax database, carefully transcribes it as dictated, and the report is then automatically faxed to that number. Worst case scenario, it is not Dr. Flintstone's office but instead a gas station. As ugly as that gets, it could get even worse because now that the wrong fax number is in the database, more reports may be sent daily to that same wrong number whenever a copy is requested to be sent to Dr. Flintstone. And to make it really a mess, no one at the gas station notified the organization that they had been receiving these faxes in error until several months later.

We can point fingers at whom to blame in the fax situation, but despite good technologies the process was not good enough to avoid a catastrophic situation. That is where written policies and training serve as essential components in good security. This could have been avoided with a policy such as this:

- When a new fax number is provided, flag the report so that the supervisor can verify that the fax number provided is accurate before it is entered into the database.

- Then with this policy, as a precaution, information technology (IT) would restrict privileges from remote users to add new numbers (or revise numbers) in the fax database. Thus, the only people who have privileges to make changes in the fax database would be those designated to do so (per written policy).

- The supervisor would then verify that fax number by sending a test document with no PHI, and not send any PHI to that fax number until the accuracy of the information has been confirmed as valid for that physician.

While all of this sounds like a lot of fuss, just remember the mess that occurred by faxing to the wrong number and how it needed to be carefully unraveled in order to proceed with breach risk analysis, reporting, and notification. For what is spent on policy, process development, and its related training, it would save time and money on fixing problems and, at times, repairing the organization's tarnished reputation.

Another potential risk to consider is the home-based office for the remote worker. Decades ago when the MTs working for hospitals were first allowed to work from home, the office space in their home was a huge issue. The hospitals had strict requirements, such as an ergonomic chair and desk, a room dedicated as an office and remote from the family activities, a door with a lock on it, adequate task lighting, no electrical cords allowed on the floor in the path where one would be walking, and good electrical surge protection. Before an MT was allowed to work at home, the home office was inspected by the MT supervisor. Some supervisors took room dimensions to create a diagram and captured pictures of the room to prove the home office was compliant with their established policies.

Things have definitely changed. Today many MTs work in their remote offices while never meeting (face to face) anyone from the organization they work for, and they never report specifics related to their home office, how it is equipped, what security is used, or its location within the home.

With the greater potential risks related to the remote workforce, it is definitely time to reevaluate home office security. While on-site inspections are likely not feasible for an MT service that has hundreds of MTs across the country, or healthcare facilities that may have dozens or more, there are definitely some requirements that make sense to implement, and some could be easily confirmed with digital photography.

Limiting access to the home office makes sense for lots of reasons—from the obvious potential security issues to the reduction of distractions for the MT when working on confidential patient documentation. It would be my expectation that all those who work remotely have already seen the wisdom in an ergonomic chair and desk, good task lighting, and electrical surge protection along with an uninterruptible power supply.

To skimp on these basics is only going to cause pain, physically and financially, either when suffering from repetitive stress injuries or redoing work that was lost when the electricity spiked near the end of a very long report that was not yet saved on the system. Having the right work environment is essential to good work habits and processes that promote security whether on-site in a hospital, in a business office, or in a home.

The medical transcription industry has carefully balanced many formidable challenges related to HIPAA compliance requirements with the enormous amount of data that is handled, stored, and transmitted on a daily basis, along with a large number of remote workforce scattered in many geographic locations. Other healthcare professions (i.e., coding and medical billing) that are transitioning to remote-based staffing would be well served to adopt some of the technologies and practices used in the medical transcription industry as a model for success. Our healthcare system and the patients we serve expect and deserve no less.

Pause for Reflection

1. What types of things have to be taken into consideration when performing a risk analysis for each MT business?
2. Who within an MT business should be included in developing a risk analysis?
3. What is the goal or purpose of encryption?
4. What measures are typically employed to ensure that remote transcription is secure?
5. Discuss issues related to MT-owned versus company-owned PCs.
6. What procedures can be implemented to ensure that reports containing PHI are not inadvertently faxed to wrong numbers?

Productivity Tools
Abbreviation Expansion Software
by Georgia Green

Experienced transcriptionists work smarter, not harder. That phrase has been used so much it's become cliché, but it's still true. There are a variety of productivity tools that smart MTs and SREs can use to improve or ensure the quality of their work and their productivity. Foremost among these is an abbreviation expander software or application.

Expanders improve your typing speed and efficiency while you are working in word processing software. Programmers work with a great deal of repetitive text entry and make use of these tools. If you make certain that your expansions have no typos, an abbreviation expander can improve the quality of your work. There are also ergonomic benefits—less stress on your hands, fingers, shoulders, and posture plus productivity benefits with increased output—because expanders allow you to produce many lines of text with fewer keystrokes.

An abbreviation expander is a program or part of a program that allows you to type abbreviations ("short forms" or "shortcuts") and produce longer words, phrases, or blocks of text. An abbreviation expander is sometimes referred to as a typing engine, speed typing program, keystroke saver, productivity software, or (somewhat incorrectly) a macro program.

Word processing software, such as MS Word, Word-Perfect, and OpenOffice include expander-like tools—AutoCorrect and QuickCorrect. These features can be turned off and on, contain a number of default entries that may or may not be helpful, and you can add and delete individual entries quickly and easily. (While working on this chapter, MS Word insisted on "correcting" EHR to HER each and every time it was used.) However, AutoCorrect and QuickCorrect are primarily designed to automatically correct spelling mistakes and to insert blocks of texts. While they can be used as abbreviation expanders while you are learning medical transcription, you will probably want more robust software when you are on the job.

For example, if I typed *The patient had a history of chf*, this would expand into *The patient had a history of congestive heart failure*. The beauty of an abbreviation expander really hits you when you realize that I could also have typed *Tp had a hx of chf* or even *tpho chf* and have it expand to *The patient had a history of congestive heart failure*.

FEATURES COMMON TO ALL ABBREVIATION EXPANDERS

1. They save keystrokes and improve speed.
2. They promote better quality.
3. They correct habitual typos and spelling errors. Note: A spelling error is corrected faster by an abbreviation expander than a spell-checker.
4. They make difficult-to-type expressions easy to type, e.g., expressions with numbers or special characters.
5. They Incorporate keyboard commands for problem characters. For example, in *x-ray*, the hyphen should be a hard hyphen to prevent the word from breaking at the end of a line; this can be done with an abbreviation expander. Frankly, you can achieve all of these goals with even the most limited abbreviation expander. That doesn't mean you won't want or need the bells and whistles offered by some products.

To reiterate the point, it is not just traditional medical abbreviations that can be expanded. You can also take advantage of the techniques used by professional stenographers who abbreviate just about everything.

The expander programs available today are almost too numerous to count. Some programs were conceived by companies that never heard of medical transcription. Anyone who uses a keyboard can use an abbreviation expander.

Some of these programs are straightforward expanders and some are text analyzers. In the former category, you create the abbreviations yourself (or import a list created by someone else). In the text analyzer model, you can instruct the software to process a selection of documents you specify and create an abbreviation list (or glossary) for you. This will produce lots of phrases that you type all the time—and the software will suggest sentence endings for you.

There are pros and cons to each type of expander. Let's move on to what is common to all expanders and how you can best use them (and avoid misusing them).

Formatting commands can be imbedded in the expansion. Formatting can also be determined by the abbreviation itself or by formatting commands as you transcribe. For example, if you used *abbj* as the shortcut for the word *abbreviation*, typing in lowercase will expand it to abbreviation, with caps lock down to ABBREVIATION, and with an initial capital letter (*Abbj*) to *Abbreviation*. Some expanders have the ability to imbed programming commands (your word processor's command to save a document, for example) within an expansion. This is analogous to what you can do with Windows hot keys.

You can even incorporate commands that will pause an expansion to allow you to insert some unique text or value. For example, you could create a shortcut for a *CBC* (*complete blood count*) and have the expansion pause after *hemoglobin, hematocrit, white blood count,* etc., so that you can insert the dictated value.

Some expander programs use pop-up windows or menus so you can see a list of short forms before you type them; otherwise they remind you that you have used an expansion after you type it. Some programs allow you to import your short forms from other expanders or from a list of abbreviations and expansions. Other features of some expanders include line counting, statistics, formatting options, and incorporation of macros, as noted above.

Abbreviation expanders can be a boon in terms of production on the job *if* used knowledgeably and responsibly. We've touched on only some aspects of word expander software; many programs have very advanced features. Only you can decide which program is best for you. Do your homework. Research available software, talk to users, and ask for trial products. The software should be easy to learn, and it should be relatively easy to create your expansions.

As with almost everything we humans invent to improve our lives, there are disadvantages. You can make a typo or misremember a shortcut and insert the wrong expansion in a report. If you fail to catch the error during proofreading, it can have serious consequences. You will need a well-designed naming system for creating shortcuts to help you remember your abbreviations and avoid expansion errors. You will find additional guidelines on the Downloads page of **www.hpisum.com**.

The Transcriptionist's Notebook

From day one in the medical transcription class, students need to keep a notebook (handwritten or electronic) with important words and phrases, do's and don'ts, special terms and procedures, geographic references, and so on—information they want easy access to.

Li'l Red Notebook (LRN) is an inexpensive productivity tool that organizes frequently needed and difficult-to-find information, keeping it available at your fingertips. It replaces a traditional word and phrase/reference notebook but is much more convenient to use than a spreadsheet. It stores information in color-coded tabbed lists that are alphabetized automatically. You can create an unlimited number of lists and display them in any order.

LRN's main feature is its ability to float over your existing application so you can see its contents while you work, without leaving your active document or resizing your current window. If you prefer not to see LRN until you need it, a keystroke toggles it between visible and invisible mode. It offers full hot-key control to search for entries and copy them to your document, as well as to add new entries. You can import, export, and/or print lists to back them up or share resources with friends, coworkers, or employees.

In addition to organizing words and phrases, you can store staff lists, individual dictator preferences, and style and formatting guidelines for different accounts. If an account has an approved abbreviation list or a hospital formulary, keep it in LRN. You can even use it to write reminders to yourself instead of filling up your work space with sticky notes.

LRN is compatible with any version of Windows and works alongside any transcription platform. It is available from **www.horusdevelopment.com**.

WHAT IS IN YOUR NOTEBOOK?

A good MT notebook includes :

- Words and phrases by medical specialty
- Drug lists
- Terms used by specific dictators or accounts
- Alpha or numeric staff lists
- Names and addresses of referring facilities
- All the cities in a particular state
- Terms that don't appear in other references
- Terms that are hard to find
- Study lists organized by chapter or specialty
- Abbreviations and their expansions
- Grammar and punctuation rules
- And anything that improves quality and productivity

Pause for Reflection

1. What is an abbreviation expander?
2. What are the advantages of using an abbreviation expander?
3. What are some of the features, besides expanding simple abbreviations, of some expander programs?
4. What types of information should you keep in your MT notebook?

Spotlight On

Ergonomics: It's All in the Tushie

by Renee M. Priest

It starts out as an isolated creak or squeak now and then, mildly irritating, but nothing to get all excited about. Insidiously, day by day, that squeaking gradually gets louder, more obtrusive, and one day, just as you delicately poise yourself above the seat and lower the derriere down to its comfortable, well-worn place . . . the darn chair BREAKS! I have watched in awe as seemingly sensible, calm, mild-mannered MTs have thrown incredibly spectacular temper tantrums when this astonishing phenomenon occurs.

Of course this does not receive much publicity, but it is a sad, sad truth that right now, all over the United States, MTs are shamelessly abusing chairs—plopping those heinies down way past the time limit per day that the manufacturer recommends for sitting; exceeding the optimum weight limitation while transcribing with a *Dorland's*, three word books, and a couple of drug books piled in the lap; endlessly fiddling with all the screws, wing nuts, and levers that manipulate height, armrest position, and back support. This tragic and truly pitiful condition has been appropriately dubbed the WT (wear and tear) syndrome. Do not make the mistake of believing that press release the chair manufacturers recently sent out. This absolutely does not have anything to do with size, shape, or poundage of the posterior in question.

Consider the length of time it takes to properly squash, mash, wriggle, and baptize that chairseat with assorted liquids and foodstuffs into just the proper configuration for maximum comfort. Is it any wonder that when this dreaded breakdown occurs the MT is amazed to learn that the favored chair was long ago officially classified as a chair "dinosaur," no longer manufactured, irreplaceable! A designation that is guaranteed to provoke a frenzied rooting through junk drawers by those hapless MTs searching for Krazy Glue, duct tape, even looting the garage to locate the husband's welder. (Okay, okay, I will admit that some MTs are thrifty,

which just might have a little something to do with this frantic behavior.)

Nevertheless, there comes a time when, despite all resuscitation efforts, the MT is forced to admit that the pile of fabric, wood, and ball bearings sitting on the floor in front of the computer is simply not repairable anymore.

The search for just the right chair can rapidly evolve into a quest that takes on mythic proportions, sort of like the search by Indiana Jones and his father for the Holy Grail—with one tiny difference. Instead of outsmarting sneaky archaeology thieves, snakes, bats, and the odd camel or two, the MT quickly finds that he/she is engaged in a battle of wits with that most heinous of hucksters—the chair salesman on commission. The search for just the right headset, transcriber, or keyboard with the perfect touch simply pales by comparison with the convoluted chair-testing process. When one's tushie is going to grace the seat in question for hours and hours and hours, no effort should be too elaborate when it comes to choosing the "creme de la creme" of chairs.

I find it handy to assemble a simple assortment of testing devices before entering any office store to peruse the tempting array of chairs on display. This will help to minimize that impulse buy—"Oh look, the color of the seat cushion matches the rug in my office," resulting in the salesman whisking you out the door with the chair conveniently crammed into a 2" x 2" box, needing only "minimal assembly" once home.

One of my oversized baskets for harvesting vegetables works quite well to hold the implements I consider essential for a true test of a chair's suitability. Just ignore that nasty look the salesman is giving you as you whip out the tape measure to "size up" the width of the backside and compare it to the chair seat. Remember, it is no longer possible to allow that half-inch or so of overhang space when measuring. Chair manufacturers strategically place

(continued)

Spotlight On Ergonomics: It's All in the Tushie, page 2

those armrest supports closer and closer to the seat cushion in a subliminal effort to undermine one's tushie self-esteem, thus provoking the desire to pay more money for the deluxe-size chair. Be aware that a salesman might attempt to tackle you as you are getting ready to douse that chair with a generous sampling of Coke or coffee. Wave that chair label claiming to be water- and stain-resistant at him and pour away.

Bringing children along is always a good idea. If necessary, borrow a few for the afternoon. Ages four through eight have proven the most successful for me. This will enable you to judge just how quickly you can restore all those ergonomic knobs and levers back to the optimum settings for ultimate comfort once the child is done spinning around in circles as fast as possible. This is also a good test of how quickly one can sponge that seat clean of the resultant eruption of stomach contents without any of it sinking into the foam padding. Do be sure to bend over and listen closely for the telltale squealing of ball bearings as those kids see how far and fast they can push

those chairs from the desk, utilizing the "feet off the top drawer" maneuver as leverage. This will give one a very reasonable estimate of the rolling life of the ball bearings.

Animals also come in handy, and they fit in that basket quite nicely. Cats, guinea pigs, perhaps birds, especially ones who like to make deposits in strategic places. Trust me, if that fabric can hold up to the canines of a teething puppy, it's a keeper.

I really should warn you that the final test in my arsenal is not for the squeamish or the faint of heart. Those salesmen really become uncontrollable when one is bringing out the heated backpad to line the chair with; the vibrating massage mat for back and "glutes"; the icy cold orthopedic pads for sciatica; and the test of all tests . . . the donut. It is most important to make sure that the chairseat can accommodate that donut easily because sitting in a chair for eight hours, afflicted with external hemorrhoids, is a lesson in endurance that will quickly separate the truly dedicated (or extremely demented) MT from those who have common sense.

Exercises

Chapter Review

Instructions: Choose the best answer.

_____ 1. Health IT functionality built into an EHR that gives providers general and person-specific information, intelligently filtered and organized, to enhance health and healthcare is _____
   A. electronic medical record.
   B. clinical decision support.
   C. clinical quality measures.
   D. computerized provider order entry.

_____ 2. Which of the following is a difference between an EHR and an EMR?
   A. The EHR can be shared electronically, the EMR cannot.
   B. The EHR is an accumulation of data from multiple patient encounters while the EMR is the record of one encounter.
   C. The EMR is the patient's record of healthcare over a lifetime; the EHR consists of just those visits that occurred at a single facility.
   D. The EMR is just specific information like dictated reports and diagnostic study results, but the EHR includes everything, including nursing notes, pharmacy records, and progress notes.

_____ 3. NIST guidelines for encryption of data are _____
   A. 128-bit or 256-bit.
   B. 64-bit or 128-bit.
   C. 256-bit or higher.
   D. 128-bit combined with password protection.

_____ 4. The probability distribution of words the speaker may use based on the speaker profile is _____
   A. an algorithm.
   B. FE-SRT.
   C. BE-SRT.
   D. a language profile.

_____ 5. CMS standards for an EHR technology in order for healthcare providers to qualify or financial incentives or avoid penalties are called _____
   A. clinical quality measures.
   B. clinical decision support.
   C. meaningful use.
   D. computerized provider order entry.

_____ 6. A system that keeps computer information safe by checking who the user is and checking that the information has not been changed is _____
   A. encryption.
   B. authentication.
   C. file transfer protocol.
   D. integrated transcription platform.

_____ 7. An Internet pipeline or entry point in which data is encrypted in both directions is called _____
   A. role-based limited access.
   B. secure web portal.
   C. virtual private network.
   D. integrated transcription platform.

_____ 8. One type of file extension for identifying digital voice or audio files is _____
   A. wma.
   B. jpg.
   C. png.
   D. docx.

_____ 9. Secure transfer of dictation via the Internet to remote transcriptionists can be accomplished using _____
   A. FTP.
   B. SRT.
   C. BE-SRT.
   D. USB.

___10. Which statement is true?
A. SRT will replace MTs.
B. SRT turns voice into text.
C. SRT needs no editing.
D. SRT saves money and time.

___11. The government organization that has established standards and criteria for the certification of EHR technology is _____
A. CMS.
B. HIMSS.
C. ONC.
D. HHS.

___12. A process to ensure the protection of PHI during all its movements through an organization carried out by a team including individuals from information technology (IT), operations, transcription, etc., is _____
A. meaningful use.
B. computerized provider order entry.
C. dictation-transcription integration.
D. security risk analysis.

___13. A method for securing these files that renders them unusable, unreadable, or undecipherable to unauthorized individuals is _____
A. authentication.
B. encryption.
C. file transfer protocol.
D. role-based limited access.

___14. A complex password consists of _____
A. a combination of more than 8 characters, numbers, and symbols.
B. a combination of more than 16 characters, numbers, and symbols.
C. a combination of more than 32 characters, numbers, and symbols.
D. a code generated by a security token.

___15. Some medical transcription organizations provide computers to their remote workforce in order to _____
A. get a tax write-off.
B. ensure loyalty and retention.
C. mitigate their potential risks.
D. track the individual's use of the computer.

___16. A reasonable practice to ensure that the remote workforce is complying with security policies and procedures is to _____
A. administer a periodic written test on security P&Ps.
B. observe the MTs via a live camera while they are working.
C. require photographs of the MT's work space or home office.
D. make periodic home visits to inspect the MT's office.

___17. A common and serious breach of PHI occurs when _____
A. a patient's report is sent to the wrong fax number.
B. MTs allow their personal computers to be used by the rest of the family.
C. an MT sells medical information about a famous person to a tabloid.
D. MTs use the Internet for research purposes while transcribing.

___18. A tool that can improve typing speed and efficiency is _____
A. Microsoft Word.
B. abbreviation expansion software.
C. a personal MT notebook.
D. an ergonomic keyboard.

___19. Transcriptioinists who work at home should invest in all of the following EXCEPT _____
A. an ergonomic chair and desk.
B. up-to-date antivirus software.
C. a small refrigerator for the office.
D. surge protectors and uninterrupted power supply.

___20. An often overlooked tool for the student and the working transcriptionist is _____
A. the transcriptionist's notebook.
B. abbreviation expansion software.
C. antivirus software.
D. firewall protection.

Abbreviations

Instructions: Expand the following healthcare documentation technology abbreviations. You may not need to transcribe these abbreviations, but you do need to know what they mean because they are essential to understanding healthcare industry communications.

1. BE-SRT _____

2. CAH _____

3. CMS _____

4. CPOE _____

5. CQMs _____

6. EHR _____

7. FE-SRT _____

8. FTP _____

9. HHS _____

10. HIMSS _____

11. ONC _____

12. SRE _____

13. SRT _____

14. TAT _____

Medical Transcription Practices

4

Learning Objectives

▶ Describe the auditory discrimination and editorial activities that take place in the dictation-transcription process.

▶ Select, evaluate, and use print and electronic references for healthcare documentation.

▶ Identify Internet resources and evaluate them for usefulness in healthcare documentation.

▶ Use efficient search strategies for finding useful and accurate information on the Internet.

▶ Identify and use proofreading and editing strategies in traditional and speech editing.

▶ Explain the transcriptionist's or speech editor's role in risk management.

▶ Identify and apply productivity strategies without jeopardizing quality.

Medical Transcription Practices

Introduction

This chapter explores a variety of best practices in medical transcription. These practices relate to the interpretation, deciphering, editing, proofreading, and productivity techniques that you will apply to your transcription practice in the medical specialty chapters and, to an even greater extent, to your work after you complete your program. Much of the content of this chapter will have greater meaning and impact once you begin the specialty chapters.

You will want to refer to this chapter again and again as you proceed through the program. If you are using a print version of the textbook, we suggest that you use Post-It "flags" or Post-It notes to mark sections to which you may want to return. If you are using an electronic version of this textbook, bookmark important sections.

There are certain interpretation and deciphering techniques that are required in order to transcribe an accurate and complete report that conveys what the dictator meant as opposed to what the dictator said. Both auditory and intellectual discrimination skills must be developed, and in order to do that, one must understand what interpretation of the spoken word entails.

"Dictation and Transcription: Adventures in Thought Transference" is aptly named. Read it carefully. Understanding all the factors that impact "thought transference" is the basis for developing the critical thinking skills necessary for success in healthcare documentation. In fact, this chapter, and this article in particular, may be the most valuable chapter in this textbook to help you develop the ability to analyze and understand the disembodied sounds of dictation and turn them into meaningful text.

As you read Dr. Dirckx's essay, reflect on how the pronunciation issues and other conscious and unconscious editing processes he discusses can impact your transcription practice and the importance of being focused on the meaning of what you are transcribing. Return to this article and re-read it periodically throughout the remainder of this course. Each time you re-read it, you will find that you will have a greater understanding of the thought transference process.

This chapter also includes guidance on developing research skills using reference books and the Internet.

Being able to translate the sounds you hear phonetically is an important component of being a good researcher, and learning which resource to use will save you time and minimize frustration.

You'll also learn the basics of editing traditional transcription and speech editing, proofreading, and specific transcribing techniques. Soon, you'll be on your way to becoming a great medical transcriptionist.

Professional Readings

Dictation and Transcription: Adventures in Thought Transference

by John H. Dirckx, MD

> The pronunciation is the actual living form or forms of a word, that is, the word itself, of which the current spelling is only a current symbolization.
> . . .
>
> General Explanations,
The Oxford English Dictionary

Every time I read this passage, I am struck anew by the realization that the sequences of letters we put down on paper are not words, but only visible representations of those evanescent sequences of vocal sound that are the only true words. When we speak of "the written word," we are indulging in metaphor: words are heard but not seen. Indeed, most of the world's 3,000 languages are exclusively spoken languages having no writing systems.

I offer these reflections to introduce an inquiry into the nature of the **dictation-transcription process**, a form of communication unique among human activities. The dictator expresses thoughts in speech (which is electronically recorded) and the transcriptionist puts those thoughts on paper by converting sounds heard to conventional symbols.

The product of the transcriptionist's effort is not, however, a mere phonetic record of what is heard but rather a rendering of the dictator's thoughts in finished English prose. That is, instead of making a perfectly faithful record of speech sounds heard, the transcriptionist performs various analytic and interpretive functions and modifies the record by a complex series of deletions, additions, alterations, and adaptations. Moreover, this editorial activity is performed simultaneously at several levels: *phonetic* (recognition and interpretation of speech sounds and their correct representation in writing), *conceptual* (monitoring of word choice, grammar, and style), and *formal* (punctuation, consistency of form, appropriate units of measure).

Even at what I have called the phonetic level, the transcriptionist constantly discriminates and adjusts on the basis of context, so that even here there is nothing mechanical or automatic about the transcription process.

Silent letters may not be the most difficult feature of English spelling, but they are surely the most paradoxic. For a phonetic writing system to include symbols that are essential to the spelling of certain words, and that nevertheless represent no sounds heard in those words, is a palpable absurdity. Yet there is hardly a letter in our alphabet that does not figure in the spelling of some word without being represented in its pronunciation.

Suffice it to say that the relation between speech sounds and the symbols that convention requires us to use to represent them is erratic, almost haphazard. That is why the transcriptionist cannot simply match a symbol to a sound heard, as in making a stenographic (shorthand) record, where, for example, *f*, *ph*, and *gh* (in *enough*) are all represented by the same symbol, while the *b*'s of *doubt* and *subtle* are not represented at all.

The same, only different. A frequent source of difficulty in transcription is the existence of homonyms or, more precisely, of homophones. **Homonyms** are two or more words that are spelled and pronounced the same but differ in meaning—for example, mole "small mammal"; mole "pigmented nevus"; mole "uterine neoplasm"; mole "breakwater"; mole "unit of measure based on molecular weight."

Strictly speaking, a set like this should cause no trouble, because even if the transcriptionist should mistake the meaning, the spelling would be the same.

Similarly, **homographs** (words spelled the same but pronounced differently) should create no ambiguity in dictation. A special kind of homograph results from variation in placement of syllable stress: *tínnitus-tinnítus, ángina-angína, fácet-facét*. The American transcriptionist may sometimes be startled by a British dictator's placement of stress in such words as *cervícal, éphedrine, labóratory*, and *skelétal*.

But it is **homophones** that demand alertness and judgment—words that sound the same but are spelled differently. Sometimes the difference is plain from the context ("I guessed he was a guest when he discussed his disgust") and sometimes it is not ("Dr. Templeton is losing his patience/patients"). Many homophone pairs

are created by our custom of reducing unaccented vowels to a neutral "uh" sound. We hear this sound, for example, in the second syllables of both *callus* and *callous, mucus* and *mucous, villus* and *villous*. Only the context tells the transcriptionist whether to type the noun form in *-us* or the adjective form in *-ous*. In the same way, *instillation* may be indistinguishable from *installation, perineal* from *peroneal, have* from *of*.

Styles of pronunciation that are characteristic of certain regional or ethnic dialects may create homophones in the dictation of some speakers. One person may fail to distinguish between *finally* and *finely*, another between *then* and *than*, a third between *his* and *he's*, a fourth between *long* and *lung*. The practice of dropping final *l* or *r* or both can erase the differences between such pairs as *sulfa/sulfur* and *femoral-popliteal/femoropopliteal*, and place the transcriptionist in peril of creating such monstrosities as *musculo-dystrophy* and *normal tensive*.

In my part of the country, a sizable segment of the populace practices *itacism*. This term, originally denoting an analogous dialectal variation in Greek, refers to a raising of the short *e* sound in a tonic (stressed) syllable so that it sounds like short *i*. Thus, for example, *attend, get, men*, and *shelter* are pronounced as if they were spelled *attind, git, min*, and *shilter*.

Although this causes little or no inconvenience in the examples I have used, the wholesale disappearance of tonic short *e* does create some ambiguities that must be averted by further modifications of the language. For instance, persons who pronounce *pen* exactly like *pin* customarily distinguish the former word by saying *inkpen* (pronounced "inkpin"). (Less than a week after making notes for the above paragraph, I saw in a local antique shop a box of old fountain pens labeled "Inkpins $1.00.")

Homophony is not confined to pairs of words. A phrase may sound almost exactly like another phrase of entirely different, even opposite meaning. Two notorious examples—*had no carcinoma* for *adenocarcinoma* and *prepped and raped* for *prepped and draped*—have passed into legend. Whole books of such blunders, many of them no doubt spurious, have been published. A frequent source of difficulty is the unaccented *a* at the beginning of words: *atonic bladder* vs. *a tonic bladder, a symmetric swelling* vs. *asymmetric swelling*.

Besides discriminating between homophones, the transcriptionist performs a variety of what might be called normalizing operations, that is, recognizing variant pronunciations and reducing them to their conven-

---

MISHEARS

"Mishears" are not always individual words. They can be adjacent words heard as a single word or breaking adjacent sounds in the wrong places.

Mishears can be entire phrases. For example, one student, in the hospital course section of a clinical resumé, began a sentence with "Early postop" (editing what she heard as "postop early" when "postoperatively" was dictated). At the end of the report when the patient was being discharged, she put "denied experiencing complications" for "did not experience any complications." The student was a former nurse and usually someone who exhibited excellent critical thinking skills. She apparently was either distracted or just not "in the zone," a term MTs use when they're focused in on content and meaning.

I gave the student my usual feedback (analyze the similarities and differences between what was said and what you heard. Try to figure out not only why you misheard it but how you might avoid such situations in the future).

As another example, once when I was working as an independent contractor, keeping long odd hours due to volume of work and delivery and pickup schedules, I was transcribing around 4 a.m. and very tired. I transcribed "The patient's 24-hour eyes and nose were monitored" when what was dictated was "The patient's 24-hour I's and O's (for intakes and outputs) were monitored." Fortunately, the error was caught before the report went to the client.

Ellen Drake

---

tional forms before putting them on paper. The range of such deviations is enormous. Some result from congenital or acquired speech impediments such as tongue-tie or obstruction of the nasal passages by hypertrophic adenoids or chronic allergic rhinitis. Some are due to dialectal variations (a few of which I have already mentioned) or to speech habits learned in childhood, such as substituting a glottal catch (momentary closure of the vocal cords) for *t* at the end of a syllable.

A large number of deviant pronunciations arise from the structure of the human vocal apparatus and the difficulty or awkwardness of producing certain sound sequences. The omission of the first *d* sound in *Wednesday* and the rearrangement of sounds in *comfortable* (="comftorble") are examples of such changes. In rapid speech, *cysts* and *tests* often come out "cyss" and "tess." We also tend to insert extraneous sounds into our speech to smooth certain transitions. Some of these inserted sounds are virtually standard (*compfort, intsulin*), some are dialectal (*hematoma-r of the rectus sheath, mower* [=more]), and some are decidedly substandard (*athaletic, drownding*).

Frank mispronunciations include both the mishandling of English phonetics by non-native speakers and isolated errors (most of them acquired by imitation) such as *phalynx, larnyx, ishium,* and *meninjocele.* Here may also be mentioned certain recurring deviations from correct pronunciation that have been adopted as an affectation by certain speakers. Among these are the bizarre plurals *abscesses, processes,* and other words pronounced to rhyme with *neuroses,* and the compulsive gallicization of words having no connection with French (*centimeter, centrifuge, difficile,* and *mitrale*).

To recapitulate, in turning a phonetic (speech) record into a written one, the transcriptionist inserts "silent" letters, suppresses extraneous sounds (including "uh"), selects the correct one of several alternative spellings, and recognizes deviant pronunciations—all in the light of a sustained monitoring of the context and a thorough understanding of medicine, medical terminology, dictating conventions, and human frailty.

In other words. Although nearly everyone takes it for granted that the kinds of editing I have been discussing thus far are part of the transcription process, many question the propriety of the transcriptionist's judging and altering the factual content of a dictation, correcting the dictator's grammar and syntax, and touching up the style to improve clarity and coherence. Yet such adjustments are manifestly necessary, not only in dictation by non-native speakers of English but in the vast majority of all dictations.

By choosing to dictate a document rather than write it out, the dictator not only sidesteps many of the mechanical tasks associated with composition but implicitly delegates these tasks to the transcriptionist. No dictators have such perfect powers of concentration that they never accidentally repeat themselves, never inadvertently substitute one word for another, never leave a sentence unfinished. Sooner or later the most alert and cautious dictator makes each of these mistakes, and others besides. Clearly these normal human lapses ought not to be reproduced in the transcript, and just as clearly the duty of identifying and correcting them devolves on the transcriptionist.

Just as mispronounced words and names must be spelled correctly by the transcriptionist, erroneous spellings supplied by the dictator must be ignored.

When the intrusive word sounds something like the right one, it is called a *malapropism* (after Mrs. Malaprop, a character in an eighteenth-century comedy by Sheridan). Some malapropisms evidently result from momentary lapses: *pericardial infusion* (for *effusion*). Others are permanent features of the dictator's vocabulary, as was the case with Mrs. Malaprop: *melanotic* (for *melenic*) *stools*; *with regards* (for *regard*) *to*.

One of the medical transcriptionist's greatest challenges is dealing correctly with **slang terms** used by dictators. These terms vary in propriety; some may be left in the record while others must be replaced with more formal terminology. The transcriptionist must therefore not only distinguish the acceptable from the inappropriate but also understand the latter and be able to supply suitable alternatives.

Among the few vestiges of grammatical inflection in modern English are changes in the form of nouns and verbs to signify whether they are **singular or plural**: *one stitch, two stitches*; *he stitches, they stitch*. Not surprisingly, most of the purely grammatical errors committed by dictators are faults of subject-verb agreement. Such errors are common in everyday speech and even writing. As the mind constructs a sentence phrase by phrase, grammatical forms are apt to be selected on the basis of ideas rather than of words. Often a singular noun is used when the speaker is actually "thinking plural" and goes on to use a plural verb: "The right and left lung (lungs) are congested." "No definite site of his occult GI bleeding were (was) identified."

A permanent medical document dictated by one professional and transcribed by another is expected to conform to certain norms of precision, clarity, coherence, and taste. Where the dictator's competence or diligence falls short, the transcriptionist must supply the deficiency. Again the task requires a broad base of knowledge about the subject of the dictation and considerable skill in composition and editing. Most transcriptionists perform this operation so deftly and unobtrusively that the majority of dictators never even suspect that their dictation has undergone revision (or that it needed it).

A matter of form. The third level at which the transcriptionist exercises a discriminating and editorial function is that of **format or layout**, including punctuation and consistency in the use of abbreviations, numerals, and units of measure. In general the transcriptionist's decisions on these points are unrelated to anything heard in the dictation. It is true that dictators often supply directions for formatting and punctuation, but many of these (such as calling each new line a "paragraph" or separating complete sentences with a "comma") must simply be ignored by the transcriptionist. Other directions, while not actually incorrect, may violate the canons of English composition or introduce inconsistencies.

Armed with basic keyboarding skills and a knowledge of the rules of punctuation, the transcriptionist creates the format of a report and supplies commas and periods as needed in the very act of transcribing the dictation. Numerals and units of measure are typed according to established conventions and in consistent fashion regardless of how they occur in the dictation. Thus "six tenths" becomes 0.6 and "four and a half milliliters" becomes 4.5 *mL*.

No one can master the lore of a craft so perfectly as never to be at a loss for a word, a meaning, a rule, a spelling. A crucial requirement for the practice of most professions is knowing where to look up what one doesn't remember or can't understand. The medical transcriptionist depends heavily on dictionaries, drug references, word books, and personal files or notebooks to supply authoritative answers to questions raised by the dictation.

While it is all too easy for transcriptionists and dictators alike to take it for granted that transcription is "writing down what somebody said," it should be evident from my remarks that it is only by penetrating and sharing the dictator's thoughts that the transcriptionist can produce an accurate and otherwise fully satisfactory transcript.

Fuller awareness of the breadth, intricacy, and difficulty of medical transcription should heighten the respect of dictators and others outside the profession for those who practice it. Transcriptionists themselves can be proud of their hard-won and socially valuable competence in a field demanding both technical and intellectual virtuosity.

Pause for Reflection

1. Reflect on the statement, "The product of the transcriptionist's effort is not, however, a mere phonetic record of what is heard but rather a rendering of the dictator's thoughts in finished English prose." What does a transcriptionist do?

2. Describe the three levels of editorial activity in the dictation-transcription process that the transcriptionist performs.

3. Reflect on the statement, "...the relation between speech sounds and the symbols that convention requires us to use to represent them is erratic, almost haphazard." List several areas in which the phonetic representation of a word may cause problems for the MT.

4. Do you think Dr. Dirckx supports a transcriptionist judging and altering the factual content of a dictation, correcting the dictator's grammar and syntax, and touching up the style to improve clarity and coherence? Justify your answer.

5. What other editing processes discussed by Dr. Dirckx take place in the dictation-transcription process?

Basic Research Skills

by Ellen Drake

Medical transcriptionists are known for their love of words and their use of medical references. Today, unlike 15–20 years ago, there are many excellent references (both printed and electronic) available for the medical transcriptionist—medical dictionaries, medical specialty word and phrase references, medical abbreviation references, and medical style manuals. No medical transcription practitioner or student should be without up-to-date reference sources.

Each type of reference fills a particular need. A **medical dictionary** confirms correct spellings and provides definitions to help the medical transcriptionist differentiate between similar-sounding words; however, it does not contain many specialty words, abbreviations, and surgical instruments. Medical **specialty word and phrase references** contain terms from one medical specialty or a group of related specialties and include slang, surgical instruments, drugs, new and unusual terms, abbreviations, and laboratory tests for particular specialties.

These types of references are also called **spellers** or simply **word books** because they do not contain definitions. *Their usefulness for students and inexperienced transcriptionists is limited.* If you use them to find the spelling of an unfamiliar word, be sure to look up the word in a dictionary or electronic reference and make sure that the meaning fits the context before using the term. **Medical abbreviation references** contain common and unusual abbreviations and their expansions from all medical specialties. **Medical style manuals** give suggestions on how to handle questions of format, punctuation, grammar, spelling, and style in medical reports.

Your reference shelf. A basic library should include a full-sized medical dictionary, an English dictionary, a current drug reference that includes indications and dosages, laboratory and diagnostic studies reference books, and an abbreviation book. Specialty and surgical word and phrase books can be added as necessary.

Electronic spell-checking programs, if sufficiently extensive and specialized, can help avoid misspellings of both technical and nontechnical words but cannot distinguish between **homophones** (*discreet/discrete, their/there*) or identify a correctly spelled but incorrectly used word. If allowed to use spell-checkers, students should use them only as a last step in the proofreading and editing process.

As a rule, we recommend that students not use spell-checking programs while they are training. It's important to look up words in references as you transcribe, and then to proofread carefully after completing each report.

Not all unfamiliar dictated words are medical. It is important to remember that many physicians have extensive vocabularies and may dictate English words that are new to the transcriptionist. Thus, an English dictionary is an essential reference.

Evaluating reference books. Learn to evaluate reference books for quality and appropriateness by examining the contents. For example, are words extracted from a preexisting large database (unauthored books) or researched and compiled by experienced transcriptionists? The former types of books may not include as many phrases and cross-referencing as the latter. Some unauthored books are, however, reviewed by a team of practicing MTs, and these would be preferable to those with no MT input.

Check the **copyright date**. This is important in references where the terminology changes rapidly, especially drug and surgery references. Who are the authors, editors, contributors, and what are their credentials? Is the publisher known for publishing quality references, and does it have a special division for medical transcription? What are the organizational features of the book? Is it user-friendly?

Become completely familiar with the **front matter** of every reference you use or acquire. Pay special attention to any instructions on how to use the book. Do you know the meanings of standard reference terms such as *see* and *see also*, *q.v.* (which see) and *cf.* (compare)? Check the table of contents, appendices, indexes, and other features of each reference book. These features, too, can help you evaluate whether the reference book you are using is a good one or not.

A word about drug references. Drug reference books are an important resource for medical transcriptionists. It is critical that medical transcriptionists be familiar with drugs, their indications and dosages, and how to research new or unusual drug names in drug reference books. If a reference book cannot provide the answer to a drug question, the medical transcriptionist may even seek help from a pharmacist.

Medical transcriptionists typically use several types of drug references frequently. Some contain short lists of drugs in alphabetical order, while others are much more comprehensive. The experienced medical transcriptionist has at least two types of drug references available: a quick-reference A to Z drug book, and a comprehensive book that gives **indications** and **dosages**. Most drug references in print or on the Internet do not follow the recommended capitalization or style for healthcare documentation. They will put all drug names in all caps or they may show both generic and brand name drugs with an initial capital letter. It is important that the MT be able to distinguish between generic and trade names in order to apply appropriate style.

Pharmaceutical companies use three different names to describe a drug: the **chemical name** (which is a complicated formula describing the drug's molecular structure), the **generic name** (a shorter name assigned to the drug chemical), and the **trade** or **brand name** (the copyrighted name selected by the pharmaceutical company).

The brand name is easy to pronounce, may indicate what the drug is used for or how often it is taken, and is selected for its appeal to prescribing physicians. A generic drug may have several trade names copyrighted by different manufacturers. Generic drug names are always written in lowercase letters, while trade name drugs have an initial capital letter. Some trade name drugs also have internal capitalization (such as pHisoHex), although in most instances it is acceptable to type such words with initial capitalization only (Phisohex).

A word of caution. Many word and phrase books include both the nonpreferred and the preferred spelling of a term. Often the nonpreferred spelling comes first alphabetically. Never choose a word from a speller unless you are sure of the meaning and that you have the preferred spelling. Similarly, identify and translate abbreviations correctly. *You must consider context.* If you cannot be sure of the translation of an abbreviation, draw a blank line and put the abbreviation in parentheses.

When you look up a term, don't just check the spelling and type or paste it into your document. There are way too many soundalikes in medical language. Check the definition to make sure you have chosen the correct term. Never put a word whose meaning you do not know into a report. Learn to identify and take the time to read the etymology (origin) of a word. Often this will help you create a mnemonic for remembering it.

When word searching, do not guess at a word just to fill in a blank. A blank does not reflect poorly on the medical transcriptionist who has thoroughly researched the question. Leaving a blank is the correct thing to do when all reference books and other sources have been exhausted. Remember, the integrity and accuracy of the medical record is far more important than never leaving a blank. The latter is not a realistic goal, even for experienced medical transcriptionists.

In class or at work, learn to use even the references you're not fond of. You may be stuck sometime and that may be all you have.

The following suggestions will help you develop research skills that will serve you well as a student and on the job. These suggestions focus on spelling and locating terms as well as on selecting and evaluating reference books.

Honing your research skills. You need to understand phonics and know which sounds are represented by which letters or combinations of letters. Most medical and English dictionaries have guidelines for pronunciation but that's not enough. You need to know that every vowel can sound like almost every other vowel. Consonant sounds fall into groups of letters that are formed in different ways, depending on the way the letters are formed in the mouth. For example, *b*, *d*, *p*, and *t* can be difficult to distinguish from one another as can *b* and *v* or *s* and *f*. *X* is pronounced like a *z* at the beginning of a word (*xiphoid*). How many letters or combinations of letters can you think of that make a *k* sound? Which ones can make an *s* sound?

Remember that a fair number of words contain silent letters (the final *e* on many words is silent) and may even begin with a silent letter. Examples of words with silent letters include *pneumonia, psychiatric, psyllium, ptosis* (all silent *p*); *mnemonic* (silent *m*); *phthisis* ("tysis"); *gnathodynia* (silent *g*); *rhinorrhagia* and *rhonchi* (silent *h*); *euphoria* (silent *e*), and *scybala* (silent *c* ["SI-ba-la"]).

When you find words with silent letters, especially at the beginning, you might write these words in the margins of the dictionary or appropriate word and phrase book at the place it would be located if it were spelled as you thought it was spelled (like "tosis" in the T's for the correct spelling *ptosis*). Be sure to write it correctly spelled, however! A final spelling stumbling block is doubled letters. Examples are *desiccate, parallel, diarrhea* (doubled *r* and a silent *h*).

Try to think of memory aids (mnemonic devices) to help you remember the spelling. In *parallel*, for example, the two *l*'s might remind you of parallel bars used in gymnastics. If you can't think of a mnemonic (speaking of silent letters—the *m* is silent), typing the word correctly 10, 20, or 50 times will help you learn the correct spelling.

Medical dictionaries rarely list every form of a word. You need to understand spelling rules well enough to be able to correctly add plural, noun, adjective, adverb, and sometimes verb endings when only one form of a word can be found.

Learn to recognize and keep a list of **coined** (made-up) **words** (nouns turned into verbs and adjectives or vice versa), **slang terms**, and **brief forms**. Some coined words are acceptable if they follow the rules for forming words and there is no simple, ready substitute. For example, *coumadinize* has become a fairly standard term. Other coined words are not so acceptable. The footnotes in the transcript keys will help you identify which is which.

Slang usually consists of unacceptable brief forms such as syllables taken from the end of a longer word (*lytes* for *electrolytes*), brief forms that can have more than one meaning (*dig* for *digoxin* or *digitalis*), and syllables or letters taken from the middle of a longer word (*tic* for *diverticulum*). These words are not acceptable because they are either obscure, can have multiple meanings, or the brief form has been pulled from the middle or end of a longer term.

Learn to break sounds into appropriate syllables and words. Breaking the sound into syllables, writing the syllables phonetically, and analyzing by comparing to known word parts (prefixes, suffixes, and root words) can help. In your medical terminology course, pay particular attention to how these word parts are combined and which combining vowels are used, if any, to connect one part to another. There are no exact rules for putting two root words together, but often, in anatomy at least, root words are put together proximal to distal (*glenohumeral*), anterior to posterior (*anteroposterior*), or cephalad (top) to caudal (bottom) (*esophagogastroduodenoscopy*).

Medical dictionaries and most spellers do not supply the **part of speech** of a term. Learn to recognize parts of speech by word endings and clues in the definition. For example, a definition that begins with an article (**a, an**, or **the**) will be a noun. If the definition begins with *to*, it will be a verb. If it begins with **pertaining to** or **relating to**, it will be an adjective. Knowing which suffixes make a word a noun, an adjective or adverb, or a verb will also help in determining the correct spelling of a word and which part of speech fits the context.

Identify the **preferred spelling** when more than one spelling is given. When a term has an alternative spelling, it is customary to use the spelling accompanied by the definition. If both spellings are accompanied by definitions, either may be used. Some dictionaries, especially English dictionaries, may put two spellings separated by a comma as the main entry. In that case, the first spelling is preferred. So, if you look up a word and the definition says "See [another spelling]," the *see* spelling is the one you'd use. If there is a complete definition with both spellings, then usually either spelling is acceptable.

Learn to recognize what type of word you're looking for so that you will know which reference book to use first. Context will help you determine whether the word is a drug, a surgical instrument, a laboratory test, or x-ray procedure, etc. While all specialties can be touched upon in a single history and physical examination, contextual clues (including format headings) should help you determine which specialty word book to choose for symptoms and diseases.

Learn to distinguish among trade (brand), generic, and chemical names of drugs, and also to distinguish between drug names and drug classes. This will save time if your main drug reference is the *Physicians' Desk Reference (PDR)*. Memorize the spellings of the 200 most-prescribed drugs and their indications. A list can be found on the Internet. This will save you hours of research time.

Find lists of the most commonly misspelled English and medical words and memorize the spellings and definitions. Study lists of English and medical homophones (soundalikes) and know which to use when.

Distinguish between Latin and English anatomical terms. English adjectives precede the noun, but in Latin the noun comes first. This is important because when you look up a phrase, you want to look up the noun first. For example, to find *bullous emphysema*, look under *emphysema* (the noun), *not* bullous. To find *Parkinson disease*, look under *disease*. The adjectives will be subentries below the noun.

In Latin phrases, the noun is followed by the adjective: *tensor fasciae latae, ligamentum flavum*. Look under the first word. Another exception is bacterial names: the genus is given first, followed by the species: *Clostridium difficile, Neisseria gonorrhoeae*. Look under the genus to find the species.

If you are looking for the name of a muscle, look under both *musculus* and *muscle*. Other Latin/English entries include *ligamentum* and *ligament, fissura* and *fissure, arteria* and *artery*.

Learn the **synonyms** for main entries. For example, a doctor might dictate a disease, but you cannot find the term under *disease* in the dictionary; try *syndrome*. *Test* and *sign* are often interchangeable, as are *sign* and *reflex*. *Procedure* and *operation* may be interchanged. *Tendons* and *ligaments* may be named for the bones or muscles to which they are attached.

Learn Latin/English equivalents too: *bone* and *os, muscle* and *musculus, nerve* and *nervus*. Sometimes English and Latin are mixed as in the *rectus abdominis muscle*. *Abdominis* doesn't sound like an English word, so you can assume it's Latin and look under *musculus* to find the correct spelling.

Learn the uses and limitations of the Internet. If you cannot find a term or phrase after consulting the appropriate reference books, a Google (or other search engine) search may be the next best choice. Know that there is no such thing as style on the Internet. Words are capitalized, hyphenated, closed, or open without regard to correctness. Misspellings are rampant. The Internet is lawless. It can be a remarkable research tool and resource, but it's not infallible. Books aren't either, but at least they've been edited and proofread in an attempt to make them as accurate as possible. It's a good idea, once you find a term you've been searching for on the Internet, to see if you can now find it in an appropriate reference.

Pause for Reflection

1. Discuss the types of references that should be included in the MT's reference library and the use of each.
2. What should the transcriptionist consider in evaluating medical reference books?
3. What are the disadvantages of spell-checking software?
4. Discuss the suggestions provided for improving your research and word deciphering skills.

Searching the "Wild, Wild Web"
by Ellen Drake and Georgia Green

Research is the lifeblood of what we do. To meet the demands of our profession, we must educate ourselves on the job throughout our careers. We learn by doing research, and in a perfect world, we would be free to research as much as we felt was necessary. But the reality of the production environment intrudes on our perfect world: we must find the information we need quickly, with as little effort as possible. We must be efficient researchers.

The Right Tool for the Job. The books in your library may be updated only every few years and may not have all the information you need. There isn't always one best tool for every circumstance, but you can narrow your choices to the ones most likely to yield results. Where do you go when your books let you down?

To the Internet: The "Wild, Wild Web"! Yes, filled as it is with inaccurate and questionable content, the Internet can be a useful tool—if you know its limitations, how to evaluate your sources, and how to use it efficiently. Note the translation of **www**—it's only half in jest, as you will see in a moment.

In 1998 the first Google index already had 26 million pages; by 2000 it had reached the one billion mark. Last year Google hit a milestone: 1 trillion unique URLs on the Web at once! Add in duplicates and related links, and the count is over 8 trillion. It's hard to really understand that number, but if you clicked on a new link every second of every day around the clock for a lifetime of 80 years, you might come close to surfing the entire Web.

Don't get us wrong. The Internet can be a great resource if you know how to evaluate the content and use it efficiently. But let's face it, many MTs think the Internet is a wonderful, free resource that means they no longer need any reference books. How cheap is the Internet, though, if it sucks up productive time? And in a production environment, time is money—right? And if you fail to evaluate your source and plug in a wrong word, you can have a far bigger problem than just loss of productivity.

Efficiency in research impacts productivity more than how well you use your expander, word processor, or anything else! It's probably pretty obvious that the single largest factor that inhibits your productivity as an MT is when you take your hands off the keyboard—to use your mouse or to pick up a reference.

Evaluating the Web. There is a famous Steiner cartoon published in the *New Yorker* (July 5, 1993) with two dogs sitting before a terminal looking at a computer screen; one says to the other, "On the Internet, nobody knows you're a dog." In a similar vein, Andrew Keen wrote a book called *The Cult of the Amateur: How Today's Internet is Killing Our Culture* (2007). The Internet has opened up the world to millions of people. It has given them a voice, a way to connect with others who think like them (or don't), and it has made available a wealth of information and misinformation. There are some real "dogs" out there, but there's also great treasure.

What does this teach us? *Discernment is critical.* Books can have errors and be inconsistent, but books are generally proofread and edited. Their errors should be fewer and more minor. Medical journals are peer-reviewed. There is no editing or peer review for most of what you'll find on the Internet. It's important to be able to research more than just spelling.

Being forewarned is forearmed. Knowing the limitations of the Internet will make you a more informed user of all that's good about it. Performing a Google search or using any search engine is somewhat like eating Bertie Bott's Every Flavor Beans. You may get what you want—but you're just as likely to get what you don't want. That is, *unless* you know what you're doing when you research. To put it another way, using and citing information found over the Internet is a little like swimming without a lifeguard. You shouldn't do it unless you're a really good swimmer.

There is an extremely wide variety of material on the Internet, ranging in its accuracy, reliability, and value. Unlike most traditional information media (books, magazines, organizational documents), no one has to approve the content before it is made public. It's your job as a researcher, then, to evaluate what you locate, in order to determine whether it suits your needs. In evaluating information on the Internet, it is important to take into account the following factors.

- Authority: What are the credentials of the person(s) providing the information?
- Affiliation: Who is the sponsor? What is its agenda?
- Currency: How current is the information? When was the site last updated? Copyright date on a Web page is not relevant.
- Purpose: Is the information provided for entertainment or education?
- Audience: Is it prepared for patients or clinicians?
- Accuracy: Does information on the site contradict itself or other sites? Is the site well-developed, free of typos and English usage errors? And, finally . . .
- Verifiability: Is there a bibliography or are there other resources provided? Where did the provider get its information?

Rather than take up a lot of space going into detail about how to evaluate Web resources, we will instead point you to a couple of excellent resources that will take you through the process quickly and easily. The first is Georgia Green's article, "Critical Literacy," which goes into detail about how to evaluate the integrity of a website (**http://www.hpisum.com/Downloads.aspx**).

Another is "Evaluating Web Pages: Techniques to Apply & Questions to Ask" from the UC Berkeley—Teaching Library Internet Workshops (**http://www.lib.berkeley.edu/TeachingLib/Guides/Internet/Evaluate.html**).

To summarize, information exists on many levels of quality and reliability. You may have heard that "knowledge is power, " or that information—the raw material of knowledge—is power. But the truth is that only some information is power: reliable information. The determination of information quality is something of an art. That is, there is no single perfect indicator.

Register as a professional. When a website requires that you register in order to access more detailed information, always register as a professional. You don't have to register as a doctor. You can usually register under "other health professionals" or "medical student." You may want to set up a separate e-mail account through Google mail (gmail), Yahoo, etc., to use exclusively for registering on websites.

Internet research techniques. Choosing a search engine is akin to knowing which book to use when. Different search engines are appropriate for different tasks. Google is currently the most popular search engine, and to its credit, it generally lists the most worthwhile pages near the top of its search results—but not always. Google searches blog posts, wiki pages, group discussion threads, and various document formats that are not Web pages per se (e.g., PDFs, Word or Excel documents, PowerPoints). Most of these resources, with the exception perhaps of PDFs which are often journal articles or pure research, are not the sources you want to use for reliable information.

To avoid unwanted websites, you can use the Advanced Search feature or simply follow your search phrase with any unwanted page type preceded by a minus sign or hyphen, e.g., -blog, -forum, .ppt, -wiki, -xls. If you use more than one operator, you do not need to separate them with commas as we have here.

Other useful Google searches include Image search. An Image search brings up photos, drawings, graphics—helpful if you need to see where the navicular bone is, for example. You can avoid certain types of results (like blog posts, wiki pages, and discussion threads) by using Google's Scholar search. These specialized Google searches will help you not only to limit your searches but also to qualify their reliability and accuracy.

There are other search engines. **Ask.com** is trying hard to compete with Google by giving you a pop-up preview of the page(s) cited before you actually click on the link. You can also Google "most popular search engines" and see what features each touts and which one appeals to you. **Scirus** is a scientific search engine and **Intute** has a health and life sciences specialized search; it's based in the UK, so watch for British spellings.

Research is not one of those skills that just come naturally. Even if you are very familiar with an English dictionary and a variety of nonmedical electronic references, there are some differences in using medical references that must be learned. This is even more true for medical information on the Internet. It's like searching

for that elusive needle in a haystack. You can't begin to evaluate the integrity of information, however, until you are dealing with a manageable amount of information. You can avoid this problem by learning to use a search engine judiciously.

Customize: You can customize your preferences and save them, so that, for example, only Web pages in English are searched, and when you click on a link, it always opens in a new window or tab.

To maximize your search, you should learn how to construct an advanced search using Boolean logic. **Boolean** refers to a system that combines key words and certain "operators" (**connecting terms**) that show relationships between your keywords, enabling you to search a large database (which is what the Internet is) quickly. When multiple terms are entered for a search using no Boolean operators, a default operation takes place. Whether results include documents with all the words or any of the words in a search string depends on the search engine's default settings. The search engine's "help" feature or FAQs pages will tell you what the defaults are and teach you how to construct effective searches. You can use the search engine to find out how to construct a Boolean search as well.

Specific searching tips. Google is a good search engine to use when you don't have enough information to construct a more specific search or when you're not sure how to spell a term. For example, an MT heard "senopalatine block." Putting that string into the Google search box resulted in Google asking, "Did you mean: 'sphenopalatine block'?"

Truncation is not available on Google but sometimes happens by accident and is worth trying. An MT heard "___gada syndrome" and Google came up with a page that contained Brugada syndrome. What happened here is that the text on the Web page broke *Bru-gada* at the end of a line. It's a long shot, but it sometimes works.

Google Scholar provides a simple way to broadly search for scholarly literature. From one place, you can search across many disciplines and sources: peer-reviewed papers, theses, books, abstracts and articles, from academic publishers, professional societies, preprint repositories, universities and other scholarly organizations. It's still a better place to search than regular Google in some ways. You can eliminate a lot of irrelevant hits if, for example, what you're searching for is an eponym, like *Brugada*. You won't retrieve geneal-

ADVANTAGES OF THE INTERNET

It's cheaper than buying a library of word books.

It can be faster than looking through books.

Information can be more up-to-date.

It's electronic, so you can copy and paste.

It's accessible from almost anywhere.

And man, there's a lot of information there.

LIMITATIONS OF THE INTERNET

It can be slower.

It's contradictory.

It can be a big distraction.

It's unedited and unreviewed.

It takes a lot more discernment.

Information can be outdated and irrelevant.

And man, there's a lot of information there.

THE BIGGEST DISADVANTAGE OF ALL IS . . .

You lose the chance for serendipity. That is, you lose the ability to browse and learn other words and related concepts to the term you're looking for. Many MTs can't look up a word in a dictionary without devouring the other entries on the page and then end up moving from page to page, looking up other terms. Sometimes, when you're searching for a difficult spelling, browsing is the only way to find it.

Of course, you can also find interesting rabbits to chase on the Internet; it's just that more often than not, those rabbits adversely affect your productivity and don't improve your knowledge for job-related tasks.

ogy, political, community news, obituaries, and business sites that may also carry the eponym. But Google Scholar doesn't take the place of **PubMed** because it isn't medicine specific.

You can also use Google to search for a missing word in a phrase by entering several key words surrounding the missing term into the Google search box. For example, suppose you couldn't hear the word "upstroke" in the following sentence, "Neck exam reveals no jugular venous distention, normal carotid upstroke, no carotid bruits." Entering the sentence without the missing word and no quotation marks can bring up a sentence containing the missing word. You have to play around with this type of search. Sometimes, the more key words you use, the better. Other times, the fewer key terms yields better results. Many search engines automatically provide suggestions for completing your search phrase as you type it in. Often, these provided suggestions will give you the word or phrase you're looking for. If auto-completion is not on by default, it may be a choice in settings.

Caveat: There are lots of sample medical reports on the Internet; don't assume that what you find is necessarily correctly spelled.

OneLook.com. OneLook is an online search engine that, as of this writing, indexes 13,549,061 words in 1009 dictionaries. You can set preferences for the results in OneLook by clicking on Customize. The customizing features are powerful: you can choose whether you want the results displayed as verbose or compact; set the category for the type of dictionaries you want to be displayed first to medicine rather than English; tell it whether to display results in the same window, another window or a separate frame; and choose to have results include single words or words and phrases, among other preferences. Often the definition for the term you need is displayed on the results page, and you need look no further.

OneLook has a very robust wild card search feature that is clearly explained on the home page. You can also search a number of medical dictionaries and glossaries including *Dorland's* and *Stedman's*. With its wild card feature, it's an invaluable resource. And, like Google, if you spell a term incorrectly, it will suggest an alternative spelling.

Caveat. If you are searching for a term and only a few obscure dictionaries come up in the results, you should question what you are hearing and the results of the search. OneLook is not useful for researching drugs or surgical instruments.

Books: Who needs 'em? We hope your answer to this question is, "We do!" Let's not throw away our books just yet. You may prefer electronic references over paper and ink references, but either way there's still a place for books. But books are not always the best resource, as noted above. We hope this article has helped you make better choices about which resource to choose when and to be a more efficient and astute researcher when the Internet is your chosen resource.

Pause for Reflection

1. What does the discussion about the volume of information and the examples of errors on the Internet teach the user about the Internet's value for research?
2. List the factors one should take into account when evaluating the usability of information found on the Internet.
3. Discuss the concepts "knowledge is power" and "information is power."
4. What types of pages would you want to avoid or ignore that might come up in a typical Google search?
5. What should you do to maximize your search results?
6. How can the website **OneLook.com** be useful?

AN ATTORNEY'S PERSPECTIVE ON EDITING AND PROOFREADING

Editing and proofreading are necessary to good risk management. An attorney speaking at a medical transcription professional meeting wanted to emphasize how important quality transcription is. She held up a large posterboard with an excerpt from a medical report that contained a typo magnified in eight-inch letters and said, "When you make a mistake, this is what we make it look like in court."

Indeed, attorneys for the plaintiff in a suit make as big an issue as possible of anything that will make the defendant look bad. If typos can influence a jury in a malpractice or liability case, grammar errors, garbled sentences, and, most damaging of all, medical content errors should be avoided at all costs.

Proofreading Skills

by Ellen Drake

Proofreading in medical transcription is not the same as proofreading an essay or a research paper written for school or an article written for a professional publication. First, healthcare documentation style differs greatly from publication styles or the style you would use for an essay, thesis, or research paper. In addition, while grammar and punctuation are important for ease of communication, they take a back seat to accuracy of medical content and word choice.

On the job, most transcriptionists do not have the luxury of proofreading as a separate step from transcription; they proofread on-screen as they transcribe. It takes practice and considerable focus to read what you have just transcribed while you type what you just heard and are listening to the next few words or phrases that you are about to transcribe. Fortunately, as a student, you do not have to do it all at once.

As a student, you can and should spend more time researching, more time transcribing, and more time proofreading. Do you want to work on your speed? Of course! But in the beginning at least, take the time to perfect all the separate steps involved. As you gain knowledge and experience, you will find that your speed will increase and you'll be able to proofread and transcribe at the same time. Proofreading skills are also critically important for speech recognition editors. This is not a transcription practice that you want to treat lightly.

It may be helpful for you to print out your reports for proofreading at first, but you will want to, at some point, start proofreading on-screen because that is what you will need to be able to do on the job. Similarly, it may be helpful to double-space for the purpose of proofreading and even to use a larger font size, for example 18- or 24-point. Errors really show up when they're enlarged. Even if you are permitted to use a spelling checker, do not spell-check your work before proofreading! Proofread first.

Take a break. You should put some time between transcribing and proofreading. It is very difficult to spot your errors when you have just finished transcribing a report. A good idea is to transcribe one day and proofread the next. If you do not have that luxury, you should wait at least one-half to one hour before proofreading. When you return to the report, you will have fresh eyes and will see what's really on the page, not what you expect to see.

Proofread slowly. Don't skim. Don't rush. You should put as much time into proofreading as you do transcribing, at least at first. Proofread at least four times. First, proofread without sound, read for meaning. Proofread a second time without sound, checking punctuation, grammar, capitalization, and formatting. Proofread by reading the report aloud. It is amazing the errors you can pick up when you read aloud. Finally, proofread with the audio, listening for each word but also listening again for meaning.

COMMON PROOFREADING ERRORS

Homophones/Soundalikes, both English and Medical
    to/two/too; there/their; peroneal/perineal; ilium/ileum
Omitted words or doubled words
    The patient was to rehab. The patient was sent to rehab.
Subject-verb agreement errors
    There was no rib fractures noted on PA and lateral chest x-ray.
Typos, inverted letters
    ehr; teh; recieved

Analyze your errors. In your MT notebook, create a section for errors. Make a note of both the types of errors you make (spelling, punctuation, capitalization, wrong words, soundalikes, etc.). Why did you make the error? What can you do to avoid making the same error in the future?

Spell-check if you are permitted to do so. Do not assume that the word suggested by the spelling checker is the correct word or the correct spelling or style. Look up all words, except obvious typos, that the spelling checker stops on. Watch out for soundalikes and keep context in mind at all times. Analyze the errors caught by your spelling checker. This will help you assess and improve your proofreading skills. Again, why did you make the error, and why did you miss it in proofreading? What can you do to avoid the same thing happening again?

Transcribe again. Once you have a corrected report, have analyzed your errors, and developed a way to avoid repeating the errors, take a break as you did before proofreading. Then, re-transcribe the report without looking at your corrected transcript. Repeat each step until you have a chartable report. What is a chartable report? A report without any wrong or misspelled words that is neat and well-formatted.

Pause for Reflection

1. How is proofreading in medical transcription different from proofreading essays or term papers?
2. What suggestions are offered to improve your proofreading skills?

Traditional Editing

by Ellen Drake

"Editing and transcription practices are the single most important area of concern to medical transcriptionists," wrote Sally C. Pitman, then editor of *Journal of the American Association for Medical Transcription*, in the Fall 1983 issue. Thirty years later, these are still important issues that are brought up at every gathering of transcriptionists.

Rationales for editing. Physicians do not dictate as they would write (neither would we, if we had to dictate). Most editing is done so unobtrusively that the majority of dictators never suspect that their dictation has undergone revision, or that it needed it. Those who do discover that dictation has been edited appreciate the improvement. Physicians do not appreciate tampering, altering medical content incorrectly, or obliterating their style, but most appreciate being made to look good.

The goal of medical transcription is the communication of medical information about a patient as clearly, concisely, and accurately as possible. On the most basic level, this requires constant decision-making regarding syntax, punctuation, and grammar. At the phonetic level, producing an accurate document involves discriminating among sounds which convey meaning and those that don't (background noises, asides, and the like), analyzing dialects and accents, and constantly choosing between various soundalikes and near-soundalikes. Producing a quality medical document becomes most difficult when dictation is garbled, unclear, incomplete, or medically inaccurate. And it is this latter area that creates the greatest controversy in editing.

It is nearly impossible to transcribe dictation without inadvertent editing. The omission or addition of articles, prepositions, and other minor words represents only a small part of the unconscious editing that takes place everywhere at all times. Recognizing the necessity and inevitability of altering the dictated document makes thoughtful, purposeful editing much more logical and desirable.

The number of variations heard for a given dictated expression is directly proportional to the number of pairs of ears listening. Everyone hears something different. Did the dictator say "adnexa were thickened, nodular" or "thick and nodular." Some may hear, "She has some dorsal asymmetry in the nose." Others hear "There was some dorsal . . ." These examples illustrate variations that make little or no difference in meaning.

On the other hand, you may transcribe something that sounds okay but on listening again hear something different that also sounds okay but significantly changes the meaning. For example, on the recent certification exam, one transcriptionist heard the phrase "I wondered if . . ." but on listening again during proofreading heard, "I warned her that if . . . ."

It is shocking that there are still supervisors, attorneys, and risk management personnel who direct transcriptionists to "type exactly what the doctor says."

Let's look at some of the less controversial editing practices of most quality-minded transcriptionists: choosing and manipulating format, recognition and interpretation of sounds, supplying punctuation and correcting grammar and style, and minor editing of content.

Choosing and manipulating format. Physicians rarely specify format. Sometimes those that do are overruled by an institution's preferences. It is up to the transcriptionist to choose the appropriate format for a report, using the guidelines established by the institution or department. The transcriptionist is usually the one who decides what dictated information goes with which headings and when to paragraph.

Recognition and interpretation of sounds. The phonetic rendering of the sounds the transcriptionist hears is based on the recognition and interpretation of those sounds. This is editing and requires that the transcriptionist select those sounds that have meaning from those that don't, insert silent letters, analyze dialects and accents to select appropriate spellings, recognize and correctly transcribe mispronounced words, differentiate between preferred and less preferred spellings, remember medical words that change spelling as they change form, and choose the appropriate spelling from among soundalike words

Soundalikes cause many of the errors made by experienced and inexperienced transcriptionists alike. Choosing the wrong word is not editing; it's a transcription error and should be studiously avoided. Is it *peroneal* or *perineal*, *breech* or *breach*, *Buerger's disease* or *Berger's disease*? When the physician dictates *malignment* (libel), is *malalignment* (out of alignment) intended?

Quality-conscious transcriptionists should study lists of English and medical soundalike words, such as those published in style manuals and textbooks for medical transcriptionists.

A transcriptionist should never type a word whose meaning is unfamiliar, even if certain of the spelling.

One inexperienced transcriptionist had to be threatened with being fired before she would give up her favorite word book. The book listed many soundalikes as well as less preferred spellings, and she was forever choosing the wrong word or the less preferred spelling because she was too lazy or in too much of a hurry to check unfamiliar words in the dictionary. Naturally, the wrong word or less preferred spelling seemed to be the one that appeared first alphabetically.

Even these routine functions, often undertaken unconsciously by the transcriptionist, may have significant impact on the meaning of the report. Physicians sometimes dictate non-words, especially by using an incorrect prefix or suffix. For example, a physician who dictates *nonsensible* may mean *nonsensical* or *insensible* (a major difference in meaning). If *varicoces* is dictated, the physician may mean *varicocele* or *varices*. The transcriptionist must use the context of the report to determine which word is intended.

A common dictation error of this type is the dictation of a word like *nonavoidable* (not in any dictionary) for *unavoidable*. Some non-words are actually mispronounced words, such as *reoccur* (recur), *reoccurence* (recurrence), *recannulization* (recanalization). The words in parentheses are the correct choice.

Punctuation. Although some physicians dictate punctuation, most do not. The transcriptionist must determine if dictated punctuation is correct and alter it if it is not. Punctuation not dictated must be supplied. There are times when it may be difficult to tell if a clause or phrase belongs at the end of a preceding sentence or the beginning of the next one. The transcriptionist must analyze the context of the report and determine the position and punctuation associated with that phrase.

Look at the following sentences about trusted sources: "Dictionaries are a very good source, but I have found errors in even the most respected. Next are textbooks, although I am finding that they too often have errors." How is the meaning changed by merely adding a comma before and after *too*?

A physician at one hospital who did dictate punctuation was especially fond of semicolons. Almost every sentence he dictated included at least one and many included two, three, and sometimes more. Transcribing the punctuation as dictated made his reports difficult to read and understand, often requiring the re-reading of a sentence several times. Changing many of his dictated semicolons to periods contributed to the clarity of his reports.

Agreement errors frequently cause problems, particularly for the foreign dictator, and subject-verb agreement errors are probably the most common dictation error corrected by transcriptionists. These errors are often due to separation of the subject from the verb by prepositional phrases or intervening clauses. The transcriptionist must catch in real-time proofreading what the ear of the dictator does not catch when talking. When the physician dictates, "The edema in both legs have not yet responded to diuretics," the transcriptionist should correct the verb to *has*. Another example: "There do not appear to have been any associated eye blinking or other automatisms" should be edited to "There does not appear" to make the verb agree in number with the subject "eye blinking."

Another common dictation error is the lack of agreement between pronouns and their antecedents and the failure to have an easily identifiable antecedent for a pronoun. For example, a physician dictated, "The dog was removed from the house with no change in his symptoms." Is it the dog's symptoms the physician is concerned with or the patient's? "His" should be edited to "the patient's" for clarity. A more subtle case of agreement appears in this sentence: "Neutrophils have several different names, all derived from the fact that their cell nucleus is lobulated into segments." Multiple neutrophils have multiple nuclei, so "cell nucleus is" should be edited to "cell nuclei are."

Foreign physicians sometimes misplace modifiers by putting them in the position they would occupy in the physician's native language. For example, "The patient tolerated well the procedure." While the meaning of this sentence is abundantly clear, the physician looks much more knowledgeable (and to some, competent) if the transcriptionist moves the adverb to the end of the sentence.

In summary, the editing of grammar, punctuation, and syntax requires that the transcriptionist have excellent English skills and knowledge. Mistakenly editing grammar or punctuation that is already correct results in edicts like "no editing, ever."

Minor editing of content. Minor editing decisions made by transcriptionists that do not affect meaning include the following: deleting redundancies, differentiating between brief forms and slang, and translating slang forms.

Slang, especially, should be translated into acceptable forms, as slang may make the dictating physician appear careless, sloppy, and unprofessional. Differentiating between brief forms and slang may include some gray areas, but in general, acceptable brief forms are taken from the beginning of the word they represent and are easily recognizable (*rehab* for *rehabilitation*); slang forms, while sometimes taken from the beginning of a word, may also be taken from the middle or end of a word and are not easily recognizable (*lytes* for *electrolytes*).

Investigating and correcting inconsistencies. These types of changes are necessary for clarity and conciseness. Inconsistencies, such as left/right discrepancies, gender discrepancies, and inconsistencies in lab results or medication dosages, should be investigated. If it is possible to determine what is correct, that is what should be transcribed. If the discrepancy cannot be resolved, or if it constitutes a major problem, the report should be flagged and a note written to the dictator.

Major editing of medical content. While most practitioners accept the kinds of editing described above (even when they say they don't), controversy continues over editing changes that alter medical content or produce major revisions in structure, grammar, or style. **Students and inexperienced transcriptionists should *never* perform major editing**. It is discussed here for the purposes of being thorough and for preparing you for future employment. When you have questions about the content of a transcription practice report, discuss them with your instructor. Your instructor may ask what you would do if you were to make an edit and give you feedback accordingly, or the instructor may suggest an appropriate edit in order to help develop your decision-making skills. On the job, substantial editing of a dictation may need to be discussed with a supervisor, should always be done with great care, and should be flagged for the dictator's approval.

The greatest controversy in editing involves the substitution of a different word based on contextual meaning and the substantial editing of medical content. Following are examples of word substitution:

D: Vitamins are given to *supply* a deficiency.
T: Vitamins are given to *correct* a deficiency.

D: In *lieu* of the patient's high fever, antibiotics were continued.
T: In *view* of the patient's high fever, antibiotics were continued.

Editing medical content requires a superior fund of knowledge in the areas of medical terminology, anatomy and physiology, pharmacology, laboratory medicine, surgery, and pathology. Editing of medical information should be done only when the transcriptionist can give a sound explanation of the reasoning behind the changes and support that reasoning in medical reference books. For example, if "forced ventilatory capacity" is dictated, editing to "forced vital capacity" could be justified because that is the name of the test. However, if there is any doubt as to the exact intended meaning, no editing should be attempted, and the dictation in question should be brought to the attention of the supervisor or dictator for clarification.

Muddled sentences, dangling modifiers, and other awkward phrasing should be rearranged or rephrased. Consider this sentence: "Visual acuity in her right eye was light perception only and improved to at least 20/40+ in the left eye with correction." At a first reading, it may appear that the physician is saying, "Visual acuity in the right eye . . . was improved to at least 20/40+ in the left eye" which, of course, makes no sense. Moving the prepositional phrase "in her right eye" to follow "light perception only" probably accurately reveals the intended meaning. Thus, "Visual acuity was light perception only in the right eye and improved to at least 20/40+ in the left eye with correction." Is this change necessary? Some would say not; others would insist that it is. Still others would insist that it is impossible to be sure what the physician meant and that the statement should be flagged for clarification by the dictator.

To quote Vera Pyle:

In editing dictation, we do not go charging in, doctoring up reports in an aggressive way, in an intrusional way. It has to be done so subtly, so delicately, so carefully, that we get a favorable response from the dictator. . . . We must be so involved with what we are transcribing that we know what is going on and can detect something that is dictated that does not make sense, that does not flow, that does not add up. We must listen with an educated ear, with an intelligent ear, so that we can produce an accurate, intelligent, clear document, always remembering the fine line between editing and tampering.

That fine line, unfortunately, is a moving target. It is unlikely that there will ever be unanimous agreement on what is or is not tampering. Perhaps that's good, because as long as people disagree, they can never become complacent. Editing will never be a routine, mindless task as long as the discussion about what's right and what's wrong, what's proper or not, is open.

Pause for Reflection

1. How do physicians feel about having the transcripts of their dictation edited?
2. What is involved in making the communication of medical information about a patient as clear, concise, and accurate as possible?
3. Identify some of the less controversial editing practices of most quality-minded transcriptionists.
4. Give some examples of minor editing of content.
5. How should the need for major editing be handled?

Speech Recognition Editing

by Audrey Kirchner

Automated speech recognition (or **ASR**, as it is known within the medical transcription industry) was supposed to be the way to eliminate most medical transcriptionists from the picture ultimately.

As the speech recognition technology has evolved, one thing has become evident. Medical transcription cannot survive without MT editors. However, doing medical transcription with voice or speech recognition is a whole different ballgame than how we transcribed before!

Let's take a look at some of the changes but more importantly, I'll give you some tips that you can start applying today that will make you better at your job and also hopefully increase your paycheck!

Understanding speech recognition and how it works. In order to improve at doing anything, you have to understand the mechanics of what you're trying to learn. Even if you've been doing medical transcription for 35+ years as I have, speech editing is a whole new world.

For almost all dictators now throughout the medical industry, speech recognition is the dictation tool of choice. Rather than dictating into phones somewhere in a hospital, healthcare providers dictate from anywhere they can . . . on cell phones, mobile devices, etc. These files are almost across the board now run through a speech engine, converting their voice into text.

That's where the medical transcriptionist comes in. As smart as the speech engines are, very few documents

STYLE RULES IN SPEECH RECOGNITION

The style rules that apply for traditional transcription do not apply in most facilities that use SRT. The report you edit will be almost verbatim other than some light editing where necessary.

In traditional medical transcription, accepted style is to expand an abbreviation on first use in a report; thereafter, the abbreviation may be used. Speech recognition, however, cannot be trained to define an abbreviation only once in a report.

Once an abbreviation gets expanded by 100 transcriptionists in 100 reports, SRT will do it every single time thereafter. Everywhere. Thus, most facilities now tell the MTs to leave abbreviations as dictated and not to expand them, even in a diagnosis. For example, it would be incorrect to have *COPD* expanded to *chronic obstructive pulmonary disease (COPD)* every time it is used whether once, twice, or ten times. And not only in that one report but in every report thereafter.

The same thing is true with dates and names. If 8-11 is edited to August 11 in one report, then when a dictator dictates a lab value of 811, SRT would expand it to August 11. Doctors aren't too happy to see a glucose value of August 11. It would also be illogical to substitute "the patient" when the dictator gives the patient's name.

But what about content errors? In an operative report, the dictator states, "With the patient in the dorsal supine following adequate epidural anesthesia." The editor adds the word *position* after "dorsal supine." The dictator also says, "The uterine was closed in a continuous locking suture...." The editor adds the word *incision* after *uterine*. SRT editors are taught to edit for clarity.

The lesson is that edits that are unique, like adding *position* after dorsal supine and *incision* after uterine, are not going to affect the "learning" of the speech engine, but edits like expanding abbreviations and dates that are repeated over and over will "teach" the engine to always make that edit. It's not just about expansion; it's about any repetitive edit that is not unique.

Ultimately, the focus in speech recognition editing is to make sure the right words are correctly spelled and in the right place—which, in the end, should also be the focus of traditional transcription as well.

(probably none) come out perfectly. What the speech engine perceives as "text" and what is supposed to be text are often two entirely different things. Some MTs have a much harder time than others adapting to this new technology.

Increased critical patient safety errors and major errors. Speech recognition is supposed to be a means to eliminate human error and reduce critical patient safety errors. However, it has done just the opposite. Critical patient safety errors have been shown to be increased in this technology, even though it has now been in place for several years.

Why? Traditional medical transcription was a procedure whereby MTs listened to the voice, thought about it, then typed the dictation onto the page. They then reviewed it quickly, going on to the next few spoken words. Today that has all changed with SRT. Now the words are already on the page for the MT and it is not a matter of "hear it, type it" but rather "read it, listen to it, verify it matches what the voice dictated," and then send it through as complete.

The problem with the new method of transcription or editing is that the brain doesn't always catch up with what the MT is seeing. The brain somehow blindly reads something and does not see that it doesn't make any sense while the eye is telling the brain that indeed, the information on the page is accurate. It may be accurate in terms of spelling, grammar, etc., but in fact, it can be 100% incorrect. Consequently, if the MT editor does not catch the mistake, the error has now become part of a patient record. Frightening!

The major drawback to this new methodology for medical transcription is that it is extremely labor intensive. The most glaring problem seems to revolve around one human attribute that can rear its head unexpectedly even in the face of the most disciplined medical transcriptionist—inattention or lack of concentration whether momentary or many times over the course of the day.

In the nanosecond that it takes to look away from the screen to move your mouse, you can miss a word. Likewise, in the snap of two fingers, you can add a critical patient safety error to a report because you weren't paying enough attention when your mind drifted off.

There are some techniques that can help all MTs increase their accuracy while doing their job. No MT or editor sets about to do sloppy transcription or to make errors. Most MTs are usually perfectionists and want to see an error-free report. However, the potential for error is so high that it seems some days you're all thumbs or that your eyes are betraying you right and left.

How can we cut down on these errors and strive for better quality when it comes to patient records?

Proper tools and equipment. First and foremost, in order to do a good job, anyone performing a job needs the proper tools. Consider investing in these if you don't have them already:

• Flat screen monitor, the largest you can afford cuts down on glare and helps you see clearly what you are editing.

• High-quality USB headset with volume control; you can't interpret accurately what you can't hear properly so invest in the best headset that you can find with the most variability in ranges and with volume control.

• Proper lighting for your work area.

• Keep your working environment distractionless; reduce noise and anything else that tempts your concentration to stray.

• Proper desk equipment including keyboards and chairs; you want to be comfortable when working for long stretches

ASR techniques, tips, and tricks. Once you have the proper work environment, now you're ready to explore some of the tricks and tips that will keep you focused on your reports and hopefully also increase your productivity while decreasing your error rates.

Synchronize the text cursor to the audible voice file. This means that the cursor should be following along from left to right as the voice file is playing in your headphones.

Tip: Do not take your eyes off the cursor for any reason. If you do, stop the voice file and resume when you are ready. Follow the cursor from left to right like the bouncing ball on *Sing Along With Mitch* from the 1950s. This is the best and only way not to miss dictation. Most critical patient safety errors are errors of omission or not catching an incorrect word substitution. If you're watching word for word, that can't happen.

Scan through the document before even putting your foot on the pedal and check such things as document type, dictator, patient information, dates, etc. Have a quick look through the document to see what may need to be changed and even change it before you start, such as headings, etc.

If there are expansions or templates needed, add them before you begin so you will not forget to do so

later. But have a care that you add only what was spoken and remove anything else in templates, expansions, etc. Failure to do this is another error-prone area with the new technology.

Concentrate, concentrate, concentrate. Matching the auditory file with the printed version requires focused concentration and is the only way to eliminate errors. If your mind is wandering, you will make serious errors.

A good rule of thumb for researching blanks is allowing no more than 3 minutes per blank. Take the time to review samples or use the Internet to research phrases. Build a library of difficult dictators or procedures and have them close at hand for references.

Spell check! If it is not automatic, do it anyway! There is no room in this day and age for misspelled words but especially in a medicolegal document.

Before you decide to send your report off into the EHR world, have a care and review the document before you submit it. Make sure one final time that you have produced the cleanest, most accurate document possible!

Practice makes perfect when it comes to ASR. Learn **keyboard shortcuts** to eliminate or cut down on the use of the mouse. This not only increases your speed, but it also cuts down on the potential for errors as noted above. Every time you look away from your screen for a second and disengage from the text, you create the potential for an error.

It might seem cumbersome and like just one more thing to add to a long day, but in the end, if it increased your production and made your job easier (it is much easier on hands, wrists, and arms to use keyboard shortcuts), wouldn't it be worth it?

Check out the Microsoft Word keyboard shortcuts and practice until you can literally do these without looking. Keyboard shortcuts that help most are:

Navigation (moving you around in the document without touching your mouse): keys like Home, End, Arrow.

Text selection (for moving text with keyboard commands, again mouseless): keys like Ctrl+End or Ctrl+Right.

Deleting or moving (to copy and paste without touching the mouse): keys like Ctrl+A or Ctrl+V.

Undo and redo. These will save you lots of time and keystrokes: Ctrl+Z and Ctrl+Y.

Pause for Reflection

1. What are some of the issues or problems with speech recognition (SR) and speech editing discussed by the author?
2. What environmental and equipment issues should be addressed when engaging in SR editing?
3. What tips does the author suggest for improving the quality of your editing?
4. What final piece of advice does the author offer?

What MTs Do That Speech Recognition Cannot

by Ellen Drake

When most people hear the words **risk management**, they probably think about botched operations, patient relations, medical record chart review, attorneys, and maybe malpractice complaints. Rarely does anyone think about medical transcription and those who are responsible for producing it—anyone, that is, except medical transcriptionists.

Medical transcriptionists are acutely aware of the role they play in the limitation of hospital risk by producing timely and accurate reports. Many, however, are

TIPS ON DICTATING AND TRANSCRIBING SPEECH RECOGNITION REPORTS

The techniques for best practices are somewhat different when dictating to a medical transcriptionist vs. dictating to a speech recognition (SR) engine for future editing by an MT. For example, in the past when dictating, I've spelled out the name of a doctor, a local town, or a medication that I'm not certain the MT will be familiar with (after all, the MT may not know how to spell Tamarac).

With SRT, it's pointless to spell out words. The software attempts to form words out of the letters you're saying and comes up with a string of meaningless garbage. In addition, if you need to go back to add, delete, or change something you said four paragraphs prior, the SR software isn't going to do this for you. It just keeps rolling right along typing what you said, and you have a whole bunch of confusing nonsense smack in the middle of your report. A human being, on the other hand, will recognize that you've made a correction, find the section of the report to which you referred, make the correction, go back to where you left off, and pick up seamlessly.

The clinicians who are dictating don't know if they're dictating to a human or to an SR engine and wouldn't know how to adjust their dictation styles even if they did.

On the transcription side, typing a document from scratch and editing an SR-generated document requires totally different skill sets. Good MTs get "in a zone" when they're transcribing a report, mak-

ing certain critical decisions and judgments. The human who has to edit the garbage put out by the SR program requires more alertness, more attention to detail, more knowledge, more critical thinking skills. Did the doctor really mean left or right? Did the doctor say Zoloft or Zocor? Celebrex or Cerebyx?

When the document is in front of you for SR editing, although you don't have to physically type an entire document, you are forced to decipher whether what is there is correct because the SR software can't. Then you need to make the corrections, which often involves deleting long strings of junk but may involve changing only one or two letters.

Aside from the obvious danger of wrong medications in the patient record, there are some errors that will escape the editor because they're insidious. For example, the dosage is the same for two medications, so a flag won't go up if you're just skimming the document and not paying close attention because it "looks" correct. Standard doses of Flexeril and Dulcolax are 10 mg. Lamictal and Pyridium are both dosed at 100 mg. These medications do not sound or look alike, but they were incorrectly interpreted by SR software. And were you alert to the fact that the patient in the report you're working on is a man, but it says he's on *oxytocin*, which is a drug intended to induce or assist labor in pregnant women? The SR software "heard" that rather than *doxazosin*.

Sherry Roth

unaware that their role in risk management can and should go beyond that.

What is risk management? Risk management is the reporting, analyzing, and tracking of atypical things that happen in a hospital. In medical transcription, risk management may involve the reporting of inconsistencies within a report, inflammatory or derogatory remarks by the dictator, or the mention of an incident that may not have been reported. Dictations containing potential risk management problems should be routed through the transcription supervisor and department head to the risk management team.

Risk management issues can include any of the following:

- Mention of any incident even though the dicctator states an incident report was completed.
- Derogatory statements referring to another physician, a hospital employee, or the hospital.
- Comments regarding injury to a body structure during the performance of an operative procedure or untoward complications as a result of anesthesia or the procedure.
- Aborted procedures or operations due to inadequate preparation of the patient or difficulties performing the procedure.
- Report of hospital-incurred incidents such as drug overdose, wrong drug administered, or patient injury.
- Inappropriate comments about the patient.
- Comments about patient dissatisfaction with personnel or treatment.
- Tests performed or drugs administered that were not ordered by the physician.
- Positive test results that may not have been on the chart or which the physician failed to note prior to the patient's discharge.

Where to begin. Risk management begins even before the first line of a report is transcribed. It begins with meticulous attention to the correct spelling of the patient's first and last names, entering the correct patient number in the report, correctly spelling and entering the physician's name in the report, and entering the correct dates of admission, discharge, or procedure.

While new technology makes retrieving this information and inserting it into the report easier, it also introduces new ways to make mistakes. Lack of attention while performing what may constitute an "automatic" procedure could mean incorporating a "Jr" when the report is really on "Sr," or mother's number instead of daughter's when their names are the same, or even

the name of someone completely unrelated to the patient.

Transcriptionists should be alert to names that may be either first or last names and should check for both in the master patient index when in doubt. For example, the physician may dictate a name like James Dean, when the patient is actually Dean James. It is not inconceivable that both names could appear in the master patient index because they are two different people. Social Security number (if known), birthdate (if given), date of admission, age, and admitting physician should be checked whenever there is a question concerning the patient name.

Hyphenated names, nicknames (e.g., Meg or Peg for Margaret; Bill, Billy, Will for William, which may not be nicknames but actual given names), soundalikes (e.g., Ellen, Helen, Elaine, and Allen), and foreign names (e.g., Hasus, Jesus) can all be sources of error carried on indefinitely in the patient's health record. Unusual first names (such as Syphyllis, Ranellen, Butch, Angel, Princess, and Doc) need to be verified as to spelling and authenticity (real first name or nickname?).

It is not unusual for a transcriptionist to find multiple entries with different patient numbers but with the same or only slight variations in spelling, and on closer examination, dates of birth, gender, and other demographic data appear to be the same. These should be reported and an effort made to determine whether they are indeed the same patient or different people. As noted above, parents and children with identical names also present opportunities for error in the patient health record.

Omit inappropriate comments. Slang or vulgar terms used disparagingly to refer to patients should be removed from the record. Physicians may utter such comments in anger or frustration, but they really do not intend for offensive or off-color remarks to be entered in the patient's record and preserved permanently.

Neither should disparaging remarks referring to nursing or allied health staff members, management, or other physicians be allowed to remain in a record. One internist who performed the history and physical examinations on patients in the eating disorders unit of a hospital would frequently question the judgment of the psychiatrist who was in charge of the unit, and more than once called him a "fat slob." He seemed to feel that it was intolerable that an overweight physician should be responsible for an eating disorders unit!

While most MTs would not think of transcribing "fat slob" or something like that, administrators and risk managers may never know of that physician's attitude—a dangerous attitude if both physicians were named in the same malpractice case—toward another medical staff member unless such dictation is reported. This is not gossip but, properly reported, is looking out for the best interests of the hospital and even the offending physician.

Another physician who frequently dictated the admitting history and physical within earshot of his patients was dictating about one patient's anxiety and altered mental state in the patient's presence, and recommended a psychiatric consult. Within 10 or 15 minutes of completing the report, the physician came on the dictation lines again, dictating a "correction" to the previously dictated report and asked that the references to the patient's mental state be removed. The patient had become quite angry at the physician's implications that the patient was "crazy" and demanded that a new report be dictated. At the second dictation, the transcriptionist could hear the patient complaining angrily in the background. This unhappy patient could easily imagine receiving poor, inadequate, or even incompetent care culminating in a malpractice complaint.

One transcriptionist received considerable criticism because a patient had received a copy of a report in which she was consistently referred to as *he*. The patient took immense offense and felt that the report was implying that her sexual orientation was equivocal. The patient actually threatened a lawsuit. The physician dictator had been foreign, and foreign doctors often confuse feminine and masculine pronouns. The patient's name was one that could have been a male or female, and the transcriptionist either had not noticed that the sex was inconsistent within the report or had not checked the health record to be certain of the sex.

Not only are the latter two examples risk management problems but also patient relations problems. It would be in the best interests of the hospital to have any ancillary departments that are involved or implicated in some way contacted by the supervisor about such problems.

These types of inflammatory comments are inappropriate and could increase the hospital's and physician's risk of a malpractice judgment should the case end up in court for any reason.

Watching for inconsistencies. The transcriptionist is expected to remain alert throughout the entire transcription of any given report in order to detect inconsistencies within the report, but access to the patient's chart is needed to verify and correct most inconsistencies. When the transcriptionist can access the patient's pharmacy and laboratory records via the appropriate databases on the mainframe, many inconsistencies can be avoided. If one of these routes is not available, the report should be "flagged" to the attention of the physician to make the necessary corrections.

In some cases, the areas of inconsistency within a report may be widely separated. The original statement at the beginning of the report (saying, for example, that the patient was admitted with pain in the *left* knee) may not be contradicted until the very end of the report (for example, Discharge Diagnosis: Dislocation, *right* knee).

The following are excerpts from actual physician dictation. Each contains an inconsistency.

This patient developed a persistent lesion on the inner aspect of the left upper lip. This lesion was at the junction of the vermilion and mucous membrane. A punch biopsy was obtained of this 1 cm lesion and was read as a probable verrucous squamous cell carcinoma of the lower lip.

He was referred to our office for evaluation recently and was noted to have a normally positioned urethral meatus but a persistent ventral hood with deficient ventral penile foreskin. Testes were bilaterally descended. He is to be admitted on an elective basis at the convenience of his parents' schedule. The plan is for removal of the dorsal hood, artificial erection to rule out chordee, and circumcision.

The patient is approximately one week prior to the onset of her menstrual period. The ultrasound shows a complex cystic ovary on the right side. Left ovary is deep into the cul-de-sac area, but is essentially normal with a small 1.5 cm follicle. Pelvic examination reveals the uterus to be retroverted, mobile. Both adnexal areas reveal no masses or thickening. The right adnexal area is slightly tender. Cannot appreciate the complex cystic ovary on the left side on bimanual examination.

In the first example, the physician dictates *upper lip* in the first sentence and *lower lip* in the last sentence. In the second example, the patient has a *ventral hood* and later a *dorsal hood*. In the final example, the ultrasound report notes a cystic ovary on the *right* side, but on physical examination, the physician states he cannot appreciate the cystic ovary on the *left* side.

Note errors and incomplete dictation. Transcriptionists are also expected to detect erroneous or incomplete drug dosages, laboratory values, and other measurements and to correct these (if the correct value can be clearly ascertained) or to flag the report to the attention of the physician for further clarification. Should charts with inaccurate or incomplete information end up in court, the opposing attorneys could have a field day. The following examples of actual physician dictation contain such errors.

The patient's physical examination revealed a 2 x 1 x 1 mass in the right upper pole of the thyroid.

Lasix 20 q. day, Micro-K 10 q. day, Zantac 150 p.o. b.i.d.

In the first example, it cannot be known whether the measurements are in millimeters or centimeters or even inches. The report should be flagged asking the physician to clarify. In the latter example, the measurements are again omitted, but consultation with a comprehensive drug reference or a pharmacist would provide the usual units used for each of these medications—milligrams (mg) for Lasix and Zantac, and milliequivalents (mEq) for Micro-K.

In some cases, risk management involves recognizing when the dictation is not an error, is not slang, is not inflammatory, and letting the work remain as dictated. Each of the following excerpts contains dictation that a transcriptionist might mistakenly believe was an error in the dictation.

She gives a history of shooting crank. Since that time, the left antecubital space has been infected.

The blistering is typical of strep. I would go ahead and give her 2 million units q.6h. of penicillin and modify therapy according to culture report.

The patient underwent an intravenous pyelogram to rule out obstruction caused by tumor or stone. The urogram was negative.

In the first example, a transcriptionist might think *crank* should be *crack*, but *crank* is a different street drug from *crack*. In the next, 2 million (units) of penicillin may seem excessive to an inexperienced transcriptionist who might think the physician meant milligrams or milliliters, but it is a standard dose for the problem indicated. In the last example, *pyelogram* and *urogram* are used interchangeably.

At times, the physician must indicate that the results of a procedure cannot be found, or that an unusual test result was artifactual in nature or the result of an error in the testing process. These remarks should not be edited as they form an important part of the record with legal implications. *These excerpts demonstrate remarks that should never be deleted.* They should, however, be reported to risk management to see if the problems noted can be resolved.

EKG showed sinus bradycardia with no acute ischemic changes. Repeat EKG showed a right bundle branch block with first-degree AV block. The pattern on this EKG was so different it may not have actually been the same patient.

Chemistry panel showed a BUN of 26 with a creatinine of 1.6, a calcium of 11.7, SGOT of 271, LDH of 690, alkaline phosphatase of 69. Urinalysis on admission cannot be found in the chart.

Remarks regarding the administration of an overdose or an unprescribed drug are important to the health record in that the patient's subsequent treatment may be affected by the incident and the information should never be deleted from the report. Failure to include the report of such incidents in a document could also appear to be an attempt to hide incriminating material from the court should the situation result in litigation.

The following example should be reported to the risk management department and/or health information management director by way of the supervisor.

Gastroscopy Report: Premedication: Demerol 50 mg, Vistaril 25 mg IM. The patient was also given Versed 10 mg IM by mistake, and was quite well sedated at the time of the procedure.

Students and inexperienced MTs cannot be expected to spot all risk management issues. However, you must always be focused on context and alert to inconsistencies, omissions, and anything else that elicits a question in your mind. *Never edit* if you are not absolutely certain that the change is acceptable and that it does not affect medical content. *Do ask questions* and while you are learning and gaining experience, seek the input of your instructor. Once on the job, seek out a more experienced MT or supervisor.

Pause for Reflection

1. What is risk management, in general and as it relates to medical transcription?
2. Give at least 5 examples of reportable risk management issues.
3. What is the first area of concern for a transcriptionist when it comes to risk management?
4. Give some examples of report content that caused risk management issues.
5. What type of editing is inappropriate for students and inexperienced MTs?

Productivity

Feeling the Need for Speed

by Georgia Green

Which is more important to success in the medical transcription field: quality or production? The answer should be obvious. It doesn't matter how many reports you can produce in an hour, a day, or an entire pay period if those reports contain medical inaccuracies or if misspellings, typos, and errors in grammar and punctuation compromise their readability. That doesn't mean productivity is not an issue.

Speed does count when it comes to the size of a paycheck based on production wages and even more so when mandated minimum production requirements determine whether you will continue to be employed. So how can a medical transcription student increase production without jeopardizing quality?

Proceed with caution. This article gives specific suggestions for improving your productivity, but these suggestions must be prefaced with this cautionary note: Speed should be the furthest thing from your mind until the last stages of training. Traditional speed-building techniques work by eliminating redundancies, but it is these same redundancies that are an essential element of fundamental transcription training. Taking shortcuts of any kind undermines the learning process, with the end result being decreased overall production and quality. Looking up the same term for a second, third, or fourth time is not a wasted effort but an investment in building your fund of medical knowledge.

Until you have committed to memory the widest possible range of medical concepts and associated vocabulary, avoid spell-checkers, macros, expanders, or templates. Electronic references that link terms with their definitions are fine for student use. If you keep a quick reference word list, manual or electronic, jot down a brief definition with each entry to reinforce these connections in your mind every time you consult the list.

After completing the entire *Healthcare Documentation: Fundamentals & Practice* course, transcribing each report twice and achieving an acceptable accuracy score on the final attempt, you can focus your attention on speed-building techniques in random practice sessions before moving to more advanced training.

Defining terms. It is important to understand the difference between *production* and *productivity*. Your total output, whether lines, characters, or number of reports, during your regularly scheduled workday is your production. Productivity, on the other hand, is a measure of your rate of production over a standard unit of time, e.g., lines per hour. If you work more hours per day, you increase your production but not your productivity. However, as your proficiency as an MT improves, you can increase both your productivity AND your production.

Let's look at a student whose productivity is 100 lines per hour. If that student's total production for a particular 8-hour workday is only 400 lines, there is a discrepancy of 4 hours. Perhaps it was necessary to slow down in order to accommodate a difficult dictator or two or three. But there is still a large chunk of time spent with an idle keyboard. Some of this downtime is a necessary part of the job—researching new terms, reviewing instructions for format and style, overcoming the occasional problem with hardware or software, and time spent mastering a new work procedure or productivity technique.

When it is appropriate to turn your attention to increasing your speed, keep a notepad next to your keyboard and keep track of time away from the keyboard so you can analyze it later. Use a chart with columns to designate various types of "down time"—word research, technical problems, consulting another person, and so on—and then just make check marks in each column to indicate each 5-minute block spent in an activity away from the keyboard.

Investment in your fund of medical knowledge. Even the clearest dictation can stump you if you encounter a term that is unfamiliar. And if you don't understand the concept behind a term, you can't be sure that what you are hearing is correct. A deficit in your internal medical knowledge database correlates directly with both the amount of time you spend researching unfamiliar terms and the number of mistakes you will make in selecting the right term. The best defense is a well-rounded program of study that includes academic coursework in the structure and function of the human body, human diseases, physical diagnosis and treatment, pharmacology, laboratory medicine, and more.

Practice makes perfect. There are so many different ways to express the same idea, and for each of these variations in expression there are hundreds of ways for an individual dictator to render a passage containing that idea in a nearly incomprehensible manner. The only way you can gain a reasonable level of competency is to engage in as much practice as possible, transcribing each report as many times as necessary to achieve mastery not only of the content but also the nuances of a particular dictator's voice and style, many of which are missed on a single pass at a report.

Once you enter the workplace, you lose this wonderful opportunity for true mastery unless you are lucky enough to encounter a supervisor or mentor who understands this concept and makes work assignments that include enough repetition to allow you the opportunity for continued mastery. While you are still a student, it is crucial that you understand the role of retranscription in "training your ear." Never take shortcuts here.

Comma chameleon. Does your understanding of grammar and punctuation allow you to supply necessary commas or correct verb tense as you transcribe, without consulting a style guide each time? Sometimes a dictator does mangle a sentence beyond saving, but most of the time you should be able to make minor fixes without interrupting your rhythm. If this isn't a problem for you, this is one productivity leak you don't have to worry about. If it is a problem, don't worry—you can overcome it with some remedial work in grammar.

Grammar guides are invaluable and you should study them—not just a review of rules but plenty of exercises, including bare-bones sentence diagramming. When you really get a solid understanding of sentence structure and why words and phrases are arranged the way they are, punctuation will fall into place much more easily. Search for a website that can guide you through the basics of sentence diagramming.

Capital Community College (**www.ccc.commnet. edu/**) hosts a comprehensive grammar site. It provides a section on diagramming sentences, but be sure to click the links for quizzes and for PowerPoint presentations and see everything the site has to offer.

If you are enrolled in a formal program of study, don't forget to ask your instructor for advice. Your school may offer a nuts and bolts grammar course, and your instructor can help you find the course that is right for you.

Plug all the leaks. Close your eyes for a moment and imagine this scenario: You are transcribing along without a hitch, then all of a sudden you come to a grinding halt. Either you didn't hear something at all or what you heard didn't make sense. What do you do? Back it up and play again. And again. And again. Slower. Faster. Reread the sentence, the paragraph. Scan the whole report. Play the dictation forward and finish the paragraph or even the report. Should you grab a book? Which book? Should someone else listen?

The answer may be "all of the above" or "none of the above," depending upon the circumstances, but developing an efficient process can contribute greatly to your productivity at the latter part of your training and as you transition to the work environment.

An "efficient process" might also be referred to as "time management" as it refers to how you handle the inevitable constant interruptions in work flow that occur when you must pause on an unclear word or phrase, replay it, research it, ask for help, etc. If you waste 10 minutes at a time on only a dozen words during your transcription session, that totals two hours in lost production. Could that time have been cut down to one hour or even to just half an hour if your process was more efficient? When you are producing high-quality lines but far less than anticipated, this is usually the area that needs attention.

Most experienced productive MTs have an efficient process in place even if they aren't consciously aware of it and cannot explain it to you, and MTs have their own twists that make that process unique. There is no single "one size fits all" process, but you can start with a guideline and gradually develop the process that you find most efficient for you.

Here is a process you can use as a starting point and customize it to meet your own style and available resources:

1. When you have stopped on a word, relisten to it one or two times.

2. Stop and ask yourself why you can't decipher it—is it mumbled, too fast or too slow, obscured in some way, or is it a term you think you can hear clearly enough but just don't know? If you can hear it but don't know it, skip down to #5.

3. If appropriate, speed up and slow down the dictation to see if this makes a difference. If the word was said too rapidly, say it aloud yourself syllable by syllable, fast and slow. Write down a phonetic equivalent and look at it. Does anything come to mind?

4. Reread the sentence the term occurs in or even the paragraph to develop a context. Ask yourself what kind of word should go here if you had to guess—is it a drug name, a body part, an English word?

5. Choose the right reference book for the job. If it is a drug name, go to a drug book; if it is an English word, try *Webster's*; if it is a body part go to your full-size medical dictionary. If you think it is a new term or if you have already checked your medical dictionary, check *Vera Pyle's Current Medical Terminology* (new, difficult, and hard-to-find terminology with definitions). Go to the appropriate specialty word book or general phrase index to narrow down your choices after consulting the medical dictionary—and then come back to the medical dictionary to confirm the meaning. Context is everything.

6. If you didn't hear enough of the word to look it up and you have an electronic reference, try a wild card search (refer to your software for instructions).

7. If the term seems to be part of a phrase, look up the parts you do hear as the term may appear as a cross-reference. If it is the name of a ligament, look also under *muscle* and *tendon* as you may find clues there.

8. STOP—don't spend more than five minutes researching in your books. Leave a blank (with a phonetic "sounds like") and finish transcribing. Then come back to it. Many terms are repeated later in the report.

9. At the end of the report go back to any missing terms and see if you understand them now since you know the full context of the report and are more familiar with the dictator's voice.

10. If you come up empty, now is the time where judgment is required. Does it seem reasonable to leave a blank? This depends on both the expectations for your performance (is this practice dictation, a test, on the job under full QA review, or are you on your own?) and the circumstances of the dictation itself. Ask yourself if a more skilled MT would have been able to fill in this blank. If the dictation truly is garbled, very heavily accented, or obscured in some way, any MT may have had trouble. Leave the blank. Did you leave too many blanks in this report and how many blanks constitute too many? Again, consider your expectations. If you feel you are not ready to abandon the search for the term, give yourself 10 more minutes and include any Internet research within this time limit.

11. Make a note about how the term sounded and its context so you can research it later if no feedback is forthcoming from your teacher or supervisor.

Developing good judgment. The ability to make independent judgments grows out of a combination of confidence in your skills and awareness of your limitations—and definitely impacts your "process," as noted above. This can't be taught from a book per se but can be enhanced through the use of critical thinking exercises. Consider the old adage about giving a man a fish versus teaching him how to fish. If you learn not just how to solve a problem in a particular situation but instead develop a mental framework for addressing problems in varying circumstances, you are able to think independently and will be able to exercise reasonable MT judgment without a teacher standing by. A good source of critical thinking exercises can be found in *H&P: A Nonphysician's Guide to the Medical History and Physical Examination* available at **www.hpisum.com**.

Smoking those keys. One of the first things you learn when you begin transcribing is that your keyboarding speed on a copy-typing exercise has little to do with the speed at which you will transcribe. In fact, the faster your raw typing speed, the greater the percentage of speed loss. A 100-wpm typist will feel much more discouragement than a 45-wpm typist. Nevertheless, good keyboarding skills are prerequisite for any MT. Generally, keyboarding speed picks up naturally over time, but if it doesn't, this area may need attention. One has to be able to move quickly through dictation that flows smoothly to make up for time lost on the more challenging parts. Keyboarding speed in and of itself should be assessed periodically apart from actual transcribing speed, and any deficits that are discovered should be addressed. Luckily, an inexpensive software program can add 20 wpm onto your baseline keyboarding speed in just a couple of weeks.

Adding to your MT toolbox. As you near the end of training and *after* you have addressed all the impediments to production discussed in this article, it is time to look at the myriad of tools used by experienced medical transcriptionists to enhance their productivity. Abbreviation expansion tools built into your word processing program or obtained through third-party software can dramatically increase your production—after you have mastered all the basics presented here.

Making the Most of Your Studies

by Ellen Drake

Preparing to transcribe. Chapter 5 is all about style and formatting of medical reports. It is primarily a reference chapter that you will use while you are transcribing the practice dictations that accompany the specialty chapters. With Chapter 6, you will enter the world of medical transcription for real, and you will start to put into practice the techniques and practices you learned in this chapter.

Transcription practice will be unlike any other exercise or activity that you have encountered up to now. Study each specialty chapter carefully and complete all the exercises, both the end-of-chapter exercises and the on-line exercises, *before* you try to transcribe the practice dictations. Read the sample reports at the end of the chapters and look up any unfamiliar terminology. Listen to the on-line audio sample reports while reading the transcripts (your instructor will tell you how to access the transcripts). Again, look up any unfamiliar terms and put them in your notebook. Relisten to difficult passages until you can say with certainty that you hear what you are reading in the transcript.

Occasionally you may encounter a dictation that seems too challenging for you at the moment. Sometimes, especially with repetitive sections of a report like the review of systems, the physical examination, and the opening and closing sections of operative reports, you may have to listen several times and study similar reports before you can decipher all the words and phrases that are difficult to hear. Even good dictators may rush through routine sections of a report, but some dictators may seem impossible to you at first. For that reason, we have purposely included multiple dictations by the same dictators for this unit. Some of the on-line

audio samples are also by the more difficult dictators in the transcription practice dictations.

You should engage in transcription practice the same way you would engage if you were working as a medical transcriptionist. When you are ready to work on the practice dictations, the first thing you need to do is to make sure that you organize your work space for efficiency, to minimize distractions, and for comfort. Review the document "Transcription Techniques" each and every time you sit down to transcribe.

Before transcribing the first line, listen to the full report, paying attention to the dictator's tone and rhythm and any unusual speech characteristics or accent. Does the dictation flow or is it choppy? Does the dictator seem organized or does he or she stumble around and make a lot of corrections? Make a note of words you don't know and look them up. Then transcribe each report carefully, stopping as often as necessary to look up new and unfamiliar words for spelling and meaning.

Each time the physician dictates, different words will be clearer. On the job, medical transcriptionists often have access to templates or "normals" and "boiler-plate" paragraphs that help them decipher difficult dictators. As a student, you too can begin to create similar "normals" and "boiler-plate" paragraphs. As you identify difficult passages for a particular voice, make a note of it. When you hear that dictator again, dictating a similar passage, you should be able to decipher a bit more than you did on the previous attempt.

Relistening to and retranscribing difficult dictation will also help you build skill in deciphering hard-to-understand phrasing. Sometimes you may need to listen to a single word over and over, but you should learn to recognize routine phrasing and patterns in dictations and transcribe in phrases rather than word-by-word.

During your training is the time to take advantage of all the luxuries you won't have when you are on the job: the luxury of extensive research, not just for words themselves but background information so that you understand what is going on in the report; the luxury of transcribing a report more than once so that you can learn to identify repeated words and phrases and anticipate what's coming next, building speed and accuracy through this process; the luxury of proofreading—multiple times, with and without the audio and by just reading the report aloud to yourself.

You may find that you are unable to understand a word the first time you encounter it, or you may not be able to find it in your references. When this is the case, leave a blank (or blanks) and continue with the transcription. The dictator may use the word in question a second time, enabling you to determine the appropriate term or context. These clues may eventually help you decipher the term.

Your ultimate goal is to produce a first-time final copy without the use of a draft copy. The standard of quality you are striving for is that which you will produce in your future employment as a medical transcriptionist—a neat, accurate, and complete report that may be placed in the patient's medical chart as a permanent record of healthcare.

However, this is just the beginning. Keep your goal in mind but don't get discouraged as you begin to transcribe. Do, however, strive to prepare a document that is free of wrong words and misspellings, that is, a report that is "chartable." Make your goal "the right word, correctly spelled, in the right place."

When you have finished a report, take a break (at least 30 minutes). Then, go back and listen to the dictation again while proofreading your transcript. Check the correctness of your transcript and attempt to fill in any blanks you left earlier. Transcriptionists often find they can decipher a difficult word after listening to it again at a later time.

After you have compared your transcript to the transcript key or received a graded transcript back from your instructor, look up all the words you missed. Write them, correctly spelled, in a journal or notebook (an electronic journal is ideal for ease of searching) along with their definitions and two or three sentences that illustrate the correct use of the term. Include the sentence from the report as well.

In addition, *analyze the reason for your error.* Was it simply inadequate research or did you do a lot of research but fail to find the term? If you failed to find the term, was it because you had spelled the word incorrectly or used an inappropriate reference? Was your misspelling due to not hearing the word clearly or failure to apply rules of phonics? Did you use a soundalike and fail to verify the definition?

There are many more questions you can ask yourself about why you misspelled a word, transcribed the wrong term, or left a blank. Once you determine why you made the mistake, you should develop a strategy for avoiding that kind of mistake in the future. If you need help in analyzing your errors or developing avoidance strategies, talk with your instructor.

Finally, if your transcript contained content errors (wrong words or seriously misspelled medical terms), transcribe the report again and follow the above processes until you have produced a report free of content errors. Once you have corrected, accurate transcripts, you can use these as sample reports to help you decipher difficult dictators in the next section of reports that you transcribe.

Soon, you will be transcribing dictations like a pro if you incorporate the transcription practices you learned in this chapter into your repertoire. But don't place unreasonable expectations on yourself in the beginning. Medical transcription can be very challenging to learn but also very rewarding. Keep your eyes on the goal and keep practicing.

Spotlight On

Editing on the Fly

by Renee M. Priest

It really does not take much to tickle the funny bones of MTs who work with words all day long. The slip of a tongue ("the patient had a sinkable episode"), the unconscious transposition of a crucial consonant or vowel ("performed a slaplingotomy"), the inadvertent addition of a syllable or two ("patient was rotototated")—these simple faux pas have been known to trigger helpless mirth and frivolity in many transcription pools or at-home offices.

Often it is not the words themselves (all perfectly valid, with easily understood meanings located in a dictionary), but the mental picture they conjure up that will start the giggling:

"The floor was full so patient was placed on telemetry." Try as I might, I cannot get past the picture of patients, packed in like sardines, lying head-to-toe all over the floor of a hospital ward, with one lone patient perched uncomfortably on top of a telemetry unit!

"The patient's dressing is falling apart, but is otherwise intact." I have to wonder if the Mummy has risen and is stalking about the waiting room trying to locate all the fragments of its dressing as they fall off on the floor.

"The patient was scoped and a very large rectal polyp was discovered in the office." Can't you just see the nurses and the physician jumping all over the office trying to trap that escaping polyp with a butterfly net?

An MT has no need of movies or television programs to provide mental stimulation and often colorful mental imagery:

"Patient is a 4-year-old male who voluntarily gave up his driver's license a few years ago."

"The patient's primary care provider recommended she be sent to a competent ophthalmologist, so she was inadvertently sent to me."

"The patient is pregnant and his wife is due in 6 weeks, so he is under some stress."

"Date of death 04/15, the patient will be sent to an assisted-living facility for further rehabilitation."

"The patient's mother and sister have prostate cancer."

And it never fails that on a day when one least suspects it, a dictator who is a frustrated creative writer will pepper his dictation with things like "Patient describes the diarrhea as being usually of a chocolate pudding consistency, but sometimes more watery, a bit like sauce or beef gravy, but never quite as thin as soup."

MTs are trained to transcribe many things in a "politically correct" manner. Perhaps my favorite of all descriptions for a deceased patient that follows the true precepts of "politically correct" is this sentence posted in an Internet message forum: "Patient failed to achieve wellness potential."

Some of the most creative mental pictures are provided by what is known as "doctorisms"—made-up words that may or may not exist in a dictionary but are perfectly valid for use in medical reports. An individual MT or patient may have never seen or heard them, but they are words that are commonly used, sometimes even in journal articles, that other dictators will understand without any problem at all:

"The patient almost syncopized in the restroom." This means the patient almost fainted, but it leaves one with visions of a patient unsuccessfully trying to get those feet moving in the same rhythm as the rest of the bathroom chorus line!

"The patient was primatized." I have to admit that at first I took this to mean that the patient, by some arcane sort of medical treatment, was converted into a primate, but I was indignantly informed that this meant the patient received a treatment of Primatene Mist.

Of course, it is not always the dictator's mistakes that cause a report to come back across our desks with great big red circles and exclamation points on it. It is just as likely to be the MT who hits that crucial wrong key or "hears" something that is a tad off: "Some of the glands exhibit secretary material"; "... performed a total abdominal hysterectomy and bilateral slaplingo-oophorectomy."

All in all, I tend to look at all this as *slaplingopathy*—the practice of slapping one's thigh and laughing uproariously. (Or would that be "ridiculopathy"?)

Exercises

Chapter Review

Instructions: Choose the best answer.

____ 1. Correcting a dictator's misspeak would be an example of which of the following editing activities?
   A. Deletion.
   B. Addition.
   C. Alteration.
   D. Adaptation.

____ 2. In "Adventures in Thought Transference," Dr. Dirckx discusses editorial activity being performed at all of the following levels EXCEPT _____
   A. formal.
   B. informal.
   C. phonetic.
   D. conceptual.

____ 3. At the phonetic level of the dictation-transcription process, the transcriptionist inserts "silent" letters, _____, selects the correct one of several alternative spellings, and recognizes deviant pronunciations.
   A. corrects misspeaks
   B. verifies and corrects discrepancies
   C. suppresses extraneous sounds
   D. supplies omitted words and phrases

____ 4. Many question the propriety of the transcriptionist _____
   A. judging and altering the factual content of a dictation.
   B. correcting the dictator's grammar and syntax.
   C. touching up the style to improve clarity and coherence.
   D. all of the above.

____ 5. Successfully translating the dictation of those who are foreign-born requires one to become familiar with the _____
   A. speech patterns of various nationalities.
   B. the alphabet of foreign languages.
   C. as many foreign languages as possible.
   D. culture of the dictator.

____ 6. *Mole* meaning "small mammal" and *mole* meaning "pigmented nevus" are examples of _____
   A. homographs.
   B. homonyms.
   C. homophones.
   D. slang.

____ 7. *Tínnitus* and *tinnítus* are examples of _____
   A. homographs.
   B. homonyms.
   C. homophones.
   D. slang.

____ 8. *Patience* and *patients* are examples of _____
   A. homographs.
   B. homonyms.
   C. homophones.
   D. slang.

____ 9. The recognition and interpretation of speech sounds and their correct representation in writing is a _____ editorial process.
   A. phonetic
   B. cultural
   C. conceptual
   D. formal

____ 10. Monitoring of word choice, grammar, and style is a _____ editorial process.
   A. conceptual
   B. cultural
   C. formal
   D. phonetic

___ 11. Insertion or editing of punctuation, ensuring consistency of format, and using appropriate units of measure is a _____ editorial process.
A. conceptual
B. cultural
C. formal
D. phonetic

___ 12. A basic library for a medical transcriptionist should include all of the following EXCEPT _____.
A. an English dictionary.
B. full-sized medical dictionary.
C. word and phrase books for individual specialties.
D. a current drug reference that includes indications and dosages.

___ 13. The usefulness of word books or spellers for students and inexperienced transcriptionists is limited because _____

A. they do not contain definitions.
B. they often include nonpreferred spellings.
C. it is difficult to distinguish between homophones.
D. all of the above.

___ 14. An important element in evaluating reference books is _____
A. authorship.
B. number of pages.
C. the inclusion of appendices.
D. number of stars by reviewers.

___ 15. If you cannot be sure of the word you are hearing, you should _____
A. just leave it out.
B. leave a blank.
C. make an educated guess.
D. none of the above.

___ 16. Slang words are not acceptable because they are either obscure, can have multiple meanings, or the brief form has been pulled from the _____
A. beginning of a longer term.
B. the first letter of each syllable.
C. middle or end of a longer term.
D. all of the above.

PEARSON
myhealthprofessionskit™

To access the online exercises for this chapter, go to **www.myhealthprofessionskit.com**. Select "Medical Transcription," then click on the title of this book, ***Healthcare Documentation: Fundamentals & Practice***.

Comic Relief

Absurdity Recognition

by Diane Guyer

Some people are convinced that there will soon be no need for medical transcriptionists. They think that voice recognition technology will make our jobs obsolete and that we will soon be as marketable as blacksmiths.

I am not worried, especially since receiving some interesting e-mails from editors who chuckle as they correct the outrageous things that are sometimes generated by speech recognition technology (SRT). For instance, a doctor with a bit of a choppy accent said, "she can range up to a . . ," but the SRT apparently heard "chicken range up to . . ." Another interesting example that was reported to me was an SRT interpretation of "back to bras and fusion" for "bacterial broth infusion." Another was "patient is being admitted for further violation" instead of "patient is being admitted for further evaluation."

Human systems have such an advantage over SRT! Although both may sort out sounds much the same way, humans filter the possible interpretations through our trusty gray matter and recognize absurdity when we hear it. For instance, it only takes a moment to figure out that what we heard as "a 50-cent, pea-sized lesion" is more likely to be "a 50-centpiece-sized lesion," and for the sake of clarity, we may even change it to "a lesion the size of a 50-cent piece." We quickly reinterpret what sounds like "the patient is experiencing quite a bit of discomfort at the sight [site] of his appendectomy incision." It is obvious to us that we should choose "increasing in size" over "increasing in sighs" or "increasing incise," even though all three sound the same. We are not tricked into transcribing "patchless" for "patulous," and we know the difference between "a neuroma" and "an aroma." We automatically eliminate any reference to lunch meat whenever we hear anything involving "below-knee."

I should add, though, that sometimes what sounds absurd is true. I thought for sure that I was hearing wrong when a local doctor dictated: "Patient comes in with several infected wounds after being gored by an antelope." I listened again and tried to make the dictated words sound like something else. I thought maybe the doctor was trying to say that the patient was eating a gourd and a cantaloupe, or perhaps that he was guarding an envelope, or that he was ignored when an aunt eloped, but no matter how hard I tried, all I could hear was "gored by an antelope." It wasn't until we got to Social History that I could breathe a sigh of relief. The patient was an animal handler at a zoo.

Then there is the issue of what we hear but *don't* transcribe. I am referring to the times when a physician is still working on a coherent thought and verbally tries out variations of what he or she wants to say. Just for fun one day, I saved a quotation to prove that human transcriptionists are still necessary.

There is no dominant mass in either breast, but there is dense fibroglandular breast tissue bilaterally, upper outer quadrants, both breasts, especially on the left side, 3 o'clock position, but—no, actually 1 o'clock position I should say, upper quadrants of both sides, especially left greater than right, but no dominant masses bilaterally.

This leads me to wonder how SRT handles the instructional and parenthetical remarks made by dictating physicians. I'm sure that "close parentheses" and "quote-unquote" have shown up more than once as "clothespin disease" and "caught in coat." I wonder if there are medical reports out there somewhere, not edited by humans, that contain words like, "Have I been saying 'left' all this time? It's really on the right, so go back and replace all the 'lefts' with 'rights.' Sorry. Thanks."

No SRT, no matter how advanced, can recognize the absurdity of accurate statements that are awkwardly expressed. Only a human editor can fix statements such as "The patient had his hernia surgery here, but his appendix was in Kansas."

Without good editing, even perfect verbatim transcription can be inaccurate. Although our jobs may change dramatically in the years ahead, there will always be a need for our valuable language skills. So, my friends, keep on keeping on. There is nothing to fear. Except maybe antelopes.

Perspectives on Style

5

Learning Objectives

▶ Define, spell, and use English words commonly used in healthcare documentation.

▶ Recognize and correctly spell commonly misspelled and misused English words.

▶ Recognize, correctly spell, and use common English soundalikes.

▶ Correctly use Arabic numerals, Roman numerals, and units of measure.

▶ Transcribe abbreviations, acronyms, and brief forms.

▶ Apply the rules of punctuation to ensure clarity and accuracy of communication.

▶ Correct sentences that may be inverted or fragmented.

Transcription Guidelines

Grammar, punctuation, and style are frequently discussed as a single unit. There are, however, distinctions.

Grammar consists of the rules by which words are combined to construct and arrange sentences. It includes determining agreement between subject and verb, pronoun and antecedent, and adjective and noun; using the parts of speech appropriately; and spelling correctly and using words properly according to their meaning. Grammar rules are the least flexible and have few exceptions. Dictators often compose their thoughts "on the fly," so to speak, and may make frequent errors in grammar. It is the job of the medical transcriptionist (MT) to correct those errors.

Punctuation consists of symbols used as pointers in sentences and to enhance meaning. There is some flexibility in punctuation rules and more exceptions than in grammar rules. One of the skills MT students must learn is to apply punctuation to the spoken word as they transcribe. This can be difficult. MTs also often have to correct a dictated punctuation mark when it is wrong. At times, dictated sentences do not conform to standard sentence structure, making editing necessary and punctuation difficult to determine.

Style, on the other hand, is very flexible. A clear style contributes to clarity of meaning. Style varies according to context. Spoken language, formal written language, literature, journalism, medical journals, and medical reports all use different styles. Even two medical journals may differ in their style preferences. Preference is a good word to associate with style because that's what style is—a preferred way of writing or speaking. It is useful for institutions and organizations to have their preferences standardized in writing for uniformity and consistency in appearance.

Each institution, facility, or transcription service has its own guidelines for MTs. Some adopt a published style reference and add their own guidelines. Others may have their own in-house style guide. Still others may have nothing in writing, and MTs find out by trial and error what the quality assurance department requires. The guidelines in this chapter are for your use in transcribing dictation accompanying this book. The styles and practices you encounter on the job may differ.

The following guidelines are not intended to be comprehensive but are general guidelines for the accurate transcription of the dictations accompanying this textbook. A medical transcription student or practicing MT should always have a comprehensive style guide, such as *The Book of Style for Medical Transcription*, latest edition (Modesto, CA: AHDI, Association for Healthcare Documentation Integrity), which we have used as our primary style reference.

You should read through this section before beginning to transcribe the dictations and again after you have transcribed a specialty. These guidelines will make more sense after you have transcribed a few reports.

Format and style. A variety of medical report formats and styles exist. See Chapter 2 for an overall review of report types and formats. The transcription samples at the end of the specialty chapters and the transcription keys for transcription practice demonstrate several different acceptable formats but by no means all of them. In general, we have followed the ASTM standard for medical report formats. The physician's dictating style may determine the appropriate format, or a particular medical facility may mandate certain format standards. Thus, various report formats may vary from dictator to dictator, report to report, and setting to setting.

We acknowledge that many stylistic factors determine proper editing, punctuation, and grammar, that our way is not the only way, and that respected reference materials vary and may even contradict one another and themselves. Additionally, the employer of the transcriptionist may mandate specific rules of style, grammar, and format, and in that case the transcriptionist should follow the employer's requirements.

Style issues. Speech recognition editing is having a major impact on style guidelines as well as the amount and kind of editing that is done. It is not within the scope of these guidelines to address the differences between speech recognition editing and the preparation of transcribed medical reports. For simplicity's sake, the transcript keys and these guidelines reflect the practices and standards used in **traditional transcription**.

Abbreviations

Abbreviation practices vary from institution to institution. In the past The Joint Commission spelled out rules for the use of abbreviations. Today its only policy concerning abbreviations is in regard to those that have been designated as "dangerous" or "error-prone." Some departments and companies have lists of acceptable abbreviations and their translations. Others use such nebulous guidelines as "Do not use any abbreviations that are not widely known or immediately recognized by the reader."

It is a good idea for students to spell out most abbreviations (except for laboratory, diagnostic, and radiology tests and metric units of measure) so that they learn the proper expansions. On the job, abbreviation expanders will no doubt handle the required expansions, but you still need to know the proper translation in order to create your expansion initially and in order to know that you have correctly interpreted the letters in the abbreviation. *H&P* sounds very much like *HNP*, but they do not mean the same thing and are not interchangeable.

In doctors' office notes, abbreviations are used much more liberally than in hospital and clinic records. As students, however, you should make an effort to know the correct translation of every abbreviation you transcribe and follow these general rules.

Abbreviations in Dosages

When abbreviations are used with numbers for medication dosage times, use periods.

q.4 h. (every 4 hours)
Note the space after the number.

Abbreviations That Need Not Be Expanded

Some abbreviations are rarely or never expanded. In rare instances, the translation of abbreviations may cause confusion rather than achieve clarity. This is particularly true for many laboratory, radiographic, and other diagnostic procedures as well as department or unit name abbreviations. These abbreviations and others like them do not need to be translated; if dictated in full, however, they should be transcribed as dictated.

ALT (alanine aminotransferase)
AST (aspartate aminotransferase)
CBC (complete blood count)
CT scan (computed tomography scan)
ECG, EKG (electrocardiogram)
ED (emergency department)
ICU (intensive care unit)
IM (intramuscular)
IV (intravenous)
IVP (intravenous pyelogram)
KUB (kidneys and urinary bladder) x-ray
L5-S1 (5th lumbar vertebra and 1st sacral vertebra)
MRI (magnetic resonance imaging)

PT (prothrombin time)
PTT (partial thromboplastin time)
VDRL (Venereal Disease Research Laboratory)
WBC, WBCs (white blood count *or* white blood cells)

Note: Do not use abbreviations that can be translated more than one way (for example, CVA or PND) unless the abbreviation has been translated in the report already.

Some terms that appear to be abbreviations may not be readily translatable or may be brand names. The following abbreviations fall in this category:

DDD pacemaker
ST depression
T.E.D. hose

Body of the Report

Expand most abbreviations on first use in the body of the report and place the abbreviation itself within parentheses. Subsequent uses of the abbreviation in the same report may be transcribed as dictated.

D: The patient was admitted with DOE and chest pain.
T: The patient was admitted with dyspnea on exertion (DOE) and chest pain.

D: Eyes: PERRLA. EOMI.
T: Eyes: Pupils equal, round, reactive to light and accommodation (PERRLA). Extraocular movements intact (EOMI).

Diagnoses

Expand almost all abbreviations for diseases, syndromes, and symptoms and operative procedure titles, in diagnoses, impressions, and assessments; place the abbreviation in parentheses after the expansion. If the abbreviation is repeated in the body of the report, transcribe as dictated.

D: ADMITTING IMPRESSION
COPD.
T: ADMITTING IMPRESSION
Chronic obstructive pulmonary disease (COPD).

D: FINAL DIAGNOSIS
Status post CABG.
T: FINAL DIAGNOSIS
Status post coronary artery bypass graft (CABG).

Error-Prone Abbreviations

The Institute for Safe Medication Practices (ISMP) publishes a list of error-prone abbreviations related to the prescribing and administering of drugs that are considered dangerous because they could be misread. From this list, The Joint Commission has identified a "minimum list" of abbreviations that are *not* to be used. In addition, each organization must identify and apply at least three other "do not use" abbreviations, acronyms, and brief forms. Eventually, avoidance of the entire list will be implemented.

Listed below are the abbreviations you should avoid using in transcription of the *Healthcare Documentation: Fundamentals & Practice* reports. A complete list of error-prone abbreviations can be found at **www.ismp.org/**

If Dictated	Transcribe
AD	right ear
AS	left ear
AU	each ear
AZT	zidovudine
cc (cubic centimeters)	use *mL* with drug dosages and liquid measurements

If Dictated	Transcribe
D/C or DC	discharge or discontinue
HCTZ	hydrochlorothiazide
h.s.	at bedtime
IU	unit
microgram	mcg
OD	right eye
OS	left eye
OU	each eye
per os	p.o., by mouth, *or* orally
q.d., QD	daily *or* every day
q.h.s.	nightly *or* at bedtime
q.o.d., QOD	every other day
/ (slash mark)	use *per* to separate doses
subq, sq, or SC	subcu
U (for unit)	unit
zero to right of decimal	Do not insert a zero after the decimal (3.0) unless dictated as part of a lab value.
zero to left of decimal	Always insert a zero before the decimal when the value is less than 1 (0.5).

Measurements

Abbreviate all metric and SI (International System of Measuring Units) units of measure when used with numerals. Expand English units of measure, except when used in tables. Expand metric and SI units of measure when not preceded by a numeral.

8 mEq	10.8 mV
5 cm	height 5 feet 6 inches
a few milliliters	several millimeters
6 mL	weight 120 pounds

When a measurement is dictated but the unit of measure omitted, it should be added if it can be done with certainty.

D: Height five six
T: Height 5 feet 6 inches

D: Decadron 0.75
T: Decadron 0.75 mg

Note: When *foot* is dictated for *feet*, transcribe *feet*.

Plural Abbreviations

To make an abbreviation plural, simply add a lowercase *s* with no apostrophe if the abbreviation is in all capital letters.

IVs were ordered to run to keep open (TKO).
The patient stated she had had 6 BMs in less than 3 hours.
The urinalysis revealed too-numerous-to-count WBCs.

Report Headings

Expand abbreviations used in report headings and subheadings.

D: CC
T: CHIEF COMPLAINT

D: HPI
T: HISTORY OF PRESENT ILLNESS

D: Neuro
T: NEUROLOGIC

Note: It is acceptable to transcribe the abbreviation HEENT as a subheading.

Style for Abbreviations

Medical abbreviations are written several ways. The three most common include all capital letters, a combination of capital and lowercase letters, and all lowercase letters with periods (primarily Latin terms used with drug dosages).

Today periods are rarely used in all-capital abbreviations unless it is a stated preference of an association or organization. Use periods in lowercase drug-related Latin abbreviations (b.i.d.) but not in non-Latin lowercase abbreviations (rbc/hpf). Generally speaking, although the style is acceptable, it is best to avoid lowercase abbreviations other than Latin abbreviations (p.r.n.) and units of measure (cm). The reason for this is that the lowercase abbreviations get lost in the text.

ACLS (advanced cardiac life support)
b.i.d. (twice a day)
CBC (complete blood count)
mmHg (millimeters of mercury)
mV (millivolt)
pCO2, PCO2, pO2 (no subscripts in transcripts)
pH
p.o. or PO (by mouth; orally)
p.r.n. (as needed)
q.i.d. (four times a day)
RBC (red blood cells)
rbc/hpf (red blood cells per high power field)
TED (thromboembolic disease)
T.E.D. stockings (a brand name)
t.i.d. (three times a day)
WBC (white blood cells)

Note: Special styles used in publishing, such as small caps and subscripts or superscripts, are rarely used in transcription because special characters do not transmit well electronically.

Uncertain Abbreviations

Never expand an abbreviation in a report if you are uncertain of the translation in the context of the report. If you cannot translate an abbreviation with confidence in its correct meaning, use the abbreviation and flag the report to the dictator's attention.

Examples of abbreviations with multiple translations:

CVA (cerebrovascular accident)
CVA (costovertebral angle)
CVA (cardiovascular accident) (rarely)

PND (paroxysmal nocturnal dyspnea)
PND (postnasal drip)

D: CHIEF COMPLAINT
PND.
T: CHIEF COMPLAINT
_____ (PND).

Note: There are many such abbreviations that can be confused. Always proceed with caution when translating abbreviations.

Words or Phrases Dictated in Full

Do not abbreviate a word or phrase dictated in full; transcribe as dictated. An exception is metric units of measure, which are routinely abbreviated when used with numerals (3 cm, 10 mg).

Apostrophes

Apostrophes are used to show possession, indicate omitted letters or numbers, and occasionally to form plurals of single lowercase letters and numbers.

Eponyms

The stylistic trend is away from using the possessive form with eponyms. It is important to note, however, that use of the possessive form remains an acceptable alternative if dictated and/or if indicated as the preference by employer or client.

Apgar score	Alzheimer disease
Babinski sign	Down syndrome
Gram stain	Hodgkin lymphoma
McBurney point	Mohs technique
Janeway lesions	Osler nodes

The possessive form is preferred when the noun following the eponym is omitted although it is understood.

He was treated for a possible Wernicke's.
He has Alzheimer's but is otherwise in good health.

If *a*, *an*, or *the* precedes an eponym, do not use the possessive form.

She was placed in the Trendelenburg position.
The Bassini hernia repair was accomplished
without difficulty.

Do not use an apostrophe to show possession in hyphenated eponyms.

> Abbe-Estlander operation
> Osgood-Schlatter disease
> Jackson-Pratt drain

Do not use the possessive when referring to surgical instruments and medical devices.

> Fogarty catheter (not Fogarty's catheter)
> DeBakey clamp (not DeBakey's clamp)
> St. Jude valve (not St. Jude's valve)

Missing Elements

Use apostrophes to indicate missing letters or numbers. The use of contractions in medical reports is not recommended, except when quoting a patient.

> *Acceptable*:
> The patient described shortness of breath present since the '90s.
> The patient complained, "I'm not passing any urine."

> *Not acceptable*:
> We won't know the results of the biopsy until Thursday.

Plurals

Do not use apostrophes to form the plurals of abbreviations or numbers, except to avoid confusion when lowercase letters or symbols are made plural.

> serial 7's   x's and y's
> +'s   4 x 4's
> WBCs   ABGs
> 40s   1990s

Possession

Use an apostrophe to form the possessive of a unit of time. Add an apostrophe and *s* ('s) to singular nouns and after the *s* on plural nouns.

> The uterus is 16 weeks' size.
> 1 hour's time
> 2 hours' time
> 3 days' time

Use an apostrophe to show possession with nouns.

> the patient's chart
> the patient's clinical presentation
> the recovery room's capacity
> the RN's pen
> the parents' concerns
> the nurses' opinions
> 2 cents' worth

Brief Forms and Slang

Brief forms are shortened forms of legitimate words that can be documented in a dictionary or have come into acceptance through usage. Brief forms can be confused with medical slang. A slang term is either not listed in a dictionary or is designated as slang. Sometimes it is difficult to differentiate between a slang word and a new term that may become standard usage with time. In the Quick-Reference Word List, slang terms are listed in quotation marks, indicating they must be expanded in medical reports ("lytes" = electrolytes).

Physicians commonly use medical slang when discussing a patient's condition, but that does not mean the same slang term is acceptable in the medical transcript. Avoid transcribing slang that disparages patients or staff. Physicians do not intend for offensive or off-color remarks to be entered into a patient's health record.

Medical slang should be avoided in medical documents for several reasons. A slang term may be obscure and might not clearly or accurately convey the intended meaning. Additionally, a slang term may be open to varied interpretations by different readers of the record, particularly obvious when a health record is subpoenaed for use in legal actions. It may be difficult to replace a slang term with an appropriate nonslang term. Flag the report if you cannot edit the term appropriately. In diagnoses and impressions, brief forms and abbreviations should be expanded.

See box, next page, for a list of terms that are currently deemed acceptable or equivocal and others that are unacceptable. Acceptable or equivocal means they are acceptable in some settings but not in others, or acceptable in some less formal reports like chart notes but not in others. Unacceptable are brief forms and medical slang that may be confused with similar terms and thus must be written out in medical transcription for clarity. A good rule to remember is, "When in doubt, write it out."

BRIEF FORMS AND MEDICAL SLANG

ACCEPTABLE BRIEF FORMS

ab, Ab	abortion
bands	banded neutrophils
basos	basophils
cardio	cardiology
chemo	chemotherapy
consult (n.)	consultation
C-section	cesarean section
C-spine	cervical spine
eos	eosinophils
exam	examination
lab	laboratory
LS spine	lumbosacral spine
lymphs	lymphocytes
monos	monocytes
neuro	neurology, neurologic
NICU ("nick-yoo")	neonatal intensive care unit
ortho	orthopedic(s)
PACU ("pack-yoo")	postanesthesia care unit
Pap smear	Papanicolaou smear
path	pathology
polys	polymorphonuclear leukocytes
postop	postoperative
preop	preoperative
prepped	prepared
pro time	prothrombin time
rehab	rehabilitation
segs	segmented neutrophils
strep	streptococcal
subcu	subcutaneous
T-spine	thoracic spine

UNACCEPTABLE MEDICAL SLANG

A fib	atrial fibrillation
alk phos	alkaline phosphatase
amp	ampule, ampicillin
appy	appendectomy
bili	bilirubin
BP	blood pressure
CA, ca	carcinoma
cabbage	CABG (coronary artery bypass graft)
cath, cath'd	catheter, catheterized
chole	cholelithiasis
circ	circumflex artery
coags	coagulation studies

crit	hematocrit
cysto	cystoscopy
D/C, D/C'd	discontinue(d), discharge(d)
diff	differential
dig ("dij")	digitalis
echo	echocardiogram
epi	epinephrine
fib	fibula, fibrillation
fib-flutter	fibrillation-flutter
fluoro	fluoroscopy
H&H	hemoglobin and hematocrit
H. flu	H. (*Haemophilus*) *influenzae*
kilo	kg (kilogram)
lap	laparoscopy, laparotomy
lap chole	laparoscopic cholecystectomy
lytes	electrolytes
med, meds	medication(s)
mets	metastases
Metz	Metzenbaum scissors
mills	millimeters
multip	multipara
nitro	nitroglycerin
osteo	osteomyelitis
path	pathology
peds	pediatrics
pentam	pentamidine
primip	primipara
procto	proctoscopy
psych	psychiatric
quads	quadriceps
retic	reticulocyte
Rx; script	prescription
sats	(oxygen) saturation
satting	saturating
tab	tablet
tabby	therapeutic abortion
tach	tachycardia
temp	temperature
tib	tibia
tib-fib	tibia-fibula
tic	diverticulum
T max	maximum temperature
trach	tracheostomy
trich	trichomonas
V fib	ventricular fibrillation
V tach	ventricular tachycardia
XRT	radiotherapy

Capitalization

Classifications and Stages

Do not capitalize words that denote categories or classifications.

> Bruce protocol
> Child class C
> class III cardiac failure
> grade 1/6 murmur
> grade 1 to 2 internal hemorrhoids
> stage I
> TIMI grade 3 flow
> type 2 diabetes
> type IIb hyperlipidemia

Department Names and Specialties

Do not capitalize a term denoting a specialist, a specialty, or a department within a medical facility.

> ophthalmology, ophthalmologist
> physical therapy, physical therapist
> emergency department
> infectious diseases

Do capitalize department names and specialties if they are referred to as people or entities.

> The patient will be seen by Pulmonology in the morning.
> I have asked Neurology to see the patient prior to and after surgery.
> Physical Therapy will plan a rehabilitation program for this patient after surgery.

Directions

Do not capitalize the first letter of points on a compass unless referring to geographical regions or for clarity.

> The clinic is east of the hospital.
> The patient is from the Southeast.
> The patient is on 3 East.
> He just moved to the West Coast.

Diseases and Anatomical Landmarks

Do not capitalize diseases or anatomic landmarks unless they are eponyms (named for a person).

> chronic obstructive pulmonary disease
> Alzheimer disease

Eponyms and Capitals

Capitalize the person's name that is the basis of an eponym.

> Gram stain
> Lyme disease
> Rovsing sign
> Stargardt disease

Do not capitalize an eponym made into an adjective or verb.

> cushingoid facies
> gram-negative bacteria
> malpighian bodies
> parkinsonian
> jacksonian seizure

Headings

Capitalize all letters in main headings (CHIEF COMPLAINT), unless instructed otherwise. Only the initial letter of each word in a subheading is capitalized, except in the physical exam of an H&P, where the subheadings are listed vertically and in all capitals.

Capitalize the first word following a colon in a heading or subheading, if the narrative format is used. See **Formats** for more information on headings.

Race, Ethnicity, Skin Color

Capitalize a person's race, ethnic or national origin, but not skin color. Hyphenating compound modifiers indicating national origin is no longer recommended.

Caucasian female	white female
African American male	black male
Asian female	Hispanic male

Titles and Degrees

Capitalize titles such as *RN, CMT, CMA, RHIT,* and academic degrees such as *MD, DO, PhD, BA, MA, and MEd. Doctor* is correctly abbreviated as *Dr.* When transcribing a medical doctor's name, do not use both *Dr.* and *MD.* Abbreviations of degrees and professional ratings are often unpunctuated, but if periods are used, do not space between the letters.

MD, M.D.	PhD, Ph.D.
MA, M.A.	MEd, M.Ed.

Trademarks

Trademarked and registered terms (devices and drugs) are generally transcribed with an initial capital letter. Mixed capitalization may be used, if known. However, manufacturers will often show their trademarks in all capital letters, a marketing technique to make the name stand out in advertisements and press releases. This practice is inappropriate for medical reports as it draws undue attention to the term.

As with eponyms, derivatives of trademarked terms are not capitalized. With few exceptions, common nouns (blade, suture, device, stapler, etc.) used with trademarked terms are not part of the trademark and are not capitalized.

Some terms may sound like they're trademarks but aren't. You cannot trust Google results for proper capitalization, style, or spelling of trademarked terms, so it's always a good idea to confirm a trademarked term, either in a reputable reference or on the manufacturer's website.

> Angelchik ring prosthesis
> Bovie cautery, but bovied
> collodion dressing
> Endo Catch bag
> Endoloop suture
> Epifoam
> Gore-Tex mesh
> Harmonic Scalpel (Scalpel is part of the trademark)
> Medipore tape
> PerFix Marlex plug
> Polysorb suture
> Port-A-Cath
> ProTack fixation device
> Savary esophageal dilator
> squeegied (from Mr. Squeegy)
> Steri-Strips, but steri-stripped
> Tegaderm dressing
> Tylenol with Codeine No. 3 tablets
> Ventralex sheet

Tip: Newer drugs and trademarked devices often have a dedicated web page, and you can put the term correctly spelled into the URL box followed by **.com** and hit Enter to get more information about a drug or device.

Eponyms

Eponyms are capitalized, but the nouns they modify are not. Derivatives of eponyms are not capitalized. The use of the apostrophe plus s ('s) to form a possessive eponym is acceptable when dictated. When the eponym is used alone without the accompanying noun, the possessive is retained. The reports in this unit were transcribed as dictated, and the 's was used when the physician dictated the possessive form.

> Barrett esophagus *or* Barrett's esophagus
> Cooper ligament *or* Cooper's ligament
> Crohn disease *or* Crohn's disease
> McBurney point *or* McBurney's point
> jacksonian seizure (from Jackson)
> Jackson-Pratt drain
> lactated Ringer's
> Meckel diverticulum *or* Meckel's diverticulum
> spigelian hernia
> subscarpally
> Scarpa fascia *or* Scarpa's fascia
> Scarpa's was reapproximated …
> Trendelenburg position

Format

There are many acceptable formats for the setup of medical and surgical reports. Many facilities use templates for each report type that contain the standard or required headings. The transcriptionist just types the dictated text following the appropriate heading, adding headings to the template or deleting them based on the dictator's style and facility specifications. See the sample template for an H&P at the end of this chapter. Using the sample H&P template as a guide, you can create your own templates using the content descriptions of the various report types discussed in chapter 2.

In addition, there are alternative acceptable forms for the same sentence, depending on whether the format calls for a narrative such as might be contained in a discharge summary, subheadings such as in a consult or office note, or main headings as in the physical examination portion of an H&P. The following examples represent just a few of such variations in format.

D: Extremities unremarkable.
T: (as dictated or)
   The extremities are unremarkable.
   (Narrative paragraph format.)

T: EXTREMITIES: Unremarkable.
   (Formal Physical Examination with separate paragraphs for each subheading.)

T: EXTREMITIES: The extremities are unremarkable.
   (Formal Physical Examination with separate paragraphs for each subheading.)

Note: If full sentences are dictated and headings need to be added, add the heading and transcribe the full sentence. Don't lop off the subject of the sentence as a heading and start the text with a verb or phrase.

Paragraphing

Transcribe paragraphs as dictated unless paragraphing would alter medical meaning or continuity. Paragraphing may be added where appropriate to break up long reports, to delineate headings, and to separate the findings from the details of the procedure in an operative report. In a long operative report, a good place to add paragraphs is when the dictator says something like "Attention was then turned," or "Next, …"

Headings

The transcriptionist may add headings and subheadings as appropriate. If a physician dictates the singular form *Diagnosis* when more than one diagnosis is provided, the transcriptionist may transcribe either *Diagnosis* or *Diagnoses*.

The transcriptionist should be alert for important headings that are not dictated but are a vital part of the report. These include the Final or Discharge Diagnosis in a Discharge Summary; the Diagnosis or Impression in a History and Physical and a Consultation; and the Preoperative and Postoperative Diagnoses and Title of Operation in an Operative Report. If any of these are not dictated, the transcriptionist should supply them as appropriate or flag the report to the attention of the dictator.

Abbreviations and brief forms should be expanded in headings and subheadings.

Diagnoses and Lists

When the dictator says *Same* for a discharge diagnosis or postoperative diagnosis, copy and paste the diagnosis to which the dictator is referring; do not transcribe the word *Same*. Dictators may or may not dictate numbers; however, diagnoses should be transcribed in a numbered vertical format if more than one diagnosis is dictated. Medications may be transcribed as a vertical list or in a horizontal narrative style. On the job, facility specifications would dictate how lists should be transcribed, including any special formatting for diagnoses.

MEDICATIONS
Patient is on the following medicines:
1. Albuterol inhaler 2 puffs 4 times a day.
2. Lortab 7.5/500 one tablet p.r.n. for pain.
3. Prednisone 5 mg once a day.
4. Theophylline 300 mg twice a day.
5. Atrovent inhaler 2 puffs 4 times day.

Misplaced Modifiers

With the trend toward verbatim transcription and the widescale adoption of speech recognition, misplaced modifiers and awkward phrasing have become less troublesome to many and are rarely edited. *However, when a sentence is extremely awkward or provokes unintended humor or when the meaning is unclear, judicious editing is recommended.*

D: CT evaluation on several occasions of her abdomen revealed …
T: (As dictated or) CT evaluation of her abdomen on several occasions …

D: Once it was freed completely, it appeared to be a lipoma with a nodule which was felt to be *later* fat necrosis.
T: (As dictated or) Once it was freed completely, it appeared to be a lipoma with a nodule which *later* was felt to be fat necrosis.

From a colonoscopy report:
D: No source of bleeding was seen until *I* was coming out and was sitting in the transverse colon when she got very upset …
T: No source of bleeding was seen until *the scope* was coming out and was sitting in the transverse colon when she got very upset …

D: Pneumoperitoneum was allowed to develop, and evaluation with the camera revealed no evidence of harm to *our* abdominal contents.
T: Pneumoperitoneum was allowed to develop, and evaluation with the camera revealed no evidence of harm to abdominal contents.

D: Dr. _____ performed the *cystocele* first, which is dictated under a separate note.
T: Dr. _____ performed the cystocele *repair* first, which is dictated under a separate note.

Numbers

At Beginning of Sentence

Avoid beginning a sentence with a numeral. Either write out the number or alter the beginning of the sentence.

D: 2 mL of Xylocaine was given.
T: Xylocaine 2 mL was given.

D: 45-year-old black male
T: A 45-year-old black male *or*
    This is a 45-year-old black male *or*
    This 45-year-old black male (if verb follows)

D: ... then the abdomen was reclosed. #1 Prolene was used in a running fashion, starting at both ends and meeting in the center.
T: ... then the abdomen was reclosed. A #1 Prolene was used in a running fashion, starting at both ends and meeting in the center.
                        or
T: ... then the abdomen was reclosed; #1 Prolene was used in a running fashion, starting at both ends and meeting in the center.
                        or
T: ... then the abdomen was reclosed. No. 1 Prolene was used in a running fashion, starting at both ends and meeting in the center.

D: Twenty milliliters of 0.5% Marcaine with epinephrine was used as field block.
T: Then 20 mL of 0.5% Marcaine with epinephrine was used as a field block.

D: ...subcuticular suture. 15 cc of half percent Marcaine with epinephrine...
T: Half-percent Marcaine 15 mL with epinephrine
T: ... subcuticular suture; 15 mL of 0.5% Marcaine with epinephrine was . . .

The wound was then packed open after assessment for hemostasis; 30 mL of 0.5% Marcaine with epinephrine was used as field block . . .

Note: If the preceding sentence is related, you can use a semicolon instead of a period and transcribe as dictated.

When a quantity and unit of measure immediately follow a heading such as estimated blood loss at the beginning of an operative report, however, transcribe the numerals.

D: Estimated blood loss 10 mL.
T: ESTIMATED BLOOD LOSS
    10 mL.

Fractions

Fractions should be transcribed as decimals when they are used with metric units of measure, and decimals should be converted to fractions when they are used with standard units of measure.

English fractions may be spelled out or transcribed as numbers, depending on style preferences; quarter-inch Penrose drain or 1/4-inch Penrose drain are both acceptable. Do not allow Autocorrect to convert English fractions (1/4, 1/2, 3/4) into single-digit numbers (¼, ½, ¾) as these characters may not transfer correctly to another computer system.

0.25 cm   1/4 inch   3.5 mL

Note: Dictators almost always dictate metric fractions the same way they dictate English fractions: one-half is 0.5 in metric, 1/2 in English; one-quarter is 0.25 in metric, 1/4 in English.

Metric numbers less than one should be preceded with a zero and a decimal point (0.5) to avoid the decimal being lost and the number interpreted as a whole number rather than a fraction, whether or not the zero was dictated. If the physician dictates a whole number with a decimal point and a zero (3.0), retain the decimal and the zero if the value refers to a laboratory test result or dimensions or volume in surgery and pathology. If the value refers to a drug dose, do not place a decimal and a zero after the whole number.

0.5 mm in diameter
3 cm in length *but* 3 inches
10 mg of diazepam

Adjacent Numbers

Spell out one of the numbers to avoid the juxtaposition of two numbers.

three 2-0 Ethibond sutures
figure-of-8 #0 Maxon *or*
0 Maxon figure-of-8 suture
three 1 to 1.5 cm stab injuries
series of two #2 silks
Two #1 PDS sutures were placed.

Inexact Numbers

In general, spell out inexact values and the unit of measure. However, if the article *a* is used to represent the number *1*, transcribe the numeral.

D & T: several centimeters

D & T: I was able to clear away a centimeter plus in diameter circumferentially around the opening.

D: It was approximately a centimeter in diameter or less.
T: It was approximately 1 cm in diameter or less.

D: The hole itself was approximately a centimeter and a half or so in diameter.
T: The hole itself was approximately 1.5 cm or so in diameter.

D: … we had been in the operating room already an hour and a half….
T: …. we had been in the operating room already 1-1/2 hours…

Plural Numbers

Do not add an apostrophe when pluralizing multi-digit numbers; do add an apostrophe when making single-digit numbers plural.

100s   4 x 4's

Suture, Blade, and Drain Sizes

A number sign may or may not be dictated. As a general rule, transcribe as dictated. When the size is a whole number, the number sign may be added for clarity. A size zero suture may be dictated and transcribed as 0 or 1-0. Multiples of 0 should be expressed with a number and hyphen before the zero.

0 suture *or* 1-0 suture
2-0 Dexon suture
#1 Tevdek suture
#10 Blake drain
#11 blade (the word *number* is dictated)
an 11 blade (*number* not dictated)

Punctuation

Standard punctuation is followed in these transcripts. Where the physician dictates punctuation marks, you should transcribe as dictated, unless the punctuation is incorrect or results in an error in meaning. Punctuation marks may be added or changed to clarify meaning and assist in reading.

Colon/Capitalization

Capitalize the first word following a colon in a heading or subheading.

HEART: The heart sounds are strong on auscultation.

Comma

The comma is probably the most misused punctuation mark in the written English language. Misuse includes inserting too many commas, too few, or using them inappropriately so that the meaning of a sentence is unclear or easily misconstrued. In medical transcription, this can have serious consequences by changing medical meaning.

Absolute Phrases

Use a comma before or after an absolute phrase—a noun or pronoun followed by a participle and possibly other words—when it appears at the beginning or end of a sentence.

A DNR order having been signed, the patient was taken off life support.
The patient was subsequently discharged, having received maximum benefit of hospitalization.
Given the penetration of the capsule of the pancreas overlying the pancreatic head, we elected to leave a Blake drain.

Adjectives Following the Noun

When even a single adjective follows a noun, as often happens in diagnoses, separate the noun and the adjective(s) with a comma.

Questionable osteomyelitis, right calcaneus.
Chronic otitis media, left ear.
Left hemiparesis and hemiplegia, status post cerebrovascular accident (CVA).
She did have a hemiarthroplasty, bipolar type, of the left hip.

Adjectives in a Series

Use a comma to separate adjectives in a series, but do not put a comma between the last adjective in a series and the noun that follows it.

> Fat pads were taken from the nasal, central, and lateral compartments of each lower lid.

Use a comma to separate paired coordinate adjectives that have no relationship to each other.

> Gross examination revealed ratty, discolored tissue.

Tip: If you can substitute *and* for the comma or change the order of the adjectives, and the sentence sounds natural, it is usually safe to use the comma.

Do not use commas between cumulative adjectives, which are adjectives that build upon one another. In most writing, it is considered bad form to use more than three or four adjectives in a row, but it happens quite often in medical transcription. Should the order of the dictated phrase vary, you would generally not edit to a different order but transcribe as dictated.

> The dissection revealed a dark green muddy fluid behind the pancreas.

> bilateral lower extremity TED hose

When the patient's race is given, consider it to be part of the noun and not an adjective.

> The patient is a frail, disoriented 70-year-old Caucasian female.

Adverbs in a Series

Do not use a comma to separate an adverb from the adjective or other adverb it modifies. The adverbs are in bold.

> The patient had a **very** large, protruding, pendulous mass.
> The patient was **mildly hemodynamically** unstable while in the emergency department but stabilized on the floor.

Appositives

Use commas to set off an appositive—a noun or phrase situated next to or near a word that it expands upon or explains. While often nonessential, an appositive is sometimes essential, in which case no commas would be used.

> Marion Bartley, MD, was asked to come to the surgery suite to stent the ureters.

> After reviewing the patient's morning labs, including CBC, PT, and PTT, the procedure started.
> The patient had a very large mass, the size of an orange, filling most of the right atrium.
> Patient was despondent over his social situation, details of which were not provided by the patient.

Aside or Afterthought

These terms are used here to identify late-coming explanations, usually adverbial phrases or clauses, and usually appearing at the end of a sentence.

> He subsequently was placed in rehabilitation where he improved, only to later show a decline in his walking.
> Femoral pulses were diminished in both right and the left, somewhat more on the left side.
> It was evident that the patient had a large prolapsing hemorrhoid, too large for rubber banding, and it was considered appropriate for a standard hemorrhoidectomy operation.
> He was given IV Ancef for infection prophylaxis, the presacral area prepped and sterilely draped in the customary fashion.
> Colonoscope was then removed, patient taken to the recovery room in stable condition.

Note: In some of the examples the phrase set off by commas appears at the end of an independent clause, although it is not at the end of the sentence.

Clauses in a Series

Three or more independent clauses (complete sentences) that are clearly meant to be one sentence where the final two clauses are joined by a coordinating conjunction are punctuated with commas.

> The wound was irrigated and inspected, sutures were placed, and a bandage was applied.

Commas and Compound Sentences

Use a comma to separate two independent clauses (complete sentences) joined by a coordinating conjunction (*and, but, for, nor, or, so, yet*).

> The patient complains of difficulty finding the right word, but he denies any extremity weakness.
> The patient's condition improved, and he was transferred from ICU to a regular bed.
> The patient's cardiac catheterization revealed only moderate stenosis of the left circumflex, and we will treat him conservatively.

If the two independent clauses—each a complete sentence—are short (fewer than four or five words long) and closely related, a comma is optional.

> He had tried chemotherapy but it was not tolerated well.

Note: Compound coordinating conjunctions (*either . . . or*) do not require a comma to separate the clauses.

> Either the chemistry panel results are erroneous or this patient's electrolytes are completely off the scale.

Do not insert a comma before a coordinating conjunction like *but* that is not followed by both a subject and a complete verb (including helping verb).

> *Incorrect:* Dermatitis apparently cleared after 34 days of ketoconazole and Augmentin, but recurred after 2 weeks off antibiotics.
> *Correct:* Dermatitis apparently cleared after 34 days of ketoconazole and Augmentin but recurred after 2 weeks off antibiotics.

> *Incorrect:* No adventitious lung sounds were noted, and no congestion identified.
> *Correct:* No adventitious lung sounds were noted and no congestion identified.

Note: In this latter example, there is a subject and a verb after the conjunction, but the verb is incomplete (*was identified* would make it complete).

Commas in a Series

Commas are used with nouns, adjectives, phrases, and clauses in a series according to the *a, b, and c rule* or the *a, b and c rule*. The use of the final comma before the words *and* or *or* in any list is optional if it does not distort medical meaning.

Essential Elements

Do not use commas to set off elements that are grammatically essential to the sentence. In addition to the examples below, adjectival phrases beginning with *that* are not set off with commas.

> The patient whom you sent over to my office on Wednesday never showed up.
> (What patient? The patient whom you sent.)
> The dog that bit the boy was tested for rabies.
> (Which dog? The dog that bit the boy.)

Insertions

Set off nonessential insertions with commas.

> The patient, surprisingly, recovered without intervention.
> Examination showed greater saphenous vein reflux at, at least, three or four calf sites.
> The patient, however, insisted on being discharged immediately.

If the rhythm or flow of the sentence is not significantly affected by the insertion, no comma is needed.

> He underwent subtotal resection of his acoustic neuroma but unfortunately also suffered injury to the brain stem and cerebellum.
> He subsequently was placed in rehabilitation where he improved.

Introductory Remarks

Use a comma after an introductory clause (an expression that includes a verb), interjections, and the words *yes* or *no*. However, there is precedent in current usage for omitting the comma after introductory transitional words or phrases and other short introductory phrases of less than five words.

> When the patient arrived in the emergency department, he was already in extremis.
> Approximately a year and a half ago, she developed a persistent and intensely pruritic dermatitis.
> Neurologically, he is grossly intact regarding motor, sensory, and cerebellar function.
> Consequently, it was decided not to admit Mr. Smith at this time.

Commas are optional in the following sentences.

> As a result, we felt that the patient was not a candidate for cardiac bypass.
> As a result we felt that the patient was not a candidate for cardiac bypass.

> On palpation, there is some tenderness in the left inguinal area.
> On palpation there is some tenderness in the left inguinal area.

> Otherwise, he will return to see me in a month.
> Otherwise he will return to see me in a month.

Hyphen

The trend in contemporary usage is to avoid the use of hyphens when they are not required for clarity. The use of hyphens with metric abbreviations is discouraged by the SI Committee. The hyphen is retained, however, with nonmetric units of measure.

> 7 cm mass
> 3 cm incision
> 1–inch scar
> 18–gauge needle
> 5– to 6–inch kitchen knife
> 3– to 4–year history
> 49-year-old man (*not* 49-years-old man)

Hyphens are still used in other compound nouns, verbs, and adjectives, however. Check with a reputable reference to determine whether a compound noun is one word, two words, or hyphenated. Here are a few examples from the dictations.

> The artery was suture-ligated … (compound verb)
> but
> A suture ligature was placed. (adjective modifying a noun)
> The artery underwent suture-ligation … (compound noun)
> double-clamp technique (compound adjective modifying a noun)
> Each of these was double-clamped … (compound verb)
> abdominal-perineal resection (compound adjective)
> ultrasound-confirmed communicating right hydrocele (compound adjective containing past participle)
> nonhealing, chronic-draining area (compound adjective containing present participle)
> extra-large Marlex plugs
> low-residue diet
> low-lying rectal cancer
> high-grade dysplasia
> a several-month history
> left-sided opacity
> through-and-through anterior fascial stays of 2-0 Prolene
> self-inflicted stab wounds
> ovoid-shaped incision
> frog-leg position
> a xiphoid-to-umbilicus incision

> a side-to-side fashion
> wet-to-moist gauze dressing

Note: You cannot replace the word *to* with a hyphen in the last few examples. Hyphens replace the word *to* in number ranges, not words. The expression is not a range; it indicates a directional relationship from one structure to another structure.

> 1 to 1.5 cm stab injuries
> 15 skin blade
> 6 mm polyp

Prefixes and Suffixes

Most common prefixes (*pre, re-, non-, un-,* etc.) are not followed by a hyphen unless they precede a proper noun, an abbreviation, or a phrase. Hyphens are no longer used in common words like reexamine and reexplored.

Generally, a hyphen is added only when there are three vowels (*salpingo-oophorectomy*) or when needed for pronunciation (*de-emphasize*) or meaning (*re-treat* versus *retreat*).

The list of prefixes that are almost always followed by a hyphen is short (*self-, ex-, all-, half-*). Similarly, suffixes are not preceded by a hyphen with rare exception, *-like* and *-type* being two of the most common in medical reports.

A hyphen is sometimes added for clarity, so that a reader doesn't stumble over the meaning or pronunciation of a term.

> Postoperatively he defervesced for several days; however, he began to re-spike fevers.
> The patient was re-prepped and draped.
> The Port-A-Cath had been pre-flushed with saline.

The prefix *post* is generally not hyphenated. When used as an adjective before a noun, *post* is connected to the root word without a hyphen. When it functions as a preposition (meaning after), it stands alone.

> The postoperative assessment was negative.
> The patient is status post cholecystectomy.
> The patient was taken to the postanesthesia care unit.

When *like* or *most* appears as a suffix, it is attached to the root word without a hyphen, unless the root word is multisyllabic or failure to hyphenate would affect quality.

sphincter-like	seizure like
uppermost	lateral most

The use of hyphens with *mid* varies. The prefix *mid* may stand alone as an adjective (*mid and left chest*) or combine with a root word without a hyphen (*midchest, midline, midlateral*). *Mid* may be hyphenated if used with a phrase or if it precedes a word that begins with another prefix (*mid-epigastric region*).

Like most prefixes, *non-* is not hyphenated in most combinations (*nonobstructed*), except when it precedes an eponym (*non-Hodgkin*), an abbreviation (*non-HIV*), or a phrase (*non-insulin-dependent*), although with the latter you may see *noninsulin-dependent*. Many dictators use *non-* before words where *un-* would be a better choice, as with *nonresectable*, but we do not generally edit this usage.

Single Letters

A hyphen is not needed to connect a single letter and noun combination such as *J tube*, *J wire*, and *T tube*; however, a hyphen is used to join a single letter and noun when they function as a compound adjective (*Y-shaped incision*, *T-tube cholangiogram*).

Ethnicity

Compound designations of Americans identified by ethnicity, race, or nationality are no longer hyphenated, either as nouns or adjectives.

> Japanese American male
> Mexican American female

When Not to Use Hyphens

Most prefixes are joined to roots without the use of a hyphen unless doing so would duplicate letters (for example, *non-native* needs a hyphen for clarity).

Prefixes that generally don't need to be hyphenated include *ante, anti, bi, co, contra, counter, de, extra, infra, inter, intra, micro, mid, non, over, pre, post, pro, pseudo, re, semi, sub, super, supra, trans, tri, ultra, un,* and *under*.

Hyphens may be used to avoid misreading or mispronouncing and if the prefix is followed by a proper noun, an abbreviation, or a phrase.

The following suffixes are not preceded by a hyphen unless it would create an awkward combination of repetitive letters: *-fold, -hood, -less, -like, -wise*.

Period

A period should be placed at the end of each line following a heading, even if it does not represent a complete sentence. The period indicates that the line is complete and nothing has been omitted.

> PREOPERATIVE DIAGNOSIS
> Umbilical hernia, incarcerated.
>
> POSTOPERATIVE DIAGNOSIS
> Umbilical hernia, incarcerated.
>
> PROCEDURE PERFORMED
> Repair of incarcerated umbilical hernia.

Question Mark

When a physician dictates a question mark, it indicates that a finding or diagnosis is uncertain. Transcribe the question mark; do not spell out the words. Note that there is no space between the question mark and the word following it. If the question mark follows the finding, it can be placed in parentheses for clarity.

> D: PREOPERATIVE DIAGNOSIS
>   Carcinoma of the liver; query metastatic, query primary.
> T: PREOPERATIVE DIAGNOSIS
>   Carcinoma of the liver; ?metastatic, ?primary.

> D: PREOPERATIVE DIAGNOSIS
>   Question mark axillary mass, left side.
> T: PREOPERATIVE DIAGNOSIS
>   ?Axillary mass, left side.

> D: There also appeared to be a possible ruptured ovarian cyst question mark, but that was not certain.
> T: There also appeared to be a possible ruptured ovarian cyst(?), but that was not certain.

Quotation Marks

Quotation marks should not be used in a medical report unless the physician is directly quoting the patient or dictates quotation marks. In the following examples, the physician dictated quotation marks.

> The 12 mm port was closed under direct vision using the Endo Close device and 0 Vicryl, closing the "endoabdominal fascia."

He had evidently had a "fullness" that had gone superiorly.

Semicolons

Use a semicolon to separate two independent clauses that are closely related in meaning. A period is also acceptable, as each independent clause is a complete sentence.

> The pylorus and first and second parts of the duodenum were then carefully examined; no evidence of injury here. The lesser sac was entered; there was no evidence of injury to the posterior wall of stomach or body of pancreas.
>
> We could not see the left anterior descending; presumably it was intramyocardial.
>
> Cystoscopy was then performed; the findings were noted above.

Use a semicolon to punctuate two independent clauses joined by a conjunctive adverb or transitional phrase (*consequently, for example, furthermore, however, in addition, indeed, in fact, moreover, nevertheless, then, therefore, thus*). Place a semicolon before the conjunctive adverb or transitional phrase and a comma after it.

> The stomach was free of any evidence of penetrating injury; however, along the lesser curvature of the stomach, there was penetration with a hematoma overlying the head of the pancreas.
>
> We continued to dissect this; however, it became evident that the tumor was locally invasive into the trachea.
>
> The 2 cm nodule was easily palpated in the lower aspect of the upper lobe, and it was not on the surface; therefore, it was elected to do an excisional biopsy utilizing the TA-90 stapler.

Note: In the last example there are three independent clauses, the first two joined by *and*, and the third joined by *therefore*.

Use a semicolon to separate a series of words, phrases, or clauses when separate internal elements are already separated by commas.

> The pericardium was opened vertically; T'd horizontally superiorly and inferiorly; and retraction sutures were placed in the pericardial edges.
>
> Procardia 10 mg 1 t.i.d.; nitroglycerin 0.4 mg p.r.n., to take one at onset of pain, a second one in 5 minutes, and a third 5 minutes later, and if no relief, go immediately to the emergency department; and Coumadin 2.5 mg Mondays, Wednesdays, and Fridays and 5 mg on Tuesdays, Thursdays, and Saturdays.

Redundancies

When an exact or near-exact redundancy is dictated, edit out the redundant statement. However, be careful not to remove text intended for emphasis or to change the dictator's style.

D: The patient was brought to the operating room where, after the institution of general endotracheal anesthesia, the abdomen was prepped and sterilely draped in the customary fashion. Once I saw the abnormal appendix at exploration, he was given IV for infection prophylaxis. The abdomen was prepped and sterilely draped in the customary fashion.

T: The patient was brought to the operating room where, after the institution of general endotracheal anesthesia, the abdomen was prepped and sterilely draped in the customary fashion. Once I saw the abnormal appendix at exploration, he was given IV for infection prophylaxis.

Subject-Verb Agreement

Subject-verb agreement errors occur frequently in medical dictation, and it is the medical transcriptionist's responsibility to correct such errors. The number of the subject determines the number of the verb. Use a plural verb with a plural subject and a singular verb with a singular subject. Compound subjects joined by the conjunction *and* take a plural verb, even if each of the subjects is singular. If a compound subject is joined by the conjunction *or*, the verb must agree with the subject nearest it. Delayed subjects, as in sentences that begin with *there*, can be particularly tricky. Phrases beginning with *including* or *as well as* are not considered part of the subject and do not influence the number of the verb. In the examples in this section, the subjects are in **bold italics**, the verbs are in **bold** type.

Collective Nouns

Not all style guides agree about whether to use a singular or plural verb with a collective noun. Generally, if the sense of the noun is plural, the verb will be plural.

The patient's *family* **understand** that the patient's outlook is grim; **they** all **agree** with the "Do Not Resuscitate" order.

A **majority** of the healthcare team **agree** that further inpatient care is needed for this patient.

Tip: The use of *they* in the first example is a clue to the choice of the plural verb with the collective noun *family*. In the second example, the article *a* in front of the collective noun *team* makes it plural (each member of the team is considered separately), while placing *the* in front of the noun would have made it singular (those agreeing would be considered collectively).

Compound Subject Joined by *And*

A plural verb must be used even if the word closest to the verb is singular.

Lab *results* and chest *x-ray* **were** both normal.
Febrile *agglutinins* and white blood *count* **were** elevated.

Compound Subject Joined by *Or*

Make the verb agree in number with the closest noun.

No definite adenopathy or *masses* **were** felt.
No definite masses or *adenopathy* **was** felt.
On chest x-ray no new suspicious masses or *change* in old density of suspicious nature **has occurred**.
No clustered microcalcifications, skin thickening, or nipple *retraction* **is** present.

Objects of Prepositions

Confusion of the object of a preposition with the subject of the sentence is probably the second most frequent occurrence of subject-verb agreement errors. The object of a preposition does not influence the number of the verb except when the subject is a word that indicates a portion—*percent, fraction, part, majority, some, all, none, remainder, portion*, etc. Then you must look at the object of the preposition to determine whether to use a singular or plural verb. If the object of the preposition is singular, use a singular verb. If the object of the preposition is plural, use a plural verb.

D: A new interstitial infiltrate in both mid lung zones with some shagging of the cardiac borders are evident on chest x-ray.

T: A new interstitial *infiltrate* in both mid lung zones with some shagging of the cardiac borders **is** evident on chest x-ray.

Note: The intervening prepositional phrases do not affect the number of the verb because the subject is not a fractional concept.

Some of the stones **were** little more than gravel. [Stones is the object of the preposition and is plural, so the verb is plural since it's a portion of the stones.]

Some of the specimen **was** so friable, it could not be saved for frozen section. [On the other hand, specimen is the object of the preposition here and specimen is singular, so the subject *some* represents a singular amount.]

Sentences Beginning with *There*

Perhaps the most frequent occurrence of subject-verb agreement errors happens in sentences or clauses beginning with *there*. Because the verb precedes the subject in this construction, care must be taken to identify the correct subject(s). Even in sentences beginning with *there*, if the compound subjects are joined by *or*, the subject closest to the verb determines the number of the verb. It is often helpful to turn the sentence around and read it with the subject or subjects first, but if the subject is compound, be sure to keep the same subject closest to the verb.

At rest, there **are** some occasional theta activity *ripples* in both temporal regions.
There **are** three small *ulcers* on the anterior wall of the stomach.
There **is** no *thrush* or oral lesions.
There **are** no oral *lesions* or thrush.
There **are** no *stridors* or meningismus.
There **is** no *meningismus* or stridors.
There **were** copious *amounts* of urine draining from the vaginal vault.
There **was** approximately *200 mL* of blood.

D: There is scattered hyperkeratotic lesions that the patient states are similar to the lesion resected on his right forearm.

T: There **are** scattered hyperkeratotic *lesions* that the patient states are similar to the lesion resected on his right forearm.

D: There are no definite palpable cervical, supraclavicular, axillary, epitrochlear, or inguinal adenopathy.

T: There **is** no definite palpable cervical, supraclavicular, axillary, epitrochlear, or inguinal *adenopathy*.

D: There were no adenopathy appreciated.

T: There **was** no ***adenopathy*** appreciated.

D: There was no nodules palpable in the area other than the liver proper.

T: There **were** no ***nodules*** palpable in the area other than the liver proper.

Subject Farther from Verb

The farther (more distant in space) the subject is from the verb, the more difficult it is to identify. Words, phrases, and clauses separating the subject from the verb are frequent causes for subject-verb agreement errors. Read the sentence without the intervening expression and choose the verb accordingly. Expressions such as *with*, *as well as*, *in addition to*, *including*, etc., frequently follow the subject in medical dictation but do not change the number of the subject or the verb, although objects of prepositions that intervene between a collective noun and the verb may affect the verb.

D: There is, on examination of the skin over the abdomen, well-approximated incision margins without erythema, crepitus, fluctuancy, or induration and mild inconsistent left mid and lower quadrant tenderness without definite rebound.

T: There **are**, on examination of the skin over the abdomen, well-approximated incision ***margins*** without erythema, crepitus, fluctuancy, or induration and mild inconsistent left mid and lower quadrant *tenderness* without definite rebound.

D: No definite findings of egophony or rhonchi, wheezes, or rub was noted.

T: No definite ***findings*** of egophony or rhonchi, wheezes, or rub **were** noted.

D: The carotid sheath containing the carotid artery, internal jugular, and vagus nerve were then exposed and retracted.

T: The carotid ***sheath*** containing the carotid artery, internal jugular, and vagus nerve **was** then exposed and retracted.

No ***evidence*** of any thrombosis of the distal vessels, including popliteal, posterior tibial, peroneal, anterior tibial, and saphenous veins, **was** seen.

Wound care instructions, as well as a prescription for Tylox q.4 h. p.r.n., #15, **were** given to the patient.

Verbal Phrases as Subjects

It may be difficult to identify the subjects of sentences if the subjects themselves are verb forms. The verbals (*ing* forms) functioning as subjects are in **bold italics**, and the verb is in **bold** type.

D: Driving or operating heavy machinery are to be avoided while on this medication.

T: ***Driving or operating*** heavy machinery **is** to be avoided while on this medication.

Symbols

The symbol ***x*** may be used to represent the word *times*. It is also used to represent *by* in measurements. Do not use *x* for *times* when it means *for*.

> sponge and needle counts reported as correct x2
> DRAINS: Jackson-Pratt (JP) x4.
> 3 x 5 cm
> diarrhea and constipation for 10 days
> (not, x10 days or times 10 days)

The **percent** symbol (%) should be used with numerals; in a range, the symbol should be repeated with each value in a range.

> 0.25% Marcaine
> 10% to 20%

The **degree** symbol ° does not transmit well electronically, so it is recommended that degrees be spelled out in medical reports. If the temperature scale (Fahrenheit, Celsius, centigrade) is also dictated, write it out as well, changing centigrade to the preferred metric scale, Celsius.

In medical reports where the degree symbol is used, the abbreviation *F* is used for *Fahrenheit* and C for *Celsius* and *centigrade*. Do not insert a space after the degree symbol or a period after the abbreviation for the scale.

37°C	37 degrees Celsius
98.6°F	98.6 degrees Fahrenheit

The **virgule or slash** (/) mark means equivalence or duality. It is sometimes misused by dictators when a comma, semicolon, or period is all that is needed.

D: OPERATION
Exploratory laparoscopy, cholecystectomy with cholangiograms/difficult dissection.

T: OPERATION
Exploratory laparoscopy, cholecystectomy with cholangiograms; difficult dissection.

T: OPERATION
Exploratory laparoscopy, cholecystectomy with cholangiograms. Difficult dissection.

Syntax or Sentence Structure

Where warranted, the transcriptionist may add conjunctions (*and, or, but*), prepositions (*of, to, with*), articles (*a, an, the*), pronouns (*it, she, her, he, him*), and verbs (including helping verbs) to complete a sentence. Such editing may be considered superfluous in a strict verbatim environment, and the MT should avoid altering the dictator's style.

It should also be noted that certain parts of a report (the physical exam for example) may be defined by clipped sentences, phrases, and single words. However, if full sentences are dictated and a heading needs to be added, add the heading and retain the complete sentence to maintain the dictator's style. Do not turn a complete sentence into an incomplete sentence by lopping off the subject and making it the heading.

D: No tenderness present over chest.
T: No tenderness is present over the chest.

D: 25-year-old male presents to the office for routine examination.
T: This 25-year-old male presents to the office for routine examination.

D: The heart has a regular rate and rhythm. (on a physical examination)
T: Heart: The heart has a regular rate and rhythm.
not
Heart: Has a regular rate and rhythm, *or*
Heart: Regular rate and rhythm.

Units of Measure

It is customary to abbreviate metric measurements when associated with a numeral in medical reports (3 cm). When indefinite values are dictated (several centimeters), spell out both the value and the unit of measure.

Abbreviations for metric measurements contain no periods and are in the same form for both singular and plural usage. For example, *cm* is the abbreviation for both *centimeter* and *centimeters*.

Standard English units of measure (inch, foot) contain so few letters that they are usually spelled out

mg (milligrams)
mmHg (millimeters of mercury)
several centimeters

Metric measurements in this transcription unit follow the recommendations of the SI system (Système International d'Unités); for example, *cm* (centimeters), *mL* (milliliters), and *g* (gram).

In a series of metric measurements, do not repeat the unit of measure unless it varies for the different values or its absence would confuse the reader.

D: 3.3 cm x 1 x 4
T: 3.3 x 1 x 4 cm
But: 2.5 mm x 2 cm

D: a centimeter and a half
T: 1.5 cm

Use a singular form of a verb with units of measure.

Approximately 10 mL of fluid was aspirated from the abdominal cavity.

Usage

Medical transcriptionists are expected to correct inappropriate grammar, such as subject-verb agreement errors, use of the wrong part of speech, incorrect pronouns, and incorrect usage. Be careful not to edit grammar that is already correct.

D: She will follow up with *myself* in 2 weeks. (reflexive pronoun)
T: She will follow up with *me* in 2 weeks. (objective pronoun)

D: The patient was appraised of the risks and benefits of surgery.
(*Appraise* means to evaluate or place a value on.)
T: The patient was apprised of the risks and benefits of surgery.
(*Apprise* means to make aware of.)

D & T:
Once we had this complete, we assured that we had adequately dissected the mesentery free.

Note: Although *ensured* is more common in the above context, *assure*, *ensure*, and *insure* all mean "to make secure or certain." Although *ensure* and *insure* are generally interchangeable, *insure* is now widely used in American English in the commercial sense of "to guarantee persons or property against risk" (insurance). *Assure* is also used with reference to a person in the sense of "to set the mind at rest": "We assured the patient that the tumor was benign."

D: We aspirated the irrigation …
   (Irrigation is the act of irrigant.)
T: We aspirated the irrigant …
   (An irrigant is the fluid used to irrigate.)

D: The umbilicus was then dissected free by placing 2 single skin hooks and using a #10 blade used to incise the skin along with sharp scissor.
T: The umbilicus was then dissected free by placing 2 single skin hooks and using a #10 blade used to incise the skin along with sharp scissors.

Note: Forceps and *scissors*, though singular in nature, are regarded as plurals; they take a plural verb unless the subject is *pair*.

A pair of scissors was used.
Scissors were used.

Verb Tense

As a rule, all parts of a History and Physical and Consultations, except for ongoing symptoms and the physical exam, are *generally* dictated in past tense; the findings on a physical exam are often dictated in the present tense. Discharge Summaries and Operative Reports are generally dictated in the past tense, although some surgeons dictate in the present tense. However, it is possible to correctly use every tense within a single paragraph. Some physicians dictate in the present tense, some in the past, and some switch back and forth. While some dictators expect the transcriptionist to edit to the appropriate tense, other dictators insist that the report be transcribed as dictated. When the dictator's preference is not known, the transcriptionist may transcribe as dictated. Editing tense is tricky, and the transcriptionist should be very certain that an edit is needed before making one.

Vernacular/Medspeak

Doctors frequently speak in a clipped, abbreviated manner. There's a fine line between slang and colloquial and what is acceptable or not. It's often quite difficult to define. For example, they may use only the first word of an adjective-noun phrase. In addition, doctors are fond of coining words—that is, making up new words. Many of these coined words cannot be verified. After making sure that you are hearing the word correctly and that no similar word with the intended meaning exists, you may spell a coined word using the techniques you learned in your medical language course. When uncertain about the spelling or whether you're hearing the term correctly, it's a good idea to flag.

In the following examples, what was dictated and transcribed and what the dictator actually *meant* are provided.

D & T: Labs were stable.
Meant: Laboratory test results were stable.

D & T: The area was checked for bleeders and any were cauterized with bipolar.
Meant: bipolar cautery

D & T: This [lesion] was electrocauterized and the specimen sent to Pathology for routine fixation and study.
Meant: The lesion was removed with electrocautery.

D & T: … 3-0 Vicryl intracutaneous interrupteds were used …
Meant: interrupted sutures

D & T: Cricomyotomy.
Meant: Cricopharyngeal myotomy.

D & T: de-serosalization
Meant: The serosa was torn or taken off.
(The hyphen was added for ease of pronunciation)

D & T: … fat was then removed in a crescenteric pattern.
Meant: crescent-shaped pattern

D & T: A total of 300 mL of lipoaspirate was suctioned.
Meant: the material aspirated by liposuction

D & T: Bovie electrocautery was used to carry the dissection down to Scarpa fascia and then angled upward subscarpally.

Meant: below Scarpa's fascia

Word Forms

Alternative Spellings

Some words have more than one acceptable spelling, and the preferred spelling may vary from reference to reference.

> curet, curette
> long standing, long-standing
> mammaplasty, mammoplasty

> *Note:* Although *mammaplasty* appears to be the preferred spelling in medical dictionaries and in PubMed citations, *mammoplasty* follows the more traditional construction with its use of the combining vowel *o*.

Combined Forms

Physicians frequently dictate combined forms. It is acceptable to use either the combined form or the standard (often hyphenated) form when it is uncertain which is dictated.

> | | | |
> |---|---|---|
> | femoral popliteal | *or* | femoropopliteal |
> | inferior lateral | *or* | inferolateral |
> | tracheal bronchial | *or* | tracheobronchial |

> lateralmost margin
> superiormost

Plurals

Generally, medical words derived from Latin or Greek are pluralized according to guidelines in the recommended references. However, some physicians prefer to pluralize Latin terms in the same way that English words are pluralized. Transcribe as dictated unless incorrect.

> | | | |
> |---|---|---|
> | cannulas | *or* | cannulae |
> | fistulas | *or* | fistulae |
> | lumens | *or* | lumina |

> condyloma   condylomata (pl.)

Tricky Spellings

Beware of words spelled differently when their form changes.

> fascia lata, tensor fasciae latae
> inflamed, inflammatory

> lateralmost margin
> superiormost

Sample Report Template

HISTORY AND PHYSICAL EXAMINATION

CHIEF COMPLAINT
*

HISTORY OF PRESENT ILLNESS
*

PAST MEDICAL HISTORY
* [Add subheadings, initial capital letters followed by colon, if dictated. Otherwise, use narrative style.]

MEDICATIONS
*

ALLERGIES
*

REVIEW OF SYSTEMS
* [Add subheadings, initial capital letters followed by colon, if dictated. Otherwise, use narrative style.]

PHYSICAL EXAMINATION
VITAL SIGNS: * [Vital signs may be separated by periods or commas.]
GENERAL APPEARANCE: *
HEENT: *[Subheadings may be dictated, but use only if dictated. Otherwise, use narrative style.]
NECK: *
CHEST: * [Add subheadings for heart and lungs only if dictated. Use narrative style.]
ABDOMEN: *
PELVIC: * [For women. Do not use heading if male patient.]
GENITALIA: * [For men generally. May be dictated for women if full pelvic exam is not done.]
EXTREMITIES: *
NEUROLOGICAL: *

IMPRESSION
* [List and number if more than one impression is dictated.]

_____

Signature   date/time

D: [date; time]
T: [date; time]
Dictator's initials/Transcriptionist's initials

NOTE: Demographic blocks vary; the one at the top of this report is just an example. An impression, assessment, admitting diagnosis (or equivalent expression) heading must be included, even if not dictated. Major headings are on lines by themselves and the text starts underneath. Most H&Ps are treated as a single report.

Spotlight On

A Little Bit of Comma Sense

by Richard Lederer, Ph.D.

Are you confounded by commas, addled by apostrophes, and queasy about quotation marks? Do you believe that a bracket is just a support for a wall shelf, a dash is something you make for the bathroom, and a colon and semicolon are large and small intestines? If so, I'm pleased to tell you I'm about to be the father of a bouncing baby about mastering punctuation.

In *Comma Sense: A Fun-damental Guide to Punctuation* (St. Martin's Press, 2005), humorist John Shore and I present what we hope will be hilarious portraits of American icons and connect each one to a mark of punctuation. We hope that while you're laughing your head off over the weird but instructional examples, you'll master everything you need to know about punctuation through simple, clear, and right-on-the-mark rules.

Punctuation can make an enormous difference in meaning. Which dog has the upper paw?: "A clever dog knows its master." "A clever dog knows it's master." The second sentence, of course. Why do so many people insert a squiggle before the *s* in the possessive *its*?

Which speaker beheld a monster?: "I saw a man eating lobster." "I saw a man-eating lobster."

Note the effect of the missing apostrophe in this sentence: "The butler stood in the doorway and called the guests names." And in this classified ad: "WANTED: Guitar for college student to learn to play, classical non-electric, also piano to replace daughters lost in fire."

Note the startling result of the absence of hyphens in this headline: FATHER TO BE STABBED TO DEATH IN STREET.

Behold the effect of the missing serial comma (the one that should go before the "and") in this book dedication—"To my parents, the Pope and Mother Teresa." And in this sentence—"At summer camp I missed my dog, my little brother, the odor of my dad's pipe and my boyfriend."

Now have a look at the difference between these two love notes:

My Dear Pat,

The dinner we shared the other night—it was absolutely lovely! Not in my wildest dreams could I ever imagine anyone as perfect as you are. Could you—if only for a moment—think of our being together forever? What a cruel joke to have you come into my life only to leave again; it would be heaven denied. The possibility of seeing you again makes me giddy with joy. I face the time we are apart with great sadness.

John

P.S.: I would like to tell you that I love you. I can't stop thinking that you are one of the prettiest women on earth.

My Dear,

Pat the dinner we shared the other night. It was absolutely lovely—not! In my wildest dreams, could I ever imagine anyone? As perfect as you are, could you—if only for a moment—think? Of our being together forever: what a cruel joke! To have you come into my life only to leave again: it would be heaven! Denied the possibility of seeing you again makes me giddy. With joy I face the time we are apart.

With great "sadness,"

John

P.S. I would like to tell you that I love you. I can't. Stop thinking that you are one of the prettiest women on earth.

The power's in the punctuation, baby! The first letter is a clear (albeit clunky) profession of undying affection; the second is sure to sweep Pat onto her feet. The only thing separating one document from the other is, of course, punctuation, which can mean the difference between a second date and a restraining order.

Exercises

Apostrophes

Instructions: Insert apostrophes as appropriate in the following sentences.

1. Its too bad that the hospitals policy prohibits patients access to their own medical records.

2. Two sonograms were compatible with a fetus of 30 weeks gestation.

3. On x-ray examination, the femur showed a fracture in its most distal portion of approximately 2 weeks duration.

4. Dr. Howards consultation was received 2 days before the patients surgery was scheduled.

5. Although its clear that the genus has been identified, the species has not.

Brief Forms and Medical Slang

Instructions: In the following examples, decide which contain brief forms that do not need to be changed and which contain medical slang that must be translated. Make the appropriate translation.

1. LABORATORY DATA: Her crit was 35.

2. A procto was done to help identify the pathology on the right side of her anus.

3. Her Pap smear showed carcinoma in situ.

4. The patient was cath'd and the urine specimen showed 1+ bacteria.

5. LABORATORY FINDINGS: The patient had a white count of 12,500 with a diff of 68 segs, 1 band, 13 lymphs, 17 monos, and 1 eo.

Capitals

Instructions: Correct the capitalization errors in the following sentences.

1. She will be seen by our Orthopedic Consultant, DR. Ortega, tomorrow.

2. LABORATORY DATA: WHITE BLOOD COUNT 14,000.

3. The culture grew out staphylococcus aureus, sensitive to Ampicillin.

4. She has Cushing's Syndrome and has developed a Cushingoid facies.

5. Heart: Positive Grade 2/6 systolic murmur.

Commas

Instructions: Insert commas where appropriate in the following sentences, and circle the commas.

1. He is showing more comedo formation and a higher proportion of pustular lesions than before and he now has a scattering of cysts over his upper back.

2. He was started on treatment with ephedrine Periactin and Sinequan and his hives are almost but not completely gone.

3. It is suspected that the cyst will recur and if it does the cyst will be excised.

4. The patient had a total protein of 5.4 albumin level was 3.2 chloride was 106 and a total bilirubin was 1.2.

5. He is to take prednisone 40 mg q.a.m. for 3 days 20 mg for 3 days 10 mg for 3 days 5 mg for 3 days 2.5 mg for 4 days and then off.

6. He will be seen by social services rehabilitative medicine and by his private cardiologist.

7. His angina however will continue until he undergoes a bypass procedure in the near future.

8. This patient as far as I can see is ready for rehabilitation.

9. She was discharged on Cardizem diuretics nitroglycerin and Atromid-S.

10. The improvement if any is very slight.

11. Her CPK levels however continued to remain within the normal range.

12. He has been instructed in the use of a low-salt diet; however it is doubtful that he will comply.

13. Her symptoms included dyspnea on exertion diaphoresis and a crushing chest pain.

14. The patient is a 72-year-old Asian female with no complaints of angina today.

15. Her hypertension is controlled with Dyazide and seems to be relatively stable.

16. The surgery was completed without complication and the patient was taken to the recovery room in satisfactory and stable condition.

17. She is scheduled for coronary artery bypass graft on September 15 2014 and she will be admitted for preoperative testing on the preceding day.

Eponyms

Instructions: Circle the correct eponym in the following sentences.

1. The patient experienced a (Jacksonian, jacksonian) seizure last week.

2. X-ray examination revealed (Osgood-Schlatter, Osgood-Schlatter's) disease.

3. We then inserted a (Rush's, Rush) rod into the tibia.

4. The abdomen was opened through a (Bevan, Bevan's) incision.

5. A (Jackson-Pratt, Jackson-Pratt's) drain was inserted for drainage.

Format

Instructions: Answer *True* or *False* to the following statements.

___ 1. Many medical facilities have instituted standard format outlines (templates) for each type of report dictated.

___ 2. If important headings are not dictated, the transcriptionist should supply them.

___ 3. Transcriptionists should type abbreviated major report headings (such as HPI) as dictated when physicians take shortcuts in dictation.

___ 4. Transcriptionists should always type the diagnoses in paragraph form even if the physician says to list and number diagnoses vertically.

___ 5. Paragraphing may be added by the transcriptionist to break up long reports appropriately.

Hyphens

Instructions: Supply hyphens as needed in the following sentences.

1. This well developed and well nourished 13 month old boy was referred to the pediatric clinic for follow up.

2. She complains of a continual stabbing like pain over a 3 week period.

3. This 25 year old woman was admitted with a history of pain in the shoulder over the last 24 hour period.

4. The x ray demonstrates an intra articular fracture.

5. The patient's pain medication was self administered as needed.

Numbers

Instructions: Find and correct the errors involving numbers and units of measure.

1. Laboratory data showed a total bilirubin of .5 mg.

2. She is 5.5 feet tall and weighs 160.5 pounds.

3. A 2 cms nodule is noted in the left lower lung.

4. There is another mole several mm away from the malignancy that we will need to check periodically.

5. The patient's blood pressure is 160 over 82 millimeters of mercury.

Semicolons

Instructions: Supply semicolons as needed in the following sentences.

1. His respirations remain labored however he continues to produce copious amounts of sputum.

2. Cross-clamp time was 1 hour and 18 minutes cardiopulmonary bypass time 2 hours and 10 minutes lowest esophageal temperature was 24°C.

3. Left ureteral stricture was dilated there were no stones apparent.

4. I have examined her underwear today they are of a heavy stretch type, they contain 12% spandex, and portions of her bra panels contain 16% spandex.

5. Her medications include Medrol 4 mg 1 tablet daily, Lasix 20 mg daily, Micro-K 10 mEq daily, #28, as well as Zantac 150 mg p.o. b.i.d., #14, doxycycline 100 mg p.o. daily for 14 days, verapamil 80 mg, #30, and Proventil inhaler 2 puffs q.i.d., 2 inhalers, 6 refills.

Soundalikes

Instructions: Circle the correct soundalike from the words in parentheses.

1. Moderate exercise would certainly (complement, compliment) the patient's post-CABG therapy.

2. The patient had a (discrete, discreet) mass in her left breast.

3. She was unwilling to sign the contract as a matter of (principal, principle).

4. To (affect, effect) a cure requires compliance from the patient.

5. There are multiple side (affects, effects) to this treatment.

6. If the trauma (affects, effects) the emotions, then the reactions, the attitude, and the patient's performance will suffer.

7. During the hospitalization, the patient's (affect, effect) became more appropriate.

8. We could not (elicit, illicit) a response from the patient who reportedly took an (elicit, illicit) drug.

9. The (pallet, palate) was noted to have a high arch.

10. The indication for C-section is failure of (descent, dissent).

Spelling and Usage

Instructions: Circle words that are spelled incorrectly and correct them.

1. He has had recurence of the catching feeling when he trys to breath, usualy at night.

2. The following dictations are breif examples of dictated labortory test results.

3. His speech is slured, and he has some tingleing and weakness in the right arm.

4. He has moderate wekness of the extremities both distaly and symetricaly.

Subject-Verb Agreement

Instructions: Review the guidelines on correct subject-verb agreement in this chapter, and complete the following exercise. Circle either the singular or plural form of the verb or pronoun in the pairs in parentheses to demonstrate correct subject-verb agreement.

1. No evidence of congestive heart failure and edema (is, are) seen on chest x-ray.

2. The occlusions in the region of the left anterior descending artery (appears, appear) to be significant.

3. We have no way of telling what the exact relationship of his pathology to his symptoms (is, are).

4. There (is, are) minimal episodes of arrhythmia seen on the EKG.

5. No episodes of angina (was, were) noted by the patient.

6. The age and sex of a patient (cause, causes) variation in the normal range of laboratory values.

7. Finger-to-nose test and heel-to-shin test (is, are) normal.

8. Inspection of the upper extremities (show, shows) some scattered small abrasions over the dorsal aspects of the hands.

9. No evidence of mucosal ulcerations or polypoid filling defects (was, were) seen.

10. Some hypertrophy of the facet joints (is, are) noted at this level.

11. A moderate exudate of polymorphonuclear leukocytes (is, are) seen.

12. Acute blood clot and old organized and degenerate blood clot (is, are) observed.

13. His BUN was within normal limits, as (was, were) his sodium and potassium.

14. No fecalith or perforations (is, are) identified.

15. Cardiac and respiratory compensation (was, were) used.

16. The endocervical canals are patent, and each (connect, connects) with (its, their) respective (uterus, uteruses). (*Note*: The patient was didelphic.)

17. Examination of sections of both right and left lungs (show, shows) severe vascular congestion but (is, are) otherwise unremarkable.

18. Sections of the remaining breast tissue (show, shows) atrophy without evidence of additional tumor.

19. The wound was explored for foreign bodies, none of which (was, were) found.

20. The compression of the renal pelvis and deviation of the left upper ureter (is, are) essentially the same as seen on the intravenous pyelogram.

21. The nodules in the left lower lobe (has, have) not changed in size.

22. Approximately 10 mL of straw-colored fluid (was, were) obtained and sent for appropriate microbiologic studies.

23. We have no way of telling what the exact relationship of this mass to the subclavian vein and subclavian artery (is, are).

24. The sulci in the region of the temporo-occipital area on the right side (is, are) slightly effaced.

25. There (is, are) minimal degenerative change in the articular facets.

26. No definite adenopathy or mass (is, are) seen in the chest or around the chest wall or axilla.

27. Multinuclear giant cells and nuclear changes consistent with herpes or other viral infection (is, are) encountered.

Psychiatry

Learning Objectives

▶ Spell and define common psychiatric terms.

▶ Identify types of questions a physician might ask about mental health symptoms during the review of systems.

▶ Identify common psychiatric diseases and describe their typical cause, course, and treatment options.

▶ Identify and define psychiatric diagnostic procedures.

▶ List common psychiatric laboratory tests and procedures

▶ Identify and describe common psychiatric drugs and their uses.

▶ Demonstrate knowledge of medical, pharmacological, adjectival, and soundalike terms by accurately completing the exercises in this chapter.

Transcribing Psychiatric Dictation

Introduction

Disorders of perception, mood, and behavior have always been placed in a separate category from other illnesses, by both physicians and laity. Except for a few conditions obviously caused by organic disease or injury of the central nervous system (alcoholic dementia, inability to speak after head injury or a stroke), mental illnesses were long thought to result from failure of normal personality development, inadequate adaptation to life stresses, acquired distortions of thought processes, and other vague and intangible factors. The specialty of **psychiatry** came into being as a field concentrating on disturbances of mood and thought for which no organic basis could be found.

Within the past few decades, psychiatric theory has undergone remarkable changes in orientation. With important exceptions, most modern psychologists and psychiatrists believe that all mental disorders are due to **structural**, **chemical**, or **electrical abnormalities** in the brain. This idea is supported by abundant evidence from diverse sources. Genetic studies show that many mental disorders run in families, and some have actually been traced to specific chromosomal abnormalities.

Biochemical research has established a correlation between the distribution of neurotransmitters such as **serotonin**, **dopamine**, and **norepinephrine** in the central nervous system and certain disorders of **cognition**, **mood**, and **behavior**. A chemical basis has been found for the way in which many drugs help in mental disorders, and new drugs designed with specific chemical goals have attained their object of providing improved control of anxiety, depression, and other common disorders. Although **drug therapy** may still be considered an adjunct to counseling and other forms of psychotherapy, for many disorders it is currently the most rapid, effective, and predictable mode of treatment.

Psychiatrists are physicians concerned with the diagnosis and treatment of mental disorders. **Clinical psychologists** are professionals concerned with the nonmedical treatment of mental disorders; a clinical psychologist ordinarily does not hold a medical degree.

Vocabulary Review

adjustment disorder A persistent state of emotional or physical distress triggered by a major life event or situation, such as the death of a loved one, interper-

> MENTAL HEALTH TREATMENT
> The playwright Jerome Lawrence is quoted as having said, "Neurotics build castles in the air, psychotics live in them, and psychiatrists collect the rent." The cost of mental health, of course, is no laughing matter when one considers the billions of dollars spent annually to treat mental disorders.

sonal conflict, divorce, financial problems, or loss of employment.

affect One's prevailing mood or emotional state, pleasant or unpleasant, particularly as perceived by the examiner: basic emotional state, and emotional content of responses to examiner (apathetic, blunted, depressed, elated, euphoric, flat, inappropriate, labile).

His affect was blunted and consistent with a depressed mood.

amnesia Loss of memory.

aversion therapy A form of behavior therapy that associates an objectionable or undesirable pattern of behavior with an unpleasant experience or consequence, so as to reduce or extinguish the behavior.

behavior (behavioral) therapy Any type of psychotherapy that focuses on the alteration or correction of undesirable behavior, including such responses to external stimuli as anxiety, depression, and physical symptoms of emotion (tachycardia, muscle tension, sweating). Behavior therapy uses conditioning, muscle relaxation techniques, meditation, breathing retraining, biofeedback, guided learning, and other methods.

client The recipient of psychotherapy; a term preferred to "patient" when the therapist is not a physician.

client-centered therapy A form of psychotherapy in which the client is encouraged, with a minimum of direction by the therapist, to discover the sources of distressing mental symptoms and means of resolving them.

cognitive therapy A form of psychotherapy based on promoting the client's rational understanding of the source of distressing emotions, thought patterns, and

CURVE BALLS

by Mary Ann and Elizabeth D'Onofrio

Psychiatry presents unique challenges requiring formats and knowledge not demanded by the other specialties. Psychiatrists, and especially psychologists, administer many tests of intellectual, reasoning, and perception skills, the results of which must be displayed in specific format.

General medical transcriptionists are ever so familiar with the ubiquitous laboratory data section of the discharge summary wherein multiple tests with their results are described by the physician dictator. These results, at least, can be transcribed in a narrative format. However, the person who transcribes psychological evaluations must, for the most part, detail the results of the client/patient's tests in tabular form. Since each of these tests has its own unique set of parameters, varying at times in wording from psychologist to psychologist, the process of setting up the test results is tedious and laborious. A time-saving device for transcriptionists is the use of templates for this repetitive display of test data.

In addition, the content of many psychiatric reports goes so far as to leave the vocabulary of medicine altogether and enter the world of popular culture. This is especially true in the area of chemical dependency. Psychiatric transcriptionists must know how to spell desipramine and Prozac; however, they may also be expected to spell whiffledust, roofies, or K2 when psychiatrists and psychologists repeat the street drug slang used by some patients.

The impact of popular culture is also markedly apparent when one transcribes reports about adolescent patients, whose influences come predominantly from music, television, and video games. Psychiatric transcriptionists without children or grandchildren around to keep them "hip" would do well to have the phone number of a local video or game store on hand or be very adept at Internet searches.

The correct spelling of a rock star's name may seem frivolous, but there is a world of difference between Eminem and the chocolate candy. Musical groups or singers are notorious for inventing unique spellings for their names, for example "Florida" (Flo Rida) or "Will I Am" (will.i.am). Conversely, LMFAO is spelled exactly as it is pronounced, in all caps. Even common names can require verification. It is useful to know that Bieber is spelled with an "ie," not an "ei."

Video games, too, find their way into psychiatric transcription. Should a transcriptionist hear "wee," in the context of video games, the dictator is most likely referring to "Wii." And only the pop-culturally aware transcriptionist will know that the first word in the title of the anime/manga series "Fruits Basket" is always plural.

Child psychology presents another challenge. In one projective attitude test, the therapist poses the so-called "magician question": into what animals would the child, if endowed with magical powers, change family members? The answers reveal a lot about the child's perceptions, feelings, and attitudes toward the family. Exposed to the multimedia environment of today, children are very sophisticated in their knowledge of unusual animals. Exotic names we encountered in dictation recently included cockatiel, peccary, and lemur.

Although most demographic information has been removed from the transcription practice reports that accompany this textbook, full names, dates, and locations are common, especially in psychiatric dictation. Maps of Europe, the Middle East, and Asia may be especially helpful when veterans name the places where they have served.

Accurate medical reports are the key to success in this field. In psychiatry and psychology, the pool of terminology floods over the borders of the merely medical and encompasses words and experiences from all walks of life. The challenge to the psychiatric transcriptionist is to maintain the field's high standards of accuracy in form and content by hitting the "curve balls" as well as the straight pitches.

> **LAY AND MEDICAL TERMS**
>
> | | |
> |---|---|
> | fear | phobia |
> | manic depressive | bipolar disorder |
> | mood | affect |

undesirable behaviors, and correction of these by adoption of more mature, balanced, and realistic attitudes.

compensation (overcompensation) A mechanism by which one covers up a defect or weakness by exaggerating or overdeveloping some other property or faculty.

confabulation Invention of stories about one's past, often bizarre and complex, to fill in gaps left by amnesia; a typical feature of Korsakoff syndrome in chronic alcoholics.

CPT (Physicians' Current Procedural Terminology) A formal classification of diagnostic and therapeutic procedures published by the American Medical Association and revised annually, in which each procedure is assigned a five-digit code. CPT codes are universally used in billing third-party payers for medical services.

cyclothymia Abnormal lability of mood, which varies between excitement and depression without becoming severe enough to be called bipolar disorder.

delusion A false belief or wrong interpretation of observed facts, sometimes associated with hallucinations. May be categorized as delusions of **grandeur** (believing that one is a monarch or other celebrity), **reference** (a false perception that the words or actions of others refer to oneself), or **persecution** (thinking one is the target of official surveillance or a hostile plot).

denial A mechanism by which one refuses to believe, remember, or accept an unpleasant fact or circumstance, such as a past painful experience or the fact of being ill.

Diagnostic and Statistical Manual of Mental Disorders (DSM) A description and classification of mental disorders based on objective criteria. Recognized as a diagnostic standard and widely used for reporting, coding, and statistical purposes, *DSM* is published by the American Psychiatric Association.

The current (fifth) edition (DSM-V) appeared in 2013. See box, *Multiaxial Assessment.*

dysphoria A general feeling of mental or emotional discomfort.

dysthymia A depressed mood, usually chronic or recurrent, that is not severe enough to be called major depression.

eating disorders See *anorexia nervosa* and *bulimia nervosa* under Common Diseases.

encephalopathy Any organic disease or damage of the brain, particularly the cerebral cortex, that causes impairment of mental or physical functioning; often due to degenerative diseases (Alzheimer disease, Creutzfeldt-Jakob disease) or chemical intoxications (alcohol, lead).

facies Distinctive facial expressions associated with specific medical conditions.

He is fearful lest he cause trouble, and the facies is tense and anxious.

family therapy Psychotherapy that treats the family as a unit and seeks to promote understanding and correction of pathologic attitudes and relationships among members of the unit.

group therapy Psychotherapy administered to several persons at once, making use of sharing of perceptions, experiences, and feelings, group dynamics, and mutual understanding and support.

She actively participated in individual and group therapy sessions and was able to bring up conflictual issues such as anger, dependence, and poor self-esteem, and was able to begin to deal with these issues effectively.

guilt A sense of having done wrong, of having failed to meet one's own or others' expectations or standards, or of being inferior or inadequate; as used in psychiatry and psychoanalysis, guilt is a distinct concept from moral guilt, which arises from deliberate violation of ethical principles or civil law.

hallucination A sensory perception for which no basis exists in fact. Hallucinations may affect any one or more of the five senses (visual, auditory, tactile, olfactory, or gustatory); a typical feature of schizophrenia, delirium tremens, and some seizure disorders.

histrionic Referring to a style of speech and behavior in which the subject acts in an excessively dramatic fashion, as if performing on stage.

hypnosis A technique by which the therapist places the client into a sleeplike trance in which outside stimuli are reduced to a minimum, the subconscious is more directly accessible, and the client is more susceptible to the influence of the therapist's suggestions and advice.

identification A mental process whereby one takes on the properties or actions of another with whom an emotional tie exists (a boy walking and talking like his father; a woman dressing and behaving like a movie idol).

libido Sexual desire or drive; often, more generally, the totality of pleasure-directed energy or activity.

loose associations A breakdown of thinking in which logical connections between related concepts are no longer perceived; characteristic of schizophrenia.

mechanism (also defense mechanism, ego-defensive mechanism, mental mechanism, unconscious mechanism) An automatic, unconscious mental process whereby repressed emotions (painful feelings, sexual urges) generate new beliefs or attitudes to protect the ego from a sense of guilt, inadequacy, or other negative feelings. See *compensation, identification, projection, rationalization, repression, sublimation.*

narcissism Extreme self-love; excessive preoccupation with oneself and one's own concerns and needs, to the exclusion of normal emotional ties with others.

neurosis A mental disorder in which the patient experiences, and gives evidence of, emotional distress, but remains in touch with reality at all times.

neurotransmitter A normal chemical substance produced in minute quantities by nerve tissue and involved in the transmission of electrical impulses from one nerve cell to another. The effect of a neurotransmitter may be to stimulate or inhibit the nerve cell on which it acts. Well-known neurotransmitters include acetylcholine, dopamine, epinephrine, gamma-aminobutyric acid (GABA), norepinephrine, and serotonin.

oppositional defiant disorder (ODD) A pattern of deviant behavior in children and adolescents charac-

> MULTIAXIAL ASSESSMENT
> A comprehensive diagnostic formulation of mental illness that includes consideration of five distinct domains or axes.
>
> Axis I refers to formal psychiatric diagnoses other than personality disorders and mental retardation, which are included in Axis II.
>
> Axis III comprises nonpsychiatric medical diagnoses such as neurologic disease, infections, neoplasms, and diabetes mellitus.
>
> Axis IV focuses on psychosocial and environmental issues, including those related to family and other interpersonal relationships, education, employment, housing. finances, access to healthcare, and interaction with the legal system.
>
> In Axis V the clinician records a global assessment of functioning. Although this reporting configuration has been dropped from DSM-V, it remains in wide use.

terized by recurrent disobedience and displays of anger, resentment, or hostility toward authority figures, particularly parents. Diagnostic criteria listed in DSM include persistence for at least six months and resulting significant distress for family or interference with academic or social functioning.

oriented in all spheres A standard phrase indicating that the subject is aware of **time** (date, day of week, season), **person** (identity of self and others), **place** (state, city, address), and **situation** (at home, at a relative's home, in a hospital).

paranoia (adj. paranoid) An abnormal mental state characterized by delusions, especially delusions of persecution.

pharmacotherapy Treatment of disease with drugs, as contrasted with methods such as counseling, diet, and surgery.

play therapy A form of psychotherapy used with children, in which structured or unstructured play settings with dolls and other toys enable the therapist to identify and correct false or unhealthy attitudes and behavior patterns.

projection A mechanism whereby one unconsciously attributes one's own thoughts and attitudes (usually negative or unpleasant) to others as a means of dealing with a sense of guilt or inadequacy.

psyche A vague term roughly equivalent to "mind." Pronounced "psy-key." Do not confuse with the slang term *psych* (psychiatry or psychology).

psychiatrist A physician who practices **psychiatry**, the medical specialty concerned with the diagnosis and treatment of mental disorders.

psychoanalyst A mental health professional (psychiatrist or clinical psychologist) who practices **psychoanalysis**, a form of psychotherapy developed by Sigmund Freud (1856–1939). Psychoanalysis seeks to uncover deep-seated (subconscious) sources of mental illness through free association, hypnotism, dream interpretation, and other techniques.

psychodrama A type of group therapy in which clients resolve conflicts and distressing emotional states by acting out their fantasies and fears in the setting of a dramatic performance before an audience of fellow clients.

psychologist A person with academic training in **psychology**, the branch of science devoted to the study of the mind and its functions. A **clinical psychologist** specializes in mental disorders and may be licensed as a counselor or psychotherapist.

psychosis A mental disorder in which, in addition to emotional distress, the patient experiences a break with reality, manifested by delusions, hallucinations, and grossly bizarre or socially inappropriate behavior.

The patient has had personality difficulties all of his life, as well as severe somatic and psychosomatic disorders. He developed an extremely acute psychotic episode here. There was no euphoria at any time.

psychotherapist A health professional trained to diagnose and treat mental disorders without the use of drugs.

The patient received regular individual psychotherapy and various group psychotherapies that were available on the unit.

rational therapy A form of treatment in which mental disorders, which are thought to result from misinformation, wrong belief systems, and distorted logic, are improved by the therapist's use of direct, positive teaching and advice.

rationalization A mental process of justifying some act or omission through logical reasoning or argumentation, usually as a means of reducing feelings of guilt or inadequacy.

reality testing An individual's ability to perceive reality as it is, not as distorted by abnormal thought processes, disorders of perception, delusions, or hallucinations.

repression The mental process of thrusting out of consciousness impulses or desires that are perceived as incompatible with one's own standards or sense of fitness, and that therefore generate unpleasant emotions; repressed material occupies a large part of the subconscious.

subconscious (mind) Elements of one's personality (feelings, attitudes, prejudices, desires, behavior patterns) of which one is unaware; a general and somewhat vague term including but not always identical to what Freud called the *unconscious*.

Mood is depressed, tearful, constricted affect. No evidence of any overt psychosis or hypomania. She does have passive death wishes, however, denies any active suicidal intentions or thoughts. Insight and judgment questionable.

suicidal ideation Thoughts of committing suicide as a relief from mental distress, without actual attempts at suicide.

sublimation Diversion of sexual energy or impulses into higher or more socially acceptable activities.

tangentiality A disorder of thinking characterized by the tendency to digress from one topic to another in speech ("to go off on a tangent") or to give oblique or irrelevant answers to questions; indicative of loosened associations, and a cardinal feature of schizophrenia.

therapist One who treats; in mental health, anyone administering psychotherapy.

titrate To adjust the dosage of a drug up or down to maintain maximum effectiveness or to reduce side effects.

transference The development, on the part of the client, of an emotional bond (positive or negative) with the therapist.

1. Discuss historical and modern opinions regarding the cause of mental disorders.
2. List the neurotransmitters that are thought to correlate to certain disorders in mood, cognition, and behavior.
3. List and briefly describe at least 4 forms of therapy for mental health disorders.
4. Distinguish among the following conditions: cyclothymia and dysthymia; neurosis and psychosis; dysphoria and euphoria.
5. What is recognized as a diagnostic standard and widely used for reporting, coding, and statistical purposes? Briefly describe it.

Medical Readings

History and Physical Examination
by John H. Dirckx, MD

Review of Systems. The psychiatric part of the review of systems is often omitted. The psychiatric history is even more intimate and sensitive, if possible, than the sexual history. A person with severe psychiatric impairment makes a most unreliable historian. For example, there is usually not much point in asking someone about a history of hallucinations or delusions, for these terms are used only by persons who are convinced of the unreality of the experiences.

A person with even a mild mood or personality disorder frequently resists talking about it. Hence part or all of the psychiatric history may have to be obtained from the patient's family or friends or from medical records.

At times it is hard to distinguish between psychiatric history-taking and psychiatric examination, since both make use of the same basic tool—interviewing the patient. When the patient's chief complaint is not psychiatric, inquiries about past or present mental illness or emotional disturbance are more clearly historical in intent. The interviewer asks about any prior diagnosis of mental, emotional, or nervous illness (anxiety, depression, social phobia, panic attacks, obsessive-compulsive disorder, bipolar disorder, schizophrenia, alcoholism, drug addiction) and treatments used, including counseling, group therapy, drug therapy, hospitalization, and electroshock.

A general notion of the subject's mental and emotional health history can be obtained by inquiring about family and marital harmony, school performance, job stability and satisfaction, social contacts, sleep pattern, drug and alcohol use, and general sense of well-being, self-esteem, and purpose in life.

Mental Status Examination. The formal mental status examination consists of the following parts:

Mental status examination demonstrates loose associations, poverty of content of thought, paranoid delusions, and auditory hallucinations.

Appearance: Dress, grooming, makeup, hair care, jewelry or other adornments; slovenly, unkempt, bizarre, mismatched, or incongruous garments or adornments.

Sensorium: Responsiveness to visual, auditory, and tactile stimuli; alertness, attention span; ability to recognize and classify objects.

Activity and Behavior: Gait, posture, level of motor activity, speech; bizarre or compulsive actions, mannerisms, or posturings.

Mood (Affect): Basic emotional state, and emotional content of responses to examiner (apathetic, blunted, depressed, elated, euphoric, flat, inappropriate, labile).

Thought Content: Unconventional thoughts, fantasies, phobias, obsessive ideas, delusions, hallucinations, poverty of imagination.

Intellectual Function: Speed, coherence, and relevance of abstract reasoning; mental arithmetic, interpretation of idioms ("time on your hands") and proverbs ("a rolling stone gathers no moss").

Orientation: Awareness of time (time of day, day of week, date, season, year), place (state, city, exact present location), person (ability to identify self, relatives, friends).

Memory: Recall of recent and remote events; general information ("How many cents in a quarter? Who is the president?").

Judgment: Competence in analyzing situations, solving problems, taking practical action ("What would you do if the house across the street caught fire?").

Insight: The patient's awareness of being ill or impaired, and a recognition of the nature and implications of the illness.

On initial mental status examination, the patient presented without psychotic signs or symptoms, and there was no evidence of any organicity. She had multiple symptoms of depression including insomnia, loss of appetite with weight loss, crying spells, anhedonia, difficulty concentrating, withdrawal, isolation. She also complained of multiple anxieties.

Orientation, memory, and judgment are often called the organic triad because they are commonly affected in organic dementia.

There is a certain overlapping of material between parts of the mental status examination. Some of the observations pertain to the field of neurology rather than psychiatry. In addition to the mental status examination outlined above, the patient may be asked to complete one or more formal standardized tests of intelligence and personality.

Pause for Reflection

1. How does psychiatric history-taking and physical examination differ from that for nonpsychiatric illnesses?
2. Briefly list and describe the components of the mental status examination.
3. What is the organic triad and its significance?
4. In addition to interviewing, what other modalities may be used to assess a patient's psychiatric condition?

Depression

by John H. Dirckx, MD

We all experience periods of sadness or grief in response to losses, disappointments, or failure to attain specific goals or wishes. The diagnosis of "major" or "clinical" depression, however, implies a more severe and lasting degree of distress and disability than these normal low tides in our emotional life.

The criteria for a major depressive episode include either a marked reduction of interest or pleasure in virtually all activities, or a depressed mood, or both, most or all of the time, for at least two weeks. In addition, three or more of the following must be present: gain or loss of weight, increased or decreased sleep, increased or decreased level of psychomotor activity, fatigue, feelings of guilt or worthlessness, diminished ability to concentrate, and recurring thoughts of death or suicide. Chronic depression that is not severe enough to meet the criteria for major depression is called **dysthymia**.

The first episode of depression typically occurs before the age of 40. Recurrences are common, and later episodes tend to be more frequent, more severe, and more lasting. Besides being more common in women, the disease runs in families. Other risk factors include drug or alcohol abuse, chronic physical illness, stressful life events, social isolation, and a history of being sexually abused.

Not only is depression one of the most commonly diagnosed mental disorders in our society today, but undoubtedly many cases go unrecognized. About 10% of men and 25% of women will experience **clinical depression** at some time in their lives. The negative impact of the disease on the economy of this country is estimated at $16 billion yearly.

Modern psychiatry is moving toward the position that virtually **all mental disorders are organically caused**. The familial clustering of many disorders and the striking gender differences in the incidence of some of them make it likely that the tendency to develop them is genetically determined. In persons with an inherited predisposition to mental illness, biochemical and physiologic responses to environmental factors and life stresses are thought to induce persisting imbalances or malfunctions in certain brain centers.

Biochemical investigations have shed light on the role of neurotransmitters in normal and abnormal mental function. Neurotransmitters are naturally occurring chemical substances that, when released at nerve endings, stimulate or inhibit the function of adjacent nerve cells.

Two **neurotransmitters**, dopamine and serotonin, are thought to play roles in the genesis of depressive disease. **Dopamine** is the chemical precursor of norepinephrine, the hormone that acts on alpha- and beta-adrenergic receptors in the sympathetic nervous system and is the body's principal vasoconstrictor agent. Dopamine, which itself has vasoconstrictor activity, acts as a neurotransmitter or regulator in the CNS. Dopamine appears to be deficient or inactive in certain parts of the limbic system in patients with depression.

Serotonin, also called 5-hydroxytryptamine or 5HT, has an even broader range of functions. Formed in chromaffin cells of the central nervous system (CNS), peripheral neurons, the gastrointestinal mucosa, and the pineal gland, it constricts blood ves-

Both mother and father and maternal uncle have suffered from depression in the past but not to the point where they have needed to be on medication. There is no history of schizophrenia or bipolar disorder in the family.

sels, inhibits gastric secretion, stimulates smooth muscle, promotes the release of pituitary hormones, and serves as a precursor of the pineal hormone melatonin (which regulates the sleep-wakefulness cycle), besides acting as a neurotransmitter in the CNS.

Depression appears to be closely linked to the action of serotonin at synapses in the limbic system. It may reflect abnormalities in the sensitivity of receptors to serotonin, or in the feedback system that normally regulates serotonin production and release, or both. Besides having low levels of CNS serotonin, persons with major depression also have elevated levels of serum cortisol which are not suppressed by the administration of dexamethasone, a synthetic corticosteroid.

A number of highly effective drugs are available to treat depression. These include the older tricyclic compounds (amitriptyline, imipramine), the selective serotonin reuptake inhibitors (SSRIs or serotoninergics) (escitalopram, fluoxetine, sertraline), monoamine oxidase inhibitors (pargyline, phenelzine), and other agents (bupropion, nefazodone, trazodone, venlafaxine).

Many patients experience troublesome side effects (drowsiness, headaches, dry mouth, disturbances of gastrointestinal or sexual function). Some of these tend to diminish or disappear with continued use, but about 15% of patients discontinue antidepressant medicine because of side effects. Hence the total pharmacologic profiles of these drugs need to be taken into consideration in individualizing treatment. Patients taking monoamine oxidase inhibitors (MAOIs) must carefully avoid many medicines (decongestants, antihistamines, antihypertensives), foods (cheese, sausage, chocolate), caffeine, and alcohol because of the risk of fatal hypertensive crisis.

The neurotransmitters dopamine and norepinephrine belong to the monoamines class. Monoamine oxidase is a naturally occurring enzyme that breaks down these substances immediately after they have exerted their effects. By blocking this breakdown, MAOIs boost levels of dopamine and norepinephrine at critical sites.

Typically it takes 4–6 weeks for full control of depression to be achieved. Antidepressant therapy is ordinarily continued for at least one year after symptoms improve. Counseling and other forms of **psycho-**therapy may be useful in hastening remission and reducing the risk of relapse.

In **seasonal affective disorder (SAD)**, exposure to high-intensity light for 1-3 hours a day has been shown to abolish symptoms in many patients. While advocates of the cognitive theory of depression may use drug treatment to relieve symptoms, they emphasize other therapeutic strategies: avoidance of depressing people, places, or situations; correction of drug or alcohol problems; improved socialization; assignment of gradually more challenging daily tasks; search for pleasurable activities; and correction of distorted or maladaptive thinking patterns. For severe depression that does not respond to either drug or **cognitive-behavioral therapy**, electroshock therapy is sometimes beneficial.

Pause for Reflection

1. Distinguish between the sadness or grief in response to upsetting life events or loss and major or clinical depression.
2. What is the term for chronic but less severe depression?
3. Describe the two neurotransmitters thought to play roles in the genesis of depressive disease.
4. What other biochemical substance may be a factor in depression?
5. Correlate drugs used to treat major depression with dopamine and serotonin.
6. What other therapeutic strategies besides drugs may be used to treat patients with major depression?

Insomnia

by John H. Dirckx, MD

Insomnia has been defined as the inability to sleep long enough or deeply enough at night to maintain optimum central nervous system (CNS) health and function during the day. Since sleep requirements vary markedly from person to person, no quantitative definition (so many minutes or hours in such-and-such a stage of sleep) is feasible. Moreover, the diagnosis of insomnia is generally based on the patient's own observations, and extensive studies have shown that these observations are often unreliable.

Insomnia is regarded as a significant and widespread public health problem. The prevalence of chronic insomnia (defined as inadequate sleep at least three nights a week for at least one month) may be as high as 15% in the general population. Besides leading to day-time drowsiness, difficulty concentrating, impairment of memory, irritability, and restlessness or anxiety, insomnia is believed to be responsible for much poor job performance and many industrial and automobile accidents.

Insomnia is not a single disorder but rather a symptom with numerous possible causes. Various patterns of sleep disturbance occur. Difficulty in falling asleep (prolonged sleep latency) can result from mental preoccupation, emotional upset (anxiety, anger), ingestion of a large meal or use of CNS stimulants (caffeine, nicotine, or various medicines) shortly before bedtime, physical distress (pain, nausea), symptoms aggravated by recumbency (cough, gastroesophageal reflux, orthopnea), or disruption of the sleep-wake rhythm (jet lag, shift work, daytime napping).

Another type of insomnia, which consists of failure to attain sleep stages 3 and 4, with frequent awakenings during the night, can also be due to emotionally induced restlessness or to physical factors such as chronic musculoskeletal problems (osteoarthritis, fibromyalgia) and nocturia due to urinary tract disease.

A third type, called terminal insomnia, isn't as serious as it sounds. This refers to awakening in the early morning (two to three hours before intended rising time) with inability to fall back asleep. Terminal insomnia is a cardinal feature of clinical depression but may occur in other conditions as well.

Alleviating insomnia begins logically with an attempt to find and eliminate its cause. Treatment of physical or emotional illness or correction of an unhealthful lifestyle may lead to improvement in sleep. Many medicines (decongestants, antidepressants, antihypertensives, nicotine patches prescribed to facilitate smoking cessation, even some antibiotics) can delay the onset of sleep or impair its quality. Changing medicines or dosage times may restore a healthy sleep pattern.

Pause for Reflection

1. Define insomnia and describe two issues that complicate diagnosis.
2. Explain the statement: "Insomnia is not a single disorder but rather a symptom with numerous possible causes."
3. How is insomnia treated?

Drug Dependency
by John H. Dirckx, MD

Many drugs, particularly those used to treat pain, anxiety, and depression, can temporarily induce pleasant emotional states, varying from carefree serenity to euphoria and exhilaration. Even when such a feeling is not part of the intended therapeutic effect of the drug, it can exercise such an appeal that the patient becomes *habituated* to the drug—that is, craves another dose as soon as the effect of the previous dose begins to wear off.

Narcotic analgesics, barbiturates, amphetamines, and benzodiazepine tranquilizers are among the prescription drugs most commonly associated with habituation, but habituation to alcohol, caffeine, and nicotine is even more prevalent. The nature of habituation is not fully understood. There appears to be a genetic tendency to alcoholism and perhaps to some other types of drug habituation.

Some habituating drugs also produce physical *dependence*. That means that after repeated dosing, the body adapts neurologically or biochemically in such a way that withdrawal of the drug can induce physical symptoms such as diaphoresis, restlessness, dysphoria, and even seizures. The development of withdrawal symptoms reinforces the craving due to psychological habituation. In fact, the victim of drug dependence may keep repeating doses not so much to get "high" over and over as just to reverse withdrawal symptoms and feel normal again.

Drug habituation can be further complicated by the development of *tolerance*—that is, the need to increase dosage continually in order to achieve the desired effect. One type of tolerance occurs when a drug stimulates an increase in the production of a cytochrome P-450 enzyme that is involved in its own breakdown. The more drug taken, the more enzyme produced; and the more enzyme, the less drug effect from a given dose.

Addiction is variously defined; some have advised abandonment of the term (as well as of *drug abuse*) because of acquired judgmental connotations. The usual meaning of addiction is a severe, disabling preoccupation with the use of a drug involving habituation, dependency, and tolerance. Drug addicts, like alcoholics, often drop out of the workforce and out of society, and some are driven to crime in order to feed their habits.

Many drugs that were formerly approved for use in this country, such as heroin and phencyclidine ("angel dust"), are now illegal because of their high potential for habituation or addiction, and the use of some other

This is a 20-year-old male with no previous psychiatric history who developed symptoms of paranoia in the aftermath of having a difficult experience using LSD.

agents, such as amphetamines and cocaine, has been sharply restricted for the same reason. Cocaine is a potent coronary vasoconstrictor and has been responsible for many deaths of young persons from acute myocardial infarction.

Alcohol abuse. By far the most prevalent form of substance abuse in our culture is the excessive consumption of alcohol. About 30% of adults drink to excess at least occasionally, and 3–5% of women and 10% of men have chronic problems with excessive drinking.

Alcoholism is a behavioral disorder characterized by habitual or recurrent intoxication, often accompanied by both physical dependency and tolerance, and typically associated with deterioration of social and occupational functioning and impairment of mental and physical health.

Alcoholism tends to run in families, and as many as 40% of chronic alcoholics manifest abnormal drinking behavior before age 20. Chronic alcohol abuse decreases life expectancy by about 15 years. Alcoholics are more likely than non-alcoholics to be involved in automobile accidents and to commit violent crimes, including spousal and child abuse and homicide.

Persons with chronic drinking problems are often also dependent on nicotine and other drugs of abuse and suffer from anxiety, depression, and other mental health problems, including denial of alcohol dependency and resistance to therapy.

Treatment must be tailored to the needs of the individual and includes detoxification, long-term counseling of both patient and family, pharmacologic measures to enforce abstinence, and attention to nutrition and other aspects of physical health. Support groups such as Alcoholics Anonymous are highly successful.

Pause for Reflection

1. Differentiate between habituation and dependence.
2. List prescription drugs and other substances most commonly associated with habituation.
3. Distinguish between tolerance and addiction.
4. Define alcoholism.

Common Diseases

Anxiety Disorders

A group of mental disorders characterized by chronic worry or fear. **Anxiety disorders** are the most common ones seen by psychiatrists; often anxiety accompanies other disorders (depression, schizophrenia).

Cause: Probably a malfunction in the part of the brain called the reticular formation. This system regulates sleep and wakefulness as well as many autonomic and endocrine functions. Persons with chronic anxiety have abnormal levels of certain neurotransmitters (norepinephrine, serotonin, gamma-aminobutyric acid [GABA]) in brain tissue.

History: Persisting or recurring feelings of apprehension, uneasiness, worry, or fear (with or without a clearly defined object) that is out of proportion to any actual danger or threat. The sense of dread may become so absorbing as to distract the patient's attention from personal, social, and occupational activities. Anxiety may be triggered by a wide variety of settings and circumstances. Besides the mental condition of constant worry or dread, the patient usually experiences physical signs of autonomic and endocrine response: heightened muscle tension, rapid pulse, hyperventilation, sweating, insomnia, problems with appetite and sexual function. *DSM-IV* lists specific criteria for 14 anxiety disorders. Five of these are described here.

Generalized Anxiety Disorder. An abiding state of excessive, distressing, and disabling worry about a number of issues, associated with restlessness, muscle tension, irritability, abnormal fatigue, and insomnia. The condition is twice as common in women and often accompanies depression.

Social Phobia. The most common anxiety disorder. A **phobia** is an irrational fear of some object or situation, with resulting efforts to avoid it. While recognizing that the fear is unfounded or out of proportion to any actual danger, the victim of a phobia is unable to overcome it. The victim of social phobia experiences an exaggerated and persistent fear of embarrassment or humiliation in a social setting, or when appearing or performing in public. This can lead to severe social, educational, or occupational disability. Many persons with this disorder also suffer from depression or alcoholism.

Agoraphobia. An intense fear of being alone or being in a public place from which escape might be difficult, or help unavailable, in case of sudden incapacitation (such as passing out or having a heart attack).

FEELING BETA NOW?

Does your heart pound and your mouth get dry when you have to speak in public? Do your palms get sweaty when you're about to shake hands with a VIP? Does looking forward to an unpleasant encounter give you butterflies in the stomach? That's not social phobia—it just shows you're human. Even professional speakers and virtuoso performers experience at least some degree of stage fright throughout their careers.

Musicians, including singers, are uniquely vulnerable to performance anxiety. Whether a soloist or an ensemble player, every musician knows that a single wrong note, or the right note at the wrong time, can blow an audition, ruin a concert, perhaps wreck a career.

In various surveys, around one third of professional musicians queried have admitted using beta-adrenergic blocking agents (beta blockers) such as propranolol to allay performance anxiety. Many take the medicine daily, others only before performances. While the majority of users obtain their beta blockers by prescription from personal physicians, a significant number get their supplies from illegal sources.

Although beta blockers are not approved by the U.S. Food and Drug Administration for this indication, drugs of this class have been shown in controlled studies to reduce various forms of physical distress associated with performance anxiety. Musicians who use beta blockers regularly report that they feel more comfortable and self-confident while performing, and thus more able to focus on the task in hand. But some admit that the drug seems to rob their work of inspiration and sparkle.

Because beta-adrenergic blockade also tends to limit peak energy output, beta blockers have found no place in competitive athletics, with one exception. In archery and marksmanship, these drugs can unquestionably contribute to steadiness of aim. They are accordingly banned by the International Olympic Committee, and the detection of propranolol in a urine sample cost one pistol marksman a couple of medals in the 2008 Olympics.

Victims of agoraphobia avoid open spaces, crowded enclosures such as stores or churches, tunnels, elevators, and public transportation.

Panic Disorder. Recurring sudden spontaneous attacks of intense anxiety, lasting minutes or hours, and accompanied by marked physical symptoms such as chest pain, tachycardia, dyspnea or choking, sweating, faintness, tremors, and tingling in the extremities. Because of the type and severity of physical symptoms, panic disorder is sometimes mistaken for a heart attack or other life-threatening emergency by both the victim and others, including physicians. Although either agoraphobia or panic disorder can occur by itself, the two are often associated in the same patient.

Obsessive-Compulsive Disorder (OCD). A chronic anxiety disorder in which the patient suffers from both obsessions and compulsions. An **obsession** is a recurring or persisting idea, thought, or image that is perceived as intrusive, distracting, and repugnant, but that the victim is unable to ignore or suppress. Examples are recurring thoughts of harming oneself or others; fear of contamination or infections; and worry about losing or throwing away something that is or may later become important. A **compulsion** is an urge to repeat a ritualistic or stereotyped form of behavior that is recognized by the victim as irrational but that cannot be omitted without an increase of anxiety. Examples include excessive, repetitive handwashing; rigid attention to order or symmetry; repeated checking of locks, switches, or clocks; and performance of everyday actions in a ritualized fashion.

Treatment: The treatment of an anxiety disorder depends on the exact nature of the disorder, its source, and its symptoms. Individual or group **psychotherapy** can provide emotional support, help the patient to gain insight into the nature of the problem, encourage psychic growth and maturation, and teach positive attitudes and goal-directed behavior. Most anxiety disorders respond well to short-term or long-term drug treatment. Agents that reduce the level of uneasiness and worry are called **anxiolytics**. Most of the anxiolytics in current use belong to the benzodiazepine class (alprazolam, oxazepam). Certain drugs used in the treatment of depression (fluoxetine, fluvoxamine) are useful in obsessive-compulsive disorder. Paroxetine is beneficial in social anxiety disorder and panic disorder. Beta-adrenergic blocking agents such as propranolol can control the autonomic component of performance anxiety, social anxiety disorder, and panic disorder (tachycardia, sweaty palms, tremors).

Bipolar Disorder (Manic-Depressive Disorder)

A type of depressive illness in which the patient's mood oscillates between depression and mania.

Cause: Apparently a malfunction of the limbic system. Susceptibility to this disorder has been traced to a gene on chromosome 18. Half of patients have at least one parent with an affective disorder.

History: Alternations of mood between **mania** and **clinical depression**, with variable intervals of normal mood in between. A **manic episode** is a period of abnormal elevation of mood, irritability, or restlessness that lasts at least one week and is accompanied by some or all of the following: inflated self-esteem, hyperactivity, **flight of ideas**, abnormal talkativeness or **pressured speech** (rapid, strained speech as if the subject's mouth can't keep up with the flow of thoughts), reduced need for sleep, short attention span, and reckless behavior. Unlike anxiety and simple depression, bipolar disorder may include a loss of touch with reality; that is, it may be a true psychosis. During either the manic or the depressive phase, the patient may experience delusions or hallucinations, or may display grossly bizarre behavior.

Treatment: Drug therapy with lithium salts, carbamazepine, or valproic acid usually controls the manic phase of bipolar disorder and helps to prevent recurrences of mania. **Tranquilizers** and **antidepressants** may also be used. Mania generally causes severe impairment of social and occupational functioning and may require hospitalization. Some patients, especially those in creative careers, refuse treatment for their mania because they feel that it interferes with their ability to create.

Schizophrenia

A chronic or recurring **psychosis** due to a disorder of thought processes.

Cause: Susceptibility to schizophrenia is probably inherited as a complex of variations affecting several genes. Neurophysiologic studies have shown abnormally small size of the part of the brain called the thalamus, as well as changes in signal intensity in adjacent white matter.

History: Gradual onset, usually before age 40, of cognitive malfunctions—disturbances of perception and thinking characterized by **delusions, hallucinations**, gross distortion of mental function, or all of these. These basic features of schizophrenia are usually accompanied by reduced energy level, flat or depressed affect, **anhedonia** (inability to experience pleasure

DIAGNOSIS
Schizophrenia, catatonic, in partial remission.

from normally pleasurable activities), and **abulia** (diminished ability to make decisions). Virtually all patients display impoverished thought content, social withdrawal, and impairment of occupational functioning. Even with intensive psychotherapy and drug treatment, about 25% of persons with schizophrenia require custodial or institutional care.

Schizophrenia is divided, on the basis of dominant clinical manifestations, into the following types:

- **disorganized (hebephrenic) schizophrenia**: severe breakdown of mental function and incongruous or silly behavior.
- **paranoid schizophrenia**: prominent delusions of persecution or grandeur, often reinforced by hallucinations.
- **catatonic schizophrenia**: statue-like posturing, rigidity, or stupor.
- **undifferentiated schizophrenia**: without defining features.
- **residual schizophrenia**: history of schizophrenia but only mild, nonpsychotic residual impairment of mental function.

Treatment: Psychotherapy is inconsistently effective in helping patients overcome disordered thinking and improving social functioning. The modern treatment of schizophrenia depends heavily on the use of drugs known as **neuroleptics** or **antipsychotics**. The older members of this class belong to the group known chemically as **phenothiazines** (chlorpromazine, fluphenazine, trifluoperazine).

Patients treated with these drugs frequently develop **parkinsonian symptoms**, including tremors, rigidity, and **akathisia** (extreme restlessness, inability to remain seated). These may be adequately controlled with drugs used to treat parkinsonism (benztropine, trihexyphenidyl). A few suffer from **tardive dyskinesia**, an irreversible neurologic disorder causing twitching and writhing movements, particularly in the lips and tongue. Neuroleptics in other classes (clozapine, haloperidol, risperidone) are useful alternatives but have their own side effects. Fluphenazine and haloperidol can be given as long-acting injections to patients who have trouble complying with daily oral medicine regimens.

Alzheimer Dementia

Dementia is a general term for deterioration of memory, judgment, and orientation that is severe enough to interfere with activities of daily living and social functioning. Dementia is usually but not always associated with aging; most patients are over 60. Alzheimer disease (see ■ Figure 6-1) is the most common type of dementia, accounting for about three fourths of cases.

Cause: Degeneration of cortical neurons typically beginning in middle life, usually due to inherited abnormality of brain chemistry but sometimes acquired.

History: Usually gradual onset of steady deterioration in certain mental functions: short-term memory loss, inability to understand spoken or written language and to express oneself in speech and writing, diminished or distorted sensory perception, inability to perform purposeful actions, personality changes with irritability and depression, deterioration of impulse control.

Course: Dementia is irreversible and progressive, usually culminating in death within 5–10 years.

Treatment: Acetylcholinesterase inhibitors (donepezil, galantamine, memantine, rivastigmine, tacrine) produce improvement in cognitive function. Anxiolytics, neuroleptics, and antidepressants may be used to control disorders of mood and behavior. Behavioral therapy is sometimes successful in reinforcing acceptable behavior and extinguishing unacceptable

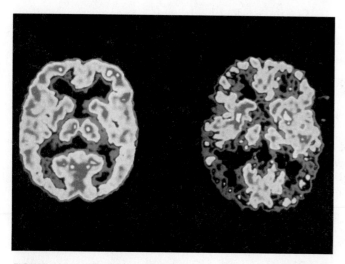

FIGURE 6-1. PET scans showing differences in cerebral glucose metabolism between a healthy brain (left) and the brain of a patient with Alzheimer dementia (right). Source: Dr. Robert Friedland, Photo Researchers, Inc.

behavior. A comfortable, secure environment (preferably home, unless the patient is too disruptive or the burden of care too taxing for the family), with familiar faces and a simple, steady routine, provides a setting in which the patient's impairments are least distressing and disabling. Support and counsel for the family are of major importance.

Other Dementias

Dementia is a feature of several conditions other than Alzheimer disease. Early differentiation among these is valuable for prognosis and in avoiding inappropriate therapy, but most forms of dementia are not only irreversible but progressive despite treatment.

The second most prevalent type, **vascular (multi-infarct, post-stroke) dementia**, results from scattered infarcts throughout the brain due to thrombosis or hemorrhage of small arteries. Symptoms depend on the areas involved and may be highly diverse and complex.

Lewy bodies are aggregations of the protein alpha-synuclein that are found in the basal ganglia of persons with parkinsonism, where they interfere with the metabolism of the neurotransmitter dopamine. **Dementia with Lewy bodies (DLB)**, which occurs when these aggregations occur in the cerebral cortex, is characterized by sleep disorders and visual hallucinations. Dementia may also be a feature of classical parkinsonism.

Frontotemporal dementia includes a group of non-Alzheimer disorders occurring in middle life and featuring malfunction of the frontal and temporal lobes of the cerebral cortex. Personality changes and problems with language use are characteristic.

Severe memory loss is the dominant feature of **Korsakoff syndrome**, which is due to deficiency of thiamine (vitamin B1) and is most often seen in chronic alcoholism. Dementia also occurs in certain **genetic disorders** (Huntington disease, Down syndrome) and **infections** affecting the central nervous system (tertiary syphilis, Creutzfeldt-Jakob disease).

The term **mixed dementia** is applied when more than one form of organic disease underlies impairment of brain function. Often this refers to cases of Alzheimer disease developing in persons already affected with vascular dementia, or vice versa.

Attention-Deficit Hyperactivity Disorder (ADHD)

A chronic behavioral disorder, most striking in children, involving hyperactivity, short attention span, and impulsiveness.

Cause: The disease runs in families, and about 25% of patients have at least one parent who is similarly affected. It is three to eight times more common in boys. Magnetic resonance imaging has shown abnormalities in the corpus callosum, the band of fibers connecting the two cerebral hemispheres. The theory that sugar and food colorings or other additives trigger hyperactivity is entirely without scientific support.

History: Often there is evidence of behavioral disturbance in infancy, and the full-blown disorder is typically recognizable by the age of six. The three cardinal features of ADHD are **inattentiveness** (short attention span, distractibility, inability to complete tasks undertaken, difficulty in following directions, tendency to lose personal articles, disregard for personal safety), **impulsiveness** (blurting out one's thoughts without adequate reflection, butting in front of others in waiting lines), and **hyperactivity** (restlessness, fidgeting, or squirming instead of sitting or standing still, excessive talking). Children with this disorder have a high incidence of academic failure, conflict with parents, teachers, and law enforcement officials, antisocial behavior, and substance abuse.

Treatment: Central nervous system stimulants (dextroamphetamine, methylphenidate, and pemoline) are usually successful in enhancing learning ability and improving social functioning. These medicines are taken early in the day so as to avoid nighttime insomnia. When improvement in academic achievement is the chief goal of treatment, the patient may be given "drug holidays" on weekends and during school vacations.

Anorexia Nervosa

A compulsive reduction of body weight to an unhealthful level by rigorous dieting, often supplemented by strenuous exercise, self-induced vomiting, or the use of diuretics or laxatives (see ■ **Figure 6-2**).

Most patients are women with perfectionistic, obsessional personalities and distorted body image (**body dysmorphic disorder**). Onset typically occurs at or just after puberty. Steady loss of subcutaneous fat and wasting of muscle mass can lead to severe emaciation. Chronic nutritional deficiency induces abnormalities in body chemistry and physiology including amenor-

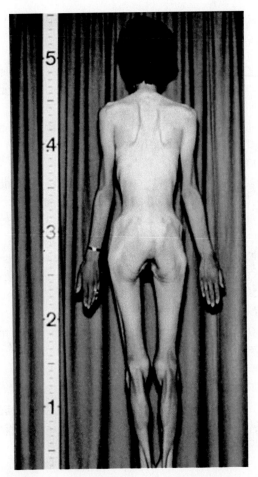

FIGURE 6-2. A woman with anorexia nervosa. Source: NMSB, Custom Medical Stock Photo.

rhea, bradycardia, hypotension, electrolyte imbalance, anemia, and dry skin with increased pigmentation and downy hair growth (lanugo).

Treatment often requires intensive counseling, pharmacotherapy, and even hospital confinement with intravenous alimentation.

Bulimia Nervosa

A common behavioral disorder of young women characterized by recurrent episodes of binge eating.

The typical patient engages in uncontrollable gorging with high-carbohydrate food several times a week. Resulting anxiety about weight gain usually leads to self-induced vomiting or purging with laxatives. Unlike anorexia nervosa, this disorder is not usually associated with marked weight loss or amenorrhea.

Repeated vomiting may result in erosion of dental enamel, chronic throat irritation, or esophageal injury. Treatment includes counseling and pharmacotherapy.

1. Distinguish among the generalized anxiety disorder, social phobia, agoraphobia, panic disorder, and obsessive-compulsive disorder.
2. List three categories or classes of drugs that are used to treat anxiety disorders and give an example of each.
3. Characterize bipolar disorder, that is, describe the behaviors a patient with bipolar disorder displays over an extended period of time. How is bipolar disorder treated?
4. Distinguish among the dominant clinical manifestations of schizophrenia. How is schizophrenia treated and what are some of the side effects of these drugs?
5. Describe the behaviors associated with the three major characteristics of attention deficit-hyperactivity disorder.
6. Distinguish between anorexia nervosa and bulimia.
7. What are the treatment options for Alzheimer's disease?

Diagnostic and Therapeutic Procedures

brain biopsy Removal of a specimen of brain tissue for histologic study; particularly valuable in confirming a clinical diagnosis of Alzheimer disease but also useful in identifying lesions of infectious or neoplastic origin.

Brief Symptom Inventory (BSI) A brief questionnaire-based survey used to screen psychiatric patients and monitor their progress during treatment. Analysis of patient-reported data helps to identify anxiety, depression, hostility, somatization, and other mental conditions, to estimate the severity of the patient's distress, and to provide a basis for treatment.

cerebrospinal fluid (CSF) analysis Diagnostic evaluation of a specimen of spinal fluid obtained by lumbar puncture is routine when certain organic diseases of the central nervous system are suspected. Testing CSF for three markers (amyloid beta 1-42, total tau protein, and p-tau181p) identifies 90% of persons with Alzheimer disease but also yields positive results in one third of normal persons.

electroconvulsive (electroshock) therapy Delivery of controlled electric shocks to the brain to alter electrochemical function, primarily in depression. The treatment, administered only by a physician, causes convulsions and loss of consciousness; the patient awakens in a state of disorientation. Several treatment sessions may be necessary before improvement is noted.

General Practitioner Assessment of Cognition (GPCOG) A nine-point test of cognitive function used in primary care to screen patients for dementia. It assesses temporal and spatial orientation, ability to draw a clock face, and awareness of a current news event.

Global Assessment of Functioning (GAF) A subjective rating by a mental health professional, on a scale of 0–100, of the social, occupational, and psychological functioning of an adult subject. The scale is published in *DSM*.

Mini-Cog A simple screening test for dementia. The subject is required to identify three objects in the room, draw the face of a clock from memory, and then recall the three objects previously identified.

Mini Mental State Examination (MMSE) (Folstein test) A 30-point questionnaire used to identify and differentiate dementias. The subject is required to demonstrate temporal and spatial orientation, count backward, identify familiar objects, repeat common phrases, perform elementary procedures involving numbers and language, and exercise basic motor skills.

MMPI (Minnesota Multiphasic Personality Inventory) The most widely used and widely researched test of adult psychopathology. Used by clinicians to assess major symptoms of social and personal maladjustment and the selection of appropriate treatment methods. It is also used in chronic pain management and substance abuse programs, in marriage and family counseling, and to support college and career counseling recommendations.

Oswestry Disability Index An assessment of functional impairment by chronic low back pain based on a self-administered questionnaire.

positron emission tomography (PET) scan Creation of tomographic (thin-slice) images by computer analysis of positrons emitted when radioactively tagged substances are incorporated into tissue. Unlike other imaging procedures, PET assesses metabolic activity and tissue function rather than structure. PET scanning of the brain with stereotactic surface projection has yielded 90% accuracy in the diagnosis and differentiation of Alzheimer and frontotemporal dementias (see ■ Figure 6-1). It has also proved useful in assessing parkinsonism, Huntington disease, epilepsy, neoplasms, and acute stroke.

therapeutic blood level Tests the amount of measurable drug in the serum. Many drugs have optimum levels where they are most effective (therapeutic range).

titrate To adjust the dosage of a drug up or down to maintain maximum effectiveness or to reduce side effects.

toxicology screen A panel of blood tests for toxic substances and drugs of abuse including alcohol, amphetamines, barbiturates, benzodiazepines, cannabinoids, cocaine, opiates, and others. Urine tests for some of these substances are also available. Screening may identify the cause of some cases of coma, delirium, or dementia.

WAIS (Wechsler Adult Intelligence Scale) A testing instrument designed to assess intellectual functioning in specific cognitive domains, including verbal comprehension and reasoning ability, and to provide a measure of general intellectual capacity. The current edition is WAIS-IV.

WMS (Wechsler Memory Scale) A specialized instrument for the assessment and differentiation of various memory functions. The fourth edition (WMS-IV) was designed to be used in parallel with WAIS-IV.

Pharmacology

It is estimated that nearly 50% of all hospital admissions are in some way related to a mental health problem such as anxiety, depression, suicide, postpartum depression, psychosis, psychosomatic illness, attention-deficit hyperactivity disorder (ADHD), panic attacks, social phobias, obsessive-compulsive disorder (OCD), posttraumatic stress disorder (PTSD), drug addiction, or alcoholism. Drugs, as well as psychotherapy, behavior modification, or educational programs, are used to treat these diseases.

The treatment of neurosis involves the use of antianxiety drugs, also known as anxiolytic agents or minor tranquilizers. The term **minor tranquilizer** is somewhat of a misnomer in that it carries the connotation that this class of drugs is somehow less effective in treating symptoms than the **major tranquilizers** (used to treat psychosis), or that the minor tranquilizers are only major tranquilizers given at a lower dose. In fact, **minor tranquilizers are completely unrelated chemically to major tranquilizers.** They are extremely effective drugs of great importance with specific therapeutic action in treating neurosis.

Tranquilizers (Anxiolytics)

The **benzodiazepines** are by far the most commonly prescribed drugs for the treatment of **anxiety** and **neurosis**. They bind to several different types of receptor sites in the brain to provide sedation. They affect thought processes, they affect emotional behavior by their action in the limbic area of the brain, and they also decrease the muscle tension that comes with anxiety. All of the benzodiazepines are Schedule IV drugs (which have a lower potential for abuse than other controlled drugs).

  alprazolam (Niravam, Xanax)
  chlordiazepoxide (Librium, Reposans-10)
  clonazepam (Klonopin)
  clorazepate (Tranxene)
  diazepam (Valium)
  halazepam (Paxipam)
  lorazepam (Ativan)
  oxazepam (Serax)

Antidepressants

Frequently prescribed **antidepressant drugs**, whose mechanisms of action vary, include:

  bupropion (Wellbutrin)
  buspirone (BuSpar)
  doxepin (Sinequan)
  escitalopram (Lexapro)
  hydroxyzine (Atarax, Atarax 100, Vistaril)
  meprobamate (Equanil, Miltown)
  paroxetine (Paxil)
  prochlorperazine (Compazine)
  sertraline (Zoloft)
  trimipramine (Surmontil)
  venlafaxine (Effexor)

Drugs Used to Treat Psychosis

The symptoms of **psychosis** include a loss of touch with reality with resulting delusions, hallucinations, inappropriate mood, and bizarre behaviors. Psychotic symptomatology may be based in part on an overactivity of the neurotransmitter dopamine in the brain either from overproduction of dopamine or from hypersensitivity of dopamine receptors.

The treatment of psychosis involves the use of antipsychotic drugs, which are also known as **major tranquilizers** or **neuroleptics**. These drugs block dopamine receptors in many areas of the brain including the limbic system, which controls emotions. Antipsychotic drugs decrease psychotic symptoms of hostility, agitation, and paranoia without causing confusion or sedation. Unlike some antianxiety drugs, none of the antipsychotic drugs are addictive; they are not scheduled drugs or controlled substances.

Phenothiazine drugs used to treat psychosis include:

chlorpromazine (Thorazine)
fluphenazine (Permitil, Prolixin)
mesoridazine (Serentil)
perphenazine (Trilafon)
prochlorperazine (Compazine)
promazine (Sparine)
thioridazine (Mellaril)
trifluoperazine (Stelazine)

Other **antipsychotic drugs** frequently prescribed include:

carbamazepine (Tegretol)
clonazepam (Klonopin)
clozapine (Clozaril)
fluoxetine (Prozac)
haloperidol (Haldol)
risperidone (Risperdal)
thiothixene (Navane)

Drugs for Attention Deficit Disorder (ADD)

Drugs used to treat ADD include **amphetamines** and other related CNS-stimulating drugs. They have a paradoxical reverse effect in that they do not overstimulate but actually reduce impulsive behavior and lengthen the attention span.

Amphetamines used to treat ADD/ADHD are classified as Schedule II drugs. They have the highest potential for abuse and addiction of any drugs used medically.

amphetamine and dextroamphetamine (Adderall)
atomoxetine (Strattera)
dexmethylphenidate (Focalin)
dextroamphetamine (Dexedrine, Dexedrine Spansules, Dextrostat)
fluoxetine (Prozac, Prozac Weekly)
methamphetamine (Desoxyn)
methylphenidate (Concerta, Metadate CD, Metadate ER, Methylin, Ritalin, Ritalin-SR)

Drugs Used to Treat Insomnia

Drugs used to induce sleep are termed hypnotics after *hypnos*, the Greek word for *sleep*.

acecarbromal (Paxarel)
chloral hydrate (Aquachloral Supprettes)
estazolam (ProSom)
eszopiclone (Lunesta)
flurazepam (Dalmane)
glutethimide (Doriden)
lorazepam (Ativan)
quazepam (Doral)
temazepam (Restoril)
triazolam (Halcion)
zaleplon (Sonata)
zolpidem (Ambien, Ambien CR)

Over-the-counter (OTC) sleep aids commonly contain the antihistamine diphenhydramine. These sleep aids use the antihistamine's side effects of drowsiness as the therapeutic effect to treat insomnia.

Bufferin AF Nite Time
Compoz Nighttime Sleep Aid
Excedrin P.M., Excedrin P.M. Liquigels
Nytol
Sominex
Extra Strength Tylenol PM
Sominex, Sominex Pain Relief

COMMONLY ABUSED DRUGS from National Institute on Drug Abuse, **www.drugabuse.gov**

Category	Name	Examples of Commercial and Street Names
alcohol	ethyl alcohol	Found in liquor, beer, and wine
cannabinoids	hashish	bhang, boom, gangster, hash, hash oil, hemp
	marijuana	blunt, dope, ganja, grass, herb, joint, bud, Mary Jane, pot, reefer, green, trees, smoke, sinsemilla, skunk, weed
club drugs	flunitrazepam	*Rophypnol*: forget-me pill, Mexican Valium, R2, roach, Roche, roofies, roofinol, rope, rophies
	GHB	*gamma-hydroxybutyrate*: G, Georgia home boy, grievous bodily harm, liquid ecstasy, soap, scoop, goop, liquid X
	MDMA	ecstasy, Adam, clarity, Eve, lover's speed, peace, uppers
dissociative drugs	dextromethorphan (DXM)	Found in some cough and cold medications: Robotripping, Robo, Triple C
	ketamine	*Ketalar SV*: cat Valium, K, Special K, vitamin K
	PCP and analogs	*phencyclidine*: angel dust, boat, hog, love boat, peace pill
	Salvia divinorum	Salvia, Shepherdess's Herb, Maria Pastora, magic mint, Sally-D
hallucinogens	LSD	*lysergic acid diethylamide*: acid, blotter, cubes, microdot, yellow sunshine, blue heaven
	mescaline	buttons, cactus, mesc, peyote
	psilocybin	magic mushrooms, purple passion, shrooms, little smoke
opioids	heroin	*diacetylmorphine*: smack, horse, brown sugar, dope. H. junk, skag, skunk, white horse, China white; cheese (with OTC cold medicine and antihistamine)
	opium	*laudanum, paregoric*: big O, black stuff, block, gum, hop
other compounds	anabolic steroid	*Anadrol, Oxandrin, Durabolin, Depo-Testosterone, Equipoise*: roids, juice, gym candy, pumpers
	inhalants	*solvents (paint thinners, gasoline, glues); gases (butane, propane, aerosol propellants, nitrous oxide); nitrites (isoamyl, isobutyl, cyclohexyl)*: laughing gas, poppers, snappers, whippets
stimulants	amphetamine	*biphetamine, Dexedrine*: bennies, black beauties, crosses, hearts, LA turnaround, speed, truck drivers, uppers
	cocaine	*cocaine hydrochloride*: blow, bump, C, candy, Charlie, coke, crack, flake, rock, snow, toot
	methamphetamine	*desoxyn*: meth, ice, crank, chalk, crystal, fire, glass, go fast, speed
tobacco	nicotine	Found in cigarettes, cigars, bidis, and smokeless tobacco (snuff, spit tobacco, chew)

Transcription Tips

1. Confusing terms: Some of these terms sound alike; others are potential traps when researching. Memorize the terms and their meanings so that you can select the appropriate term for a correct transcript.

   allusion—an indirect reference
   illusion—an unreal or misleading image or perception
   delusion—a false belief in spite of evidence to the contrary

   The patient made frequent allusions to childhood molestation by her father.

   He made allusion to a history of some kind of tropical disease.

   The patient was suffering from the illusion that there were insects crawling all over him.

   The patient suffered from the illusion of being weightless and transparent.

   The patient had the delusion that his parents had been replaced by alien doppelgangers.

2. Slang terms. Transcribe the slang term *psych* as either *psychiatric* (adjective) or *psychiatry* (noun), selecting the meaning that is appropriate to the context of the report. Not to be confused with *psyche* ("psy-kee") (the mind).

3. Spelling. Many words in this medical specialty begin with a silent *p*: psychiatry, psychiatrist, psychology, psychologist, psychoanalysis, psychogenic, psychomotor, psychoneurosis.

4. Note the challenging spellings of these common psychiatric drugs.

   The antidepressant drug *Asendin* allows patients to ascend from the depths of depression; note, however, that the spelling of *Asendin* does not include the *c* in *ascend*.

5. Be careful when expanding abbreviations.

   The abbreviation *SAD* (seasonal affective disorder) should not be confused with the emotion of sadness.

6. Dictation Challenges

   A common phrase in psychiatry is "the patient is oriented in three spheres," meaning the patient is oriented to time, person, and place. This is the same as "oriented times three," which is transcribed as "oriented x3." Occasionally, you may here "oriented in four spheres"; the fourth sphere is generally assumed to be situation (at home, at a relative's home, in a hospital).

   The chief complaint in a psychiatric history is often quoted in the first person.

   Chief Complaint: "I'm here because I can't stop crying."

Spotlight On

War Souvenirs

by Linda C. Campbell

Bill was a good family friend. A kind, clever, handsome man, he had nonetheless neglected his teeth for years. The state of decay was to the point where his teeth were quite literally rotting out of his mouth. We had assumed the obvious: Bill had a dental phobia. He was afraid of the dentist. What never occurred to any of us, including his wife, was that his mouthful of rotten teeth was a result of deliberate self-neglect. It took a dentist to figure out that Bill's mouth was not primarily a dental problem; it was a psychiatric problem.

Penny, Bill's wife, had recently reached a milestone with her husband. Throughout their marriage, Bill had refused to see a dentist. Penny had been after him for years to please, please do something. Seemingly out of the blue, for the first time in 20 years, Bill told his wife that maybe it was time for him to go to the dentist and see about getting his remaining teeth pulled and replaced with dentures. Penny made the phone call immediately to set him up with an appointment.

Bill and Penny anticipated that it would be a very long appointment. To their surprise, the dentist spent only a few moments looking in Bill's mouth. Then he asked to speak with both of them in his office.

The dentist began to ask questions that had nothing to do with dental work. Did Bill see a psychiatrist regularly? No, Bill replied, but he had talked to a counselor over at the Veterans Administration a couple of times. Next question to Penny: How did she feel about Bill seeing a counselor? Penny said laughingly that she didn't know what her husband had to talk about with a psychiatrist, but as long as it wasn't about her, she was fine with it. Back to Bill: You ever been given medication for anxiety? None. Wait; he was prescribed Librium once when he was having trouble sleeping, but it made him feel loopy and he stopped taking it. Ever use illegal drugs? No. Then more probing questions that had nothing to do with dentistry. Did you serve in the military? Yes. Are you a war veteran? Yes. Were you deployed? Yes, to Vietnam.

A war veteran, Bill claimed that he never spoke to anyone except his wife about what went down in 1960s 'Nam. Penny was quick to point out that Bill never talked about the war, and that she was always careful not to press him about details that he was uncomfortable or unwilling to discuss.

Bill became quiet and stopped responding to the dentist's line of questioning. Penny, assuming the dentist had overstepped the boundaries of acceptable questioning, offered her arm to her husband to help pull him out of the chair. Bill pushed her arm away and leaned back into the chair. "The nightmares are back," he said. His story continued. Something awful had happened in the Mekong Delta, Bill said. He had recurrent nightmares about it for several years, but when the bad dreams went away, he figured he had come to grips with it and made a conscious decision never to talk about it, never remember it, never acknowledge it. The dreams were held at bay until a few weeks ago.

Bill and three of his fellow soldiers had been slogging through the Mekong Delta, a murky wetland with heavy jungle growth. It provided shade from the hot sun and camouflage for the soldiers, but that worked for both Bill's troop as well as the enemy's. The four men were marching single-file through the forested pathway. A voice hollered out a warning an instant before Bill heard a loud explosion. The lead soldier had accidentally tripped an enemy landmine, and Bill had watched frozen with horror as his three buddies were blown up right in front of him. Bill sustained shrapnel wounds but he had survived the explosion. Physically, he survived.

The dentist opinioned that, emotionally, Bill carried unresolved feelings about surviving when the other men had died. Furthermore, he believed that Bill's neglected teeth were a manifestation of a subconscious effort to experience suffering. It's called "survivor's guilt, the dentist explained. (The Oscar-winning 1980 film *Ordinary People*, directed by Robert Redford, well illustrates the concept of survivor's guilt.)

The dentist's diagnosis of survivor's guilt was difficult for Bill to accept. He didn't believe the poor condition of his teeth had anything to do with his mental state. Being afraid to go the dentist didn't

Spotlight On

War Souvenirs *(continued)*

mean he was crazy. Penny tended to agree with Bill. They were both reluctant to face issues that within two years would become a crisis.

Two years after the dentist's assessment, Bill was still having nightmares and now daytime flashbacks of the slaughter. His ability to cope with simple activities of daily living became problematic. He had to be talked into taking a shower, and then further talked into using soap in the shower. Whereas once they had been a social couple, Bill no longer wanted friends over. He had started to hoard useless items and stopped throwing things away.

We didn't see Bill and Penny again as a couple. They ended up divorcing, and Penny died unexpectedly soon after. Prior to her death, I ran into her

at the grocery store and she gave me an update on Bill. "He broke down and went to a shrink at the Veterans Administration," she said. They had diagnosed him at the V.A. with PTSD (posttraumatic stress disorder). Progress had been slow, Penny said, too slow to save the marriage, but she thought Bill was making some headway with private counseling and group therapy and the new antidepressant drugs. His nightmares didn't occur nearly as often. The hoarding was still a problem, though. Bill could control inanimate things; his stuff didn't go away unless Bill decided it was going away. Not so with people. The last I heard from Bill, he said he felt great. He was going to VFW dinners and dances and meeting new people. He had joy in his life again. He never missed a counseling session or a pill. But doggone, Bill never did get his teeth fixed.

PIPELINE DREAMS

When Alzheimer's disease was first identified and for many years after, the only way to definitively prove the diagnosis was by means of a postmortem examination of the brain. As of this writing, clinical diagnosis (based on the history and physical exam) is still the method of diagnosis. There are no definitive diagnostic imaging studies or laboratory tests for biomarkers that can confirm the diagnosis.

However, researchers following participants enrolled in the Women's Health and Aging Study II (WHAS-II), a longitudinal, population-based study of healthy women aged 70 to 80 years living in Baltimore, Maryland, think they may have found a way to predict Alzheimer's disease before it becomes severe.

A link between high serum ceramide levels and memory impairment and hippocampal volume loss had been found in previous studies. Researchers questioned whether high serum ceramide levels are associated with increased risk for Alzheimer's disease. The study showed that higher baseline serum ceramides were associated with increased risk of Alzheimer's.

The women, none of whom had dementia at baseline, were followed for at least 6 visits over a 9-

year period. It was found that those in the middle third of the higher serum ceramide levels had a tenfold increased risk of developing Alzheimer's than those at the lowest levels. Women in the top third were 7.6 times more likely to develop Alzheimer's. The small study needs to be replicated in a larger study, which is under way with more than a thousand people and 4500 blood samples.

Flutemetamol, a new imaging agent, could soon make it possible to identify patients with Alzheimer's sooner and start treatment sooner. Flutemetamol is used in PET scanning to identify beta amyloid, the brain plaque associated with suspected Alzheimer's disease. Flutemetamol has a two-hour half-life, meaning that the tracer can be manufactured elsewhere and shipped to an imaging center for use in PET scanning.

Two other tracers, florbetapir F 18 and florbetaben, are also in late-stage clinical trials for PET scan imaging for Alzheimer's disease.

Source: Fran Lowry, *Medscape Medical News*, July 24, 2012. Whitney L.J. Howell, *Diagnostic Imaging*, July 25, 2011.

Exercises

Medical Vocabulary Review

Instructions: Choose the best answer.

_____ 1. When using words such as "apathetic, blunted, depressed, elated, euphoric, flat, inappropriate, labile," the dicatator is mostly like describing the patient's _____
A. affect.
B. behavior.
C. delusions.
D. cognitive state.

_____ 2. _____ is a form of psychotherapy directed toward helping the patient understand the reasons for distressing emotions, thought patterns, and undesirable behaviors and correct them by adopting more mature, balanced, and realistic attitudes.
A. Aversion therapy
B. Behavioral therapy
C. Cognitive therapy
D. Rational therapy

_____ 3. _____ refers to a labile mood, varying between excitement and depression, not severe enough to be called bipolar disorder.
A. Delusions
B. Dysthymia
C. Confabulation
D. Cyclothymia

_____ 4. Multiaxial assessment is a method of categorizing psychiatric and medical diagnoses that is part of the _____
A. MMSE.
B. DSM-IV.
C. CPT code.
D. WAIS-IV.

_____ 5. In multiaxial assessment, the axis that lists psychosocial and environmental factors that may be contributing to the psychiatric diagnoses is _____
A. Axis I.
B. Axis II.
C. Axis III.
D. Axis IV.
E. Axis V.

_____ 6. A word meaning a general feeling of mental or emotional discomfort is _____
A. neurosis.
B. euphoria.
C. dysphoria.
D. dysthymia.

_____ 7. Unconsciously attributing one's own thoughts and attitudes to others as a means of dealing with guilt or inadequacy is _____
A. projection.
B. sublimation.
C. identification.
D. rationalization.

_____ 8. The primary distinction between neurosis and psychosis is _____
A. the neurotic patient is not paranoid.
B. the psychotic patient has violent tendencies.
C. the neurotic patient stays in touch with reality.
D. the psychotic patient has hallucinations.

_____ 9. The part of the mental status examination that questions the patient about fantasies, phobias, obsessive ideas, delusions, hallucinations, and poverty of imagination is _____
A. sensorium.
B. behavior.
C. thought content.
D. intellectual function.

___10. On the mental status examination, the "organic triad" refers to all of the following EXCEPT _____
A. orientation.
B. insight.
C. judgment.
D. memory.

___11. An instrument used to assess a patient's pain and disability is the _____
A. Mini-Cog.
B. Oswestry Disability Index.
C. Brief Symptom Inventory.
D. General Practitioner Assessment of Cognition.

___12. All of the following are instruments used by the examiner to assess dementia EXCEPT _____
A. Mini-Cog.
B. Brief Symptom Inventory.
C. Mini Mental State Examination.
D. General Practitioner Assessment of Cognition.

___13. Which of the following is the most accurate statement with respect to the distinction between minor and major tranquilizers?
A. Minor tranquilizers are less effective than major tranquilizers.
B. Minor tranquilizers are just major tranquilizers given at a lower dose.
C. Minor tranquilizers are related chemically to major tranquilizers.
D. Minor tranquilizers are extremely effective drugs of great importance with specific therapeutic action in treating neurosis.

___14. Which of the following drugs would most likely be prescribed to a patient with persisting or recurring feelings of apprehension, uneasiness, worry, or fear that is out of proportion to any danger or threat?
A. Ativan (lorazepam).
B. Serentil (mesoridazine).
C. Haldol (haloperidol).
D. Risperdal (risperidone).

___15. Tardive dyskinesia is NOT a side effect of _____
A. prochlorperazine (Compazine).
B. methylphenidate (Ritalin).
C. risperidone (Risperdal).
D. trifluoperazine (Stelazine).

___16. Drugs used to treat psychosis may be referred to as _____
A. anxiolytics.
B. neuroleptics.
C. tranquilizers.
D. amphetamines.

___17. Which of the following drugs does NOT belong in the group with the others?
A. Tegretol (carbamazepine).
B. Haldol (haloperidol).
C. Risperdal (risperidone).
D. Thorazine (chlorpromazine).

___18. Frequently prescribed antidepressant drugs include all of the following EXCEPT _____
A. Prozac (fluoxetine).
B. Zoloft (sertraline).
C. Lexapro (escitalopram).
D. Wellbutrin (bupropion HCl).

___19. Drugs that have the highest potential for abuse and addiction of any drugs used medically are _____
A. amphetamines used to treat ADHD.
B. phenothiazines used to treat psychosis.
C. benzodiazepines used to treat anxiety and neurosis.
D. major tranquilizers used to treat anxiety and neurosis.

___20. All of the following drugs are used to treat ADD/ADHD EXCEPT _____
A. Prozac (fluoxetine).
B. Concerta, Ritalin (methylphenidate).
C. Permitil, Prolixin (fluphenazine).
D. Adderall (amphetamine and dextroamphetamine).

Dissecting Medical Terms

Instructions: As you learned in your medical language course, words are formed from prefixes, combining forms (root word plus combining vowel), and suffixes. Combining vowels (usually o but not always) are used to connect two root words or a root and a suffix. By analyzing these word parts, you can often determine the definition of a term without even looking it up (if you know the definition of the parts, of course!). Being able to divide and analyze the words you hear into their component parts will also improve your auditory deciphering ability and spelling and help you research those words that you cannot easily spell or define. It will also help you decipher, define, and spell coined words that may not appear in reliable resources.

For the following terms, draw a slash (/) between the components and then write a short definition based on the meaning of the parts. Remember that to define a word based on its parts, you start at the end, usually with the suffix. If there's a prefix, that is defined next and finally the combining form is defined. The actual definition of medical words does not always equal the sum of their parts because of changes in meaning over time; when this is the case, adjust your final definition to fit today's use.

Example: normocephalic

Divide & Analyze: normocephalic = normo/cephal/ic = pertaining + head + normal
Define: normal (shape and contour) of the head

1. Term   antecubital
   Divide   _____
   _____
   Define   _____

2. Term   dysthymia
   Divide   _____
   _____
   Define   _____

3. Term   edentulous
   Divide   _____
   _____
   Define   _____

4. Term   encephalopathy
   Divide   _____
   _____
   Define   _____

5. Term   hydrocephalus
   Divide   _____
   _____
   Define   _____

6. Term   introverted
   Divide   _____
   _____
   Define   _____

7. Term   neuropathological
   Divide   _____
   _____
   Define   _____

8. Term   polypharmacy
   Divide   _____
   _____
   Define   _____

9. Term   psychophysiological
   Divide   _____
   _____
   Define   _____

10. Term   schizophrenia
    Divide   _____
    _____
    Define   _____

Spelling Exercise

Instructions: Review the adjective and adverb suffixes in your medical language textbook. Test your knowledge of **adjectives** by writing the adjectival form of the following psychiatric words. Consult a medical dictionary to verify your spelling.

Noun	Adjective
1. arouse	_____
2. assess	_____
3. delusion	_____
4. excess	_____
5. face	_____
6. intellect	_____
7. introvert	_____
8. narcissism	_____
9. repeat	_____
10. trauma	_____

Abbreviations Exercise

Instructions: Expand the following common psychiatric abbreviations and brief forms. Then memorize both abbreviations and definitions to increase your speed and accuracy in transcribing psychiatric dictation.

Abbreviation	Expansion
1. CNS	_____
2. DTs	_____
3. GAF	_____
4. LSD	_____
5. mEq	_____
6. PT	_____
7. THC	_____
8. WAIS	_____
9. WMS-IV	_____

Transcript Forensics

This section presents snippets of transcribed dictations from clinic notes; history and physical examinations and consultations; procedure notes; and discharge summaries. Explain the passage so that a nonmedical person can understand it. Pay particular attention to terms that are in bold type. Sample responses are available to your instructor.

Example

Excerpt: Patient shows significant **psychomotor retardation** but no **agitation**. She speaks in a very low volume voice. She is alert and **oriented in all three spheres**. Memory grossly intact in all modalities. Speech is coherent.

Explanation: The patient's *mental and physical activity is restricted* but she does not seem *upset*. She is able to *think clearly* and knows *people, places, and date and time*. *Recent and remote memory* seems okay on general questioning. Her speech is *understandable*.

1. **Excerpt:** Mood is depressed, tearful, **constricted affect**. No evidence of any **overt psychosis** or **hypomania**. She does have **passive** death wishes, however, denies any active suicidal intentions or thoughts. **Insight and judgment** questionable.

Explanation: _____
_____
_____
_____
_____

2. **Excerpt:** Thought processes **linear and coherent**. Thought content shows no recurrent **psychotic symptoms**. No suicidal ideation or plans. No **homicidal ideation** or plans. The patient does not appear to be reacting to **internal stimuli** and denies auditory or visual hallucinations. Cognitive functions: **Oriented x3**. Remote, recent, and immediate recall is intact.

Explanation: _____
_____
_____
_____
_____
_____
_____

3. Excerpt: At the time of discharge, the patient is alert and **oriented x4**. Mood **euthymic**. **Affect** is appropriate and no longer **blunted or flat**. Memory intact. Insight and judgment good. He denies any suicidal or homicidal ideation.

Explanation: _____
_____
_____
_____
_____
_____
_____

4. Excerpt: Patient responded well to individual and group **psychotherapy, milieu therapy**, and **psycho-pharmacologic** management. Family therapy was also begun and will continue after discharge.

Explanation: _____
_____
_____
_____
_____
_____
_____

5. Excerpt: FAMILY PSYCHIATRIC HISTORY: She has a son with **ADHD**. Her mother and a maternal aunt have been diagnosed with major depression; the mother may have a component of **mania**. The mother abuses **marijuana** and alcohol primarily, but other drugs as well. Her great grandmother on her father's side has **Alzheimer's disease**.

Explanation: _____
_____
_____
_____
_____
_____
_____

6. Excerpt:
DIAGNOSES:
AXIS I **Major depression**, recurrent, severe. Rule out **panic disorder**.
AXIS II **Avoidant personality disorder**.
AXIS III Diabetes mellitus, hypercholesterolemia, obesity, hypertension, obstructive sleep apnea.
AXIS IV Moderate to severe. Financial difficulties, limited support, other psychosocial problems.
AXIS V **GAF**: 45, current. Highest in past year: 50.

Explanation: _____
_____
_____
_____
_____
_____
_____
_____
_____

7. Excerpt: MEDICATIONS: Alprazolam ODT 0.25 mg t.i.d.; Effexor XR 37.5 mg b.i.d.; trazodone 50 mg at bedtime; Ambien 5 mg at bedtime; Ativan 1 mg p.r.n. (Note: Include the drug categories and indication in your explanation.)

Explanation: _____
_____
_____
_____
_____
_____
_____

Sample Reports

Sample psychiatric reports appear on the following pages, illustrating a variety of reports. Fictional names are provided for illustration of proper format, and no resemblance to actual persons is intended. Sample transcripts were prepared according to *The Book of Style for Medical Transcription* (AHDI).

Discharge Summary

AMADOR, ANDREA
Hospital #256243
Admitted: May 1, [add year]
Discharged: May 14, [add year]

CHIEF COMPLAINT
The patient was transferred from the emergency department where she was treated after deliberate suicide attempt on multiple medications.

HISTORY OF PRESENT PSYCHIATRIC ILLNESS
This was the first acute psychiatric hospitalization for this 45-year-old divorced white female, who was admitted to the locked unit on an involuntary commitment status for treatment of depression. The patient attempted suicide by taking an overdose of Asendin, lithium, Xanax, Elavil, and Zoloft. The patient was admitted with the following diagnoses: (1) Major depression with possible psychotic features. (2) Paranoid personality features. (3) Rule out subclinical dementia.

HOSPITAL COURSE
The patient was initially admitted to the locked psychiatric unit on May 1 and was started on Elavil 25 mg p.o. at bedtime and Ativan 1 mg p.o. h.s. p.r.n. insomnia. The patient received regular individual psychotherapy and various group psychotherapies that were available on the unit. After several days of stabilization in the locked psychiatric unit, she was transferred to the acute adult psychiatric unit, where psychiatric treatment continued.

The patient was seen in consultation by her family physician, as described above. Since the patient continued to complain of sleep difficulties, the dose of Elavil was increased to 75 mg, which she tolerated without any side effects. The patient was started on Zoloft on May 9, which she tolerated without side effects during her hospital stay. The dosage of Elavil was further increased to 100 mg p.o. at bedtime on May 10. The patient remained quite depressed, tearful, anxious, and insecure during her hospitalization, especially during the first 5 days. The patient was allowed to hold individual therapy sessions with her outpatient psychotherapist during the last 2-3 days of her hospitalization. Since the patient remained quite anxious, she was started on Librium 5 mg p.o. daily on May 11.

(continued)

Discharge Summary *(continued)*

AMADOR, ANDREA
Hospital #256243
Page 2

The patient was cooperative and compliant with all therapeutic assignments and expectations. She actively participated in individual and group therapy sessions and was able to bring up conflictual issues such as anger, dependency, and poor self-esteem, and was able to begin to deal with these issues effectively. The patient successfully completed the treatment program and was discharged on May 14.

Evaluation prior to discharge revealed that the patient did not have any acute suicidal ideation, intent, or plan. Her mood at the time of discharge was significantly less depressed, with appropriate affect. She denied any feelings of hopelessness or helplessness.

The patient was discharged with prescriptions for Eskalith CR 45 mg p.o. daily, dispense 20; Ogen 1.25 mg p.o. at bedtime, dispense 20; Synthroid 0.1 mg p.o. daily, dispense 20; Elavil 100 mg p.o. at bedtime, dispense 20; Zoloft 50 mg p.o. daily, dispense 20; Librium 5 mg p.o., dispense 20; and Bentyl 20 mg p.o., dispense 20, without refill. The patient had an appointment at the clinic the following day for outpatient followup. She was also strongly advised to obtain medical followup by her family medical doctor after discharge.

DISCHARGE DIAGNOSES
1. Major depression, severe, single episode.
2. Mixed personality disorder with schizoid, hostile-dependent, and passive-aggressive features.

RICHARD KAHN, MD

RK:hpi

D: 5/15/[add year]
T: 5/16/[add year]

Letter

June 25, [add year]

Department of Social Services
Disability Evaluation Division
1992 Golden Gate Boulevard, Suite 9
San Francisco, CA 94132

Re: SENG, RATHANY #123-45-6789

Dear Staff:

Thank you for referring to me the case of Ms. Seng for psychiatric evaluation. The patient was examined in psychiatric consultation on June 22 with the aid of an interpreter. No physical examination was given. No psychological testing was given. All past medical records provided were noted and reviewed.

HISTORY OF PRESENT ILLNESS
Ms. Seng is a 44-year-old Cambodian refugee. She lives in an apartment with her husband and three children. She describes feeling sick all the time, too weak and tired, dizzy and depressed, to do anything except "rest." Currently, she is taking a combination of five different medications under the care of two different physicians. She takes Proventil inhaler for relief of asthma-like symptoms, analgesics, decongestants, and two different forms of tricyclic antidepressants. She feels that the medications are helping her. She is not receiving any formal psychiatric treatment with or without medication.

MENTAL EXAMINATION
The patient is a clean, neatly dressed, well-groomed Asian female. She understands English and responds to questions before they are translated. There is no evidence of any ambulatory difficulties or speech impediments. There is no evidence or history of alcoholism or illicit drug use. She is oriented to time, place, persons, and events. There is no evidence of any delusion or hallucinations at the present time and no history of such in the past. There is no evidence of any paranoia such as feelings of being persecuted or plotted against. Thought content is generally well organized, coherent, and relevant, without flight of ideas or loose associations.

Depression is manifested by occasional crying periods, usually occurring every other day. There is fitful sleep. There are occasional nightmares. There is no suicidal ideation or history of any suicidal attempts. Energy level is described as poor, with description of fatigue with minimal exertion.

Memory for recent and remote events, she feels, is impaired. She cannot recall her Social Security number. She can recall her address and phone number. She can do simple arithmetic such as addition and subtraction between the sums of 1 and 10. General information and knowledge appear to be average.

(continued)

Letter *(continued)*

Re: SENG, RATHANY #123-45-6789
June 25, [add year]
Page 2

DIAGNOSIS

AXIS I
Factitious disorder, not otherwise specified. Rule out posttraumatic stress disorder.

AXIS II
Diagnosis deferred.

AXIS III
No known documented physical illness.

AXIS IV
Degree of psychosocial stressors cannot be evaluated.

AXIS V
Highest level of adaptive functioning cannot be evaluated because of the factitious disorder.

It is my medical opinion that Ms. Seng's impairments regarding her ability to carry out work-related activities cannot be assessed because of the factitious disorder.

Very truly yours,

SARAH KATEN, MD

SK:hpi

Comic Relief

The doctor as humorist:

The patient said her husband took "downers" and she took "uppers" and the relationship didn't work out.

The husband brought the patient to the emergency department because she was unresponsive in bed.

The patient has visions of becoming an expert locksmith and then either having his own business or becoming a burglar. Because of his poor contact with reality, I have doubts that he could function in any of these fields.

He thinks he might have poor memory; however, he cannot remember any details.

It was our opinion that the patient could return to his usual work. The patient was not of the same opinion.

She said she had married the patient for better or for worse. However, she stated she did not expect that there would be so much worse.

Mr. Blank is a giant of a man who appears to be roughly 24 months' pregnant.

The patient says she had an ovary but it died.

The patient says he is already too screwed up to try drugs.

He states he is unable to lift anything heavier than a bottle of beer without causing pain.

Dermatology

7

Learning Objectives

▶ Describe the structure and function of the skin.

▶ Spell and define common dermatologic terms.

▶ Identify dermatology vocabulary that might be used in the review of systems.

▶ Describe the negative and positive findings a physician looks for on examination of the skin.

▶ Describe the typical cause, course, and treatment options for common diseases of the skin.

▶ Identify and define common diagnostic and surgical procedures of the skin.

▶ List common dermatology laboratory tests and procedures.

▶ Identify and describe common dermatology drugs and their uses.

▶ Demonstrate knowledge of anatomical, medical, pharmacological, adjectival, and soundalike terms by accurately completing the exercises in this chapter.

Transcribing Dermatology Dictation

Introduction

Hair, skin, nails . . . these structures comprise the **integumentary system**. Most women and a great many men pay particular attention to and a lot of money for the care and upkeep of these anatomic structures.

Dermatology is the medical specialty concerned with the study, diagnosis, and treatment of the skin and its accessory structures (hair, nails, surface glands). Medical doctors are schooled during their residencies in skin conditions and their attendant treatments, but for serious or hard-to-treat skin disorders, they may refer a patient to a **dermatologist**. Physicians who are dermatologists have advanced training in this art and science. Other subspecialties include **dermatopathology** and **immunodermatology** which are involved with the microscopic evaluation of cutaneous diseases.

Most dermatologists diagnose and treat a whole range of dermatologic conditions, from benign inconveniences such as acne and warts to unidentified or suspicious lesions. Dermatologists are often the first line of defense in identifying and treating skin cancer, a disease that is all too common in sun worshipers, tanning salon aficionados, and fair-skinned people who have had frequent sun exposure.

Most dermatology practices offer aesthetic dermatologic services, that is, the treatment of aging or damaged skin. **Aesthetic dermatology** includes such procedures as chemical peels, microdermabrasion (removing surface skin with a friction device), injectable fillers (collagen) or muscle relaxants (Botox), laser hair removal, laser vein removal, laser resurfacing, and sclerotherapy (injection of a vasoconstricting drug, such as saline, to close off spider veins and varicose veins). **Skin rejuvenation** is a term used to encompass medical treatment or minimally invasive procedures performed to improve the appearance of the skin. Aesthetic procedures have become commonplace in the United States for men as well as women.

Anatomy Review

The **skin** is the largest organ of the human body and accounts for about 15 percent of total body weight. The skin protects the body from injury and provides the first line of defense against disease-causing microbes. It also helps to regulate body temperature and keeps the body from drying out through evapora-

> ### FAST FACTS
>
> Estimates are that the average person sheds up to 500 million cells per day. Because the cells of the epidermis are so easily shed, they are often left behind in crime scenes and can be used to profile a person's DNA.
>
> An average adult's skin spans 21 square feet, weighs 9 pounds, and contains more than 11 miles of blood vessels.
>
> Tattoo artists use a needle that penetrates the epidermis and deposits ink in the dermal layer of the skin; thus, "a tattoo is forever."
>
> A fingernail or toenail takes about 6 months to grow from the base to tip.
>
> The average human scalp has about 100,000 hairs.
>
> Over $5 billion a year is spent on nail services in the U.S.

tion (**thermoregulation**). The skin consists of two layers: the outer epidermis and the inner dermis or true skin (see ■ Figure 7-1).

The **epidermis** is the outer or surface layer that we see when we look at our skin. It has several sublayers: from the most superficial to the deeper layers, they are the **stratum corneum, stratum lucidum, stratum granulosum, stratum spinosum**, and **stratum basale** (basal layer). Dermatologists who perform microscopic examinations of excised specimens may refer to these layers in dictation.

The top layer of the epidermis is composed of dead, flat squamous cells that are shed. These squamous cells are arranged in layers, or **strata**, called **stratified squamous epithelium**. The dead cells are replaced by new cells made in the stratum basale. As these new cells push upward from the stratum basale toward the skin surface, they die and become filled with the protein **keratin**. Because the cells of the epidermis are so easily shed, they are often left behind in crime scenes and can be used to profile a person's DNA.

Melanocytes are the cells that produce **melanin**. They are located in the deeper layers of the epidermis and give skin its coloring (**pigmentation**). The more melanin that is expressed, the darker the skin color. Melanin that is unequally distributed produces scattered dots of darker skin color called **freckles**.

Beneath the epidermis is the middle layer of skin, known as the **dermis** or **corium**. The dermis lies safely

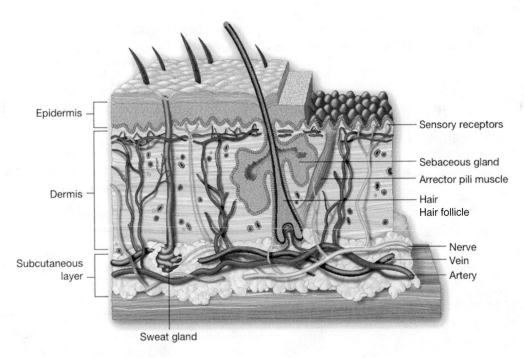

Epidermis

Dermis

Subcutaneous
layer

Sweat gland

Sensory receptors

Sebaceous gland

Arrector pili muscle

Hair
Hair follicle

Nerve
Vein
Artery

FIGURE 7-1. Cross-section of skin and a hair follicle

beneath the epidermis and does not shed. The **dermis** contains a variety of structures. Tiny blood vessels (**capillaries**) carry nourishment form the blood to the dermis. Fibers of **collagen**, an elastic tisue, allow the dermis to stretch (necessary in growth) and retract (when a person loses weight, for example). The older the person, the less elastic these fibers become, leading to "sagging" skin.

Specialized **nerve endings** in the dermis send signals to the brain for the perception of light touch (tactile sensation), pressure, pain, and temperature. Most of the voluntary muscles of the face are anchored to bone and inserted in the dermis, providing for the expression of emotion. Involuntary muscles acting on hair follicles cause "goose pimples" and "hairs standing on end" in response to cold or certain emotions.

Lymph vessels in the dermis transport lymph fluid from tissues into the blood. **Hair follicles** and the **sweat (sudoriferous)** and **oil (sebaceous) glands** are also located in the dermis.

The lowest layer of the skin is the **subcutaneous fascia** or **hypodermis**. It is composed of fibrous connective tissue and fat. **Lipocytes**, which are **fat cells**, are located here. Fat is needed to protect the deeper tissues and act as insulation. Heavier people have more "insulation" and tend to perceive the environmental temperature as warmer than those who are thin. The subcutaneous fascia is attached to the underlying muscles of the body.

Scalp hair serves a purpose other than to adorn the face. It protects the head from sunburn and helps the body retain heat (most body heat is lost through the top of the head). The hair also acts as a net to catch falling or airborne debris, keeping it out of the eyes, nose, and mouth. **Body hair** can be present on every part of the body except the palms of the hands and soles of the feet. It serves the same purpose as scalp hair but is more coarse and thick in the axillary and pubic areas. Eyelashes, for example, protect eyes from foreign bodies, and nose hair, which is often thick and whisker-like, helps trap dust, pollen, even viruses and bacteria.

Hair is made of **keratin**, which is a protein. Only the **base** of the hair (**follicle**) where it inserts into the dermis has nerve endings. It hurts when someone pulls your hair but not when it is cut because the **shaft** of the hair contains no nerves. Small children are often afraid at their very first haircut because they don't understand the difference between pulling and cutting hair; their experiences tell them that hair hurts when brother or sister yanks it. Within the dermis of the hair are blood vessels which nourish the hair follicle.

Nails protect the otherwise vulnerable tops and tips of the fingers and toes.

The surface skin glands are the **sebacous glands** and **sweat glands**. The sebaceous glands secrete an oily substance called **sebum** which moisturizes and protects the skin surface. The sweat glands produce a fluid called **sweat**, a watery, somewhat salty substance that helps cool the body. Sebum and sweat are carried from the glands to the body surface through tiny holes in the skin called **pores**.

Pause for Reflection

1. Distinguish between the dermis and the epidermis.
2. Squamous cells in the epidermis are arranged in layers called _____.
3. What accounts for variations in color of the skin?
4. Most of the cells of the epidermis are _____ containing a horny material called _____ which imparts mechanical toughness to the skin.
5. Unequally distributed melanin produces scattered dots of darker skin color called _____.
6. Elastic tissue that allows the dermis to stretch and retract is called _____.
7. Another word for sweat glands is _____ glands and another word for oil glands is _____ glands.
8. What bodily functions are associated with or provided by the skin?

Vocabulary Review

abscess   A collection of pus in any part of the body that, in most cases, causes swelling and inflammation around it. Pus forms in a tissue space walled off from surrounding tissues by fibrin, coagulated tissue fluids, and eventually fibrous tissue.

alopecia   Local or widespread loss of scalp hair.

avulsion   The ripping or tearing away of a part.

blepharitis   Inflammation of one or both eyelids.

bulla (pl. *bullae*) A blister; a fluid-filled epidermal sac larger than a vesicle.

carbuncle   A spreading lesion made up of furuncles communicating by subcutaneous passages.

cellulitis   A type of infection occurring in soft tissues, including the skin, whose cardinal features are diffuse and spreading tissue swelling, redness, pain, and fever; often caused by streptococci.

cicatrix (scar)   A zone of fibrous tissue occurring at the site of a healed injury or inflammatory or destructive lesion extending into the dermis.

conchal bowl (or **concha**) The cartilage that is situated right near the ear canal and looks like a bowl.

crust   A hard, friable, irregular layer of dried blood, serum, pus, tissue debris, or any combination of these adherent to the surface of injured or inflamed skin; a scab.

cryoprobe   A cryosurgical instrument containing a circulating refrigerant, which can be rapidly chilled so as to deliver subfreezing temperature to tissues.

decubitus ulcer   An erosion of the skin and subcutaneous tissues due to prolonged pressure, occurring chiefly in immobile persons confined to bed. Also known as a *bedsore* or *pressure ulcer*.

Physical examination reveals a very large decubitus ulcer in the area of his right hip. This ulcer is very deep and has required a great deal of debridement and will require much more.

---

dermatitis   Inflammation of the skin. See *photodermatitis* (abnormal skin reaction to sunlight).

dermatographism   The property of abnormally sensitive skin by which strokes or writing with a pointed object are reproduced on the skin surface as raised red lines. Also *dermographism*.

dermatome 1) An instrument used to obtain thin slices of skin for grafting. 2) An area of skin that is mainly supplied by a single spinal nerve (dermatome distribution).

dermatosis   A general term for any abnormal condition of the skin, but usually excluding inflammatory conditions, which are called dermatitis.

discoid Consisting of small, flat plaques.

eczema Superficial dermatitis of unknown cause accompanied by redness, vesicles, itching, and crusting.

erosion   A surface defect in the epidermis produced by rubbing or scratching.

eschar   The crust that forms on a burn.

exacerbation   An increase in the severity of a disease, particularly when occurring after a period of improvement (remission).

excoriation   Abrasion of the epidermal surface by scratching.

fissure A linear defect or crack in the continuity of the epidermis.

friable Crumbly; fragmenting or bleeding easily on touch or manipulation; said usually of diseased tissue.

furuncle A deep, solitary abscess; a boil.

hypertrophic Overgrown, usually as a result of increase in the size of cells.

keloid A firm, nodular, irregular, often pigmented mass of fibrous tissue representing a hypertrophic scar.

lichenification Thickening, coarsening, and pigment change of skin due to chronic irritation, usually scratching.

macule A flat patch or mark differing in color from surrounding skin.

malar Pertaining to or situated on the cheeks.

nevus (1) A pigmented lesion of the skin. (2) A skin lesion present since birth (birthmark).

papule A small elevated zone of skin.

pit A small depression in the skin resulting from local atrophy or scarring after trauma or inflammation.

plantar (*not* planter) Pertaining to the sole of the foot.

pruritus, pruritic Itching.

pustule A small, elevated, circumscribed lesion of the skin that is filled with pus.

pyoderma General term for any purulent (pus-forming) infection o f the skin.

rhinophyma Enlargement and deformity of the external nose, usually as a result of rosacea.

scab See *crust*.

scale A flake of epidermis shed from the skin surface.

scar See *cicatrix*.

telangiectatic Pertaining to telangiectasia; a permanent dilatation of small blood vessels (capillaries, arterioles, venules), visible through a skin or mucous surface.

ulcer A cutaneous defect extending into the dermis.

vector An animal that transmits a pathogenic organism from one host to another.

venous stasis (ulcer, discoloration) Cessation or impairment of venous flow, initially causing skin discoloration but may lead to a skin ulcer.

LAY AND MEDICAL TERMS

athlete's foot	tinea pedis
baldness	alopecia
bruise	contusion
blackhead	comedo
blister	vesicle
cold sore/fever blister	herpes simplex
common wart	verruca vulgaris
hives	urticaria (or wheals)
jock itch	tinea cruris
pimples	acne vulgaris
shingles	herpes zoster
wrinkles	rhytides
zit	(acne) pustule

vesicle A small thin-walled sac containing clear fluid.

wheal (weal, welt) A small zone of edema in the skin, which may be red or white and may appear or disappear abruptly; typically accompanied by intense itching. Local or generalized eruptions of wheals are called hives (urticaria).

Medical Readings

History and Physical Examination
by John H. Dirckx, MD

Review of Systems. Skin. The patient is questioned about prior diagnosis of severe or chronic cutaneous disease and any treatments used for them in the past or at present. The more common skin complaints include local or general eruptions or rashes, itching, dryness or scaling, pigment changes, and solid tumors of various kinds. Disorders of the **hair** (abnormal appearance of the hair, excessive hair, hair loss) and **nails** (deformity, discoloration) are also part of the dermatologic history.

The physician questions the patient about the duration of the problem; whether it comes and goes, remains unchanged, or is gradually getting better or worse; whether it is spreading from one area to others; whether the patient can suggest any reason for the problem; and

Skin: No history of itching, rash, nonhealing sores, or pigmented lesions.

whether anything seems to make the problem better or worse.

Physical Examination. Cutaneous diagnosis depends on a consideration of many factors: the type, number, grouping, and location of lesions; combinations of features occurring together; signs of evolutionary change, secondary infection, or the effects of treatment; and the presence of associated symptoms such as fever, headache, or pain in the joints or abdomen. While many skin problems (acne, warts, poison ivy, ringworm) arise in the skin and stay there, many others (hives, the eruptions of chickenpox and lupus erythematosus) are signs of systemic disease.

In assessing the skin, the physician ensures adequate exposure of the surface by removing clothing, dressings, bandages, and ointments and by using bright natural or artificial light and, as needed, a magnifying lens.

Examination of the skin is not carried out by inspection alone. The examiner palpates any area of skin that appears abnormal and observes its temperature, texture, tenseness or laxness, moistness or dryness, and also looks for tenderness and crepitation.

Turgor is the degree to which tissue spaces, particularly in the skin and subcutaneous tissues, are filled with extracellular fluid. When a zone of normally lax skin, such as on the abdomen, is gently picked up between thumb and finger and then released, it should flatten out again immediately. Failure to do so (**tenting**) indicates poor skin turgor, a sign of significant dehydration.

In evaluating skin color, the examiner considers the intensity and distribution of normal **pigment** (melanin) and any abnormal coloration, including cyanosis (blueness), erythema (redness), jaundice (yellowness), and bronzing. Localized or generalized loss of pigment is also noted, as well as any tattoos and surgical or traumatic scars. When local or diffuse redness is present, a diascope can be used to distinguish capillary dilatation from other causes. A **diascope** is a small flat piece of clear glass or plastic, which is pressed firmly against the reddened skin. **Blanching** (fading of redness) on pressure indicates that redness is probably due to dilatation of skin capillaries. Redness that is due to hemorrhage or abnormal pigmentation will not fade on pressure.

Pause for Reflection

1. List three common skin complaints.
2. Examination of the skin is carried out by means of what techniques?
3. What is *turgor* in reference to the skin?
4. What is *tenting*?
5. Explain *blanching* and its significance.

Perspectives on Dermatology

by John H. Dirckx, MD

Pity the dermatologist!

Colleagues in other branches of medicine never tire of accusing the specialist in skin diseases of *making rash judgments*, of *not looking beyond the surface*, of *running a skin game* . . . and much more along the same lines.

And it gets worse. Among the hoary axioms of medical lore, none are so deeply ingrained as those that state that a dermatologist's patients never get better and never die; that dermatologists don't have to take night or weekend call because there are no cutaneous emergencies; that the diagnosis of skin disease poses no mysteries, because the evidence is all out in the open; that classing dermatology as a branch of internal medicine is therefore preposterously paradoxical; that the diagnostic labels assigned to cutaneous lesions are chiefly descriptive because their essential nature remains unknown; and that the whole of dermatologic therapy is summed up in one simple formula: if it's wet, dry it; if it's dry, wet it; and if that doesn't work, try steroids.

Let's take a closer look at these belittling views of cutaneous medicine and see how well they stand up under scrutiny.

The dermatologist's patients never get better, and they never die.

This double-barreled slur implies not only that skin disorders are all relentlessly chronic and only slightly responsive to treatment, but that they're so trivial that they pose no threat to life.

It's true that some of the more common skin disorders, such as psoriasis, seborrheic dermatitis, and atopic eczema, are stubbornly persistent, their treatment mainly symptomatic, their victims doomed indefinitely to repeated visits to the dermatologist.

But nearly every kind of specialist has a captive clientele of patients who keep coming back over the

Examination today reveals an acute eczematous dermatitis which for the first time shows a fairly definite pattern over her buttock area, low midback, and shoulders.

years because of chronic conditions. In cardiology it's hypertension and coronary artery disease; in pulmonology, asthma and chronic bronchitis; in gastroenterology, irritable bowel syndrome and inflammatory bowel disease; in rheumatology, more than twenty varieties of arthritis; in psychiatry, anxiety and depression.

Besides, many cutaneous maladies (bacterial and fungal infections, contact dermatitis) clear up completely and permanently with appropriate treatment. Others (infantile eczema, adolescent acne, pityriasis rosea) resolve spontaneously with the passage of time.

The view that there are no lethal skin disorders is utterly false. Cutaneous melanomas cause 9000 deaths yearly in this country. Squamous cell carcinomas, much less likely to metastasize but also much more common, account for another 3000 deaths annually.

Pemphigus vulgaris is a blistering dermatosis caused by autoimmune destruction of a tissue substance that binds epithelial cells together. The dermatologist must not only recognize this disorder but institute prompt immunosuppressive treatment, without which the disease has a significant mortality rate. Most deaths are due to staphylococcal infection. Because immunosuppression inhibits the inflammatory response to infection, the treating physician must be particularly alert for subtle signs that antibiotic therapy is also indicated.

Equally fallacious is the belief that **there are no dermatologic emergencies**.

One survey found that 5% of emergency department visits were for skin complaints; at a pediatric emergency department the figure was 31%. These numbers must not be taken too seriously, however. As most of us are aware, only a minority of emergency department visits nowadays are for truly urgent problems.

But several disorders with cutaneous manifestations are recognized as life-threatening emergencies. These include fulminating infections such as meningococcemia, necrotizing fasciitis, and toxic shock syndrome, and severe allergic reactions such as toxic epidermal necrolysis and Stevens-Johnson syndrome. Each of these requires rapid, accurate recognition and aggressive, specific therapy. Each can prove lethal within 24 hours if misdiagnosed or mismanaged.

Is it true that **the basis for a dermatologic diagnosis is plainly evident to the eye**?

Hardly. As in other specialties, dermatologic diagnosis begins with the history—the onset, duration, and progression or spread of cutaneous signs, the presence of itching or burning, possibly relevant family, occupational, or travel history, recent or current use of medicines, and associated symptoms such as fever, chills, nausea, or muscle or joint pain. In arriving at a diagnosis, the dermatologist may consider the results of laboratory studies—smear, culture, biopsy, blood studies—and the response to treatment.

You can count on your ten fingers the so-called **primary lesions of cutaneous disease**: macule, papule, nodule, vesicle, bulla, pustule, plaque, wheal, petechia, purpura. Even fewer are the secondary lesions, which arise through the evolution of primary lesions or from external factors such as scratching, infection, or treatment: erosion, ulcer, excoriation, crust, scale, lichenification, atrophy. More than a thousand named diseases or conditions of the skin consist of various combinations and permutations of these few basic elements. Merely recognizing them is as easy as distinguishing among pieces of fruit in a basket, but recognition is only the beginning.

What is the exact shape of the lesions? Are they round, oval, ring-shaped, bull's-eye-shaped, scalloped, dimpled, wholly irregular? Is their color due to dilated capillaries, extravasated blood, deposits of pigment, lipid, or other materials? Is the color evenly distributed? Are lesions isolated, grouped in linear or anular array, or randomly distributed?

Are they limited to certain skin surfaces (flexor/extensor, hairy/hairless, sun-exposed/sun-protected, scalp, finger webs, bilaterally symmetrical)?

Collecting and sorting the data, weighing one piece of evidence against another, perceiving interrelations, interpreting subtle signs, discarding red herrings—all these go into finding the correct solution. The very essence of dermatologic diagnosis is the ability to discern a unifying pattern that fits one diagnosis and no other, a skill that takes years of experience to develop.

How can dermatology be classed as a branch of internal medicine? To answer that, we must trace the history of the expression *internal medicine* (German *innere Medizin*) to its origins in the nineteenth century, when the modern medical specialties began to emerge. Until then the average physician dealt with the entire range of human ills, and practiced surgery, dentistry, obstetrics, and pharmacy as the occasion arose.

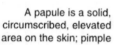

A macule is a discolored spot on the skin; freckle

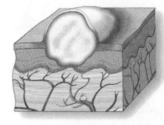

A pustule is a small, elevated, circumscribed lesion of the skin that is filled with pus; varicella (chickenpox)

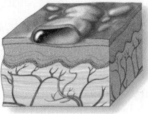

A wheal is a localized, evanescent elevation of the skin that is often accompanied by itching; urticaria

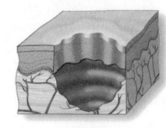

An erosion or ulcer is an eating or gnawing away of tissue; decubitus ulcer

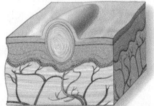

A papule is a solid, circumscribed, elevated area on the skin; pimple

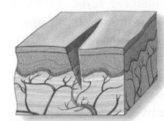

A fissure is a crack-like sore or slit that extends through the epidermis into the dermis; athlete's foot

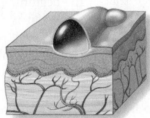

A vesicle is a small fluid-filled sac; blister. A bulla is a large vesicle.

FIGURE 7-2. Primary skin lesions

The development of ophthalmology, otorhinolaryngology, orthopedics, and other fields dealing with specific body areas left a broad residue of practice that was called internal because it was concerned largely with disorders of the thoracic and abdominopelvic viscera. A more apt term, found in the modern medical lexicon, is *systemic*.

Numerous systemic diseases have cutaneous manifestations, which can tip off the astute diagnostician to their presence before more obvious and ominous signs and symptoms appear. Unlike ivy dermatitis and plantar warts, the classical childhood febrile exanthems (measles, rubella, varicella, roseola, and scarlet fever) are systemic infections with prominent cutaneous features. Other infectious diseases are accompanied by dis-

tinctive dermal signs, such as erythema chronicum migrans in Lyme disease, the rose spots of typhoid fever, and the notoriously protean (variable) skin manifestations of secondary syphilis.

Several autoimmune disorders elicit characteristic cutaneous reactions (the palpable petechiae of vasculitis, the butterfly rash of systemic lupus erythematosus, and the heliotrope rash of dermatomyositis). Cutaneous markers of internal malignancy include acanthosis nigricans, extramammary Paget disease, and Peutz-Jeghers syndrome.

Primary care providers may perhaps be excused for misdiagnosing some of these as allergic or nonspecific skin reactions and zapping them with topical steroids. But the special skill of the dermatologist consists precisely in the ability to recognize and interpret these skin signs and deduce their significance accurately.

The inclusion of dermatology as a branch of internal medicine thus reflects the perception that the skin is a mirror of "internal" disease, and that the dermatologist's diagnostic focus is not confined to a few millimeters of integument.

The names of skin diseases are purely descriptive, because nobody knows what causes most of them.

Before the fields of dermatopathology, microbiology, and histochemistry came into being and furnished precise explanations for them, skin conditions were indeed given purely descriptive names such as *dermatitis exfoliativa, erythema anulare centrifugum, lichen planus, pityriasis rosea,* and *pyoderma gangrenosum.* After all, some kind of distinctive labels were needed, and what more logical than to base those labels on visual features?

If many of these terms remain in use today, like the much older and entirely misleading *cholera, influenza,* and *malaria,* that is simply because they had become deeply entrenched in daily use and codified in hundreds of books and articles long before their genetic, infectious, degenerative, or malignant bases had been discovered.

If it's wet, dry it; if it's dry, wet it; if all else fails, prescribe steroids.

That may sound like a waggish epigram by Oscar Wilde, but it happens to sum up, with perfect accuracy, the basics of dermatologic therapy. Virtually all textbooks agree that wet, oozing lesions should be treated with topical astringents and other drying agents. They also agree that dry, scaly lesions should be hydrated and lubricated with wetting agents and emollients. Moreover, the selection and dosage of topical (sometimes systemic) **corticosteroids** in the management of skin disease (including, when appropriate, their omission) became one of the defining elements of the art of dermatology during the second half of the twentieth century.

Clearly it is inappropriate to dismiss dermatology as a branch of medicine dealing with trivial but persistent nuisances limited to the body surface, for which the specialist has only picturesque names and a rigidly simplistic and minimally efficacious therapeutic armamentarium. **Cutaneous medicine** is a reputable and indispensable specialty, whose practitioners are uniquely equipped to face many diagnostic and therapeutic challenges.

Pause for Reflection

1. Using the text, refute each of the following statements.
   a. Dermatology patients never get better, and they never die.
   b. There are no dermatologic emergencies.
   c. The basis for a dermatologic diagnosis is plainly evident to the eye.
2. Summarize the basics of dermatologic therapy.

Advanced Wound Therapy

Negative Pressure Wound Therapy
by John H. Dirckx, MD

Most of the recent advances in medical science have involved creating things that never existed in nature, such as synthetic antibiotics and radiopharmaceuticals. But sometimes real progress is made simply by finding ways to aid and abet the natural healing power of living tissues or to exploit natural forces such as gravity and osmotic pressure. And occasionally what seems like a cutting-edge development turns out to be the reinvention or rediscovery of a principle or technique that is hundreds or thousands of years old.

The application of **oral suction** to snakebites and certain other superficial lesions must surely go back very far into human prehistory. The practice of **cupping** (creating a partial vacuum within a cup-shaped vessel of horn or metal placed over a lesion or incision to draw out blood or other material) was well established before the beginning of the Christian era. Rubber bulbs, syringes, aspirators, suction pumps, and vacuum drainage devices have been integral features of medicine and surgery for decades or centuries.

Negative pressure wound therapy (NPWT) is therefore not so much the exploitation of a newly discovered principle or property of nature as a refinement of existing knowledge and techniques. NPWT is the intermittent application of a partial vacuum to a wound, ulcer, or other surface lesion by means of a motorized pump, appropriate tubing, and a dressing of spongelike synthetic material held in place by an occlusive drape.

Within the past decade, NPWT has shown promise in promoting the healing of acute and chronic wounds, partial-thickness burns, diabetic and pressure ulcers, and skin grafts. An environment of controlled negative pressure increases local vascularity and oxygenation of tissues while evacuating edema fluid, exudate, extravasated blood, and bacteria.

The use of polyurethane foam with a mechanical vacuum pump was approved for wound care by the U.S. Food and Drug Administration (FDA) in 1995. In this method a sterile, resilient, open-cell polyurethane foam dressing material is trimmed to fit a surface lesion or to fill a wound or ulcer. The dressing is held in place and its margins sealed with a drape that has an acrylic adhesive coating.

The application of negative pressure to the occluded foam causes its cells to collapse and exert a continuous suction on the covered tissues. A manometer at the pump measures the degree of vacuum within the system. Drainage is collected in a canister. The use of a Y-connector makes it possible to treat more than one lesion simultaneously with a single pump.

NPWT removes interstitial fluid and infectious materials and maintains a closed, warm, moist environment for wound healing. Animal and limited human studies suggest that negative pressure assists in the development of granulation tissue, with wound contracture and neo-epithelization, by mechanically stimulating cell proliferation and angiogenesis (capillary formation).

Negative pressure wound therapy can be applied in a hospital or nursing facility or in the patient's home. Selected patients can remain ambulatory and even resume employment with a battery-operated portable pump worn on a belt around the waist. Dressings are normally left in place for 48 hours between changes. More frequent changes may be appropriate in the presence of infection or when close monitoring of wound status is necessary. Foam is not bioabsorbable and must be completely removed at each dressing change.

Current treatment guidelines call for a negative pressure of 125 mmHg to be applied for 5-minute periods separated by 2-minute intervals of normal pressure. These recommendations are based on empirical observations that a stronger vacuum or a continuous vacuum is associated with reduced rather than increased blood flow.

Vacuum therapy has been applied successfully to a wide variety of lesions, including deep, complicated, nonhealing wounds of mixed etiology, dehiscent surgical wounds, neuropathic and ischemic ulcers, and pressure ulcers (**bedsores**). It has permitted the use of simple techniques for soft-tissue reconstruction and wound closure that formerly required complex pedicled or microsurgical free flaps.

Some surgeons routinely employ NPWT both before and after skin grafting. Application of negative pressure to a thoroughly debrided wound promotes formation of a richly vascularized bed of granulation tissue for grafting. After graft placement, a vacuum foam dressing serves as a bolster, conforming to the contours of the graft and keeping it in contact with its bed, and further enhances the probability of a successful take by continuously removing edema fluid or exudate from beneath the graft and reducing the microbial population. Foam that has been impregnated with ionic silver may be preferred for treating colonized or infected lesions or to reduce the risk of infection in skin grafts.

Contraindications to the use of NPWT include the presence within the treatment zone of severely ischemic, necrotic, or malignant tissue; uncontrolled infection; exposed organs, bone, or blood vessels; and a non-enteric fistula or sinus tract. All devitalized or necrotic tissue must be debrided, necessary surgical revascularization must be performed, and infection must be controlled with antibiotic therapy or by excision of osteomyelitic bone before application of negative pressure therapy. Grafting over exposed organs, blood vessels, tendons, nerves, bone, or implanted hardware requires the surgical interposition of natural tissues or the creation of a complete barrier with fine-meshed collagen or synthetic material.

The potential for significant hemorrhage with vacuum therapy must be considered in the immediate postoperative period, in patients with fresh vascular grafts, and in those on anticoagulants. Poor patient compliance, such as may occur in dementia, negates the benefits of the treatment and contraindicates it.

Although employed with increasing frequency and supported by favorable anecdotal reports, NPWT has not been extensively studied in randomized clinical trials, and compelling evidence of its effectiveness in some applications is lacking. Large and rigorously controlled trials are under way and may eventually provide strong endorsement of NPWT. Meanwhile, health insurance carriers including Medicare have recognized it as medically necessary and reimbursable for certain conditions.

Pause for Reflection

1. What is the mechanism by which negative wound pressure therapy works?
2. Discuss the medical applications for which vacuum pressure is suitable.
3. Discussion contraindications for the use of NWPT.

Hyperbaric Oxygen Therapy

by John H. Dirckx, MD

The combination of elevated atmospheric pressure and the breathing of pure oxygen constitutes **hyperbaric oxygen therapy (HBOT)**. Although first used to treat decompression sickness, HBOT has found application in many other acute and chronic conditions. The basis of its effectiveness in most of those other conditions appears to be its ability to raise the concentration of oxygen in tissues.

HBOT achieves this result by two unrelated mechanisms. First, breathing pure oxygen under hyperbaric (higher than atmospheric) pressure virtually saturates hemoglobin, the constituent of red blood cells that transports oxygen in loose chemical combination from the lungs to the tissues. Breathing 100% oxygen at normal atmospheric pressure cannot achieve anything like this saturation.

Second, under increased atmospheric pressure, more oxygen gas is dissolved in the plasma (the fluid component of circulating blood). Although under normal conditions the transport of dissolved oxygen by the plasma is far less significant than its transport by hemoglobin, with HBOT the contribution of plasma transport to tissue oxygenation increases enormously. In fact, breathing pure oxygen at three times normal atmospheric pressure results in a 15-fold increase in the concentration of oxygen dissolved in plasma. That is a concentration sufficient to supply the needs of the body at rest even in the total absence of hemoglobin!

Increasing the oxygen supply to damaged or infected tissue promotes healing by stimulating angiogenesis (the formation of new capillaries) and enhancing the proliferation of fibroblasts (cells that produce collagen fibers for the repair of injury). These effects can be of critical importance in certain conditions, including wounds that refuse to heal because of severe mechanical damage, vascular compromise, or diabetes.

Delivery of oxygen to tissues at high concentrations can have beneficial effects beyond those noted. A rise in tissue oxygen causes vasoconstriction, which reduces edema in crushed or burned tissues and decreases intracranial pressure in acute head trauma and intracranial abscess. It also suppresses the growth of anaerobic bacteria (which prefer an environment low in oxygen) in gas gangrene and of some aerobic organisms involved in necrotizing soft tissue infections.

Although tissues, particularly those involved in superficial infections and nonhealing wounds, absorb some oxygen directly from a hyperbaric environment, the principal effect of HBOT is achieved through augmentation of oxygen delivery by the lungs. Local treatment of superficial lesions with oxygen applied through a topical unit under slightly elevated pressure is not HBOT and is only marginally effective.

In hospital settings, multiplace chambers provide room for several patients as well as for physicians or medical attendants. Inside such a chamber both patients and medical staff breathe from flexible, transparent soft plastic helmets or tightly fitting aviators' masks, which supply pure oxygen. A multiplace chamber is equipped with means of removing exhaled carbon dioxide and water vapor from the atmosphere. In addition, exhaled oxygen must be continuously extracted from the atmosphere to reduce the risk of fire. The largest hyperbaric chamber in the U.S. is a 6,000-square-foot facility built at the Mayo Clinic in 2007 with a seating capacity of 24.

One standard atmosphere (1.0 atm), the pressure exerted by the atmosphere at sea level, is defined as 760 torr (mm of mercury, mmHg), 29.92 inches of mercury (mmHg), 14.696 psi (pounds per square inch), 1013.25 millibars, or 101.325 kPa (kilopascals). In HBOT parlance, a pressure of 1.0 atm is referred to as 1.0 ATA (for "atmosphere absolute").

A typical HBOT session consists of 90 to 120 minutes of pure oxygen breathing at 2.0 to 2.5 ATA. HBOT sessions may be referred to as "dives," with patients being said to have "arrived at depth" and being "brought to surface" at specified times. The duration, frequency, and total number of sessions of HBOT for various indications have not yet been standardized. For most conditions, treatments are administered once daily. For acute disorders such as decompression sickness and carbon monoxide poisoning, one or two sessions may suffice. For chronic disorders such as diabetic ulcers, therapy may be continued for 50 or more sessions. A session can cost up to $1000, depending on the facility.

A QUESTIONING MIND

It's easy to let your mind wander while transcribing and start transcribing what you hear rather than what the dictator is saying. Staying alert is essential to avoid transcribing something like "you stitch" when you hear "U stitch," referring to the suture pattern.

Sometimes, you'll hear some strange expressions, such as "patient arrived at depth" and "patient was brought to the surface," or "brought to sea level." While these expressions are typical of hyperbaric oxygen treatment reports, the lesson here is that some things you'll hear may not make sense but other things that you hear may make some kind of sense to you.

It's always a good idea to have a questioning mind. Question anything you hear that is new, odd, different than what you expect to hear. If you can't document a term or expression, ask for help or leave a blank.

Portable HBOT chambers made of nonrigid materials can achieve pressures of about 1.3 ATA. These less expensive units may be found in smaller healthcare facilities and are also used in homes.

Hyperbaric oxygen therapy is not without its discomforts and dangers. The commonest adverse effect is pain in the ears due to stretching of the tympanic membranes by the pressure difference between the middle ear and the surrounding atmosphere. This is similar to what happens when you drive through the mountains or travel by air. Although many people are able to equalize pressures by wiggling their jaws or performing some variation of the Valsalva maneuver, some cannot. For these, surgical placement of ventilating tubes in the tympanic membranes may make the difference between a successful series of HBOT sessions and no treatment.

The maximum pressure for HBOT is 3.0 ATA, because oxygen toxicity, with pulmonary edema or seizures, can occur at pressures above that limit. Even below 3.0 ATA, a patient wearing a helmet or mask for HBOT may be instructed to remove it occasionally and breathe atmospheric air to permit the partial pressure of oxygen in the blood to drop. These intervals of breathing room air are called air breaks (not "air brakes"!). In a monoplace chamber that is filled with pure oxygen under pressure, the patient must breathe through a mask providing ordinary air in order to take an air break.

Pause for Reflection

1. How does HBOT aid in the healing of chronic wounds?
2. Describe a typical HBOT session.
3. What are some of the dangers of HBOT?

Common Diseases

Atopic Dermatitis (Eczema)

A chronic pruritic condition of the skin.

Cause: Unknown. Most patients have a personal or family history of allergy. May be exacerbated by irritants, emotional stress.

History: Recurrent itching, particularly affecting the back of the neck and the antecubital and popliteal areas, usually causing constant scratching.

Physical Examination: Patches of redness, sometimes with weeping, scaling, or vesiculation. Excoriations and lichenification from scratching. Sometimes evidence of secondary infection.

Diagnostic Tests: Scratch tests and RAST may be positive for many allergens.

Course: Chronic, with remissions and exacerbations. Secondary infection may result from scratching, and very chronic lesions may progress to fibrosis or pigmentation.

Treatment: Avoidance of known allergens, irritants, strong soaps, excessive wetting of skin, and excessive bathing. Moisturizers to restore texture of skin, and topical adrenocortical steroids to reduce itching and inflammation.

Contact Dermatitis

Dermatitis resulting from contact with an irritant or allergen.

Cause: Numerous substances, including industrial chemicals, cosmetics, toiletries, and household products, can cause either an irritant or allergic-type of contact dermatitis. Irritant contact dermatitis results from direct chemical attack on the skin and typically produces symptoms within minutes of exposure. Allergic contact dermatitis occurs only in sensitized persons, and there may be a latent period of 2-5 days between exposure and appearance of symptoms.

History: Itching, burning, stinging, with variable amounts of swelling, redness, and other physical signs, on parts of the skin that have been exposed to the causative agent.

Physical Examination: Redness, swelling, vesicles or bullae, weeping, crusting. Signs of damage from scratching or of secondary infection may be present.

Course: Secondary infection may occur.

Treatment: Avoidance of the cause, soothing applications, topical or even systemic adrenocortical steroids.

Impetigo

A spreading bacterial infection of the skin causing itching and crusted sores.

Cause: Staphylococci, sometimes streptococci. Infection may begin in a trivial cut or abrasion. Impetiginization refers to the development of impetigo in an area of skin already damaged by a noninfectious dermatitis. Scratching and poor personal hygiene, particularly among children, lead to rapid spread of lesions and often transmission to household contacts, schoolmates, or playmates.

History: Itching and crusted sores, especially on the face.

Physical Examination: Macules, vesicles, bullae, pustules, and copious gummy purulent exudate forming honey-colored crusts on an erythematous base. In severe infection there may be fever.

Diagnostic Tests: Smear and culture can identify the causative bacteria.

Course: Without treatment, increasing spread often occurs. Systemic effects (toxemia, dehydration) may occur in children, particularly those already debilitated by disease or malnutrition. A severe form of impetigo known as ecthyma may leave scars.

Treatment: Strict attention to personal hygiene; isolation may be appropriate. For most cases of impetigo, the antibiotic mupirocin applied as an ointment is curative. In the presence of extensive disease, fever, or toxemia, antibiotics are administered systemically.

Tinea Corporis (Tinea Circinata, Ringworm of the Body)

Superficial fungal infection of the skin.

Cause: Fungi of the genera *Epidermophyton*, *Microsporum*, and *Trichophyton*. Transmission from infected persons or animals sometimes occurs. Moisture and friction favor invasion of skin.

RINGWORM
The long-established lay term *ringworm* causes much misunderstanding and consternation. Skin diseases known by this name are not due to worms, and physicians never thought they were. The word *ring* in *ringworm* refers to the circular shape of the lesions, with central clearing. *Worm* is just a metaphorical allusion to the "moth-eaten" appearance of skin infected by various superficial fungi. Clothes-eating moth larvae are incorrectly called worms. *Tinea*, the Latin term for ringworm, also means "moth."

History: One or more slowly expanding round or oval patches of red, scaly skin, usually on exposed surfaces, with a variable amount of itching. There may be a history of recent new exposure to domestic animals or to persons with similar lesions.

Physical Examination: Lesions are pink, red, or tan, round or oval and sharply circumscribed, and covered with fine scales. The outer border of a lesion is raised slightly, and with continuing expansion of the margin, the skin near the center of the lesion gradually clears and assumes a normal appearance.

Diagnostic Tests: Scrapings of scales heated with potassium hydroxide (KOH) often show fungal material on microscopic examination. Culture on Sabouraud's medium may be required to confirm the presence of fungi. Examination with Wood light shows characteristic fluorescence only when infection is due to species of *Microsporum*.

Course: Tinea may become chronic and widespread, with extension to scalp, hair, and nails. Secondary bacterial infection may complicate diagnosis and treatment. In some persons an autoimmune phenomenon called a **dermatophytid** or **id reaction** may cause eruption of vesicular lesions on areas not infected with fungus, particularly on the hands.

Treatment: Numerous antifungal medicines are effective in topical form. Topical adrenocortical steroids may also be used if inflammation and itching are severe. Systemic antifungal treatment may be needed when infection is severe or resistant to topical treatment.

Other Superficial Fungal Infections of the Skin

The fungal organisms responsible for tinea corporis can also cause more localized infections. In **tinea capitis (ringworm of the scalp)**, infected hairs break off at the scalp surface, leaving patchy areas that appear bald, often with black dots representing the roots of broken-off hairs. Mild itching and scaling may occur. Treatment is with oral antifungals such as griseofulvin and selenium sulfide shampoo. **Kerion** is a complication, with boggy edema and exudation of pus though hair follicle openings.

Tinea pedis (athlete's foot) causes erythema, itching, scaling, fissuring, maceration, and vesicle formation of varying degree, particularly between the toes. **Tinea cruris (jock itch)** is a similar infection of the groin. **Tinea versicolor**, caused by *Malassezia furfur*, consists of variable numbers of white to tan macules with very fine scales. Patches are lighter than surrounding tanned skin, but darker than surrounding untanned skin, hence the name *versicolor* "changing colors." Tinea pedis, tinea cruris, and tinea versicolor usually respond to topical antifungals.

A wet mount preparation revealed short batlike hyphae, confirming the diagnosis of tinea versicolor.

Tinea unguium (onychomycosis) is probably the most important chronic nail disease. Fungal infection of fingernails and toenails causes discoloration, deformity, splitting, crumbling of nails, and separation from nail beds, generally without other symptoms. Oral antifungal treatment, usually for several months, is standard. Topical methods and even avulsion of infected nails are sometimes used.

The left and right 1st, 2nd, and 3rd toenails show onychomycosis.

Candidiasis

Candidiasis (or candidosis; infection of skin and mucous membranes with the yeastlike fungus *Candida albicans*) causes shiny, sharply delineated patches of intense erythema with itching or burning. Infection is more common in diabetics and typically occurs on areas where two skin surfaces are in apposition, with trapping of moisture: under the breasts, in the anogenital area, and in skin folds of obese persons. Diagnosis is confirmed by microscopic examination for hyphae or culture. Infections in the mouth (called **thrush**) and the vagina are treated with either topical or systemic antifungals.

Herpes Simplex

Local viral infection of skin or mucous membranes, causing vesicular lesions, typically recurrent.

Cause: Herpesvirus type 1 (oral, labial, facial herpes) and type 2 (genital herpes). Transmission is by direct contact with an infected person, not necessarily with visible lesions. Genital herpes is a sexually transmitted disease. The virus may lie dormant for months or years before causing symptoms. Viral activation, with ensuing skin eruption, may be triggered by physical or emotional stress, fever or respiratory infection (hence the lay terms "cold sore" and "fever blister"), sun exposure, and menstruation.

History: Clusters of small, painful vesicles about the nose or lips or on the genitals. These often recur in the same place, at greater or lesser intervals, in response to triggering factors mentioned above, or for no apparent reason. Vesicles may ulcerate. Women with genital herpes may have severe pain on urination. The first episode of infection is typically the most severe.

Physical Examination: A cluster of 4-6 small vesicles or ulcers on an erythematous, edematous base. With a first episode there is often fever and regional lymphadenitis. Secondary infection may cause pustule formation, crusting, and even **impetigo**.

Diagnostic Tests: Viral culture yields proof of herpes infection.

Course: An episode of infection typically runs its course in about a week. Secondary bacterial infection may lead to exacerbation of symptoms. Intrauterine infection is associated with abortion or fetal damage. A child delivered through an infected birth canal may acquire localized or widespread neonatal infection, typically severe. Ocular infection with herpes simplex virus causes **herpetic (dendritic) keratitis**, a severe ulcerative disorder of the cornea that can lead to visual impairment.

Treatment: Analgesics and topical applications to control pain. Topical or (preferably) systemic treatment with antiviral drugs (acyclovir, penciclovir, valacyclovir).

Herpes Zoster (Shingles)

A reactivation of varicella-zoster infection, with local involvement of nerves and skin.

Cause: After recovery from chickenpox, the varicella-zoster virus remains in the body for life, lying dormant in cells of the dorsal spinal nerve roots or in ganglia of cranial nerves. Reactivation of the virus leads to the clinical syndrome known as **zoster**.

History: Stinging or burning pain, almost always in the distribution of a single dorsal nerve root; usually on the trunk but occasionally on the face or in the ear. Before or after the onset of pain, a rash appears within the **dermatome (skin distribution)** of a single nerve root. On the trunk, this is a band 6-8 cm in width, running around half of the body from back to front. Pain and rash are both in the same dermatome, but not necessarily in exactly the same places within that dermatome.

Physical Examination: Fever is generally absent. Skin lesions are highly typical, consisting of one or more clusters of vesicles, each cluster surrounded by a zone of erythema. Involvement of the geniculate ganglion of the facial (seventh cranial) nerve can lead to facial paralysis and lesions of the outer ear.

> *Her herpes zoster is still quite active with numerous vesicles. However, there are no new blisters evident.*

Diagnostic Tests: Diagnosis is clinically evident. Fluid from vesicles gives a positive **Tzanck test.**

Course: Symptoms are more severe in persons over 40. Pain and skin lesions usually resolve within 2-6 weeks. However, one-half of patients over 60 develop postherpetic neuralgia, with chronic pain that can persist for months or years.

Treatment: Mild cases in younger persons are treated symptomatically. In severe disease, in older or immunodeficient persons, or when there is involvement of the eye or ear, antiviral agents (famciclovir, valacyclovir) shorten the duration of symptoms and reduce the risk of postherpetic neuralgia.

Verruca Vulgaris (Common Wart)

Virally induced coarse papules of the skin and mucous membranes.

Cause: Human papillomavirus (HPV), of which about 80 types have been identified by immunologic means. Most types preferentially affect particular areas (**plantar warts** on soles of the feet, **genital warts** on the external genitalia or uterine cervix). Transmission is by

---

HERPES ZOSTER

When the rash of zoster appears on the trunk of the body, it is so distinctive that the diagnosis can hardly be missed. Even many laypersons can accurately recognize it. When fully developed, the cutaneous eruption looks like a belt or sash running around half of the body.

Zoster is a Greek word for "belt." Another is *zone*, which in its latinized form *zona* was formerly used as a name for this condition. The lay English term *shingles* is a corruption of Latin *cingulum*, which also means "belt, girdle."

---

direct contact. Genital warts are transmitted sexually. Scratching and picking at lesions causes **autoinoculation** (implantation of infective viral material at new sites, with spread of lesions).

History: One or more papules on skin surface, or on anogenital mucosa. Mild itching may occur, and occasionally bleeding.

Physical Examination: One or more coarsely textured papules, varying from flat (on the sole of the foot or the face) to elevated (on the hands or the genitals). Typical genital warts are narrow-based, raised, and tend to come to a point; lesions of this type are called **condylomata acuminata** (singular, **condyloma acuminatum**). There may be evidence of excoriation or damage from scratching, picking, or crude attempts at removal. Secondary infection may occur.

Diagnostic Tests: Suspicious lesions treated with dilute acetic acid become chalky gray or white (acetowhitening) if they are warts. Diagnosis is usually clinically evident, but biopsy can provide histologic confirmation. **Wart virus** cannot be cultured. Cervical infection produces characteristic changes on Pap smear, but the Pap smear is not an adequate screening test for HPV infection. DNA typing of HPV present on the cervix can identify types associated with risk of malignant change.

Course: Without treatment most HPV infections resolve within 18-36 months, but meanwhile the condition may have been transmitted to others. Cervical infection with certain types of HPV is the leading cause of **cervical carcinoma,** usually after a latent period of more than 10 years.

Treatment: Depending on the site of infection, surgical excision, electrocautery, laser ablation, and **cryotherapy** (freezing with liquid nitrogen or a cryoprobe) are currently the most popular methods. Others include destruction with caustic chemicals such as salicylic acid, bichloracetic acid, and podofilox, application of the immune response modifier imiquimod, and injection of interferon directly into lesions.

Acne Vulgaris

A chronic eruption of comedones, papules, pustules, and cysts occurring primarily in adolescence.

Causes. The ultimate cause is unknown. There may be a genetic predisposition (identical twins are equally affected). The disease tends to be worse in males but does not occur in castrated males. It comes on about the time of puberty and typically resolves within 5-8 years, but may persist into the middle and late 20s or beyond. Acne or acneform lesions develop in Cushing syndrome, including the type induced by treatment with adrenocortical steroids; in women with hyperandrogenism of any cause; and in persons exposed to certain chemicals (chloracne, due to industrial exposure to chlorine; iodism, due to medicinal administration of iodide). Acne typically gets worse during times of emotional stress.

The lesions of acne develop in oil (**sebaceous**) glands, apparently as a result of heightened sebum production that leads to retention of sebum and plugging of gland ducts. Plugged, enlarged glands are called **comedones** (singular, **comedo**). These are colloquially called **whiteheads** when closed, and **blackheads** when the gland orifices are open, exposing sebum plugs, which darken as a result of chemical changes (not dirt). Very large comedones form cysts. Retained sebum is broken down by bacteria (*Propionibacterium acnes*) or spontaneous chemical changes to form fatty acids, which cause local inflammation and induce a foreign body reaction. Surface bacteria (staphylococci) invade inflamed tissue to produce pustules. Symptoms are aggravated by application of greasy or oily cosmetics and by repetitive picking or squeezing of lesions. Healing of pustules may be protracted and may leave pits or scars.

History: Appearance of lesions varying in type (blackheads, whiteheads, papules, pustules, cysts), number, distribution, and severity on the face, upper back, and chest; rarely elsewhere.

Physical Examination: Essentially as above.

Diagnostic Tests: Culture may be useful to identify unusual organisms causing secondary infection. Other laboratory studies may disclose underlying or contributing causes.

Course: Eventually, spontaneous remission occurs. This can take years, however, and in the meantime the patient may suffer severe emotional distress. The course of cystic acne may be especially protracted, and any severe case of acne is likely to leave some scarring.

Treatment: Vigorous skin hygiene with greaseless soaps and cleansers is the foundation of treatment. Topical drugs include benzoyl peroxide, azelaic acid, retinoids (adapalene, tazarotene, tretinoin), and antibiotics (clindamycin, erythromycin). Antibiotics such as tetracycline, minocycline, and erythromycin may also be administered orally for long periods. Expression of sebum from comedones with a comedo extractor by a physician may reduce symptoms. Injection of adrenocortical steroid into lesions may also help by lessening local inflammation.

In women, cyclical hormone therapy with an oral contraceptive containing norgestimate and ethinyl estradiol often provides long-term control. Isotretinoin taken orally for 4-6 months induces lengthy, usually permanent resolution of acne, but it is reserved for severe cases because of side effects (peeling of lips in 90%; elevation of blood cholesterol in 15%; abnormal liver function tests; grave risk of fetal damage if taken by a pregnant patient).

Rosacea (Acne Rosacea)

A reddish facial eruption occurring in the middle-aged and elderly.

Cause: Unknown. Occurs more commonly in persons with migraine headaches. Responds to antibiotic treatment. A rash similar to rosacea sometimes results from prolonged application of potent topical adrenocorticosteroids to the face.

History: Burning and flushing of the face, with patchy or diffuse rosy tint, papules, and sometimes pustules or excessive sebum production.

Physical Examination: As noted above. The cheeks, nose, and chin show a faint to bright inflammatory blush. Papules, pustules, **telangiectases** (visible patches of dilated skin vessels), and oiliness are usually present to some degree. Inflammation of the eyelids and even the cornea may occur. In some patients marked hyperplasia of the tissues of the nose (rhinophyma) eventually develops.

Course: Rosacea is highly chronic, but treatment provides a fair degree of control.

Treatment: Topical metronidazole or other antibiotics provide improvement in symptoms. Oral antibiotics and topical corticosteroids may be required.

Lasers can obliterate telangiectases. For severe rhinophyma, plastic surgery is required.

Urticaria (Hives)

An acute, often transitory eruption of intensely itchy papules or wheals (see ■ Figure 7-2).

Cause: Urticaria is caused by a release of histamine from mast cells in the dermis, with resultant local edema, capillary dilatation, and stimulation of nerve endings. Many factors can incite this reaction: allergies to food (shellfish, strawberries), medicines (aspirin, penicillin), insect bites or stings (bee stings), nonallergic sensitivity to medicines (atropine, codeine), parasitic infestation, sunlight, cold, heat (cholinergic urticaria), and even, in susceptible individuals, simple stroking of the skin (dermographism).

History: Sudden onset of a localized or generalized eruption of intensely itchy wheals or papules, which may be transitory.

Physical Examination: Wheals (raised white or red papules) surrounded by erythema. Wheals may be round or scalloped and confluent. Signs of scratching may be evident.

Diagnostic Tests: Blood studies and allergic screening may indicate the underlying cause, but usually do not.

Course: Urticaria often occurs in attacks at intervals of a few hours, but typically resolves within 1-2 weeks unless continued exposure to the causative agent occurs. Urticaria persisting beyond one month may point to occult infection or malignancy. Complications: Secondary infection due to scratching.

Treatment: Severe urticaria responds to intramuscular epinephrine. Antihistamines such as diphenhydramine or hydroxyzine may be given orally or by injection to control an acute attack. Regular use of antihistamines prevents or mitigates further attacks. The nonsedating antihistamines fexofenadine and loratadine may be useful prophylactically, even though they are ineffective in other forms of pruritus. Doxepin, a tricyclic antidepressant, is also effective either orally or topically. In severe cases, topical and systemic corticosteroids may be used.

Psoriasis

A chronic skin disorder characterized by scaly plaques.

Cause: Increased proliferation of epidermal cells. Evidently an autoimmune disorder, to which some persons are genetically predisposed.

History: Plaques of scaly thickening of the skin, particularly the scalp, knees, and elbows, with moderate itching. Nails and joints may also be affected.

Physical Examination: Reddish-purple thickened plaques of skin covered with silvery, firmly adherent scales. Pitting or stippling of nails and inflammation of joints, particularly the distal interphalangeal joints, may also be noted. In guttate psoriasis the plaques are small and numerous. **Koebner phenomenon** (formation of lesions at sites of trauma) may be noted.

Diagnostic Tests: Skin biopsy (usually unnecessary) shows characteristic changes in the epidermis.

Treatment: Topical steroids, calcipotriene, tar ointments; tar shampoos to the scalp. UVB (ultraviolet B); PUVA (psoralen + ultraviolet A). Oral methotrexate, etretinate, cyclosporine.

Pityriasis Rosea

A mild, benign, self-limited scaly eruption.

Cause: Possibly viral. More common in spring and fall. The male to female attack ratio is 2:3. Person-to-person transmission has not been demonstrated.

History: Appearance of a solitary scaly patch (herald patch) on the skin, followed in 1-2 weeks by a generalized eruption of similar but smaller lesions. Itching is mild or absent.

Physical Examination: A widespread eruption of oval fawn-colored macules with fine scales on the trunk and proximal extremities. The hands, face, and feet are typically spared. Trunk lesions follow a segmental distribution, especially on the back, giving a "Christmas tree" appearance.

Diagnostic Tests: Because pityriasis simulates secondary syphilis, a serologic test for syphilis is often done to rule out that possibility.

Course: Lesions disappear spontaneously in about 6 weeks.

Treatment: Ultraviolet treatments, oral erythromycin, and topical or oral steroids may hasten clearing, but treatment is seldom needed since itching is mild, affected body parts can easily be covered by clothing, and spontaneous resolution within weeks is virtually certain.

Basal Cell Carcinoma

A slowly growing, waxy or pearly papule with telangiectatic vessels, appearing usually on parts of the body exposed to sunlight, particularly the face (see ■ Figure 7-3). Most appear in the middle-aged or elderly. Ulceration and widespread erosion may occur if treatment is

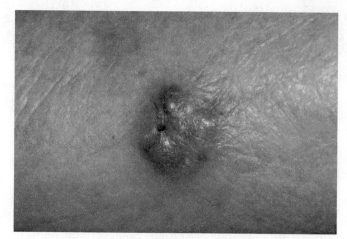

Figure 7-3. Basal cell carcinoma

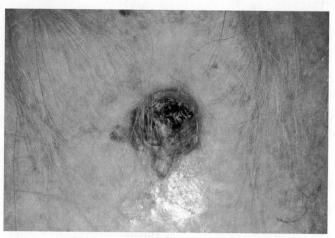

FIGURE 7-4. Squamous cell carcinoma

delayed, but metastasis is rare. Treatment is by surgical excision, including Mohs chemosurgery and cryotherapy.

Squamous Cell Carcinoma

A hard red nodule appearing on sun-exposed skin, usually in a middle-aged or elderly person (see ■ Figure 7-4). The lesion may develop in a preexisting actinic keratosis and may rapidly ulcerate. Metastasis is uncommon. Treatment is by excision.

Melanoma

A pigmented malignancy of the skin that develops in persons of all ages, progresses rapidly, metastasizes widely, and is fatal without treatment. Among malignancies melanoma ranks ninth in incidence, and incidence is increasing. At least some cases are due to sun exposure. It is estimated that, for a person under age 30, visiting a tanning parlor 10 or more times a year increases the risk of melanoma sevenfold. The risk is also higher in persons of white race, persons with many

The patient was noted to have a large hyperpigmented nevus of the right breast just at the interface of the areola with the skin margin at the lower outer quadrant of the breast. This lesion measured 0.8 x 0.6 cm, and a question of a malignant melanoma or atypia was raised due to the appearance of the lesion. It was recommended to the patient that this lesion be removed for permanent pathology as well as a resection of an additional suspicious lesion along the right upper abdomen which measured 0.3 x 0.3 cm.

Excisional biopsy revealed a Clark level IV malignant melanoma.

pigmented nevi, and persons with a family history or prior personal history of melanoma.

Melanoma can arise anew or develop from a previously benign pigmented nevus. Features of a pigmented lesion that suggest malignancy are irregularity of shape or border, uneven distribution of pigment, pink, blue, or black color, bleeding or ulceration, and rapid enlargement.

Treatment is by excision. Prognosis depends on the thickness of the tumor (**Breslow classification**) or the depth of invasion (**Clark classification**). In metastatic disease, radiation and chemotherapy may prolong survival.

Thermal Burns

Thermal burns are caused by contact of skin or mucous membrane with hot objects, liquids, or vapors. The amount of injury depends on the degree of heat and the extent and duration of contact. High heat induces an intense inflammatory reaction with leakage of fluid into tissues. It also coagulates protein and destroys tissues by vaporization or carbonization.

Skin burns are classified as **first degree** (redness of the surface without blistering), **second degree** (redness and blistering), and **third degree** (redness, blistering, and charring). First and second degree burns normally heal without scarring unless they become infected. In third degree burns, the nature and depth of injury usually lead to scarring. Deep burns can destroy tissues below skin level: subcutaneous fat, muscles, nerves, tendons, and even bone.

Extensive burns, even when only first degree, typically cause severe biochemical imbalance, due to sequestration of fluid in the burned area with proportionate reduction of blood volume. Dehydration, shock, toxemia, and severe local or systemic infection may complicate any severe burn.

Treatment is aimed at correcting fluid and electrolyte imbalances, relieving pain, and preventing or treating infection. Third degree burns often require grafting.

Cold Injury

The harmful local effects of intense cold (frostbite) are similar to those of heat: local inflammation, often with blistering and tissue destruction. Treatment is similar to that for burns. Exposure to atmospheric cold, or prolonged immersion in cold water, can induce systemic hypothermia, a drop in the rectal (core) temperature below 35ºC. The basic treatment is rewarming. Severe hypothermia can lead to profound derangement of physiologic functioning, including cardiac and respiratory arrest. Vigorous resuscitation efforts may be necessary.

Pause for Reflection

1. Distinguish among atopic dermatitis, contact dermatitis, and urticaria.
2. Distinguish among impetigo, tinea corporis, and candidiasis.
3. List and briefly define four other fungal skin infections.
4. Distinguish between herpes simplex and herpes zoster.
5. What is another name for *warts* and what causes them?
6. The medical name for a chronic eruption of comedones, papules, pustules, and cysts occurring primarily in adolescence is _____. Plugged, enlarged glands are called _____ (singular, _____).
7. Describe acne rosacea and its treatment.
8. Distinguish among basal cell carcinoma, squamous cell carcinoma, and melanoma.
9. How are burns classified?

Diagnostic and Surgical Procedures

ablation Total removal of a part, normal or abnormal, by surgical or chemical means.

biopsy, excisional Complete excision or removal of a lesion. In addition, some adjacent normal-appearing tissue is also removed for comparison.

biopsy, incisional Partial removal of a lesion by making an incision into the lesion and removing a section of it as well as some adjacent normal-appearing tissue for comparison.

biopsy, punch Removal of one section of a lesion using a sharp surgical instrument known as a punch.

A punch biopsy was obtained of this 1 cm lesion and was read as a probably verrucous squamous cell carcinoma of the lower lip.

Punch biopsy of the lip lesion was consistent with verrucous squamous cell carcinoma.

biopsy, skin Removal of all or part of a skin lesion. The tissue is sent to the pathology laboratory for histologic diagnosis and to determine whether it is malignant.

bx Abbreviation for *biopsy*.

cryosurgery The application of liquid nitrogen (at a temperature of -196° C) to destroy superficial skin lesions.

cryotherapy Local treatment of neoplasms or other lesions by freezing.

debridement Successive scraping away of dead skin down to viable tissue that bleeds from a wound or burn to prevent infection and promote healing.

diascopy Inspection of red or purplish lesions through a transparent plastic or glass plate, which compresses the skin. If the color is due to dilated blood vessels, it blanches (fades) with compression; color due to deposition of pigment, including blood pigment, in tissues is not altered by surface pressure.

electrodesiccation See *fulguration*.

fulguration The application of an electrical current to destroy superficial skin lesions.

graft See *skin graft.*

hemostasis, methods of obtaining: electrocautery, cautery, bipolar cautery, Bovie cautery, needlepoint electrocautery, microtip Bovie. Bovied is a coined term that has gained acceptance over time.

irrigation and debridement (I&D) A procedure in which an open wound or burn is bathed with a solution to achieve wound hydration, remove deep debris, and aid visual examination. Cellular debris and surface pathogens contained in wound exudates or residue are irrigated away. Dead skin can then be scraped away down to viable tissue to prevent infection and promote healing.

skin graft, full-thickness A skin graft consisting of the epidermis and the full depth of the dermis.

skin graft, split-thickness A skin graft consisting of the epidermis and a portion of dermis, or a mucosal graft consisting of only a partial thickness of mucosa.

Wood light An ultraviolet lamp with a filter that selects wavelengths under which certain funguses infecting skin or hair fluoresce brightly.

Laboratory Procedures

culture and sensitivity (C&S) Laboratory test that grows a colony of bacteria removed from an infected area in order to identify the specific infecting bacteria and then determine its sensitivity to a variety of antibiotics.

intradermal test The injection into the dermis of a chemical or other type of substance known to produce an allergic reaction in sensitive individuals. This creates a **wheal** which is outlined with a pen and/or measured. The area is examined again in 30 minutes. A reddened, enlarged area at the site of the injection indicates a positive allergic reaction to that chemical or allergen.

patch test The application to the skin of a piece of filter paper containing a chemical or other type of substance known to produce an allergic reaction in sensitive individuals. Many patches are taped to the skin and labeled. After 24-48 hours the skin underneath is examined. A reddened, raised area of skin indicates sensitivity to the substance applied.

RAST (radioallergosorbent) test A blood test that measures IgE antibodies to allergens. It can measure

many allergens with just one blood sample. It is an alternative to skin tests.

scratch test The application, to a superficial scratch made in the skin, of a chemical or other type of substance known to produce an allergic reaction in sensitive individuals. Many scratches are made in the skin, and the area is examined again in 30 minutes. A reddened, raised area of skin indicates sensitivity to the substance applied.

Tzanck test Microscopic examination of stained ulcer scrapings or fluid from a vesicle or bulla for multinucleated giant cells, observed in pemphigus vulgaris and some lesions caused by viruses (varicella, zoster, herpes simplex, cytomegalovirus).

Pharmacology

Because of the superficial nature and location of most dermatologic diseases, they respond well to topical drug therapy. Mild cases of skin diseases such as acne, psoriasis, poison ivy, contact dermatitis, superficial infections, herpes simplex infections, lice, and diaper rash can be successfully treated with topical agents. However, systemic drugs may be necessary when dermatologic problems become widespread or particularly severe.

Acne Drugs

Acne vulgaris is the most common form of acne, usually seen in adolescence. Topical creams, lotions, liquids, and gels are used to remove oil and dead skin (keratolytic action), to close the pores (astringent action), to inhibit the growth of skin bacteria (antiseptic action), and to kill skin bacteria (antibiotic action).

Topical prescription antibiotics may be used to treat more serious cases of acne vulgaris.

azelaic acid (Azelex, Finevin)
chlortetracycline (Aureomycin)
clindamycin (Cleocin T, C/T/S)
erythromycin (A/T/S, Emgel, EryDerm, Erygel, Staticin, T-Stat)
meclocycline (Meclan)
tetracycline (Achromycin, Panmycin, Sumycin, Tetracyn, Tetralan)

Tetracycline may be prescribed orally for systemic treatment of acne vulgaris, and severe cystic acne that is unresponsive to antibiotic treatment may be treated topically with a form of vitamin A such as tretinoin

(Retin-A) or systemically with isotretinoin (Accutane). These drugs cause epithelial cells to multiply more rapidly. This rapid turnover prevents pores from becoming clogged and infected and decreases cyst formation.

Psoriasis Drugs

Psoriasis is treated with coal tar lotions, gels, shampoos, and bath liquids to decrease the rate of epidermal cell production, correct abnormalities of the keratinocytes, cleanse away dead skin (keratolytic action), and decrease itching (antipruritic action).

> Aqua Tar
> Balnetar
> Denorex, Extra Strength Denorex
> Estar
> Neutrogena T/Derm, Neutrogena T/Gel
> Tegrin for Psoriasis, Tegrin Medicated,
>   Tegrin Medicated for Psoriasis
> Zetar

The red, scaly patches of psoriasis are caused by abnormal keratinocytes within the skin. Synthetic vitamin D-type drugs such as calcipotriene (Dovonex) are applied topically to activate vitamin D receptors in the keratinocytes and slow the abnormal cell growth.

Psoralens for Psoriasis

Severe, disabling psoriasis may also be treated by exposure to ultraviolet light in combination with a drug that sensitizes the skin to the effects of ultraviolet light. Drugs such as methoxsalen (Oxsoralen-Ultra, 8-MOP) are collectively known as **psoralens**. This combined treatment damages cell DNA and decreases the rate of cell division. The combination therapy of methoxsalen and ultraviolet light is known as **PUVA** (psoralen/ ultraviolet wavelength A).

Topical Corticosteroids

Both over-the-counter and prescription corticosteroids are used to relieve contact dermatitis, poison ivy, and insect bites. They are also used to treat psoriasis, seborrhea, and eczema.

Topical corticosteroids come in several strengths and in several forms (ointment, gel, lotion, cream, and aerosol). Some common over-the-counter and prescription topical corticosteroid drugs are:

> alclometasone (Aclovate)
> amcinonide (Cyclocort)

> **TEN MINUTES TO SAVE YOUR LIFE**
>
> Free cancer screenings throughout the country are provided by the American Academy of Dermatology. A skin cancer screening is a visual inspection of your skin by a medical professional. If the screening is in a private setting, a full-body screening can be provided. If the screening is in a public setting with very limited privacy, only exposed areas (face, neck, arms, hands, etc.) will be visually inspected for skin cancer.

> betamethasone (Alphatrex, Betatrex, Diprolene, Diprolene AF, Diprosone, Luxiq, Maxivate, Psorion, Teladar)
> clobetasol (Cormax, Olux, Temovate)
> clocortolone (Cloderm)
> desonide (DesOwen, Tridesilon)
> desoximetasone (Topicort, Topicort LP)
> dexamethasone (Decadron, Decaspray)
> diflorasone (Florone, Florone E, Maxiflor, Psorcon E)
> fluocinolone (Derma-Smoothe/FS, Flurosyn, Synalar, Synalar-HP)
> flurandrenolide (Cordran, Cordran SP)
> fluticasone (Cutivate)
> halcinonide (Halog, Halog-E)
> halobetasol (Ultravate)
> hydrocortisone (Cortaid Intensive Therapy, Cortaid with Aloe, Cort-Dome, Cortizone-5, Cortizone-10, Dermacort, Dermolate, Hycort, Hytone, Lanacort 5, Lanacort 10, Locoid, Maximum Strength Bactine, Maximum Strength Caldecort, Maximum Strength Cortaid, Maximum Strength KeriCort-10, Pandel, Scalpicin, T/Scalp, Westcort)
> mometasone (Elocon)
> prednicarbate (Dermatop)
> triamcinolone (Aristocort, Aristocort A, Flutex, Kenalog, Kenalog-H)

Topical Antibiotics

Used to treat minor, superficial bacterial skin infections. They act to inhibit the growth of or kill bacteria by blocking their ability to maintain a cell wall. Topical antibiotics are manufactured as gels, lotions, creams, ointments, and sprays.

> bacitracin (Baciguent)
> clindamycin (Cleocin T, Clinda-Derm)
> erythromycin (A/T/S, T-Stat)
> gentamicin
> mupirocin (Bactroban, Bactroban Nasal)
> neomycin (Myciguent)

Drugs for Fungus and Yeast Infections

Fungal infections such as ringworm (tinea corporis), athlete's foot (tinea pedis), jock itch (tinea cruris), and fungal infections of the nail (onychomycosis) can be effectively treated with topical antifungal drugs. These drugs alter the cell wall of the fungus and disrupt enzyme activity, resulting in cell death. These drugs are manufactured in cream, ointment, lotion, and shampoo forms.

Over-the-counter topical antifungal drugs include Desenex, miconazole (Micatin, Monistat-Derm), and tolnaftate (Aftate, Tinactin). Prescription drugs for fungus infections include:

> butenafine (Mentax)
> ciclopirox (Loprox, Penlac Nail Lacquer)
> clotrimazole (Cruex, Desenex, Lotrimin, Lotrimin AF 1%)
> econazole (Spectazole)
> haloprogin (Halotex)
> ketoconazole (Nizoral, Nizoral A-D)
> miconazole (Lotrimin AF 2%, Micatin, Monistat-Derm, Prescription Strength Desenex, Ting)
> naftifine (Naftin)
> nystatin (Mycostatin, Nilstat)
> oxiconazole (Oxistat)
> sulconazole (Exelderm)
> terbinafine (Lamisil AT, Lamisil DermGel)
> triacetin (Fungoid, Fungoid Creme, Fungoid Tincture)

Severe topical fungal skin infections may be treated with oral drugs such as griseofulvin, itraconazole, ketoconazole, and terbinafine. Yeast infections of the skin, caused by *Candida albicans*, are treated with topical drugs such as miconazole (Monistat-Derm) and ketoconazole (Nizoral), such as those used for fungi.

Drugs Used to Treat Itching

Topical corticosteroids inhibit inflammation and itching, and antihistamines inhibit inflammation, redness, and itching caused by allergic reaction and the release of histamine. As a group, these drugs are also known as *antipruritics*. (*Pruritus* means *itching*.) These combination drugs are applied topically:

> Bactine Antiseptic Anesthetic (benzalkonium, lidocaine)
> benzocaine (Americaine Anesthetic, Bicozene, Dermoplast, Lanacane, Solarcaine, Solarcaine Medicated First Aid)
> Caladryl (calamine, diphenhydramine)
> Caladryl Clear (diphenhydramine, zinc oxide)
> Calamycin (benzocaine, calamine, pyrilamine, zinc oxide)
> Cetacaine (benzocaine, butamben, tetracaine)
> EMLA (lidocaine, prilocaine)
> lidocaine (Solarcaine Aloe Extra Burn Relief, Unguentine Plus, Xylocaine, Zilactin-L)
> Medi-Quik (benzalkonium, lidocaine)
> Ziradryl (diphenhydramine, zinc oxide)

For severe itching, these antihistamines may be given orally:

> cyproheptadine (Periactin)
> diphenhydramine (Benadryl)
> hydroxyzine (Atarax, Vistaril)

Transcription Tips

1. Confusing terms related to the integumentary system: Some of these terms sound alike; others are potential traps when researching. Memorize the terms and their meanings so that you can select the appropriate term for a correct transcript.

   Ace (wrap)—a trademarked term for a type of bandages

   ACE (inhibitors)—abbreviation for angiotensin-converting enzyme

   Allis (clamp)—an eponym applied to a variety of surgical instruments

   Alice—a woman's first name.

   aphthous—pertaining to aphthae, small painful ulcers of the oral mucosa

   abscess—a localized collection of pus

   atopic—allergic (in the context of dermatology), as in atopic dermatitis

   ectopic—located away from normal position or arising in an abnormal site or tissue

   callus (noun)—synonym: callosity; a local growth of hard, horny epithelium, such as that on a toe from ill-fitting shoes; also, a meshwork of bone growth over a fracture site, a sign of healing on x-rays

   callous (adj.)—usually refers to an uncaring, insensitive personality; some dictionaries include *calloused* and *callused* which also mean pertaining to a callus.

   carbuncle—a cluster of boils (furuncles), usually caused by a *Staphylococcus aureus* infection.

   caruncle—a small fleshy eminence, which may be normal or abnormal

   furuncle—a boil, usually caused by a *Staphylococcus aureus* infection.

   canker ("KANG-ker")—an ulceration, especially of the oral mucosa; an aphthous ulcer

   chancre ("SHANG-ker")—a primary cutaneous lesion seen at the site of inoculation of infection, associated with various infections

   donor (*not* doner)—a person or site on the body that supplies living tissue for grafting or transplantation

   eminence—a prominence or projection, especially upon the surface of a bone

   imminence—something about to occur

   fungal—pertaining to a fungus, including mushrooms, yeasts, and molds

   fundal—pertaining to the bottom or base of an organ

   lichen—any of a number of skin diseases characterized by small, firm papules set close together, as in lichen planus

   liken—to describe as similar, equal or analogous; to compare.

   melanotic—pertaining to melanin or melanosis (excessive pigmentation due to disturbance in melanin production)

   melenic—pertaining to melena, passage of tarry black stools resulting from gastrointestinal bleeding

   psoriasis—a skin disorder characterized by scaly plaques (Note: The *p* is silent.)

   cirrhosis—a chronic liver disease.

   tinea ("TIN-ee-uh")—a fungal infection, as in tinea versicolor,

   tenia (taenia) ("TEH-nee-uh")—a bandlike structure or tapeworm.

2. Spelling: Memorize the spelling of these difficult-to-spell terms. Note silent letters, doubled letters, and unexpected pronunciations

   aphthous ("AF-thes")

   blepharochalasis ("BLEF-a-ro-kal-e-sis")

   desiccate (one *s*, two *c*'s)

   dyskeratotic (*dys*, not dis)

   eczema (pronounced "EK-ze-ma" or "EGG-zem-a")

   Mohs (rhymes with "toes") surgery (named for Dr. Frederic Mohs). Not possessive.

   onychomycosis

   pruritus (itching; mistakenly thought to end in *-itis*, meaning inflammation)

   psoriasis, psoriatic (silent *p*)

   verrucous (two *r*'s, 1 *c*)

   xanthoma (*x* sounds like *z*)

   Xeroform (bandage material)

   Tzanck ("tsangk" or "zangk") smear

Transcription Tips

3. Note the challenging spellings or unusual capitalization of these common dermatology drugs.

   Akne-Mycin (brand name)
   Benzamycin (brand name)
   clindamycin (generic ends in –mycin)
   erythromycin (generic ends in –mycin)
   gentamicin (generic ends in –micin)
   interferon alfa-2b
   pHisoHex (patterned after pH)
   Xylocaine ("z" sound at the beginning)
   Zyrtec

4. Tricky abbreviations. Some abbreviations are acronyms and pronounced as a word; others have soundalike letters. Listen carefully and know the translation in order to choose the correct abbreviation. Although some abbreviations do not need to be expanded, know what they mean in order to choose the correct one.

   ATA—atmosphere absolute
   HBO—hyperbaric oxygen
   MRSA ("mersa")—methicillin-resistant *Staphylococcus aureus*

5. Dictation Challenges

   There is no plural form for *decubitus* because it is an adjective. However, it is sometimes used alone in place of the noun. When the erroneous "decubiti" is dictated, edit to *decubitus ulcers*.

   There is no official brief form for the terms *subcutaneous* or *subcuticular*. If the brief form *subcu* is dictated, it may be translated if the correct term is known; otherwise, *subcu* should be transcribed as dictated. Do not use a brief form unless it is dictated. Do not use *subq* for *subcu*.

   Bipolar cautery is electrocautery in which both active and return electrodes are incorporated into a single handheld instrument, so that the current passes between the tips of the two electrodes and affects only a small amount of tissue. Do not transcribe "by polar cautery."

   Do not confuse *dactinomycin* (an antibiotic antineoplastic for various tumors, carcinomas and sarcomas) with *daptomycin* (an antibiotic for complicated skin infections).

Spotlight On

What Is Vulgar?

by Ellen A. Drake

Imagine encountering the term *acne vulgaris* or *verruca vulgaris* for the first time. *Vulgaris* looks a lot like our English word *vulgar*, doesn't it? It brings to mind the meaning "crude, indecent," as in "a vulgar joke."

Vulgaris is a Latin adjective (from the noun *vulgus*, "the crowd, the masses") meaning "common, pertaining to the common people," or "ordinary, shared by all." This is the meaning that applies to the Latin Vulgate Bible of the 4th century, referring to the common speech of a people, the vernacular.

The word *vulgar* is an example of pejoration, a linguistic term applied when the meaning of a word changes for the worse over time. The only Latin sense reminiscent of our modern word was in the idea of "general sharing," i.e., "sexually promiscuous."

Our word *vulgar* appeared in English in the late 14th century, still with the meaning it carried in Latin. Perhaps due to the lack of opportunity for education and refinement and the perceived ill manners of the common people, it began to take on connotations similar to those we associate with the word today. By the 17th century, it was found to mean "deficient in taste," making explicit what, over time, had become implicit in its meaning.

However, the medical terms *acne vulgaris* and *verruca vulgaris* still carry the original meaning of "common"—common acne, common warts. You can see how people might have a completely different concept of a medical term than the one intended if they fail to consider the origin and evolution of a word's meaning. In this example, the danger is even more likely, considering negative cultural attitudes toward acne and warts!

Exercises

Medical Vocabulary Review

Instructions: Choose the best answer.

___ 1. Hemostasis is obtained during surgery using which surgical procedure?
A. Electrocautery.
B. Electrodesiccation.
C. Electrofulguration.
D. Cryosurgery.

___ 2. A deep solitary abscess is a _____
A. bulla.
B. carbuncle.
C. furuncle.
D. decubitus ulcer.

___ 3. An area of skin that is mainly supplied by a single spinal nerve is a _____
A. dermatome.
B. fissure.
C. wheal.
D. nevus.

___ 4. If a condition or the cause of a condition is not obvious or hidden but sometimes able to be inferred from indirect evidence, the dictator might say that it is _____
A. occult.
B. discoid.
C. hypertrophic.
D. telangiectatic.

___ 5. Superficial dermatitis of unknown cause accompanied by redness, vesicles, itching, and crusting is _____
A. pruritus.
B. eczema.
C. cellulitis.
D. dermatographism.

___ 6. A hard, friable, irregular layer of dried blood, serum, pus, tissue debris adherent to the surface of injured or inflamed skin is _____
A. a keloid.
B. a cicatrix.
C. an eschar.
D. a crust or scab.

___ 7. A flat patch or mark differing in color from surrounding skin is a _____
A. papule.
B. macule.
C. pustule.
D. wheal.

___ 8. Another word for a skin erosion is _____
A. ulcer.
B. fissure.
C. vesicle.
D. excoriation.

___ 9. An increase in the severity of a disease, particularly when occurring after a period of improvement, is _____
A. an excoriation.
B. an exacerbation.
C. lichenification.
D. dermatographism.

___ 10. _____ is the degree to which tissue spaces, particularly in the skin and subcutaneous tissues, are filled with extracellular fluid.
A. Tone
B. Edema
C. Turgor
D. Blanching

___ 11. Candidal infections in the mouth are called ____
  A. thrush.
  B. impetigo.
  C. id reactions.
  D. herpes simplex.

___ 12. _____ are visible patches of dilated skin vessels.
  A. Dermatoses
  B. Decubitus ulcers
  C. Telangiectases
  D. Excoriations

___ 13. In squamous cell carcinoma, the thickness of the tumor is classified using the _____ classification.
  A. Breslow
  B. Clark
  C. Dukes
  D. Broders

___ 14. Burns that extend into subcutaneous fat, muscles, nerves, tendons, and even bone are classified as _____
  A. first-degree burns.
  B. second-degree burns.
  C. third-degree burns.
  D. partial-thickness burns.

___ 15. The ripping away of a part is _____
  A. an avulsion.
  B. an abrasion.
  C. an erosion.
  D. a fissure.

___ 16. Which generic drug is a topical corticosteroid?
  A. clindamycin.
  B. methoxsalen.
  C. dexamethasone.
  D. sulconazole.

___ 17. Which of these generic drugs does not belong in the group with the others?
  A. cyproheptadine.
  B. diphenhydramine.
  C. hydroxyzine.
  D. lidocaine.

___ 18. Which generic drug is NOT used to treat fungal or yeast infections?
  A. mupirocin.
  B. miconazole.
  C. ciclopirox.
  D. clotrimazole.

___ 19. A physician might prescribe which one of these generic drugs for acne?
  A. calcipotriene.
  B. methoxsalen.
  C. clocortolone.
  D. tetracycline.

___ 20. The class of drugs used to treat severe itching is called _____
  A. psoralens.
  B. antipruritics.
  C. antibacterials.
  D. corticosteroids.

Diagnostic and Surgical Procedures

Instructions: Match the following diagnostic and surgical procedures to their descriptions or definitions. Some answers may be used more than once.

___ 1. excisional biopsy

___ 2. cryosurgery

___ 3. debridement

___ 4. electrocautery

___ 5. electrodesiccation

___ 6. incisional biopsy

___ 7. fulguration

___ 8. full-thickness skin graft

___ 9. punch biopsy

___ 10. Wood light

A. Removing a section of a lesion as well as some adjacent normal-appearing tissue for comparison

B. Removal of one section of a lesion using a specifically designed round knife

C. An ultraviolet light with a special filter for examining funguses on the skin

D. Complete removal of a lesion, sometimes with adjacent normal-appearing tissue for comparison

E. Compressing the skin using a transparent plastic or glass plate through which red or purplish lesions can be examined

F. Application of liquid nitrogen to destroy superficial skin lesions

G. A skin graft consisting of the epidermis and a portion of dermis

H. Successive scraping away of dead skin down to viable tissue that bleeds

I. Application of an electrical current to destroy superficial skin lesions

J. A skin graft consisting of the epidermis and the full depth of the dermis

K. A method for obtaining hemostasis during surgery

L. Local treatment of neoplasms or other lesions by freezing

Laboratory Procedures

Instructions: Match the following laboratory procedures to their descriptions or definitions. Some answers may be used more than once.

___ 1. culture and sensitivity

___ 2. intradermal test

___ 3. patch test

___ 4. scratch test

___ 5. Tzanck test

___ 6. radioallergosorbent test

A. Microscopic examination of stained fluid from a vesicle or bulla

B. Application to the skin of a piece of filter paper containing a chemical or other type of substance known to produce an allergic reaction in sensitive individuals

C. Application to a superficial scratch made in the skin of a chemical or other type of substance known to produce an allergic reaction in sensitive individuals

D. A test in which an allergen is injected to determine sensitivity to the allergen

E. Laboratory test that grows a colony of bacteria for the purpose of identifying them and determining which antibiotic will effectively treat the infection

F. Blood test that measures IgE antibodies to allergens

Dissecting Medical Terms

Instructions: As you learned in your medical language course, words are formed from prefixes, combining forms (root word plus combining vowel), and suffixes. Combining vowels (usually **o** but not always) are used to connect two root words or a root and a suffix. By analyzing these word parts, you can often determine the definition of a term without even looking it up (if you know the definition of the parts, of course!).

Being able to divide and analyze the words you hear into their component parts will also improve your auditory deciphering ability and spelling and help you research those words that you cannot easily spell or define.

For the following terms, draw a slash (/) between the components and then write a short definition based on the meaning of the parts. Remember that to define a word based on its parts, you start at the end, usually with the suffix. If there's a prefix, that is defined next, and finally the combining form is defined.

Example: cheilitis

Divide and Analyze:
cheilitis = cheil/itis = inflammation + lip
Define: inflammation of the lips

1. thromboangiitis
   Divide _____
   _____
   Define _____

2. dyskeratotic
   Divide _____
   _____
   Define _____

3. lymphadenectomy
   Divide _____
   _____
   Define _____

4. intracuticular
   Divide _____
   _____
   Define _____

5. intraepithelial
   Divide _____
   _____
   Define _____

6. lymphopenia
   Divide _____
   _____
   Define _____

7. preauricular
   Divide _____
   _____
   Define _____

8. subcuticular
   Divide _____
   _____
   Define _____

9. submental
   Divide _____
   _____
   Define _____

10. supraclavicular
    Divide _____
    _____
    Define _____

Abbreviations Exercise

Instructions: Expand the following common abbreviations and brief forms. Then memorize both abbreviations and definitions to increase your speed and accuracy in transcribing dictation

Abbreviation	Expansion
1. BCC	_____
2. C&S	_____
3. EBL	_____
4. HBO	_____
5. HPV	_____
6. KOH	_____
7. MAC	_____
8. MRSA	_____
9. PUVA	_____
10. RAST	_____

Transcript Forensics

Instructions: This section presents snippets of transcribed dictations from clinic notes; history and physical examinations and consultations; operative reports and procedure notes; and discharge summaries. Explain the passage so that a nonmedical person can understand it.

Example
PROCEDURE
Excision of left **preauricular nevus sebaceus**.

Explanation: Complete removal of a lesion consisting of hyperplastic oil (sebaceous) glands and hair follicle in front of the ear.

1. PROCEDURE: Excision of right **posterior** neck **lipoma**.
   Explanation: _____
   _____
   _____

2. The patient had a recent left inguinal **lymph-adenectomy** and is now admitted to the hospital with left **groin cellulitis**. Examination was remarkable for the presence of **erythema** and tenderness in the left groin area.
   Explanation: _____
   _____
   _____

3. PROCEDURE: Excision of **basal cell carcinoma** on the right ear, with **frozen section and full-thickness skin graft** taken from the right **supraclavicular region** for coverage.
   Explanation: _____
   _____
   _____

4. Biopsy showed recurrent **superficially invasive squamous cell carcinoma**, which was totally removed by the **punch biopsy** with an **intra-epithelial** squamous cell extending to the punch biopsy margin.
   Explanation: _____
   _____
   _____

5. The area of **partial thickness denudation** is increased in size. There is minimal to no drainage. There is no **erythema**. There is **induration** proximal to the wound, but with less tenderness and with no **fluctuance**.
   Explanation: _____
   _____
   _____

6. IMPRESSION: Scalp **abscesses**. Rule out **MRSA**.
   Explanation: _____
   _____
   _____

7. The patient is showing more **comedo** formation and a higher proportion of pustular lesions than before with numerous **blackheads** and **whiteheads** over the chin and along the jaw line and over the forehead. The lesions show some **inflammatory** reaction, and some deep cysts are now palpable on the forehead and over the scapulae.
   Explanation: _____
   _____
   _____

8. The patient was first seen in the dermatology clinic and was thought to have infected **eczema** or a gram-negative toe web infection and possible **contact dermatitis** secondary to Neosporin use.
   Explanation: _____
   _____
   _____

9. One asymptomatic wartlike lesion of a 1 cm size on the medial aspect of his right knee was removed and turned out to be **benign**. The second lesion, a growing **freckle** approximately 2.5 x 1 cm on the anterior aspect of his chest, was removed and revealed **malignant melanoma, Clark's level III**.
   Explanation: _____
   _____
   _____

10. Physical examination showed, covering most of the back and also the medial central buttocks, **confluent, erythematous, scaly plaques** with some **crusting**. Similar plaques were also present on the anterior lower legs. (Can you guess the diagnosis?)
    Explanation: _____
    _____
    _____

Sample Reports

Sample dermatology reports appear on the following pages, illustrating a variety of reports. Fictional names are provided for illustration of proper format, and no resemblance to actual persons is intended. Sample transcripts were prepared according to *The Book of Style for Medical Transcription* (AHDI).

History and Physical Examination

JESSUP, JENNIFER
#652145

DATE OF ADMISSION
July 24, [add year]

HISTORY
This 17-year-old was admitted via the emergency department. She gives a history of shooting crank. Since that time the left antecubital space has been infected.

PAST HISTORY
The patient has been shooting for at least a year. She denies use of drugs other than crank. The patient has a 2-year-old child and a 3-week-old child and has been in the hospital only for that. Denies accidents, injuries, and other infections.

SOCIAL HISTORY
The patient is a 17-year-old IV drug user.

PHYSICAL EXAMINATION
VITAL SIGNS: Temperature 102.2 degrees. Pulse 112. Respirations 20. Blood pressure 104/60.
GENERAL: Well-developed, well-nourished, English-speaking Caucasian 17-year-old female.
EENT: No gross abnormalities. Pupils constricted. Fair dental repair.
NECK: Supple, no palpable nodes.
CHEST: Lungs are clear.
HEART: Heart regular, not enlarged, no murmurs.
BREASTS: Breasts normal.
ABDOMEN: Soft. No palpable masses.
PELVIC AND RECTAL: Not done.
EXTREMITIES: Examination of the left antecubital space reveals there is a generalized area of tender cellulitis with a moderate amount of swelling on the left as compared with the right.

(continued)

History and Physical Examination *(continued)*

JESSUP, JENNIFER
#652145
Page 2

DIAGNOSES
1. Chronic intravenous drug user.
2. Cellulitis, left arm.

PLAN
The patient should be admitted to the hospital for IV antibiotics and possible opening of the wound.

ROSALIND SKINNER, MD

RS:hpi
d: 1/24/[add year]
t: 1/24/[add year]

Discharge Summary

WERNIG, INGE
#98765

DATE OF ADMISSION
June 10, [add year]

DATE OF DISCHARGE
June 11, [add year]

ADMISSION DIAGNOSES
1. Left lower leg cellulitis.
2. Left lower leg ulceration.
3. Diabetes mellitus.
4. Possible psoriasis.

DISCHARGE DIAGNOSES
1. Left lower leg cellulitis.
2. Left lower leg ulceration.
3. Diabetes mellitus.
4. Lichen simplex chronicus.

BRIEF HISTORY
This is a 48-year-old white female with obesity and diabetes who has had a smoldering left lower extremity cellulitis for the past 2-3 months. It is possibly related to her pruritus and psoriasis. She has been treated in the past with Coumadin and IV antibiotics. On the day of admission she presented to my office with worsening of the cellulitis and a new 2 cm ulceration, and was admitted for IV antibiotics and further evaluation.

EXTREMITIES
Extremities revealed bilateral edema 1 to 2+ to the knees, with erythema and diffuse excoriations with erythema from the ankle to the midshin area on the left lower extremity. She had a 2 x 2 cm superficial ulcer on the lateral aspect of the ankle.

LABORATORY
Labs on admission revealed sodium was 138. Electrolytes were normal. BUN and creatinine were normal. The creatinine was 1.4, which is probably acceptable for this obese woman. PT was slightly elevated at 15.6, PTT was normal. A subsequent chemistry panel was essentially normal. CBC revealed a white blood cell count of 6,000, hemoglobin 12, hematocrit 35, with 345,000 platelets and a normal smear.

(continued)

Discharge Summary *(continued)*

WERNIG, INGE
#98765
Page 2

DISCHARGE MEDICATIONS
Glyburide 2.5 mg daily, Keflex 500 mg p.o. q.i.d., Lasix 20 mg daily, Mellaril 50 mg nightly, Topicort cream
to affected areas b.i.d., and normal saline and dressing changes for wound care.

DARREN WHINERY, MD

DW:hpi
d: 6/10/[add year]
t: 6/11/[add year]

Hyperbaric Treatment Note

FLETCHER, STEPHEN
#868668

DATE OF TREATMENT
May 23, [add year]

TREATMENT
Number 6 of 20.

INDICATION AND DIAGNOSIS
Type 2 diabetic ulcer, controlled. Ulcer of the foot/toe.

WOUND EVALUATION
Measurements essentially unchanged from May 18. Please see that note for details. There is more granulation tissue now and less fibrinous tissue. We continue with current dressings of Aquacel Ag.

PRETREATMENT VITAL SIGNS
Blood pressure 126/70, pulse 74, respiratory rate 18, temperature 98.6. Blood sugar 142. Pain assessment zero. The patient had the ability to clear his ears. Tympanic membranes are intact bilaterally. Lungs are clear and equal bilaterally.

MEDICATIONS
Reviewed. There are no changes.

The patient does not have a cold; there are no respiratory allergy tests taken. Safety procedures were reviewed with the patient. The patient was educated on the use of the air-break mask. Information from the previous HBO sessions had been reviewed.

Time start of pressurization 0625 hours. Rate set to bring patient to ATA was 2.0. Time patient arrived at depth 0635 hours. Treatment continued to a depth of 2.0 ATA. Air breaks were not used. Treatment time of 110 minutes was used, which was calculated from the time pressurization began to the time the patient was brought up to surface. The patient was brought up to surface at 0815 hours.

POSTTREATMENT VITAL SIGNS
Blood pressure 130/76, pulse 80, respiratory rate 20, temperature 98.1. Blood sugar 139. Pain assessment remained at zero. The patient continued to have the ability to clear his ears. Tympanic membranes were intact bilaterally. There was no blood or evidence of any swelling or pressure. Lungs remained clear and equal bilaterally.

Patient tolerated the treatment without complications. I was in attendance at all times during the procedure.

ERIC SCHONE, MD

ES:hpi d: 5/23/[add year] t: 5/23/[add year]

Consultation

RUBIN, WILLIAM
#253695
Date of Consultation: 11/25/[add year]

Attending Physician: Nathan E. Day

The patient was admitted to the hospital for treatment of a leg ulceration. Consultation was requested specifically for an eruption on the back and legs, which the patient states has been present 3 months. No treatment has been given for this. The nurses report that the area had been oozing on the back, but since the start of oral Keflex, the oozing has stopped. The patient is not a good historian and states only that the eruption started about 3 months ago, and it is occasionally pruritic.

Physical examination showed, covering most of the back and also the medial central buttocks, confluent, erythematous, scaly plaques with some crusting. Similar plaques were also present on the anterior lower legs.

IMPRESSION
My impression is confluent psoriasis which had been secondarily infected.

PLAN
1. The Keflex should be continued to treat the secondary infection.
2. The psoriasis will be treated with a combination of 10% LCD and 0.1% triamcinolone cream.

LAWRENCE RICHARDS, MD

LR:hpi

d: 11/25/[add year]
t: 11/26/[add year]

Comic Relief

Dictation and transcription mistakes are common occurrences in dermatology dictation. Here are some favorites.

Correct	**Incorrect**
Cicatrix on the chin.	Six pricks on the skin.
Kwell lotion was applied daily during her hospital stay.	Kwell lotion was applied gaily during her hospital stay.
Keratosis removed from forearm by desiccation.	Keratosis removed from forearm by defecation.
He has an ulceration on the lower third of his left leg.	He has an ulceration on his left lower third leg.
The skin was closed with vertical mattress sutures.	The skin was closed with vertical massive sutures.
Carbuncle.	Car bump.
Allergies were denied.	Orgies were denied.
Marked atypical changes.	Marked A to pickle changes.
Patient was treated with 100% oxygen.	Patient was treated with under the sun oxygen.

Family Medicine

8

Learning Objectives

▶ Describe the structure and function of the head, eyes, ears, nose, and throat.

▶ Spell and define common otorhinolaryngology and pediatric terms.

▶ Identify otorhinolaryngology and pediatric vocabulary that might be used in the history and review of systems.

▶ Describe the negative and positive findings a physician looks for on pediatric exam of the head, eyes, ears, nose, and throat.

▶ Describe the typical cause, course, and treatment options for common diseases of infants and children as well as ears, nose, and throat diseases in adults.

▶ Identify and define common diagnostic and surgical procedures of family medicine practice.

▶ List common laboratory tests and procedures in family medicine practice.

▶ Identify and describe common otorhinolaryngology drugs and their uses.

▶ Demonstrate knowledge of anatomical, medical, pharmacological, adjectival, and soundalike terms by accurately completing the exercises in this chapter.

Transcribing Family Medicine Dictation

Introduction

In classical antiquity, professional physicians apparently treated all comers, young and old, for whatever ailed them, from battle wounds and migraine headaches to epilepsy and periodic fevers (usually malaria). It's true that at various times and places itinerant and often unlearned practitioners set fractures, pulled teeth, and lanced boils. And throughout most of human history, babies were delivered by midwives. But members of the medical profession typically took a holistic and generalized view of healing.

During the nineteenth century, advances in biochemistry, histopathology, microbiology, and pharmacology led to an immense growth in the scientific database of medicine. The development of sophisticated diagnostic and surgical instruments, the increasing urbanization of society, and the multiplication of regional medical centers with teaching programs favored the emergence of the earliest medical specialties—otorhinolaryngology, ophthalmology, obstetrics-gynecology, and dermatology.

By 1939 American specialty boards had been established for internal medicine, pediatrics, general surgery, orthopedic surgery, urology, psychiatry, radiology, and pathology. Fewer and fewer physicians chose to enter general practice, opting for narrower limits of clinical responsibility, greater prestige, and higher income.

Around the middle of the twentieth century the proliferation of specialties and subspecialties led to increasing fragmentation of medical practice, a shift of focus from patients to diseases, a gradual loss of traditional standards of caring and personal interest that had characterized professional health care in earlier times.

Meanwhile, the explosion of information in fields such as nuclear medicine, diagnostic imaging studies, electron microscopy, and genetics made it increasingly difficult for those physicians who went into general practice to achieve a basic mastery of the entire field of medicine after completing medical school and a one-year rotating internship.

The time was ripe for a major change in the structure of American medicine. In 1969 the American Board of Family Practice (ABFP) became the twentieth specialty board to be recognized by the American Board of Medical Specialties. Board certification currently requires successful completion of a three-year residency in family practice at an approved institution. Continu-

ing medical education is mandatory for board members, as is periodic recertification through completion of a formal examination.

Unlike other boards, ABFP does not contribute to the body of technical or scientific information, but rather builds on a core of knowledge derived from other specialties. Residency training emphasizes a style of practice that is continuing, comprehensive, evidence-based, preventive, proactive, and family-centered.

In this country, nearly one fourth of all office visits are made to family physicians. Like the general practitioners of decades ago, today's family physicians provide a range of medical services, often including obstetrics. In addition to diagnosing and managing acute and chronic illnesses, they offer preventive care, including routine checkups, health-risk assessments, immunizations and screening tests, and counseling on maintaining a healthful lifestyle. In particular, their role is crucial in delivering medical care to underserved and rural populations.

Family physicians treat more children than pediatricians, and provide more care for patients with ear, nose, and throat complaints than otorhinolaryngologists. This chapter on Family Medicine focuses on pediatrics and ENT (ears, nose, and throat).

ARE YOU SMARTER THAN A FIFTH GRADER?

Children are not miniature adults, although their wisdom can sometimes rival the most intellectual of "grown-ups." The story is told of a tall truck that got stuck under a low bridge. Dozens of people stopped to help push, but the truck didn't budge. A tow truck tried to pull the truck out, but despite all efforts, it didn't move an inch.

The best minds in the community decided to either dismantle the truck or remove a piece of the bridge. Equipment was brought in to begin the process. As a crowd gathered to watch, a child pushed his way to the front and asked, "Why don't they just let the air out of the tires?"

Children tend to think in the here and now. Playing "pretend" or "make believe" is an important step in learning to understand the consequences of certain choices. Their thinking is black and white with few shades of gray, unlike adults. Perhaps that is why the solution to the truck-bridge dilemma eluded the adults but was obvious to the child.

Pediatrics

Introduction

Pediatric medicine (or **pediatrics**) is the branch of medicine devoted to the health of children in illness and wellness. Pediatricians treat individuals throughout the period of their greatest growth and development—from newborn to adolescent.

A special sensibility is needed to work with babies and children who cannot verbalize their medical complaints with much more than a wail. A disease or disorder in a child may present differently than the same malady in an adult, and extra training in a pediatric residency is undertaken by physicians who expect to become board certified in pediatrics.

To evaluate and treat children in general, one does not need to be a **board-certified pediatrician**. The family doctor, a physician assistant, or a family nurse practitioner might be selected by the patient's parent to follow the child. These individuals have the education, training, and experience that may make them an ideal choice to treat children.

Neonatology is the study and care of newborns (*neo-* meaning new, *natal-* pertaining to birth, and *-ogy* meaning study of), especially those born too early. Premature infants often have more than one complication because their time in utero is cut short and development is not yet complete.

> *This infant was born at 34 weeks and had a grade 2 heart murmur that on echocardiogram revealed a small atrial septal defect.*

A **neonatologist** is board-certified in pediatrics and has additional specialized training in diagnosing and treating disorders of the newborn. Premature babies and full-term newborns with complications are evaluated and treated by neonatologists in pediatric critical care units in medical centers. These units are staffed by physicians, nurses, and others who have specialized training and credentials.

A child with a disease or condition that proves baffling might be referred to a specialist. A child with recurrent abdominal pain could be referred to a gastroenterologist who treats both adults and children, or a pediatric gastroenterologist if one is available.

Adolescent medicine physicians tend to set up their practices in major cities. They work with children who are going through a most difficult emotional period—the preteen and teenage years. Children in this age group are either prepubescent (before puberty), pubescent (going through puberty), or postpubescent (puberty complete or nearly complete). Knowledge of both child and adult disorders is required since bodies undergo major developmental changes between the onset of puberty and its completed process.

A pediatrician might agree to see a longstanding patient into adulthood, but most encourage their patients to "graduate" to a family medicine specialist when the patient turns 18.

Otorhinolaryngology

Introduction

The ears, nose, and throat (ENT) are adjacent to one another anatomically, similar in histologic structure, and subject to many of the same diseases. Diseases, injuries, and abnormalities of the ears, nose, and throat are the special field of the **otorhinolaryngologist**.

Some refer to the specialty simply as head and neck surgery. Practitioners are called and professionally designated by the more accurate term **otolaryngologists**–head and neck surgeons, as specialists trained in otolaryngology are experts in surgical conditions of the head and neck.

Most otorhinolaryngologists provide a full range of medical and surgical services for pediatric and adult patients with head and neck disorders and diseases.

Otolaryngologists are medical doctors (MD, DO) who, in the United States, complete at least five years of surgical residency training. This is composed of one year in general surgical training and four years in head and neck surgery.

Anatomy Review

Each ear has three parts (see ■ **Figure 8-1**):

The **outer ear**, consisting of the **pinna** (the cartilaginous appendage on either side of the head, which collects sound waves like a funnel) and the **external auditory meatus** (a tube that conducts sound waves from the pinna to the middle ear). The meatus is lined with skin that secretes **cerumen** (earwax), a mildly antimicrobial substance that traps dust and other particulate foreign material.

The **middle ear**, a cavity in the temporal bone separated from the external auditory meatus by the **tympanic membrane**, which vibrates in response to sound waves and imparts the vibration to a series of very small

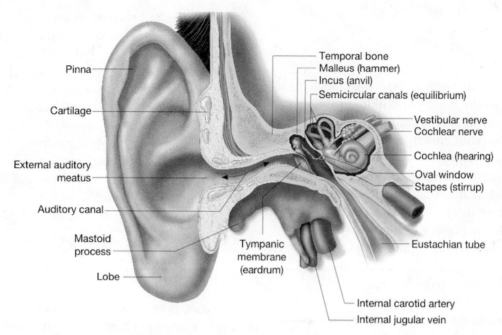

FIGURE 8-1. The ear and its anatomic structures

bones (**malleus**, **incus**, and **stapes**), which in turn transmit them to the inner ear.

The **inner ear**, consisting of the **cochlea** (an organ shaped like a snail shell, in which sound vibrations are converted to nerve impulses to be sent through the eighth cranial, or **vestibulocochlear**, **nerve**) and the vestibular system, the organ of balance (containing minute position sensors in a fluid medium, which send information about head position to the balance center in the brain, also through the eighth cranial nerve).

The middle ear communicates with the pharynx by a minute passage called the **auditory (eustachian)** tube,

which serves to equalize air pressure between the middle ear and the atmosphere. It also communicates with epithelium-lined air cells within the skull, called **mastoid air cells.**

The external **nose** (see ■ Figure 8-2) is supported by a framework of cartilage and covered by skin. The **nostrils** (anterior **nares**) open into paired passages separated by a cartilaginous **septum** and lined with **mucous membrane**, which is rich in serous and mucous glands and blood vessels. The lining membrane of these passages is closely attached to convoluted ridges of bone called

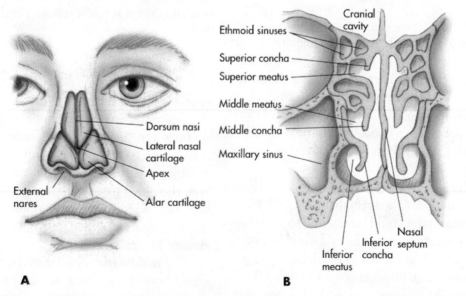

A   **B**

FIGURE 8-2. Nose and nasal cavity, (A) Nasal cartilages and external structure. (B) Meatus and positions of the entrance to the ethmoid and maxillary sinuses.

turbinates (three on each side), which increase the surface area of membrane that is exposed to inspired air.

Adjacent to the nasal passages, and communicating with them by narrow orifices, are the **paranasal sinuses**. These are cavities within the bones of the skull, somewhat variable in size and shape, and lined with mucosa like that of the nose. The nasal passages end at the **choanae**, or posterior nares, where they enter the **nasopharynx**, the uppermost part of the pharyngeal cavity. The nasal passages warm and moisturize inspired air, and particulate matter in the air is trapped in the mucus film lining them.

The throat, or **pharynx** (see ■ Figure 8-3), is a cavity lined with mucous membrane that conducts air from the nose and mouth into the trachea, and food and drink from the mouth into the esophagus. It consists of three portions: the **nasopharynx,** on a level with the

nasal passages and communicating with them; the oropharynx, on a level with the mouth and communicating with it; and the **hypopharynx** or **laryngopharynx**, which lies below the **oropharynx** and gives entry to the esophagus and the larynx.

The **tonsils** and **adenoids** are masses of lymphoid tissue surrounding the zone between the mouth and the oropharynx. At the boundary between the oropharynx and the hypopharynx lies the **epiglottis**, a flexible valve that closes the respiratory passage during swallowing of food or drink.

The lining of the pharynx secretes **mucus**, which keeps the surface moist, traps inhaled particles, and supplements the saliva as a lubricant for food. **Lymph glands** in the front and back of the neck receive lymphatic drainage from the throat and adjacent structures.

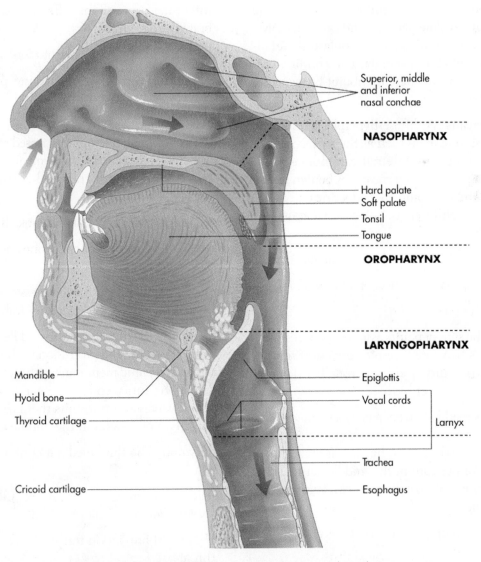

FIGURE 8-3. Structures of the oral cavity, pharynx, and esophagus

Pause for Reflection

1. Name and define the structures of the outer, middle, and inner ear.
2. What is cerumen and what is its purpose or function?
3. What is the purpose or function of the auditory or eustachian tube?
4. Name and define the primary structures of the nose.
5. Name and define the primary structures in the mouth and throat.

LAY AND MEDICAL TERMS

dizziness	vertigo
eardrum	tympanic membrane
earwax	cerumen
hammer, anvil, stirrup	malleus, incus, stapes
strep throat	streptococcal pharyngitis
tongue tie	ankyloglossia

Vocabulary Review

ABO incompatibility A hemolytic disease in which a mother makes antibodies against her baby's blood when her blood type is different from the baby's. The antibodies can cross the placenta and cause hemolytic disease of the newborn or erythroblastosis fetalis, resulting in jaundice and anemia. This condition can also be caused by Rh incompatibility between the mother and baby.

acanthosis nigricans A diffuse hyperplasia and darkening of the skin in areas such as the axilla or groin. One form accompanies internal carcinomas and is called *malignant acanthosis nigricans*. A benign nevoid form in adults may accompany endocrine diseases. A benign form in children is called *pseudoacanthosis nigricans*.

ad lib. According to pleasure (Latin *ad libitum*).

aneurysm Abnormal dilatation of a blood vessel.

ankyloglossia Tongue tie.

Apgar scores The sum of points assigned on assessment of a newborn's heart rate, respiratory effort, muscle tone, reflex irritability, and color, usually calculated at 1 and 5 minutes after birth.

atelectatic otitis media See *tympanic membrane atelectasis*. A narrow passage between the middle ear and the pharynx by which equilibrium is maintained between the air pressure in the middle ear and that of the atmosphere. Also called the *pharyngotympanic* or *eustachian tube*.

auricle The protruding flap of the external ear, also known as the *pinna*.

Battle's sign Postauricular mastoid ecchymosis, a sign seen in basilar skull fractures.

bilirubinemia The presence of bilirubin in the blood. Hyperbilirubinemia is an excessive amount of bilirubin in the blood, evidenced by jaundice (yellowing of the skin and mucous membranes).

brawny Thickened or hardened as a result of severe inflammatory response. Examples: brawny edema, brawny erythema.

bulla (pl. **bullae**) A blister or bleb.

ceruloplasmin A copper-carrying protein in blood plasma that is absent in Wilson disease.

cholesteatoma A benign but locally invasive growth of the tympanic membrane caused by prolonged negative pressure (partial vacuum) in the middle ear. It contains cholesterol, hence the name.

conchal bowl (or **concha**) The cartilage that is situated right near the ear canal and looks like a bowl.

diastasis Dislocation of two bones normally attached to each other.

decibel A measure of the loudness of sound; one tenth of a *bel* (named for Alexander Graham Bell).

eardrum Strictly speaking, the middle ear. In everyday usage, both lay and professional, the term refers only to the tympanic membrane, a thin, tough layer of tissue at the inner end of the ear canal that receives sound waves and transmits them to the inner ear by the chain of ossicles in the middle ear.

endolymph The fluid medium contained in the inner ear.

glottic Pertaining to the larynx. Glottal or glottic spasm is *laryngospasm*.

HEENT Abbreviation for head, eyes, ears, nose, and throat.

Hz Abbreviation for *hertz*, a measure of the frequency of a vibration, particularly one producing sound; equivalent to one cycle (or double vibration) per second. The normal human ear can detect sounds ranging in pitch from 20 to 20,000 Hz.

impaction Plugging of an orifice with a dense mass of some material, as cerumen (earwax) in the external auditory meatus.

larynx The voice box, containing the **vocal cords** (see ■ Figure 8-4) and situated between the laryngopharynx (the lowermost part of the throat) and the trachea (windpipe).

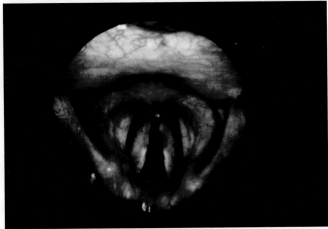

FIGURE 8-5. Vocal cords

malaise A vague sense of being unwell.

mucopus Mucus mixed with pus.

nystagmus Rhythmic, involuntary, jerky movements of both eyes, usually from side to side.

ossicles The small bones of the middle ear—the malleus (hammer), incus (anvil), and stapes (stirrup).

otoscope An instrument that directs a light into the ear through a conical speculum, and is equipped with a magnifying lens.

patent ("PAY-tent") (1) Open, unobstructed. (2) Apparent, evident.

polyps, nasal Massive overgrowths of chronically inflamed mucosa.

purulent Containing or consisting of pus.

recalcitrant (1) Stubborn, not responding as desired (said of an illness). (2) Defiant of authority or guidance (said of a child).

red reflex A luminous red appearance seen when a beam of light is projected into the eye onto the surface of the retina.

refractory Resistant to treatment; not responding to stimulus.

rhinitis Inflammation of the nasal mucous membrane.

rhinoscope An instrument for examining the interior of the nose.

serous effusion Noninfected fluid in the middle ear space; fluid behind the eardrum.

serous gland One producing a thin, watery secretion, not containing mucus.

situs solitus The normal position of organs.

speculum An instrument for inspecting a body cavity or orifice, often equipped with a light source, a magnifying lens, or both.

stenosis Abnormal narrowing of a passage or vessel.

syndactyly Webbing of the fingers or toes, the most common congenital anomaly of the hands and feet.

TMJ Temporomandibular joint.

tongue tie (ankyloglossia) A condition in which the bottom of the tongue is attached to the floor of the mouth. This restricts a patient's ability to freely move the tip of the tongue. The surgical correction of the condition is called *frenuloplasty*.

tympanic membrane atelectasis A complication of chronic serous otitis media in which the middle ear contains a viscous fluid and the tympanic membrane (eardrum) has become thin, atrophic, retracted, and adherent to middle ear structures; there is usually conductive hearing loss.

topical Referring to a medicine applied directly to skin or mucous membrane.

Valsalva maneuver Attempt at forced expiration, with the lips and nostrils closed; this drives air into the auditory tubes unless they are obstructed.

vasoconstrictor A medicine that constricts blood vessels, either when applied topically or through systemic action.

Medical Readings

History and Physical Examination: Head, Eyes, Ears, Nose, Throat, Mouth, Teeth (HEENT)

by John H. Dirckx, MD

Review of Systems. Head. The head is not a system but an anatomic region. In this part of the history the physician records any diseases or injuries of the scalp, skull, and brain and any significant history of headaches. Alternatively, conditions affecting the brain may be taken up in the neurologic history, and disorders of the hair and scalp may be recorded as skin conditions. The organs of special sense (eyes and ears, including balance centers), the upper respiratory tract (nose, sinuses, pharynx), and the mouth and teeth are treated as separate "systems." (See ■ Figure 8-5.)

Full details of any significant head injury (concussion, skull fracture), no matter how remote in time, are included in the past medical history. Of cardinal importance is the establishment of a clear picture of any headache problem, acute or chronic. Headache can be a symptom of life-threatening disease. Moreover, several common types of headache are ordinarily diagnosed on the basis of history alone.

In questioning the patient about headaches, the physician seeks to learn their nature, location, frequency, severity, and duration; associated symptoms such as nausea, vomiting, watering of the eye on the affected side, or aching or stiffness in the neck; triggering factors such as fatigue, stress, menstrual periods, hunger, or certain foods; aggravating factors such as coughing, straining, or bending forward; and alleviating factors such as rest, analgesics, or an ice bag. A migraine headache is often preceded by a warning (aura) consisting usually of flashes of light perceived by the patient before the headache begins.

Eyes. A thorough review of ocular history elicits information about past or present symptoms such as blurring of vision, double vision, partial or complete loss of vision, or difficulty of near adaptation; seeing spots or flashes; seeing halos or rings around lights; undue visual impairment with reduced illumination; pain in, on, or behind the eyeball; redness, discharge, watering, or abnormal sensitivity to light; swelling, drooping,

Severe headaches lasting about half an hour occur several times a day and occasionally awaken him at night. The pain seems to be in or behind the right eye and is accompanied by watering and redness of the eye.

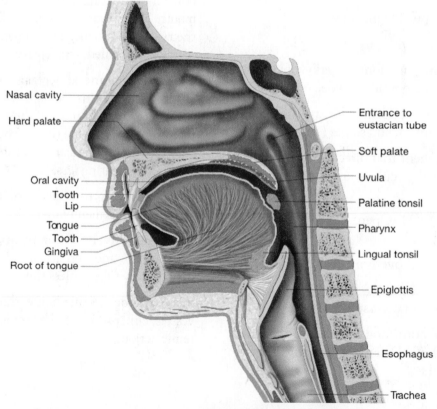

FIGURE 8-5. Head and neck anatomy

itching, or crusting of lids; and full details about the use of glasses or contact lenses and the date of the most recent eye examination. Eye symptoms can indicate neurologic or systemic rather than purely local disease, as in the case of loss of vision due to a brain tumor or retinopathy due to diabetes.

No ocular symptoms or visual deficits.

Ears. The examiner inquires about the duration, degree, and pitch range of **hearing loss** in one or both ears; ringing, popping, or other abnormal sounds heard by the patient; pain, pressure, itching, swelling, bleeding, or discharge; history of occupational, avocational, or military exposure to loud noises; history of injury to the ear, particularly **perforation of the tympanic membrane**; possible effects of air travel or scuba diving on the ears; any ear surgery; and use of a hearing aid. Pain felt in the ear can result from a wide range of non-otic diseases, including pharyngitis, laryngeal cancer, mumps, and brain tumor.

Vertigo and **dysequilibrium**, suggesting disease of the inner ear, are usually dealt with here also. The distinction between these two symptoms is sometimes difficult to make; lay persons refer to both as "dizziness." **Vertigo** is a constant or intermittent feeling that one is spinning ("like I just got off a merry-go-round"). In contrast, **dysequilibrium** means difficulty maintaining one's balance when standing or walking. Vertigo is usually accompanied by some degree of dysequilibrium, but dysequilibrium often occurs alone. Several drugs can produce temporary impairment of hearing or balance, and a history of their use may be significant.

No history of infection, earache, or hearing loss.

Nose. The nasal history includes mention of any acute or chronic pain, swelling, obstruction, or discharge affecting the nose; sneezing, nosebleeds, or frequent colds; seasonal or occasional allergies; sinus infections; disturbance of the sense of smell; history of fracture or other injuries; submucous resection for deviated septum, removal of polyps, cautery for nosebleeds, or other surgical procedure; and regular or long-term use of decongestants or antihistamines for nasal symptoms, particularly inhalers, drops, or sprays.

The common cold is a universal human experience. Members of the laity often apply the generic term *cold*

WHY CHILDREN GO TO A DOCTOR	
1. Colds	11. Skin injuries
2. Coughs	12. Head injuries
3. Croup	13. Arm or leg injuries
4. Sore throat	14. Abdominal pain
5. Pus or drainage from eyes	15. Headache
	16. Constipation
6. Earache	17. Unexplained crying
7. Diarrhea	18. Immunization reactions
8. Vomiting	
9. Wheezing	19. Hives
10. Fever	20. Unexplained rashes

Denies frequent colds, epistaxis, or nasal fracture. No history of trauma, obstruction, nosebleed, or discharge.

or *sinus* (*trouble*) to any condition characterized by nasal obstruction and discharge. Hence careful and detailed questioning may be needed to elicit clues to nasal allergy, chronic irritation from dust or smoke, or obstruction due to a tumor. The lay meaning of **congestion** usually diverges from the correct technical sense, "swelling due to engorgement of blood vessels."

The patient has a 4-day history of purulent rhinorrhea, bilateral nasal obstruction, and a sensation of fullness in the periorbital regions.

Throat: The throat includes not only the **pharynx**, the common channel shared by the respiratory and digestive tracts, but also the **larynx**. Important historical points include **sore throat** (the most common presenting symptom in many outpatient practices), postnasal drip, choking, and difficulty swallowing; atypical throat pain, which may be due to foreign body, abscess, tumor, or neurologic disease; hoarseness or other change in the voice; and history of tonsillectomy or other throat operation. Pain, swelling, or mass in the neck is included here for convenience.

Sore throat is worse in the morning and evening but very mild or absent during the day.

She has clear nasal discharge, sneezing, and itching of the nasal mucous membranes, worse when around cats or dust.

Mouth and Teeth. These are not the exclusive province of the dentist. The oral and dental history can have important health implications. Chronic, painful conditions of the mouth, gums, or teeth can severely impair nutrition. Many systemic diseases are reflected in oral and dental symptoms. A recent history of dental work may provide a clue to bacteremia with ensuing infective endocarditis. The complete oral and dental history includes soreness, swelling, or ulceration of the lips, gums, or tongue; excessive salivation or excessive dryness of the mouth; abnormal taste or absence of taste; bleeding gums; frequent toothache or sensitivity of teeth to sweet, hot, or cold food or drinks; dental caries; loose, damaged, or missing teeth; regularity of dental care; and wearing of orthodontic braces, dentures, or other appliances.

The patient wears a bite plate prescribed by an oral surgeon for TMJ syndrome.

Pause for Reflection

1. In the Review of Systems why is it important for a doctor to get detailed information about any type of headache?
2. Why should a family physician get a clear history about eye problems the patient may be having?
3. Distinguish between vertigo and dysequilibrium.
4. What must a doctor do when a patient complains of a "cold" or "sinus trouble"?
5. What is the most common presenting symptom in many family practices?
6. Why are the mouth and teeth important to the family physician?

Physical Examination of the Head, Face, and Neck.

The head is symmetrical and normally developed, without exostoses or traumatic lesions.

Head and Face. The physician usually begins the examination with the head and face, since they are normally uncovered by clothing and are the parts at which one naturally looks first in viewing or studying another person. The examiner notes the size, shape, and symmetry of the skull, palpating for swellings, lumps, or tenderness. Deformities of the skull can be congenital (as a feature of many inherited deforming syndromes) or acquired (as in acromegaly and Paget disease).

The amount, distribution, texture, and color of scalp hair are observed, as well as the pattern of any hair loss. The scalp is inspected for scaling, dermatitis, signs of acute or past trauma, and other lesions. Any tremors or involuntary movements of the head are noted.

A mere glance at the **face** will usually suffice to tell the examiner whether the patient is alert or somnolent, anxious or apathetic, angry or euphoric. The face not only registers the patient's current emotional state but often reflects systemic disease as well. Parkinsonism, myxedema, acromegaly, myasthenia gravis, allergic rhinitis, and Cushing syndrome each produce characteristic changes in facial features.

Generalized changes in skin color (pallor, flushing, cyanosis, jaundice, abnormal pigmentation) are apt to be noted first in the face because it is uncovered by clothing and seen first. Color changes may, however, be largely confined to the face, as with the circumoral pallor of scarlatina and the malar flush of tuberculosis.

Facial configuration and symmetry can be distorted by various congenital syndromes. Paralysis due to peripheral neuropathy (Bell palsy) or stroke can also cause facial asymmetry, as a result of impaired mobility of one part of the face. The examiner may instruct the patient to perform various movements such as wrinkling the forehead, showing the teeth, and pursing the lips to whistle, in order to test for facial muscle weakness or paralysis.

Cutaneous eruptions may be largely confined to the face (acne, rosacea, the malar rash of lupus erythematosus) or may appear there as part of a general exanthem (varicella). The lips are subject to conditions that seldom affect other parts of the skin. Masses or cutaneous nodules are carefully evaluated for signs

This 14-year-old is seen for followup of his acne. There has been no improvement with topical treatment; in fact, he has more comedo formation and a higher proportion of pustular lesions than before, with a scattering of cysts over his upper back.

of malignancy. The examiner notes the presence and character of any facial hair. A mustache or beard may be worn to conceal surgical or traumatic scars or other lesions; these must be looked for.

Subtle degrees of swelling may not be apparent if the examiner has had no previous acquaintance with the patient. Facial swelling can be diffuse or can affect certain areas more than others—the eyelids in infectious mononucleosis, the cheeks in Cushing syndrome, the lips in angioneurotic edema. Swelling over a paranasal sinus can indicate underlying infection. Swelling of the parotid gland occurs in mumps and obstruction of a salivary duct, but may also represent a tumor. The physician carefully palpates any facial swelling or mass to assess its consistency, tenderness, and other significant features.

Pain in the lower **jaw** or difficulty in chewing or speaking will prompt an assessment of the mandible, the temporomandibular joints, and the muscles of mastication for mobility, spasm, swelling, crepitus, or tenderness.

The **neck** is not simply a column for supporting the head. Through it pass all nerve connections between brain and body, all inspired oxygen and exhaled carbon dioxide, all swallowed food and drink, and all blood supply to the brain, which consumes 25 percent of the body's oxygen intake. Because subtle abnormalities of the neck can herald life-threatening developments, the region is carefully assessed.

Neck: The neck is supple without palpable masses or venous distention.

The neck is subject to many musculoskeletal injuries and disorders, some of which can affect its configuration and mobility in obvious ways. The examiner tests neck mobility by gently grasping the patient's head and putting it through a range of movements, noting any restrictions due to joint stiffness, muscle spasm, or pain.

Any swellings or masses are palpated for size, shape, consistency, mobility, pulsatility, and tenderness. Additionally, the entire neck is felt for **enlarged lymph**

The thyroid is diffusely enlarged, smooth, and nontender.

nodes, which may appear in any of several locations. Each anatomic group of nodes "drains" (receives lymphatic channels from) a specific region of the head, face, neck, or thorax. The **thyroid gland** is felt and its size and consistency assessed. For this examination the physician may ask the patient to swallow in order to move the gland up and down under the palpating fingers. The larynx and the uppermost part of the trachea are also felt and any lesions or lateral deviation noted.

The pulsations of the **carotid arteries** are gently palpated and compared. The physician applies a stethoscope over each carotid in turn to listen for **bruits**—harsh sounds synchronous with the pulse, caused by passage of blood through a vessel narrowed by arteriosclerosis.

Carotid pulses are full and equal; no carotid bruits are heard.

The **external jugular veins** at the sides of the neck are normally not distended with blood when one is in an upright position, but can be seen to be filled with blood in the recumbent position. The physician can judge the patient's venous pressure by noting the height to which the upper body must be raised from the horizontal before the external jugular veins are no longer visibly distended. Increased venous pressure, which occurs in cardiac failure, may cause the jugular veins to remain filled even in the erect position. Pressure over the liver may cause the level of blood in the external jugular veins to rise in congestive heart failure (hepatojugular reflux). The internal jugular veins are not visible, but they can impart faint pulsations to the soft tissues of the neck that are coordinated in a complex way with cardiac function.

Jugular venous pulses are seen at 60° elevation.

Neck veins are elevated to the angle of the jaw at 90°.

Physical Examination of the Ears. The diagnostician has full access to the external ear, very limited access to the middle ear, and none at all to the inner ear except through testing of hearing and equilibrium.

Examination of the ear begins with inspection of the **pinna** for deformity, inflammation, injury, and abnormal masses. The **external ear** is subject to many developmental anomalies, some of which have more than cosmetic importance. Malformations of the external ear occur as part of various inherited syndromes that include faulty development of other structures as well. They may also indicate congenital renal disease. There is a high correlation between diagonal earlobe creases and coronary artery disease in middle-aged and elderly men.

The framework of the pinna is cartilage, a tissue with poor healing potential. Hence severe or repeated trauma to the ear or severe infection can result in permanent deformity. The pinna is a frequent site for the tophi of gout. The earlobe is subject to sebaceous cysts. Piercing of the **pinna or earlobe** for ornaments sometimes results in infection, hypertrophic scarring, or keloid formation.

> *The tympanic membranes were reddened, and shotty nodes were present in the right and left side of the neck.*

Inspection of the ear canal and **tympanic membrane** is generally performed with an **otoscope** (see ■ Figure 8-6), a handheld instrument with a light source, exchangeable cone-shaped specula of various sizes, and a magnifying lens. (A specialist may prefer to use a head mirror or headlamp and handheld specula.) In order to get an adequate view of the tympanic membrane, the examiner must straighten the ear canal by pulling the pinna back and up with one hand while positioning the otoscope with the other. Because otoscopic examination can be performed with one eye only, there is no true depth perception. Accumulated wax (**cerumen**) or exudate, foreign material, swelling of the ear canal, and inability of the patient to tolerate the insertion of the speculum can all render adequate otoscopic examination difficult or impossible.

Under ideal conditions the examiner inspects the ear canal for injection, edema, impacted cerumen, exudate, blood, and foreign material. The normal tympanic membrane appears gray or opalescent and nearly flat, but with recognizable landmarks. Behind it the **manubrium** (handle) of the **malleus** (hammer) can just be seen. Possible abnormalities are injection, bulging, retraction, or perforation of the tympanic membrane; discoloration by blood in the middle ear, which can result from basal skull fracture; a fluid level, bubbles, or both behind the tympanic membrane, indicating **serous fluid** in the middle ear; and tumors, such as cholesteatoma. Prior infections or perforations may have left scars on the tympanic membrane. A **polyethylene** (PE) ventilatory tube (**grommet**) placed in the tympanic membrane for chronic infection will be visible to the examiner.

Otoscopes are made to two basic designs (see ■ Figure 8-6). The open or operating otoscope is so constructed that the physician can insert instruments through it into the ear canal. When the closed, or pneumatic, otoscope is in position, its interior forms a closed space continuous with the ear canal. Pressure and suction alternately applied to this space by means of a short rubber tube attached to a rubber bulb (or inserted in the physician's mouth) will move the tympanic membrane in and out unless the membrane is fixed by disease. This method is principally useful in children. The mobility of the tympanic membrane can also be tested by having the patient swallow while pinching the nostrils together or perform the Valsalva maneuver.

Hearing can be tested in various ways. Pure-tone audiometry with sophisticated electronic equipment in a soundproof booth is the method used by otologists, and may also be a part of school and industrial hearing testing, but it is not included in a standard physical examination. A rough notion of auditory acuity can be obtained by testing the examinee's ability to hear the spoken and whispered voice at various distances, with first one ear and then the other occluded. The patient's ability to hear a ticking watch held at various distances from the ear can also be compared with that of a person having normal hearing. Auditory discrimination can be tested by noting how well the patient can distinguish pairs of words differing in only one consonant, such as *back/bat* and *cool/pool*.

Hearing loss can be of two types: **conductive** and **neurosensory**. Conductive hearing loss results from disease or injury of middle ear structures, neurosensory loss from malfunction of the acoustic nerve due to aging

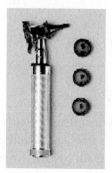
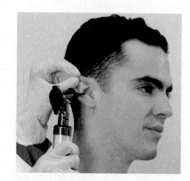

FIGURE 8-6. Otoscope

The tympanic membrane is slightly injected and deeply retracted.

(presbycusis), noise exposure, or certain drugs and chemicals. Both conductive and neurosensory hearing loss can exist together in varying degrees. Two tests of value in distinguishing types of hearing impairment are the **Rinne** and the **Weber test**, both requiring the use of a tuning fork.

In the **Rinne test**, the examiner notes whether the patient can hear the sound of the vibrating fork better (that is, longer, as it gradually ceases to vibrate) by **air conduction** or by **bone conduction**. Air conduction is tested by placing the prongs of the vibrating fork near the external auditory meatus. Bone conduction is tested by placing the shank of the vibrating fork against the **mastoid process** (the bony prominence behind the external ear). With an intact acoustic nerve, the vibrations of the fork will still be audible by air conduction even when they can no longer be heard by bone conduction. When this is not the case, conductive hearing loss rather than neurosensory loss is likely.

In the **Weber test** the examiner touches the shank of the vibrating fork to the middle of the patient's forehead. If the sound of the fork seems louder in the ear whose hearing is impaired, the impairment is conductive. If the sound of the fork seems fainter in the impaired ear, the impairment is neural.

The Weber lateralizes to the right.

The assessment of **equilibrium** is usually performed by observing the patient's **gait**, particularly when walking a line (heel-to-toe walking), and testing the ability to stand erect with eyes closed without swaying or falling (**Romberg test**). The sensitivity of the Romberg test can be enhanced by having the patient stand with one foot in front of the other (tandem Romberg).

Another test of **vestibular function** requires the patient to observe the location of some object (such as the examiner's forefinger), close the eyes, and touch the object. **Past-pointing** (failure to touch the object) suggests vestibular disease in a patient with normal coordination. The **caloric test** is occasionally used to assess vestibular function. Warmed or chilled water is gently injected with a syringe into the ear canal, one side being tested at a time. The sensation of vertigo and observable nystagmus indicate an intact vestibular apparatus on the side being tested. Persistence of this response for several minutes suggests abnormal sensitivity of the balance center to stimulation.

Examination of the Nose, Throat, Mouth, and Teeth.

Examination of the **nose** begins with external inspection for developmental abnormalities, traumatic deformities, enlargement (rhinophyma), nodules, ulcers, and other cutaneous lesions. The interior of each nostril is then viewed with a beam of light from a head mirror or other source. When a head mirror is used, the nostril is gently dilated with a **bivalve nasal speculum**. Alternatively, a **cone-shaped speculum** larger than those used for ear examination can be attached to an otoscope.

Nose: Nasal passages are clear and no lesions are noted.

The interior of the nose is inspected for **septal deviation** or perforation; mucosal edema, injection, ulcers, erosions, or polyps; discharge, hemorrhage, foreign bodies, and tumors. The sense of smell can be tested if necessary by having the patient try to identify familiar substances such as coffee or cinnamon by smell alone.

The **paranasal sinuses** are irregular cavities within certain bones of the skull. They are lined with mucous membrane and communicate with the nasal cavity by very small openings. They cannot be examined directly, but thickening of their lining membranes and accumulations of fluid due to infection can sometimes be detected by **transillumination**. If a small electric light is placed against appropriate parts of the head and face or inside the mouth in a darkened room, a deep ruddy glow can be seen through the skin. The examiner can judge from the intensity and configuration of this glow whether the sinus cavities are filled with air, as they should be, or with mucus or pus. (This method is far inferior to x-ray, CT scan, and MRI for diagnosis of sinus disease.)

Transillumination shows relataive opacification of the left maxillary antrum, sinus.

For the examination of the **oral cavity**, the patient is instructed to open the mouth widely (see ■ Figure 8-7). The physician directs a beam of light into the mouth, gently using a tongue depressor to move lips

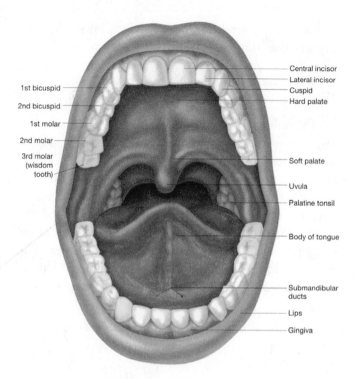

1st bicuspid
2nd bicuspid
1st molar
2nd molar
3rd molar (wisdom tooth)

Central incisor
Lateral incisor
Cuspid
Hard palate
Soft palate
Uvula
Palatine tonsil
Body of tongue
Submandibular ducts
Lips
Gingiva

FIGURE 8-7. The oral cavity

or tongue as needed to improve the view. The buccal mucosa, the palate, and all surfaces of the tongue are inspected for petechiae, ulcers, tumors, leukoplakia, and signs of injury. The upper surface of the tongue is observed particularly for abnormal roughness or smoothness, furrowing, fissuring, or dilated papillae. When the tongue is protruded for inspection, any tremulousness or lateral deviation due to neurologic disease can be noted.

Dental: The teeth are in good repair and the gums are healthy.

The examiner observes the number, shape, and alignment of the **teeth** and any mottling, staining, caries, cavities, or restorations (fillings). Note is made of chipped, cracked, or missing teeth, as well as any dental appliances (bridges, plates, retainers, orthodontic braces) in use. Occlusion (bite) can be assessed by having the patient bring the teeth together while the lips are held apart with a tongue depressor. The gums are inspected for swelling, inflammation, ulceration, abnormal coloring, hypertrophy, or retraction.

Inspection of the **pharynx** is performed by having the patient say "ah," which raises the **soft palate** and otherwise dilates the **oropharynx**, while the examiner presses down gently on the back of the tongue with a

The uvula rises in the midline on phonation.

The tongue protrudes in the midline.

tongue depressor. Adjustments in the position of the examiner's head and in the light source permit assessment of the soft palate and **uvula**, the root of the tongue, the faucial pillars, the tonsils if present, and the posterior wall of the oropharynx. Mucosal lesions, paralysis of the soft palate, edema, injection, exudate, and postnasal discharge or hemorrhage can thus be noted.

This part of the physical examination may be the most convenient opportunity for the examiner to note any abnormal odor of the patient's breath. Besides dental and oral disease, infection in any part of the respiratory tract can impart a **foul odor to the breath**. Certain metabolic disorders (ketosis, uremia, hepatic failure) can impart characteristic odors to the breath due to excretion of abnormal gases by the lungs. Alcohol and paraldehyde as well as certain foods and condiments can also be detected in the breath as they are excreted by the lungs.

Inspection of both the **nasopharynx** and the **larynx** can be performed with an angled mirror inserted through the mouth into the oropharynx. These examinations are not routine but may be indicated in certain circumstances and are easily performed if the patient can cooperate. Sometimes the pharynx and palate are sprayed with topical anesthetic to prevent gagging during the examination.

Indirect laryngoscopy is performed with an angled mirror much like a dentist's mirror but with a longer handle. Light is provided by a head mirror or other adjustable source. The examiner inserts the mirror into the posterior pharynx, being careful to avoid contact with the soft palate or pharyngeal walls, and views the vocal cords while the patient says "eeee" in a high-pitched voice. Tumors, paralysis, or inflammatory lesions of the cords can be seen. In addition, foreign bodies or tumors of other parts of the hypopharynx can be noted.

A smaller mirror is used to examine the nasopharynx (**posterior rhinoscopy**). The technique is largely the same but the mirror is directed upward to enable the examiner to see the choanae, the adenoids if present, and the orifices of the eustachian tubes.

Masses and other lesions in the mouth and pharynx can be palpated if necessary, the examiner donning a rubber glove and gently inserting one or two fingers to assess consistency or tenderness.

1. List 3 features that a physician makes note of in examining the head and face.
2. List 3 things that a physician makes note of on examination of the neck.
3. What is the examiner looking for on inspection of the ear canal?
4. Ears: A fluid level, bubbles, or both behind the tympanic membrane is an indication of _____.
5. Distinguish between conductive and neurosensory hearing loss.
6. Distinguish between air conduction and bone conduction.
7. How are the patient's equilibrium and vestibular function assessed?
8. List 3 things that the examiner looks for on external and internal examination of the nose.
9. What technique is used to examine the paranasal sinuses?
10. What does the physician look for on examination of the mouth?
11. What is the physician examining when asking the patient to say "ah" while pressing down the back of the tongue with a tongue depressor?

Pediatric History and Physical Examination

by John H. Dirckx, MD

The history and physical examination of an infant differ substantially from those of an older child or adult. The entire history must be obtained from sources other than the patient. Parental factors and antenatal events loom large in the history; indeed, a newborn has no other history. The physician must be alert for developmental anomalies and disturbances of nutrition, growth, and maturation that are not diagnostic considerations in later life. On the other hand, degenerative diseases and most kinds of malignancy simply do not occur. Examination techniques are limited to those requiring no cooperation from the patient. Sizes, shapes, textures, and levels of function that would be abnormal in an adult may be perfectly normal in a baby, and vice versa.

A newborn undergoes a thorough examination within a few hours after birth. Periodic well-baby checks are part of routine pediatric care. When an infant is admitted to the hospital, a history and physical will be done. Although these examinations vary in scope and emphasis, certain basic points of similarity can be noted. My purpose here is to sketch briefly the pediatric history and physical examination with particular attention to variations from diagnostic procedures used for older children and adults.

The physician precedes the recording of the pediatric history by identifying the informant or informants, their relation to the child, and any emotional or other factors that may affect the accuracy of their information. The chief complaint and history of present illness for a small child are necessarily stated from the viewpoint of the informant.

The past history begins before the child's conception with the health history of the parents and their families and of any older siblings, particularly with respect to hereditary diseases or abnormalities. Pertinent circumstances of the mother's pregnancy include any drug or chemical exposures; use of alcohol, tobacco, or caffeine; exposure to ionizing radiation; maternal infections, particularly rubella or genital herpes; toxemia, hemorrhage, or abnormal weight gain. As full an account as possible is obtained of the labor and delivery, with specific inquiries about gestation time, length of labor, any complications, use of forceps, Apgar scores, the child's birth weight, and evidence of congenital anomalies. The child's health during the neonatal period is reviewed, with particular attention to jaundice, respiratory distress, feeding difficulties, fever, or seizures. The nutritional history (breast or bottle feeding, vitamin supplements, weight gain) is reviewed.

An important feature of the pediatric history is an account of the child's growth and development. Any available data on height and weight at various ages are collected. Teething history is recorded. Psychomotor development is traced in terms of "milestones" such as acquisition of head control, speech, walking, and toilet training. Social responses and adjustments of the older infant and toddler are evaluated.

The physician attempts to learn something of the family's living circumstances (family income, level of

REFLEXES OF INFANTS

A reflex is an inborn behavior or innate ability. Babies are assessed shortly after birth by a pediatrician or other attending physician to check if the following reflexes are present:

suck reflex: Necessary in order to drink milk or formula. Babies without an adequate sucking reflex may have to be tube-fed formula.

rooting reflex: Touching one side of the baby's face will cause it to turn its head in that direction.

grasp or palmar reflex: The baby closes its fingers around an object when the palm is stimulated by an object or the examiner's finger.

Moro or startle reflex: The baby moves its arms and legs in an outward direction when startled.

tonic neck reflex: When the baby's head is moved in one direction, the corresponding arm and leg on that side extend and on the opposite side bend.

Babinski or plantar reflex: The normal finding of the Babinski reflex in a newborn is different from that of a young child or adult. In a normal newborn, stroking the bottom of the foot from the heel to ball of the foot with a finger causes the toes to point up (upgoing toes); in an adult, the normal finding is just the opposite—downgoing toes.

blink reflex: The child blinks when the examiner shines a light in the eyes.

step or walk reflex: When the newborn is held upright, the neonate's legs move as if trying to walk.

intelligence and responsibility of parents, marital harmony and stability, social environment), being particularly alert for any evidence of child abuse or neglect. In the past medical history, attention is given to routine immunizations against childhood diseases.

The examination of a small child calls for much patience and skill. The physician usually solicits the help of a parent or nurse to hold and comfort the child during the examination and to restrain it as needed. Every effort is made to keep the child calm and relaxed because little can be learned by palpating a patient who is writhing or by auscultating one who is screaming.

The child's temperature is taken rectally, and blood pressure is determined with a suitably sized cuff. Height (length) and weight are recorded, as well as the circumferences of the head and the chest. Throughout the examination the physician is particularly alert for evidence of congenital or developmental abnormalities. The skin is evaluated for jaundice, rashes, or signs of dehydration. Any deformity or abnormal enlargement of the head is noted, and the fontanels are palpated.

The eyes are examined for strabismus, congenital cataract, and signs of infection. Vision can be tested in preschool children with an eye chart consisting entirely of E's printed in various positions. The child uses three fingers to show which way the crosspieces of each E are pointing.

Examination of ears, nose, and throat is often a trying experience for both examiner and patient. Assistance is essential. Auscultation of the lungs of a crying child may have to be confined to the inspiratory phase of respiration. The heart is examined for evidence of congenital anomalies. Palpation of the abdomen is performed carefully to detect malignant tumors, which occasionally occur in quite small children, and umbilical or inguinal hernias. Examination of the genitalia and rectum is generally limited to external inspection unless disease or injury of these structures is suspected.

In the orthopedic examination, the physician looks for evidence of congenital malformations or injuries, and pays particular attention to the hip joints, legs, and feet. The neurologic examination of a small child includes tests for **reflexes** that are present in normal infants but not in older children or adults. These include the Moro (startle), grasp, rooting, and tonic neck reflexes. Alertness, muscle tone, and general responsiveness to stimuli are assessed with due consideration of the child's age.

Pause for Reflection

1. What limitations are incurred in obtaining the history and performing a physical exam on an infant?

2. What is different about the past history for a newborn or infant as compared to an older child or adult?

3. In addition to the usual vital signs (blood pressure, temperature, pulse), what other parameters are included in the initial exam of a newborn or infant?

4. List 4 specific abnormalities that a physician looks for on full exam of a newborn or infant that are not as relevant in an older child or adult.

Common Diseases

Otitis Externa (Swimmer's Ear)

Infection of the external auditory meatus.

Causes: Infection with bacteria (*Proteus, Pseudomonas*) and sometimes fungi (*Aspergillus*). Predisposing causes include water exposure (swimming, showering), excessive cerumen, mechanical trauma (probing with paper clip), foreign body (cotton, pencil eraser), diabetes mellitus, and immune compromise.

History: Earache, itching in the external auditory meatus, purulent discharge. **Hearing loss** if the meatus is occluded by swelling or exudate.

Physical Examination: Redness and swelling of the meatus, sometimes with complete occlusion; purulent exudate, perhaps with excessive cerumen or foreign body visible. Tenderness on manipulation of the pinna.

Course: Generally benign, but in diabetes mellitus and AIDS an external ear infection may resist conservative treatment and become chronic, perhaps invading the skull or brain, with resulting neurologic damage.

Treatment: After gentle cleansing and removal of any foreign material, cerumen, or exudate, topical antibiotics (ear drops), often with hydrocortisone to combat local inflammation, are instilled several times a day. Sometimes a gauze wick is inserted to facilitate penetration of ear drops when edema of the meatus is extreme. In invasive infections, intravenous antibiotics and even surgery may be required.

Otitis Media

Bacterial infection of the middle ear and adjoining mastoid air cells (see ■ **Figures 8-8, 8-9**).

Cause: Infection by *Streptococcus pneumoniae, Haemophilus influenzae, Streptococcus pyogenes,* and other bacteria. Otitis media commonly occurs as a sequel to a viral upper respiratory infection. Obstruction of the auditory tube by edema leads to pressure changes within the middle ear and secretion of mucus and serous fluid, which becomes infected by bacteria already present in the tissues. Otitis media is often bilateral. It is commoner in infants and small children than in adolescents and adults, accounting for one third of all pediatric office visits.

History: Pain and pressure in one or both ears, hearing loss, sometimes fever.

Physical Examination: Redness of the **tympanic membrane**, sometimes with formation of bullae. Immobility of the tympanic membrane, reflecting malfunction of the auditory tube. Occasionally **bulging of the**

membrane. If spontaneous rupture occurs, blood or purulent exudate in the external auditory meatus.

Course: It is estimated that 20–80% of all cases of otitis media will resolve spontaneously without treatment. When there is fever or severe pain, antibiotic treatment is usually prescribed because of the risk of serious complications in a few patients. Neglect of the infection, its failure to respond to standard initial treatment, or a series of recurrent infections can lead to chronic otitis media, typically due to different organisms (*Proteus, Pseudomonas,* staphylococci) than acute infection.

Complications of chronic otitis media include spontaneous rupture of the tympanic membrane, with chronic purulent drainage; destruction of the bones within the middle ear that transmit sound; invasion of

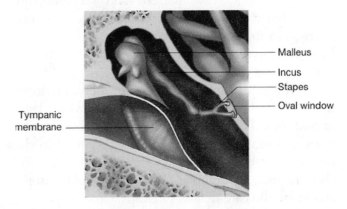

FIGURE 8-8. The ossicles of the middle ear along with the oval window and tympanic membrane

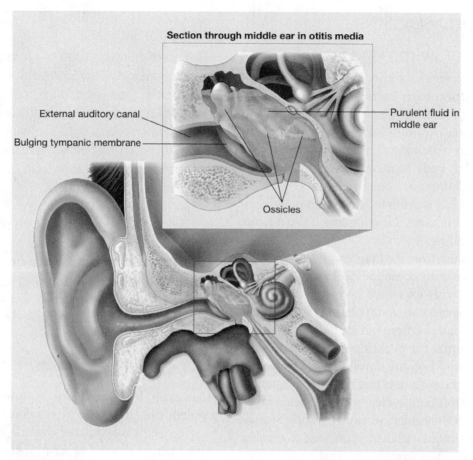

Section through middle ear in otitis media

External auditory canal

Bulging tympanic membrane

Purulent fluid in middle ear

Ossicles

FIGURE 8-9. Acute otitis media, showing the tympanic membrane bulging and purulent fluid in the middle ear

mastoid air cells (**mastoiditis**), skull bones, and even the central nervous system by infection; formation of **cholesteatoma**, a benign but locally invasive growth of the tympanic membrane caused by prolonged negative pressure (partial vacuum) in the middle ear. Chronic otitis media can lead to permanent conductive hearing loss and, in small children, speech defects because of inability to hear speech sounds properly.

Treatment: In the absence of fever and severe pain in patients over age two, analgesics and observation are preferred to antibiotic treatment. For selected patients, systemic antibiotics (amoxicillin with or without clavulanic acid, erythromycin, trimethoprim-sulfamethoxazole), decongestants, analgesics.

If tympanic membrane rupture threatens, **myringotomy** (surgical puncture of the membrane, with release of pus). In children with recurrent or refractory infections, polyethylene (PE) tubes may be placed in the tympanic membrane(s) to aerate the middle ear(s) and allow for escape of purulent secretion. Cholesteatoma and mastoiditis are treated surgically. Chronic perforation of the tympanic membrane requires surgical repair (**tympanoplasty**).

Vertigo

A sense of motion (spinning, falling, floor tipping) when no such motion is occurring.

Causes: Labyrinthitis, often following respiratory infection and hence often called viral. Degenerative changes in the balance-sensing mechanism of the inner ear. Increased pressure within the endolymphatic sac (Ménière disease). Vascular or neoplastic disease of the inner ear or temporal lobe of the cerebral cortex. Diplopia, head injury, multiple sclerosis, drugs, alcohol.

History: A feeling of spinning or falling to one side, or a sense that the floor is tipping or rotating, coming on suddenly, often with head movement, and lasting seconds, minutes, hours, days, weeks, or months. When severe, vertigo may make it impossible for the patient to stand or walk and may be accompanied by nausea and vomiting. There may also be tinnitus and hearing loss.

Physical Examination: May be essentially normal. The **Romberg test** (patient standing with eyes closed) may indicate inability to maintain equilibrium. Eyes may show nystagmus.

Treatment: May be limited to treatment of the underlying cause. In **Ménière disease**, salt restriction and diuretic therapy may help by reducing the pressure of the endolymph. Medicines such as meclizine and dimenhydrinate may diminish or abolish vertigo temporarily. In some cases of positional vertigo, head manipulation can reduce symptoms by promoting reorientation of the balance mechanism.

Hearing Loss

Reduction, often permanent, in the acuity of hearing in one or both ears. Hearing loss is divided into three types depending on the location of the abnormality.

Conductive hearing loss: Disease or abnormality in the outer or middle ear: cerumen impaction, otitis media with effusion, hardening of the tympanic membrane (otosclerosis), injury or disease of the ossicles.

Sensory hearing loss: Disease of the cochlea: acoustic trauma, ototoxicity (aminoglycosides, loop diuretics, cisplatin), aging.

Neural: Eighth nerve lesions; cerebrovascular disease. Hearing loss is assessed by audiometry and the Weber and Rinne tests.

Treatment is that of the underlying cause, if possible. Generally no treatment is effective.

Coryza (Common Cold)

A common, mild rhinitis caused by viruses.

Causes: Any of numerous viruses spread readily from person to person. Risk of catching colds may be heightened by exposure to severe winter weather (especially whole-body chilling), drying of indoor air by heating systems, or crowding indoors during the winter.

History: Headache, nasal stuffiness, runny nose, sneezing, throat irritation, malaise. Occasionally fever, chills, anorexia, and muscle aching.

Physical Examination: Erythema and edema of nasal mucosa. Temperature may be slightly elevated.

Course: Generally self-limited. Sometimes complicated by sinusitis, otitis media, pharyngitis, bronchitis.

Treatment: Purely symptomatic. Oral decongestants are moderately effective. Aspirin, acetaminophen, or ibuprofen relieve discomfort. Rest, fluids. Antihistamines do not decongest, antibiotics do not kill cold viruses, and nasal decongestant sprays may cause rebound congestion worse than the disease.

Allergic Rhinitis (Hay Fever)

A recurrent, often seasonal inflammation of the nasal mucous membrane caused by allergy to inhaled materials.

Causes: Sensitivity to pollens, grasses, mold spores, dust mites, animal dander, second-hand cigarette smoke, and other inhalant allergens.

THE USUAL CHILDHOOD DISEASES

"The usual childhood diseases" are not so common anymore thanks to modern medicine. Immunizations have spared much human misery and even human life.

A simple series of vaccinations have controlled diseases such as diphtheria, pertussis, and tetanus (DPT); measles, mumps, and rubella (MMR; German measles); poliomyelitis; hepatitis A and hepatitis B; meningococcus; pneumococcus; and varicella (chickenpox).

The first vaccines are given to an infant anywhere from one to six months of age, depending upon the manufacturer's recommendation. These are followed by booster shots at regular intervals thereafter until the series has been completed (usually three or four sessions). An influenza vaccine (flu shot) is recommended annually for children over six months of age.

A relatively new vaccine (Gardasil) has been developed to prevent infection with certain types of the human papillomavirus (HPV) infection (a sexually transmitted disease), which is linked to cervical cancer. The HPV vaccine is recommended for girls ages 9 to 17 and women ages 18 to 26.

History: Recurrent or constant nasal congestion and irritation, with copious watery discharge, itching, sneezing (often many times in a row), and itching and watering of the eyes. Symptoms may occur consistently at certain seasons (spring, fall) or, especially when due to house dust, may be perennial.

Nasal passages are clear and no lesions are noted.

The nares are patent.

Physical Examination: Watery, red eyes. Pale or bluish, markedly swollen nasal mucosa. **Polyps** (massive overgrowths of chronically inflamed mucosa) may be present.

Diagnostic Tests: Nasal smear shows eosinophils. Skin testing or RAST (radioallergosorbent testing) can identify causative allergens.

Treatment: Decongestants, antihistamines, nasal corticosteroid spray. Avoidance of known allergens when possible. Use of air filters as appropriate. Continued administration of desensitizing antigens often markedly reduces symptoms.

Epistaxis (Nosebleed)

Bleeding from the nose may be due to nasal trauma, irritation of the mucosa by dust or dry air, upper respiratory infection or allergic rhinitis, or coagulation defect.

Treatment of acute nosebleed is by application of direct pressure and, if necessary, topical vasoconstrictor. If bleeding persists or recurs, cautery with silver nitrate or anterior nasal packing may be necessary.

Rarely, bleeding comes from the posterior nares (usually in middle-aged or elderly patients with hypertension or arteriosclerosis) and requires a posterior nasal pack.

Nose: The middle and inferior turbinates are pale and boggy, with watery secretions.

Prevention of further nosebleeds may include use of lubricating applications to the mucosa, humidification of air, and avoidance of dusts and other irritants.

Sinusitis

Infection of one or more paranasal sinuses (see ■ Figure 8-10).

Cause: Usually occurs as a complication of viral or allergic rhinitis. Swelling of the nasal mucosa leads to blockage of the sinus openings, with accumulation of purulent secretion within the sinuses affected. Attacks may occur repeatedly in some persons, and sinusitis may become chronic.

Nose: Denies frequent colds, epistaxis, or nasal fracture. No history of obstruction or discharge.

History: Pressure or pain in one or more sinus cavities, often aggravated by bending forward. Pain may be manifested as a severe headache or may radiate into the teeth. Purulent nasal or postnasal discharge may be present. Occasionally fever, chills, and malaise.

Physical Examination: Edema and erythema of nasal mucosa. Purulent discharge in nasal passages or oropharynx (postnasal drip).

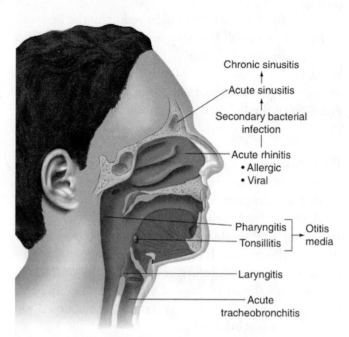

FIGURE 8-10. Chronic sinusitis to laryngitis and tracheobronchitis

Diagnostic Tests: In chronic sinusitis, x-ray or other diagnostic imaging shows thickening of sinus membranes and often presence of fluid within cavities.

Treatment: Decongestant, analgesic. A short course of nasal decongestant spray may help to open and drain sinuses. Control of allergic component if present. When symptoms (severe, persistent pain) or clinical picture (fever, bloody discharge) suggests bacterial infection, an oral antibiotic (amoxicillin, trimethoprim-sulfamethoxazole) is prescribed. Chronic sinusitis may respond to prolonged antibiotic therapy (ciprofloxacin). Surgical procedures can be used to correct anatomic lesions predisposing to sinusitis, or to improve drainage of a chronically infected sinus.

Acute Pharyngitis (Sore Throat)

Acute inflammation of the throat due to infection.

Cause: Usually viruses, including the Epstein-Barr virus, which causes infectious mononucleosis. Occasionally bacteria such as *Streptococcus pneumoniae* and Group A beta-hemolytic *Streptococcus pyogenes* ("strep throat"), or fungi such as *Candida*. Infection with cold viruses may predispose to bacterial infection. Sore throat is more prevalent in cold weather.

History: Pain, irritation, or a sense of fullness or swelling in the throat, accentuated by swallowing and often radiating to the ears. Fever, painful glandular swelling in the neck.

Physical Examination: May be essentially normal. Fever is often present. Edema and erythema of the

ASSESSMENT
Recurrent streptococcal pharyngitis.

oropharynx, often involving the tonsils, soft palate, and uvula, occur in most bacterial and many viral throat infections. Severe infections, including streptococcal pharyngitis (**strep throat**) and infectious mononucleosis, cause formation of white or gray exudate (consisting of dead tissue, white blood cells, and bacteria) on pharyngeal walls and especially on the tonsils.

A firmly adherent exudate is characteristic of *Candida* infection (**thrush**). The presence of vesicles or ulcers suggests viral infection (herpes simplex virus, **coxsackievirus**). Severe pain and swelling may cause a hollow or "hot potato" voice, and may make swallowing virtually impossible, so that the patient drools to avoid swallowing saliva, and becomes dehydrated from lack of fluid intake. Extreme swelling may compromise the airway. Cervical lymph glands may be swollen and tender. Some strains of beta-hemolytic streptococci cause a widespread red rash (**scarlet fever, scarlatina**).

Diagnostic Tests: Throat culture or **strep screen** may identify the causative organism. Blood studies (white blood cell count and differential, ASO titer, heterophile antibodies) help to diagnose strep throat and infectious mononucleosis. Smears or scrapings of exudate can confirm presence of *Candida*.

Course: Viral sore throat runs its course within a week or two. Occasionally it becomes complicated by streptococcal infection, which may lead to acute rheumatic fever. It may also progress to otitis media, acute or chronic tonsillitis, or lower respiratory infection. **Peritonsillar abscess** (quinsy) is a severe bacterial infection developing above and behind one tonsil and causing extreme pain and swelling, with deviation of the uvula away from the affected side.

Treatment: Acute **viral pharyngitis** requires no treatment except analgesics, gargles, soothing lozenges, and perhaps a soft diet. If **streptococcal infection** is diagnosed, a 10-day course of an antibiotic known to be able to eradicate streptococci (such as penicillin V, erythromycin, or cephalexin) is mandatory. Candidal oropharyngitis (**thrush**) is treated with topical antifungal medicine. The treatment of **peritonsillar abscess** is surgical drainage.

Pause for Reflection

1. Distinguish between otitis externa and otitis media.
2. Describe complications that may accompany chronic otitis media.
3. What surgical procedure is performed in otitis media if tympanic membrane rupture is threatened? In chronic perforation of the tympanic membrane?
4. How is vertigo treated?
5. Differentiate the 3 types of hearing loss.
6. What is the treatment regimen for coryza or the common cold and what types of treatment will not help?
7. What diagnostic tests may be used to help diagnose allergic rhinitis?
8. What is epistaxis?
9. How does sinusitis differ from allergic rhinitis?
10. What are the causes of pharyngitis?
11. What is thrush?
12. Compare the treatment for viral pharyngitis and streptococcal infection.

Diagnostic and Surgical Procedures

AOE (automated otoacoustic emission) testing A hearing test done usually on newborns. A small earpiece is placed into a baby's outer ear which sends out gentle clicking sounds. If a baby has a functioning middle and inner ear, an echo response will be generated that can be measured by a computer.

ABR (auditory brainstem response) A hearing test done on newborns or infants. It measures activity in the brainstem in response to sounds. Three small sensors are placed on the baby's head and neck and headphones on the ears. Clicking sounds are played and the brain's response is recorded by a computer. Also, BAER (brainstem auditory-evoked response).

audiography A precise measurement of the faintest loudness (in decibels) that the patient can hear, each ear tested separately at each of several pitches (for example, 250, 500, 1000, 2000, 3000, 4000, 6000, and 8000 Hz); this can be performed by a trained technician with carefully calibrated testing equip-

HAVE YOU HAD YOUR TONSILS OUT?

In the 1950s and early 1960s, it was not unusual to have a child's tonsils removed after a few bouts of pharyngitis, tonsillitis, or sore throat. Tonsillectomy was performed routinely, even in the doctor's office, long before outpatient surgery became the norm. A common question one child asked another was, "Have you had your tonsils out yet?" The promise of "all the ice cream you can eat" after surgery was very enticing—after all, what was a little postoperative pain when you could eat ice cream to your heart's delight?

Some felt that tonsils were actually the cause of sore throats because they were a breeding ground for viruses and bacteria. The expectation was that your tonsillectomy was just a sore throat or two away.

In the late 1960s the practice of routine tonsillectomy came to an end when it was proposed, then widely accepted, that tonsils should not be removed unless absolutely necessary because they are composed of lymphoid tissue, and lymphoid tissue assists with immune function.

Today tonsils are removed only in severe cases of recurrent strep infection or obstruction. Even very large "kissing tonsils" are considered better in than out. Tonsils shrink with age, and most adults "outgrow" frequent tonsillar infections. (Sore throats caused by allergies and sinus drainage are common and not related to strep or other bacteria.)

ment, or by automated machinery activated by the patient.

BiliBlanket A portable phototherapy device for the treatment of neonatal jaundice (hyperbilirubinemia) It uses fiberoptics and represents advanced technology in phototherapy treatment given in the hospital or at home. See also *phototherapy*.

ethmoidectomy A surgical procedure to remove the partitions between the ethmoid sinuses in order to create larger sinus cavities.

frenuloplasty Surgical repositioning of an abnormally attached lingual frenum, the restraining structure under the tongue. Also called *frenoplasty*. Used to correct *tongue tie*.

I&D (incision and drainage) A procedure used to open and drain an abscess that has not been responsive to conservative measures.

insertion of collar button (ventilation) tubes Surgical placement of tiny tubes in the eardrum to prevent chronic ear infections. See *myringotomy tubes*.

myringotomy A surgical procedure in which a tiny incision is created in the eardrum to relieve pressure caused by excessive build-up of fluid, or to drain pus from the middle ear.

myringotomy tubes (often called **ear tubes**) Small tubes that are surgically placed into a child's eardrum by an ear, nose, and throat surgeon. The tubes may be made of plastic, metal, or Teflon and are placed to help drain the fluid out of the middle ear in order to reduce the risk of ear infections.

otoscopy Inspection of the external auditory meatus and tympanic membrane with an otoscope; mobility of the tympanic membrane can be assessed when the patient swallows or performs the Valsalva maneuver (or when, in children, the examiner blows a puff of air into the ear).

phototherapy Light treatment is the process of using light to eliminate bilirubin in the blood of newborns. These light waves are absorbed by the baby's skin and blood and change bilirubin into products which can pass through their system. See also *Biliblanket*.

pneumotympanometry Assessment of the mobility of the tympanic membrane by applying pressure to its outer surface with a device fitting tightly in the external meatus.

polypectomy, nasal A surgical procedure to remove polyps that are located in the nasal passages.

posterior rhinoscopy Inspection of posterior nares with angled mirror placed in the oropharynx.

pulse oximetry A noninvasive method of assessing arterial oxygen saturation of hemoglobin by passing a beam of red and infrared light through a pulsating capillary bed. Slang: *pulse ox*.

rhinoplasty Surgical correction of nasal deformities for functional or cosmetic purposes ("nose job").

Rinne test The sound of a vibrating tuning fork positioned so that the tines are near the pinna (**air con-**

duction) should be heard by the patient even after the sound sensed when the shank of the tuning fork is placed on the mastoid process behind the ear (**bone conduction**) can no longer be heard. When bone conduction is heard longer than air conduction in an ear with reduced hearing, the hearing loss is due to obstruction of the meatus or disease of the middle ear.

septoplasty A corrective surgical procedure to straighten the nasal septum, the partition between the two nasal cavities. Ideally, the septum should run down the center of the nose. When it deviates into one of the cavities, it narrows that cavity and impedes airflow. Often the inferior turbinate on the opposite side enlarges, which is termed *compensatory hypertrophy*. Deviations of the septum can lead to nasal obstruction.

septorhinoplasty A procedure similar to rhinoplasty, but it not only improves the appearance of the nose but removes any internal obstructions that may be blocking nasal breathing.

spirometry Measurement of the breathing capacity of the lungs, as in pulmonary function testing.

submucous resection of inferior turbinates A surgical procedure in which the bone expanding the turbinates on the inside is shaved down, allowing for significant long-term reduction in the size of the turbinates. This procedure is often performed in conjunction with septoplasty when there is a deviated septum and nasal obstruction is significant.

tonsillectomy and adenoidectomy (T&A) Surgical removal of the palatine tonsils and adenoids in the throat due to recurrent episodes of infection and chronic hypertrophy. Also called *adenotonsillectomy*.

tympanotomy Incision of the tympanic membrane. See *myringotomy*.

tympanic membrane Same as *eardrum*.

tympanostomy Incision of the tympanic membrane with insertion of a tube for drainage.

Weber test A vibrating tuning fork placed against a bony surface of the head at the midline sends vibrations through the bones of the skull. These should be heard equally in the two ears. If there is hearing loss due to blockage of the external auditory meatus or to injury or disease of the middle ear, the tone of the fork will be heard louder in the affected ear. In hearing loss due to damage to the inner ear or acoustic nerve, however, the tone will be heard louder in the more normal ear.

x-ray To identify foreign bodies, masses, or abnormalities of the airway due to injury or disease.

Laboratory Procedures

arterial blood gases (ABGs) Unlike most blood tests where blood is drawn from a vein, this test requires that blood be drawn from an artery. It measures the pH and the levels of oxygen (O_2) and carbon dioxide (CO_2) in the blood from an artery. It is a measure of lung function (how well your lungs move oxygen into and carbon dioxide out of the blood). Values include partial pressure of oxygen (PaO_2), partial pressure of carbon dioxide ($PaCO_2$), pH (normal values are between 7.35 and 7.45), bicarbonate (HCO_3), oxygen (O_2) content and saturation.

ASO titer A test to detect and measure antistreptolysin O in serum. This antibody is present during and shortly after streptococcal infections. The value is measured in Todd units.

capillary blood gas Capillary blood gas (CBG) samples may be used in place of samples from arterial punctures or indwelling arterial catheters to estimate acid-base balance (pH) and adequacy of ventilation of newborns and infants. A puncture or small incision is made with a lancet or similar device at a highly vascular area (heel, finger, toe). As the blood flows freely from the puncture site, the sample is collected in a heparinized glass capillary tube.

nasal smear Examination of a stained smear of scrapings from the nasal mucosa for evidence of infection (neutrophilic leukocytes) or allergy (eosinophilic leukocytes).

PPD (purified protein derivative) A tuberculin skin test for tuberculosis. The abbreviation does not need to be expanded in medical reports.

rapid strep test (RST) The most rapid in-office test done by a clinician to test for streptococcal pharyngitis (strep throat), a group A streptococcal infection of the pharynx.

RAST (radioallergosorbent) test A blood test that measures specific serum IgE antibodies to allergens. Used as an alternative to skin tests to determine sensitivity to suspected allergens. Many allergens can be tested with a single blood specimen.

serology Blood tests used to measure serum antibody titers in infectious disease and to detect antigens. Example: Serology was negative for syphilis, HBsAg, Chlamydia, gonorrhea, and HIV. Also, *serologic test*.

serum-specific IgE antibodies See *RAST*.

strep screen Faster than a culture, but detecting only beta-hemolytic streptococci. "Strep" is an acceptable brief form for streptococcus.

throat culture To identify bacterial pathogens.

Pharmacology

Decongestants

Decongestants act as vasoconstrictors to reduce blood flow to edematous tissues in the nose, sinuses, and pharynx. They produce vasoconstriction by stimulating alpha receptors in the smooth muscle around the blood vessels. Decongestants decrease the swelling of mucous membranes, alleviate nasal stuffiness, allow secretions to drain, and help to unclog the eustachian tubes. Decongestants are commonly prescribed for colds and allergies. They can be administered topically as nose drops or nasal sprays, or can be taken orally. Decongestants are often combined with antihistamines in cold remedies.

> desoxyephedrine (Vicks Inhaler)
> oxymetazoline (Afrin, Dristan, Duration, Sinex)
> phenylephrine (Neo-Synephrine, Nostril)
> pseudoephedrine (Drixoral, Sudafed)
> tetrahydrozoline
> xylometazoline (Otrivin)

Antihistamines

Antihistamines exert their therapeutic effect by blocking **histamine H_1 receptors** in the nose and throat. Histamine is released by the antibody-antigen complex that occurs during allergic reactions. Histamine causes vasodilation, which causes blood vessels and tissues to become engorged, swollen, and red. Histamine also irritates these tissues directly, causing pain and itching. Antihistamines block the action of histamine at the H_1 receptors. Antihistamines dry up secretions, shrink edematous mucous membranes, and decrease itching and redness. A significant side effect of early antihistamines was drowsiness; however, newer antihistamines have a different chemical structure that does not produce drowsiness.

> azatadine (Optimine)
> brompheniramine (Dimetane)
> cetirizine (Zyrtec)
> chlorpheniramine (Chlor-Trimeton)
> clemastine (Tavist)
> dexchlorpheniramine (Polaramine)
> diphenhydramine (Benadryl)
> fexofenadine (Allegra)
> loratadine (Claritin)
> phenindamine (Nolahist)
> promethazine (Phenergan)

Mast Cell Inhibitors

Mast cell inhibitors act to stabilize the membrane of mast cells and prevent them from releasing histamine. This prevents edema of the nasal passages in patients with allergic rhinitis. Example is cromolyn (Nasalcrom).

Corticosteroids

Corticosteroids act by inhibiting the body's inflammatory response by decreasing vasodilation and edema of the mucous membranes. Corticosteroids have no antihistamine effect. Corticosteroids have no effect on the common cold. They are administered intranasally to treat allergic and nonallergic rhinitis. Corticosteroids for the nose include:

> beclomethasone (Beconase, Vancenase)
> budesonide (Rhinocort, Rhinocort Aqua)
> flunisolide (Nasalide)
> fluticasone (Flonase)
> mometasone (Nasonex)
> triamcinolone (Nasacort, Tri-Nasal)

Corticosteroids can be applied topically as a paste to treat mouth ulcers and inflammation. Example is triamcinolone (Kenalog in Orabase).

Antibiotics

Antibiotics are not effective in treating the common cold which is caused by a virus; however, they are prescribed for infections caused by bacteria, particularly streptococci. Antibiotic solutions may be prescribed for topical application in the ears to treat external otitis media and other infections.

> chloramphenicol (Chloromycetin Otic)

Corticosteroids and antibiotics are often combined in a single solution for topical application in the ear.

Antitussive Drugs

Antitussive drugs decrease coughing by suppressing the cough center in the brain or anesthetizing the stretch receptors in the respiratory tract. Their main purpose is to stop nonproductive dry coughs. They are not prescribed for a productive cough that generates sputum because it is important for the patient to cough up this sputum. Some antitussives are narcotics, such as codeine and hydrocodone; these are prescription schedule drugs. Over-the-counter antitussives contain the non-narcotic dextromethorphan or diphenhydramine.

> benzonatate (Tessalon Perles)
> codeine
> dextromethorphan (Benylin DM, Pertussin ES, Robitussin, Sucrets, Vicks Formula 44D)
> diphenhydramine (Benylin Cough)
> hydrocodone (Hycodan)

Expectorants

Expectorants reduce the viscosity or thickness of sputum so that patients can more easily cough it up.

> guaifenesin (Humibid L.A., Robitussin)
> terpin hydrate

Combination ENT Drugs

A number of trade name drugs contain various combinations of decongestants, antihistamines, antitussives, expectorants, and the pain relievers acetaminophen or ibuprofen.

COMMON DRUGS WITH CHALLENGING SPELLINGS OR UNUSUAL CAPITALIZATION

Contac (*not* Contact)
Dimetane
Dimetapp
NasalCrom
Neo-Synephrine
NyQuil
PediaCare
Tessalon Perles (*not* pearls)
Singulair
Skelaxin
Sudafed
Symbicort
pseudoephedrine (the *p* is silent)
Zithromax Z-Pak
Zyrtec

Antifungal and Antiyeast Drugs

Yeasts, which are closely related to fungi, grow easily in the warm, dark environment of the mouth, particularly in immunocompromised patients. *Candida albicans* yeast infections are alternatively known as oral candidiasis, moniliasis, or thrush. Systemic treatment of Candida with oral fluconazole (Diflucan) has largely replaced the use of topical agents such as clotrimazole and nystatin. Antifungal drugs are applied topically as a solution (the patient is told to "swish and swallow") or supplied as a troche (to suck on as a lozenge). Nizoral is also available as an oral tablet that acts systemically.

Transcription Tips

1. Confusing Terms: Some of these terms sound alike; others are potential traps when researching. Memorize the terms and their meanings so that you can select the appropriate term for a correct transcript.

   abscess—a collection of pus

   aphthous—pertaining to an ulcer

   adhesion—an abnormal fibrous band or structure between organs or tissues

   adhesive—a substance used to make things stick together

   aural—pertaining to the ear or hearing

   oral—pertaining to the mouth or speaking

   buccal—pertaining to the cheek

   buckle—a shape distorted by twisting or folding; the fastener on a belt

   caudal—pertaining to the tail, situated near or directed toward the tail of something

   coddle—indulge; cook in nearly boiling water

   cuttle—short for cuttlefish

   Cottle—eponym for a surgical elevator

   cerumen—earwax

   serum—the clear portion of blood or other bodily fluid

   distention—enlargement (Note: The spelling *dis-ten-sion* is not preferred)

   dissention—disagreement

   effusion—an exudate or discharge

   infusion—injection of a fluid or medicine

   facial—pertaining to the face (facial recess)

   fascial—pertaining to fascia, the tissue covering muscles and other organs (fascial graft)

   faucial—pertaining to the passage from the mouth to the pharynx (faucial tonsils)

   fornix—arch-shaped roof of an anatomical space

   pharynx—the throat (often mispronounced as "fair-nix" which accounts for the soundalike above)

   gait—the manner in which one walks

   gate—an entrance or opening in a fence or wall

   hear—to listen

   here—at this point or place

   hoarse—low, rough, harsh-sounding voice

   horse—a quadruped equine animal that one rides

   lingual—pertaining to the tongue

   lingula—a tongue-like structure

   malleus—a bone of the middle ear

   malleolus—a bone in the ankle

   naris ("na-ris", short *i*)—nostril, singular

   nares ("na-reez")—nostrils, plural (Note: *Naris* should be transcribed as the singular form.)

   palate—the roof of the mouth

   palette—a board artists use to mix their paints, a range of colors

   pallet—a platform for storing or moving heavy objects; a temporary bed

   scutum—a bony plate that divides the tympanic cavity and mastoid air cells

   sputum—expectoration

   serous—pertaining to or resembling serum, as in serous otitis media

   serious—grave or of great consequence

   vallate—having a wall or rim; cup-shaped

   valet—a person who parks the car

2. Slang Terms. Expand these slang brief forms when encountered in dictation.

bicarbs	bicarbonates
sats (oxygen)	saturations
satting	no simple edit for this slang

3. Spelling. Memorize the spelling of these difficult-to-spell terms. Note silent letters, doubled letters, and unexpected pronunciations.

   abutting

   ankyloglossia

   anulus (one n)

   asymmetric

   bicortical (*not* by cortical)

   bipolar (*not* by polar)

Transcription Tips

3. Spelling (*continued*)

buccal
choana (pl., choanae)
chorda tympani (nerve)
cochleariform (process)
cricopharyngeus
eustachian
fontanel phlegm
piriform sinus
rhinitis
rhinoconjunctivitis
sagittal (1 *g*, 2 *t*'s)
syndactyly
tensor tympani
tarry (resembling black tar)
trismus
uncinate

4. Tricky Abbreviations. Some abbreviations are acronyms and pronounced as a word; others have soundalike letters; *B, D, P,* and *V* can all sound alike, as can *T* and *D, F* and *S, N* & *and.* Although some abbreviations do not need to be expanded, you do need to know what they mean in order to choose the correct expansion.

ABR (auditory brainstem response)
CNS (central nervous system), not to be
    confused with C&S (culture and sensitivity)
CRP (C-reactive protein)
EBL (estimated blood loss)
ET (endotracheal)
GBS (group B streptococcus)
GERD (gastroesophageal reflux disease)
    ("gurd")
hCG (human chorionic gonadotropin)
    (the *h* can sound like the number *8*)
I&D (incision and drainage)
IMF (intermaxillary fixation)
MDI (metered dose inhaler)
NICU (neonatal intensive care unit)
    (pronounced "nick-yoo" or spelled letter-
    by-letter, NICU can be difficult to decipher)

PE (pressure equalization or polyethylene) (no
    expansion required)
PDS (trademarked suture, no expansion)
PMI (point of maximum impulse)
PPD (purified protein derivative) (tuberculosis
    test, no expansion required)
PSA (prostate specific antigen) (no expansion
    required)
T&A (tonsillectomy and adenoidectomy)
UVC (umbilical vein catheter)

AD, AS, AU (right ear, left ear, and each ear) are traditional abbreviations that are on the list of error-prone abbreviations. Although physicians continue to dictate these abbreviations, The Joint Commission directs that they be expanded in medical transcripts to avoid confusion with similar abbreviations. Thus, even if dictators use these abbreviations, medical transcriptionists should translate them and place the abbreviation in parentheses following the translation. Note that *AU* is often incorrectly translated as both ears.

5. Dictation Challenges

When the term *mental* is used in ENT dictation, it refers to the *mentum*, or chin—not to thought processes.

The term *alveolar* in ENT dictation refers to a bony ridge in the oral cavity—not to the alveoli of the lungs.

Stapes ("stay-peez") is sometimes mispronounced as if it is one syllable.

Don't confuse the soundalike prefixes *oro-* (mouth) and *auri-* (ear).

Both the Latin *auri-* (aural) and the Greek *oto-* (otic) mean ear.

Both the Greek *tympano-* and Latin *myringo-* refer to the eardrum or tympanic membrane.

Spotlight On

Who Nose?

by Susan M. Turley

If Bo knows football and baseball, then it might be correct to say that I now know noses. Recently I had the chance to see surgery from the other side—the patient's side.

After many years of extreme nasal stuffiness, I gathered my courage and decided to have a surgical correction. The plastic surgeon confirmed that my turbinates were grossly hypertrophied and were the cause of my inability to breathe. After we agreed that a turbinectomy would be beneficial, he then asked delicately if I had considered having any plastic surgery at the same time. "Hey," I said, "I have a list!"

We started with number one on the list: a nose job. It was painful hearing him brutally describe the unacceptable aspects of my nose—bulbous tip, uneven width, drooping tip, drooping underside, excessive length—even though I had seen all these problems myself in the mirror.

Then there were finances to consider. My insurance would pay for the functional nasal surgery (turbinectomy and cartilage graft) but not for any cosmetic surgery. I would be responsible for the surgeon's fee, hospital's fee, and anesthesiologist's fee that pertained to the cosmetic part of the surgery.

On the morning of surgery, I found myself first paying the hospital's bill in full with my VISA card. The anesthesiologist came in and started an IV in my right hand. I had no doubts, though, that he would return, and he did. With my right hand, I then laboriously wrote out a check to him for $700. Question: Did the first patient to undergo a rhinoplasty coin the phrase "paying through the nose"?

After the anesthesiologist left, the plastic surgeon arrived to mark my nose and cheeks with a skin marking pen. I gave my checkbook (thank goodness, no one else needed to be paid) and glasses to the nurse and was wheeled into the operating room.

The temperature in surgery was no warmer than 50 degrees, it seemed. Even the nurses were complaining of the cold. They gave me lots of warm blankets, though, and I was comfortable. Someone said, "How're you doing?" "Who, me?" I answered. Without my glasses I couldn't tell if the staff was talking to me or just chitchatting among themselves. "Me? I feel fine." That was all she wrote, as they say. I never felt drowsy; I never even knew when I fell asleep. That's what I call a smooth induction.

The next thing I knew I was in the recovery room. Disembodied voices kept calling my name and saying the surgery went fine. A nurse asked me how much pain I was having, and I said my nose felt like when I slammed my hand in the car door. She promptly provided a shot of Demerol and Compazine. (I had dry heaves for what seemed like hours.) I was very chilly, and the nurses wrapped warm blankets around me, even putting them on my head so that I could pretend I was hibernating in a warm cave.

When my husband and son were allowed into the recovery room to see me, they maintained a respectful distance, not quite sure how to react to my extensively bruised face. From my eyebrows down to my cheekbones, the skin was pitch black, as if some prankster had poured indelible black ink all over my face. Later at home, my husband regained his sense of humor and cheerfully told well-wishers on the phone that I looked as if I had gone several rounds with Mike Tyson. Actually I thought I looked *worse* than that. But within five days, the bruising was barely noticeable.

The week following surgery had its own set of annoying problems. My glasses did not sit right over the nasal splint and, with my eyelids still swollen, it was nearly impossible to enjoy the new mystery I had purchased especially for the occasion. My nose was filled with packing so that I mouthbreathed, snored, and coughed without getting much sleep for nearly a week. One small blessing was that some nasal packing now used is absorbable and does not need to be painfully pulled out of the nose.

As the swelling went down and the nasal splint came off, I began breathing more fully than I had in years, and I really liked my new nose. Would I do it again? Sure. By the way, where is that list?!

Exercises

Medical Vocabulary Review

Instructions: Choose the best answer.

____ 1. Ossicles is a collective term used to refer to
_____
  A. septum and turbinates.
  B. tonsils and adenoids.
  C. small bones in the skull.
  D. malleus, incus, and stapes.

____ 2. Rhythmic, involuntary, jerky movements of
both eyes, usually from side to side, is ____
  A. laryngospasm.
  B. nystagmus.
  C. Battle's sign.
  D. acanthosis nigricans.

____ 3. Cerumen plugging the external ear canal
may be referred to as _____
  A. mucopus.
  B. an impaction.
  C. serous effusion.
  D. serous otitis media.

____ 4. The procedure used to correct ankyloglossia
is _____
  A. a frenuloplasty.
  B. a rhinoplasty.
  C. a septoplasty.
  D. a rhinoscopy.

____ 5. A baby born to a mother with ABO or Rh
incompatibility may exhibit _____
  A. serous effusion.
  B. grunting and flaring.
  C. jaundice and anemia.
  D. pseudoacanthosis nigricans.

____ 6. The tube that connects the middle ear to
the pharynx is the _____ tube.
  A. eustachian
  B. auricular
  C. vestibular
  D. refractory

____ 7. The medical term for tongue tie is ____
  A. atelectasis.
  B. brawny edema.
  C. ankyloglossia.
  D. glottic spasm.

____ 8. The normal fluid medium contained in the
middle ear is called _____
  A. otitis media.
  B. endolymph.
  C. mucopus.
  D. serous effusion.

____ 9. An invasive growth of the tympanic
membrane caused by prolonged partial
vacuum in the middle ear is _____
  A. atelectasis.
  B. cholesteatoma.
  C. syndactyly.
  D. an aneurysm.

____ 10. Which of the following is NOT a hearing
test performed on an infant or child?
  A. AOE test.
  B. ABR test.
  C. Audiography.
  D. Apgar score.

____ 11. Neonatal jaundice or hyperbilirubinemia
may be treated with _____
  A. incision and drainage.
  B. myringotomy tubes.
  C. phototherapy.
  D. tympanostomy.

___ 12. Serous otitis media may be treated with all
of the following EXCEPT _____
   A. otoscopy.
   B. tympanotomy.
   C. tympanostomy.
   D. myringotomy.

___ 13. Which procedure is performed to correct
tethering of the tongue?
   A. Septoplasty.
   B. Frenuloplasty.
   C. Rhinoplasty.
   D. Ethmoidectomy.

___ 14. Which procedure is performed to assess air
conduction or bone conduction in a patient
with hearing loss?
   A. Rinne test.
   B. Weber test.
   C. AOE test.
   D. ABR test.

___ 15. The part of the throat that contains the
vocal cords is the _____
   A. trachea.
   B. pharynx.
   C. larynx.
   D. laryngopharynx.

___ 16. Complete this sentence: Examination of the
right ear revealed a normal eardrum with no
fluid behind it and a _____ ventilation tube.
   A. retracted
   B. patent
   C. refractory
   D. purulent

___ 17. Complete this sentence: Mucous membranes
of the nose were erythematous and inflamed;
the patient has chronic _____
   A. diastasis.
   B. malaise.
   C. otitis media.
   D. rhinitis.

___ 18. Complete this sentence: The patient is
autistic and it was felt that a _____ test
rather than skin testing would be the best
way to determine what he is allergic to.
   A. RAST
   B. Rinne
   C. Weber
   D. ABR

___ 19. Complete this sentence: The patient's
refractory _____ was treated by cauterizing
the nasal vessels with silver nitrate.
   A. rhinitis
   B. epistaxis
   C. sinusitis
   D. coryza

___ 20. Complete this sentence: Examination
revealed a viscous fluid behind a tympanic
membrane that was thin, atrophic, retracted,
and adherent; a diagnosis of _____ was
made.
   A. Ménière disease
   B. chronic otitis externa
   C. adhesive serous otitis media
   D. tympanic membrane atelectasis

Diagnostic and Surgical Procedures

Instructions: Match the following diagnostic and surgical procedures to their descriptions or definitions. Some answers may be used more than once.

____ 1. ABR (auditory brainstem response)

____ 2. adenotonsillectomy

____ 3. AOE (automated otoacoustic emission) testing

____ 4. audiography

____ 5. ethmoidectomy

____ 6. I&D (incision and drainage)

____ 7. myringotomy and tubes

____ 8. nasal polypectomy

____ 9. otoscopy

____ 10. pneumotympanometry

____ 11. posterior rhinoscopy

____ 12. pulse oximetry

____ 13. rhinoplasty

____ 14. Rinne test

____ 15. septoplasty

____ 16. spirometry

____ 17. T&A (tonsillectomy and adenoidectomy)

____ 18. tympanostomy

____ 19. tympanotomy

____ 20. Weber test

A. Noninvasive method of assessing arterial oxygen saturation of hemoglobin by passing a beam of red and infrared light through a pulsating capillary bed

B. A hearing test done on newborns that generates an echo response that can be measured by a computer

C. A hearing test to evaluate whether hearing loss is due to injury or disease of the middle ear or acoustic nerve

D. A surgical procedure that improves the appearance of the nose and removes any internal obstructions to breathing

E. A surgical procedure to remove massive overgrowths of chronically inflamed mucosa in the nasal passages

F. Assessment of the mobility of the tympanic membrane

G. Corrective surgical procedure to straighten the partition between the two nasal cavities

H. Hearing test done on newborns or infants that measures activity in the brainstem in response to sounds

I. Hearing test of air conduction and bone conduction

J. Incision of the eardrum with insertion of a tube for drainage

K. Incision of the eardrum

L. Inspection of posterior nares with angled mirror placed in the oropharynx

M. Inspection of the external auditory meatus and tympanic membrane with a lighted instrument equipped with a magnifying lens

N. Measurement of the faintest loudness (in decibels) that the patient can hear

O. Procedure used to open and drain an abscess

P. Removal of the palatine tonsils and adenoids

Q. Removal of the partitions between the sinuses to create larger sinus cavities

R. Shaving down of the bone of the inferior turbinates

S. Surgical correction of nasal deformities for functional or cosmetic purposes

T. Measurement of the breathing capacity of the lungs

Laboratory Procedures

Instructions: Match the following laboratory procedures to their descriptions or definitions. Some answers may be used more than once.

___ 1. arterial blood gases

___ 2. ASO titer

___ 3. capillary blood gases

___ 4. PPD

___ 5. rapid strep test

___ 6. RAST

___ 7. serology

___ 8. serum-specific IgE antibodies

___ 9. strep screen

A. A measure of how well the lungs move oxygen into and carbon dioxide out of the blood

B. A test specifically for beta-hemolytic streptococci

C. An immunoglobulin created in the blood in response to allergens

D. Blood test that measures specific serum IgE antibodies to allergens

E. Blood tests used to measure serum antibody titers in infectious disease and to detect antigens

F. Method to estimate pH and adequacy of ventilation of newborns and infants

G. Test to detect and measure an antibody that is present during and shortly after streptococcal infections

H. Tuberculin skin test for tuberculosis

I. Used to test for group A streptococcal infection of the pharynx

Pharmacology

Instructions: Choose the best answer.

___ 1. Which of the following generic drugs is a decongestant?
A. guaifenesin.
B. beclomethasone.
C. diphenhydramine.
D. pseudoephedrine.

___ 2. Which of the following drugs does not belong in the group with the others?
A. Mycostatin, Nilstat (nystatin).
B. Neo-Synephrine, Nostril (phenylephrine).
C. Benylin DM, Pertussin ES (dextromethorphan).
D. Humibid L.A., Robitussin (guaifenesin).

___ 3. Which of the following generic drugs suppresses coughing?
A. triamcinolone.
B. clotrimazole.
C. dextromethorphan.
D. terpin hydrate.

___ 4. If a patient had thick sputum and a productive cough, you might expect the physician to prescribe which one of the following drugs?
A. Humibid L.A., Robitussin (guaifenesin).
B. Benylin Cough (diphenhydramine).
C. Rhinocort, Rhinocort Aqua (budesonide).
D. Chloromycetin Otic (chloramphenicol).

___ 5. External otitis media and other ear infections may be treated with topical applications of _____
A. decongestants.
B. antitussives and expectorants.
C. antibiotics and corticosteroids.
D. antihistamines and mast cell inhibitors.

Dissecting Medical Terms

Instructions: As you learned in your medical language course, words are formed from prefixes, combining forms (root word plus combining vowel), and suffixes. Combining vowels (usually **o** but not always) are used to connect two root words or a root and a suffix. By analyzing these word parts, you can often determine the definition of a term without even looking it up (if you know the definition of the parts, of course!).

Being able to divide and analyze the words you hear into their component parts will also improve your auditory deciphering ability and spelling and help you research those words that you cannot easily spell or define.

For the following terms, draw a slash (/) between the components and then write a short definition based on the meaning of the parts. Remember that to define a word based on its parts, you start at the end, usually with the suffix. If there's a prefix, that is defined next, and finally the combining form is defined.

Example: tonsillitis

Divide and Analyze:
tonsillitis = tonsil/itis = inflammation + tonsils
Define: inflammation of the tonsils

1. Term   adenotonsillar hypertrophy
   Divide   _____
              _____
   Define   _____

2. Term   rhinoconjunctivitis
   Divide   _____
              _____
   Define   _____

3. Term   angioedema
   Divide   _____
              _____
   Define   _____

4. Term   ankyloglossia
   Divide   _____
              _____
   Define   _____

5. Term   antrostomy
   Divide   _____
              _____
   Define   _____

6. Term   avascular
   Divide   _____
              _____
   Define   _____

7. Term   cholesteatoma
   Divide   _____
              _____
   Define   _____

8. Term   cochleariform
   Divide   _____
              _____
   Define   _____

9. Term   edematous
   Divide   _____
              _____
   Define   _____

10. Term   endotracheal
    Divide   _____
              _____
    Define   _____

11. Term   erythematous
    Divide   _____
              _____
    Define   _____

12. Term   frenuloplasty
    Divide   _____
              _____
    Define   _____

13. Term   gingivobuccal
    Divide   _____
              _____
    Define   _____

14. Term   intermaxillary
    Divide   _____
              _____
    Define   _____

15. Term   lymphadenopathy
    Divide   _____
              _____
    Define   _____

16. Term   malocclusion
    Divide   _____

    Define   _____
             _____
17. Term   mucoperiosteal
    Divide   _____

    Define   _____
18. Term   myringotomy

    Divide   _____

    Define   _____
19. Term   osteotomy
    Divide   _____

    Define   _____
20. Term   postauricular
    Divide   _____
             _____
    Define   _____
21. Term   septorhinoplasty
    Divide   _____

    Define   _____
22. Term   supraglottic
    Divide   _____

    Define   _____
23. Term   transconjunctivally
    Divide   _____

    Define   _____
24. Term   tympanoplasty
    Divide   _____

    Define   _____
25. Term   zygomaticomaxillary
    Divide   _____

    Define   _____

Spelling Exercise

Instructions: Review the adjective suffixes in your medical language textbook. Test your knowledge of adjectives by writing the adjectival form of the following words. Consult a medical dictionary to verify your spelling.

Noun	Adjective
1. cartilage	_____
2. cerumen	_____
3. cochlea	_____
4. columella	_____
5. cortex	_____
6. ellipse	_____
7. epilepsy	_____
8. erythema	_____
9. exudate	_____
10. mandible	_____
11. mastication	_____
12. maxilla	_____
13. mucus	_____
14. necrosis	_____
15. obstruction	_____
16. ossicle	_____
17. parasymphysis	_____
18. perichondrium	_____
19. pharynx	_____
20. vestibule	_____

Forming Plurals

Instructions: Review the rules for forming plurals. Test your knowledge of plurals by writing the plural form of the following terms. Consult a medical dictionary to confirm your spelling.

Singular	Plural
1. antrostomy	_____
2. choana	_____
3. cortex	_____
4. conjunctiva	_____
5. ecchymosis	_____
6. naris	_____
7. myringoplasty	_____
8. osteotomy	_____
9. petechia	_____
10. sinus	_____

Abbreviations Exercise

Instructions: Expand the following common abbreviations and brief forms. Then memorize both abbreviations and definitions to increase your speed and accuracy in transcribing dictation

Abbreviation	Expansion
1. ABR	_____
2. AOE	_____
3. CNS	_____
4. CRP	_____
5. CSF	_____
6. dB	_____
7. EBL	_____
8. EOMs	_____
9. ET (tube)	_____
10. GBS	_____
11. GCF	_____
12. GERD	_____
13. hCG	_____
14. I&D	_____
15. IMF	_____
16. JVD	_____

Abbreviation	Expansion
17. LS (spine)	_____
18. MCL	_____
19. OC (junction)	_____
20. ORIF	_____
21. PE (tubes)	_____
22. PPD	_____
23. T&A	_____
24. TM	_____
25. URI	_____

Transcript Forensics

Instructions: This section presents snippets of transcribed dictations from clinic notes; history and physical examinations and consultations; operative reports and procedure notes; and discharge summaries. Explain the passage so that a nonmedical person can understand it.

Example

This is a 9-month-old female who has a history of **neonatal jaundice**. She was born at **36 weeks**, normal spontaneous vaginal delivery, and weighed 5 pounds 14 ounces.

Explanation: This somewhat premature baby had elevated bilirubin levels in the blood as evidenced by yellowing of the skin shortly after birth. Her delivery and birth weight were normal.

1. Patient was delivered by cesarean section, secondary to **maternal herpes**. He had a fair initial respiratory effort with crying, was warmed, suctioned, and stimulated. Infant continued to develop respiratory distress with **flaring and grunting**. He was **retracting** and had a respiratory rate in the 60s to 70s. He continued to sound like he had a **pleural effusion**.

Explanation: _____

_____

_____

_____

_____

_____

2. Chief Complaint: A 4-year-old white female who has had chronic **middle ear effusions**. This has failed to resolve despite antibiotic therapy.

Explanation: _____
_____
_____
_____
_____
_____

3. DIAGNOSTIC IMPRESSION: **Acute otitis media** of his right ear with **spontaneous rupture of the tympanic membrane** and **URI**.

Explanation: _____
_____
_____
_____
_____
_____

4. This is a 7-year-old male with a long-standing history of **ankyloglossia**. The **risks, benefits, and alternatives** to **frenuloplasty** were discussed with the patient and his parents, and **informed consent** was obtained.

Explanation: _____
_____
_____
_____
_____
_____

5. ASSESSMENT: Patient with **near-syncope** who passed out while in the bathroom She said she had some **black tarry stool**, but is on a vitamin with iron, and a rectal exam was **heme negative**. Additionally, her **hemoglobin and hematocrit** and her **blood pressures are normal**. She probably has a viral illness.

Explanation:_____
_____
_____
_____
_____
_____
_____

6. INDICATIONS FOR OPERATION
The patient presents with **persistent serous effusions**, recurrent infections. He is a **Down child** with associated abnormalities. He had failed **AOE testing**. We elected to go ahead with an **ABR**. Risks, benefits, and options, particularly given his underlying health history, were discussed in detail.

Explanation: _____
_____
_____
_____
_____
_____

7. PREOPERATIVE DIAGNOSIS
   Masticatory dysfunction, secondary to **mandibular horizontal hypoplasia**.

   Explanation: _____
   _____
   _____
   _____
   _____
   _____

8. The patient was **extubated** in the operating room and transported to the recovery room in a stable condition. **Estimated blood loss was 300 mL. Prognosis** is good with expectation for full recovery.

   Explanation: _____
   _____
   _____
   _____
   _____
   _____

9. (From a myringotomy with tubes operative report)
   After removal of **cerumen** under microscopic guidance, radial **myringotomy incision** was made in the anterior inferior quadrant. The middle ear **effusion was suctioned**, and an Armstrong Teflon beveled **tympanostomy tube** was placed.

   Explanation: _____
   _____
   _____
   _____
   _____
   _____

10. PREOPERATIVE DIAGNOSIS
    Pulmonary failure with need for **tracheostomy**, on **mechanical ventilator**, unable to **wean off**.

    Explanation: _____
    _____
    _____
    _____
    _____
    _____

Sample Reports

Sample family medicine reports appear on the following pages, illustrating a variety of reports. Fictional names are provided for illustration of proper format, and no resemblance to actual persons is intended. Sample transcripts were prepared according to *The Book of Style for Medical Transcription* (AHDI).

Operative Report

BLACK, CHARLES
#690838

DATE OF OPERATION
December 17, [add year]

PREOPERATIVE DIAGNOSIS
Recurrent otitis media.

POSTOPERATIVE DIAGNOSIS
Recurrent otitis media.

NAME OF PROCEDURE
Bilateral tympanotomy tube insertion.

SURGEON
ERIC HALL, MD

DESCRIPTION OF PROCEDURE
A 1-year-old taken to the operating room and put under general anesthesia using inhalation anesthetic agents. Wax removed from external ear canals. Incision made in the anterior-inferior portion of both tympanic membranes and Armstrong silicone tubes placed bilaterally. Only scant fluid present at this point in time. Estimated blood loss less than 1 mL. Patient taken to the recovery room in satisfactory condition.

ERIC HALL, MD

EH:HPI

d: 12/17/[add year]
t: 12/18/[add year]

Emergency Department Note

LEE, THOMAS
#780172

DATE OF VISIT
January 30, [add year]

CHIEF COMPLAINT
A 37-year-old male patient who comes in with right ear pain. It started tonight, about an hour ago. He had cold symptoms for a few days, cough and congestion. Denies any other symptoms. He is allergic to sulfa, takes no medications. Does not smoke or drink.

PHYSICAL EXAMINATION
VITAL SIGNS: Afebrile, vital signs stable, uncomfortable.
GENERAL APPEARANCE: A 37-year-old male patient with above history with right ear pain.
HEENT: Normal except for dull red bulging of right tympanic membrane and nasal congestion. He also had spontaneous rupture of the tympanic membrane with some drainage.
NECK: Supple.
LUNGS: Clear.
HEART: Normal.
ABDOMEN: Benign.
SKIN: Without rash.
NEUROLOGIC: Exam was nonfocal.

HOSPITAL COURSE
He is to take 2 Vicodin orally and 2 to go, and amoxicillin 1000 mg orally.

DIAGNOSTIC IMPRESSION
Acute otitis media of his right ear with spontaneous rupture of the tympanic membrane and upper respiratory infection (URI).

DISCHARGE INSTRUCTIONS
Amoxicillin, Vicodin, and followup.

DEREK PREGLER, MD

DP:hpi

d: 1/30/[add year]
t: 1/31/[add year]

Operative Report

MASTERSON, MEGAN
#912093

DATE OF PROCEDURE
April 4, [add year]

PREOPERATIVE DIAGNOSES
1. Nasal septum deviation.
2. Inferior turbinate hypertrophy, bilaterally.

POSTOPERATIVE DIAGNOSES
1. Nasal septum deviation.
2. Inferior turbinate hypertrophy, bilaterally.

PROCEDURES
1. Septoplasty.
2. Bilateral submucosal resection of the inferior turbinates.

SURGEON
Robert Martinez, MD

ANESTHESIOLOGIST
Christian Dear, MD

ANESTHESIA
General.

COMPLICATIONS
None.

ESTIMATED BLOOD LOSS
Less than 20 mL.

INDICATIONS
An 18-year-old with chronic nasal obstruction.

FINDINGS
The findings are a marked right septal spur on the right side totally spanning the nasal airway, and enlarged turbinates, particularly on the left side.

(continued)

Operative Report *(continued)*

MASTERSON, MEGAN
#912093
Page 2

OPERATIVE PROCEDURE
Consent was obtained. Patient underwent general anesthesia. The table was rotated 90 degrees; the head was straight. In the nose, a topical decongestant with epinephrine-soaked neuro patties was placed. The septum and turbinates were injected with 2% lidocaine with epinephrine. A left hemitransfixion incision was made in the mucoperichondrium; periosteal flaps were elevated. The osseocartilaginous (OC) junction was divided. A portion of the posterior cartilage was removed, approximately 1 cm to 1.5 cm.

The contralateral mucoperiosteum was elevated. Jansen-Middleton forceps were used to make a sagittal cut through the perpendicular plate in the inferior portion and the spur was removed. The chisel was used to remove a portion to deflect the maxillary crest posteriorly. The incision was closed with 4-0 chromic. The membranes were coapted with 4-0 plain gut. Stab incisions were made in the inferior turbinates and the mucosa elevated with a Cottle elevator. Submucosal resection with a microdebrider was performed. The incisions were closed with 4-0 chromic and the turbinates outfractured. The nose and nasopharynx were suctioned. The patient was transferred to the recovery room in stable condition.

ROBERT MARTINEZ, MD

RM:hpi

d: 4/4/[add year]
t: 4/5/[add year]

Comic Relief

The following gaffes were created by speech-recognition software.

Incorrect	**Correct**
The patient presents with a cute tiny penis.	The patient presents with acute tinea pedis.
I would like urine put on this.	I would like your input on this.
There were problems in violating the patient secondary to cooperation.	There were problems evaluating the patient secondary to cooperation.
The patient's father works as attacks analyst.	The patient's father works as a tax analyst.
We will refer this youngster to an off the mall adjust.	We will refer this youngster to an ophthalmologist.
Two hundred fifty grand Catholics were ministered.	Two hundred fifty milligrams of Keflex was administered.

PEARSON
myhealthprofessionskit™

To access the online exercises and transcription practice, go to **www.myhealthprofessionskit.com**. Select "Medical Transcription," then click on the title of this book, *Healthcare Documentation: Fundamentals & Practice*. Then click on the Family Medicine chapter.

Internal Medicine

Learning Objectives

▶ Describe the structure and function of the endocrine system.

▶ Identify and describe formed elements of blood.

▶ Differentiate between benign and malignant tumors and explain the diagnostic and therapeutic modalities used in oncology.

▶ Discuss the consequences of aging and the role of end-of-life care.

▶ Spell and define common vocabulary terms in the subspecialties of internal medicine.

▶ Describe the negative and positive findings an internal medicine specialist looks for on the review of systems and physical examination.

▶ Describe the typical cause, course, and treatment options for common endocrine diseases, blood disorders, and cancers.

▶ Identify and define diagnostic, surgical, and therapeutic procedures in internal medicine.

▶ List common laboratory tests and procedures used in internal medicine.

▶ Identify common internal medicine drugs and their uses.

▶ Demonstrate knowledge of anatomical, medical, pharmacological, adjectival, and soundalike terms by accurately completing the exercises in this chapter.

Transcribing Internal Medicine Dictation

Introduction

Internal medicine is the medical specialty dealing with the prevention, diagnosis, and treatment of adult diseases. Physicians specializing in internal medicine are called **internists**. They are especially skilled in the management of patients who have undifferentiated or multisystem disease processes.

The American Board of Internal Medicine recognizes many subspecialties of internal medicine, including **endocrinology**, **hematology**, **oncology**, and **geriatrics** which are covered in this chapter.

Endocrinology

Endocrinology is the study of the glands that make up the endocrine system. These glands are located in different areas of the body, and many important hormones are produced by endocrine glands (also called ductless glands because their secretions pass directly into the circulation) (see ■ **Figure 9-1**).

Endocrine literally means "internal secretion." The endocrine glands are described below. Some of these endocrine glands (for example, the pancreas and the gonads) perform nonhormonal functions as well.

The **pituitary gland**, or **hypophysis**, situated on the undersurface of the brain, consists of two distinct masses of endocrine tissue. The anterior pituitary (**adenohypophysis**) produces hormones that regulate the development and function of other endocrine glands: **thyroid-stimulating hormone (TSH)**, **adrenocorticotropic hormone (ACTH)**, which stimulates the adrenal cortex, and the gonadotropins: **follicle-stimulating hormone (FSH)** and **luteinizing hormone (LH)**, which regulate gonadal functions. The anterior pituitary is also the source of **growth hormone (somatotropin)**, which regulates the natural growth process, and **prolactin** (required for lactation after pregnancy).

The posterior pituitary (**neurohypophysis**) is in direct continuity with the part of the brain called the **hypothalamus**. It produces two hormones: **oxytocin**, which stimulates uterine contractions in labor, and **vasopressin (antidiuretic hormone, ADH)**, which helps to control water balance by promoting reabsorption of water by the kidneys.

The **thyroid gland**, whose name means "shield-shaped," is situated in the front of the neck overlying the junction of the **larynx** and **trachea**. The thyroid

Past medical history is significant for diabetes and coronary artery disease. Patient is status post coronary artery bypass surgery, hyperlipidemia, hypertriglyceridemia, chronic renal failure, congestive heart failure, and insomnia.

gland produces two iodine-containing hormones, **thyroxine (T_4)** and **triiodothyronine (T_3)**, which circulate in the blood bound to a plasma protein (**thyroid binding globulin, TBG**). These hormones influence general metabolism, chiefly by regulating gene transcription of body proteins (including growth hormone).

The four **parathyroid glands** are so-called because they lie on or in the capsule of the thyroid gland. These glands produce **parathyroid hormone (PTH)**, which regulates the serum calcium level within narrow limits. Calcium control is important for proper maintenance of bones and teeth; more critically, the level of calcium in the serum and in tissue fluids exerts a potent influence on nerve and muscle function. Parathyroid hormone maintains the level of calcium in serum by moving calcium ions out of the bones, reducing the renal clearance of calcium, and increasing the rate of intestinal absorption of calcium. **Calcitonin**, a hormone produced by the thyroid gland, is also involved in regulation of serum calcium.

The **adrenal glands** are two crescent-shaped caps of endocrine tissue, one situated on top of each kidney. Each adrenal gland consists of two essentially different bodies of endocrine tissue: the outer **cortex** and the inner **medulla**.

The adrenal cortex produces three classes of hormones, two of which play crucial roles in the control of sugar, protein, and mineral metabolism. The **glucocorticoids** (principally **cortisol**) increase glucose production by the liver, affect protein and fat metabolism, help to regulate blood pressure, mediate many of the responses of the body to stress, and tend to suppress immune and inflammatory responses.

The **mineralocorticoids** (principally **aldosterone**) regulate electrolyte and water balance by promoting renal retention of sodium ions of potassium, hydrogen, and ammonium ions. **Adrenal androgens** play a minor role in reproductive physiology in both men and women. They are chiefly of interest as a cause of hirsutism and virilization in certain adrenal diseases.

The **adrenal medulla** is part of the **sympathetic nervous system**. Cells of the adrenal medulla are stim-

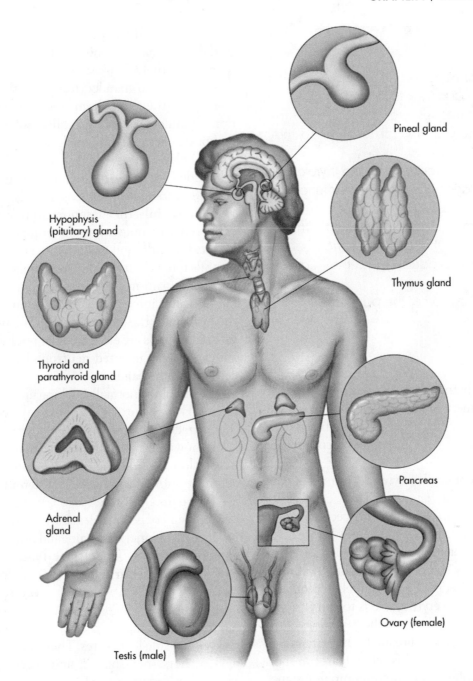

Hypophysis
(pituitary) gland

Thyroid and
parathyroid gland

Adrenal
gland

Testis (male)

Pineal gland

Thymus gland

Pancreas

Ovary (female)

FIGURE 9-1. Primary glands of the endocrine system

ulated directly by sympathetic nerve endings to produce **epinephrine**, **norepinephrine**, and **dopamine**, which although not essential to life play a critical part in the body's response to severe stress. These hormones affect many tissues, increasing the rate and force of cardiac contractions, relaxing the smooth muscle of the bronchi, constricting some blood vessels and dilating others, stimulating liver and muscle tissue to produce and release glucose, and controlling fat breakdown and insulin production.

The **pancreas** is an **endocrine** gland as well as an **exocrine** one (one that produces a secretion released

through a duct). The endocrine function of the pancreas is performed by the **islets of Langerhans**, tiny aggregations of endocrine cells interspersed among the exocrine secretory elements.

The **B** or **beta cells** of the islets of Langerhans produce insulin, which increases glucose utilization and exerts other complex influences on the metabolism of carbohydrates, proteins, and fats. The **A** or **alpha cells** produce **glucagon**, an inhibitor of glucose activity, and the **D** or **delta cells** produce somatostatin, which inhibits secretion of growth hormone by the anterior pituitary.

Hematology

Hematology is the branch of medicine concerned with diagnosis and treatment of disorders of the **formed elements of the blood** (red blood cells, white blood cells, platelets) (see ■ Figure 9-2) and of **blood coagulation** (see ■ Figure 9-12).

Red blood cells or **erythrocytes** are formed in bone marrow by repeated divisions of large cells called erythroblasts. Developing erythrocytes become gradually smaller, finally losing their nuclei just before being released into the circulation. The circulating erythrocyte is a round disk with both sides slightly hollowed, so that when seen on edge it has a dumbbell profile.

The function of the erythrocyte is to carry oxygen from the capillaries of the lungs to the capillaries of the rest of the body, and carbon dioxide from the tissues to the lungs for excretion. This chemical transport depends on **hemoglobin**, an iron-containing substance that is responsible for the red color of blood. An erythrocyte survives for about 120 days after entering the circulation. Then it disintegrates and is removed from the blood, principally by phagocytes in the spleen, which conserve and recycle its iron content.

White blood cells (leukocytes) are larger than erythrocytes and much less numerous in circulating blood, the ratio being about 600:1. Unlike erythrocytes, which perform their only function in circulating blood, leukocytes appear in the blood only when in transit from their point of production to their destination in tissues. All leukocytes have nuclei. They are divided into two major classes on the basis of the sites where they develop.

Although all leukocytes arise from precursor cells in the bone marrow, only myeloid leukocytes develop to maturity there. Leukocytes of myeloid origin are further divided into granulocytes, which show conspicuous granules in their cytoplasm, and monocytes, which do not. Granulocytes are also called **polymorphonuclear leukocytes** because their nuclei are typically divided by shallow clefts into two to five lobes. Granulocytes are subdivided according to the staining properties of their granules into neutrophils, eosinophils, and basophils.

Neutrophils, the most numerous of all white blood cells, have granules that show approximately equal affinity for acidic and basic stains. The function of neutrophils is to engulf and digest devitalized tissue, invading microorganisms, and other foreign material. Within minutes after injury, neutrophils begin to migrate from the blood into the affected tissue. The nuclei of immature neutrophils are elongated but not lobed. Such cells are called **unsegmented neutrophils, stab cells, band cells,** or simply **bands**.

Eosinophils, normally making up no more than 5% of circulating white blood cells, have coarse granules that attract eosin and other acid dyes. Their function is unknown but their numbers increase in parasitic infestation and allergic disorders, and decrease after administration of adrenocortical steroid drugs.

Basophils constitute 1% or less of circulating leukocytes. Their coarse granules stain with basic dyes. They produce histamine, serotonin, and other biochemically active substances. These three types of granulocytes (**polymorphonuclear leukocytes**) are formed in bone marrow by differentiation of precursor cells called **myelocytes.**

Monocytes are large cells that make up 5–8% of total circulating leukocytes. Their nuclei are large, kidney- or horseshoe-shaped, and eccentrically placed. Monocytes function as phagocytes in tissues and are perhaps identical with histiocytes.

Lymphocytes are white blood cells that develop from precursor cells in bone marrow but migrate to other tissues before maturing. They can be found in both lymphoid tissue (spleen, lymph nodes) and in the blood, where they normally make up about 25% of circulating white blood cells. Lymphocytes are slightly larger than erythrocytes and have relatively large, dark-staining nuclei. Their function is to produce antibodies, to modulate immune processes, and to perform other protective functions. Lymphocytes are divided into two major populations, designated **B** and **T**, whose activities are closely related.

B cells (B lymphocytes) migrate in an immature state from the marrow to lymphoid tissue. Here they undergo differentiation and maturation before moving to other lymphoid tissues via the bloodstream, where they constitute 5–15% of circulating lymphocytes. A mature B cell can synthesize antibodies in small amounts, but these remain attached to the cell surface. Under appropriate circumstances, however, B cells evolve into plasma cells, which produce antibodies in large amounts and release them into the circulation.

T cells (T lymphocytes) migrate from the marrow to the thymus for maturation before proceeding to other lymphoid organs and tissues. They make up 55–65% of circulating lymphocytes. On the basis of their surface proteins, T cells are subdivided into several types, each with its specific function.

Helper (or inducer) **T cells** stimulate or augment the production of antibody by B cells and plasma cells. Suppressor T cells modify or curb this production. **Cytotoxic** (killer) **T cells** destroy cells they recognize as antigenic.

A few large granular lymphocytes that are neither B nor T cells are known as **null cells**. Their functions are unknown, but some of them seem to operate as natural killer cells, attacking foreign cells directly without any true immune response.

Platelets are very small round or oval bodies found in circulating blood. They are formed in bone marrow

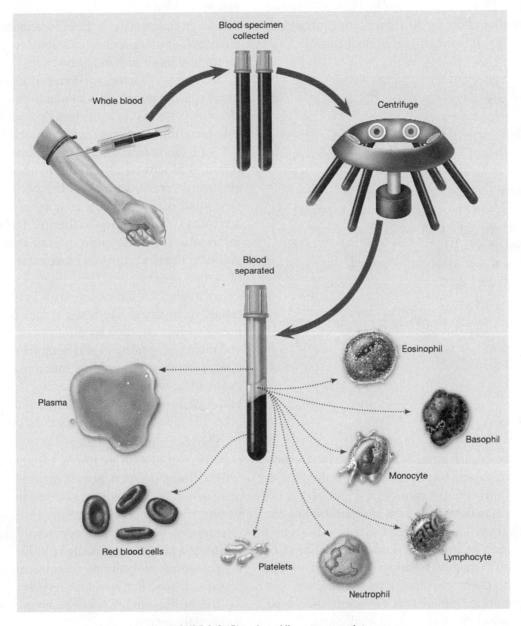

FIGURE 9-2. Blood and its components

as extrusions from the cytoplasm of giant cells with lobed nuclei called megakaryocytes. Platelets are not cells and do not have nuclei. They function in blood clotting.

Blood coagulates (clots) when the soluble plasma protein fibrinogen is converted to insoluble fibrin. Normally this occurs after another plasma protein, prothrombin, is converted to thrombin. Activation of prothrombin can come about through a number of alternative biochemical pathways, variously involving platelets, tissue factors, and plasma proteins other than prothrombin and fibrinogen. All known coagulation mechanisms require the presence of calcium. In addition, Factor V (labile factor), Factor VII (stable factor, proconvertin), Factor VIII (antihemophilic globulin, AHG), Factor IX (Christmas factor), Factor X (Stuart-Prower factor), and Factor XI (plasma thromboplastin antecedent) are all necessary for normal coagulation.

Pause for Reflection

1. What is another name for red blood cells and what is their function? What substance is responsible for the color of red blood cells and what is its function?
2. What is another name for white blood cells? List the different types of white blood cells and their function.
3. Explain the following terms: B cells and T cells.
4. What are null cells?
5. What are platelets?
6. Besides platelets, name two plasma proteins that are important in coagulation of blood.

Oncology

Oncology is the branch of medicine devoted to the prevention, diagnosis, and treatment of malignant disease. An **oncologic surgeon** specializes in the partial or complete excision of malignant tumors and surrounding tissues to which they may have spread, as well as the repair or reconstruction of structures damaged by tumors or their treatment. A **medical oncologist** treats many types of cancer using chemotherapy, hormone therapy, and immunomodulating therapies. A **radiation oncologist** administers radiotherapy to treat malignancies.

Neoplasia refers to any growth of cells or tissues that is erratic, not in accord with normal bodily needs or patterns of growth and development, and not under the control of normal regulatory mechanisms. Neoplasia results in the formation of a neoplasm (growth, tumor).

Neoplasms are divided into two large classes: **benign** and **malignant**. A malignant tumor, or cancer, is one that, if unchecked, tends to cause death; a benign tumor has no such inherent tendency. Histologic examination of a malignant tumor shows cells that are more primitive, undifferentiated, or anaplastic than those composing a benign tumor. A malignant tumor enlarges by infiltrating and invading adjacent tissues, whereas a benign tumor simply gets bigger. A malignant tumor can spread by **metastasis**—transmission of malignant cells or groups of cells by the bloodstream, the lymphatic channels, or other routes to establish new foci of malignancy at remote sites in the body.

A variety of factors are currently recognized as capable of causing neoplasia. Cellular mutation, induced by chemical toxins (carcinogens), radiation, chronic inflammation, or certain infections, can lead to formation of a clone or colony of cells whose internal structure and biochemical nature are aberrant or atypical and whose proliferation and behavior do not respond to normal controls. Many tumors are triggered by the activation of oncogenes—inherited bits of genetic misinformation capable of promoting erratic cell growth and development and responsible for familial clusters of certain cancers.

A malignant tumor can arise in virtually any cell, tissue, or organ of the body. It can cause death in a broad variety of ways: by outgrowing its blood supply and undergoing necrosis and hemorrhage, by producing toxic substances, by eroding into a major blood vessel, by invading or metastasizing to a vital organ such as the brain, or by impairing nutrition, immunity, or some other life-sustaining biochemical function.

Diagnosis of malignancy. The signs and symptoms of malignant disease are highly variable. Many kinds of cancer (lung, pancreas) cause no symptoms until they have invaded surrounding tissues or spread by metastasis and have become essentially untreatable. Cancer screening is the testing of apparently healthy persons for subtle indications of malignant disease. The following screening procedures are currently advised for all persons, at specified ages or intervals:

Breast: Examination of the breasts by a physician, and mammography.

Uterine cervix: Pap smear.

Colon and rectum: Digital examination, sigmoidoscopy or colonoscopy, and examination of stools for occult blood.

When cancer is suspected, prompt and vigorous diagnostic evaluation is in order, unless the age or general health of the patient makes this inappropriate. Imaging techniques (x-ray, MRI, CT, ultrasound, nuclear imaging) can provide highly specific information about the nature, location, and extent of malignant disease. Blood tests that detect or measure immunologic or biologic markers (abnormal tumor products, immunoglobulins) can provide valuable further information.

The diagnostic procedure par excellence for malignant disease is **biopsy**, the removal of a specimen of tissue for histologic examination by any of various techniques including a **needle** inserted through the skin, endoscopy, laparoscopy, or open surgery.

A fine-needle biopsy was done after mammograms which showed a suspicious lesion. Fine-needle was reported out as probably infiltrating ductal carcinoma. The patient opted to go for a modified radical mastectomy rather than lumpectomy and followup radiation.

A biopsy specimen is examined by a pathologist, first grossly and then (after fixation, embedding in a medium such as paraffin, thin sectioning, and staining) microscopically to determine whether it contains malignant cells, from what type of normal cells they have arisen, how undifferentiated they are, what tissue abnormalities they show (cyst formation, abortive attempts at organization, tissue death), and how far they have extended or invaded. For certain types of cancer (**breast cancer**), pathologic examination of surgically removed material can be performed immediately (before the surgical wound is closed) by the **frozen section technique**, which substitutes freezing of tissue for the more time-consuming paraffin process.

Diagnostic information obtained about a cancer is generally formulated according to a rigorous and highly specific scheme.

The **type** of a cancer is its histologic nature: what kind of cells (squamous epithelium, gland tissue, duct tissue) have undergone malignant change?

The **grading** of a cancer is a measure of its degree of malignancy, based on the proportion of undifferentiated cells that it contains. The higher the grade, the greater the probability of invasion and metastasis.

Staging is a measure of the extent of a malignant disease at the time of evaluation, expressed in arabic numerals (1, 2, 3 ...) with or without qualifying letters. Staging takes into account the type, size, and extent of the primary tumor; the degree of lymph node involvement, if any; and the number and location of any distant metastases. The presence of associated symptoms, such as weight loss and fever, may be relevant to the staging of certain malignancies.

A basic framework used in expressing the staging of a wide variety of malignancies is the T-N-M (tumor, nodes, metastases) classification. In this system, numbers indicate the extent of involvement, according to criteria that are specific for each type of tumor. Thus, T2 might represent a primary tumor that is larger than 5 cm in diameter but has not invaded locally; N2, involvement of lymph nodes at two distinct sites; M0, no evidence of distant metastasis.

Arriving at an accurate prognosis for a malignant tumor depends on precise typing, grading, and staging; on other diagnostic information (imaging and laboratory studies); and on due consideration of the patient's age and general health. The compilation of cancer statistics by national and international **tumor registries** has made possible the publication of survival information for each type of tumor depending on grade and stage. The **five-year survival rate** is a familiar index of prognosis. If a given type, grade, and stage of tumor has a five-year survival rate of 56% with a given treatment, that means that 56% of persons with such a tumor who undergo such a treatment will still be living after five years.

Treatment of malignancy. The goals of treatment in malignant disease are to effect a cure when possible and to conserve the patient's comfort in all cases, with due attention to nutrition, hydration, and control of symptoms such as pain, nausea, and dyspnea.

Surgery has always been the principal method of treating cancer. Complete **resection** of a primary tumor that has not spread or metastasized usually proves to be curative. But adequate resection may involve damage to or removal of much normal tissue, while conservative surgery may fail to remove all cancer cells. When curative surgery is not feasible, a **palliative procedure** may be undertaken to reduce the volume of the tumor (**debulking**) or to remove devitalized, necrotic, bleeding, or infected tissue. In some types of malignancy, a palliative effect may be achieved by **surgical removal**

CANCER

The term *cancer,* the Latin word for 'crab,' was used for malignant ulcerations by the Roman medical writer Celsus (1st century AD). Much earlier, Greek writers including Hippocrates used the Greek word *karkinos,* also meaning 'crab,' and its derivative *karkinoma,* for malignant disease.

The association between malignancy and crabs has been variously explained. One theory is that malignant tumors were thought to gnaw or erode tissue like the claws of a crab. According to another view, the dilated veins on the surface of a cancerous breast seemed to suggest the outline of a crab with outstretched claws.

Cancer nomenclature is highly complex and constantly changing. Two main types of malignant tumor are distinguished on the basis of their tissues of origin. **Carcinoma** (by far the more common) develops from epithelium, either glandular (adenocarcinoma) or squamous (squamous carcinoma). **Sarcoma** (from a Greek word meaning 'to become fleshy') denotes a tumor arising from connective tissue (muscle, bone).

after treatment, red and white blood cell counts and other diagnostic tests are performed regularly to monitor drug effects and detect severe bone marrow depression or other toxic effects of the drugs on normal tissues.

A course of chemotherapy typically includes three or more drugs given according to a precise regimen or **protocol**. The drugs used in such combinations are represented by their first letters in initialisms such as MOPP (mechlorethamine, Oncovorin, procarbazine, and prednisone); note that Oncovorin is a brand name for vincristine.

Because rapidly proliferating tissue is particularly subject to damage by ionizing radiation, x-ray and other forms of radiation have long been used as an adjunct to surgery and chemotherapy in the treatment of many malignant tumors. The dose and delivery site of **radiation therapy** must be carefully adjusted to ensure maximal therapeutic response with minimal side effects and risk of delayed complications.

Pause for Reflection

1. Define *neoplasm.*
2. The mechanism by which malignant tumors spread to distant sites is referred to as _____.
3. What diagnostic methods are employed when cancer is suspected?
4. Distinguish between *grading* and *staging.*
5. Explain the T, N, M system of cancer classification.
6. Briefly describe the three methods of treating cancer.

of certain endocrine glands: the testes in metastatic carcinoma of the prostate, the ovaries in breast cancer.

During the past generation, **chemotherapy** of cancer with a wide variety of agents has become firmly established as a valuable and often curative resource. Useful cancer drugs include alkylating agents (nitrogen mustard, chlorambucil, busulfan), antimetabolites (methotrexate, 5-fluorouracil, 6-mercaptopurine), antibiotics (doxorubicin, dactinomycin, mithramycin), plant alkaloids (vinblastine and vincristine from periwinkle), hormones (adrenal corticosteroids, estrogens, androgens), monoclonal antibodies (cetuximab, trastuzumab), and others (enzymes, platinum complex).

Most of these agents are toxic to cancer cells, and most of them can also damage normal cells and tissues. Because cancer is a life-threatening disease, a higher risk of severe side effects is considered tolerable. Most cancer chemotherapy must be administered by injection and continued over a period of weeks. During and

Geriatrics

Just as no one would define pediatrics as "the medical care of very short people," geriatrics is not simply "the treatment (Greek *iatrike*) of people who are old (*gerontes*)." Aging imparts entirely new dimensions to human physiology, pathology, psychology, and pharmacology. The specialty of geriatrics seeks to understand those dimensions and adapt medical theory and practice so as to deal with them in positive and productive ways.

On purely statistical grounds, the risk of degenerative, autoimmune, and malignant diseases rises steadily as one grows older. **The elderly are particularly prone to hypertension, coronary and cerebrovascular** arteriosclerosis, **chronic obstructive pulmonary disease (COPD), degenerative joint disease (DJD), osteoporosis, and cancers of the skin, breast, prostate, lung, and colon.** For that reason, the screening of asymptomatic persons for early indications of treatable diseases becomes an increasingly important part of medical care with advancing years.

Many factors associated with aging have a negative impact on the quality of life: impairment of hearing and vision, memory loss, cognitive impairment ranging from occasional mild confusion ("senior moments") to frank dementia, reduction in dexterity and mobility due to arthritis or the sequelae of injuries or strokes, difficulty in obtaining nourishing and palatable meals regularly, and social alienation (see ■ **Figure 9-3**).

Many older persons live with chronic anxiety and depression, often due to a combination of stressors such as forced retirement, death of a spouse, shrinking income from pension or savings, living alone, loss of a driver's license, and loss of autonomy through dependence on caregivers who, even though they may be close relatives, don't really care. Withdrawal and hypoactivity resulting from depression in the elderly are too often mistaken for signs of dementia and basically ignored.

The effects of advancing age influence many aspects of medical care for the elderly. Several new symptoms occurring in a person under 40 usually turn out to have a single cause. No such assumption can be made in a person over 60, by which age **co-morbidity** (the simultaneous presence of more than one disease) is the rule rather than the exception.

As diagnoses accumulate, so do the bottles of pills. It is by no means unusual for an **elderly person to be taking ten or more prescription medicines every day.** Drowsiness, loss of appetite, confusion, and other symptoms noted by physicians or caregivers are often traced to the effects of medicines. **Polypharmacy** (prescribing many drugs for the same person) presents a considerable challenge to the patient with intact faculties; one with cognitive impairment or memory loss may take medicine erratically, or not at all.

An older patient is likely to be seeing several specialists (urologist, ophthalmologist, dermatologist, rheumatologist, cardiologist, gastroenterologist) on a regular basis, each of whom may prescribe one or more medicines without being aware of other medicines the patient is already taking. Interactions between medicines taken together inappropriately are a common cause of severe symptoms and of emergency department visits.

The longer one lives, the more complex does one's medical history (illnesses, injuries, diagnostic tests, operations, medicines) become, and the harder it gets to reconstruct it from the memories of patient or family and from written records, which grow ever more elusive with the passing years. When the situation is further complicated by difficulties in communication or cognitive impairment, just establishing the history of the present illness may become a major undertaking.

Medical problems arising in young or middle-aged people are typically self-limited, and any honest physician will tell you that most of them will eventually

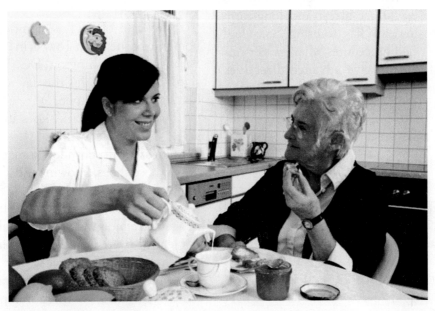

FIGURE 9-3. A geriatric nurse assisting a patient with activities of daily living. Source: Gina Sanders, Shutterstock.

resolve without any treatment whatsoever. Conversely, medical problems of the elderly tend to become chronic even with treatment, which may be purely symptomatic, and often proves quite ineffective.

The health professional caring for older patients needs a strong, positive outlook and a cheerful disposition that sheds light and warmth into lives growing dim and frosty. You've heard this before, but it bears repeating. Getting old may not be any picnic, but it doesn't seem quite so bad when you consider the alternative.

End-of-Life Care

Although the principal goal of all health care is to preserve and prolong life, it is often appropriate, in the presence of terminal illness, to abandon futile attempts at cure and to direct medical and nursing efforts toward **palliative treatment**, with adequate control of pain and other distressing symptoms, emotional and spiritual support, and preservation of the patient's autonomy and dignity. End-of-life care is a **multidisciplinary approach** to meeting the needs of persons with terminal cancer, end-stage renal or pulmonary disease, and other conditions.

The **hospice movement** provides formal programs and facilities to meet the needs of dying persons for comfort and care and also to afford support and counsel for caregivers and family members during and after the patient's final illness.

Features of formal end-of-life programs include patient-controlled analgesia and anesthesia systems and advance dialog about the patient's wishes with respect to **life-extending care**, including resuscitation in the event of respiratory or cardiac arrest and long-term preservation after brain death has occurred. State legislatures have established procedures whereby persons nearing the end of life can give **advance directives** regarding the provision or withholding of such care in the event that they become incompetent or comatose.

Pause for Reflection

1. What is the goal of geriatrics?
2. What factor(s) makes diagnosis more difficult in the aging patient?
3. Describe some of the problems associated with medications for the elderly.
4. Discuss the concept of end-of-life care.

A Caregiver's Perspective: My Last Two Years with Marion

by Linda C. Campbell

My mother, Marion Bartley Campbell, was a most practical woman. In fact, her practicality far exceeded any vanity she may have had. She did not think highly of her looks or her talents. Interestingly, this tendency to devalue herself (for she was beautiful and talented) made it possible for her to endure the last two years of her life, which were spent in utter dependency.

A near-lifelong smoker from the age of 16 until 15 years before her death in 2003, the cigarettes took a silent, undetected, immense toll on the arteries of her legs. With the circulation to her lower extremities severely compromised, it was necessary, the surgeon informed us, for Marion to undergo a surgical femoral-popliteal bypass in both lower extremities to "save her legs." Part of the saphenous vein in her lower leg would be harvested and that vessel sewn into place to act as a conduit around the damaged, clotted-off part of the artery. This "new" vessel would carry limb-sustaining, nourishing blood to both legs.

We thought this was the nightmare. We were wrong.

The surgery was a dismal failure. We later discovered that the surgeon who performed the surgery had lost his credentials as a vascular surgeon several years before. Why didn't I notice all the amputees in this surgeon's office? Why did the insurance company insist that this general surgeon with no training in thoracic or vascular surgery be selected to carry out such delicate vascular surgery?

The date of 9/11 is significant for the senseless bombing of the Twin Towers in New York City and the Pentagon in Washington, DC. This date is even more significant for me. It's the day my mother lost both of her legs above the knee.

I had put Marion's shoes in the trunk of my car when she first went into the hospital and we expected her to leave with both legs intact. It was heart-rending to see those shoes, knowing she would never need them again.

Marion accepted this horrible turn of events with her usual humor and aplomb. Her practical nature did not let her down. There was nothing she could do about the outcome of the surgery; her legs would not grow back, and prosthesis was not a practical alternative for her 74-year-old weak thigh stumps.

It took a lawyer to uncover the real reason she became an amputee. The hospital wasn't talking. The medical staff wasn't talking. The nursing notes revealed no details of Marion's pulseless legs. It took a year of legal work to finally determine that the surgeon did not bypass the clots properly. He stitched the new vessels into the old clotted areas. The intraoperative angiograms later obtained by the malpractice attorney confirmed this, but there was no mention of it in Marion's medical record. (The lawsuit was eventually dropped. Our interest was in getting to the truth.)

I understand why people put their parents in nursing homes and healthcare facilities. Often there is no choice. **Employment and the sheer responsibility of caring for a parent with a catastrophic condition may make it impossible to care for a parent at home.** Even with the availability of home health nurses, caring for a sick or injured parent is emotionally wracking. It can be physically disabling for the caretaker. (My back sustained significant disk narrowing as a result of transferring my 100-pound mother from the bed to her wheelchair.)

I majored in nursing back in college in the 1970s. It was a "technical nursing" program that jammed four years of nursing education and practice into two years of study. Its graduates were awarded a Registered Nurse credential upon successful completion of the program and passing the credentialing exam.

Turned out, nursing wasn't really for me. I completed nearly all of the two-year program but became diverted by other, more interesting studies. I never forgot my days as a student nurse, though. Those experiences are remarkably green in my memory. I could not have anticipated that the skills I learned in nursing school would help prepare me to care for my mother.

I was incredibly fortunate. The company president for whom I worked was sympathetic to my situation and had known my mother well. My employer endured my lack of production as I learned—or tried to learn—to balance caretaking and the newly necessitated home-based employment. Without her incredible generosity, my mother would have been just one more statistic in a nursing home.

I learned to do so many near-impossible tasks those last two years of my mother's life. Marion was confined to bed most of the day because she could not get around on her own. To keep her mobile, we would transfer her from bed to wheelchair, which she could push around the house. The insurance company would not provide a motorized wheelchair. Apparently they felt that a short 75-year-old woman with no legs should be able to balance herself in a little seat and push herself around.

She could not take care of her own toileting. We kept a bedpan nearby which was well utilized several times a day. She could not wipe herself. She had to wear "adult diapers." She could not transfer herself from wheelchair to tub. She was completely dependent on us for her personal needs.

But Marion was practical, remember. She had my brother build her some shelves that surrounded the bed where she stored books, cassette tapes, snacks, even an electric skillet that she used to cook her favorite shredded potatoes. There was no keeping her down, and she kept this valiant spirit to the end of her life.

There are so many things I wish I had known—things one would expect to find on the Internet in this age of information. Not so. What was there centered around younger people with a single amputation and learning to walk with a prosthesis. There was precious little about an aged woman with no legs, who couldn't do for herself and never would again.

What lessons did I take away from this experience?

I learned that I should have hired a malpractice attorney right away instead of waiting an entire year. We didn't believe in frivolous lawsuits. We didn't believe it was right to sue a doctor. I still believe that. What we learned is that the only way to find out what really happened in the operating room was to hire a lawyer. The lawyer couldn't restore Marion's legs but was instrumental in revealing the truth. And the truth was, this doctor should never have been allowed to perform delicate vascular surgery. The attorney also discovered that this surgeon had numerous lawsuits against him which had all been settled out of court so as not to appear on his record.

I learned that phantom pain is real. Marion endured increasing "pings" of pain in both legs that progressed in intensity with the march of time. The brain uses a feedback mechanism that sends messages to the legs to function. If the legs don't return the ping, the brain sends out increasingly stronger pain messages to get a response. No legs, no response. We were told the pain would eventually go away. It didn't. We should have insisted on stronger pain medicine to increase her comfort and manage her very real pain.

I would have requested that my mother undergo a simple loop colostomy so that she wouldn't have to worry about defecating on herself. She had a tendency toward loose stools, and once when I was taking her for a "walk" in the wheelchair, she suddenly had to move her bowels. They moved—all over her and all over the wheelchair. It was a horrible mess, and to my everlasting shame, I cried in despair as my mother watched me.

I would have set my alarm every four hours during the night so that I could put the bedpan under my mother. In retrospect, I know there had to be many a night where she lay awake in discomfort while trying to hold her urine. The humiliation of wearing an adult diaper only increases when that diaper is wet.

Good insurance is everything. Most of Marion's medical expenses were paid by Medicare and her HMO. However, the insurance company gave her an uncomfortable, clackety manual wheelchair. I would have insisted they provide a motorized wheelchair with a comfortable seat cushion. I would have insisted that they pay for the Chux we used several times a day to put under my mother's bottom. I would have insisted they buy a decent mattress for the electric bed that I purchased. I would have insisted on a quality bedside commode. (Marion couldn't balance on the cheap one they provided.) I kept a good record of our out-of-pocket expenses. They surpassed $50,000. There went my 401K.

I learned that home health aides weren't very effective in helping my mother. Most of them were tiny foreign women who, despite their best efforts, could not move or bathe a 100-pound woman with a poor sense of balance, and they were often difficult to communicate with.

One of the hardest lessons to learn (because it is not apparent at the time) is that **a parent who is handicapped, handicaps the caretaker**. My mother had intact mental faculties, but she was afraid of being left alone. In an emergency, she knew that she would not be able to vacate the house or even move from the bed. I was with her pretty much 24/7. I gave up every scheduled activity for those two years, including church, and I had to stop the music lessons for my adolescent girls. I simply could not leave the house because of the time I would be away. That was my mother's one fear, and it was justifiable.

This true story has an unbelievable ending. Marion was admitted to the hospital at my insistence because she was having problems breathing. She was put on Coumadin, a blood thinner, because her heart was in atrial fibrillation and would not convert to a normal rhythm. She was transferred to a skilled nursing facility at the insistence of the insurance company until she could be moved back home. It was at this skilled nurs-ing facility that she was given an overdose of Coumadin. When she started hemorrhaging from her nose, mouth, and under her fingernails, she was given a blood transfusion. Unfortunately, they gave her type A blood. Marion was type B. She was dead the next day. The death certificate listed "coagulopathy" as third in a list of medical conditions. We knew better.

The time I spent with my mother had its challenges, but we bonded in a way that we never expected. Today I look back on those two years I spent caring for her as a privilege, not a duty.

Vocabulary Review

acromegaly Abnormal growth of the body, especially facial features and extremities due to excess of pituitary growth hormone.

adenocarcinoma of the prostate The most common malignancy of the prostate, it arises from glandular epithelium. Like benign prostatic hyperplasia (BPH), prostate cancer is an overgrowth of hormone-sensitive secretory cells.

alopecia Hair loss.

amino acid A relatively simple nitrogen-containing organic compound. Of the 20 amino acids that are essential to human metabolism, half can be manufactured in the body and the others must be obtained in the diet.

anemia Deficiency of red blood cells.

blood type A genetically determined and permanent characteristic of a person's red blood cells based on the presence of certain antigens. Two blood type systems of clinical importance are the ABO (comprising types A, B, AB, and O) and the Rh (comprising Rh-positive and Rh-negative).

body mass index (BMI) A measure of the proportion of fat to lean body mass.

bruit A vascular hum synchronous with heartbeat, heard with a stethoscope.

calorie A measurement of the energy released by food.

carbohydrate One of three basic food types, it is the source of energy in the diet which is consumed in the form of starches and sugars.

Chvostek sign Twitching of the face after percussion over the facial nerve in front of the ear, a sign of latent tetany due to hypocalcemia.

clotting factors See *factors, blood clotting.*

corticosteroid Cortisol or aldosterone (hormones of the adrenal cortex), or any synthetic drug having similar effects.

dependent edema Edema of the lower extremities, aggravated by the dependent (downward hanging) position.

diaphoresis Sweating.

Duke bleeding time See *bleeding time.*

dyslipidemia Any of various disorders characterized by abnormally high levels of lipids (cholesterol, triglycerides) in the blood.

dyspnea Shortness of breath.

edema Swelling due to the presence of fluid in tissue spaces.

essential amino acids Amino acids that cannot be made in the body and must be obtained from diet.

euthyroid Normal thyroid.

exophthalmos Bulging or protrusion of one or both eyes (see ■ Figure 9-7).

factors, blood clotting Substances present in the blood that participate in the clotting process.

    Factor I fibrinogen
    Factor II prothrombin
    Factor III tissue thromboplastin
    Factor IV calcium
    Factor V labile factor (proaccelerin)
    Factor VI (term not currently in use)
    Factor VII stable factor (proconvertin)
    Factor VIII antihemophilic globulin (AHG)
    Factor IX Christmas factor
    Factor X Stuart-Prower factor
    Factor XI plasma thromboplastin antecedent
    Factor XII Hageman factor
    Factor XIII fibrin-stabilizing factor

fat One of three basic food types, also called *lipid.* It is an oily or greasy substance built up of fatty acids (long, straight-chain organic acids).

Gleason score A numerical indicator of the malignant potential of prostatic carcinoma, determined by adding the grades of the two least differentiated biopsy specimens. Example: Gleason score 1+2 for a score of 3/10.

glucose A 6-carbon sugar that is the most plentiful in the blood and the principal fuel of cellular energy metabolism.

goiter Enlarged thyroid gland (see ■ Figure 9-4).

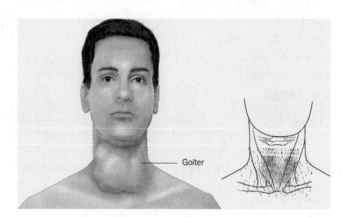

FIGURE 9-4. Goiter of thyroid gland

Hashimoto thyroiditis Chronic autoimmune form of thyroiditis; results in hyposecretion of thyroid hormones.

hormone A chemical messenger or mediator produced by a cell, tissue, or gland.

hyperglycemia Elevated blood glucose.

hyperkalemia Elevation of serum potassium.

hypersecretion Excessive hormone production by an endocrine gland.

hypertension Elevation of blood pressure.

hyperthyroidism Overactive thyroid gland.

hypoglycemia Low level of blood glucose.

hypotension Abnormally low blood pressure.

hypothyroidism Underactive thyroid gland.

infarction Death of tissue due to interruption of its blood supply.

ischemia Inadequate blood supply.

Keith-Wagener-Barker changes Abnormal signs in the retina and retinal vessels due to hypertension and arteriosclerosis, using Roman numerals I through IV.

ketoacidosis, diabetic Accumulation of ketone bodies in the body tissues and fluids from abnormal metabolization of fat.

left shift See *shift to the left.*

LAY AND MEDICAL TERMS

high blood pressure	hypertension
losing hair	alopecia
"mets" (slang)	metastases
sex drive	libido
sugar diabetes	diabetes mellitus
sweating	diaphoresis
swollen feet	dependent edema
water pill	diuretic

lid lag Slowness of upper eyelids to move with eye movements, noted in exophthalmos.

lipid Fat.

myelofibrosis A disorder of the bone marrow, in which the marrow is replaced by scar (fibrous) tissue.

myxedema Abnormal swelling of the skin due to deficiency of thyroid hormone (see ■ Figure 9-6).

nocturia The need to rise from bed to urinate during the night.

non-Hodgkin lymphoma Cancer of the lymphatic tissues other than Hodgkin lymphoma.

normochromic MCHC is in the normal range.

normocytic anemia Erythrocytes normal in size but decreased in number.

nutrition The intake and use of foods by the body.

orthostatic hypotension Low blood pressure brought on by a sudden change in body position, most often when shifting from lying down to standing.

peripheral edema Edema of the extremities.

peripheral neuropathy Damage to the nerves in the lower legs and hands as a result of diabetes mellitus. Symptoms include either extreme sensitivity or numbness and tingling.

The patient has a fairly severe diabetic neuropathy causing postural hypotension. He has decreased pin sensation, stocking-glove fashion, up to about the wrist and the hands, to just about the knees and the legs. This was for pain sensation. Joint position sense appears to be intact.

petechia (pl., petechiae) A very small spot of hemorrhage under the surface of skin or mucous membrane, usually multiple, due to a local or systemic disorder.

pitting edema Edema that retains the mark of the examiner's fingers after release of pressure.

poikilocytosis An abnormally wide variation in the shapes of red blood cells as seen in a stained smear.

polydipsia Excessive thirst.

polyphagia Excessive hunger.

polyuria Excessive urination.

postprandial After meals.

protein One of three basic food types, made up of long strands of amino acids, proteins are responsible for maintenance and repair of tissues and organs, and for production of intracellular enzymes, hormones, and other substances.

ptosis Sagging.

releasing hormone Promotes release of a specific hormone into the circulation.

sella turcica The saddle-shaped bony depression in which the pituitary rests.

shift to the left An increase in the relative number of immature neutrophils, as detected in a differential white blood count. The various types of cells were formerly recorded on forms arranged in columns, the more immature neutrophils being recorded at the extreme left of the form.

sickle cell (sickling) An abnormal red blood cell found in persons with sickle cell anemia; the cell assumes a sickle or crescent shape at reduced oxygen levels (see ■ Figure 9-5).

somatostatin A hormone that inhibits production and release of growth hormone.

spherocytosis Abnormal spherical shape of red blood cells as noted in a stained smear of whole blood on microscopic examination.

staging tumors The process of classifying tumors based on their degree of tissue invasion and the potential response to therapy.

thyromegaly Enlarged thyroid gland.

TNM staging system T refers to the tumor's size and invasion, N to lymph node involvement, and M to

Normal red blood cells

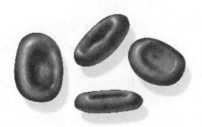

Sickled cells

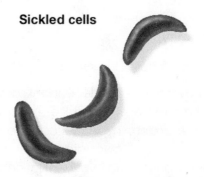

FIGURE 9-5. Comparison of normal-shaped erythrocytes and the abnormal sickle shape noted in patients with sickle cell anemia

the presence of metastases of the tumor cells. Example: T2N0M0 (no spaces between numbers).

tropic hormone Stimulates the cells of a remote gland to produce its secretion.

Trousseau sign Spastic contraction of the hand after application of a constricting cuff to the arm, a sign of latent tetany.

vascular Pertaining to one or more blood vessels.

vasculitis Inflammation of blood vessels.

vitamin An organic compound normally present in many foods that the human body needs in trace amounts, usually to serve as boosters or catalysts in essential metabolic processes.

Medical Readings

History and Physical Examination

by John H. Dirckx, MD

Review of Systems. The physician asks if there are problems with the patient's vision (bulging eyes may be a sign of thyroid disease; loss of vision could indicate retinopathy secondary to diabetes mellitus). Difficulty swallowing or swelling in the neck could be due to thyroid disease. Excessive thirst or urination might indicate diabetes mellitus. Heat or cold intolerance and hair changes might be symptomatic of thyroid disease.

Physical Examination. The amount, distribution, texture, and color of the scalp hair are observed, as well as the pattern of any hair loss. The patient's face not only registers current emotional state but often reflects systemic disease as well. **Myxedema, acromegaly**, and **Cushing syndrome** each produce characteristic changes in facial features.

Any swellings or masses in the neck are palpated for size, shape, consistency, mobility, pulsatility, and

tenderness. The **thyroid gland** is felt and its size and consistency assessed. For this examination the physician may stand behind the patient and have the patient swallow in order to move the gland up and down under the palpating fingers.

Normally the patient sits upright for the eye examination. The orbital margins are inspected for swelling. The lids are observed for evidence of deformity and swelling. Bulging or protrusion of one or both eyes (**exophthalmos**) can result from the type of hyperthyroidism called **Graves disease**.

Metabolism and Nutrition

Metabolism is a general term for the sum of all the chemical and electrical processes that occur in the living body. A principal part of metabolism is the **oxidation** of foods so as to release energy in tiny amounts that are usable at the cellular level. Most metabolic processes are at least partially under the control of hormones.

A **hormone** is a chemical messenger or mediator produced by a cell, tissue, or gland. Hormones are released into the circulation and perform their functions at sites remote from their origins. Some hormones stimulate cellular functions, while others inhibit them. A **tropic hormone** stimulates the cells of a remote gland to produce its secretion, and a **releasing hormone (relin)** promotes release of a specific hormone into the circulation.

Nutrition. Nutrition refers to the intake and use of foods by the body. Each of the three main types of food (**protein, fat, carbohydrate**) has its own function in human nutrition.

A normal adult requires one gram of **protein** per kilogram of body weight per day to supply sufficient materials for maintenance and repair of tissues and organs, and for production of intracellular enzymes, hormones, and other substances. Proteins are built up

HAZARDS OF OBESITY

What's so bad about being overweight?

Obesity is known to be an independent risk factor for many life-threatening and life-shortening conditions (hypertension, hypercholesterolemia, type 2 diabetes mellitus, myocardial infarction, obstructive sleep apnea, and hypoventilation syndrome) as well as for others capable of causing severe distress or disability (osteoarthritis and other orthopedic disorders, infertility, lower extremity venous stasis disease, gastroesophageal reflux disease, and urinary stress incontinence).

Certain common malignancies (cancer of the colon, rectum, and prostate in men, and of the breast, cervix, endometrium, and ovary in women) occur more commonly in obese persons than in those of normal weight.

Lesser degrees of obesity can constitute a significant health hazard in the presence of diabetes mellitus, hypertension, heart disease, or other risk factors. Distribution of excess body fat in central depots (abdominal or male pattern, with an increased waist-to-hip ratio) rather than in peripheral ones (gluteal or female pattern) is associated with higher risks of many of these disorders.

Obese persons are more liable to injury than persons of normal weight. Because they move more slowly, they are more likely to be hit while crossing a street. A larger body is more unwieldy: obese persons are more likely to fall on stairs or in the shower.

An overweight person is more difficult for a physician to examine. Palpation of masses in the abdomen, breasts, or subcutaneous tissues may be virtually impossible. Excess fat also disperses x-rays and renders other imaging techniques less useful. Overweight persons are notoriously poor candidates for thoracic and abdominal surgery, and have a much higher incidence of unsuccessful outcomes, complications, and intraoperative and postoperative mortality.

Not least among the adverse consequences of obesity are social stigmatization, poor self-image, low self-esteem, and the anxiety and depression resulting from them. Overweight persons face occupational discrimination, social rejection, and derision from persons of normal weight, including friends and relations, who are apt to attribute their obesity to a lack of self-discipline or even to moral degeneracy.

The obese tend to have higher rates of unemployment and a lower socioeconomic status, and this is only partly related to their inability to qualify for certain jobs because of size or weight restrictions.

In public they are often the target of rude and disparaging remarks and other tokens of hostility from ignorant and ill-disposed strangers. They can't travel comfortably in compact cars, be accommodated comfortably in restaurants, or fit comfortably into seats in theaters, sports arenas, buses, or airplanes (all of which are designed to cram the maximum number of paying customers into the available space).

Excessive size of trunk and limbs makes for clumsiness in performing many of the activities of daily living. Bathing and personal hygiene may be awkward or impossible for the overweight, particularly in public facilities. Physical exercise, part of any rational program for the treatment of obesity, is often far more difficult for the obese than for persons of normal weight.

Their choice in clothing is sharply limited. Euphemisms used by manufacturers and vendors of clothing who cater to overweight persons (*stout, portly, stocky, corpulent, full-figured, large framed*) can seem almost as offensive as intentionally derogatory street terms.

Surely it must be evident to even the slenderest intelligence that obesity, besides being a very prevalent condition, poses harrowing health risks and generates devastating psychological trauma.

of long strands of **amino acids**, which are relatively simple nitrogen-containing organic compounds that serve as building blocks for all the complex proteins of the human organism. About half of these can be synthesized in the body; the rest, called **essential amino acids**, must be obtained from the diet.

Carbohydrate (consumed in the form of **starches** and **sweets**) is the most important source of energy in most diets. Carbohydrate foods are chemically degraded in the digestive system to simple sugars, especially **glucose**, a 6-carbon sugar that is the most plentiful in the blood and the principal fuel of cellular energy metabolism.

Fats (lipids) are oily or greasy substances built up of **fatty acids** (long, straight-chain organic acids). Fats in the diet come mainly from animal foods, but the term *fat* is often extended to include oils of plant origin.

All three basic types of food can be and are burned in the body as fuel. The amount of energy that a foodstuff can supply can be determined by burning the food outside the body in a **calorimeter** (a small furnace equipped with a sensitive means of measuring heat production). The energy released by food is measured in calories per gram (cal/g). The large calorie or kilocalorie (kcal, 1000 calories) is a more convenient unit of measure in nutrition; in modern parlance, **kilocalories** are usually called simply **calories**.

Whereas proteins and carbohydrates both supply about 4 calories (kcal) per gram, fats supply about 9. The active adult requires 2500–4000 kcal/day: 1200–1800 kcal to meet the energy demands of basic life processes, plus those needed for physical exertion. In the average middle-class American diet, 50% of calories come from carbohydrates, 35% from fat, and 15% from protein.

Water, Minerals, and Vitamins. By convention, the subject of nutrition also includes materials usually not thought of as foods: water, minerals, and vitamins. **Water** is the most abundant substance in the body and the principal constituent of blood. **Intracellular fluid** accounts for about 40% of total body weight, **interstitial fluid** (in tissue spaces, outside of cells) another 15%, and **plasma** (the fluid part of blood) about 5%. The water content of plasma, and indirectly that of the intracellular and interstitial compartments, is regulated within narrow limits by a complex system of checks and balances involving the sensation of thirst, perspiration, gastrointestinal fluid loss, renal excretion and reabsorption of water and electrolytes, and other chemical processes.

Essential dietary **minerals** include iron (needed for the production of red blood cells and as a catalyst in many metabolic processes), calcium (a principal constituent of bones and teeth), sodium, potassium, zinc, magnesium, and many more.

Vitamins are organic compounds, normally present in many foods, that the human body needs in trace amounts, usually to serve as boosters or catalysts in essential metabolic processes.

Disorders of nutrition are relatively common and have many causes, among them overeating, alcoholism, stringent dieting, anorexia nervosa, malabsorption due to inherited abnormalities or to gastrointestinal disease or surgery, and any severe chronic disease including metastatic carcinoma. Specific vitamin deficiencies occur but are rare in our culture. Most nutritional deficiencies are complex and occur as part of a more general pattern of illness.

The most common nutritional disorder, except among the extremely poor, is not undernutrition but **obesity**, an excess of subcutaneous fat in proportion to lean body mass.

> *Endocrine: She says she recently lost 30 pounds by avoiding sweets. She did it because of her diagnosis of diabetes.*

Body Mass Index (BMI) is the weight in kilograms divided by the body surface in square meters, a useful measure of the proportion of fat to lean body mass. The National Institutes of Health (NIH) has defined obesity as a BMI of 30 or more, and overweight as a BMI between 25 and 30. By these criteria, about two thirds of adults in the United States are either overweight or obese, and the prevalence of obesity is increasing in both children and adults. The cause of obesity is unknown, but in most cases it appears to be genetically determined. **Most obese persons do not have faulty eating habits or endocrine disease.**

Obesity is an independent risk factor for hypertension, hypercholesterolemia, type 2 diabetes mellitus, myocardial infarction, some cancers, osteoarthritis, gastroesophageal reflux disease, and a number of other conditions.

> *She also has a history of hypertension, currently controlled. She has mild type 2 diabetes mellitus, which has been controlled with diet.*

Weight reduction leads to reduction in many of these risks, but cannot repair damaged arteries or joints. Most safe and effective weight-reduction programs include a diet low in fat and in total calories and 30 minutes of strenuous physical exercise on most or all days of the week. Other methods include the use of behavior modification therapy, hypnosis, or drugs to suppress appetite, and gastrointestinal surgery to reduce the size of the stomach or diminish intestinal absorption of food.

Pause for Reflection

1. List the 3 main types of food and discuss their role in metabolism and nutrition.
2. The amount of energy that a foodstuff can supply is measured in _____.
3. Discuss the role of water, minerals, and vitamins in metabolism and nutrition.
4. What is one way in which obesity is defined?
5. Discuss the effects of obesity and weight loss on one's health.

Common Endocrine Diseases

Hypothyroidism

A syndrome resulting from deficiency of circulating thyroid hormone. When the disorder appears at birth or in early infancy, it is called **cretinism**; hypothyroidism occurring after early childhood is called **myxedema** (see ■ Figure 9-6).

Causes: Congenital absence or hypoplasia of the thyroid gland; intrinsic thyroid disease (**Hashimoto thyroiditis**); deficiency of dietary iodine; goitrogenic foods, or medicines; deficiency of pituitary thyroid-stimulating hormone.

History: Weakness, lethargy, myalgia, constipation, depression, intolerance to cold, polymenorrhea, weight gain, hoarseness.

Physical Examination: Dry, sallow skin, brittle hair and nails, thinning of scalp hair and outer thirds of eyebrows, puffy face, sluggish speech, bradycardia, nonpitting edema. A **goiter** (see ■ Figure 9-4) may be present when disease is due to iodine deficiency, antithyroid agents, or thyroiditis.

Diagnostic Tests: The T_4 and other measures of thyroid hormone are depressed, the TSH level elevated (except when disease is due to pituitary TSH deficiency). There may be reduction of red blood cells, blood sugar, and sodium, and elevation of cholesterol. Antibody to thyroid may be found in Hashimoto thyroiditis.

Course: With treatment the prognosis is excellent. Complications of untreated disease include coronary artery disease, congestive heart failure, heightened susceptibility to infection, psychosis, and coma.

Treatment: Deficiency of thyroid hormone can be corrected by administration of levothyroxine. Maintenance treatment must be continued indefinitely unless a treatable cause of hypothyroidism can be found and eliminated.

Hyperthyroidism (Thyrotoxicosis)

A syndrome resulting from excessive thyroid hormone in the circulation.

Causes: The principal cause is autoimmune disease of the thyroid gland, with production of thyroid-stimulating immunoglobulin by the immune system. This condition (**Graves disease**) (see ■ Figure 9-7) is eight times more common in women and usually comes on between ages 20 and 40. Graves disease may be accompanied by other autoimmune disorders (pernicious anemia, myasthenia gravis, diabetes mellitus). Less common causes of hyperthyroidism are acute thyroiditis and inappropriate administration of thyroid hormone.

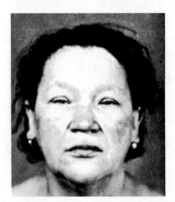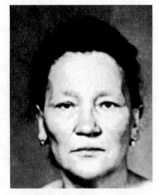

FIGURE 9-6 . (Left) Myxedema of the face, with somnolent look. and stiff hair. (Right) After 3 months of treatment with thyroxine. Source: Pearson Education, PH College.

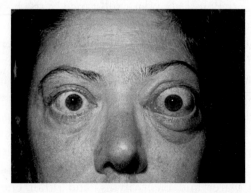

FIGURE 9-7 . A woman with exophthalmos (Graves disease). Source: Chet Childs, Custom Medical Stock Photo.

History of Graves disease about 30 years ago with significant and severe exophthalmos to the point that she cannot even close her eyes fully. She is status post multiple decompression surgeries for exophthalmos as well as other plastic surgery-type procedures to try to get her eyes to close without success.

History: Restlessness, nervousness, fatigue, intolerance to heat, sweating, cardiac palpitations, weight loss, frequent bowel movements, menstrual irregularities, enlargement of thyroid gland (goiter). In Graves disease, bulging of eyes, conjunctival drying or irritation.

Physical Examination: Tachycardia, warmth and moistness of skin, resting tremor of hands, hyperactive deep tendon reflexes, loosening of nails. In Graves disease, diffuse or nodular enlargement of thyroid, sometimes with arterial **bruit** (a vascular hum synchronous with heartbeat, heard with a stethoscope); **exophthalmos** (undue prominence of eyes due to edema of orbital contents), staring gaze, **lid lag** (slowness of upper eyelids to move with eye movements).

Diagnostic Tests: The levels of T_3 and T_4 are elevated, and TSH is depressed. The radioactive iodine uptake is increased. Thyroid-stimulating immunoglobulin is present in the serum. Antinuclear antibody may also be present. There may be mild anemia and hypercalcemia.

Course: Complications include atrial fibrillation, paralysis, and hypercalcemia.

Treatment: End-organ effects of thyroid hormone (tachycardia, tremor, restlessness) can be reduced by beta-blocker treatment. Glandular hyperactivity can be reduced by antithyroid medicines (propylthiouracil, methimazole), radioactive iodine, or thyroidectomy.

She has had a thyroidectomy and multiple thyroid surgeries. She has had multiple eye surgeries for exophthalmos.

Hypoparathyroidism

Causes: The most common cause is accidental removal of the parathyroid glands during thyroidectomy. Rarely the parathyroid glands may be damaged by trauma, infection, neoplasm, or chemical poisons, or by autoantibodies, which may be formed in the polyglandular autoimmune syndrome.

History: With acute onset, tetany, tingling of face, hands, and feet, muscle cramps, **carpopedal spasm** (painful cramps of wrists and ankles), laryngospasm with respiratory obstruction, seizures. With more chronic onset, mental retardation, abnormalities of bones and teeth, cataract, parkinson-like disorder due to calcification of basal ganglia.

Physical Examination: The skin may be dry and coarse. Deep tendon reflexes are hyperactive, and the **Chvostek sign** (twitching of face after percussion over facial nerve in front of ear) and **Trousseau sign** (spastic contraction of the hand after application of a constricting cuff to the arm) are present.

Diagnostic Tests: The serum calcium is low and the serum phosphorus is high. Excretion of phosphorus in the urine is reduced. The level of parathyroid hormone in the serum is low.

Treatment: Calcium replacement, intravenously in acute tetany, and vitamin D. Treatment must be continued indefinitely.

Adrenal Insufficiency (Addison Disease)

An acute or chronic **deficiency of cortisol** and related hormones from the adrenal cortex.

Causes: Degeneration of the adrenal cortices, usually as an autoimmune phenomenon sometimes involving other endocrine glands as well. Other diseases (infection, malignant tumors) may account for destruction of the adrenal glands in rare cases. Deficiency of pituitary ACTH also causes some adrenal insufficiency, but not the full-blown clinical picture of Addison disease. Adrenal crisis may be precipitated by severe physical stress (surgery), systemic disease (meningococcemia), or by sudden withdrawal of steroid therapy.

History: Weakness, easy fatigability, anorexia, nausea, vomiting, diarrhea, abdominal pain, amenorrhea, emotional lability. In addisonian crisis, fever, confusion, collapse, coma.

Physical Examination: Weight loss, wasting, hypotension, sparseness of axillary hair; increased pigmentation of skin, especially over pressure points, skin creases, and nipples. In crisis, severe hypotension and evidence of dehydration.

Diagnostic Tests: The eosinophil count is elevated. The serum sodium is low, the potassium and BUN (blood urea nitrogen) elevated. Serum cortisol is abnormally low and does not rise in response to administration of ACTH. Chest x-ray shows a small vertical heart.

The patient is a 40-year-old woman with autoimmune-induced Addison disease. She also has severe migraine headaches.

Course: Without treatment, steady progression is likely. Addisonian crisis can be rapidly fatal. Fluid and electrolyte depletion, wasting, cardiovascular collapse.

Treatment: The basic treatment is replacement of missing corticosteroids. Supportive treatment and elimination of any identifiable underlying or precipitating cause are important. In crisis, intravenous fluid and electrolyte replacement may be lifesaving.

Cushing Syndrome (Hyperadrenocorticism)

A syndrome due to prolonged elevation of adrenal cortical hormones in the circulation (see ■ Figure 9-8).

Causes: The most frequent cause of Cushing syndrome today is medicinal administration of adrenocortical hormones. The condition can also result from production of excessive adrenocortical hormones by a neoplasm of the adrenal cortex, from medicinal administration of ACTH, or from production of ACTH-like substances by other neoplasms (such as bronchogenic carcinoma). When excessive adrenal cortical activity results from an elevated level of ACTH from a tumor (basophil adenoma) of the pituitary, the condition is called Cushing disease.

History: Increasing obesity, stretch marks (especially on trunk and thighs), acne, easy bruising, impaired wound healing, weakness, thirst, headache, amenorrhea or impotence, increased body hair, personality change.

Physical Examination: Truncal obesity, moon face, **buffalo hump** (soft tissue prominence over upper back), protuberant abdomen with purple striae (stretch marks), hirsutism, acne, hypertension.

Diagnostic Tests: Blood glucose is elevated and potassium is low. The serum level of cortisol is high and does not fall after administration of dexamethasone, a synthetic corticosteroid. Urinary excretion of cortisol is also increased. In Cushing disease and other disorders due to excessive ACTH, the blood level of ACTH is elevated. Otherwise the ACTH level is subnormal, its production by the pituitary having been suppressed by high circulating levels of corticosteroid. An adrenal tumor may be shown by abdominal CT scan. Tumor of the pituitary is identified by cranial MRI.

Course: Depends on the origin of the problem. Untreated Cushing syndrome can be complicated by osteoporosis, nephrolithiasis, psychosis, heightened susceptibility to infection, and consequences of hypertension and diabetes mellitus; it is generally fatal within a few years.

Treatment: Discontinuance of corticosteroid treatment, or reduction of dose. Surgical removal of a causative pituitary or adrenal neoplasm. Ketoconazole or metyrapone can be used to suppress cortisol levels when surgery is not feasible.

Type 1 Diabetes Mellitus

Cause: A lack of insulin in the circulation due to failure of pancreatic B cells to respond to normal stimuli to insulin production (see ■ Figure 9-9). Failure of insulin production may be due to toxic, infectious, or autoimmune damage to B cells in genetically predisposed persons.

History: **Polyuria** (increased output of urine), **polydipsia** (excessive thirst), **polyphagia** (excessive appetite), weakness, and weight loss, coming on gradually or suddenly, usually in a person under 40 years of age. With fulminant onset, type 1 diabetes mellitus may present as **ketoacidosis** with dyspnea, drowsiness, collapse, and coma.

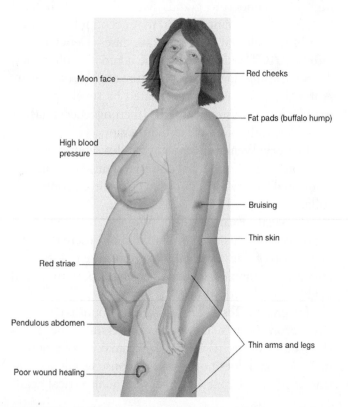

Moon face

Red cheeks

Fat pads (buffalo hump)

High blood pressure

Bruising

Thin skin

Red striae

Pendulous abdomen

Thin arms and legs

Poor wound healing

FIGURE 9-8 . Cushing syndrome caused by hyperadrenocorticism

IMPRESSION:
Diabetes mellitus, type 2. Hypoglycemia secondary to oral hypoglycemic agents in the face of renal insufficiency, leading to hypoglycemia. Hyperkalemia, acute, secondary to her renal insufficiency and being on ACE inhibitors.

Physical Examination: Unremarkable in uncomplicated diabetes. In ketoacidosis: tachypnea, tachycardia, hypotension, flushing, fruity breath, and stupor or coma. Symptoms of cardiovascular, neurologic, or ocular complications may be evident in long-established or neglected disease.

Diagnostic Tests: Fasting blood sugar is over 140 mg/dL, and 2-hour postprandial blood sugar is over 200 mg/dL. Sugar is present in the urine. Serum cholesterol is often elevated. In ketoacidosis, ketones are found in the serum and the urine, and there is chemical evidence of metabolic acidosis (low blood pH, low blood HCO_3). Glycosylated hemoglobin (HbA_{1c}) reflects blood sugar levels over the preceding few weeks and is used to monitor control. Laboratory studies may also show evidence of systemic complications (infection, renal disease).

Course: Type 1 diabetes mellitus is a lifelong derangement of carbohydrate metabolism. In most patients, careful attention to diet and general health and proper use of insulin permit good control of blood sugar and fair protection against complications. Diabetes predisposes to numerous other conditions, including hypercholesterolemia, atherosclerosis, ocular cataracts and retinopathy, renal disease, infections of the urinary tract, skin, and other tissues, neuropathy, and microvascular disease in the extremities.

Treatment: Type 1 diabetes mellitus is by definition a disease that must be treated with insulin as a condition of the patient's survival. The mainstay of treatment, however, is diet, with limitation of total calories and restriction of carbohydrate and cholesterol. Increased fiber helps to stabilize carbohydrate metabolism, and artificial sweeteners are substituted for sugar. Injections of insulin are given 1–4 times a day. The patient monitors plasma glucose level by self-testing of fingerstick blood with a portable electronic glucometer. A variety of insulin products are available with different patterns of absorption and peak activity.

The proper management of diabetes requires scrupulous attention to general health, care of the skin and the feet, and vigorous treatment of complications. Regular eye examinations and periodic testing for microalbuminuria provide early detection of retinop-

athy and nephropathy respectively. Diabetic ketoacidosis is treated with intravenous fluids, insulin, and general supportive measures.

Type 2 Diabetes Mellitus

Cause: A relative deficiency of circulating insulin accompanied by insensitivity or resistance of tissues, particularly liver and muscle, to insulin effect (see ■ Figure 9-9). There is a genetic predisposition to this form of diabetes, but the mechanism of transmission is unknown. Type 2 diabetes mellitus accounts for 90% of all cases of diabetes mellitus. Most patients are over 40 and obese.

History: The condition may remain asymptomatic for months or years. Polyuria, polydipsia, and sometimes weakness or fatigue occur as in insulin-dependent disease, but weight loss and ketoacidosis do not occur.

Physical Examination: Unremarkable except for obesity, unless complications have developed. Hypertension is often present.

Diagnostic Tests: Fasting blood sugar over 140 mg/dL; 2-hour postprandial blood sugars over 180 mg/dL. There is often sugar in the urine. Ketones are not found in serum. The cholesterol is often elevated. With advanced disease there may be chemical or electrocardiographic evidence of complications.

Course: Mild type 2 diabetes mellitus may cause few symptoms, particularly with treatment. Complications are the same as those for type 1 diabetes mellitus, with the exception of ketoacidosis. Complications typically do not develop as rapidly or become as severe as type 1 diabetes.

Treatment: Dietary restriction of carbohydrate alone may suffice to control blood sugar levels and abolish symptoms of polyuria and fatigue. Cholesterol restriction is also advised. Drugs such as pioglitazone and rosiglitazone help to overcome insulin resistance. Alpha-glucosidase inhibitors (acarbose, miglitol) impede absorption of dietary carbohydrate. To achieve optimal control, the use of insulin may be required. Care of general health and avoidance of skin injury and infection are important in the management of all forms of diabetes.

Carcinoma of the Pancreas

Causes: Carcinoma of the pancreas ranks fourth among malignant tumors as a cause of death in the U.S. It is more common in men, and most cases occur after age 60. Other risk factors are obesity, cigarette smoking,

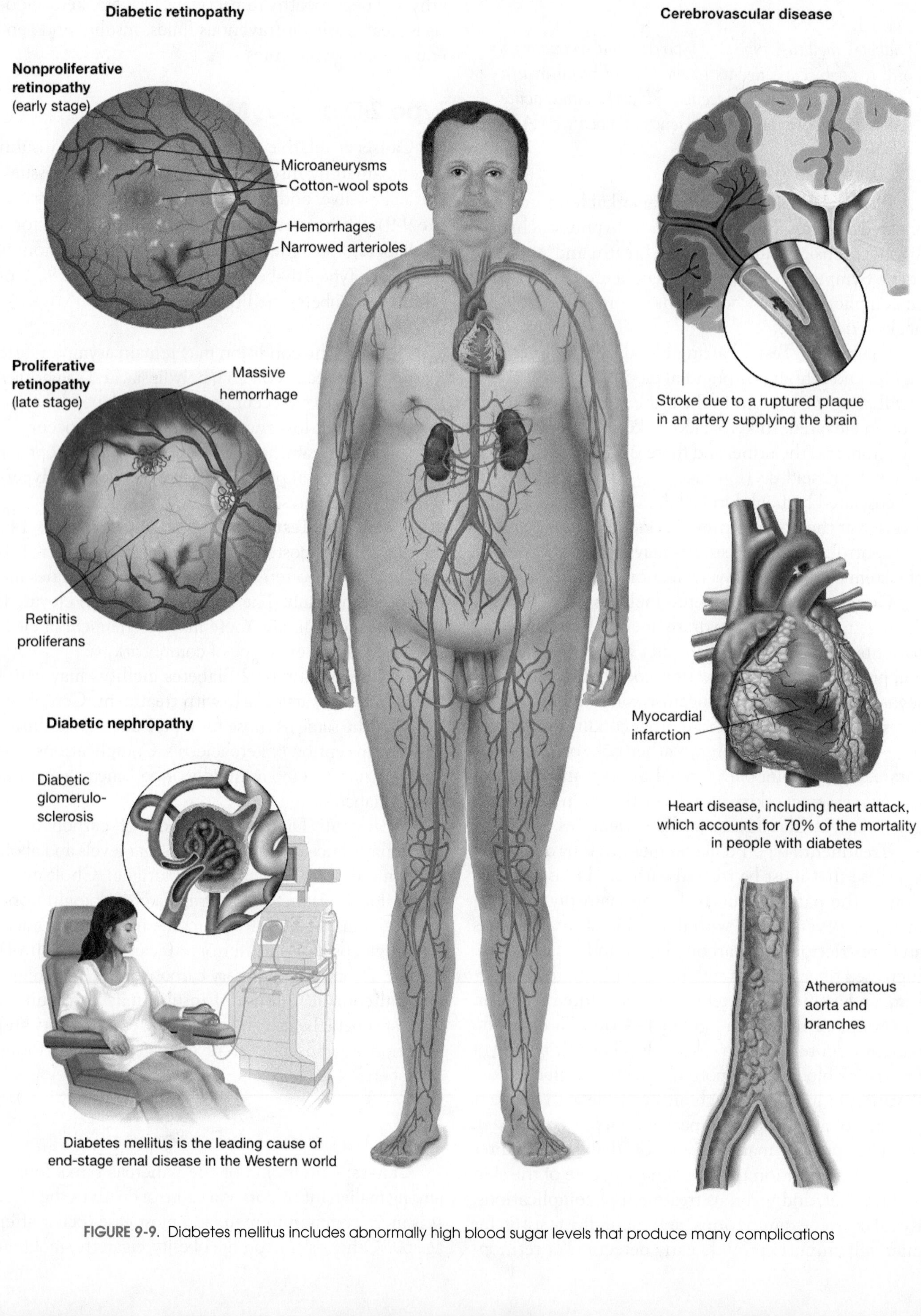

Diabetic retinopathy

Cerebrovascular disease

Nonproliferative retinopathy
(early stage)

Microaneurysms
Cotton-wool spots

Hemorrhages
Narrowed arterioles

Stroke due to a ruptured plaque
in an artery supplying the brain

Proliferative retinopathy
(late stage)

Massive
hemorrhage

Retinitis
proliferans

Myocardial
infarction

Heart disease, including heart attack,
which accounts for 70% of the mortality
in people with diabetes

Diabetic nephropathy

Diabetic
glomerulo-
sclerosis

Atheromatous
aorta and
branches

Diabetes mellitus is the leading cause of
end-stage renal disease in the Western world

FIGURE 9-9. Diabetes mellitus includes abnormally high blood sugar levels that produce many complications

and type 2 diabetes mellitus. Most tumors are **ductal cell adenocarcinomas** arising in the head of the gland.

History: Symptoms are insidious in onset and include anorexia, indigestion, weight loss, weakness, and fatigue.

Diagnostic Tests: Imaging studies (CT, MRI, ultrasound), laparoscopy, and pancreatic biopsy can provide a specific diagnosis but are often not performed early enough. Serum markers such as pancreatic oncofetal antigen (POA), alpha fetoprotein (AFP), carcinoembryonic antigen (CEA), CA 19-9, and CA 125 are often useful in following the progress of the disease once it is recognized but are too nonspecific to establish a diagnosis.

Course: By the time clear-cut indications of trouble such as abdominal pain, jaundice, ascites, and sudden onset of diabetes mellitus appear, most patients have invasion of the portal vein or the superior mesenteric artery, metastases to regional nodes, liver, adrenals, lungs, bone, and elsewhere, or tumors too large for resection.

Treatment: Such patients are candidates only for **palliative treatment** (radiation, chemotherapy, surgery to relieve biliary obstruction). Resectable tumors are treated with the **Whipple procedure** (pancreaticoduodenectomy). The overall five-year survival rate for pancreatic carcinoma is less than 3%.

Metabolic Syndrome

A combination of metabolic disorders (obesity, hypertension, insulin resistance, hyperlipidemias, and others) associated with a high incidence of cardiovascular disease and premature death.

Cause: Genetic predisposition to insulin resistance, compounded by overeating and a sedentary lifestyle.

History: Overweight, often from childhood. Inactive lifestyle. Hypertension, hyperglycemia often noted early in life. Premature symptoms of cardiovascular disease.

Physical Examination: Obesity (waist circumference over 40 inches [102 cm] in men and over 35 inches [88 cm] in women). Systolic blood pressure over 130, diastolic pressure over 85. Signs of premature

Diabetes mellitus type 1. Will continue her regular insulin per sliding scale and check her hemoglobin A1c; when she is eating, we will transition her back to some longer-acting insulin with 70/30.

Diabetes mellitus type 1 for 43 years. She describes herself as a brittle diabetic with volatile sugars up and down.

cardiovascular disease may be evident on examination of ocular fundi, heart, peripheral vessels.

Diagnostic Tests: Fasting plasma glucose of 100 mg/dL (5.55 mmol/L) or higher. High-density lipoprotein (HDL) cholesterol less than 40 mg/dL (1.04 mmol/L) in men and less than 50 mg/dL (1.30 mmol/L) in women. Triglyceride 150 mg/dL (1.70 mmol/L) or more. Elevated low-density lipoprotein (LDL) cholesterol, plasma insulin, and uric acid.

Course: Characterized by early and rapid development of the usual complications of obesity, hypertension, hyperglycemia, and dyslipidemia. Progression to type 2 diabetes mellitus is expected.

Treatment: Weight control, regular aerobic exercise. Drug treatment of hypertension, hyperglycemia, and lipid abnormalities as appropriate.

Pause for Reflection

1. Distinguish between hypothyroidism and hyperthyroidism.
2. What 2 signs may be present in hypoparathyroidism? How is hypoparathyroidism treated?
3. Distinguish between Addison disease and Cushing syndrome.
4. Distinguish between type 1 and type 2 diabetes mellitus.
5. How is pancreatic cancer treated?
6. What is metabolic syndrome?

Common Blood Disorders

Iron Deficiency Anemia

Anemia due to deficient iron stores; the most common type of anemia.

Cause: Depletion of iron stores usually results from chronic or recurring blood loss (gastrointestinal hemorrhage, menstruation, repeated blood donation). It can also occur in certain metabolic states (pregnancy, chronic infection) and, rarely, because of inadequate iron intake (vegetarians, dieters).

History: Fatigue, poor exercise tolerance, cardiac palpitation, shortness of breath. Dysphagia occurs in

A 56-year-old white female was admitted because of severe anemia. She had hypertension and hyperlipidemia which were well controlled. The stool was brown but strongly Hemoccult positive. It was felt that she had significant blood loss.

Plummer-Vinson syndrome (due to formation of esophageal webs). Pica (eating nonfood materials such as clay).

Physical Examination: Pallor, tachycardia, smooth tongue, brittle nails, **cheilosis** (chapping and fissuring of lips).

Diagnostic Tests: The red blood cell count is abnormally low. With advanced disease, cells become **microcytic** (smaller than normal; MCV reduced) and **hypochromic** (containing less hemoglobin than normal; MCH reduced). Abnormal cells, including **target cells** (cells so thin that the central portions of opposite sides touch, causing a bull's-eye appearance), may occur. The serum iron and serum ferritin are abnormally low. Administration of iron produces a prompt improvement in the red blood cell count, with elevated reticulocyte count. Diagnostic evaluation may include an aggressive search for a site of blood loss.

Treatment: Oral iron replacement continued for several months restores the red blood cell values and serum iron and ferritin to normal.

Pernicious Anemia

A chronic anemia due to deficiency of vitamin B_{12} absorption.

Cause: Pernicious anemia is an inherited autoimmune disorder that typically does not cause symptoms until after the age of 35. The biochemical cause is lack of secretion of intrinsic factor by glands in the gastric mucosa, with resultant failure to absorb vitamin B_{12}. All patients have **gastric achlorhydria** (lack of hydrochloric acid in gastric juice). Neurologic symptoms (ataxia, confusion, dementia) eventually occur.

History: Gradual onset of weakness, paresthesia in the fingers and toes, dysequilibrium, anorexia, sore tongue, and diarrhea.

The patient was noted to have a low B12 level, and it was felt that she should receive B12 replacement therapy as an outpatient. It was felt that this may have been a contributing factor to the severity of her anemia.

Physical Examination: Pallor, icterus. The tongue appears red and smooth. Ataxic gait, diminished sense of vibration and position in extremities; later, loss of perception of light touch and pinprick.

Diagnostic Tests: The red blood cell count is low. Red blood cells are large (**macrocytosis**; increased MCV) and variable in size (**anisocytosis**). The reticulocyte count is low. Polymorphonuclear leukocytes have multilobulated nuclei. Bone marrow smear shows large precursors of red blood cells with abnormal morphology. The serum indirect bilirubin is elevated. The serum vitamin B_{12} is abnormally low. The Schilling test (administration of radioactively tagged B_{12} orally before and after administration of intrinsic factor) shows an increase in the urinary excretion of B_{12}. Endoscopy shows atrophic gastritis, and chemical studies indicate achlorhydria.

Course: This is an irreversible condition requiring lifelong treatment, without which neurologic damage may become irreversible. There is a heightened risk of gastric carcinoma in persons with achlorhydria.

Treatment: Administration of vitamin B_{12} regularly throughout life.

Aplastic Anemia

Failure of marrow production of red blood cells (also white blood cells and platelets).

Cause: Damage to bone marrow by chemicals (benzene), drugs (chloramphenicol), radiation, neoplastic infiltration, or autoantibodies.

History: Gradual onset of weakness, fatigue, dyspnea, headache.

Physical Examination: Pallor, **purpura** or **petechiae**, tachycardia, oral or pharyngeal infection or ulceration.

Diagnostic Tests: The red blood cell, white blood cell, and platelet counts are abnormally low. Marrow smear shows hypoplastic or acellular marrow.

Treatment: Blood transfusion to correct anemia. Oxygen and control of hemorrhage as needed. Antibiotics for infection. Corticosteroids, immunosuppressive agents, colony stimulating factors. Marrow transplantation if possible.

Acute Lymphocytic Leukemia (ALL) (Acute Lymphoblastic Leukemia)

A rapidly progressive hematologic malignancy of children.

Cause: Mutation of lymphocyte precursor cells, possibly due to drugs, radiation, or genetic predisposition or chromosomal aberration. Onset is in childhood, usually before age five.

History: Pallor, weakness, irritability, repeated infections, bleeding tendency, bone pain, headache, stiff neck, vomiting, cranial nerve palsies and other neurologic abnormalities.

Physical Examination: Pallor, lethargy, neurologic findings, evidence of opportunistic infections, hemorrhagic phenomena.

Diagnostic Tests: The white blood cell count may be low, elevated, or normal. Anemia and thrombocytopenia are often present. Serum levels of uric acid and creatinine may be elevated. Bone marrow examination shows replacement of normal elements by infiltrations of blast cells. Cerebrospinal fluid shows lymphoblasts (extremely immature lymphocytes) in central nervous system involvement. Imaging studies including radionuclide bone scans may show abnormalities due to infiltration of organs or tissues by malignant lymphoblastic cells.

Course: The disease is ordinarily fatal in less than six months. With vigorous treatment, many patients achieve long-term survival and apparent cure. Anemia, thrombocytopenia, susceptibility to infection, invasion of the central nervous system (50%), and infiltration and damage of the liver and other organs often prove lethal.

Treatment: Chemotherapy with vincristine, daunorubicin, or asparaginase, combined with corticosteroid. For central nervous system involvement, cranial irradiation and injection of methotrexate intrathecally (into the subarachnoid space). Control of anemia (transfusions if necessary), bleeding, and infection; personal and family counseling.

Chronic Myelogenous Leukemia (CML)

A malignancy of the marrow characterized by markedly elevated levels of circulating white blood cells formed there, with immature and abnormal cells.

Cause: The **Philadelphia chromosome**, the first oncogene to be associated with a specific malignancy; this is a reciprocal translocation of strands of genes between chromosomes 9 and 22. It results in malignant proliferation of myelogenous (marrow-produced) white blood cells (granulocytes and monocytes), which, however, retain their functions for years, until the disease reaches its terminal stage. Onset generally occurs in middle life (30s, 40s, and 50s).

History: Weakness, fatigue, fever, night sweats, bone pain.

Physical Examination: Low fever, enlargement of the spleen, tenderness over the sternum due to hyperactive marrow.

Laboratory Tests: Marked elevation of the white blood cell count, with modest increases in immature forms. Other cells in the circulation are generally normal in number and form. The uric acid may be elevated. Marrow smear shows increased cellularity and increased immature white blood cells. Chromosomal studies identify the Philadelphia chromosome.

Course: Usual survival is less than five years. Long-term survival, and apparent cure, however, occur in half of patients who undergo successful bone marrow transplantation. The disease typically ends in a phase of greatly accelerated production of wholly immature and undifferentiated stem cells (blastic crisis), in which marrow dysfunction can lead to marked anemia, bleeding disorders, and toxemia.

Treatment: Largely supportive and palliative. Chemical suppressants of marrow activity (hydroxyurea, interferon alfa) lower white blood cell counts and mitigate symptoms. In the blast stage, chemotherapy protocols including vincristine, daunorubicin, and prednisone provide brief remission. Allogeneic bone marrow transplant (from a sibling or unrelated donor matched with respect to critical antigens, particularly HLA) is apparently curative in about one half of patients, and is more likely to be effective in younger patients.

Chronic Lymphocytic Leukemia (CLL)

A malignancy of B lymphocytes.

Cause: Malignant change in a B-cell precursor, with formation of a clone of abnormal immunologically incompetent cells. This results in infiltration of bone marrow and other tissues with abnormal lymphocytes and failure of immune response. Most cases occur in the middle-aged and elderly.

History: Gradual onset of weakness and fatigue, often with enlarged lymph nodes. In some asymptomatic patients the condition is discovered incidentally on routine blood testing.

Physical Examination: Enlargement of lymph nodes, liver, spleen, or all of these. Pallor or jaundice may be present.

Diagnostic Tests: Relative and absolute **lymphocytosis** (increase in the percentage of lymphocytes among white blood cells, and in their total number). The lymphocytes are small but normal in appearance.

Bone marrow may show infiltrations of lymphocytes. Red blood cell or platelet count may be reduced. There may be a deficiency of IgG in serum.

Course: Typically chronic, with mild or absent symptoms. Most patients survive 5–10 years after diagnosis. Possible complications include autoimmune hemolytic anemia, thrombocytopenia, and **lymphoma** (development of a malignant solid neoplasm of lymphoid tissue).

Treatment: Largely supportive and palliative. Chlorambucil, fludarabine, and adrenal corticosteroids may be used in severe or terminal disease. **Splenectomy** may be needed to control hemolytic anemia.

Hodgkin Disease (Lymphoma)

Cause: Unknown. Genetic influences and viral infection have been implicated, but without conclusive proof (see ■ Figure 9-10).

History: Painless enlargement of one or more lymph nodes, fever, sweats, pruritus, abdominal pain (aggravated by alcohol).

Physical Examination: Enlargement of lymph nodes, possibly spleen; fever. Infiltration of skin may occur.

Diagnostic Tests: Lymph node biopsy shows **Reed-Sternberg cells** (characteristic large cells with two nuclei).

Prognosis: The overall survival rate is about 50%; with early diagnosis and treatment, about 80%.

Treatment: Radiation, chemotherapy.

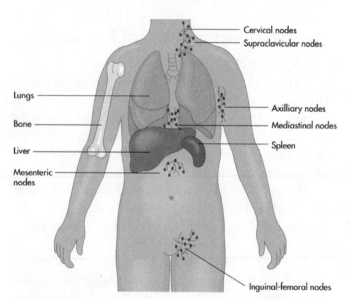

FIGURE 9-10. Lymph nodes and organs affected in Hodgkin disease in children

Non-Hodgkin Lymphoma

A variegated group of lymphocyte malignancies (see ■ Figure 9-11). Oncogenes have been identified for some types.

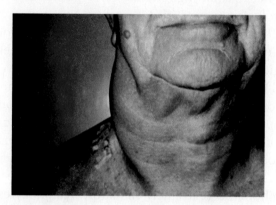

Figure 9-11. Non-Hodgkin lymphoma.
Source: Dr. P. Marazzi, Photo Researchers, Inc.

History: Painless enlargement of lymph nodes, fever, sweats, weight loss, abdominal pain.

Physical Examination: Enlargement of lymph nodes, spleen.

Diagnostic Tests: The peripheral blood may be normal. Lymph node biopsy shows characteristic malignant changes, and bone marrow biopsy shows infiltration of abnormal lymphoid aggregates. The serum LDH is elevated. Chest x-ray and CT scan of the abdomen and pelvis may show hilar and abdominal or pelvic lymphadenopathy.

Treatment: Radiation, chemotherapy, bone marrow transplantation.

Coagulation Disorders (Coagulopathies)

Deficiency or lack of any of the plasma clotting factors, including fibrinogen and prothrombin, can occur as an isolated genetic defect (see ■ Figure 9-12).

Classical hemophilia (**hemophilia A**), due to congenital deficiency of Factor VIII, is transmitted as a sex-linked recessive trait, carried by females but expressed only in males. **Hemophilia B** (Factor IX disease, Christmas disease) shows a similar pattern of inheritance. Acquired deficiency of prothrombin (**hypoprothrombinemia**) is more frequent than congenital deficiency. It can result from deficiency of vitamin K (an essential chemical building block for prothrombin), hepatic disease (particularly biliary obstruction, which blocks absorption of vitamin K by preventing passage of bile salts into the bowel), or treat-

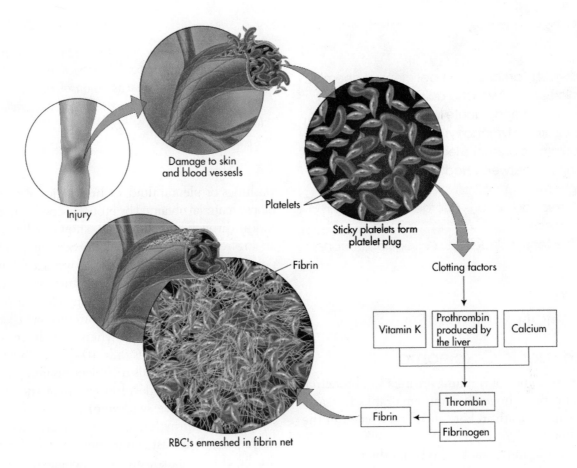

Injury

Damage to skin
and blood vessesls

Platelets

Sticky platelets form
platelet plug

Clotting factors

Fibrin

| Vitamin K | Prothrombin produced by the liver | Calcium |

Thrombin

Fibrin ← Fibrinogen

RBC's enmeshed in fibrin net

FIGURE 9-12. The clotting process (coagulation)

ment with coumarin anticoagulants. Acquired or congenital **deficiency of plasma clotting factors** causes a hemorrhagic tendency of variable severity characterized by prolonged bleeding from wounds, hematoma formation, hemarthrosis (bleeding into joints), and hematuria (blood in the urine).

Congenital or acquired deficiency of platelets (**thrombocytopenia**) is associated with **petechiae** (pinpoint hemorrhages in the skin) or **purpura** (larger skin hemorrhages). Frank or severe hemorrhage occurs less frequently. Idiopathic thrombocytopenic purpura (ITP) is an autoimmune disorder of children, usually benign and self-limited. In **thrombotic thrombocytopenic purpura (TTP)**, deficiency of platelets may be accompanied by hemolytic anemia, renal impairment, and bizarre neurologic manifestations. The acute form may progress rapidly to a fatal termination. In **Glanzmann disease** (thrombasthenia), the platelet count is normal but platelet function is impaired.

Hemorrhagic manifestations, usually purpuric, also occur in certain diseases of blood vessels. In hereditary hemorrhagic telangiectasia (**Osler-Weber-Rendu disease**), recurrent bleeding occurs from telangiectases in the skin and mucous membranes. **Von Willebrand disease** is a hereditary hemorrhagic disorder, often mild, characterized by deficiency of Factor VIII, abnormal platelet function, and vascular abnormalities. Examples of acquired vascular disorders accompanied by purpuric bleeding include **Henoch-Schoenlein purpura, Cushing syndrome**, and **scurvy**.

Disseminated intravascular coagulation (DIC), which results from imbalance between the mechanisms of coagulation and of fibrinolysis, can be induced by **infection** (meningococcemia , Rocky Mountain spotted fever, septicemia), trauma, shock, complications of pregnancy and parturition, and myelocytic leukemia. Clinical manifestations range from widespread bleeding to widespread intravascular thrombosis, and both of these may occur together.

Precise diagnosis of a **hemorrhagic disorder** depends on the results of several basic tests, which are often performed together as a **coagulation panel**: platelet count, bleeding time, clotting time, prothrombin time, partial thromboplastin time, and clot retraction. In addition, **plasma assay** for specific coagulation factors is possible.

Pause for Reflection

1. Distinguish among iron-deficiency anemia, pernicious anemia, and aplastic anemia.
2. Distinguish among acute lymphocytic leukemia (ALL), chronic lymphocytic leukemia (CLL), and chronic myelogenous leukemia (CML).
3. Distinguish between Hodgkin and non-Hodgkin lymphoma.
4. Define coagulation disorder and list three examples.
5. List the tests included in a coagulation panel.

Common Cancers

Bronchogenic Carcinoma

A malignant tumor of the lung arising from bronchial epithelium. Bronchogenic carcinoma ranks first as a cause of cancer death in both men and women in the United States.

Causes: Cigarette smoking is by far the most common cause of bronchogenic carcinoma. About 10% of regular smokers will develop lung cancer. Prolonged inhalation of second-hand smoke causes about 3000 deaths a year in the United States. Inhalation of industrial carcinogens (particularly asbestos, silica, chromium, nickel, and polyvinyl chloride) and exposure to ionizing radiation or radon are other known causes.

History: Gradual onset of cough (or change in a chronic cough), dyspnea, wheezing, hemoptysis, anorexia, weight loss, chest pain.

Physical Examination: May indicate weight loss, muscle wasting, or signs of bronchial obstruction, pneumonia, atelectasis, cavitation, or pleural effusion.

Diagnostic Tests: Chest x-ray or CT scan demonstrates a solitary nodule, infiltrate, atelectasis, cavitation, or pleural effusion. Cytologic examination of bronchial

A CT scan of the chest obtained immediately prior to admission revealed a 4.0 x 3.7 cm ill-defined pleural-based mass in the right upper lobe medially, with associated invasion and destruction of the fifth thoracic vertebra, an additional 2.0 cm lingular mass, focal bronchiectasis in the lingula, shotty mediastinal lymph nodes, and cholelithiasis.

The patient underwent a flexible bronchoscopy, right thoracotomy, right upper lobe lobectomy. The patient's preoperative diagnosis was lesion of right upper lobe. Postoperative diagnosis was carcinoma, right upper lobe.

washings or pleural fluid, or histologic examination of biopsy material obtained by bronchoscopy or needle aspiration through the chest wall, shows malignant tissue arising from bronchial epithelium. Screening of high-risk populations (for example, smokers over age 60) with low-radiation, high-resolution CT, sputum cytology, or both can often detect disease early enough for cure.

Course: Bronchogenic carcinoma is typically advanced and inoperable when first diagnosed. The five-year survival rate is only 10–15%. Obstruction of airways commonly leads to atelectasis and pneumonia. Complications include obstruction of the vena cava (superior vena cava syndrome) or esophagus, cardiac tamponade or arrhythmia, neurologic disorders (phrenic nerve palsy, **Pancoast syndrome** due to involvement of the brachial plexus), and **paraneoplastic syndromes** (Cushing syndrome, hypercalcemia) due to production of hormone-like agents by tumor cells.

Treatment: Surgery, radiation, and chemotherapy.

Breast Cancer

A malignant tumor of the female breast, arising most frequently from ductal epithelium. The commonest cancer in women, and the second-commonest cause of cancer death (after lung cancer) in women. One in eight or nine women will develop breast cancer.

Cause: Women who have no children, or whose first pregnancy occurs late in the childbearing years, are at increased risk of breast cancer. So are women who have a family history of breast cancer, particularly cancer occurring at an early age in one or more female relatives, which may be associated with the BRCA1 or BRCA2 oncogene. According to most authorities, the risk of breast cancer is slightly increased by estrogen replacement therapy after menopause.

History: A solitary, firm, nontender mass in the breast, usually discovered by the patient accidentally or during physician examination. Sixty percent occur in the upper outer quadrant of the breast. Occasionally nipple discharge is the presenting symptom. With advancing disease, swelling and local pain. Bone pain, weight loss, and jaundice are symptoms of systemic spread through metastasis.

Physical Examination: There may be enlargement or abnormal contour of one breast on inspection. The tumor is felt as a hard, ill-defined, nontender solitary mass. There may be skin or nipple retraction, fixation of the tumor to the underlying chest wall or the overlying skin, and signs of local inflammation (swelling, redness, ulceration). Axillary lymph nodes may be found enlarged if cancer cells have spread to them.

> *Her past medical history is significant for previous diagnosis of stage IIA cancer of the left breast (T2N0M0). She had a lumpectomy for this in 2001. All of her nodes were negative.*

Diagnostic Tests: Mammography (a specialized x-ray procedure) can identify changes indicative of breast cancer (calcification, mass, or both) as long as two years before a tumor becomes palpable, and is therefore a valuable screening procedure for asymptomatic women over 50, and for younger women believed to be at increased risk because of a family history of early-onset breast cancer or presence of BRCA1 or BRAC2 as detected by genetic testing. Ultrasound examination can supply valuable additional information.

Biopsy is required for confirmation of malignancy and precise identification of tumor type. A biopsy can be obtained through the skin by either a large-needle or fine-needle technique. **Excisional biopsy** (removal of the tumor followed by frozen-section examination before closure of the surgical site) is the method usually

> *BREASTS: She had evidence of prior left **lumpectomy**. Left breast tissue was a little dense, but no mass was noted. Right breast was unremarkable.*

chosen when clinical and mammographic evidence supports a diagnosis of cancer.

Course: An untreated breast cancer typically enlarges, invades surrounding and underlying tissues, and causes extensive cutaneous ulceration. **Breast cancers** spread to axillary and mediastinal lymph nodes, liver, bone, and brain. For a solitary, localized tumor, the five-year survival rate is 95% and the 10-year survival rate is 90%. The figures for disease that has become systemic before treatment is instituted are 5% and 2% respectively. Five-year and even 10-year rates do not adequately reflect the long-term mortality of breast cancer, which is eventually the cause of death in most patients, except when cancer is discovered very early by screening procedures (see ■ Figure 9-13).

Treatment: The basic treatment of breast cancer is **surgical removal of the tumor (lumpectomy).** Various further procedures, including **radical mastectomy** (removal of the entire breast as well as surrounding and underlying tissues and axillary lymph nodes) (see ■ Figure 9-13) may be appropriate with certain types and stages of cancer. Both radiation treatments and chemotherapy are usually administered after surgery.

> *Suspicious calcifications in the upper outer breasts bilaterally need biopsy. These are suspicious for malignancy.*

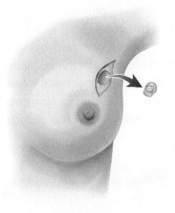

(a) Lumpectomy

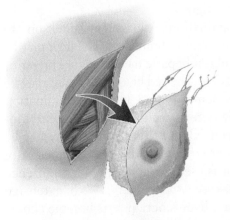

(b) Modified radical mastectomy

FIGURE 9-13. (a) Lumpectomy to remove a breast tumor. (b) Modified radical mastectomy to remove a breast tumor plus surrounding and underlying tissues and axillary lymph nodes.

Status post stage IIA cancer of the left breast, estrogen-and progesterone-receptor positive, treated with lumpectomy, chemotherapy, radiation, and tamoxifen and Arimidex.

Radiation is not usually needed after radical mastectomy, but the procedure is mutilating and psychologically devastating. In metastatic disease, elimination of estrogen stimulation through either oophorectomy (removal of the ovaries) or administration of tamoxifen, a chemical anti-estrogen, delays progression of disease and mitigates symptoms.

Adenocarcinoma of the Colon and Rectum

A malignant neoplasm arising from glandular epithelium in the large intestine. In both men and women, colon cancer ranks second as a cause of cancer deaths in the U.S. One half of all colon cancers are situated in the sigmoid colon or rectum. These tumors tend to grow slowly, but may eventually become bulky; they may encircle and constrict the bowel.

Causes: Most colon cancers arise by malignant transformation of benign polyps (**adenomas**). Several oncogenes are associated with heightened risk of developing primary cancer in the colon; some of these predispose to formation of multiple malignant tumors, which may involve organs other than the bowel. Risk factors for developing colon cancer include age over 40, a history of adenomas (benign polyps) of the colon, a family history of colon cancer, and a history of ulcerative colitis.

History: Depending on the location of the tumor, crampy abdominal pain, change of bowel habits, bloody stools, weakness, fatigue.

Physical Examination: A mass may be felt on abdominal or digital rectal examination. The liver may be enlarged or irregular if hepatic metastases are present.

Diagnostic Tests: The red blood cell count may be low as a result of hemorrhage. Chemical examination of the stool may detect occult blood. The **carcinoembryonic antigen (CEA)** titer in the serum may be elevated. This is not a reliable diagnostic indicator of colon cancer, but is useful in watching for recurrence or metastatic disease after surgery. With extensive hepatic metastases, liver function tests become abnormal. Barium enema demonstrates mucosal defects, a space-occupying lesion, or an encircling obstruction. Abdominal CT scan may provide additional informa-

tion. Endorectal ultrasound is valuable in distal lesions. Chest x-ray may show pulmonary metastases. Colonoscopy with biopsy provides definitive diagnosis.

Course: The overall survival rate in treated colon cancer is about 35%. If complete resection of primary tumor can be carried out, the survival rate is about 55%.

Treatment: The procedure of choice is **surgical resection**. **Rectal carcinoma** may require **abdominoperineal resection** (removal of the entire lower bowel, including the anus) with sigmoid colostomy. Tumors higher in the colon may be able to be resected with simple anastomosis of normal bowel above and below the surgical site. Chemotherapy and radiation therapy are valuable adjuncts to surgery in colon carcinoma.

Adenocarcinoma of the Prostate

A malignant tumor arising from glandular epithelium of the prostate gland.

Cause: Adenocarcinoma of the prostate is the most common cancer in men (31% of all cancers diagnosed). The incidence of prostatic cancer found at autopsy in men over 50 is about 40%. However, prostate cancer causes only 11% of all cancer deaths in men. The risk of developing prostatic carcinoma is higher in men with a family history of it and in those who have undergone vasectomy. The tumor is testosterone-dependent (that is, it does not occur in men who have undergone orchidectomy). **Adenocarcinoma of the prostate does not arise from benign prostatic hyperplasia.**

History: There may be no symptoms. Diminished urine flow, urinary frequency, nocturia, and dribbling of urine may occur as in benign prostatic hyperplasia. The first symptom may be bone pain due to metastasis.

Physical Examination: The prostate, as palpated on digital rectal examination, may be unusually firm, nodular, or asymmetric.

Diagnostic Tests. The level of **prostate specific antigen (PSA)** or acid phosphatase or both in the serum is elevated in many cases of prostate carcinoma, particularly when metastasis has occurred. **Transrectal ultrasound** may detect abnormally dense areas within the prostate gland, representing tumor. Transrectal biopsy discloses zones of malignant tissue. The **Gleason**

The patient is a 74-year-old man with a history of hormone-refractory prostate cancer diagnosed originally in 1999; underwent radiation therapy and developed bone metastases. He then underwent hormonal therapy with a good response.

grading system gives a histopathologic estimate of malignancy and likely future behavior. X-ray studies and radionuclide bone scans may show metastases to bones of the spine or pelvis.

Course. Progression of disease is typically slow, and most patients die of other causes before the prostatic cancer has reached a lethal stage. Metastasis to lymph nodes and to the spine or pelvis eventually occurs. Urinary obstruction may lead to urinary tract infection and even renal failure.

Treatment. Surgical excision (usually **radical prostatectomy**), radiation by external beam or implanted radioactive needles; in advanced (metastatic) disease, castration or administration of estrogen (or an antiandrogen such as flutamide) to suppress tumor growth.

Transurethral resection of the prostate (TURP)—well-differentiated adenocarcinoma of the prostate gland (Gleason score 1 + 2 for a score of 3/10).

The patient has a heavily trabeculated bladder with an enlarged occlusive prostate. Transrectal ultrasonography showed a volume of 31.9 mL with poor bladder emptying. Transrectal biopsy revealed a pathologic diagnosis of chronic prostatitis and benign prostatic hyperplasia.

Pause for Reflection

1. Describe the cause, diagnosis, course, and treatment of bronchogenic carcinoma.
2. List risk factors for breast cancer. How is it treated?
3. How is a definitive diagnosis of adenocarcinoma of the colon and rectum achieved? How is this disease treated?
4. What diagnostic procedures are used to identify carcinoma of the prostate gland?
5. How is carcinoma of the prostate treated?

Diagnostic, Surgical, and Therapeutic Procedures

biopsy, prostatic Prostatic biopsy is usually performed in conjunction with a transrectal ultrasound (TRUS) examination to assess the size and configuration of the gland.

brachytherapy A form of cancer treatment in which radioactive material is inserted into the body close to the tissues to be treated.

chemotherapy protocol A program according to which cancer drugs are administered to a given patient; specifies choice of agents, routes of administration, dosages, intervals, and duration of treatment.

DXA scan (dual x-ray absorptiometry) The preferred technique for measuring bone mineral density. Formerly called DEXA (dual-energy x-ray absorptiometry). The DXA scan is typically used to diagnose and follow osteoporosis. It is not to be confused with the nuclear bone scan, which is sensitive to certain metabolic diseases in which bones are attempting to heal from infections, fractures, or tumors.

excisional biopsy Removal of a tumor followed by frozen-section exam before closure of the surgical site.

fine-needle biopsy Sampling of a gland or organ tissue via insertion of a fine-bore needle and collecting a specimen for pathologic diagnosis.

glucometer A small portable device used to measure blood sugar.

imaging studies Imaging techniques (x-ray, MRI, CT, ultrasound, nuclear imaging) provide highly specific information about the nature, location, and extent of malignant disease.

lobectomy Surgical removal of a lobe of the thyroid gland.

lumpectomy Surgical removal of a tumor from the breast rather than removing the entire breast (see ■ Figure 9-13).

mammogram A radiographic image of the breast produced with special equipment and techniques to screen for carcinoma in women without breast symptoms.

parathyroidectomy Surgical removal of one or more of the parathyroid glands.

prostatectomy Removal of the entire prostate gland.

radiation therapy Radiation therapy uses targeted energy to kill cancer cells, shrink tumors, and provide relief of certain cancer-related symptoms. By focusing the radiation directly on the tumor, these therapies minimize the risk of common side effects associated with radiation treatment.

radical mastectomy Removal of the entire breast as well as surrounding and underlying tissues and axillary lymph nodes as appropriate with certain types and stages of cancer (see ■ Figure 9-13).

radioactive diagnostic aid for thyroid imaging Example: sodium iodide I 123 and I 125.

staging tumors The process of classifying tumors based on their degree of tissue invasion and the potential response to therapy.

surgical resection Removal of all or a portion of an organ, gland, or lobe that is cancerous.

TNM staging system T refers to the tumor's size and invasion, the N to lymph node involvement, and M to the presence of metastases of the tumor cells. Example: T2N0M0 (no spaces).

thyroidectomy Surgical removal of the thyroid gland (see ■ Figure 9-14).

thyroid scan Imaging study of the thyroid gland, using radioactive iodine to detect tumors or other pathology.

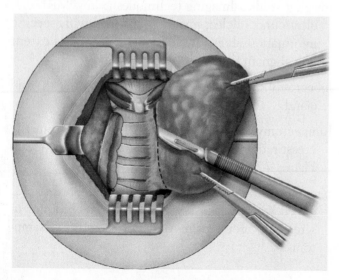

FIGURE 9-14. Thyroidectomy

transperineal implantation of radioactive isotopes Treatment for prostate cancer.

transrectal ultrasound (TRUS) An ultrasound procedure to examine the prostate gland for tumors that cannot be felt by a digital rectal exam, and to estimate the size of the prostate gland. In a prostate needle biopsy, it is used to guide the needle to the right part of the prostate gland.

Laboratory Procedures

band forms, bands Immature neutrophils whose nuclei appear as bands, in contrast to mature neutrophils whose nuclei are segmented or lobed.

basic metabolic profile (BMP) A set of 7 or 8 blood chemical tests. See *chem-7* and *chem-8* panels. Cf. *BNP*.

The basic metabolic profile shows a sodium of 138, a potassium of 3.8, the chloride is 98, the bicarbonate is 28, the BUN is 17, the creatinine is 1.8, and the random blood sugar is 179. The BNP is 80.6.

basos An acceptable brief form for *basophils*.

bleeding time The number of minutes it takes for a small incision in the skin, made with a lancet, to stop bleeding. Either the **Duke method** (puncture of the earlobe) or the **Ivy method** (puncture of the forearm) may be used.

blast forms, blasts Very immature cells, particularly leukocytes, not normally found in peripheral blood but present in acute leukemia.

B-type natriuretic peptide (BNP) A test that measures the amount of the BNP hormone in the blood. BNP is made by the heart and normally only a low amount of BNP is found in the blood. Not to be confused with "BMP"; the context of the report and the values given determine which test is meant.

burr cell An abnormal red blood cell with a jagged contour.

chem-7 panel A blood test for sodium, potassium, chloride, bicarbonate, BUN, creatinine, and glucose.

chem-8 panel Chem-7 panel plus calcium.

clotting time The time needed for a clot to form in a tube of freshly drawn blood under standard conditions. The Lee-White method is the one most often used.

coags Slang term for *coagulation studies*.

complete blood count (CBC) A group of blood tests, including counts of red blood cells, white blood cells, and platelets; a differential count of the various types of white blood cells; and a determination of hemoglobin and hematocrit.

coagulation panel Platelet count, bleeding time, clotting time, prothrombin time, partial thromboplastin time, and clot retraction. In addition, plasma assay for specific coagulation factors is possible.

comprehensive metabolic profile (CMP) A group of 14 specific blood tests including glucose, calcium, albumin, total protein, sodium, potassium, carbon dioxide or bicarbonate, chloride, BUN, creatinine, ALP, ALT, AST, and bilirubin. It is used as a broad screening tool to evaluate organ function and check for conditions such as diabetes, liver disease, and kidney disease, and to monitor known conditions such as hypertension.

differential white blood cell count A determination of the relative numbers of the six types of white blood cells normally found in peripheral blood. When the count is performed visually, a technician observes 100 white blood cells in a stained smear of whole blood and reports the number of each cell type found as a percent. The differential count can also be done electronically. The six types of white blood cells are segmented neutrophils (PMNs or segs), band neutrophils (bands, representing the immature form), eosinophils (eos), basophils (basos), lymphocytes (lymphs), and monocytes (monos).

eos Brief form for *eosinophils*.

erythrocyte A mature red blood cell. Cf. *reticulocyte*.

fasting blood sugar (FBS) A measure of the concentration of glucose in the plasma after a 12-hour fast.

free T4 test A measure of the plasma concentration of thyroxine (T4) that is free (not bound to protein).

glycated hemoglobin, glycosylated hemoglobin See *hemoglobin A1c*.

granulocytes White blood cells with conspicuous cytoplasmic granules. According to the staining proper-ties of these granules, the cells are classified as neutrophils, eosinophils, and basophils.

hemoglobin A1c (Hgb A1c, HbA1c, glycated hemoglobin) Hemoglobin in red blood cells that has united chemically with plasma glucose. The concentration of hemoglobin A1c reflects plasma glucose levels during the preceding several weeks and so serves as a measure of long-term glucose control in diabetes mellitus.

H&H Slang abbreviation for *hemoglobin and hematocrit*. The hemoglobin level is usually dictated first.

Hct, HCT Abbreviation for *hematocrit*.

hematocrit The percentage of a blood sample that consists of cells. The sample is spun in a centrifuge, which quickly drives all of the cells to the bottom of the tube. The length of the column of cells is expressed as a percent of the total length of the specimen. Red and white blood cells and platelets are all included, but red blood cells far outnumber the other formed elements.

hematocrit, central A hematocrit value determined by using a blood sample drawn from a central line catheter.

hemoglobin (Hgb, HGB) The oxygen-carrying complex of iron and protein in red blood cells. The hemoglobin level is reduced in anemia.

hemoglobin A1 Normal adult hemoglobin.

hemoglobin F Normal fetal hemoglobin, found also in adults with certain forms of anemia and leukemia.

hemoglobin S The abnormal hemoglobin found in the red blood cells of persons with sickle cell anemia.

leukocytes White blood cells (WBCs), including neutrophils, eosinophils, basophils, lymphocytes, and monocytes.

lipid profile A measure of the plasma concentrations of total cholesterol, high density lipoprotein cholesterol (HCL-C), low density lipoprotein cholesterol (LDL-C), and triglycerides.

MCH (mean corpuscular hemoglobin) The average weight of hemoglobin per red blood cell, calculated from the hemoglobin level and the red blood cell count.

MCHC (mean corpuscular hemoglobin concentration) The average concentration of hemoglobin in red blood cells, calculated from the hemoglobin level and the hematocrit.

mcL (microliters) Used in cell counts to avoid using such abbreviations as **µL** or **mm³** or **10³** because special characters and superscript numerals do not transmit well electronically.

MCV (mean corpuscular volume) The average volume of a red blood cell, calculated from the hematocrit and the red blood cell count.

microhematocrit A hematocrit measurement performed on a small specimen of blood obtained by finger stick and centrifuged in a capillary tube.

monos Brief form for *monocytes*.

myelocytes White blood cells formed in bone marrow: neutrophils, basophils, eosinophils, and monocytes.

neutrophil, segmented A mature neutrophil with a segmented or lobulated nucleus. Also called *polymorphonuclear leukocytes* or *polys*.

ovalocytosis Abnormal oval shape of red blood cells, seen in various congenital disorders of red blood cell formation, including elliptocytosis.

partial thromboplastin time (PTT) The time required for a clot to form in blood treated with certain reagents. Abnormal prolongation of this time occurs in deficiency of various coagulation factors and after treatment with heparin.

platelets Noncellular formed elements in circulating blood, produced in bone marrow and active in blood coagulation. Also called *thrombocytes*.

polymorphonuclear leukocytes (PMNs, polys) White blood cells with segmented or lobulated nuclei. An acceptable brief form is *polys*. The term is often used synonymously with *neutrophils*, although eosinophils and basophils are also polymorphonuclear leukocytes.

polys Brief form for *polymorphonuclear leukocytes*.

prostate specific antigen (PSA) A screening test that measures the amount of prostate specific antigen in the blood. High levels of PSA may indicate the presence of prostate cancer.

prothrombin time (PT, pro time) The time required for a clot to form in blood treated with certain reagents. The result, reported in seconds, is converted to an international normalized ratio (INR) by application of a factor established for the batch of thromboplastin used in the test. The prothrombin time is prolonged in deficiency of certain coagulation factors and after treatment with heparin or coumarin anticoagulants.

PT/PTT Prothrombin time and partial thromboplastin time.

RBCs (red blood cells) The most numerous cells of the blood, which carry oxygen from the lungs to the tissues, and carbon dioxide from the tissues to the lungs.

red blood cell count The number of red blood cells per cubic millimeter of blood, as counted by a technician using a microscope or by an electronic cell counter. The count may be reported either as a simple numeral (e.g., 5,300,000/mcL [microliter]) or as the product of a number less than ten and 10^6 (e.g., 5.3 x 10^6). The count may be dictated simply as 5.3 and may be so transcribed or may be expanded to 5,300,000.

red blood cells, nucleated Immature red blood cells, released from the bone marrow before disappearance of their nuclei. Mature RBCs have no nuclei.

Admission CBC values included hemoglobin 13.6, hematocrit 42.9, MCV 82.3, WBC 8.14 with 88.4% neutrophils, and platelets 200. A urinalysis on June 3 was positive for glucose, protein, and occult blood, and also revealed 1 to 3 red blood cells and 0 white blood cells. On June 4, the PT was 13.8, and the APTT 25.9. Admission blood chemistry values included BUN 16, creatinine 0.9, potassium 4.8, glucose 219, total bilirubin 0.4, alkaline phosphatase 92, AST 14, ALT 10, albumin 4.0, and calcium 9.0.

red blood cell indices Measures of the volume and hemoglobin content of red blood cells, derived by calculating from the hemoglobin, hematocrit, and red blood cell count. The red cell indices are the MCV, MCH, and MCHC.

reticulocyte An immature red blood cell whose cytoplasm contains an irregular network of degenerating nuclear material. An increase in the number of reticulocytes indicates increased red blood cell production in response to blood loss or hemolysis.

segs An acceptable brief form for *segmented neutrophils*.

stabs Another name for *bands* (immature neutrophils). The German word *Stab* means *staff* or *rod*, referring to the unsegmented nucleus of an immature neutrophil.

target cell An abnormal red blood cell with a bull's-eye appearance due to flattening of the cell with a prominent spot of hemoglobin in the center.

thrombocytes See *platelets*.

thyroid function test (TFT) Blood test to measure the levels of thyroxine, triiodothyronine, and thyroid-stimulating hormone in the bloodstream to determine thyroid function.

triglycerides, serum The level of fat in the serum, usually measured in the fasting state.

type and cross match ABO and Rh typing of a unit of blood intended for transfusion and laboratory confirmation that it is compatible with the prospective recipient's blood.

We will follow CBCs, and type and cross her for some blood in case of blood loss during surgery.

WBCs (white blood cells) See *leukocytes*.

white blood cell count (white count, white cell count) The number of white blood cells per cubic millimeter of blood, as counted by a technician using a microscope or by an electronic cell counter. The count may be reported as either a simple numeral (e.g., 7,200/mm^3 or mcL) or as the product of a small number and 10^3 (e.g., 7.2 x 10^3). In the latter case, the report may be dictated simply as 7.2 and may be so transcribed or may be expanded to 7,200.

Pharmacology

Drugs Used to Treat Endocrine Disorders

Thyroid Supplements

Thyroid supplements containing T$_3$, T$_4$, or both are used to treat hypothyroidism. They may be obtained from natural sources (beef or pork thyroid glands) or manufactured synthetically.

desiccated thyroid (Armour Thyroid, Bio-Throid, Nature Throid, NP Thyroid, Westhroid)

liotrix (Thyrolar), a 1:4 mixture of synthetic T$_3$ and T$_4$

liothyronine (Cytomel, Triostat), a synthetic product containing only T$_3$

levothyroxine (Levothroid, Levoxyl, Levolet, Levo-T, Synthroid, Tirosint), a synthetic product containing only T$_4$

Antithyroid Drugs

Antithyroid drugs, used to treat hyperthyroidism, act by inhibiting the production of T$_3$ and T$_4$.

methimazole (Tapazole, Northyx)

propylthiouracil (PTU)

sodium iodide I 131 (Hicon), a radioactive agent also used to treat thyroid cancer

Corticosteroids

Besides their role in treating adrenal insufficiency (Addison disease), synthetic **corticosteroids** are used extensively in oral, injectable, or topical formulations or by inhalation to inhibit inflammatory reactions associated with injury, infection, allergy, and autoimmune disease.

betamethasone (Celestone)

dexamethasone (Dexameth, Dexamethasone Intensol)

fludrocortisone (Florinef)

hydrocortisone (A-Hydrocort, Hydrocortone, Solu-Cortef)

methylprednisolone (A-Methapred, Medrol, Solu-Medrol)

prednisolone (Orapred, Pediapred, Prelone)

prednisone (Deltasone, Meticorten, Liquid Pred)

triamcinolone acetate (Kenalog-40)

Insulin

Regular subcutaneous injections of **insulin** are essential in the treatment of type 1 diabetes mellitus, and often prove useful in the control of type 2 as well. Natural insulins of animal origin have been largely replaced in clinical practice by synthetic insulins designed to match the chemical structure of human insulin, thus avoiding allergic reactions to foreign protein. The pharmacodynamics (onset of action, peak effect, and duration of action) of insulins can be altered by the addition of other substances (protamine, zinc). Several synthetic insulin analogs have been chemically modified so as to

INSULIN PUMP

An insulin pump is a portable or implantable electronic device that delivers insulin from a reservoir through an indwelling subcutaneous catheter. A small basal dose of rapidly acting insulin is infused continuously. In addition, bolus doses are administered manually by the patient before meals or as needed to deal with marked elevations of plasma glucose, as determined by routine fingerstick testing. Newer pumps also track blood sugar values.

achieve similar effects. Two kinds of insulin may be combined in fixed proportions to provide a desired pattern of response.

Rapid-acting insulins:
    regular insulin (Humulin R, Novolin R)
Intermediate-acting insulins:
    NPH insulin (Humulin N, Novolin N)
Mixtures of NPH and regular insulins:
    Humulin 70/30
    Novolin 70/30
Rapid-acting insulin analogs:
    insulin aspart (NovoLog, NovoPen)
    insulin glulisine (Apidra)
    insulin lispro (Humalog)
Intermediate-acting insulin analogs:
    insulin detemir (Levemir)
    insulin glargine (Lantus)
Mixtures:
    insulin aspart protamine (NovoLog Mix 50/50,
      NovoLog Mix 70/30)
    insulin lispro protamine (Humalog Mix 50/50,
      Humalog Mix 75/25)

Oral Antidiabetic Drugs

Oral antidiabetic drugs act in various ways to normalize glucose metabolism in type 2 diabetes mellitus. Contrary to popular belief, these drugs are not "oral insulin" and are ineffective in type 1 diabetes. **Sulfonylureas** lower blood sugar by stimulating the pancreas to produce more insulin. First-generation sulfonylureas, which revolutionized the treatment of type 2 diabetes during the 1950s, have now been supplanted by a second generation with smoother response and fewer side effects.

glimepiride (Amaryl)
glipizide (Glucotrol)
glyburide (Diaßeta, Glynase PresTabs)
linagliptin (Tradjenta)
nateglinide (Starlix)

Repaglinide (Prandin), which belongs to the **meglitinide** class of drugs, lowers blood glucose by stimulating the release of insulin from the pancreas.

Drugs of the **thiazolidinedione** class help to control type 2 diabetes by increasing the sensitivity of muscle and fat cells to the patient's own insulin. They do not stimulate the pancreas to produce or release insulin.

pioglitazone (Actos)
rosiglitazone (Avandia)
sitagliptin (Januvia)

Metformin (Fortamet, Glucophage), a unique agent of the **biguanide** class, is currently the most widely prescribed drug for type 2 diabetes mellitus. Besides increasing the sensitivity of muscle cells to insulin, metformin suppresses both glucose production by the liver and the absorption of glucose from the intestine.

Combinations of drugs from two of the above classes in fixed proportions improve glucose control while affording simpler dosing regimens.

glipizide and metformin (Metaglip)
glyburide and metformin (Glucovance)
pioglitazone and glimepiride (Duetact)
repaglinide and metformin (PrandiMet)
rosiglitazone and metformin (Avandamet)
rosiglitazone and glimepiride (Avandaryl)
saxagliptin and metformin (Kombiglyze XR,
  Onglyza)
sitagliptine and metformin (Janumet)

Alpha-glucosidase inhibitors impede the digestion of carbohydrate in the intestine, reducing the rise in plasma glucose that normally follows a meal.

acarbose (Precose)
miglitol (Glyset)

Drugs Used to Treat Obesity

Appetite Suppressants

Appetite suppressants reduce the craving for food that results from dietary restrictions prescribed for weight loss.

dimethylpropion (Tenuate)
lorcaserin (Belviq, "bel-VEEK")

phentermine (Adipex-P)
topiramate (Topamax)

Combinations:
bupropion and naltrexone (Contrave)
phentermine and topiramate (Qsymia,
"kyoo-sim-EE-uh").

Orlistat (Xenical), a **lipase inhibitor** that blocks the absorption of dietary fats, assists in weight loss, but the side effects of diarrhea and fecal incontinence are difficult for many to tolerate.

Drugs Used to Treat Anemia

Iron, Vitamin B$_{12}$, ATG, EPO

Acute or chronic insufficiency of red blood cells can arise from any of numerous causes. Treatments for anemia are accordingly diverse. Iron deficiency anemia is treated with **iron supplementation**, usually oral.

ferrous fumarate (Hemocyte, Femiron, Feostat)
ferrous gluconate (Fergon, Ferate)
ferrous sulfate (Feosol, Fer-In-Sol, Slow Fe)

Pernicious anemia is treated with regular supplementation of vitamin **B$_{12}$** (cyanocobalamin, methylcobalamin), aplastic anemia with **antithymocyte globulin** (ATG) (Atgam, Thymoglobulin), and sickle cell anemia with decitabine (Dacogen) and hydroxyurea (Doxia).

Drugs that **stimulate erythopoiesis** (red blood cell formation) are administered in anemia associated with chronic renal failure, which results from a deficiency of erythropoietin (EPO), a substance normally produced by the kidney.

darbepoetin alfa (Aranesp)
epoetin alfa (Epogen, Procrit)
epoetin beta (Mircera)

Drugs Used to Treat Malignant Diseases

Chemotherapeutic agents used to treat cancer fall into numerous categories on the basis of their chemical structure and mode of action. Some of these drugs are also valuable in the treatment of non-malignant diseases, particularly autoimmune disorders.

Alkylating Agents

Alkylating agents impair cell function or chemically modify DNA.

altretamine (Hexalen)
busulfan (Myleran)
carboplatin (Paraplatin)
carmustine (BCNU)
chlorambucil (Leukeran)
cisplatin (Platin)
cyclophosphamide (Cytoxan)
dacarbazine (DTIC-Dome)
ifosfamide (Ifex)
lomustine (CCNU)
mechlorethamine (Mustargen)
melphalan (Alkeran)
oxaliplatin (Eloxatin)
procarbazine (Matulane)
streptozotocin (Streptozocin)
temozolomide (Methazolastone, Temodar)
thiotepa (Thioplex)

Plant Alkaloids

Plant alkaloids are naturally occurring substances that inhibit the proliferation of malignant cells by various mechanisms.

Camptothecan analogs, from the Asian happy tree
(Camptotheca acuminata):
irinotecan (Camptosar)
topotecan (Hycamtin)
Podophyllotoxins, from May apple:
etoposide (Etopophos, Toposar, VePesid)
teniposide (Vumon)
Taxanes, from the Pacific yew tree (taxus):
docetaxel (Taxotere)
paclitaxel (Onxol, Taxol)
Vinca alkaloids, from periwinkle:
vinblastine (Velban, Alkaban AQ)
vincristine (Oncovin)
vinorelbine (Navelbine)

Antitumor Antibiotics

Antitumor antibiotics are natural products of various species of the soil fungus Streptomyces that inhibit the proliferation of malignant cells by various mechanisms.

bleomycin (Blenoxane)
dactinomycin (Cosmegen)
daunorubicin (Cerubidine)
doxorubicin (Adriamycin)
epirubicin (Ellence)

idarubicin (Idamycin)
mitomycin (Mutamycin)
mitoxantrone (Novantrone)
plicamycin (Mithracin)

Antimetabolites

Antimetabolites resemble normal cell constituents in chemical structure, but when incorporated into metabolic processes they inhibit or derange them, arresting cellular function and proliferation.

capecitabine (Xeloda)
cladribine (Leustatin)
cytarabine (Cytosar, Cytosar-U, Tarabine PFS)
floxuridine (FUDR)
fludarabine (Fludara)
5-fluorouracil (5-FU) (Carac, Efudex, Fluoroplex)
gemcitabine (Gemzar)
hydroxyurea (Droxia, Hydrea)
6-mercaptopurine (6-MP) (Purinethol)
methotrexate (Rheumatrex, Trexall)
nelarabine (Arranon)
pentostatin (Nipent)
tioguanine (Lanvis)

Monoclonal Antibodies

Monoclonal antibodies (mAb, MABs), produced by clones of immune cells derived from a unique parent cell, recognize components of malignant tumors as foreign and inhibit or destroy them. Notice that the nonproprietary names end in –mab.

alemtuzumab (Campath)
bevacizumab (Avastin)
gemtuzumab ozogamicin (Mylotarg)
ibritumomab (Tioxetan)
rituximab (Rituxan)
trastuzumab (Herceptin)

Miscellaneous Antineoplastics

Several agents have unique modes of action. Some of these are enzymes (names ending in -ase) and others inhibit (-inib) factors essential to the growth and multiplication of cancer cells.

aflibercept (Zaltrap)
asparaginase (Elspar, Kidrolase)
bexarotene (Targretin)
bortezomib (Velcade)
estramustine (Emcyt, Estracit)
gefitinib (Iressa)
imatinib (Gleevec)
lapatinib (Tykerb)
mitotane (Lysodren)
pegaspargase (Oncaspar)

Common Chemotherapy Regimens

Chemotherapy is often given in the form of combination regimens identified by acronyms, often pronounced as words rather than spelled out. Most regimens consist of generic drug names, but a brand name may be substituted in order to create a memorable or pronounceable acronym. The drugs may be given individually in a specific order at designated intervals or in combination, depending on the regimen and tailored to the individual. Common side effects of chemotherapy include bruising, bleeding, anemia, fatigue, nausea and/or vomiting, hair loss, mouth sores, peripheral neuropathy, and organ toxicity.

Example:
ABVD (Adriamycin [doxorubicin], bleomycin, vinblastine, dacarbazine). Used to treat Hodgkin lymphoma.

Transcription Tips

1. Confusing Terms: Some of these terms sound alike; others are potential traps when researching. Memorize the terms and their meanings so that you can select the appropriate term for a correct transcript.

   aphasia—inability to speak or write
   aphagia—inability or refusal to swallow

   brittle (short "i")—a brittle diabetic has easily disrupted glucose control
   bridal (long "i")—pertaining to a bride
   bridle (long "i")—a horse's harness

   callus (noun)—a hard growth of skin or bone
   callous (adj.)—insensitive, emotionless (not generally medical)

   diffuse—scattered
   defuse—reduce anger, stop bomb from exploding

   dysphasia—difficulty speaking or writing
   dysphagia—difficulty swallowing

   illicit (adj.)—illegal
   elicit (verb)—draw out

   vesicle—blister
   vesical—pertaining to the urinary bladder

2. Slang Terms. Expand these slang brief forms when encountered in dictation.

alk phos	alkaline phosphatase
CA	carcinoma
"cabbage"	CABG (acronym for coronary artery bypass graft)
coags	coagulation studies
crit	hematocrit
dig ("dij")	digoxin
H&H	hemoglobin and hematocrit
mets	metastases
mono	mononucleosis
nitro	nitroglycerin
pulse ox	pulse oximetry
rhabdo	rhabdomyolysis
sats	saturations (oxygen)

3. Spelling. Memorize the spelling of these difficult-to-spell terms. Note silent letters, doubled letters, and unexpected pronunciation.

   AccuChek glucose home test kit
   anion gap (*not* "an ion gap")
   arcus senilis (cholesterol deposits in or hyalinosis of the corneal stroma causing a white or gray ring around the cornea)
   arrhythmia (double *r*, silent *h*)
   asthma ("azma")
   bruit; bruits ("broo-ee," "brew," or "broot"; "broo-eez")
   cachexia ("kuh-kex-ee-a")
   Choice DM A1c home test kit
   coccidioidomycosis (a syllable is often omitted in pronunciation)
   crepitus
   defervescing
   dehiscence
   diarrhea (two *r*'s, silent *h*)
   dyspnea
   euthyroid (having normal thyroid function)
   fascicular (block)
   Graves disease (not possessive or plural)
   guaiac
   hematochezia
   Hemoccult (trademarked so capitalized)
   Homans sign (the *s* on *Homans* is often missed because it's followed by *sign*; not possessive)
   icterus (*not* icteris)
   livedo reticularis
   mydriasis
   pruritic, pruritus
   rhonchi (silent *h*)
   shotty (*not* shoddy), as in shotty adenopathy, means resembling buckshot

4. Note the challenging spellings or capitalization of these common drugs.

   Advair
   Arimidex
   Benadryl
   Byetta subcu injection in prefilled pen injector
   Celebrex

Transcription Tips

4. Spelling of common drugs *(continued)*

Cozaar
DiaBeta
diazepam
Diltiazem XR
Diovan HCT
Estrace
ferrous sulfate
fosinopril
Inderal (not Inderol)
Levoxyl
lisinopril
Lopressor and Minipress (two *s*'s)
NovoLog
Pneumovax
PolyMem Silver
ProAir HFA
Restoril
ReVia
Rythmol
Skelaxin
Slow-Fe ("slow eff ee")
Singulair
Synthroid (*not* Synthyroid)
Xenical ("zenikal")
VESIcare
Xopenex HFA

5. Be careful when transcribing these abbreviations. Note: Laboratory studies generally are not expanded, but you need to be able to distinguish between similar-sounding letters.

ANA (antinuclear antibody) (not A&A)
BMP (basic metabolic profile)
BNP (B-type natriuretic peptide)
CABG ("cabbage") (coronary artery bypass graft)
CK-MB (MB isoenzyme of creatine kinase; do not translate)
CMP (comprehensive metabolic profile)
CNS (*not* C&S) (central nervous system)
CPAP ("see-pap") (continuous positive airway pressure)

CVA (cerebrovascular accident)
CVA (costovertebral angle) tenderness
GTT (glucose tolerance test)
gtt (from Latin abbreviation for *drops*)
I&Os (*not* INO)—intakes and outputs
INR (international normalized ratio; do not translate)
PMI (point of maximum impulse)
PVC (premature ventricular contraction)
SP, S/P (status post)

6. Dictation Challenges

The American Diabetes Association prefers Arabic numerals (type 1, type 2) to Roman numerals when identifying diabetes mellitus. Note that *type* is not capitalized unless at the beginning of a sentence.

Chemotherapy regimens are often designated by acronyms or abbreviations sometimes pronounced as words. For example, CHOP (Cytoxan, Adriamycin, vincristine, prednisone). How is CHOP formed from that combination of drugs? A synonym for Adriamycin is 14-hydroxy-daunomycin, and vincristine is the generic name for Oncovin.

Rather than dictate a specific drug name, physicians will often say that a patient is placed on a class of antibiotics, such as aminoglycosides, cephalosporins, fluoroquinolones, macrolides. Sometimes, they will substitute the suffixes for certain classes, such as mycins and cillins. Although these are suffixes, it is acceptable to write them as words.

Sometimes more than one adjective may be used to describe anemia; the dictator is not misspeaking or stumbling.

normocytic anemia (erythrocytes normal in size but decreased in number)
normochromic (MCHC is in the normal range)
microcytic (smaller than normal; MCV reduced)
hypochromic (containing less hemoglobin than normal; MCH reduced).

Spotlight On

Check Mates

by Judith Marshall

Sharing a checking account is more intimate than sharing a bed. We did both for 29 years. The marriage was like all unions—exasperating, tumultuous, tender, erotic, depressing, joyous, and then, suddenly over. He died. Some things were easier than others. He was, after all, 24 years older than I and in failing health for years. As if that really matters.

Hospital caregivers and the funeral directors were magnificent. Friends overwhelmed me with kindness. The phone rang incessantly, the mail brought expressions of sympathy, and people came with food, cakes, and sweet remembrances. A simple wake took place in our home town and then a funeral in his New Hampshire home town. The autumn weather was spectacular, the foliage cheerfully mocking any sadness. He was laid to rest next to his beloved mother in the family plot we had visited together for decades and bedecked with wreaths and flowers. Our golden retrievers romped in the fields next to the cemetery, about a mile from where my Yankee boy was raised, the old homestead now occupied by a young professor's family who loved the history of the place. The sort of place that reminds one of *Our Town* or *Spoon River Anthology* or the music of Aaron Copland.

As all bereaved know, when the rituals have ended and the phone stops ringing, then begins the endless business paperwork. Death certificates were purchased by the dozen and even more photocopied. Surprising finds were encountered, love letters hidden for 60 years, a wedding ring from a former marriage, a dog tag from our first golden retriever, his fraternity pins and Waltham watches and pictures from his Army days in Panama, 1940–1945, things I had never seen.

I did my crying and moaning in the shower, feeling very noble and Eleanor Rooseveltian, loving him and hating him and cursing him and missing him. Some angel or fairy or demon takes over and we remember only the good things. He was an expert cook and baker and went to bartending school in his 70s. He was a beloved professor. He was a gifted carpenter, an excellent fisherman. He loved the Red Sox. He retired when we were married and began his new careers. He slept on the kitchen floor with each new puppy. We sobbed and held each other with the loss of each of our four goldens. He packed my lunches for work, packed my suitcases for travel, rubbed my feet, and brushed my hair. He could fix anything, he could untangle anything, and he never threw anything away. He loved corny jokes and *Jeopardy* on television. He loved his son and daughter and his grandchildren. He could iron and sew buttons and hems. He was my mother's girlfriend—the two of them shopping, cooking, and chattering in the kitchen. She died a few months before he did.

Each year I would go abroad and he took me to the airport and picked me up a week or weeks later. We both had a wonderful time in our separations. The craft fairs we did, the bed and breakfast inn we owned in Vermont, the concerts by the lake, the square dancing and round dancing we did. Like my father, he never used foul language. There any resemblance to my father ended.

He loved Halloween and his favorite costume was a ballerina complete with tutu and toe shoes, which he wore when he was 85. He was the last to leave the hall, still dancing while I waited, exhausted, in the car. So the WASP from New Hampshire, himself hewn from granite rock, and the Polish girl from Cleveland, despite all differences, stayed together (as we often said) for the sake of the dogs.

There was one thing I kept postponing. I did not want to go to the bank and take his name off of the account. I liked being the Mrs. in that Dr. and Mrs. It made me feel special and important. He was always very unassuming and modest and rarely used any titles. I was the pompous snob. During my grief, I was struggling with changing the names on the checking account online with Big Bank when an anonymous young man began to speak to me with great compassion and sensitivity. He said he envied me. That I must have many happy memories, and of the billions of people on the earth, many never have the experience of a partner for so many years and the joy that was surely mine in thinking of him and our life together. At that moment, I accepted my husband's death and began to heal.

Exercises

Medical Vocabulary Review

Instructions: Choose the best answer.

___ 1. Patients with diabetes mellitus who are noncompliant about taking medications and checking their blood sugars are likely to exhibit which of the following conditions?
A. Cushing syndrome.
B. hypoglycemia.
C. hyperglycemia.
D. Addison disease.

___ 2. A patient who has swelling of the lower extremities, aggravated by hanging them down over the edge of a bed or chair, has which of the following conditions?
A. Clubbing.
B. Cyanosis.
C. Hyperemia.
D. Dependent edema.

___ 3. _____ disease is another name for hyperthyroidism or overactive thyroid.
A. Addison
B. Graves
C. Cushing
D. Hodgkin

___ 4. Another term for postural hypotension or low blood pressure brought on by a sudden change in body position is which of the following?
A. Orthostatic hypotension.
B. Postprandial hypotension.
C. Postoperative hypotension.
D. Dependent hypotension.

___ 5. Which of the following is NOT a type of anemia?
A. Aplastic.
B. Sickle cell.
C. Pernicious.
D. Thrombocytopenic.

___ 6. Any of various disorders characterized by abnormally high levels of cholesterol or triglycerides in the blood may be referred to as _____
A. dyslipidemia.
B. myxedema.
C. hyperglycemia.
D. hyperkalemia.

___ 7. A physician who suspects a bleeding disorder may order any of the following tests for confirmation EXCEPT____
A. prothrombin time.
B. complete blood count.
C. Lee-White clotting time.
D. partial thromboplastin time.

___ 8. Lack of insulin in the circulation due to failure of pancreatic B cells to respond to normal stimuli is the cause of which of the following conditions?
A. Diabetes mellitus type 1.
B. Hyperadrenocorticism.
C. Adrenal insufficiency.
D. Hypoparathyroidism.

___ 9. Complications of diabetes mellitus type 2 include all of the following EXCEPT ____
A. retinopathy.
B. renal disease.
C. ketoacidosis.
D. neuropathy.

___10. Symptoms of both diabetes mellitus type 1 and 2 include all of the following EXCEPT ____
A. polydipsia.
B. polyuria.
C. polyphagia.
D. polyphasia.

Diagnostic, Surgical, and Therapeutic Procedures

Instructions: Match the following diagnostic, surgical, and therapeutic procedures to their descriptions or definitions. Some answers may be used more than once

____ 1. brachytherapy

____ 2. fine-needle biopsy

____ 3. lobectomy

____ 4. radical mastectomy

____ 5. parathyroidectomy

____ 6. TNM staging system

____ 7. thyroidectomy

____ 8. thyroid scan

____ 9. transperineal implantation of radioactive isotopes

___ 10. transrectal ultrasound (TRUS)

A. Removal of the entire breast as well as surrounding and underlying tissues and axillary lymph nodes

B. Classification of cancer based on tumor size, lymph node involvement, and whether there is metastases.

C. Surgical removal of the thyroid gland

D. A form of brachytherapy for prostatic carcinoma

E. Cancer treatment in which radioactive material is inserted into or close to the tissues being treated

F. Imaging study using radioactive iodine to detect tumors or other pathology

G. Surgical removal of a lobe of a gland or organ, such as the thyroid or lung

H. Sonographic imaging of the prostate to detect tumors or guide a needle biopsy

I. Insertion of a fine-bore needle and collection of a specimen for pathologic diagnosis

J. Removal of one or more of the glands alongside or inside the thyroid gland.

Laboratory Procedures

Instructions: Match the following laboratory procedures to their descriptions or definitions. Some answers may be used more than once

___ 1. basic metabolic profile

___ 2. B-type natriuretic peptide

___ 3. complete blood count

___ 4. coagulation panel

___ 5. comprehensive metabolic profile

___ 6. hemoglobin A1c

___ 7. lipid profile

___ 8. PT/PTT

___ 9. red blood cell indices

___ 10. thyroid function test

A. A blood test that includes platelet count, bleeding time, clotting time, prothrombin time, partial thromboplastin time, and clot retraction

B. A blood test that reflects plasma glucose levels over a period of time and so is a measure of long-term glucose control in diabetes mellitus

C. Two tests that measure clotting time of the blood

D. A test that measures the amount a hormone in the blood that is made by the heart, normally present in the blood only in small amounts, a marker for myocardial infarction

E. A panel of tests that measures thyroxine, triiodothyronine, and thyroid stimulating hormone

F. MCV, MCH, and MCHC

G. A set of 7 or 8 blood chemistry tests that includes electrolytes

H. Blood test for total cholesterol, high density lipoprotein cholesterol, low density lipoprotein, and triglycerides.

I. A panel of 14 to 20+ blood tests that includes electrolytes, glucose, calcium, kidney and liver function tests, and lipids.

J. A group of blood tests that includes hemoglobin, hematocrit, red and white blood cell counts, and white blood cell differential.

Dissecting Medical Terms

Instructions: As you learned in your medical language course, words are formed from prefixes, combining forms (root word plus combining vowel), and suffixes. Combining vowels (usually o but not always) are used to connect two root words or a root and a suffix. By analyzing these word parts, you can often determine the definition of a term without even looking it up (if you know the definition of the parts, of course!). Being able to divide and analyze the words you hear into their component parts will also improve your auditory deciphering ability and spelling and help you research those words that you cannot easily spell or define. It will also help you decipher, define, and spell coined words that may not appear in reliable resources.

For the following terms, draw a slash (/) between the components and then write a short definition based on the meaning of the parts. Remember that to define a word based on its parts, you start at the end, usually with the suffix. If there's a prefix, that is defined next and finally the combining form is defined. The actual definition of medical words does not always equal the sum of their parts because of changes in meaning over time; when this is the case, adjust your final definition to fit today's use.

Example: adenopathy
Divide & Analyze: adenopathy = adeno/pathy = disease + gland
Define: literally disease of gland but used as synonym for lymphadenopathy, disease of the lymph glands.

1. Term   adenoidectomy
   Divide _____
           _____
   Define _____

2. Term   angioedema
   Divide _____
           _____
   Define _____

3. Term   arrhythmia
   Divide _____
           _____
   Define _____

4. Term   bronchoscopy
   Divide _____
           _____
   Define _____

5. Term   cardiomegaly
   Divide _____
           _____
   Define _____

6. Term   cholelithiasis
   Divide _____
           _____
   Define _____

7. Term   conjunctivitis
   Divide _____
           _____
   Define _____

8. Term   dyslipidemia
   Divide _____
           _____
   Define _____

9. Term   endocarditis
   Divide _____
           _____
   Define _____

10. Term   epithelialization
    Divide _____
           _____
    Define _____

11. Term   hematochezia
    Divide _____
           _____
    Define _____

12. Term   hyperbilirubinemia
    Divide _____
           _____
    Define _____

13. Term   hypertriglyceridemia
Divide   _____

Define   _____

14. Term   intertrochanteric
Divide   _____

Define   _____

15. Term   microalbuminuria
Divide   _____

Define   _____

16. Term   neurocardiogenic
Divide   _____

Define   _____

17. Term   neuropathy
Divide   _____

Define   _____

18. Term   normocytic
Divide   _____

Define   _____

19. Term   prophylaxis
Divide   _____

Define   _____

20. Term   rhabdomyolysis
Divide   _____

Define   _____

21. Term   serological
Divide   _____

Define   _____

22. Term   tachyarrhythmias
Divide   _____

Define   _____

23. Term   thoracoscopic
Divide   _____

Define   _____

24. Term   thrombocytopenia
Divide   _____

Define   _____

25. Term   vitiliginous
Divide   _____

Define   _____

Spelling Exercise

Instructions: Review the adjective and adverb suffixes in your medical language textbook. Test your knowledge of **adjectives** by writing the adjectival form of the following internal medicine words. Consult a medical dictionary to verify your spelling.

Noun	Adjective
1. anxiety	_____
2. congestion	_____
3. defervesce	_____
4. enterococcus	_____
5. episode	_____
6. erythema	_____
7. expiration	_____
8. feces	_____
9. palpation	_____
10. vitiligo	_____

Abbreviations Exercise

Instructions: Expand the following common internal medicine abbreviations and brief forms. Then memorize both abbreviations and definitions to increase your speed and accuracy in transcribing dictation.

Abbreviation	Expansion
1. ACE (inhibitors)	_____
2. ANA	_____
3. AV	_____
4. BK	_____
5. BMI	_____
6. CABG	_____
7. CHF	_____
8. CNS	_____
9. COPD	_____
10. CPAP	_____
11. CVA	_____
12. D&C	_____
13. EGD	_____
14. EOMs	_____
15. EOMI	_____
16. I&Os	_____
17. JVD	_____
18. NIDDM2	_____
19. OA/DJD	_____
20. PCA	_____
21. PERRLA	_____
22. PMH	_____
23. PMI	_____
24. PT	_____
25. PVCs	_____
26. PVRs	_____
27. RA	_____
28. TEE	_____
29. TMs	_____
30. URI	_____

Transcript Forensics

This section presents snippets of transcribed dictations from clinic notes; history and physical examinations and consultations; procedure notes; and discharge summaries. Explain the passage so that a nonmedical person can understand it. Pay particular attention to terms that are in bold type. Sample responses are available to your instructor.

Example

Excerpt: HEENT: The head is **atraumatic, normocephalic**. He does have male pattern baldness. He has **earlobe creases** bilaterally. Pupils equally round and reactive to light. There is no **conjunctival irritation**. There is no **icterus**. There are no **petechiae**. The nose is normal. The mouth is unremarkable. The mucosa is dry. He does have upper plates. The tongue is slightly dry as well.

Explanation: The HEENT exam is mostly normal. There is no trauma to the head and it is normally shaped. The earlobes have a groove that may be an indication of cardiovascular risk. Pupils react normally. Conjunctivae are not red nor is there any jaundice (yellowness of the membranes), and no pinpoint hemorrhages. The dry mucosa and slightly dry tongue may indicate some element of dehydration. He has upper dentures.

1. **Excerpt:** NECK: The neck is **supple**. I could not detect any **jugular venous distention** at this point, in the Fowler position. There is no audible **bruit**. However, he does have some **rhonchi** transmitted to the neck but certainly no stridor. The thyroid is not enlarged on palpation, and the **carotid upstroke pulse is decreased** bilaterally. There is no **supraclavicular adenopathy**.

Explanation: _____
_____
_____
_____
_____
_____
_____
_____
_____

2. **Excerpt:** ABDOMEN: The abdomen is **rotund** with no tenderness on **palpation**, and I could not feel any masses. There is no **hepatosplenomegaly** to my exam at this point.

Explanation: _____

_____

_____

_____

_____

_____

_____

3. **Excerpt:** The heart tones are distant but with a **normal S1 and S2**. No associated **gallop, rub, or murmur**. The **PMI** is nonpalpable.

Explanation: _____

_____

_____

_____

_____

_____

_____

4. **Excerpt:** The lungs show **inspiratory and expiratory rhonchi**, more prominent on the left side than on the right.

Explanation: _____

_____

_____

_____

_____

_____

5. **Excerpt:** The extremities show some slight **clubbing**, but there is no **cyanosis** and there is definite **edema**, 2+ bilaterally, which is **symmetric**. There is some **erythema** on the lower extremities. There is no **purpura**. There may be some mild **ecchymotic areas** on the forearms bilaterally.

Explanation: _____

_____

_____

_____

_____

_____

_____

6. **Excerpt:** Neurologically, the patient is a bit confused. There is no **focal neurological deficit**. He is able to move all 4 extremities without much difficulty. He is certainly confused and at times does not cooperate and becomes almost **catatonic**.

Explanation: _____

_____

_____

_____

_____

_____

_____

7. **Excerpt:** The chest x-ray shows a possible right lower lobe **infiltrate**. There is certainly **flattening of the diaphragms** bilaterally and COPD changes.

Explanation: _____

_____

_____

_____

_____

_____

_____

8. **Excerpt**: Aside from having some **dyspeptic symptom**s, the primary issue is the pain that he has had postoperatively. He denies having had any **hematemesis**. He does have some nausea and occasional vomiting. There has been no abdominal discomfort in terms of diarrhea or constipation, and there have been no **black or bloody stools**.

Explanation: _____
_____
_____
_____
_____
_____
_____
_____

9. **Excerpt**: The chest is symmetric. There is a well-healed scar on the left upper lateral chest posteriorly. However, he is **exquisitely tender** upon palpation of this area. There is no evidence of infection at this point. There is no swelling, and there is no drainage, and no **hyperemia**, and there is no **vesicle**.

Explanation: _____
_____
_____
_____
_____
_____

10. **Excerpt**:
DIAGNOSIS AT THIS TIME
1. **Obstipation**; rule out **occult** gastrointestinal pathology.
2. **Status post gastric carcinoma**.
3. **Acute cystitis**.
4. Diabetes mellitus type 2.
5. Status post hypertension.

Explanation: _____
_____
_____
_____
_____
_____
_____
_____

Sample Reports

Sample internal medicine reports appear on the following pages, illustrating a variety of styles. Fictional names are provided for illustration of proper format, and no resemblance to actual persons is intended. Sample transcripts were prepared according to *The Book of Style for Medical Transcription* (AHDI).

Chart Note

CHANDLER, LAURA
Age: 42
12/14/[add year]

CHIEF COMPLAINT
Increasing fatigue, nocturia, and vaginal pruritus.

HISTORY OF PRESENT ILLNESS
Brief exam for this obese 42-year-old female with a 2-year history of mild hypertension and type 2 diabetes mellitus, controlled by diet. Medications include Ortho-Novum 10/11. The patient was started on hydrochlorothiazide 50 mg 2 weeks ago because of elevated diastolic pressures.

Blood sugar by glucose meter is 417. Urine negative for ketones. Apical pulse of 90. Blood pressures are 144/94 and 140/98. Height 5 feet 2 inches, weight 186.

PHYSICAL EXAMINATION
Unremarkable.

RECOMMENDATIONS
1. Instruction to patient to push fluids for the next several days.
2. Discontinue hydrochlorothiazide and birth control pills to end possible drug-induced hyperglycemia.
3. Start Micronase 2.5 mg every other day and Capoten 25 mg b.i.d.
4. Set up appointment on Friday for fasting blood sugar.
5. Patient to see the nurse practitioner for fitting of a diaphragm and nutritional counseling on a 1200-calorie ADA diet.

AF:hpi

History and Physical Examination

HERNANDEZ, JUANITA
#357153

DATE OF ADMISSION
August 10, [add year]

IDENTIFICATION AND HISTORY
This patient is a 67-year-old Mexican American female. She was admitted to the hospital early this morning at approximately 4 a.m. She was seen in the emergency room at approximately 3 a.m. because of diaphoresis and weakness, with subsequent diagnosis of hypoglycemia. She was admitted to the hospital and placed on the progressive care unit. She was admitted with a hemoglobin of 6.9 and a potassium of 6.2, with evidence of renal insufficiency.

It should be noted that she has been admitted to the hospital in the past because of chronic renal insufficiency and hyperkalemia. This resulted in a program which included DiaBeta 5 mg b.i.d., Inderal 20 mg 3 times a day, Quinidex Extentabs 1 b.i.d., and ferrous sulfate.

IMPRESSION
1. Diabetes mellitus, type 2.
2. Hypoglycemia secondary to oral hypoglycemic agents in the face of renal insufficiency, leading to hypoglycemia.
3. Hyperkalemia, acute, secondary to her renal insufficiency and being on angiotensin-converting enzyme inhibitors.

RECOMMENDATIONS
1. Discontinue her Vasotec.
2. Hydration with saline, since I think at least part of her renal failure is probably on the basis of prerenal azotemia secondary to her furosemide therapy.
3. Sodium bicarbonate for treatment of her metabolic acidosis.
4. Kayexalate p.o. and Kayexalate enemas.
5. Glucose infusion followed by regular insulin.

CARLOS SOBERVILLA, MD

CS:hpi

d: 8/10/[add year]
t: 8/10/[add year]

Discharge Summary

CROWELL, ELIZABETH
#779079

DATE OF ADMISSION
June 5, [add year]

DATE OF DISCHARGE
June 6, [add year]

DISCHARGE DIAGNOSES
1. Severe hypokalemia.
2. Gastroenteritis.
3. Dehydration.
4. Addison disease.
5. Chronic neck pain.
6. Chronic obstructive pulmonary disease (COPD) and emphysema.
7. Elevated hematocrit.

CONSULTATIONS AND PROCEDURES
None.

HISTORY OF PRESENT ILLNESS
The patient is a very pleasant 57-year-old lady who presented to the emergency room with a 2-day history of nausea, vomiting, and diarrhea. She was admitted to the hospital with diagnosis of hypertension and hypokalemia.

HOSPITAL COURSE
Her potassium on admission was 2.1. She was started on normal saline at 150 mL an hour with 40 mEq of potassium. She had diffuse ST-segment depression on EKG, which was obtained in the emergency room, which was attributed to hypokalemia. Hemoglobin on admission was 20.3 and hematocrit 58. The elevated hemoglobin and hematocrit were attributed to dehydration and underlying COPD. Chest x-ray was obtained on admission and revealed emphysema and left lower lobe calcified granuloma. EKG was repeated in the morning and revealed improved diffuse ST-segment depressions. The patient has Addison disease and has not been able to keep down oral medications, so she was given hydrocortisone 100 mg IV q. 12 hours and Cortef was held. She also was given morphine 2–4 mg IV q. 4 hours p.r.n. for pain control.

(continued)

Discharge Summary *(continued)*

CROWELL, ELIZABETH
#779079
Page 2

Also, the patient had elevated troponin and CK, which was attributed to ischemic changes secondary to dehydration. Urinalysis was obtained on admission and was positive for blood, leukocyte esterase, and nitrates. Patient was started on Rocephin 1 g IV. Patient has been afebrile.

DISPOSITION
Patient was discharged in stable condition with regular diet, activity as tolerated.

MEDICATIONS AT THE TIME OF DISCHARGE
1. Norvasc 10 mg 1 tablet daily.
2. Clonidine 1 mg 1 tablet p.o. twice a day.
3. Cortef 5 mg 3 tablets in the morning and 2 tablets in the afternoon.
4. MS Contin 15 mg 1 tablet p.o. at bedtime.
5. MS Contin 15 mg 1 tablet p.o. twice daily.
6. Morphine 15 mg p.o. q. 4 hours p.r.n. for breakthrough pain.
7. We will hold the lisinopril HCT for now.
8. Bactrim double-strength 1 tablet p.o. b.i.d. for 5 days.

Follow up with Dr. _____ on June 8. Should she have recurrent nausea, vomiting, fever or chills, she is to call us immediately or return to the emergency room.

LANA MEIRING, MD

LM:hpi

d: 6/7/[add year]
t: 6/7/[add year]

Comic Relief

Mishears and Mispeaks

This child will probably be shorter than he wants to be, but he should have picked different parents.

Physical examination revealed a garrulous, obese woman who was short of breath on motion but not on talking.

At 2 a.m. the patient was found dead in bed after otherwise having had a good day.

The doctor's basic suggestions were that treatment remain conservative, and that procrastination be the procedure of choice for the time being.

It should be noted that this history was obtained in the patient's broken English and my broken Spanish.

The patient celebrated her wedding anniversary last evening with a ham dinner and a tiff with her husband.

Review of her past history showed that she had had a very uneventful life.

The patient underwent radiation to both necks.

The patient was in no acute distress except when she moved.

The patient's problem started two years ago when he started seeing his doctor.

The patient performed the surgery admirably.

The patient was sent for a hematocrit because she was acting pale.

Admission blood sugar was 230 pounds.

The patient has gone on an eating rampage.

The patient was put on a 1000-dollar diet.

Despite treatment, the patient improved.

PEARSON
myhealthprofessionskit™

To access the online exercises and transcription practice, go to **www.myhealthprofessionskit.com**. Select "Medical Transcription," then click on the title of this book, *Healthcare Documentation: Fundamentals & Practice*. Then click on the Internal Medicine chapter.

Pulmonary Medicine

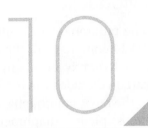

Learning Objectives

▶ Describe the structure and function of the respiratory system.

▶ Spell and define common pulmonary terms.

▶ Identify pulmonary medicine vocabulary that might be used in the review of systems.

▶ Describe the negative and positive findings a physician looks for on examination of the lungs.

▶ Describe the typical cause, course, and treatment options for common diseases of the respiratory system.

▶ Identify and define common diagnostic and surgical procedures of the respiratory system.

▶ List common pulmonary laboratory tests and procedures.

▶ Identify and describe common pulmonary drugs and their uses.

▶ Demonstrate knowledge of anatomical, medical, pharmacological, adjectival, and soundalike terms by accurately completing the exercises in this chapter.

Transcribing Pulmonary Medicine Dictation

Introduction

The pulmonary, or respiratory, system (see ■ Figure 10-1) comprises all the organs and tissues that serve to deliver oxygen to circulating blood and to remove carbon dioxide from it. The respiratory system consists of the nose, mouth, pharynx, larynx, trachea, bronchi, lungs, pleura, diaphragm, and chest wall (ribs and muscles).

An **internist**, a specialist in internal medicine, is the physician who treats patients with pulmonary disorders. A **thoracic surgeon** participates in the treatment of conditions and diseases of the respiratory system by surgical means.

Respiratory therapy is an allied health specialty that assists patients with respiratory and cardiopulmonary disorders. Duties of a **respiratory therapist** include conducting pulmonary function tests, monitoring oxygen and carbon dioxide levels in the blood, administering breathing treatments, and ventilator management.

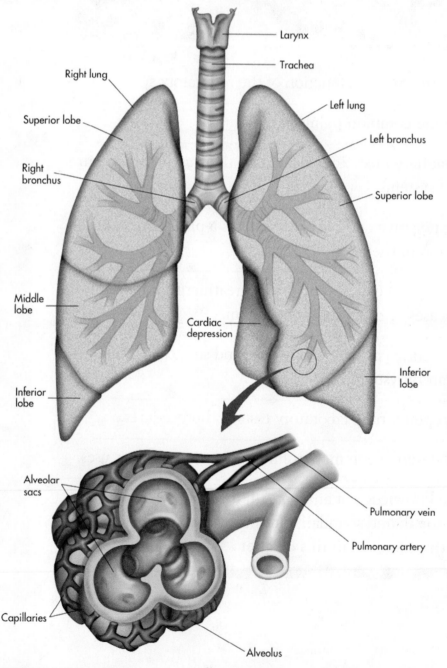

FIGURE 10-1. The respiratory system: larynx, trachea, bronchi, and lungs with an expanded view showing the structures of an alveolus and the pulmonary blood vessels

Anatomy Review

Inspiration occurs when the diaphragm moves downward and the chest wall moves outward. This creates a slight vacuum within the chest cavity, causing the lungs to expand and draw air inward through the airway (mouth and nose, throat, trachea, and bronchi) into the lung tissue proper. At the end of inspiration, the diaphragm and chest wall relax, so that the lungs passively contract and expel air. This is known as **expiration**.

During both phases of respiration, blood in pulmonary vessels takes up **oxygen** from the inspired air and releases **carbon dioxide** into the air that is about to be exhaled. Respiration is under involuntary control from a center in the brain stem. Respiratory rate varies with changes in the oxygen and carbon dioxide levels in the blood as well as in the composition and **pH** (alkalinity vs. acidity) of the serum.

The airway is lined by mucous membrane, which contains glands producing both mucous and serous secretions. The walls of the trachea and bronchi are reinforced by partial rings of cartilage, which prevent their collapse under negative pressure.

Lung tissue proper consists of numerous microscopic air sacs or **alveoli** (singular, **alveolus**), through whose extremely thin epithelial walls the respiratory gases can readily diffuse between the air within them and the blood in adjacent pulmonary vasculature. The lungs are protected by a delicate serous membrane called the **pleura**. The **visceral** layer of the pleura is closely applied to the surfaces of the lungs; the **parietal** layer lines the chest cavity. Normally the two layers are in contact, with a minute amount of serous fluid between them to serve as a lubricant as the lungs move with respect to the chest wall during respiration.

Pause for Reflection

1. The process of breathing is referred to as _____ and consists of two actions, _____ and _____.
2. During both phases of respiration, blood takes in _____ and releases _____.
3. Lung tissue is filled with tiny air sacs called _____.
4. The protective serous membrane closely applied to the surface of the lung is the _____ and the outer layer which lines the chest cavity is the _____.

SYMPTOMS AND SIGNS OF RESPIRATORY DISEASE

- Cough (dry or productive) or choking.
- Production of sputum (watery, viscous, or purulent).
- Hemoptysis (coughing up blood from respiratory passages).
- Dyspnea (shortness of breath), tachypnea (increased respiratory rate).
- Audible wheezing with respirations (inspiratory or expiratory).
- Chest pain (constant, intermittent, or synchronous with breathing). Pleuritic chest pain, the pain of pleurisy (pleuritis), is sharp, localized, and closely related to chest wall movement with breathing.
- Cyanosis (bluish color of skin, particularly lips and nail beds, due to presence of excess unoxygenated blood in the circulation).
- Respiratory distress, indicated by increased effort to breathe, pursing of lips, use of accessory muscles of respiration (neck and upper chest muscles not needed for normal breathing), intercostal retractions (sucking in of muscles between ribs on inspiration).
- Percussion of the chest may disclose hyperresonance due to a cavity within lung tissue or air in the pleural space; or dullness due to consolidation of lung tissue by infection, or neoplasm, or to fluid in the pleural space.
- Auscultation may detect rales (crackling or bubbling sounds due to passage of air through fluid in respiratory passages); rhonchi (singular, rhonchus; whistling or honking sounds due to passage of air through respiratory passages narrowed by edema, secretions, or neoplasm); a pleural friction rub (due to inflammation or scarring of adjacent surfaces of visceral and parietal pleura); or reduction or absence of breath sounds (due to pulmonary consolidation, pleural air or fluid, collapse of a lung, or neoplasm).
- Digital clubbing (enlargement of fingertips with elevation of proximal parts of nails, due to chronic pulmonary disease).

Vocabulary Review

accessory muscles of respiration Neck and upper chest muscles not needed for normal breathing.

apnea Cessation of breathing.

atelectasis Collapse of lung tissue.

auscultation Listening to the chest, particularly breath sounds, with the use of a stethoscope.

barrel chest In pulmonary emphysema the antero-posterior diameter of the chest is often increased so that the rib cage approaches a cylindrical shape (like a barrel).

basilar Pertaining to the bases (lowermost parts) of the lungs.

bronchiectasis Abnormal, irreversible dilatation of bronchi, related to chronic infection.

cachexia A general appearance of debility and malnutrition.

cavitation A pathological hollow space or place in tissues or organs such as occurs in the lungs in pulmonary tuberculosis.

Cheyne-Stokes respirations Cyclic alternations between periods of apnea or hypopnea and periods of tachypnea.

cough May be variously described as brassy, bubbling, croupy, hacking, harsh, hollow, loose, metallic, nonproductive, productive, rasping, rattling, or wracking.

CPAP (continuous positive airway pressure) A method of positive pressure ventilation to keep the airways open at the end of exhalation, increase oxygenation, and improve breathing. Often prescribed for patients with obstructive sleep apnea.

community-acquired pneumonia (CAP) Pneumonia not acquired in a hospital or a long-term care facility.

crackles Rales.

cyanosis Bluish color of skin, particularly lips and nail beds, due to presence of excess unoxygenated blood in the circulation.

cuffing, peribronchial Thickening of bronchial walls as seen on chest x-ray.

decompensation Failure to maintain a stable status of diseases or symptoms.

> **LAY AND MEDICAL TERMS**
>
> | | |
> |---|---|
> | breaths | respirations |
> | phlegm | mucous secretions |
> | sweating | diaphoresis |
> | trouble breathing | dyspnea |

---

digital clubbing Enlargement of fingertips with elevation of proximal parts of nails, due to chronic pulmonary disease.

dullness to percussion Muffling on percussion due to consolidation of lung tissue by infection or neoplasm, or to fluid in the pleural space.

dyspnea Shortness of breath.

exacerbation Worsening in severity of symptoms.

flash pulmonary edema Rapid onset of pulmonary edema (accumulation of fluid in the pulmonary tissues and air spaces) brought on by decompensated congestive heart failure, acute myocardial infarction, or mitral regurgitation.

hemoptysis Coughing up blood from respiratory passages.

hyperresonance Accentuated breath sounds on auscultation due to a cavity within lung tissue or air in the pleural space.

hypopnea Very shallow breathing.

hypoxemia Reduction of oxygen tension.

IMV (intermittent mandatory ventilation) A mode of mechanical ventilation. The patient is allowed to breathe on their own but assisted by a ventilator; the ventilator takes over (this is the mandatory part) when patient effort is not sensed. Usually followed by a number, e.g., IMV of 5, which refers to the ventilator setting.

infiltrate Diffusion of inflammatory fluid or exudate into air cavities of the lung, or their walls, producing cloudiness of lung tissue on chest x-ray.

intercostal retractions Sucking in of muscles between ribs on inspiration.

intermittent positive pressure breathing (IPPB).

Kussmaul respirations Rapid and deep respirations.

nebulizer Any of various devices used to convert water, usually containing dissolved medicine (bronchodilator, surfactant), into a fine mist that can be inhaled into the respiratory tract through a mouthpiece.

orthopnea Shortness of breath (dyspnea) relieved by assuming an upright position. Two-pillow orthopnea means the patient's shortness of breath is relieved when the upper body is supported on two pillows.

palliative Providing relief but not curative, for example, giving morphine to terminal cancer patients in doses necessary to relieve pain.

PCP Abbreviation for *Pneumocystis* pneumonia, due to *Pneumocystis jiroveci* (formerly *P. carinii*).

phthisis ("TI sis") Greek word for *consumption*, an old term for pulmonary tuberculosis. Used today to reflect the progressive body wasting associated with untreated tuberculosis.

pleura A delicate serous membrane protecting the lungs.

pleural effusion Fluid in the pleural space. Types of effusion include chylothorax (fluid from the intestine), hemothorax (blood), hydrothorax (serous fluid), and pyothorax or empyema (pus).

pleural friction rub A creaking, grating, or rubbing sound caused by friction between inflamed pleural surfaces during breathing.

pleuritic pain Sharply localized stabbing pain in the chest that is aggravated by taking a deep breath, and virtually abolished by breathholding. It typically results from irritation of the pleura due to pleurisy, pneumonia, pulmonary infarction, or chest wall injury.

production of sputum Phlegm from the respiratory passages. Can be watery, viscous, or purulent.

pulse oximetry A method of monitoring the oxygen saturation of circulating hemoglobin, as detected by a probe attached to the patient's finger or earlobe. The probe (see ■ Figure 10-2) emits two beams of light at different wavelengths and records the differential absorption of these beams by hemoglobin in the capillary circulation, providing an estimate of oxygen saturation. The oximeter is programmed to sound an alarm when pulse, blood flow, or oxygen saturation falls outside of established safe limits.

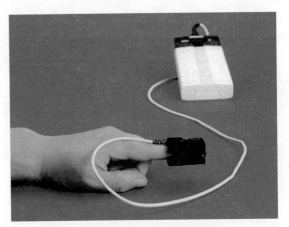

FIGURE 10-2. Pulse oximeter.
Source: Michal Heron, Pearson Education

rale An irregular discontinuous sound, like bubbling fluid, crackling paper, or popping corn. Rales are heard on auscultation of the lungs and are due to passage of air through fluid—mucus, pus, edema fluid, or blood—or to the sudden expansion of small air passages that have been plugged or sealed by mucus.

respiratory distress Indicated by increased effort to breathe, pursing of lips, and use of accessory muscles of respiration.

rhonchi (singular, **rhonchus**) Whistling or honking sounds resulting from passage of air through a respiratory passage narrowed by bronchospasm (in asthma), swelling, thickened secretions, or tumor. Rhonchi vary widely in pitch and intensity; in asthma, rhonchi of many different pitches may be heard together ("**musical chest**").

shortness of breath Feeling out of breath; breathlessness; difficulty catching one's breath.

spirometry The measurement of lung volumes and inspiratory and expiratory flow rates with a spirometer according to a standard testing protocol.

spontaneous ventilation Unaided natural ventilation or breathing, as opposed to mechanical or artificial ventilation.

sputum May be variously described as blood-streaked, bloody, clear, foul-tasting, frothy, gelatinous, green, purulent, putrid, ropy, rusty, viscid, viscous, watery, or yellow.

tachypnea Increased respiratory rate.

tension pneumothorax Accumulation of air or gas in the pleural space so that the pressure within the pleural space is greater than atmospheric pressure. This can result when the patient is on positive pressure ventilation or when the tissues around the opening into the pleural cavity act as valves, allowing air to enter but not to escape. The resultant positive pressure in the cavity displaces the mediastinum to the opposite side, with consequent interference with respiration.

wean To gradually discontinue or deprive, as in to wean off ventilation.

wheezing Whistling sound made in breathing.

Medical Readings

History and Physical Examination

by John H. Dirckx, MD

Review of Systems. The respiratory history begins with a survey of past or current diagnoses of respiratory problems such as asthma, bronchitis, pneumonia, emphysema, pleurisy, pneumothorax, tuberculosis, and lung cancer, with treatments prescribed for any of these.

Respiratory: No history of asthma, bronchitis, pneumonia, chronic cough, hemoptysis, or purulent sputum.

Lay persons often misunderstand the terms **asthma** and **bronchitis** and apply them indiscriminately and inappropriately to various pulmonary and nonpulmonary complaints. The patient is questioned about shortness of breath (intermittency, severity, inciting factors), cough, and chest pain. These three symptoms can also indicate cardiac disease. **Dyspnea** is a cardinal feature of asthma. Generally there is audible wheezing as well, and cough which may produce thick sputum.

The significant features of a **cough** are its frequency, character, factors that provoke it (such as cold air, smoke, dust, or lying down), and the character and volume of sputum produced. **Hemoptysis** (coughing up blood) of even slight degree demands careful investigation because it can indicate pulmonary malignancy, pulmonary infarction, or, less often, tuberculosis. Often the patient cannot reliably distinguish between expectorated material (brought up from the trachea or lungs) and nasopharyngeal secretions.

Sharply localized stabbing pain in the chest that is aggravated by deep inspiration and virtually abolished by breath-holding is called **pleuritic** because it typically results from irritation of the **pleura** (the membrane lining the thoracic cavity and covering the lungs) due to pleurisy, pneumonia, pulmonary infarction, or chest wall injury. The lungs themselves contain no pain-sensitive nerves. If the **smoking history** and details of any known respiratory allergies have not previously been recorded, they may be brought in here.

Patient is a 44-pack-year cigarette smoker with mild respiratory allergies to pollen, molds, and dust.

Pause for Reflection

1. Which 3 symptoms, if present, may indicate either pulmonary or cardiac disease?
2. Which symptoms elicited in the Review of Systems could be an indication of asthma?
3. What are the implications of hemoptysis?
4. Address the 2 ways that the text mentions in which patient confusion can complicate the taking of the Review of Systems.
5. What are the implications of sharply localized stabbing pain in the chest that is aggravated by deep inspiration and virtually abolished by breath-holding?

Physical Examination. The **respiratory rate** is one of the vital signs that are routinely determined during a physical examination and monitored in hospitalized patients and those receiving urgent care. Breathing is an automatic function whose rate is governed principally by the concentrations of oxygen and carbon dioxide in the blood. The normal resting rate in healthy adults is 12-16 respirations/minute.

More rapid breathing (**tachypnea**) occurs in circumstances that increase the need for oxygen, such as exercise, emotional excitement, and elevation of body temperature, and it can also be caused by most abnormal conditions that impair the ability of the heart and lungs to exchange oxygen and carbon dioxide (pneumonia, shock, congestive heart failure) or by **metabolic acidosis** (as in **Kussmaul respirations**, both rapid and deep, of diabetic coma).

Exercise brings on attacks of paroxysmal wheezing and coughing, dyspnea, and production of clear, viscous sputum.

Abnormally slow breathing (**bradypnea**) can result from respiratory depression due to drugs, stroke, head injury, or the terminal stage of any severe systemic or metabolic disorder. **Cheyne-Stokes respirations** are cyclic alternations between periods of **apnea** (cessation of breathing) or **hypopnea** (very shallow breathing) and periods of tachypnea.

If instructed to "breathe naturally," the average person finds it impossible to do so. Measurement of respiratory rate in the conscious patient is therefore performed surreptitiously—for example, while the examiner pretends to count the pulse or listen to the heartbeat. Ideally the respirations are counted for a full minute. Respiratory rate can be recorded automatically by various devices, most of them detecting respiratory movements of the thorax.

In examining the respiratory system, the physician first observes the configuration and musculature of the chest wall and the fullness and symmetry of breathing movements. Congenital deformities and injuries or diseases of the ribs or spine can alter the shape of the thorax. In pulmonary emphysema the anteroposterior diameter of the chest is often increased so that the rib cage approaches a cylindrical shape (**barrel chest**). Unless the patient is thin, the examiner will need to find some of the bony landmarks of the chest wall by palpation.

Expiration is accompanied by wheezing audible without a stethoscope.

Evaluation of the lungs is performed almost entirely by the techniques of **auscultation and percussion (A&P)**. The passage of air into and out of the lungs during normal respiration produces a characteristic sequence of sounds heard through the chest wall with a stethoscope. Structural changes in the breathing apparatus due to disease or injury cause predictable changes in the quality and loudness of the breath sounds and can induce abnormal sounds as well. The patient is instructed to breathe somewhat more deeply than normal with the mouth open (so as to avoid extraneous sounds caused by the passage of air through the nose) while the examiner listens at specific places on the front and back of the chest. Ordinarily the broad, flat diaphragm chest piece of the stethoscope is preferred for this purpose.

Normal inspiration and expiration yield a faint sighing or whispering sound called **vesicular breathing**. This sound might be compared to that of a steady, gentle breeze passing through and stirring the leaves of a tree. The inspiratory phase of vesicular breathing is slightly longer than the expiratory phase, and slightly louder. In fact, the expiratory phase may be inaudible. When the two phases of respiration are about equal in intensity, one speaks of **bronchovesicular breathing**. When the expiratory phase is louder, the term **bronchial** (or **tubular**) **breathing** is applied.

Certain abnormal conditions can superimpose **abnormal sounds** (rhonchi, rales, or rubs) on the basic inspiratory-expiratory breath sounds. A **rhonchus** is a continuous sound such as is made by a whistle or horn. Rhonchi result from passage of air through a respiratory passage narrowed by bronchospasm (in asthma), swelling, thickened secretions, or tumor. Rhonchi vary widely in pitch and intensity. In asthma, rhonchi of many different pitches may be heard together ("musical chest").

Inspiratory rhonchi are heard over the right upper chest.

A **rale** is an irregular, discontinuous sound, like bubbling fluid, crackling paper, or popping corn. Rales are due to passage of air through fluid—mucus, pus, edema fluid, or blood—or to the sudden expansion of small air passages that have been plugged or sealed by mucus. Asking a patient with rales or rhonchi to cough and then listening again to the breath sounds may supply helpful information about the character or severity of the underlying disorder. The examiner carefully notes in what part of the chest and at what part of the breathing cycle rhonchi or rales are heard or are loudest.

There are fine crepitant rales at both bases.

A **rub** is a creaking, grating, or rubbing sound caused by friction between inflamed pleural surfaces during breathing; it can indicate pleurisy, pneumonia, pulmonary infarction, or chest wall injury causing an irritation of the pleura.

Reduction or absence of breath sounds over a part of the chest wall can result from any of several conditions—collapse of lung tissue (**atelectasis**), consolidation of lung tissue due to pneumonia, presence in the pleural space of air (**pneumothorax**), blood (**hemothorax**), pus (**empyema**), or fluid (**hydrothorax, pleural effusion**), and tumor. Some of these can be differentiated by determining how well the sound of the patient's voice passes through the involved area. When the patient says "ee," the examiner hears "ee" through normal lung, "ay" through consolidated lung or air in the pleural space. Enhancement of sound transmission by consolidated lung is called **bronchophony**. Whispered pectoriloquy means that even whispered words are clearly heard through the stethoscope.

This is a 61-year-old white female with known history of COPD, who was diagnosed with pneumonia last week and started on Levaquin. She states that she has been taking this regularly without improvement. Now, she complains of substernal chest pain, worse with activity and inspiration, decreased with rest. She also reports subjective fevers, shortness of breath, orthopnea, myalgia, and wheezing.

In another test using the patient's voice, the examiner places the flat of the hand over various parts of the chest while the patient repeatedly says "bananas," "ninety-nine," or some other word or phrase yielding similar resonance and overtones. The vibration felt by the examiner, known as **vocal fremitus**, is enhanced by consolidation of lung, damped by intervening air or fluid.

Percussion of the chest, though a valuable diagnostic procedure, has been largely supplanted by x-rays. This procedure is based on the fact that structural alterations within the thorax change the behavior of sound waves that are produced when the chest wall is tapped. In the standard technique, called **mediate percussion**, the examiner places the palm of one hand with outspread fingers against the patient's chest and taps the back of the middle finger smartly with the flexed tip of the other middle finger.

The **percussion note** over normal lung tissue is described as **resonant**. In atelectasis, consolidation, or pleural effusion the note is dull or even flat; in pneumothorax or emphysema it may be hyperresonant or even tympanitic (drumlike). Percussion can be used to find the levels of the right and left hemidiaphragms in inspiration and expiration and to trace the left border of an enlarged heart.

As a rough test for obstructive pulmonary disease, the examiner may instruct the patient to blow out a match held several inches from the mouth without pursing the lips.

The patient fails match test at 3 inches.

Pause for Reflection

1. Distinguish between tachypnea and bradypnea and between Kussmaul respirations and Cheyne-Stokes respirations.
2. What external observations does the physician make in assessing the respiratory system?
3. The primary technique for evaluation of the lungs is _____.
4. Distinguish between vesicular breathing, bronchovesicular breathing, and bronchial or tubular breathing.
5. Name and define 3 abnormal sounds that may be heard on auscultation.
6. List 3 conditions that may result in reduction or absence of breath sounds. What are 2 techniques by which the examiner differentiates the cause for reduced or absent breath sounds?
7. Although largely replaced by x-rays, percussion can still be a useful technique. Explain.

Assessment of Pulmonary Function
by John H. Dirckx, MD

Acute and chronic disorders of the respiratory tract can impair the flow of air into and out of the lungs, reduce the amount of lung tissue available for gas exchange, or both. **Diagnostic spirometry** is the measurement of lung volumes and inspiratory and expiratory flow rates with a precisely calibrated instrument (**spirometer**) according to a standard testing protocol.

Spirometry is indicated in respiratory disorders causing dyspnea, wheezing, or cough when a quantitative assessment of lung volumes and flow rates is needed for diagnosis or for judging the severity of the condition or the response to treatment. Testing of respiratory volumes and flow rates is also valuable in screening smokers for early chronic obstructive pulmonary disease, in planning surgery involving removal of lung tissue, and in quantifying pulmonary disability.

The testing procedure requires the patient to breathe through a disposable mouthpiece attached by flexible tubing to the spirometer. A padded clamp occludes the nostrils to ensure that air flow occurs only through the mouth. After inhaling as deeply as possible, the patient exhales into the mouthpiece as rapidly and forcefully as possible. Several repetitions of the test may be required in order to achieve maximal measurements.

Ordinarily the results of various efforts are not averaged, but the best scores are assumed to be the most accurate.

The validity of test results depends on close adherence to standard testing protocol, accurate calibration of the instrument, and good cooperation by the subject.

The following measurements are performed during standard spirometry:

Tv (Vt) (tidal volume): the volume of air inhaled and exhaled during normal breathing, measured in liters (L).

FVC (forced vital capacity): the maximum volume of air that can be forcefully exhaled after a maximal inspiration, in liters.

FEV_1 (forced expiratory volume in 1 second): the volume of air that is exhaled during the first second of forceful exhalation, in liters.

FEV_1/FVC: the **ratio of FEV_1 to FVC**, expressed as a percent.

FEF_{25-75} (forced expiratory flow 25%-75%): the average flow rate during the midportion of a forced expiration, measured in liters per second (L/sec).

PEF (peak expiratory flow): the highest flow rate attained during forced expiration, measured in liters per second (L/sec).

Spirometry: Baseline spirometry showed significantly decreased flow volumes, the ratio suggesting a restrictive pattern, although she did have a significant 27% improvement in FEV1 after 2 albuterol + ipratropium nebulizer treatments consistent with a significant reversible airflow obstructive component consistent with asthma. Baseline FVC=1.68 (53% predicted), FEV1=1.37 (52%), FEV1%=81; post med FVC=2.00 (63% predicted), FEV1=1.74 (66%), FEV1%=87; 27% improvement in FEV1 post med.

For patients believed to have asthma, in which the bronchi are subject to intermittent constriction with resulting reduction of airflow, the testing procedure may be modified by administration of pharmaceutical agents. Inhalation of histamine or methacholine causes sharp reduction of flow rates due to **bronchospasm** in persons with hyperreactive airways. Inhalation of a bronchodilator quickly improves flow rates in a person with naturally occurring bronchospasm, or after challenge with histamine or methacholine.

The range of normal spirometry findings for a given subject depends on height, age, gender, and race. The results obtained by testing are therefore reported not only as absolute numbers but also as percents of the patient's predicted performance, based on these variables. In addition, the spirometer generates a graph plotting inspiratory and flow rates against volumes (**flow-volume loop**).

Often the coaching provided by the technician performing the test is crucial in obtaining a maximal inspiration and expiratory effort. The technician may urge the patient to exhale "as if you were trying to extinguish the sun."

Abnormal spirometric findings are basically of two types. In obstructive lung disease, a reduction in flow rate (FEV_1) occurs without a proportionate reduction in lung volume (FVC). This pattern is seen in emphysema and chronic bronchitis, which together constitute chronic obstructive pulmonary disease (COPD), as well as in asthma and acute bronchitis. In restrictive lung disease, both volume and flow rate are reduced in proportion. This type of spirometric finding occurs in pulmonary diseases causing scarring of the lungs or filling of air spaces with fluid or exudate, and also in diseases of the chest wall (pleura, ribs) impairing respiratory effort.

A compact, handheld personal spirometer to determine FEV_1 may be helpful for persons with asthma to judge the severity of acute airway compromise and the need for, or effectiveness of, medicines.

Incentive spirometry (see ■ Figure 10-3) is entirely different from **diagnostic spirometry**. It is a respiratory therapy technique applied to breathing exercises prescribed to prevent atelectasis and pneumonia due to inadequate lung expansion in postoperative patients and those with chest injuries who may fail to breathe deeply enough because of pain on breathing.

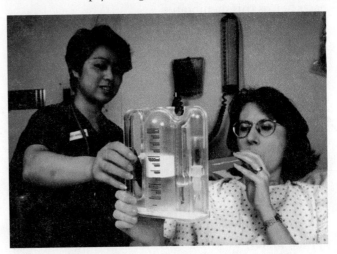

FIGURE 10-3. Incentive spirometry.
Source: Michal Heron, Pearson Education.

It is also prescribed for patients confined to bed for long periods of time.

Exercises consist of periods of deep breathing at regular intervals throughout the day. Use of a personal spirometer enables the patient to measure pulmonary flow so as to meet goals established on the basis of age, gender, and height.

The following respiratory volumes cannot be measured by spirometry. They can, however, be determined indirectly by **plethysmography** (in which the subject sits in a sealed chamber while pressure and volume changes are noted during normal breathing, maximal inspiration and expiration, and panting respirations) or determination of **total lung capacity** by tracer gas studies (in which a known concentration of nonabsorbable gas is breathed for a period of time and its concentration in expired air is then determined).

TLC (**total lung capacity**): the volume of air in the lungs after maximal inspiration.

FRC (**functional residual capacity**): the volume of air remaining in the lungs after normal expiration.

RV (**residual volume**): the volume of air remaining in the lungs after maximal expiration.

The expression **pulmonary function tests (PFTs)** is something of a misnomer, in that spirometric measurements do not really assess the function of the lungs, which is to exchange oxygen and carbon dioxide between the atmosphere and the blood. But some tests that may be performed in conjunction with spirometry do indeed measure gas exchange. The **alveolar-capillary membrane**, consisting of the walls of the pulmonary capillaries as they lie in apposition to the smallest pulmonary air sacs (the alveoli), is the anatomic site of gas exchange. **Gas diffusion tests** measure the passage of gases across this membrane.

In the **carbon monoxide diffusion capacity (D_LCO) test**, the patient takes a maximum inhalation of a mixture of air, helium, and carbon monoxide and holds it for 10 seconds. The exhaled breath is then analyzed, and from the concentrations of gases present the diffusing capacity is calculated as the volume of gas transferred per minute per millimeter of mercury of difference between the gas pressure of alveolar air and capillary blood. Normally this value is at least 25mL/minute/mmHg.

Another way of assessing pulmonary gas diffusion is the **nitrogen washout test**. The air we breathe is approximately 80% nitrogen and 20% oxygen. Breathing 100% oxygen for a period of several minutes nor-mally results in a gradual washing out of nitrogen from the lungs. For the nitrogen washout test, the subject breathes 100% oxygen and the nitrogen composition of exhaled air is determined serially. The finding of a nitrogen concentration greater than 2.5% after 7 minutes indicates erratic pulmonary gas diffusion. A variation of this test can be performed by graphing the nitrogen concentration of a single exhalation after maximal inhalation of 100% oxygen.

Pulmonary gas diffusing capacity may be significantly reduced in both restrictive and obstructive lung disease and in pulmonary embolism, and test results may also be abnormal in cardiac disease, anemia, and other conditions affecting respiratory physiology.

Pause for Reflection

1. Describe diagnostic spirometry and give examples of indications for spirometry.
2. Explain the measurements derived from spirometry.
3. What is a histamine or methacholine challenge test?
4. Explain the two types of abnormal spirometry findings.
5. What is incentive spirometry?
6. Define total lung capacity (TLC), functional residual capacity (FRC) and residual volume (RV) and explain how they are measured.
7. Briefly describe the carbon monoxide diffusion capacity (D_LCO) test and the nitrogen washout test.

Arterial Blood Gases

by John H. Dirckx, MD

Chemical measurement of arterial blood gases (oxygen and carbon dioxide) is used to assess the adequacy of **pulmonary gas exchange** in persons with respiratory or circulatory disease and those receiving oxygen therapy, with or without ventilatory assistance. Ordinarily the pH of the specimen is also determined to identify acidosis or alkalosis and to permit indirect calculation of the bicarbonate ion concentration.

The specimen for blood gas determination is drawn from an **artery**, not a vein. All room air is excluded from the specimen, heparin is added to prevent coagulation, and the specimen is stored in ice until testing is performed. Blood gases are measured in millimeters of mercury (mmHg or torr).

Arterial blood gases (ABG) on 2L showed a pH of 7.38, pCO2 of 54, pO2 87.4.

The normal **partial pressure of oxygen** (PO_2) in arterial blood is 75 to 100 torr. This level normally declines with age. The arterial oxygen may be increased in hyperventilation due to anxiety. Reduction of oxygen tension (**hypoxemia**) can result from any condition that depresses or inhibits respiratory movements (paralysis, chest injury, pneumothorax, massive obesity, central nervous system depression by drugs, trauma, or disease); any condition that prevents normal oxygen exchange in lung tissue (pneumonia, bronchitis, pulmonary edema, asthma, airway obstruction); or reduction of available oxygen in the atmosphere.

Oxygen saturation, which can be measured by **pulse oximetry**, can also be calculated from the PO_2 and the concentration of hemoglobin. The normal oxygen saturation is 95-100%. A reduction below this level has essentially the same significance as a reduction in the partial pressure of oxygen.

Eventually the patient was weaned off oxygen to the point that her saturation was 95%.

The normal **partial pressure of carbon dioxide** (pCO_2) is 35 to 45 torr. Increase in carbon dioxide tension (**hypercapnia**) may be caused by most of the same conditions that reduce oxygen (except reduction in available oxygen). Increase in carbon dioxide and bicarbonate ion also occurs in response to metabolic alkalosis. Reduction of carbon dioxide (**hypocapnia**) occurs in hyperventilation and in response to metabolic acidosis.

CO2 was 161, pCO2 of 43 and pO2 of 7.29. Blood sugar was 207.

A rise in serum pH is called **alkalosis** and a fall in pH is called **acidosis**. Either of these conditions can be respiratory in origin, resulting from a disturbance in the excretion of carbon dioxide by the lungs, or metabolic in origin, reflecting abnormalities in the levels of other ions. **Respiratory alkalosis** is due to excessive loss of

ARTERIAL PUNCTURE
Arterial puncture is more painful than venipuncture so collection of arterial blood gases is generally accompanied by anxiety on the part of the patient. Patient anxiety can be a problem because patient cooperation is essential for a successful puncture and collection. Often, it is a respiratory therapist who draws the blood for ABGs rather than the laboratory's phlebotomist, and, indeed, the blood gas analysis may even be performed in the respiratory department. This is because patients requiring an ABG are often on some type of respiratory therapy, and the test is being performed to assess the effectiveness of the therapy.

carbon dioxide via the lungs, as from hyperventilation, while **respiratory acidosis** indicates abnormal retention of carbon dioxide, as from disease of the respiratory or circulatory system that impairs pulmonary gas exchange. The causes of **metabolic alkalosis** include loss of hydrogen ions from the gastrointestinal tract through vomiting and loss of hydrogen ions from the kidneys as a result of diuretic administration, hyperaldosteronism, or Cushing syndrome.

Metabolic acidosis is divided into two types on the basis of the **anion gap** of the serum. If the sum of the cation concentrations of serum (sodium plus potassium) is compared to the sum of the anion concentrations (chloride plus bicarbonate), it will be found that the cation concentration is higher. This is because the calculation takes into account only the principal cations and anions, and the anions not included (phosphate, sulfate, protein, and various organic anions) exceed the cations not included (calcium, magnesium, and others). The difference between cation and anion concentrations when only the four principal ions are included in the calculation is called the **anion gap**, which is normally 12–20 mEq/L [12–20 mmol/L].

Metabolic acidosis with a normal anion gap may be due to loss of bicarbonate ion from the bowel through diarrhea, or from the kidney as a result of renal disease (**renal tubular acidosis**). When metabolic acidosis is accompanied by an increased anion gap, the difference in unmeasured anion is usually due to the presence of excessive anions derived from organic acids. These may be normal anions abnormally retained by a diseased kidney; anions abnormally produced in certain conditions (lactic acidosis, diabetic ketoacidosis); or extraneous substances (salicylate, methanol).

Any shift in serum pH tends to be compensated by whatever mechanism remains unimpaired. Hence, for example, metabolic acidosis leads to increased pulmonary excretion of carbon dioxide, with a resulting tendency towards respiratory alkalosis. Consequently, electrolyte imbalances are frequently complex and difficult to diagnose.

Pause for Reflection

1. What is the significance of a reduction in partial pressure of oxygen (pO_2) and oxygen saturation?
2. Define *hypoxemia, hypercapnia,* and *hypocapnia.*
3. How is the acidity or alkalinity of serum measured? What is the term for a rise in this concentration? What is the term for a fall in this concentration?
4. Distinguish between respiratory and metabolic alkalosis.
5. What is respiratory acidosis?
6. Describe the 2 types of metabolic acidosis.

Mechanical Ventilation

by John H. Dirckx, MD

Mechanical ventilation refers to any procedure whereby part or all of a person's breathing is performed by another person or by a machine. In the past, ventilation devices such as the iron lung (once crucial in the treatment of respiratory paralysis due to poliomyelitis) operated by creating a negative pressure outside the chest that sucked atmospheric air into the lungs. All ventilatory methods in use nowadays employ positive pressure, blowing air into the respiratory tract at higher than atmospheric pressure through a closed system.

The simplest form of mechanical ventilation is **mouth-to-mouth resuscitation**, an emergency procedure used to maintain air exchange in a person whose respiratory activity has ceased because of cardiac arrest, brain injury, drug or chemical intoxication, asphyxia, immersion, or any other cause.

The principal non-emergency settings in which mechanical ventilation is used are during major surgery and in providing ventilatory assistance for patients with acute or chronic impairment of breathing function. The interface between a ventilatory apparatus and the patient can be a **mask**, any of various oral, pharyngeal, and endotracheal airways, or a tracheostomy aperture.

An **endotracheal tube** (see ■ Figure 10-4), which is inserted into the windpipe and sealed in position with an inflatable cuff, is in many ways the ideal airway for mechanical ventilation. It can be introduced through either the nose (nasotracheal airway) or the mouth (orotracheal airway). It bypasses the tongue and glottis and prevents both leakage of ventilatory gas and aspiration of vomitus into the respiratory tract.

Endotracheal intubation is standard for the delivery of inhalation anesthesia in surgery because it permits close control of oxygen and anesthetic concentrations and allows the anesthesiologist to supplement the patient's breathing efforts as required by the depth of anesthesia, the effect of muscle relaxants administered, or the opening of the thorax for cardiovascular or pulmonary surgery. The anesthesiologist provides ventilatory assistance by making regular manual compressions of a rubber bag.

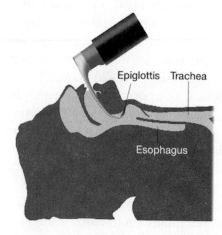
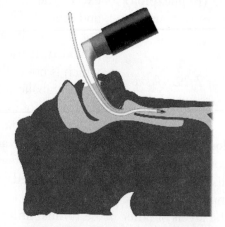
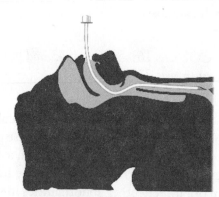

Epiglottis   Trachea

Esophagus

FIGURE 10-4. Endotracheal intubation

Short-term ventilatory support can be life-saving in acute lung injury, certain intoxications, and conditions such as Guillain-Barré syndrome that are characterized by temporary paralysis of respiratory muscles. More chronic **disorders of breathing activity** (myasthenia gravis, muscular dystrophy, irreversible brain or spinal cord injury, amyotrophic lateral sclerosis) or of **gas exchange** (chronic obstructive pulmonary disease, pulmonary fibrosis or cavitation) may impose lifelong dependence on mechanical ventilation.

Except in emergency situations and in surgery, **ventilatory assistance** is ordinarily provided by an automatic machine, commonly called a **respirator** or **ventilator**, that is programmed to deliver the desired volume of air for each breath at the desired frequency. A respirator may supply room air, an air-oxygen mixture, or 100% oxygen.

The presence of a tube in the trachea is uncomfortable for a conscious patient and usually causes coughing and retching. Irritation of the tracheal mucosa can lead to subglottic stenosis, a narrowing of the proximal trachea due to scarring. For long-term respirator use, a **tracheostomy** (see ■ Figure 10-5) is often performed to provide an interface that is more comfortable and less likely to cause complications.

Many kinds of **respirators** are available, varying in complexity and versatility. All permit the setting of volume and pressure limits, cycling times, triggering factors to initiate a breath, and the degree to which the patient's own efforts contribute to overall respiratory function. Most respirators also have built-in monitoring capabilities. These help in determining when a patient

is ready to be **weaned from a respirator**—that is, able to resume natural, unassisted breathing with adequate gas exchange.

Continuous positive airway pressure (CPAP) technology deserves brief mention here. In **obstructive sleep apnea (OSA)**, breathing is repeatedly interrupted during sleep as the airway is intermittently blocked by the soft palate or by lax or bulky pharyngeal tissues, including the tonsils. Nighttime hypoxemia and shallow, restless sleep can lead to daytime lethargy, difficulties with memory and concentration, and even personality change. A CPAP device provides a steady flow of room air at low pressure through the nose during sleep to overcome intermittent upper respiratory obstruction.

ABBREVIATIONS
Many pulmonary function terms consist of a combination of upper and lowercase letters and subscripts. If the platform or software does not permit subscripts, the numbers can be typed on the same line with the abbreviation without a space.

CO_2	or	CO2
FEV_1	or	FEV1
FiO_2	or	FiO2 (note the lowercase *i*)
pCO_2	or	pCO2
PCO_2	or	PCO2
pO_2	or	pO2
PO_2	or	PO2

pH (Note the lowercase *p*; at the beginning of a sentence add the word "The" before *pH*.)

Pause for Reflection

1. List the ways in which a patient may be connected to a respirator. Which is the best and why?
2. Why is endotracheal intubation the standard of delivery for anesthesia?
3. When and why is a tracheostomy employed in mechanical ventilation?
4. What is *weaning*?
5. What is CPAP and for what purpose is it used?

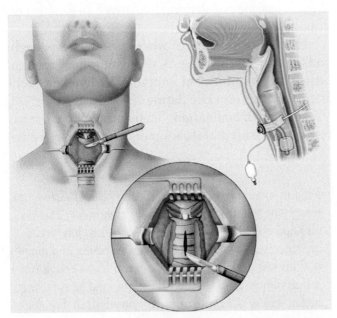

FIGURE 10-5. Tracheotomy, an incision through the trachea to assist breathing.

Common Diseases

Acute Bronchitis

Acute, self-limited inflammation of the bronchial passages.

Cause: Usually viral in origin, as a complication of an upper respiratory infection. Sometimes due to bacterial secondary infection. Can also be due to irritation by smoke or dust.

History: Cough, usually productive, occurring as a complication of a respiratory infection. When severe it may be accompanied by fever, shortness of breath, and wheezing. Cough may be worsened by the recumbent position and may keep the patient awake at night.

Physical Examination: Often no physical findings other than frequent or spasmodic coughing. The breath sounds may be bronchial, or rhonchi may be heard, chiefly on inspiration.

Diagnostic Tests: Blood studies are normal. Smear and culture of sputum may indicate bacterial infection but usually do not. Chest x-ray may show increased bronchial markings.

Course: Cough may continue for weeks or months, but resolution is eventually complete. Cough may result in rib fracture or other complications. Bronchitis lasting for three months and occurring in two successive years is termed **chronic bronchitis**.

Treatment: Largely symptomatic, with hydration, expectorants, and cough suppressants, at least for nighttime use. Many patients experience improvement when taking **bronchodilator drugs** either orally or by inhaler. Most patients are treated with **antibiotics** (clarithromycin, trimethoprim-sulfamethoxazole, tetracyclines), even though the vast majority of cases of bronchitis are due to viral infection.

Chronic Bronchitis

Chronic productive cough lasting for at least three months in each of two successive years. Chronic bronchitis is one form of **chronic obstructive pulmonary disease (COPD)**, the other being **emphysema**. The two forms may be combined in varying proportions.

Cause: Most cases occur in smokers. Air pollution, allergy, and infection may play a part in some cases. Obesity is a risk factor.

History: Severe persistent cough with copious production of bronchial mucus, particularly on arising in the morning.

Physical Examination: Wheezes and inspiratory rhonchi on auscultation of the chest. When bronchitis is severe, cyanosis may be noted.

Diagnostic Tests: The hematocrit may be slightly elevated, reflecting **polycythemia** (increase in number of circulating red blood cells) in response to diminished oxygen exchange in the lungs. Arterial blood shows reduction of oxygen and increase of carbon dioxide. Chest x-ray shows increased bronchopulmonary markings. Electrocardiogram may show right axis deviation and P pulmonale.

Course: Progressive deterioration of pulmonary function and heightened susceptibility to bacterial infection.

Treatment: Cessation of smoking and avoidance of respiratory irritants and infections are essential. Bronchodilators orally or by inhaler may improve bronchial air flow. Ipratropium by inhaler is particularly effective. Hydration, exercise, and postural drainage may assist in freeing the tract of secretions. When hypoxia is severe, home oxygen may be useful.

Asthma (Reactive Airways Disease, RAD)

A chronic or recurrent inflammatory disease of the trachea and bronchi characterized by recurrent narrowing of air passages with wheezing and shortness of breath (see ■ Figure 10-6).

Cause: Abnormal sensitivity of respiratory passages to a wide variety of triggering factors: emotional stress, airborne irritants (dust, cigarette smoke) and allergens (pollen, animal dander, dust mite protein), physical exertion (exercise-induced asthma), respiratory infection, and drugs (aspirin, beta-blockers). Asthma affects about 5% of the population; there may be a genetic predisposition.

History: Paroxysms of wheezing, dyspnea, cough, and tightness in the chest. Severe asthma may result in physical exhaustion and symptoms of **hypoxia** (deficiency of oxygen in circulating blood).

Physical Examination: Tachypnea; labored, noisy respirations with prolongation of the expiratory phase.

Mild to moderate wheeze after Ventolin and Atrovent treatment followed by a Ventolin treatment. He has also had Solu-Medrol IV. At 1223 he still has moderate wheeze. The patient was given Xopenex and magnesium sulfate IV. At 1340 he has a harsh cough but he has almost no wheeze at this time, and he is feeling better. He is not short of breath any longer. He does not have a prolonged respiratory phase.

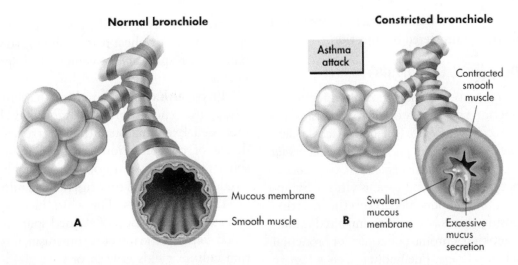

Normal bronchiole

Constricted bronchiole

Asthma attack

Contracted smooth muscle

Mucous membrane

Smooth muscle

A

B

Swollen mucous membrane

Excessive mucus secretion

FIGURE 10-6. An asthma attack, showing changes in bronchioles: (A) normal bronchiole and (B) constricted bronchiole in asthma attack

Sibilant (whistling) or **sonorous** (humming) **rhonchi** may be heard throughout the chest, particularly on expiration. In severe asthma, retraction of intercostal muscles may be noted on inspiration. The chest may be hyperresonant to percussion, and cyanosis may indicate hypoxia.

Diagnostic Tests: Pulmonary function tests indicate significant reduction in measures of air flow, particularly FEV_1 (forced expiratory volume in the first second of exhalation). When the diagnosis is in doubt, a **provocative test** (challenge of an asymptomatic patient with methacholine or histamine) will lead to reduction in air flow.

During an asthmatic attack, administration of bronchodilator by injection or inhalation leads to marked improvement in air flow measurements. In severe asthma, the blood level of oxygen may be reduced. The eosinophil count may be increased in allergic asthma, and eosinophils may be detected in sputum. Chest x-ray may show hyperinflation of the thorax.

Course: Many cases of childhood asthma are "outgrown." Asthma may persist and progress throughout life, depending on its underlying cause and triggering factors. Infection, cor pulmonale, and acute respiratory distress syndrome are possible complications.

Treatment: Avoidance of known inciting factors; smoking cessation. For intermittent symptoms and exercise-induced asthma, aerosolized bronchodilator administered by inhalation usually suffices to control symptoms. More severe or chronic disease is better treated with aerosolized corticosteroid, with bronchodilator treatment during exacerbations. The patient may be instructed to adjust the dosage of these agents

on the basis of measurements made with a simple portable peak flow meter. Other treatments include oral theophylline, mast-cell stabilizers (cromolyn, nedocromil), leukotriene antagonists (montelukast, zafirlukast), and the atropine-like drug ipratropium. In severe refractory asthma (**status asthmaticus**), oxygen is

IT'S BREATHTAKING!

Asthma is an often lifelong disease that causes wheezing, breathlessness, chest tightness, and coughing. It can limit a person's quality of life. While we don't know why asthma rates are rising, we do know that most people with asthma can control their symptoms and prevent asthma attacks by avoiding asthma triggers and correctly using prescribed medicines, such as inhaled corticosteroids.

The number of people diagnosed with asthma grew by 4.3 million from 2001 to 2009. From 2001 through 2009 asthma rates rose the most among black children, almost a 50% increase.

A rising trend in asthma prevalence was observed for non-Hispanic black children, non-Hispanic white women, and non-Hispanic black men. In 2009, asthma prevalence was greater among children than adults, and was especially high among boys and non-Hispanic black children. Prevalence among adults was greatest for women and adults who were poor.

Greater access to medical care is needed for the growing number of people with asthma.

administered by inhalation and bronchodilators and corticosteroids are administered by injection.

Pneumonia (Pneumonitis)

Inflammation of lung tissue, usually due to infection.

Cause: Infection by a variety of microorganisms, including *Streptococcus pneumoniae* (pneumococcus), *Klebsiella pneumoniae*, *Mycoplasma pneumoniae*, *Chlamydia pneumoniae*, *Legionella pneumophila*, *Staphylococcus aureus*, *Pneumocystis jiroveci*, and various viruses. Symptoms, signs, and clinical course depend on the infecting agent. Predisposing causes are debility, impaired immunity, cigarette smoking, chronic pulmonary or bronchial disease, and advanced age. Pneumonia (see ■ Figure 10-7) often occurs as a complication or extension of upper respiratory infection.

History: Fever, chills, cough, purulent or bloody sputum, **pleuritic chest pain** (stabbing, sharply localized pain with respiratory movements), dyspnea, myalgia, malaise.

Physical Examination: Most patients have fever. The pulse and respiratory rate may be markedly increased. Examination of the lungs reveals rales or evidence of **consolidation** (reduced or absent breath sounds, flat percussion note). In mycoplasmal or viral pneumonia, physical findings may be minimal.

Diagnostic Tests: The white blood count may be elevated. Examination of stained sputum shows white blood cells and the infecting organism, if bacterial. Sputum culture yields growth of bacterial agents. Bronchoscopy and bronchoalveolar washings may be necessary to obtain satisfactory sputum for examination.

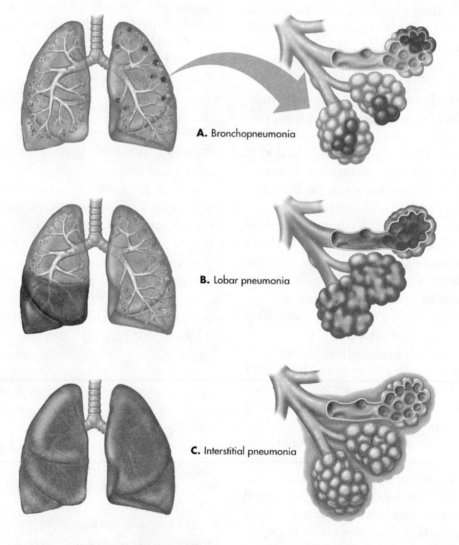

A. Bronchopneumonia

B. Lobar pneumonia

C. Interstitial pneumonia

FIGURE 10-7. (A) Bronchopneumonia with localized pattern. (B) Lobar pneumonia with a diffuse pattern within the lung lobe. (C) Interstitial pneumonia is typically diffuse and bilateral.

Chest x-ray shows evidence of pulmonary infiltrates or consolidation, atelectasis, pleural effusion.

Course: Some pneumonias, including most viral and mycoplasmal infections, resolve spontaneously. **Lobar pneumonia** due to *Streptococcus pneumoniae*, staphylococcal pneumonia, and (in immunocompromised hosts) *Pneumocystis jiroveci* pneumonia frequently progress to a fatal termination, even with treatment. Pneumonia ranks sixth as a cause of death in the U.S.

Complications: Pleural effusion, empyema, septicemia, endocarditis, arthritis, respiratory failure.

Treatment: Oral antibiotics may suffice in mild disease. Azithromycin, clarithromycin, and levofloxacin are the agents usually chosen. In more severe disease, hospitalization, intravenous antibiotics, and oxygen by inhalation may be necessary.

Influenza

Influenza is an acute respiratory infection caused by any of several related viruses.

Onset is abrupt, with fever, chills, myalgia, and cough. Inflammation of lower respiratory mucosa often progresses to pneumonitis, and bacterial superinfection is common. The disease is highly contagious and may occur in epidemics in late fall, winter, and early spring.

Influenza causes about 50,000 deaths annually in the U.S., most of them in the elderly. Vaccination confers effective protection and is recommended for all persons over 50 and for those with diabetes mellitus, immunodeficiency, and cardiac or pulmonary disease. However, vaccines must be reformulated annually because of spontaneous alteration in viral antigenic makeup.

For exposed persons who have not been immunized, prophylaxis with amantadine, rimantadine, oseltamivir, or zanamivir can prevent illness. Treatment of established infection with these agents slightly reduces the duration of clinical symptoms. Therapy otherwise is symptomatic.

Pulmonary Tuberculosis

Cause: Infection of lungs and other tissues and organs by *Mycobacterium tuberculosis* (see ■ Figure 10-8). Person-to-person spread by respiratory droplets is the usual route of infection. Primary infection may be asymptomatic but leaves a focus of infective organisms in the lung and induces a state of hypersensitivity to the infecting organism. Postprimary infection, which may result from breakdown of a primary focus or from a new dose of organisms

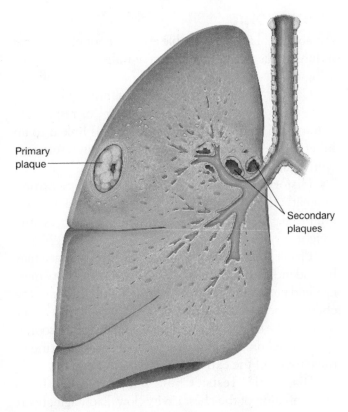

FIGURE 10-8. Pulmonary tuberculosis

from without, typically leads to significant and chronic clinical disease. The infection can also be transmitted by unpasteurized milk from infected cows. Other species, notably those of the M. *avium intracellulare* complex (MAI, MAC) may also cause tuberculosis, typically acquired through the gastrointestinal tract. Persons with AIDS are at particular risk of tuberculosis, including MAI tuberculosis.

History: Cough, purulent or bloody sputum, fever, night sweats, weakness, anorexia, weight loss.

Physical Examination: Fever, cachexia (wasting), evidence of rales, consolidation, or cavitation in the lungs.

Diagnostic Tests: The tuberculin skin test is positive. Sputum contains acid-fast organisms, and sputum culture is positive for M. *tuberculosis*. Chest x-ray may show a calcified primary focus, hilar lymphadenopathy, upper lobe infiltrates, pleural effusion, or cavitation.

Course: Prognosis with treatment is good. Complications include **phthisis** (wasting) and hemorrhage.

Treatment: Simultaneous treatment with three or four drugs (isoniazid, rifampin, pyrazinamide, streptomycin, ethambutol) for a protracted period is the standard.

Emphysema

An abnormal and irreversible enlargement of air spaces in lung tissue due to breakdown of walls of air sacs (see ■ Figure 10-9).

Cause: Cigarette smoking is a principal cause. Some cases are due to infection, allergy, or respiratory irritants. In some patients, emphysema is linked to an inherited deficiency of alpha$_1$-antitrypsin in respiratory epithelium and other tissues.

History: The onset is usually after age 50. Shortness of breath, growing progressively worse, is the dominant symptom. Some patients experience weakness and weight loss.

Physical Examination: Tachypnea and dyspnea may be evident, with activity of the accessory respiratory muscles and pursed lips. The anteroposterior diameter of the chest is increased (**barrel chest**). There is hyperresonance of the thorax on percussion, and the breath sounds are reduced on auscultation. Weakness and wasting of the muscles of the extremities are often noted.

Diagnostic Tests: Chest x-ray typically shows hyperinflation of the chest cavity (low diaphragm, heart in vertical position) and **hyperlucency** (reduced resistance to passage of x-rays) of lung tissue. X-ray may also show **bullae** or **blebs** (air-filled cavities). Blood gas studies are usually normal but may show diminished partial pressure of oxygen. Pulmonary function tests show increased total lung capacity but reduced vital capacity and rate of air exchange.

Course: Recurrent respiratory infections, congestive heart failure (right ventricular failure, cor pulmonale), progressive respiratory failure.

Treatment: Smoking cessation, bronchodilators, oxygen inhalation, antibiotics as needed, physical therapy. For cardiac failure, sodium restriction and diuretics.

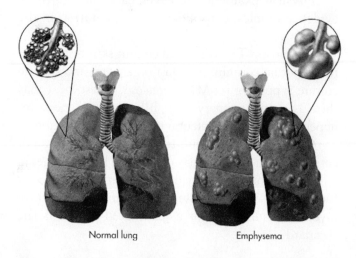

Normal lung   Emphysema

FIGURE 10-9. Emphysema

Pulmonary Embolism and Infarction

Obstruction of parts of the pulmonary arterial circulation by one or more emboli.

Cause: Thromboemboli from the deep veins of the lower extremities or pelvis passing through the right ventricle are the principal cause. Emboli may also consist of tumor material, amniotic fluid, fat, air, or injected foreign material. Predisposing causes of pulmonary thromboembolism include prolonged immobilization, surgery, childbirth, injury to venous endothelium, hypercoagulable state (cancer, oral contraceptives), congestive heart failure, obesity, and advanced age. Trapping of an embolus in a pulmonary artery results in both reflex vasoconstriction with extensive compromise of pulmonary circulation and reflex bronchoconstriction with impairment of pulmonary gas exchange.

History: Sudden onset of dyspnea, chest pain, anxiety, diaphoresis, collapse. If infarction occurs, chest pain may be pleuritic and there may be hemoptysis.

Physical Examination: Tachycardia, tachypnea, crackling rales or wheezes, pleural friction rub, cyanosis, fever.

Diagnostic Tests: The arterial oxygen tension is diminished. The electrocardiogram may show right axis deviation or right heart strain. Chest x-ray in acute pulmonary embolism may show an infiltrate or atelectasis. If infarction occurs, a wedge-shaped zone of opacification may be apparent. A **ventilation-perfusion scan** (radionuclide scan) shows areas of lung tissue that are normally ventilated (normal air flow) but not normally perfused (impeded blood flow). Pulmonary angiogram confirms and localizes pulmonary arterial obstruction. The source of the embolus may be discovered by venography, ultrasonography, impedance plethysmography, or other diagnostic modality.

Course: About 10% of patients die within the first hour, and the overall mortality rate is about 30%. Fatal outcome is usually due to right ventricular failure or cardiogenic shock.

Treatment: Vigorous supportive efforts, including oxygen and treatment for shock and cardiac failure. Thrombolytic therapy with streptokinase, urokinase, or **tissue plasminogen activator** (tPA) is often successful in dissolving the embolus. Intravenous heparin and oral warfarin are administered to prevent further thrombosis of deep veins. Passage of further emboli through the inferior vena cava may be prevented by surgical plication, ligation, or insertion of a filter. Prevention of pulmonary embolism includes use of compressive stockings in surgical and other bedfast patients, early ambulation after surgery, and use of low-dose heparin in selected medical and surgical patients.

Pleural Effusion

Presence of fluid in the pleural space as a result of local or systemic disease.

CT scan and chest x-ray consistent with right pleural effusion.

Causes: Pleural transudates (fluid relatively low in protein) occur in congestive heart failure, cirrhosis with ascites, nephrotic syndrome, myxedema, and obstructive disorders of the pulmonary circulation (superior vena cava obstruction, pulmonary embolism, constrictive pericarditis). **Pleural exudates** (fluid higher in protein and also containing LDH) are due to pneumonia and other pulmonary or pleural infections including tuberculosis, malignant disease, and uremia.

History: There may be no symptoms. With large effusions, dyspnea. With local inflammation, pleuritic chest pain.

Physical Examination: Reduced breath sounds, dullness to percussion, reduced **tactile fremitus** (transmission of vocal vibrations to the examiner's hand on the chest wall) over the effusion. In the presence of pleural inflammation, a **pleural friction rub** may be heard.

Diagnostic Tests: Chest x-ray, particularly **lateral decubitus films** (taken with patient lying on side), shows the effusion. Fluid obtained by **thoracentesis** (needle puncture of chest wall with aspiration of fluid by syringe) (see ■ Figure 10-10) is examined for protein and LDH (lactic dehydrogenase) to distinguish between transudate and exudate, and for white blood cells, pathogenic microorganisms, and malignant cells to establish an underlying cause for the effusion. Pleural biopsy, closed (needle) or open, may be required for definitive diagnosis.

Treatment: Correction of the cause of effusion, if possible.

CT scan showed a large dependent right pleural effusion with extension to the apex. No evident pneumothorax. Probable comprehensive atelectasis is noted in the right lung base. Stranding densities noted projecting into the anterior left base likely representing scar versus atelectasis.

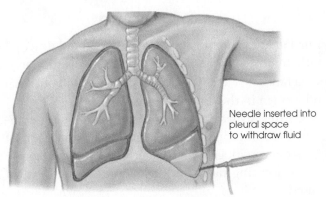

Needle inserted into pleural space to withdraw fluid

FIGURE 10-10. Thoracentesis

Spontaneous Pneumothorax

Sudden leakage of air from a lung into the pleural space (see ■ Figure 10-11).

Cause: Rupture of a bleb or bulla, which may be solitary or part of a generalized process. The condition is commoner in males and in smokers.

History: Sudden onset of chest pain and dyspnea, which may occur at rest or during sleep.

Physical Examination: Tachycardia; reduced breath sounds, hyperresonance, and reduced **tactile fremitus** over the pneumothorax.

Diagnostic Tests: Chest x-ray (inspiratory and expiratory films) shows pneumothorax.

Course: A small pneumothorax resolves spontaneously. Larger ones may severely compromise cardiopulmonary dynamics. The recurrence rate is 50%.

Treatment: Thoracostomy tube connected to a water seal bottle and suction, to withdraw air from the pleural space. **Thoracotomy** (open surgery) may be required for a continuing leak or for recurrent pneumothorax.

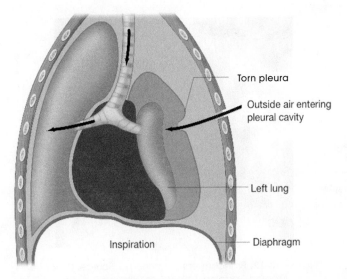

Torn pleura

Outside air entering pleural cavity

Left lung

Inspiration

Diaphragm

FIGURE 10-11. Pneumothorax

Bronchogenic Carcinoma

A malignant tumor of the lung arising from bronchial epithelium (see ■ Figure 10-12). Bronchogenic carcinoma ranks first as a cause of cancer death in both men and women in the United States.

Causes: Cigarette smoking is by far the most common cause of bronchogenic carcinoma. Inhalation of industrial carcinogens, particularly asbestos, and exposure to ionizing radiation or radon are other known causes.

History: Gradual onset of cough (or change in a chronic cough), dyspnea, wheezing, hemoptysis, anorexia, weight loss, chest pain.

Physical Examination: May indicate weight loss, muscle wasting, or signs of bronchial obstruction, pneumonia, atelectasis, cavitation, or pleural effusion.

Diagnostic Tests: Chest x-ray or CT scan demonstrates a solitary nodule, mass infiltrate, atelectasis, cavitation, or pleural effusion. Cytologic examination of bronchial washings or pleural fluid or histologic examination of tissue obtained by biopsy shows malignant tissue arising from bronchial epithelium.

Course: Bronchogenic carcinoma is typically advanced and inoperable when first diagnosed. The 5-year survival rate is 10-15%. Obstruction of airways commonly leads to atelectasis and pneumonia.

Complications include obstruction of the vena cava (superior vena cava syndrome) or esophagus, cardiac tamponade or arrhythmia, neurologic disorders (phrenic nerve palsy, Pancoast syndrome due to involvement of the brachial plexus), and paraneoplastic syndromes (Cushing syndrome, hypercalcemia) due to production of hormone-like agents by tumor cells.

Treatment: Surgery, radiation, and chemotherapy.

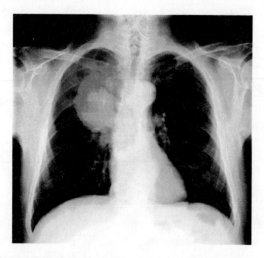

FIGURE 10-12. Bronchogenic carcinoma. Source: Du Cane Medical Imaging, Ltd., Photo Researchers, Inc.

Pause for Reflection

1. Distinguish between acute and chronic bronchitis.
2. Describe the findings on physical examination in a patient with asthma.
3. List the causes and treatment of pneumonia.
4. Describe the cause, prevention, and treatment of influenza.
5. Describe the cause and treatment for pulmonary tuberculosis.
6. Discuss the physical findings and results of diagnostic studies in emphysema.
7. What imaging studies may be used in the diagnosis of pulmonary embolism or infarction?
8. Distinguish between transudates and exudates in pleural effusion.
9. Distinguish between pleural effusion and pneumothorax.
10. List 3 complications, other than death, of bronchogenic carcinoma.
11. List 3 common diseases that are primarily attributable to smoking.

Diagnostic and Surgical Procedures

bronchoalveolar lavage (BAL) Obtaining of material from lung tissue by washing.

bronchoscopy Inspection of the interior of the trachea and main bronchi with a fiberoptic instrument. Specimens and biopsies can be taken through the instrument.

cardiopulmonary resuscitation (CPR) The use of external compression of the heart coupled with breathing techniques to revive a victim whose heart and respirations have stopped.

chest x-ray (CXR) Standard views are anteroposterior (AP), posteroanterior (PA), and lateral. An AP film shows the lungs as the x-rays pass from the front of the body (anterior) to the back (posterior). A PA film shows the lungs as the x-rays pass from the back of the body to the front. In the lateral view, the x-rays pass from side to side. Other views that may be referenced are oblique (the patient is positioned at a 45-degree angle to the film) and lateral decubitus (the patient is lying on either side). Images obtained as the patient takes a deep breath and holds it are called inspiratory x-rays; images taken after exhalation and before inspiration are called expiratory x-rays.

lung biopsy Removal of tissue from the lung for microscopic examination and diagnosis. The technique may be percutaneous (needle biopsy), by transbronchial lavage (washing) through a fiberoptic bronchoscope, transthoracic (via needle or open procedure), or aspiration (through a needle). See *pleural biopsy.*

Mantoux tuberculin skin test Skin test for tuberculosis (TB). A needle is inserted intradermally, and a small amount of purified protein derivative (PPD) from the bacterium *Mycobacterium tuberculosis* is inserted under the skin. A Mantoux test is a definitive test and is usually done to confirm a previously positive tine test. A positive reaction means the patient has or has had tuberculosis. The diameter of the indurated skin reaction (the palpable, raised, hardened area or swelling) is measured across the forearm (perpendicular to the long axis) in millimeters.

PET scan A nuclear imaging study that reveals how organs and tissues are functioning.

pleural biopsy A procedure to remove a sample of the tissue lining the lungs and the inside of the chest wall for microscopic examination and diagnosis. It may be done percutaneously (needle through the skin and chest wall) or by open technique. See *lung biopsy.*

PPD test See *Mantoux test, tine test.*

pulmonary function tests (PFTs) To measure the rate and volume of gas exchange in the respiratory system by means of finely calibrated instruments.

thoracoscopic wedge excision Resection of a small piece of lung that contains a suspicious nodule or known cancer with a margin of healthy tissue around it through a special videoscope. The procedure is usually done on patients whose lung function is such that a more invasive or extensive surgery would be contraindicated.

tine test Skin test for tuberculosis. A multiple-puncture device is used to pierce the skin and insert a small amount of purified protein derivative (PPD) from the bacterium *Mycobacterium tuberculosis*. A positive reaction is confirmed by doing a Mantoux test. The

four small blades used to puncture the skin are called tines because they resemble the tips or tines of a fork.

transthoracic needle biopsy Excision of tissue for microscopic examination and diagnosis using a needle inserted through the skin and chest wall.

tuberculin skin test See *Mantoux tuberculin skin test.*

ventilation-perfusion (V-P) scan A nuclear scan so named because it studies both airflow (ventilation) and blood flow (perfusion) in the lungs. The initials V-Q are used in mathematical equations that calculate airflow and blood flow. The purpose of this test is to look for evidence of a blood clot in the lungs, called a pulmonary embolus, that lowers oxygen levels, causes shortness of breath, and sometimes is fatal.

Laboratory Procedures

acid-fast stain A staining procedure in which sputum, tissue, or other material is exposed to fluorochrome dye and then washed with acid-alcohol. Organisms of the genus *Mycobacterium* and some others retain the dye and are said to be acid-fast.

agglutinins, cold Antibodies formed by persons with mycoplasmal pneumonia, which cause red blood cells to clump when chilled but not at room or body temperature.

agglutinins, febrile A group of antibody tests, each for a specific febrile (fever-causing) infectious disease, used as a screening procedure in patients with fever of unknown origin (FUO).

arterial blood gases (ABGs) The specimen of blood is drawn from an artery as opposed to the venous blood drawn for chemistry studies on the blood. Oxygen and carbon dioxide are the principal gases dissolved in the blood. Blood gas measurements include partial pressures of oxygen (pO_2) and of carbon dioxide (pCO_2) and oxygen saturation. From these data and the serum pH, it is possible to calculate the bicarbonate level. Alternatively, the base excess may be reported as the variation from a neutral blood pH.

basic metabolic panel (BMP) A panel of 7 or 8 chemical blood tests used as a screening tool or to assess and monitor fluid and electrolyte status, kidney function, blood sugar levels, and response to therapy. It includes sodium, potassium, chloride, and bicarbonate, or CO_2 (the electrolytes), plus BUN, creatinine (measures of kidney function), and glucose (blood sugar). Calcium may be included although not technically part of a BMP. May be referred to as a chem-7, or chem-8 if calcium is included.

chem-20 A comprehensive panel of blood chemistry tests that includes the tests included in a BMP plus liver function tests (ALT, AST, alkaline phosphatase, total protein and albumin, and bilirubin) and cholesterol (HDL, LDL, triglycerides, and total cholesterol), and LDH. The more common name is **CMP (comprehensive metabolic panel)**. May also be referred to as a chemistry panel.

electrolytes, sweat Sodium and chloride ions in the sweat, increased in persons with cystic fibrosis.

erythrocyte sedimentation rate A test that indirectly measures how much inflammation is in the body. Also called a *sed rate*.

INR (international normalized ratio) A modification of the prothrombin time test in which the test result is multiplied by a constant established for the batch of thromboplastin reagent used.

sputum smear and culture Microscopic examination of respiratory secretions for pathogenic organisms, neoplastic cells, or other abnormal findings.

Pharmacology

Respiratory diseases such as asthma (reversible obstructive airways disease), bronchitis, chronic obstructive pulmonary disease (COPD), and emphysema require medication to treat chronic symptoms as well as prevent acute attacks. Aside from the antibiotics used to treat respiratory infections, there are several classes of drugs prescribed to treat pulmonary diseases and to treat patients on ventilators, as well as to help patients stop smoking (see ■ Figure 10-13).

Bronchodilators

Bronchodilators relax the smooth muscle that surrounds the bronchi, thereby increasing air flow. This dilatation of the bronchi is due either to stimulation of $beta_2$ receptors in the smooth muscle of the bronchi, to the release of epinephrine which itself stimulates $beta_2$ receptors, or to inhibition of acetylcholine at cholinergic receptor sites in smooth muscle.

Bronchodilators are given orally as a tablet or liquid, via nebulizer as a liquid that is made into a fine mist, intravenously, or as a solution or powder released from an aerosol canister through a dispenser with a special mouthpiece. The **metered-dose inhaler (MDI)** (see ■ Figure 10-14) automatically injects a premeasured dose into the lungs as the patient inhales through

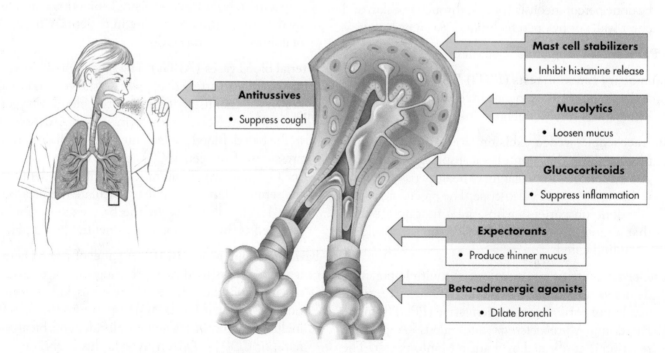

Antitussives
• Suppress cough

Mast cell stabilizers
• Inhibit histamine release

Mucolytics
• Loosen mucus

Glucocorticoids
• Suppress inflammation

Expectorants
• Produce thinner mucus

Beta-adrenergic agonists
• Dilate bronchi

FIGURE 10-13. Drugs to treat respiratory disorders

Combivent 2 puffs 4 times a day. She has been given albuterol nebulizer also to take as needed. She finds significant benefit from the nebulizer and from metered-dose inhalers.

the mouth. The dosage for MDIs is given as a number of metered sprays or **puffs**. Bronchodilators can also be given as a capsule that releases a microfine powder for inhalation when used with a Rotahaler inhalation device. Bronchodilators administered through inhalers include:

> albuterol (ProAir HFA, Proventil, Ventolin)
> aminophylline (Phyllocontin)
> bitolterol (Tornalate)
> epinephrine (Ana-Guard, AsthmaHaler Mist, microNefrin, Primatene Mist)
> fenoterol (Berotec)
> fluticasone propionate; salmeterol xinafoate (Advair HFA, Advair Diskus)
> ipratropium (Atrovent)
> isoproterenol (Isuprel)
> metaproterenol (Alupent)
> pirbuterol (Maxair Autohaler)
> salmeterol (Serevent)
> terbutaline (Brethaire, Brethine, Bricanyl)
> theophylline (Accurbron, Bronkodyl, Elixophyllin, Quibron-T Dividose, Respbid, Slo-bid Gyrocaps, Slo-Phyllin Gyrocaps, Sustaire, Theobid Duracaps, Theolair, T-Phyl, Uni-Dur, Uniphyl)
> tiotropium bromide (Spiriva)

Antibiotics

> amoxicillin
> azithromycin (Zithromax; Z-Pak)
> cefotaxime sodium (Claforan)
> clarithromycin (Biaxin)
> doxycycline (Doryx, Monodox, Vibramycin)
> levofloxacin (Levaquin)

Leukotriene Receptor Antagonists

Leukotriene is produced in the body in response to inhaled antigens and causes airway edema, bronchial constriction, and inflammation. Leukotriene receptor antagonists block the action of leukotriene at the receptor level.

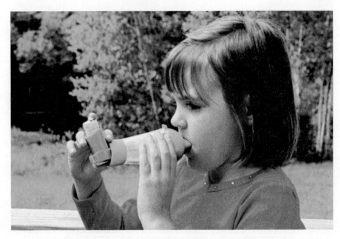

FIGURE 10-14. Metered-dose inhaler (MDI).
Source: Pearson Education, PH College.

> montelukast (Singulair)
> zafirlukast (Accolate)
> zileuton (Zyflo)

Corticosteroids

Corticosteroids (hydrocortisone and cortisone) are produced naturally by the adrenal glands. They suppress the inflammatory response of the immune system. Corticosteroids reduce inflammation and tissue edema associated with asthma and other chronic lung diseases and prevent acute attacks. They do not produce bronchodilation; they are always used in conjunction with bronchodilators. They are administered prophylactically because they are not effective during acute attacks of bronchospasm. These drugs are given by inhaler, and dosage is prescribed in numbers of puffs.

> beclomethasone (Beclovent, Vanceril)
> budesonide (Pulmicort Turbuhaler)
> flunisolide (AeroBid)
> fluticasone (Flonase, Flovent, Flovent Diskus, Flovent Rotadisk)
> methylprednisolone sodium succinate (Solu-Medrol)
> triamcinolone (Azmacort)

Mast Cell Inhibitors

Mast cell inhibitors stabilize the cell membranes of mast cells and prevent them from releasing histamine during the immune system's response to an antigen. This prevents bronchospasm in patients with bronchial asthma due to allergies. Mast cell stabilizers are not bronchodilators so they are not effective in treating acute asthma attacks but only in preventing attacks.

Note: Cromolyn is given by nebulizer or by a special device called a Spinhaler turbo-inhaler that punctures the capsule and allows the powdered drug within to be inhaled.

>   cromolyn (Intal)
>   nedocromil (Tilade)

Antituberculosis Drugs

Tuberculosis (TB) is caused by *Mycobacterium tuberculosis*, a gram-positive bacterium that is resistant to antibiotics that are usually effective against gram-positive bacteria. Treatment with a combination of antituberculosis drugs is necessary.

>   aminosalicylic acid (Paser Granules)
>   aminosidine (Gabbromicina)
>   capreomycin (Capastat)
>   cycloserine (Seromycin Pulvules)
>   ethambutol (Myambutol)
>   ethionamide (Trecator-SC)
>   isoniazid (INH, Nydrazid)
>   rifampin (Rifadin, Rimactane)
>   rifapentine (Priftin)
>   streptomycin

Combination drugs to treat tuberculosis include Rifamate (isoniazid, rifampin) and Rifater (isoniazid, rifampin, pyrazinamide).

Drugs Used to Treat AIDS Patients

Pneumocystis pneumonia (PCP) is the most common serious complication in AIDS patients and eventually affects about three fourths of all AIDS patients. *Pneumocystis jiroveci* (formerly called *P. carinii*) is a protozoan that seldom causes symptoms in healthy individuals.

>   atovaquone (Mepron)
>   Bactrim (trimethoprim and sulfamethoxazole)
>   clindamycin (Cleocin)
>   dapsone
>   pentamidine (NebuPent, Pentam 300)
>   primaquine
>   Septra (trimethoprim and sulfamethoxazole)
>   tobramycin
>   trimethoprim
>   trimetrexate (NeuTrexin)

Drugs used to treat AIDS wasting syndrome by stimulating the appetite of AIDS patients include:

>   Cachexon (glutathione)
>   cyproheptadine (Periactin)
>   dihydrotestosterone (Androgel-DHT)
>   dronabinol (Marinol)
>   marijuana
>   megestrol (Megace)
>   oxandrolone (Oxandrin)
>   sermorelin (Geref)
>   somatropin (BioTropin, Serostim)
>   testosterone (AndroGel, Theraderm Testosterone Transdermal System)
>   thalidomide (Thalomid)

Mycobacterium avium-intracellulare complex (MAC) infection is a common late-stage complication of AIDS. Drugs used to treat MAC infection include:

>   aminosidine (Gabbromicina)
>   clarithromycin (Biaxin, Biaxin XL)
>   gentamicin, liposomal (Maitec)
>   piritrexim
>   rifabutin (Mycobutin)
>   rifalazil
>   rifapentine (Priftin)
>   streptomycin

Drugs used for **respiratory syncytial virus infection (RSV)** include ribavirin (Virazole) and RSV immunoglobulin (RespiGam).

Surfactants

Natural surfactants derived from ground-up cows' lungs are used to supplement low levels of natural surfactant in the lungs of premature infants suffering from **infant respiratory distress syndrome (IRDS)**, also known as **hyaline membrane disease**. Surfactant maintains surface tension to prevent the lungs from collapsing with each breath. Surfactants are administered via endotracheal tube.

>   beractant (Survanta)
>   colfosceril palmitate (Exosurf, Curosurf, and Infasurf.

Transcription Tips

1. Confusing terms related to the respiratory system: Some of these terms sound alike; others are potential traps when researching. Memorize the terms and their meanings so that you can select the appropriate term for a correct transcript.

   consolidated—forming a mass, joined together as a whole

   consolidative—tending or causing something to form into a mass

   dieresis—the division or separation of parts normally united (pathologic or surgical)

   diuresis—increased urination, often by means of diuretic medication

   effusion—accumulation of fluid in organ or tissue

   infusion—the introduction of fluid into a vein by means of gravity

   embolism—obstruction of a vessel by an embolus (the condition)

   embolus—the plug or material that obstructs the vessel (the cause)

   mucus (noun)—secretions

   mucous (adj.)—pertaining to mucus or the membranes that produce mucus

   perfuse (the *s* sounds like a *z*)—to pour over or through

   profuse (the *s* sounds like an *s*)—abundant

   perfusion—generally, the passage of fluid through vessels of an organ, as blood perfusion through the pulmonary artery

   profusion—abundance

2. Slang Terms. Expand these slang brief forms when encountered in dictation.

a. fib.	atrial fibrillation
bicarb	bicarbonate
trach ("trake")	tracheostomy
pulse ox	pulse oximetry
regurg	regurgitation

3. Note the challenging spellings or unusual capitalization of these common pulmonary drugs.

   ASA (acetylsalicylic acid, aspirin; transcribe as dictated)

   Advair Diskus or Advair HFA

   AeroBid

   Azmacort

   Bronkaid

   ProAir HFA

   Pulmicort (Flexhaler, Respules, Turbuhaler)

   Singulair (not Singular)

   Zithromax; Z-Pak

   Zyrtec

4. Spelling. Memorize the spelling of these difficult-to-spell terms. Note silent letters, doubled letters, and unexpected pronunciation.

   larynx (not lar-*nyx*, a common mispronunciation)

   pharynx (not phar-*nyx*)

   phlegm (starts with *ph*, *g* is silent—"flem")

   oropharynx

   phthisis ("thi sis" or "ti sis"; the *ph* is silent)

   pleural (lungs) (not plural)

   pneumonia (silent *p*)

   xiphoid (*x* is pronounced as a *z*)

5. Dictation Challenges

   The respiratory term *alveolar* refers to the alveoli in the lungs. *Alveolar* is also used to describe a ridge in the oral cavity and may be heard in dental dictation or other dictation relating to the nose, mouth, and throat.

   The correct format for transcribing terms related to smoking history is as follows: . . . a 50-pack-year history of smoking (meaning a pack a day for 50 years, or 2 packs a day for 25 years, etc.)

   The unusual phrase *pulmonary toilet* refers to various measures such as postural drainage, percussion, and hydration that are used to clear secretions from the respiratory tract.

   A *Y stent* is shaped like a *Y* to fit into the bronchus where the right and left segments take off from it.

   Listen carefully for *–ive* and *–ed* endings on words like *consolidated/consolidative*. There are nuances of meaning; the two words are not synonymous.

   An acceptable abbreviation for *micrograms* is *mcg* when accompanied by a number.

Spotlight On

Confessions of an Addict

by Judith Marshall

I grew up in Cleveland under the shadow of the great steel mills. I thought the color of the sky was orange and the natural quality of air was acrid. I would wake up and hear the birds coughing. I thought all mothers and fathers, aunts and uncles, and grandparents came with cigarettes in their mouths and lived in a cloud of smoke. At age 14 I got a work permit and somehow it seemed natural that I began smoking in the basement of a hospital, desperately trying to appear sophisticated and grown up.

Over 30 years ago I began my smoking career and, oh, how I loved it. Cigarettes were my best friend, my pal, my lover, my source of strength, my comfort, delight, reward, and badge of elegance. Cigarettes were then socially acceptable and medically benign.

Smoking and medical transcription were natural together. As soon as I could bounce a *Dorland's* on my knee, I realized that I was born to smoke and to transcribe, preferably at the same time. I perfected a system of drinking coffee in the morning and cola in the afternoons along with the two packs (and later three) of cigarettes a day. My system was so full of caffeine and nicotine it was no wonder I typed two thousand words a minute.

I blamed my near-constant headaches on the dumb doctors who didn't know how to dictate. The cough and shortness of breath were more insidious in onset, and I found I could blame those on something other than cigarettes as well. All of us working in the hospital basement smoked all day long and so did the doctors. The dictation room was like Brigadoon, wafting in and out of a fog.

Each new voice on the tape called for another cigarette. Each tape completed, another cigarette. Every break in the cafeteria demanded a cigarette. There were ashes in my typewriter, in my hair, and in my shoes. I remember a little soft brush I kept in my desk so I could whisk the work before I turned it in.

My excuse was that I smoked to keep my weight down. Then one day I took a cigarette, sat in front of a mirror, and smoked it. In the mirror I saw A FAT SMOKER.

Then began the desperate search for a painless way to quit. I began asking doctors how they quit smoking. The younger ones had never started, they were quick to tell me. The older ones stressed a beatific attitude I came to despise. "Oh," they said nonchalantly, "I just threw them out the car window one day and that was that, fifteen years ago." Litterbugs! The weaker of that group took up gumballs, chocolates, mints, or chewing gum. The stronger took up scalpels. I don't trust anyone who is not addicted to something.

Hypnotism appealed to me, but its fascination was short-lived. It frightened me more than cigarettes. I was positive that once I went under, other more virulent habits would surface—I would begin eating chalk or running amok wearing banana leaves (and probably rolling them up and smoking them as well).

The bookstore was no help. There were hundreds of books on dieting but none on how to quit smoking. I discovered the powerful tobacco industry had its tendrils everywhere. I turned to popular magazines. They just made me want to smoke more. All those slender, beige, beautiful people. They were rich, well-dressed, laughing, carefree people partying on rooftops on a gorgeous summer evening. No one looked over 30.

I couldn't relate to the strong and handsome cowboys or sailors, but I did begin to collect other ads. I bought white satin pajamas and a white satin dog. I wanted that satin moment. I wanted to go a long way, baby. I wanted flowers decorating my cigarettes and a butterfly tattoo on my ankle. My favorite was the ballerina ad. She was young, slim, beautiful, and slightly damp from all those pliés. She was relaxing in the dance studio, lighting up. The message was that she could function and exercise without trouble breathing.

Spotlight On

Confessions of an Addict *(continued)*

I went to work out at the gym and it was Cardiac City. Obviously it was my fault, not the cigarettes.

Remarkable creature that I am, I can play bingo, crochet, talk, and smoke, simultaneously. So I began to choose the workplace with an eye towards the comfort and ease with which I could smoke. I shifted from hospital to doctor's office to transcription service in a ceaseless hunt for the ashtray.

I began to scour the charts looking for patients with lung cancer who had never smoked. This gave me immeasurable feelings of security. Conversely, I delighted in patients whose summaries indicated that they lived to an old age despite 80 pack years. I mentally logged this as more proof that I too could escape. Everyone has an Uncle Joe who beats the odds, smokes four packs a day, drinks a fifth of bourbon a day, and lives to 95. It helps us rationalize our habits. From my vantage point in transcription I adopted literally hundreds of Uncle Joes. It was very consoling.

Professional meetings were more appealing to me if they were dinner or luncheon meetings. I could smoke with impunity in the restaurant. And the Scotch with the cigarettes wasn't bad, either. My major concern while flying out to the national meeting in Denver in 1982 was whether the altitude would affect my smoking habit and make it less enjoyable. (It certainly did.) I was furious at that meeting because some of the morning session rooms did not have coffee, only ice water. Only a smoker can appreciate how welcome hot coffee is with a cigarette in the morning and how repulsive ice water.

What new trade would I have to learn if I quit smoking? I was positive I could not transcribe without smoking. I became angry with doctors. I wanted answers from them. "The patient was placed on a 1200-calorie ADA diet, advised to exercise and quit smoking." Pompous, unfeeling clucks. What did they know about it? I could hear the disgust in the doctors' voices as they related in the course of the discharge summary that the patient, having sustained a moderate myocardial infarction and having undergone CABG, resumed smoking upon discharge.

The answer never did come from the doctors. The postman delivered it. In the summer of 1983 an innocent-appearing postcard addressed to Occupant fluttered into my mailbox. It promised a free introductory stop-smoking session. It promised to unhook me forever from the habit of coffee-cola-cigarettes, practically painlessly. I told the counselor that if they could do all of that, I was the Queen of Romania.

Everyone calls me Your Majesty now. I quit smoking July 29, 1983. After five weeks of participation in a group, doing all my homework, using a method of gradual withdrawal and behavior modification, I graduated.

On a steaming hot Friday I put out that last cigarette and, like any rational intelligent adult, headed for the kitchen. I defrosted everything in the freezer and as soon as it was cooked, I ate it. Then I began working on the larger freezer in the basement. If I had had a microwave oven instead of having to wait, I would have cleaned out our entire year's supply of codfish balls. Finally I asked my husband to chain me inside the car, pack a suitcase for the dogs, and drive us to the Maine coast so I could sit on the rocks and breathe (without smoking or eating). I calmed down.

Our stop-smoking program recommended saving the money spent on cigarettes and putting it in a glass jar, then buying oneself a present. So far we have a new complete set of English bone china. Next is a trip to England!

Exercises

Medical Vocabulary Review

Instructions: Choose the best answer.

___ 1. Exercise, emotional excitement, fever, pneumonia, shock, congestive heart failure that increase the body's need for oxygen result in _____
   A. apnea.
   B. orthopnea.
   C. hypopnea.
   D. tachypnea.

___ 2. A chest x-ray of a patient with tuberculosis might reveal _____
   A. chylothorax.
   B. peribronchial cuffing.
   C. cavitations in the lungs.
   D. increased bronchopulmonary markings.

___ 3. A typical finding on physical examination of a patient with pulmonary emphysema is
   _____
   A. phthisis.
   B. a barrel chest.
   C. pleural friction rub.
   D. dullness to percussion.

___ 4. Irregular discontinuous sounds like crackling paper or popping corn, heard on auscultation of the lungs due to passage of air through fluid or sudden expansion of small air passages that have been plugged or sealed by mucus, are _____
   A. rales.
   B. rubs.
   C. rhonchi.
   D. wheezes.

___ 5. Among the possible symptoms experienced by a patient with bronchogenic carcinoma is _____ or coughing up of bloody.
   A. fever
   B. hemoptysis
   C. Kussmaul respirations
   D. Cheyne-Stokes respirations

___ 6. A creaking or grating sound heard on auscultation of the lungs in a patient with pleurisy, pneumonia, pulmonary infarction, or chest wall injury is a _____
   A. rub.
   B. rale.
   C. rhonchus.
   D. wheeze.

___ 7. Patients with obstructive sleep apnea are often treated with a form of mechanical ventilation, specifically a _____ device.
   A. continuous positive airway pressure
   B. cardiopulmonary resuscitation
   C. intermittent mandatory ventilation
   D. intermittent positive pressure breathing

___ 8. A patient whose asthma has worsened or become more severe in spite of treatment is said to have had _____
   A. cachexia.
   B. flash pulmonary edema.
   C. an exacerbation.
   D. an arrest of symptoms.

___ 9. On physical examination, patients with emphysema may be noted to _____
   A. use accessory muscles of respiration.
   B. be in acute respiratory distress.
   C. exhibit cachexia or phthisis.
   D. have decompensation.

___ 10. On physical examination of a patient with pneumothorax or emphysema the percussion note may be _____
   A. dull or flat.
   B. metallic or rattling.
   C. creaking or grating.
   D. hyperresonant or tympanitic.

___ 11. A method of monitoring the oxygen saturation of circulating hemoglobin, as detected by a probe attached to the patient's finger or earlobe, is _____
   A. CPAP.
   B. spirometry.
   C. pulse oximetry.
   D. arterial blood gases.

___ 12. _____ is a bluish color of skin, particularly lips and nail beds, due to presence of excess unoxygenated blood in the circulation.
   A. Cyanosis
   B. Acidosis
   C. Alkalosis
   D. Cachexia

___ 13. _____ is the presence of blood in the pleural space.
   A. Empyema
   B. Hemothorax
   C. Hydrothorax
   D. Pneumothorax

___ 14. _____ is a respiratory therapy technique applied to breathing exercises prescribed to prevent atelectasis and pneumonia.
   A. Mechanical ventilation
   B. Incentive spirometry
   C. Diagnostic spirometry
   D. Intermittent mandatory ventilation

___ 15. Which of the following is NOT able to be determined by diagnostic spirometry?
   A. Tv (tidal volume).
   B. FVC (forced vital capacity).
   C. PEF (peak expiratory flow).
   D. TLC (total lung capacity).

___ 16. Which of the following is NOT able to be determined by arterial blood gases?
   A. pH (acid-base balance).
   B. PO_2 (partial pressure of oxygen).
   C. HCO_3 (bicarbonate).
   D. PCO_2 (partial pressure of carbon dioxide).

___ 17. A rise in serum pH due to excessive loss of carbon dioxide via the lungs is called _____
   A. acidosis.
   B. alkalosis.
   C. cyanosis.
   D. effusion.

___ 18. Another name for asthma is _____
   A. pleurisy.
   B. acute bronchitis.
   C. reactive airways disease.
   D. respiratory distress syndrome.

___ 19. _____ may be performed when the diagnosis of asthma is in doubt in an asymptomatic patient.
   A. A PET scan
   B. Intermittent mandatory ventilation
   C. A sputum smear and culture
   D. A methacholine challenge test

___ 20. Severe, refractory asthma is referred to as _____
   A. palliative.
   B. an exacerbation.
   C. status asthmaticus.
   D. decompensation.

Diagnostic and Surgical Procedures

Instructions: Match the following diagnostic and surgical procedures to their descriptions or definitions. Some answers may be used more than once or not at all.

___ 1. bronchoalveolar lavage

___ 2. bronchoscopy

___ 3. lung biopsy

___ 4. Mantoux skin test

___ 5. PET scan

___ 6. pleural biopsy

___ 7. pulmonary function tests

___ 8. thoracoscopic wedge excision

___ 9. tine test

___ 10. transthoracic needle biopsy

___ 11. tuberculin skin test

___ 12. ventilation-perfusion scan

A. Intradermal tuberculin skin test

B. Resection of a small piece of lung that contains a suspicious nodule or known cancer with a margin of healthy tissue around it through an endoscope

C. A nuclear scan that studies both airflow and blood flow in the lungs

D. A procedure to remove a sample of the tissue lining the lungs and the inside of the chest wall for microscopic examination and diagnosis

E. Excision of tissue for microscopic examination and diagnosis using a needle inserted through the skin and chest wall

F. Using a fiberoptic scope through which specimens and biopsies can be taken to view the trachea and main bronchi

G. Computerized tomography scan

H. A nuclear imaging study that reveals how organs and tissues are functioning

I. External compression of the heart coupled with breathing techniques to revive a victim whose heart and respirations have stopped

J. Removal of tissue from the lung for microscopic examination and diagnosis

K. Tests that measure the rate and volume of gas exchange in the respiratory system

L. Washing lung tissue to obtain material for culture or histology

Laboratory Procedures

Instructions: Match the following laboratory procedures to their descriptions or definitions. Some answers may be used more than once or not at all.

____ 1. acid-fast stain

____ 2. arterial blood gases

____ 3. basic metabolic panel

____ 4. chem-20

____ 5. cold agglutinins

____ 6. erythrocyte sedimentation rate

____ 7. febrile agglutinins

____ 8. INR

____ 9. sputum smear and culture

____ 10. sweat electrolytes

A. Microscopic examination of respiratory secretions for pathogenic organisms, neoplastic cells, or other abnormal findings

B. A blood clotting test for monitoring patients on anticoagulants

C. Test that indirectly measures how much inflammation is in the body

D. A laboratory procedure in which sputum, tissue, or other material is exposed to fluorochrome dye and then washed with acid-alcohol

E. A panel of 7 or 8 chemical blood tests to monitor electrolytes, kidney function, and blood sugar

F. A blood test for evaluating pulmonary function by measuring pO2, pCO2, and oxygen saturation

G. A test for sodium and chloride ions in perspiration

H. A test for antibodies formed by persons with mycoplasmal pneumonia

I. A group of antibody tests, each for a specific fever-causing infectious disease

J. A comprehensive panel of blood chemistry tests that includes electrolytes, kidney function tests, liver function tests, blood glucose, and cholesterol panel

Pharmacology

Instructions: Choose the best answer.

___ 1. Which of the following drugs is an inhaled bronchodilator?
   A. Singulair (montelukast).
   B. Atrovent (ipratropium).
   C. INH, Nydrazid (isoniazid).
   D. Azmacort (triamcinolone).

___ 2. Which of the following drugs does NOT belong in the group with the others?
   A. Rifadin (rifampin).
   B. Zyflo (zileuton).
   C. Accolate (zafirlukast).
   D. Singulair (montelukast).

___ 3. Which of the following drugs is NOT an antituberculosis drug?
   A. streptomycin.
   B. Rifadin (rifampin).
   C. Myambutol (ethambutol).
   D. NebuPent, Pentam 300 (pentamidine).

___ 4. If a patient had tuberculosis due to *Mycobacterium avium-intracellulare* complex, you might expect the physician to prescribe which one of the following drugs?
   A. Priftin (rifapentine).
   B. Mycobutin (rifabutin).
   C. Rifamate (isoniazid, rifampin).
   D. Rifadin, Rimactane (rifampin).

___ 5. Patients with bronchial asthma due to allergies would likely be given a mast cell stabilizer such as _____ as prophylaxis against bronchospasm.
   A. cromolyn (Intal)
   B. clindamycin (Cleocin)
   C. albuterol (Proventil, ProAir HFA)
   D. cycloserine (Seromycin Pulvules)

___ 6. AIDS patients with *Pneumocystis* pneumonia could be treated with any of the following drugs EXCEPT _____
   A. NeuTrexin (trimetrexate).
   B. Cleocin (clindamycin).
   C. BioTropin, Serostim (somatropin).
   D. Septra (trimethoprim and sulfamethoxazole).

___ 7. Drugs that suppress the inflammatory response but do not produce bronchodilation are _____
   A. surfactants.
   B. corticosteroids.
   C. antibiotics.
   D. mast cell stabilizers.

___ 8. Which drug is a leukotriene receptor antagonist?
   A. Tilade (nedocromil).
   B. Azmacort (triamcinolone).
   C. Singulair (montelukast).
   D. Marinol (dronabinol).

___ 9. Which drug is used to treat respiratory syncytial virus infections?
   A. Virazole (ribavirin).
   B. Survanta (beractant).
   C. Capastat (capreomycin).
   D. Septra (trimethoprim and sulfamethoxazole).

___ 10. A patient with an acute asthma attack and bronchospasm would likely take _____
   A. a corticosteroid.
   B. a mast cell inhibitor.
   C. a leukotriene receptor antagonist.
   D. an inhaled bronchodilator.

Dissecting Medical Terms

Instructions: As you learned in your medical language course, words are formed from prefixes, combining forms (root word plus combining vowel), and suffixes. Combining vowels (usually **o** but not always) are used to connect two root words or a root and a suffix. By analyzing these word parts, you can often determine the definition of a term without even looking it up (if you know the definition of the parts, of course!).

Being able to divide and analyze the words you hear into their component parts will also improve your auditory deciphering ability and spelling and help you research those words that you cannot easily spell or define.

For the following terms, draw a slash (/) between the components and then write a short definition based on the meaning of the parts. Remember that to define a word based on its parts, you start at the end, usually with the suffix. If there's a prefix, that is defined next, and finally the combining form is defined.

Example: anticoagulation

Divide & Analyze:
   anticoagulation= anti/coagulat/ion = condition + against + blood clot formation

Define: something that acts to prevent blood clot formation

1. bronchodilator
   Divide _____
   _____
   Define _____

2. chemotherapy
   Divide _____
   _____
   Define _____

3. decompensation
   Divide _____
   _____
   Define _____

4. dysfunction
   Divide _____
   _____
   Define _____

5. endobronchial
   Divide _____
   _____
   Define _____

6. extubate
   Divide _____
   _____
   Define _____

7. fibromyalgia
   Divide _____
   _____
   Define _____

8. hepatosplenomegaly
   Divide _____
   _____
   Define _____

9. intrapulmonary
   Divide _____
   _____
   Define _____

10. organomegaly
    Divide _____
    _____
    Define _____

11. pathologic
    Divide _____
    _____
    Define _____

12. photocoagulate
    Divide _____
    _____
    Define _____

13. pneumothorax

Divide _____

_____

Define _____

14. supraclavicular

Divide _____

_____

Define _____

15. tachypneic

Divide _____

_____

Define _____

16. thoracoscopic

Divide _____

_____

Define _____

17. transthoracic

Divide _____

_____

Define _____

Spelling Exercise

Instructions: Review the adjective suffixes in your medical language textbook. Test your knowledge of adjectives by writing the adjectival form of the following pulmonary medicine words. Consult a medical dictionary to verify your spelling.

Noun	Adjective
1. anxiety	_____
2. base	_____
3. consolidation	_____
4. inflammation	_____
5. vein	_____
6. production	_____
7. reaction	_____
8. symmetry	_____
9. tachypnea	_____
10. thoracoscope	_____

Abbreviations Exercise

Instructions: Expand the following common abbreviations and brief forms. Then memorize both abbreviations and definitions to increase your speed and accuracy in transcribing dictation

Abbreviation	Expansion
1. CAP (protocol)	_____
2. CPAP	_____
3. COPD	_____
4. DP (pulse)	_____
5. DVT	_____
6. EOMI	_____
7. ESR	_____
8. GERD	_____
9. HPI	_____
10. LAFB	_____
11. LMS (bronchus)	_____
12. NSR	_____
13. O_2	_____
14. pCO_2	_____
15. PCP	_____
16. PE	_____
17. pO_2	_____
18. RBBB	_____
19. RRR	_____
20. VNA	_____

Transcript Forensics

Instructions: This section presents snippets of transcribed dictations from clinic notes; history and physical examinations and consultations; operative reports and procedure notes; and discharge summaries. Explain the passage so that a nonmedical person can understand it.

Example: The patient is a 55-year-old lady who presented to the emergency room complaining of acute onset of **dyspnea**, says she woke up with inability to breathe. Denies any nausea, vomiting, chest pain, chest tightness, **hemoptysis**, cough, fever, chills. Patient recently had a **pneumothorax**, which was diagnosed at the local ER.

Explanation: The patient woke up with the sudden onset of shortness of breath, unable to breathe. The symptoms listed could be associated with cardiac or pulmonary problems including heart attack, a blood clot to the major arteries in the lungs, or even pneumonia or bronchitis, but they are all negative. Hemoptysis, the spitting up of blood, could be linked to pneumonia or tuberculosis or cancer. The patient did recently have air in the membrane covering the lungs and lining the chest (pleural space), possibly from a ruptured cavity (bled) in the subpleural space.

1. PAST MEDICAL HISTORY: Asthma, early emphysema, COPD from tobacco abuse.

   Explanation: _____
   _____
   _____
   _____

2. Patient is currently on Adalat 30 mg once a day, Aciphex 20 mg once a day, Zyrtec 10 mg once a day, atenolol 50 mg 1/2 a day, potassium chloride 20 mEq 1/2 twice a day, Flonase 50 mcg one spray each side daily, and Zoloft 100 mg once a day. [*Note: Identify the conditions that the medications treat.*]

   Explanation: _____
   _____
   _____
   _____
   _____
   _____

3. Respirations: Good air entry bilaterally. Patient has decreased air entry on the right-hand side. No **wheezing**. There are bilateral basal **crackles**. Chest is **resonant to percussion** on the left side. Some **dullness to percussion** on the right-hand side.

   Explanation: _____
   _____
   _____
   _____

4. CT scan showed a large dependent right **pleural effusion** with extension to the apex. No evident **pneumothorax**. Probable comprehensive **atelectasis** is noted in the right lung base. **Stranding densities** noted projecting into the anterior left base likely representing scar versus atelectasis.

   Explanation: _____
   _____
   _____
   _____

5. This is a 61-year-old white female with known history of **COPD**, who was diagnosed with **pneumonia** last week and started on **Levaquin**. She states that she has been taking this regularly without improvement. Now, she complains of **substernal** chest pain, worse with activity and inspiration, decreased with rest. She also reports subjective fevers, shortness of breath, **orthopnea, myalgia**, and wheezing.

Explanation: _____

_____

_____

_____

_____

_____

6. This is a 59-year-old female with past medical history significant for paroxysmal atrial fibrillation, CHF, hypertension, **asthma**, alcohol/tobacco abuse, who was admitted after presenting to the emergency room in **acute respiratory distress**, was **intubated** and found to be in **flash pulmonary edema** and **CHF**. No identifiable **triggers** except for the recent resumption of smoking.

Explanation: _____

_____

_____

_____

_____

_____

7. The patient was admitted to the CCU, intubated. Originally treated for asthma **exacerbation**, however, improved substantially with **diuresis**. Was **extubated** on hospital day #2 and did well until hospital day #3 when she reaccumulated some fluid. Was treated with **CPAP** and more diuresis.

Explanation: _____

_____

_____

_____

_____

_____

8. VITAL SIGNS: Temperature 97.7. Pulse 132. Respirations 32. Blood pressure 122/64. **Oximetry** 89% on room air. He has been placed on oxygen. LUNGS: Moderate wheeze. Minimally **prolonged expiratory phase**.

Explanation: _____

_____

_____

_____

_____

_____

9. Chest x-ray showed **consolidation** of blood flow with bilateral **perihilar vascular congestion**, possibly suggestive of **cardiopulmonary edema** with a **pneumothorax**. CO2 was 161, pCO2 of 43, and pO2 of 7.29.

Explanation: _____

_____

_____

_____

_____

_____

10. PREOPERATIVE DIAGNOSIS: Pulmonary failure with need for **tracheostomy**, on **mechanical ventilator**, unable to **wean off**.

Explanation: _____

_____

_____

_____

_____

_____

Sample Reports

Sample pulmonary medicine reports appear on the following pages, illustrating a variety of reports. Fictional names are provided for illustration of proper format, and no resemblance to actual persons is intended. Sample transcripts were prepared according to *The Book of Style for Medical Transcription* (AHDI).

Consultation

SINGH, PRAKASH
#101091

Date: 12/12/[add year]

Attending: Theodore Liou, MD

This is a 32-year-old East Indian male, lifelong nonsmoker, referred to me. He complains of a less than 2-week history of dry cough associated with dull substernal discomfort and dyspnea, particularly on exertion. Otherwise, he has been remarkably free of any other associated symptoms. In particular, he denies any preceding cold or flu or allergic exposure. He denies any associated fevers, chills, night sweats, or weight loss.

He admits to having childhood asthma, but felt he grew out of this by the time he was a teenager. He has traveled extensively throughout the U.S., including travel to the California deserts and Central Valley. He has not had pneumonia vaccine. He had a TB skin test 10 years ago and a flu vaccine 3 years ago.

PAST MEDICAL HISTORY
Past medical history is remarkably negative.

PHYSICAL EXAMINATION
Blood pressure 140/80, pulse 85, respiratory rate 22, temperature 99.3. Chest exam is completely normal, with no rales, wheezes, rhonchi, or rubs. Even on forced exhalation there was no cough or prolongation. Cardiac exam showed a regular rate and rhythm with no murmur or gallop.

LABORATORY DATA
PA chest x-ray is striking for a new interstitial infiltrate seen in both midlung zones with some shagging of the cardiac borders, indicating involvement of the lingula and right middle lobe. Surprisingly, the lowest part of the lung fields and the apices appear to be spared.

Spirometry before and after bronchodilator performed in my office shows a vital capacity of 3.79 or 69% after an 11% improvement with bronchodilator. The FEV1 achieves 3.24 liters or 72% of predicted after 12% improvement with bronchodilator. The FEV1/FVC ratio was mildly increased at 85 instead of predicted 82.

(continued)

Consultation *(continued)*

SINGH, PRAKASH
#101091
12/12/[add year]
Page 2

ASSESSMENT AND PLAN
Differential diagnosis includes the following:
1. Hypersensitivity pneumonia.
2. Mycoplasmal pneumonia.
3. Less likely candidates appear to be Wegener's granulomatosis, Goodpasture's syndrome, sarcoidosis, alveolar proteinosis, and allergic bronchopulmonary aspergillosis.

RECOMMENDATIONS
1. CBC with differential, chem-20, Wintrobe sed rate, angiotensin-converting enzyme, urinalysis, and mycoplasma titers.
2. Full pulmonary function tests within 2 weeks.
3. Vibramycin 100 mg daily for 14 days.

If he still has significant symptoms and restrictions on PFTs after 2 weeks, he will have to be evaluated for one of the more chronic diagnoses, which may ultimately require open lung biopsy. Otherwise, we should hope that within 2 weeks the patient will be improved and his x-ray will have cleared.

THOMAS LEE, MD

TL:hpi

d: 12/12/[add year]
t: 12/13/[add year]

Operative Report

WERNIG, JASON
#828986

DATE OF PROCEDURE
June 10, [add year]

PROCEDURE
Fiberoptic bronchoscopy

INDICATIONS
Worsening pulmonary infiltrates in a febrile patient, unknown etiology. Rule out resistant nosocomial pneumonia.

PREMEDICATION
Versed 1 mg IV.

ANESTHESIA
1% topical Xylocaine, total of 30 mL.

INSTRUMENT
Olympus BFP10 bronchoscope.

PROCEDURE
After informed consent was obtained from the patient's mother and appropriate premedication, the bronchoscope was inserted directly through the tracheostomy tube while the patient continued to receive oxygen supplementation. The lower trachea and tracheobronchial tree were then fully examined in this fashion. There was very severe, intense tracheobronchitis noted, with very friable mucosa. Patchy areas of denudation of the mucosa were also noted, particularly along the right lateral wall. The main carina was sharp and in the midline. The right and left bronchial trees showed the same diffuse erythematous changes but no purulence and no endobronchial abnormalities. Bronchial washings were obtained from throughout the tracheobronchial tree and submitted for Gram stain, routine acid-fast bacilli, fungal smears and cultures, and cytologic review. The instrument was then removed and the procedure terminated. No complications were encountered.

DIAGNOSTIC IMPRESSION
Severe tracheobronchitis.

RODNEY KWUN, MD

RK:hpi

d: 6/10/[add year]
t: 6/11/[add year]

Comic Relief

Dictation and transcription mistakes are common occurrences in pulmonary transcripts. Here are some favorites.

Dictated	**Transcribed**
The x-ray was practically normal.	The x-ray was frantically normal.
There were no abnormal masses.	There were no admirable masses.
There was a bruit in the chest.	There was a brewery in the chest.
There were diminished breath sounds.	There were diminished breasts.
He has complained of progressive dyspnea on exertion.	He has complained of progressive dyspnea to his vision.
The chest revealed no rales or rubs.	The chest revealed no rales or ruts.
The lungs showed bibasilar rales.	The lungs showed biceps rales.
Bronchopneumonia, etiological.	Bronchopneumonia, theological.
The patient had a barrel-shaped chest.	The patient had a bell-shaped chest.
There were basilar rales noted.	There were dazzler rales noted.
The lung fields were clear.	The lung fumes were clear.

PEARSON

myhealthprofessionskit™

To access the online exercises and transcription practice, go to **www.myhealthprofessionskit.com**. Select "Medical Transcription," then click on the title of this book, ***Healthcare Documentation: Fundamentals & Practice***. Then click on the Pulmonary Medicine chapter.

Ophthalmology

11

Learning Objectives

▶ Describe the structure and function of the eyes.

▶ Spell and define common ophthalmology terms.

▶ Identify ophthalmology vocabulary that might be used in the review of systems.

▶ Describe the negative and positive findings a physician looks for on examination of the eyes.

▶ Describe the typical cause, course, and treatment options for common diseases of the eyes.

▶ Identify and define common diagnostic and surgical procedures of the eyes.

▶ List common ophthalmic laboratory tests and procedures.

▶ Identify and describe common ophthalmic drugs and their uses.

▶ Demonstrate knowledge of anatomical, medical, pharmacological, adjectival, and soundalike terms by accurately completing the exercises in this chapter.

Transcribing Ophthalmology Dictation

Introduction

Ophthalmology is a branch of medicine devoted to the prevention, diagnosis, and treatment of eye diseases. An **ophthalmologist** is a physician with specialty training and certification in the medical and surgical management of congenital abnormalities, injuries, infections, and degenerative and malignant disorders of the eyes and adjacent structures (eyelids, tear glands, and duct system).

The **evaluation of disorders of vision**, including myopia, presbyopia, and astigmatism, and their treatment with corrective lenses, form a major part of many ophthalmologic practices. **Ocular surgery** is performed to correct strabismus, cataract, glaucoma, retinal detachment, and other conditions. Because much ocular surgery is performed under local anesthesia with conscious sedation rather than under general anesthesia, recovery time is brief. For that reason, most eye operations are "same-day surgery," carried out in free-standing outpatient surgery centers rather than in hospitals.

Distinguish carefully between an **ophthalmologist** and other eye care professionals:

An **optometrist** is a doctor of optometry (OD) with graduate training and certification in the measurement of refractive errors and their treatment with corrective lenses, including contact lenses. Optometrists have an undergraduate degree as well as four years of graduate education to earn their doctoral degree in optometry. In some states optometrists also provide limited treatment for other eye disorders.

An **optician** prepares corrective lenses, including contact lenses, according to an ophthalmologist's or optometrist's prescription and fits them to the patient.

Anatomy Review

Each **eye** (see ■ Figure 11-1) is a roughly spherical structure protected on all sides except the front by the bones and soft tissues of the orbit. Blood vessels and nerves enter at the back of the eye. The **eyeball** (bulb, globe) consists of three concentric layers: the outer **sclera**, a tough coat of connective tissue; the pigment layer or **uveal tract**, a delicate, spongy, vascular membrane of pigmented cells; and the innermost layer, the light-sensitive **retina**.

Anteriorly the sclera is modified to form the transparent **cornea**, through which light rays enter the eye. The uveal tract consists of three parts: the **iris**, which

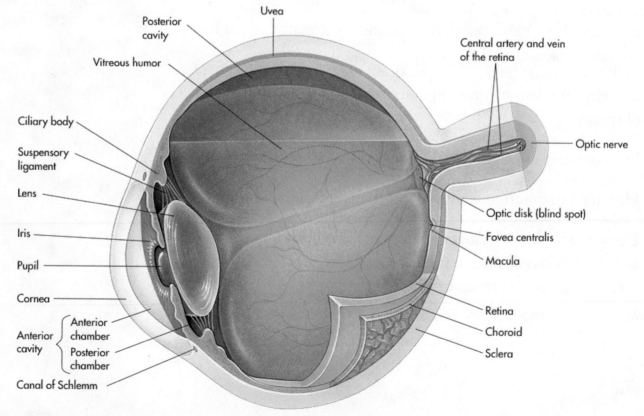

FIGURE 11-1. Anatomy of the eye

regulates the amount of light entering the eye; the **ciliary body**, which adjusts the focus of the eye; and the **choroid**, which underlies the retina. The **retina** is a layer of specialized nerve cells that are stimulated by light rays within the visible range. Nerve fibers of these cells unite to form the **optic nerve**.

The **ocular fundus** is the rear wall of the eye as viewed through the pupil with an **ophthalmoscope**. The fundus consists of the retina and its arteries and veins and the **disc** (optic nerve head). The disc appears as a round, ivory-colored plaque raised somewhat from the surrounding retina and having a shallow central depression, the **cup**. The disc lies on the nasal side of the fundus, not at its center. The central portion of the retina, concerned with central vision and hence the most sensitive, appears as a faint yellow spot, the **macula lutea**. The retinal vessels (branching arteries, each closely accompanied by a vein) emerge from the center of the disc.

The optic nerve passes back through an aperture in the orbit and crosses the optic nerve of the opposite eye, with which it exchanges some fibers. Behind the crossing, the newly assorted bundles of fibers, called the **optic tracts**, carry visual impulses into the brain.

On their way to the retina, light rays pass through both the cornea and the **lens**, a transparent structure suspended just behind the cornea. The shape of the lens can be altered by the pull of **muscles** originating in the ciliary body, and this alteration adjusts the focal distance of the eye. The **iris**, the colored part of the eye, lies between the cornea and the lens, and controls the amount of light entering the eye by changing the diameter of the **pupil**, the black-appearing round aperture in the middle of the iris.

The part of the eye lying anterior to the lens contains a watery fluid, the **aqueous humor**, which is produced by the ciliary body and drains into small veins in the anterior chamber at the "drainage angle" (the slight angle between cornea and sclera). The space occupied by the **aqueous humor** is divided into the **anterior chamber** (between cornea and iris) and the **posterior chamber** (between iris and lens). Behind the lens, the cavity of the eye is filled with a somewhat denser fluid, the **vitreous humor**. Both humors are

refractive media, participating in the transmission and refraction of light rays.

The **eyelids** are folds of skin, supplied with oil and sebaceous glands and lash follicles, that shut out light and provide a watertight seal over the eyes. The medial or nasal junction or angle between upper and lower lids is called the **inner canthus**; the lateral or temporal angle is called the **outer canthus**. The visible part of the sclera is covered by a delicate vascular membrane, the **conjunctiva (bulbar conjunctiva)**, which is continuous with the lining of the inner surfaces of the eyelids (**palpebral conjunctiva**). The conjunctiva does not extend over the cornea.

A **lacrimal gland** is situated near the front of each **orbit**, above and lateral to the eyeball. This gland produces **tears**, which moisten, lubricate, and cleanse the eyeball.

Tears flow downward and medially to drain by way of the **lacrimal puncta** (minute openings at the inner canthus) and nasolacrimal ducts into the nose.

Each eye is equipped with six **extraocular muscles**, which produce eye movement and control the direction of gaze (see ■ Figure 11-2). Three **cranial nerves** (III, oculomotor; IV, trochlear; and VI, abducens) supply these six muscles. In addition, the oculomotor nerve sends motor branches to the upper eyelid, the ciliary body (focus), and the iris (light/dark adaptation). Coordination of the movements and position of the two eyes and fusion of their images into a single three-dimensional one takes place in the brain.

Pause for Reflection

1. Describe the 3 layers of the eyeball.
2. What are the functions of the iris, the ciliary body, and the retina?
3. Describe the structures of the ocular fundus.
4. How are the focal distance and the amount of light entering the eye controlled?
5. Distinguish between the following pairs of terms: Aqueous humor and vitreous humor; anterior chamber and posterior chamber; inner canthus and outer canthus; and bulbar conjunctiva and palpebral conjunctiva.
6. Distinguish between the lacrimal gland and the lacrimal puncta.
7. What structures produce eye movement and control the direction of gaze?

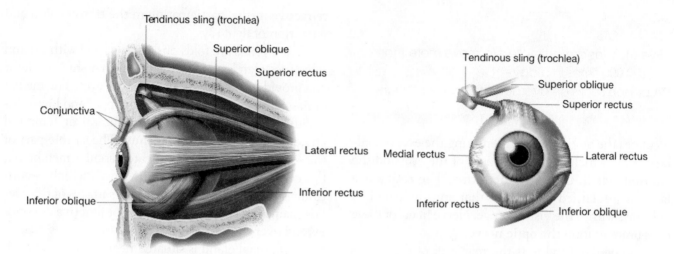

FIGURE 11-2. Eye muscles: lateral and anterior views of rectus and oblique muscles

Vocabulary Review

akinesia Temporary paralysis of the eye muscles, usually by means of a retrobulbar block.

Amsler grid A tool used in visual field testing.

aphakia (adj., **aphakic**) Absence of the lens of the eye; it may be congenital, traumatic, or as a result of cataract extraction.

AV (arteriovenous) nicking Tapering of a venule where an arteriole crosses it.

balanced saline solution (BSS) An irrigating solution commonly used during eye surgeries.

blepharochalasis Drooping eyelid skin.

blepharospasm Spasm of the eyelids, usually due to local irritation, photophobia, or both.

Bowman layer (or **membrane**) Anterior limiting lamina, a thin layer of the cornea beneath the outer layer of stratified epithelium.

canaliculus (pl., **canaliculi**) An extremely narrow tubular passage or duct; in ophthalmology, the lacrimal duct.

capsulorrhexis In cataract extraction surgery, a continuous circular tear in the anterior lens capsule to allow expression or phacoemulsification of the lens nucleus. Also, *capsulorhexis*.

C₃F₈ (perfluoropropane) gas An intraocular gas used to tamponade the retina in retinal detachment surgery or to replace intravitreal fluid that may have leaked out during other surgeries such as trabeculec-

tomy. Other gases used for similar purposes are sulfur hexafluoride (SF_6), perfluoroethane (C_2F_6).

coloboma (iridis) A congenital defect in the iris, in which a wedge-shaped segment is absent, giving a keyhole appearance to the pupil; similar defects are created by certain types of ocular surgery.

crystalline lens The natural lens of the eye.

cupping of the disc The normal optic nerve head has a slight central depression (physiologic cupping). Increase in the depth of the cup occurs with increased intraocular pressure (glaucoma) or atrophy of the optic nerve.

Descemet membrane Posterior limiting lamina, a thin hyaline membrane between the substantia propria and the endothelial layer of the cornea.

diopter (D) A unit of refractive power of lenses. For example, reading glasses may be rated as 2.25 diopters; intraocular lenses may be rated 19.0 diopters.

diplopia Double vision; seeing two overlapping two-dimensional images instead of one three-dimensional image; may result from injury or disease of one or both eyes or from failure of fusion of images in the cerebral cortex, due to alcohol, drugs, fever, infection, neoplasm, or trauma.

ectropion Eversion (turning outward) and drooping of the lower eyelid, exposing the conjunctival surface and allowing overflow of tears.

egress Escape or come out of.

entropion Inward turning of the margin of the lower eyelid, often so that the lower lashes touch the eyeball.

epiphora Chronic overflow of tears from the lower eyelid onto the cheek; may be due to blockage of the nasolacrimal duct or to deformity of the lower lid (ectropion).

exophthalmos Abnormal bulging of the eye between the lids; may be due to local disease (orbital cellulitis or neoplasm) or (when bilateral) to systemic disease (Graves disease).

flare and cells Diminished clarity of the aqueous humor due to protein leakage from the iris and swirls of inflammatory cells in the anterior chamber due to inflammation.

fornix An archlike structure or the vaultlike space created by such a structure. The inferior fornix of the conjunctiva is the the inferior line of reflection of the conjunctiva from the eyelid to the eyeball; the superior fornix is the superior line of reflection of the conjunctiva from the eyelid to the eyeball, which receives the openings of the lacrimal duct.

fundus The rear of the interior of the eye, consisting of the retina, its blood vessels, and the optic nerve head.

glaucoma Any of several related disorders in which sustained elevation of increased intraocular pressure can lead to irreversible impairment of vision.

hyaloid membrane The vitreous membrane, a delicate boundary layer enveloping the vitreous body of the eye.

hyperemia Redness due to dilatation of superficial blood vessels.

hyphema Presence of blood in the anterior chamber.

hypopyon Presence of pus in the anterior chamber.

injection (or **injected**) When pertaining to the eyes, *injection* refers to congestion or dilation of the visible vessels with blood. See also *hyperemia*.

intraocular lens (IOL) An artificial lens used to replace the native lens after cataract extraction.

keratic precipitates (KPs) Whitish deposits of inflammatory cells on the posterior surface of the cornea.

lacrimal punctum (pl., **puncta**) A minute aperture in either eyelid at the inner canthus, through which tears pass into a nasolacrimal duct.

lacrimation Tearing.

LAY AND MEDICAL TERMS

blindness	amaurosis
crossed eyes	esotropia
double vision	diplopia
farsightedness	hyperopia
lazy eye	amblyopia
nearsightedness	myopia
wall-eye	exotropia
white of the eye	sclera (pl. scleras, sclerae)

---

miosis Sustained constriction of the pupil, which may be due to ocular or nervous system disease or to the effect of drugs (pilocarpine, morphine).

mydriasis Sustained dilatation of the pupil, which may be due to ocular or nervous system disease or to the effect of drugs (atropine, cyclopentolate).

nyctalopia Marked reduction of visual acuity at night (that is, under conditions of near-darkness). Also called *night blindness*.

nystagmus A rhythmic back-and-forth movement of the eyes usually due to congenital abnormality or central nervous system disease.

papilledema Swelling of the optic disc, as observed with an ophthalmoscope; usually due to increased intracranial pressure (**"choked disc"**) (caused by intracranial hemorrhage, neoplasm, or disturbance of cerebrospinal fluid circulation) or intrinsic eye disease (**optic neuritis**). The disc appears edematous and perhaps injected, and the retinal vessels as they emerge from the swollen disc appear to be kinked (**"stepping" of vessels**).

peritomy An incision made completely around the periphery of the conjunctiva in surgical repair of a retinal detachment.

photophobia Aversion to bright light, which causes a sense of pain in the eye, usually because of irritability or spasm of the iris.

propofol A rapidly acting hypnotic used in the induction of general anesthesia and as procedural sedation for ophthalmic surgery.

ptosis Drooping of an upper eyelid that cannot be fully corrected by voluntary effort.

retinal detachment A separation of the retina from its supporting layers (see ■ Figure 11-12). Surgical treatment includes laser repair of tears or holes in the retina before detachment occurs, pneumatic retinopexy, scleral buckle, or vitrectomy.

retinitis Inflammation of the retina, the light-sensitive membrane at the back of the eyeball.

rhegmatogenous Arising from or caused by a tear, as in rhegmatogenous retinal detachment.

scotoma (pl., **scotomata**) A blind spot; a gap in the visual field of one or both eyes in which objects cannot be seen. A scotoma that appears identical in each eye is always due to a disease or condition of the central nervous system (for example, migraine headache). A scotoma may appear as a black hole or may show flashes or swirls of white or colored light.

Snellen chart A chart used to assess visual acuity.

strabismus A general term for any condition in which the direction of gaze is different in the two eyes, as noted by an observer.

tarsus A plate of connective tissue forming the framework of the eyelid. Also, **tarsal plate**.

Tenon capsule, membrane The sheath of the eyeball.

visual field defect See *scotoma*.

xerophthalmia Abnormal dryness of the eye, usually due to decreased flow of tears.

Medical Readings

History and Physical Examination

by John H. Dirckx, MD

Review of Systems. A thorough review of ocular history elicits information about past or present symptoms such as blurring of vision, double vision, partial or complete loss of vision, difficulty of near adaptation; seeing spots or flashes; seeing halos or rings around lights; undue visual impairment with reduced illumination; pain in, on, or behind the eyeball; redness, discharge, watering, abnormal sensitivity to light; swelling, drooping, itching, or crusting of lids; and full details about the use of glasses or contact lenses and the date of the most recent eye exam. Eye symptoms can indicate neurologic or systemic rather than purely local disease, as in the case of loss of vision due to a brain tumor or retinopathy due to diabetes.

The pupils are round, regular, and equal and react to light and accommodation.

Physical Examination. The eyes are subject to many acute and chronic diseases, some of which can threaten vision. Moreover, the eyes register or reflect many systemic disorders such as arteriosclerosis, diabetes, thyrotoxicosis, and diseases of the nervous system. Hence they deserve attentive examination.

Eyes: No ocular symptoms or visual deficits.

Unless some historical point has drawn particular attention to one or both eyes, the physician's evaluation will usually be limited to an inspection of the lids and lashes and the parts of the eye exposed between them, a test of the pupillary light reflexes, a rough check of ocular movements and visual fields, and an inspection of the ocular fundi. A test of vision is often included. All of these procedures can be performed quickly and easily with standard equipment, but several of them require the cooperation of the patient.

Normally the patient sits upright for the eye examination, if possible. The orbital margins are inspected for swelling or ecchymosis, and may be palpated for tenderness if any clue to recent trauma is noted. The lids are observed for evidence of deformity, swelling, discoloration, masses, crusting, or disorders of the tear glands and ducts. Bulging or protrusion of one or both eyes (**exophthalmos**) can result from hyperthyroidism or orbital disease.

The left eye is swollen nearly shut and the lids are deeply discolored.

The **anterior chamber** of the eye—the part in front of the pupil—is easily studied with the help of a hand lamp. The physician looks for opacities in the cornea and anterior chamber, abnormalities of the iris, and irregularities in the shape of the pupil, incidentally observing whether the pupil constricts when light is shone directly into the eye. This procedure also serves as a test for **photophobia** (abnormal sensitivity to light).

A check of the **accommodation** reflex may also be made by asking the patient to look at a near object and noting whether the pupils constrict. **Astigmatism**, a warping of the cornea out of its expected spherical form, can sometimes be detected by noting distortion in the reflection of some regularly shaped object on the cornea, but is more precisely determined by vision testing with refracting lenses designed for the purpose which only an ophthalmologist would normally have on hand. The location of a lesion of the cornea or iris is indicated by the **hour position** to which it would be nearest if the eye were a clock dial (e.g., 5 o'clock).

Eyes: Examination of the eyes reveals pupils that react to light in a normal manner. The optic fundi are normal. His extraocular motions are normal, and there is no nystagmus.

Abnormalities of the white of the eye can be due to discoloration or disease of the **sclera** or of the overlying **conjunctiva**, usually the latter. Mild or early jaundice is typically more evident in the sclerae than in the skin. Conjunctival swelling and discharge or **lacrimation** (excessive tearing) are noted, as well as the degree and distribution of any redness. Very thin sclerae, such as occur in some connective tissue disorders, appear blue.

The scleras are deeply icteric, jaundiced.

Imbalance of the **extraocular muscles** may or may not be readily apparent. Imbalances are called **tropias** when the eyes cannot be made to look in the same direction, **phorias** when there is a tendency to deviation that the patient habitually controls so as not to see double. Even a slight degree of tropia can sometimes be detected by observing whether the reflections of a handheld lamp appear at corresponding points on the two corneas. Tropias and phorias can also be demonstrated with the cover test. The patient gazes steadily at a distant object and the examiner covers first one eye and then the other, noting whether one or both eyes swing into a different position immediately after being uncovered. This test depends on intact vision in both eyes; however, in an uncorrected tropia, vision is eventually lost in one eye.

The physician tests the integrity of the **extraocular muscles** (the voluntary muscles, six for each eye, that control the direction of gaze) (see ■ Figure 11-2) by having the examinee follow the movements of a handheld object such as a lamp while holding the head immobile. Abnormalities of ocular movement can be due to disease or injury of the brain or of the third, fourth, or sixth cranial nerve on either side, or to orbital disease or injury affecting one or more of the extraocular muscles.

The **visual field** of an eye is that part of the space before it that it can see while held motionless. Abnormalities of visual field, which can be caused by retinal or neural disease or injury, represent partial loss of vision in the form of blind spots (**scotomata**) or narrowed range of vision. Visual fields can be roughly tested by the **confrontation method**. The subject is instructed to gaze at the examiner's nose while first one eye and then the other is covered. The examiner moves a finger or a light from the side and then from above and below into the subject's range of vision, and the subject reports when the object first becomes visible. If the examiner in turn gazes at the subject's nose (and if the examiner's own visual fields are normal), both should see the object at the same time. More elaborate equipment is needed for more precise mapping of visual fields.

The **optic fundus** is the portion of the interior of the eye that can be seen by an examiner looking through the pupil with an **ophthalmoscope**, a handheld instrument with a light source and a set of magnifying lenses that can be quickly changed.

The principal features of the fundus are the retina, the optic disc or nerve head, and branches of the central retinal artery and vein. Retinal and optic nerve disease as well as the effects of systemic conditions such as diabetes, arteriosclerosis, and hypertension, are readily observed in the fundus, provided that the examiner's view is not blocked by an opaque lens (cataract) or a hemorrhage or foreign body within the eye.

The examiner adjusts the instrument to compensate for visual deficit (**refractive error**) in the subject's eye. Since the strength (in diopters) of the lens being used can be read from a scale on the ophthalmoscope, this examination serves as a rough measure of visual acuity. Sizes and distances in the fundus can be measured by comparison with the diameter of the disc. **Edema of the disc (choked disc)** is measured by the difference between lens settings needed to focus on the disc and on the rest of the fundus. If the pupil is very small, it may be dilated with drops in preparation for ophthalmoscopic examination.

Firm palpation of the eyeball through the closed lids (which is moderately uncomfortable and slightly dangerous) can reveal undue hardness, such as occurs in acute and chronic glaucoma. In some settings, **tonometry** is a routine part of the examination of persons over 40.

Pause for Reflection

1. Explain the importance of obtaining a thorough review of systems and attentive exam regarding the eyes.
2. What is included in a routine exam of the eyes on physical exam?
3. What is the physician testing when the patient is asked to look at a near object and noting whether the pupils constrict? What is the physician testing when the examinee is asked to follow the movements of a handheld object such as a lamp while holding the head immobile?
4. Distinguish between *tropias* and *phorias*.
5. What is meant by "visual fields are normal to confrontation"?
6. How is edema of the disc (choked disc) measured?

ABBREVIATIONS

OD, OS, OU—simple, basic abbreviations for *oculus dexter* "right eye," *oculus sinister* "left eye," and *oculus uterque* "each eye," traditionally used in ophthalmology reports.

Although these abbreviations are on the ISMP error-prone list, the abbreviations should be transcribed as dictated in visual testing and measured values, e.g., visual acuity 20/20 OU.

The abbreviation "mmHg" for millimeters of mercury is used by ophthalmologists to describe intraocular pressure.

Vision Testing

by John H. Dirckx, MD

Vision (Distance and Near). Vision testing is usually performed with standard charts containing letters or words of various sizes. The eyes are tested both separately and together. For children and illiterates, charts with pictures or symbols are used.

For the assessment of distant vision, the subject is placed 20 feet from the **Snellen chart**, and visual acuity is recorded as the smallest line of type in which the subject can read more than half the letters correctly. Each line is designated by the distance at which a person with normal vision can read it. Thus, 20/20 ("twenty twenty") vision is normal, while 20/80 ("twenty eighty") vision means that the subject must be as close as 20 feet to read a type size that a person with normal distant vision can read at 80 feet.

Remember that the first number will always be "20" followed by a second, usually the same or larger, number. Once this is clear, there is no danger the transcriptionist will erroneously type "2200" or "22-100" when the physician dictates, "The patient had vision in the right eye of twenty two hundred [20/200]."

For **near vision** testing, lines or paragraphs are printed in various sizes of type (Jaeger test types) on a card that can be held in the hand. Testing may involve finding the smallest print that the subject can read at a standard distance, or finding the range of distances through which the subject can read a particular size of type.

Visual field testing is used to map areas of impaired or absent vision due to retinal disease or other ocular or neurologic abnormality. An **Amsler grid** consists of a network of lines, usually white on black, around a central point at which the subject is instructed to gaze while the examiner moves a small object through various parts of the visual field to detect defects.

Perimetry is an assessment of peripheral vision, performed by testing the subject's ability to discern moving objects or flashing lights at the extreme periphery of the visual fields.

Tests for color blindness employ printed figures made up of variously sized dots in various colors and shades (see ■ Figure 11-3). Persons with normal color vision perceive numbers against a background of differently colored dots, but color-blind persons see only a random scattering of dots.

Refraction. Refraction is the use of an instrument containing lenses of various powers to measure deficiencies of near and distant vision more precisely than is possible with vision charts alone. This procedure enables the examiner to determine the strength of the corrective lens that must be prescribed to correct nearsightedness (**myopia**) or farsightedness (**hyperopia**).

The patient's visual acuity is 20/50 in the right eye. She has visual acuity in the left eye of counting fingers on the basis of aphakia and a pupillary membrane with updrawn pupil. Her optic discs have a cup:disc ratio of 0.34 in each eye and the peripheral retinas are within normal limits.

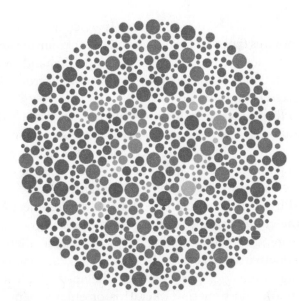

FIGURE 11-3. Color vision chart

Eye examination shows best vision of 20/50+ in the right eye and 20/200 in the left. Pupils and extraocular motility are normal. Intraocular pressures are 18. Slit lamp exam shows the eyelids in good position with weakness of the orbicularis and facial muscles. There is a clear corneal epithelium and the normal pseudophakia of the right eye and a dense nuclear cataract on the left. Fundus examination in each eye is normal.

By testing cylindrical lenses of various strengths at various angles, the examiner can also measure **astigmatism** (distortion of images by warping of the cornea out of the normal spherical shape) and prescribe appropriate correction. Refraction refers to the sum total of "refractometry," or measuring the refractive error of the eye. It is the essential component needed prior to prescribing glasses.

The refractive error in the right eye was a –0.50 + 1.00 axis 113 with a reading add of 2.25 which gave a J1 reading.

The previous sentence in the blue box describes the geometric calculations needed to establish the index of refraction for the manufacture of spectacles particular to the patient's needs. "Reading add" refers to the total dioptic power added to a distance prescription to supplement accommodation for reading

Pause for Reflection

1. What does it mean when the dictator says that a patient has vision of "twenty eighty OD"? How is this transcribed?
2. Describe 2 ways in which the visual fields may be tested.
3. How is a patient tested for color blindness?
4. What is refraction testing?

Ocular Imaging

by John H. Dirckx, MD

Several imaging techniques are available to supplement the physician's visual observation of structures within the eye. The most basic of these is **digital photography**, which can be used to record high-resolution images of the external eye, the anterior chamber and lens (**slit lamp biomicrography**) (see ◼ Figure 11-4), or the ocular fundus (**retinal photography**).

Stereoscopic images of the retina, obtained with special equipment, permit three-dimensional assessment that is not possible with a standard monocular ophthalmoscope. Digital images can be transmitted for consultation at a distance, stored for future reference, and used to monitor the progression of a disease process or the effects of treatment.

Angiography of the ocular fundus after intravenous injection of a fluorescent dye (fluorescein or indocyanine green) provides sequential images of blood flow and identifies vascular abnormalities of the choroid and retina such as arterial occlusion, capillary leakage, microaneurysms, and neovascularization. The fundus is illuminated with blue light of a certain wavelength (excitation color) while a barrier filter permits only light of the wavelength of the fluorescent dye to reach the camera. Blood vessels appear black in a series of black-and-white images obtained at intervals of about 1 second as the dye perfuses the retinal vasculature.

Optical coherence tomography (OCT) is a noninvasive imaging method that uses light waves rather than x-rays to produce cross-sectional images of living tissue. The technique is based on **interferometry**, the analysis of the pattern according to which light scatters after striking an object.

OCT has been applied to examination of various regions and tissues, including the anterior chamber of the eye. Images of the retina can be obtained with a

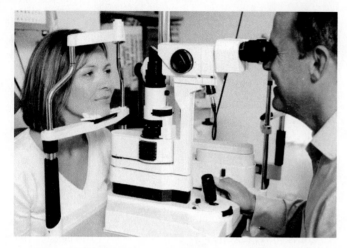

FIGURE 11-4. Slit lamp biomicrography

resolution comparable to that of a low-power microscope, permitting retinal layers to be distinguished and measured, and identifying changes of diabetic retinopathy and chorioretinitis.

Diagnostic methods to assess the corneal surface include **confocal microscopy**, which uses a pinhole light source and pinhole acquisition of images to improve resolution, and **corneal topography**, in which a computer analyzes the pattern of light reflected from the anterior surface of the cornea to produce a color-coded relief map

Pause for Reflection

1. List 3 imaging techniques used to record high-resolution images of the external eye, the anterior chamber and lens, the ocular fundus, or the vessels of the choroid and retina.
2. Describe optical coherence tomography and its uses.
3. Name and describe imaging methods used to assess the cornea.

Common Diseases

Conjunctivitis

Inflammation of the conjunctiva. (Pinkeye, referring to conjunctivitis with injection, is a lay term with no fixed medical meaning.)

Causes: Infection, allergy, injury (including injuries due to chemicals, heat, or other radiant energy), or other process affecting the anterior part of the eye.

Infection may be due to viruses (particularly certain adenovirus types) or bacteria (including chlamydia and gonococcus). Transmission is generally by hand contact. Neonatal conjunctivitis is acquired from an infected birth canal.

History: Soreness, itching, irritation, or foreign body sensation in one or both eyes, with redness of the conjunctiva, inability to tolerate contact lenses, and often a mucopurulent discharge that blurs vision, crusts the eyelashes, and glues the eyelids together during sleep.

Physical Examination: Patchy or diffuse injection of the conjunctiva, sometimes with coarsely granular appearance ("cobblestoning," typical of some allergic conjunctivitis). Lid edema, blepharospasm, lacrimation, ocular discharge, photophobia, chemosis (typically allergic), and sometimes keratitis or enlargement of preauricular lymph nodes (nodes in front of the ear). Slit lamp examination precisely locates areas of inflammation.

Diagnostic Tests: Microscopic examination of conjunctival scrapings can identify infection due to chlamydia. Culture is necessary to confirm gonococcal conjunctivitis.

Course: Seasonal or perennial allergic conjunctivitis is typically recurrent or chronic during times of exposure to allergens. Most infectious conjunctivitis is viral in origin, benign, and self-limited. Because it is highly contagious, however, epidemics are common in daycare centers and schools and among groups of persons who live or work in close proximity. Untreated gonococcal conjunctivitis can spread to the cornea, causing perforation and blindness. Chlamydial conjunctivitis is of two kinds. *Chlamydia trachomatis* types A–C cause trachoma, a severe conjunctivitis with keratitis, often leading to lid deformity and blindness. Types D–K cause a milder infection, inclusion conjunctivitis, which typically resolves without sequelae.

Treatment: Contact lens wear is discontinued as long as inflammation persists. Allergic conjunctivitis is treated with topical vasoconstrictors, mast cell stabilizers (cromolyn, lodoxamide), and corticosteroids. Systemic antihistamines and steroids may be required. Both forms of chlamydial conjunctivitis respond to systemic tetracycline, doxycycline, or erythromycin. Gonococcal conjunctivitis is treated with systemic ceftriaxone. Other kinds of bacterial infection are treated with topical sulfonamide or antibiotic drops. Although most non-allergic conjunctivitis is viral in origin and self-limited, cultures cannot reliably rule out bacterial infection; physicians therefore often choose to treat acute conjunctivitis with a topical sulfonamide or antibiotic. Careful handwashing is important in preventing spread of infection to others.

Hordeolum (Stye)

An acute staphylococcal abscess, typically small, that forms near the margin of an upper or lower eyelid. Treatment is with warm compresses and topical sulfonamide or antibiotic. Incision and drainage may be necessary.

Chalazion

A cyst arising in a sebaceous (meibomian) gland on an upper or lower eyelid. Although inflammation is seldom present, the lesion may grow large and become cosmetically objectionable. Treatment is incision and curettage.

Keratitis

Inflammation of the cornea.

Causes: Keratitis may result from injury (chemical, abrasion, erosion, puncture, contact lens wear), infection (bacterial, viral, fungal, or protozoan), or systemic disease. Bacteria causing keratitis include pneumococcus, staphylococcus, *Pseudomonas*, and *Moraxella*. Syphilitic and tuberculous keratitis (due to systemic infection) also occur. Viral keratitis may be due to herpes simplex virus or varicella-zoster virus. Keratitis in contact lens wearers may be due to the protozoan parasite *Acanthamoeba*.

History: Pain in the eye, aggravated by opening and closing the lid; lacrimation, photophobia, visual blurring. There may be a history of corneal trauma (fingernail scratch, cigarette ash, airborne foreign body) or of systemic infection (tuberculosis, syphilis).

Physical Examination: Conjunctival injection, particularly near to the corneal rim. Photophobia, lacrimation, watery or purulent discharge. **Fluorescein staining** of the cornea followed by examination with cobalt blue light shows ulceration or other epithelial defects.

Diagnostic Tests: Microscopic examination or culture of scrapings from the cornea may indicate a causative organism.

Course: Certain infections (herpes simplex virus, *Acanthamoeba*) cause progressive and severe damage if untreated, with visual loss due to corneal scarring. Thinning and bulging (descemetocele) of an inflamed zone of cornea may also occur. Corneal infection can extend to the sclera, iris, or optic nerve.

Treatment: Specific antimicrobial treatment, if available, is mandatory. Topical antibiotics usually suf-fice in bacterial keratitis. Viral infections are treated with topical idoxuridine or trifluridine and systemic acyclovir. Topical steroids are used in selected cases.

Uveitis

Inflammation of any part of the uveal tract, typically also affecting contiguous ocular tissues. One of three concentric layers of the eyeball, the **uveal tract** is a delicate, spongy, vascular membrane of pigmented cells. Anterior uveitis, which involves the iris (**iritis**) and usually the ciliary body as well (**iridocyclitis**), is the most common type (up to 90%). Intermediate uveitis occurs in the vitreous body and adjacent peripheral parts of the retina. Posterior uveitis arises in the choroid at the back of the eyeball (**choroiditis**) but generally extends to involve the overlying visual retina as well (**chorioretinitis**).

Causes: Often no cause can be found. Numerous systemic diseases, particularly those known or believed to be due to autoimmunity, can be complicated by uveitis. These include inflammatory bowel disease, ankylosing spondylitis, multiple sclerosis, and systemic lupus erythematosus. Persons with the HLA-B27 antigen are genetically predisposed to uveitis. Viral, bacterial, fungal, and parasitic infections are less common causes, but congenital infection with *Toxoplasma* or cytomegalovirus (CMV) is an important source of **chorioretinitis** in children. CMV retinitis can complicate systemic infection in persons with AIDS.

History: Blurring of vision occurs in most forms of uveitis. Other symptoms depend on the part of the uveal tract that is involved. In anterior uveitis, eye pain and photophobia result from inflammation of iris structures. When the vitreous is affected the patient may see **floaters** (opaque spots that float or drift with eye movement). Chorioretinitis causes patchy visual loss (distorted images, blind spots, loss of central vision), occasionally accompanied by flashes of light.

Physical Examination: In anterior uveitis the conjunctiva is injected and the pupil is constricted by ciliary spasm. **Slit lamp examination** (see ■ Figure 11-4) shows dilated ciliary vessels, cells and flare in the anterior chamber, and keratic precipitates on the posterior surface of the cornea. Inflammation of the vitreous body causes clumps ("snowballs") and drifts ("snowbanks") of whitish material. In chorioretinitis, examination of the ocular fundus shows retinal edema, patches of depigmentation, and blood vessel proliferation (neovascularization). In chronic disease there may be extensive retinal scarring.

Diagnostic Tests: Laboratory studies and other procedures may be undertaken to establish the underlying cause of uveitis. **Fluorescence angiography** can help to delineate vascular changes in the choroid.

Course: Acute unilateral **iridocyclitis**, often of unknown cause, may resolve spontaneously. Without treatment, however, some cases become chronic and can lead to cataract formation, glaucoma, or corneal calcification (**band keratopathy**). Involvement of the choroid and overlying visual retina typically leads to some degree of visual impairment, which may be irreversible.

Treatment: The mainstay of treatment in most forms of uveitis is the use of adrenal corticosteroids topically or systemically to suppress inflammation. Cycloplegics may be prescribed in anterior uveitis to relieve painful ciliary spasm. In refractory disease, an antimetabolite such as methotrexate or a monoclonal antibody may be used to reverse an autoimmune process. Specific therapy is indicated if an infectious cause is identified. In chorioretinitis, blood vessel proliferation can be arrested by **laser photocoagulation**.

Open Angle Glaucoma

The most common type of glaucoma (an ocular condition in which the pressure of the aqueous humor is abnormally high), consisting of a persistent elevation of intraocular pressure (see ■ Figure 11-5).

Cause: Unknown; apparently related to decreased reabsorption of aqueous humor from the anterior chamber of the eye. However, the **drainage angle** is not demonstrably narrowed, hence the name (contrast narrow-angle glaucoma). Both eyes are about equally affected, and the condition runs in families.

History: Gradual loss of peripheral vision. Appearance of halos around lights, especially at night, when intraocular tension is very high.

Physical Examination: Increased cupping of the optic disc (increased cup-to-disc ratio).

Diagnostic Tests: Intraocular tension, as determined by **tonometry** (see ■ Figure 11-6), is elevated (normal 10–21 mmHg). Visual fields are diminished.

Course: Optic atrophy, with partial to complete loss of vision within 15–20 years if untreated.

Treatment: Long-term treatment with miotics: beta-adrenergic blocking agents (timolol, levobunolol, metipranolol, epinephrine, and pilocarpine). **Laser trabeculectomy surgery** may be undertaken in refractory cases to improve drainage.

Narrow Angle Glaucoma

Acute onset of unilateral ocular pain and visual loss due to sudden obstruction of the outflow of aqueous humor (see ■ Figure 11-5).

Cause: *Predisposing*: A narrow anterior chamber angle (more common in the elderly, in persons with hypermetropia, and in Asians). *Precipitating*: Prolonged dilatation of the pupil, such as occurs in a darkened theater or after administration of certain drugs (anticholinergic medicines orally, mydriatic drops for eye examination).

History: Sudden onset of pain in one eye, with blurring of vision, halos around lights; often nausea, vomiting, and abdominal pain.

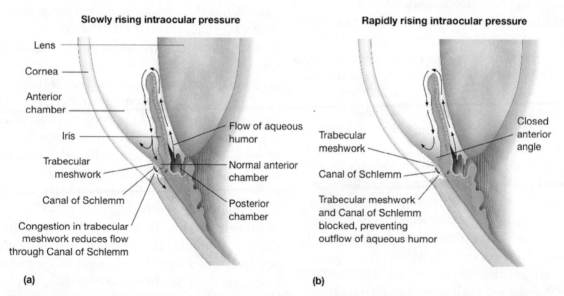

FIGURE 11-5. Glaucoma, characterized by increased intraocular pressure. (a) closed angle glaucoma (acute), (b) open angle glaucoma (chronic).

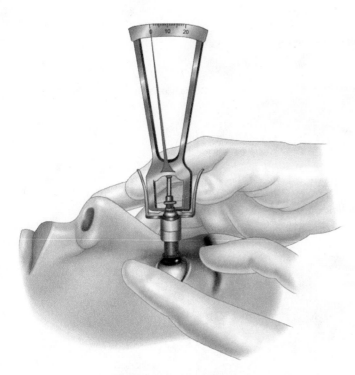

FIGURE 11-6. Tonometer to measure intraocular pressure

Physical Examination: Redness of the eye, steamy cornea, dilated nonreactive pupil.

Diagnostic Tests: **Tonometry** shows markedly elevated intraocular pressure.

Course: Severe and permanent visual loss occurs if acute glaucoma is not promptly treated.

Treatment: Intravenous acetazolamide and mannitol are administered to reduce intraocular pressure.

Laser iridectomy (destruction of a wedge of iris) permits drainage of the anterior chamber. The unaffected eye is usually operated on prophylactically as well.

Cataract

An ocular lens that has become cloudy or opaque because of intrinsic physical or chemical change (see ■ Figure 11-7).

Causes: Largely unknown. Infantile cataracts occur after maternal rubella or when the child has galacto-

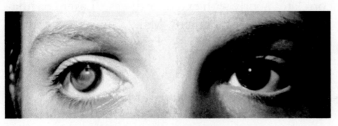

FIGURE 11-7. Cataract of the right eye.
Source: Pearson Education, PH College

semia. Cataract can occur in various systemic diseases (diabetes mellitus, hypoparathyroidism) or as a complication of other ocular disease (uveitis, glaucoma) or injury (penetrating injury of the lens, ionizing radiation). The most common type is **senile cataract**, occurring as part of aging, with onset after age 50. The risk is increased by cigarette smoking.

History: Gradual painless loss of vision, not improved by glasses, and seeing rings or halos around lights at night.

Physical Examination: Inspection confirms the presence of partial or complete opacity of one or both lenses. A fully developed cataract, with severe impairment of vision, is called "ripe." **Slit lamp examination** (see ■ Figure 11-4) gives more precise information about the type, extent, and location of lenticular opacity.

Course: Without treatment the entire lens eventually becomes opaque and vision is lost. Surgery restores vision at any stage by removing the lens.

Treatment: Surgical removal of the opaque lens by a variety of techniques, leaving the posterior capsule of the lens intact. Fragmentation with ultrasound (**phacoemulsification**) (see ■ Figure 11-8) is the standard procedure. A synthetic lens is usually implanted at the time of cataract extraction.

Retinopathy

A general term for degenerative disorders of the retina, usually accompanied by loss of vision and often due to systemic disease (see ■ Figure 11-9). Two types will be discussed here: hypertensive retinopathy and diabetic retinopathy.

Hypertensive Retinopathy

Degenerative retinal changes due to impairment of blood supply to the retina and choroid in persons with severe hypertension, with variable degrees of visual loss. Chronic hypertension accelerates the development of arteriosclerosis, and many of the physical findings are due to vascular changes. The **Keith-Wagener-Barker** classification is often used to grade funduscopic observations:

Grade I—focal or diffuse narrowing of retinal arterioles, with reduction of the arteriole-venule ratio (**AV ratio**; normally 4:5) to 3:4 or 1:2; narrowed arterioles may be described as having a **copper-wire** or **silver-wire** appearance.

Grade II—further narrowing of arterioles, with reduction of the AV ratio to 1:2 or 1:3; crossing phe-

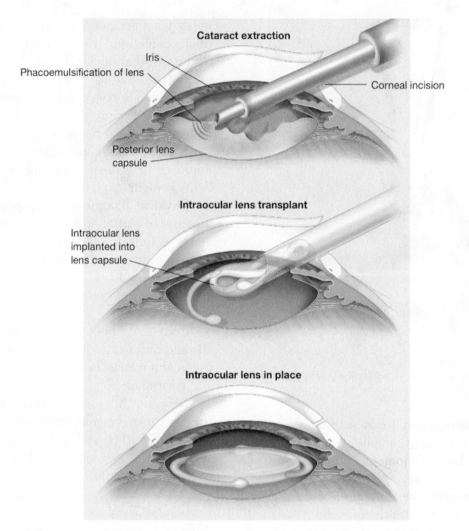

FIGURE 11-8. Phacoemulsification (cataract extraction and insertion of intraocular lens)

nomena or AV nicking (tapering of a venule where an arteriole crosses it).

Grade III—all of the above, with **"flame"** (flame-shaped) hemorrhages and **cotton wool spots** (exudates); these are fluffy opaque zones of degenerative change following microscopic infarction and hemorrhage in the retina.

Grade IV—all of the above, with papilledema. Close observation of the changes of hypertensive retinopathy is of value in judging hypertensive vascular damage elsewhere in the body. There is no treatment.

Diabetic Retinopathy

Degenerative vascular changes in the retina occurring in diabetes mellitus, particularly in poorly controlled diabetes; the principal cause of legal blindness before age 65. Two forms are recognized. In **proliferative retinopathy** there is formation of new blood vessels (**neovascularization**) in the retina, with visual loss and a risk of vitreous hemorrhage and retinal tears. The condition is detected by **fluorescein angiography** and treated by **laser photocoagulation** (occasionally, surgery).

In **nonproliferative retinopathy**, changes are limited to venous dilatation, **microaneurysms** (appearing as tiny red spots adjacent to vessels), retinal hemorrhages and **hard** (sharp-bordered) **exudates**, and retinal edema. As retinal edema resolves, it may leave folds or tucks in the retina, which appear as whitish streaks, often arranged in fanlike configurations. A complete encirclement of the macula by radially disposed streaks constitutes a macular "star figure." Visual impairment correlates poorly with extent of disease. **Laser coagulation** is the usual treatment. Maintaining good control of diabetes reduces the risk of severe retinopathy.

Strabismus

A disorder of ocular motility in which the two eyes do not look in exactly the same direction, and cerebral fusion of their images into a three-dimensional one cannot occur (see ■ Figure 11-10).

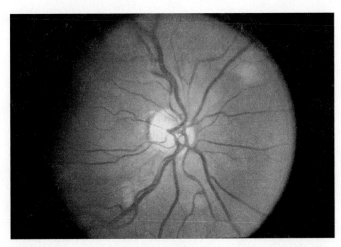

FIGURE 11-9. Retinopathy seen through an ophthalmoscope.
Source: Pearson Education, PH College.

Heterophoria is a transient deviation of one eye from the normal position with respect to the other. It may occur as a slight congenital weakness or imbalance of ocular muscles that is symptomatic only in the presence of fatigue. Other causes include fever, alcohol and drug use. Inward deviation of one eye is called **esophoria**, outward deviation is called **exophoria**, and normal positioning of both eyes is called orthophoria.

Heterotropia is a persistent deviation of one or both eyes, due to congenital ocular muscle weakness or imbalance. If one eye is consistently affected, central suppression of its image eventually occurs, with resulting **amblyopia** (dulling of vision that cannot be corrected with a lens). Treatment of heterotropia must be carried out before amblyopia has developed. Treatment consists of prismatic lenses that permit images to fuse, occlusion of one eye to preserve the vision of the other, exercises to improve strength and coordination of ocular muscles, and surgery to bring the eyes into line.

Paralytic strabismus results from paralysis of one or more eye muscles due to congenital abnormality, trauma, infection, multiple sclerosis, herpes zoster, neoplasm, or hemorrhage. Surgical treatment may be helpful in selected cases.

Nystagmus is involuntary rhythmic movements of the eyes, typically bilateral, due to congenital abnormality, multiple sclerosis, or central nervous system tumor, infection, or hemorrhage, or intoxication (chronic alcoholism). Transitory nystagmus occurs after riding on a merry-go-round or in the presence of vertigo. There is no treatment for nystagmus other than removing the cause, if it can be detected.

Visual Impairment

Emmetropia: Normal vision.

Hyperopia (farsightedness): The focus of light rays passing into the eyes lies behind the retina, due to a congenitally short anteroposterior diameter of the eyeball. Treatment is with corrective lenses.

Myopia (nearsightedness): The focus of light rays passing into the eye lies in front of, rather than on, the retina, because of a congenitally long anteroposterior diameter of the eyeball. This condition, much commoner than the preceding, shows a familial tendency and when severe it predisposes to glaucoma. Treatment is with corrective lenses.

Astigmatism: The image falling on the retina is distorted because the curvature of the cornea is not the same in all axes (that is, the cornea is not spherical). Correction is with lenses having a cylindrical curvature to neutralize the effect of corneal distortion.

Presbyopia: Loss of normal accommodation with aging, due to diminished elasticity of the eyes, with inability to focus on objects or print near to the eye. Treatment is with corrective lenses for reading. Persons with myopia as well as presbyopia require bifocals or even trifocals (often with no-line progressive lenses) to provide a choice of focal distances.

IMPRESSION
1. *Increasing myopia, left eye.*
2. *Early presbyopia.*

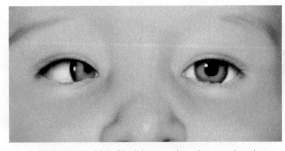

FIGURE 11-10A. Strabismus, showing esotropia.

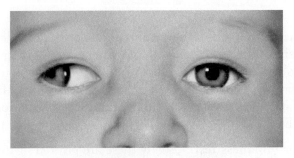

FIGURE 11-10B. Strabismus, showing exotropia.
Source: Pearson Education, PH College.

Pause for Reflection

1. Describe the physical findings of the eye in patients with conjunctivitis.
2. What is keratitis and how is it diagnosed?
3. Distinguish among the different types of uveitis.
4. Distinguish between open angle and closed angle glaucoma.
5. What is the treatment for cataract?
6. Distinguish between hypertensive and diabetic retinopathy.
7. Summarize the Keith-Wagener-Barker classification used to grade funduscopic observations in cases of hypertensive retinopathy.
8. Distinguish between heterotropia and heterophoria.
9. Define *emmetropia, hyperopia, myopia, astigmatism,* and *presbyopia.*

Diagnostic and Surgical Procedures

Amsler grid See *visual field testing.*

blepharoplasty Surgery on the eyelids to remove skin and fat and reinforce surrounding muscles and tendons to improve vision impaired by sagging eyelids (see ■ Figure 11-11).

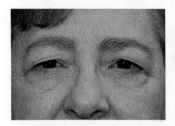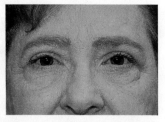

FIGURE 11-11. Blepharoplasty, upper eyelid lift, showing eyelid droop before surgery, and 6 weeks postop. Source: Bella Modella Studio.

cataract extraction Surgical removal of the clouded lens of the eye, often with placement of an artificial intraocular lens (see ■ Figure 11-7). The most common types of cataract extraction are **phacoemulsification** and **extracapsular cataract extraction (ECCE).**

color blindness test Usually these are printed figures made up of variously sized dots in various colors and shades (see ■ Figure 11-3). Persons with normal color vision perceive numbers against a background of differently colored dots. Color-blind persons see only a scattering of dots.

cryopexy Surgical treatment of retinal detachment consisting of localized freezing of the surface of the sclera to fix the retina to the choroid.

dacryorhinocystotomy A variation on dacryocystorhinotomy, passage of a probe through the lacrimal sac into the nasal cavity.

electroretinography (ERG) Instrumental determination of changes in electrical potential of the retina in response to light stimuli; identifies visual abnormalities due to retinal disease.

endodiathermy A procedure using a probe for cauterizing bleeding retinal vessels such as in diabetic retinopathy or before large and more central retinectomies. Another indication is to mark a break in **retinal detachment** surgery or in preparation for a **retinotomy.**

extracapsular cataract extraction (ECCE) Removes the lens but leaves the capsule intact for implantation of an intraocular lens (see ■ Figure 11-8).

fluorescein staining Fluorescein dye is applied to the cornea and conjunctiva, and the surface of the eye examined with a cobalt blue light, to detect injuries, ulcerations, or foreign bodies. See also *retinal arteriography.*

funduscopic examination Inspection of the fundus (the rear of the interior of the eye, consisting of the retina, its blood vessels, and the optic nerve head). The examination is performed with an **ophthalmoscope.** Also called *ophthalmoscopy.*

intracapsular cataract extraction (ICCE) Rarely performed due to a high rate of complications and the large incision required. It involves removal of the lens and capsule; an intraocular lens may be placed in the anterior chamber or sutured to the sulcus.

keratocentesis Corneal paracentesis, surgical puncture of the cornea with a needle to remove fluid and reduce intraocular pressure.

LASIK (laser in situ keratomileusis) A corneal procedure for vision correction. A flap of anterior corneal stroma is dissected, the deeper layers are partially ablated with the laser, and the hinged superficial flap is then replaced.

ophthalmoscopy See *funduscopic examination.*

orbital imaging Radiographs or MRI of the skull with emphasis on the orbit(s) to identify orbital or intraocular foreign body.

panretinal photocoagulation Use of a laser to destroy almost the entire retina to treat neovascularization, such as in diabetic retinopathy.

perimetry A means of assessing peripheral vision by testing the subject's ability to discern moving objects or flashing lights at the extreme periphery of the visual fields.

peripheral iridotomy Puncture of the iris without the removal of iris tissue to decrease intraocular pressure in patients with angle-closure glaucoma. Standard surgical instruments or a laser may be used to make the puncture, allowing the aqueous to pass directly from the posterior chamber into the anterior chamber, bypassing the pupil. A **laser peripheral iridotomy (LPI)** uses a laser beam to selectively burn a hole through the iris near its base. Either an argon laser or Nd:YAG laser may be used.

phacoemulsification Fragmentation of the lens of the eye with ultrasound (see ■ Figure 11-8).

pneumatic retinopexy Fixation of the retina in its proper position with the injection of a bubble of gas into the interior of the eye in the vitreous cavity. With proper postoperative positioning, the retina can be pushed back into proper position and then the gas will spontaneously disappear in a few weeks. Gases used in this procedure may be either perfluoropropane (C_3F_8), sulfur hexafluoride (SF_6), or perfluoroethane (C_2F_6).

PRK (photorefractive keratectomy) A vision correction procedure using computer-guided excimer laser ablation to reprofile the anterior corneal curvature. Also called *T-PRK (tracker-assisted photorefractive keratectomy).*

refraction Determination of near and distant vision more precisely than is possible with vision charts. The instruments used include a **retinoscope** and an **auto-refractor** for objective measurement, and a **phoropter** for subjective refraction. The instruments are also used in detecting and measuring astigmatism.

retinal arteriography Imaging of the retinal arteries with fluorescein injected into an arm vein. Also called *fluorescein angiography.*

retrobulbar block A type of regional anesthetic nerve block in which a local anesthetic is injected into the area located behind the globe of the eye (the retrobulbar space) providing akinesia of the extraocular muscles and preventing movement of the globe. Sensory anesthesia of the cornea, uvea, and conjunctiva is also achieved by blocking the ciliary nerves.

scleral buckle procedure The most common procedure to treat a **retinal detachment** (see ■ Figure 11-12). A piece of silicone sponge, rubber, or semi-hard plastic is sewn onto the sclera of the eye, either over the area of detachment or encircling the eyeball like a ring, pushing the sclera toward the middle of the eye and relieving traction on the retina. Other procedures may be performed in conjunction with a scleral buckle to scar the retina and hold it in place until a seal forms between the retina and the choroid to keep the retina detachment from recurring.

sclerostomy Treatment of glaucoma by means of the surgical creation of an opening through the sclera.

sclerotomy Incision into the sclera.

slit lamp examination A low-power microscope with built-in illumination projected through a narrow slit used to view a magnified cross-sectional image of the anterior structures of the eye: cornea, anterior chamber, iris, and lens (see ■ Figure 11-4).

tamponade Surgical compression by placement of a pack, a pad or plug made of cotton, sponge, or other material.

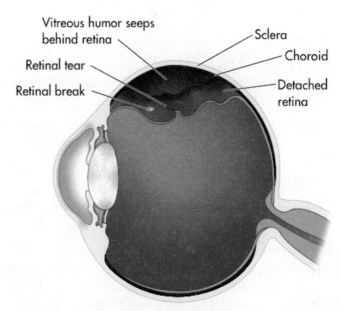

FIGURE 11-12. Retinal detachment

tonometry Determination of the pressure of the aqueous humor (intraocular pressure), to detect glaucoma. Tonometers of various types are used; one of the more common ones is the Schiøtz tonometer (see ■ Figure 11-6).

trabeculectomy Surgical removal of a portion of the trabecular meshwork to create a fistula between the anterior chamber of the eye and the subconjunctival space to facilitate drainage of the aqueous humor in glaucoma.

visual field testing Use of a black felt sheet or screen mounted on a wall to map areas of impaired or absent vision. An Amsler grid consists of a network of lines, usually white on black, around a central point at which the subject is instructed to gaze while the examiner moves a small object through various parts of the visual field to detect defects.

vitrectomy Surgical extraction of the contents of the vitreous chamber (vitreous humor, vitreous gel) of the eye. An anterior vitrectomy removes only a small amount of aqueous fluid from the front of the eye. A **posterior** or **pars plana vitrectomy** removes some or all of the fluid from the deeper portions of the eye.

wet-field cautery Irrigation of the surgical field while applying cautery to achieve hemostasis. The Wet-Field coagulator is a trademarked device "designed to provide precise episcleral, intrascleral, and intraocular hemostasis with reduced peripheral tissue trauma" but *wet-field* is generally used in a generic sense.

Laboratory Procedures

blood glucose May be ordered if arteriovenous nicking of the eye vessels occurs, to rule out diabetes mellitus.

cytomegalovirus (CMV) A herpesvirus that is often not symptomatic but can cause infections, and particularly virulent in persons with AIDS, resulting in CMV retinitis.

thyroid panel May be ordered if bulging eyes are noted, to rule out thyroid disease.

human leukocyte antigen (HLA) Patients with HLA-B27 antigen are genetically predisposed to acute anterior uveitis. HLA-A29 antigen is associated with posterior uveitis conditions such as birdshot retinochoroidopathy.

Pharmacology

Ophthalmic drugs may be applied topically to treat superficial infections or inflammations of the cornea and surrounding tissues, treat allergy symptoms in the eye, treat glaucoma, or produce anesthesia or mydriasis to facilitate examination of the eye. Some ophthalmic drugs are taken systemically for severe infection or inflammation in the interior of the eye. All drugs intended for topical application in the eye are specially formulated in solution that is physiologically similar to fluids in the eye so as not to damage the delicate eye tissues.

Antibiotic Drugs

These drugs are used to treat superficial bacterial infections of the cornea, conjunctiva, eyelids, and tear ducts. Antibiotics are not effective against viral infections. Ophthalmic antibiotics are dispensed as ointments or solutions.

bacitracin
chloramphenicol (Chloromycetin, Chloroptic)
ciprofloxacin (Ciloxan)
erythromycin (Ilotycin)
gentamicin (Garamycin, Genoptic, Gentacidin, Gentak)
levofloxacin (Quixin)
norfloxacin (Chibroxin)
ofloxacin (Ocuflox)
tobramycin (Tobrex)

Anti-infective drugs effective in treating fungal infections of the eye include natamycin (Natacyn).

Sulfonamides

Sulfonamide ophthalmic drugs are not classified as antibiotics, but they do inhibit the growth of bacteria and are used to treat infections in the eye. Examples include sulfacetamide (Bleph-10, Cetamide, Ocusulf, Sulamyd) and sulfisoxazole (Gantrisin).

Corticosteroids

Corticosteroids are used topically in the eye to treat the inflammation that results from trauma, surgery, contact with chemicals, or allergies.

dexamethasone (Decadron, Maxidex)
fluorometholone (Flarex, Fluor-Op, FML, FML Forte)
loteprednol (Alrex, Lotemax)

prednisolone (Econopred, Inflamase Forte,
  Pred Forte, Pred Mild)
rimexolone (Vexol)

Antiviral Drugs

Antiviral drugs act by inhibiting viral DNA reproduction. Topical antiviral drugs for the eye that are effective against herpes simplex virus (HSV) include:

trifluridine (Viroptic)
vidarabine (Vira-A)

Systemic antiviral drugs that are effective against cytomegalovirus (CMV) retinitis, a disease most often seen in AIDS patients, include:

cidofovir (Vistide)
ganciclovir (Cytovene, Vitrasert)
valganciclovir (Valcyte)
foscarnet (Foscavir)

Nonsteroidal Anti-inflammatories

Nonsteroidal anti-inflammatories are used topically to treat inflammation that results from surgery or allergic reactions.

diclofenac (Voltaren)
ketorolac (Acular)

Antihistamines and Mast Cell Inhibitors

Topical antihistamines relieve the symptoms of allergic conjunctivitis. These symptoms are caused by histamine released by the antibody-antigen complex that forms during allergic reactions. Histamine causes vasodilatation, which causes blood vessels and tissues to become engorged, swollen, and red. Histamine also irritates these tissues directly, causing pain and itching. Antihistamines exert their therapeutic effect by blocking **histamine (H_1) receptors** in the eye.

azelastine (Optivar)
emedastine (Emadine)
levocabastine (Livostin)
olopatadine (Patanol)

Topical mast cell inhibitors act to stabilize the cell membranes of mast cells and prevent them from releasing histamine. This prevents redness and vasodilatation in the eye.

cromolyn (Crolom, Opticrom)
lodoxamide (Alomide)

Drugs for Glaucoma

Drugs for glaucoma act either by decreasing the amount of aqueous humor circulating in the anterior and posterior chambers (to decrease the intraocular pressure) or by constricting the pupil (miosis) to open the angle of contact between the iris and the trabecular meshwork (to allow the aqueous humor to flow freely).

Direct-acting miotics cause pupillary constriction by stimulating the iris muscle around the pupil to contract and produce miosis. These were the first drugs developed for glaucoma and are used less often now. These drugs are administered topically as eye drops.

carbachol (Carboptic, Isopto Carbachol)
phenylephrine (Mydfrin, Neo-Synephrine)
pilocarpine (Akarpine, Isopto Carpine, Pilocar,
  Pilopine HS)

These drugs inhibit cholinesterase, an enzyme that normally destroys acetylcholine. As excess acetylcholine accumulates, it causes miosis.

demecarium (Humorsol)
echothiophate iodide (Phospholine Iodide)

Carbonic anhydrase inhibitors decrease the production of aqueous humor by blocking the enzyme carbonic anhydrase, which is active in the production of aqueous humor.

acetazolamide (Diamox, Diamox Sequels)
brinzolamide (Azopt)
dichlorphenamide (Daranide)
dorzolamide (Trusopt)
methazolamide (Neptazane)

Beta-blockers block the production of aqueous humor to decrease intraocular pressure. They have no effect on pupil size and therefore do not cause the blurred vision or night blindness associated with other miotics that constrict and fix the pupil. These drugs are administered topically as eye drops.

betaxolol (Betoptic, Betoptic S)
carteolol (Ocupress)
dapiprazole (Rev-Eyes)
levobetaxolol (Betaxon)
levobunolol (Betagan Liquifilm)
metipranolol (OptiPranolol)
timolol (Betimol, Timoptic)

Alpha/beta receptor agonists activate both alpha and beta receptors in the eye. This increases the flow of aqueous humor present while decreasing the overall production of aqueous humor.

apraclonidine (Iopidine)
brimonidine (Alphagan, Alphagan P)
dipivefrin (Propine)
epinephrine (Epifrin, Glaucon)
epinephryl (Epinal)

Prostaglandin F agonists mimic the action of naturally occurring prostaglandin F by combining with its receptors to increase the flow of aqueous humor. Example is latanoprost (Xalantan).

Mydriatic Drugs

Mydriatic drugs are used to dilate the pupil (mydriasis) and paralyze the muscles of accommodation (cyclo-plegia) of the iris. They block the action of acetylcholine, which normally tends to constrict the pupil. Mydriatic drugs are used to prepare the eye for internal examination and to treat inflammatory conditions of the iris and uveal tract.

atropine (Atropine Care, Atropisol,
    Isopto Atropine)
cyclopentolate (Cyclogyl, Pentolair)
homatropine (Isopto Homatropine)
hydroxyamphetamine (Paredrine)
phenylephrine (Neo-Synephrine, Mydfrin)
scopolamine (Isopto Hyoscine)
tropicamide (Mydriacyl)

Transcription Tips

1. Confusing terms related to ophthalmology: Some of these terms sound alike; others are potential traps when researching. Memorize the terms and their meanings so that you can select the appropriate term for a correct transcript.

   anisocoria—unequal pupil diameters

   anisophoria—muscular imbalance of the eyes varies with the direction of gaze

   aura—a sensation or muscular activity that precedes a neurological event, like a migraine or seizure

   ora—short for ora serrata retinae, the margin of the optic part of the retina

   buckle (scleral)—a surgical procedure to repair a retinal detachment

   buccal—pertaining to the cheek

   choreal—pertaining to chorea, involuntary rapid jerky movements

   corneal—pertaining to the cornea, the anterior part of the sclera

   instilled—placed drop by drop

   installed—placed in position; not used in the context of administering medications

   sight—vision

   site—a place

   cite—to state or reference

   recession—posterior displacement of ocular muscle insertion surgically

   resection—excision

   Tenon (membrane, capsule)—the sheath of the eyeball

   tendon—connective tissue attaching muscle to bone

   viscus—organ

   viscous—gummy, gel-like

2. Spelling. Memorize the spelling of these difficult-to-spell terms. Note silent letters, doubled letters, and unexpected pronunciation.

   accommodation (two *c*'s, two *m*'s)

   akinesia

   aqueous

   capsulorhexis *or* capsulorrhexis

   curvilinear (curvi-, *not* curva-)

   cystitome (cysti-, *not* cysto-)

   Descemet (membrane)

   fluorescein

   funduscopy (*not* -oscopy)

   hyaloid

   ophthalmology, ophthalmologic (always -phth-)

   paracentesis (pl., paracenteses)

   peritomy

   phacoemulsification (*ph* sounds like *f*)

   pseudophakia (silent *p*)

   ptosis (silent *p*)

   pterygium (silent *p*)

   rhegmatogenous (silent *h*)

   Schiøtz tonometer

   tarsus

   Vannas (scissors)

   Weck-Cel sponge

   Wet-Field cautery *or* wet-field cautery

3. Watch out for spelling changes when forming derivatives.

   The spelling *disk* (from the Greek diskos) is preferred over *disc* (from Latin discus) for all uses except ophthalmology. Use *disc* in ophthalmology unless otherwise instructed. Dictators' spelling preferences for derivatives of *disc* can be determined by their pronunciation: *diskitis* ("dis-ki-tis") or *discitis* ("dis-si-tis"); *diskectomy* ("disk-ec-tom-y") or *discectomy* ("di-sec-to-my").

4. Spelling. Note the challenging spellings or unusual capitalization of these common ophthalmology drugs.

   gentamicin

   Healon

   hyoscine

   Lacri-Lube

   Neo-Synephrine

   mitomycin C

   ofloxacin

   TobraDex

   Quixin

   VisionBlue dye

   Viscoat

   Wydase

Transcription Tips

Note that *–olol* is a common ending for beta blockers, which are used in the treatment of glaucoma (increased intraocular pressure).

5. Tricky Abbreviations. Some abbreviations are acronyms and pronounced as a word; others have soundalike letters; *b, d, p,* and *v* can all sound alike, as can *t* and *d, f* and *s, n* and *and*. Although some abbreviations do not need to be expanded, you do need to know what they mean in order to choose the correct expansion.

BSS (balanced saline solution)
I&A *or* IA (irrigation-aspiration)
IOL (intraocular lens)
IOP (intraocular pressure)

The Latin abbreviations *OU* (L., *oculus uterque*), *OS* (L., *oculus sinister*), and *OD* (L., *oculus dexter*): each eye, left eye, and right eye, respectively, are traditional abbreviations that are on the list of error-prone abbreviations. Although physicians continue to dictate these abbreviations, The Joint Commission directs that they be expanded when referencing medications to avoid confusion with similar abbreviations. However, when used with visual testing and measured values, the abbreviations should be used, e.g., visual acuity 20/20 OU. Note that OU is often incorrectly translated as both eyes.

6. Dictation Challenges

The HEENT exam can be challenging to transcribe. The abbreviation *PERRLA* (pupils equal, round, and reactive to light and accommodation) may be dictated as "per-la" rather than being spelled out letter by letter. A variation of this is *PERL* ("pearl"), which stands for "pupils equal, reactive to light." *Sclerae* and *conjunctivae* are always plural in the HEENT exam unless the dictator specifies right or left, or the patient has only one eye.

The term *injected* or *injection* when used as an adjective pertaining to the eyes refers to congestion or dilation of the visible vessels with blood. Although the American Medical Association recommends changing the term to *hyperemia* or *vasodilation* in formal publication, the terms should be transcribed as dictated in the healthcare record unless otherwise instructed.

Intraocular pressure, like blood pressure, is measured in millimeters of mercury (mmHg). If not dictated, the unit does not need to be added unless otherwise instructed.

Visual acuity at a distance, measured using the Snellen chart, is always expressed as two numbers which should be transcribed separated by a virgule (slash).

20/20   20/40   20/200

The first number will always be 20 (for the 20 feet between the vision chart and the patient). A dictated value that sounds like "twenty two hundred" or "twenty over two hundred" is correctly transcribed as 20/200. The phrase "twenty two hundred minus 2" is transcribed 20/200-2.

The *cup-to-disc (cup:disc) ratio* refers to the ratio of the diameter of the optic cup to the diameter of the optic disc; it is usually reported as a decimal fraction; "point 5" would be transcribed as 0.5.

When dictating terms that consist of several combining forms, dictators may rearrange the order of the combining forms. The spelling can usually be deduced using standard rules for combining word parts. For example, *dacryocystorhinostomy* may be dictated as *dacryorhinocystotomy*. Transcribe as dictated unless otherwise instructed.

Spotlight On

A Flock of Floaters

by Ellen A. Drake

Like Ramón y Cajal, pathologist and neuroscientist, who found the retina to be "the unfathomable mystery of life," I too find the eye to be a mystery, even after many years of undergoing diagnostic studies, treatments, and surgeries for birdshot retinochoroidopathy and other conditions of the eyes.

I was 45 when it happened. I had accepted a job as Director of Education with Health Professions Institute (HPI) in California. When we packed up and moved from Florida, I had barely recovered from a severe viral illness and bronchitis. The move was grueling and stressful, and my health continued to deteriorate. I barely noticed my worsening vision. I just assumed that I needed to have my eyes checked and my contacts replaced.

Almost a year later, I was walking down a San Francisco street with my husband and friends when I realized that I could barely see. It was as if someone had smeared Vaseline all over my contact lenses. I went to see an ophthalmologist the next week.

Thus began my adventure into the mysteries of the eye. The ophthalmologist examined my eyes and remarked that I did, indeed, have "a flock of floaters." Her diagnosis was AMPPE (acute multifocal placoid pigment epitheliopathy), which she pronounced as "amp-pee," characterized by multiple yellowish-white, flat, placoid lesions over the posterior fundus and involving the RPE (retinal pigment epithelium) where the rods and cones relating to night vision and color vision are located. I had noticed increasing night blindness and would eventually note difficulties with certain colors and tones.

The MT in me overcame my anxiety; the phrases sounded almost lyrical to me. My doctor tried to explain my condition, and to some degree I think I understood, but I soon realized that I would have to research and study on my own before I really understood what was happening to my eyes.

My ophthalmologist prescribed some corticosteroid eye drops and referred me to a retina specialist, who didn't contradict her diagnosis but added his own—choroiditis. He said that he would give me a subconjunctival injection of the corticosteroid triamcinolone into the eye as topical drops would never get to the source of the problem. "You're going to put a needle into my eye?" I asked in horror. I had imagined the eye as something like a balloon; how could you stick a needle into it without popping it, I asked myself.

He explained the procedure carefully, detailing the possible risks and complications. It was a safe procedure, as procedures go. Risks include vitreous hemorrhage, retinal tear, and retinal detachment, and a lesser risk of endophthalmitis. I signed an informed consent, and he carried out the procedure, first instilling some anesthetic drops, then bathing my eye with a surgical cleanser that left my sclera and the rims of my lids stained orange. Before the injection, he placed a Q-tip soaked in anesthetic inside my lower lid and let it stay there for several minutes. Then he used a tiny needle to instill more anesthetic in the area of the intended injection. The iodine-based cleanser and the anesthetic hurt more than the injection. Fortunately, there were no complications.

Over the next half dozen years, I received many more subconjunctival injections and several more diagnoses: uveitis, vitritis, and vitiliginous choroidopathy, also characterized by pale yellow to white lesions on the retina. After moving back to Florida, I went to see the ophthalmologist son of a woman I had worked for in high school. He was the first person to mention birdshot retinochoroidopathy (or chorioretinopathy, depending on the source) as a diagnosis, a colorful synonym for vitiliginous choroidopathy; the lesions on the retina look like birdshot to observers.

Frustrated, I said, "I've had so many different diagnoses, I've lost count. Isn't there any way to confirm the diagnosis?" He said that he could order a test called HLA-A29 (human leukocyte antigen A29), but it was expensive. A negative test did not mean that I did not have this disease, but if the test was positive, there was a 90% correlation. "I want it," I said. The test was positive, and finally I had a definitive diagnosis. Frankly admitting that he felt unqualified to treat my problem because it was so rare, he referred me to the Emory Eye Clinic in Atlanta.

Spotlight On A Flock of Floaters, page 2

By the time I got to Emory, my vision was "counting fingers" in the left eye, 20/400 in the right. I was surely facing blindness, and I don't mind saying I was very afraid. I first saw the chair of the retina department who explained that my condition is very rare and not a lot is known about it. It is believed to be an autoimmune condition, possibly triggered by a viral illness (I'm convinced of that!), but no one really knows what causes birdshot. He recommended that my primary care physician work me up for other autoimmune diseases like collagen vascular disease and sarcoidosis. My immune workup proved to be negative. The specialists at Emory agreed it was a "textbook case" of birdshot chorioretinopathy.

At the time my retina specialist was participating in a Bausch and Lomb clinical trial for a new implantable device to treat posterior uveitis. No bigger than a grain of rice, it would be placed in the eye and release minute amounts of the corticosteroid fluocinolone, putting the medicine right where it was needed. I had to have at least two failed corticosteroid injections over a six-month period before I could be eligible.

My desire to be in the trial was as motivated by curiosity as it was by the potential for a more effective treatment. The trial was to determine the effective dose of medication, one implant releasing twice the dose of the other. I was informed of possible risks and side effects: the treatment was known to cause cataracts and there was a high risk for increased intraocular pressure (glaucoma) unable to be controlled with drops. I signed the informed consent with little hesitation, knowing both cataract and glaucoma were treatable. Without the implant, I would continue to need the steroid injections each time the inflammation flared up; continued flareups almost certainly meant more vision impairment or blindness due to optic nerve damage.

Since then, all my treatments have been at Emory Eye Clinic. I am on my third retina specialist, and they have all been great. I am the poster child for birdshot—every new Fellow that rotates through the clinic gets to look deep into my eyes.

Although I was told that many if not most cases of birdshot "burn out" over time; mine has not. The most frequent complication is macular edema. The Retisert implant, now FDA approved, is designed to release medication for up to 30 months and has been replaced twice in my left eye. Between replacements, after the medication runs out, I again receive injections of triamcinolone to treat flareups.

At some point, the injections became intravitreal (deeper into the eye) instead of subconjunctival, and these clearly are a more effective treatment. I've had so many injections, I've lost count. When the injections are no longer effective, the implant is replaced. An implant placed in my right eye has long since run out of medicine, but my eye has remained stable for several years now.

I have also had the expected cataract extractions and glaucoma surgeries (trabeculectomies) in each eye. I have had several fluorescein angiograms, OCTs, two ERGs, and several visual field tests. During the postop period after the trabeculectomy on my right eye, I was found to have severe macular edema in my left eye. It was thought that I had developed a retinal vein occlusion or neovascularization with leaking blood vessels between the layers of the retina. I was treated two or three times with an injection of Avastin (bevacizumab), an angiogenesis inhibitor for treatment of colon carcinoma. A similar drug Lucentis (ranibizumab) was developed specifically for the eye, but it was newer and, therefore, much more expensive, so I was given Avastin "off label."

My adventure isn't over. I am currently one year postop for my third Retisert implant in the left eye. Much of my vision has been restored. I vary between 20/40 and 20/50 in the right eye and 20/60 to 20/100 in the left eye. My near vision is the most affected. Because of the scars on my macula and retina, I have great difficulty reading normal type. Fortunately, my computer can enlarge the view to whatever size I need. Almost all my pleasure reading is done on my iPad.

Although I have learned a lot about the eye and particularly about this disease, to me it is the most complex and remarkable organ in the human body. With Santiago Ramón y Cajal, I still experience the "shuddering sensation of the unfathomable mystery of life."

Exercises

Medical Vocabulary Review

Instructions: Choose the best answer.

___ 1. Complete the sentence. This patient has
_____, status post extracapsular cataract
extraction.
A. akinesia
B. aphakia
C. coloboma
D. exophthalmos

___ 2. _____ of the pupils will limit the ability of
an examiner to perform a funduscopy.
A. Miosis
B. Mydriasis
C. Nyctalopia
D. Photophobia

___ 3. Choked disc is another term for ____
A. blepharospasm.
B. exophthalmos.
C. photophobia.
D. papilledema.

___ 4. Seeing two overlapping two-dimensional
images instead of one three-dimensional
image is _____
A. diplopia.
B. scotoma.
C. retinitis.
D. strabismus.

___ 5. In cataract surgery, the lens is removed
through _____
A. a peritomy.
B. Descemet membrane.
C. a capsulorrhexis.
D. cupping of the disc.

___ 6. Excessive tearing is _____
A. epiphora.
B. lacrimation.
C. ectropion.
D. xerophthalmia.

___ 7. Another word for the lacrimal duct is
_____
A. sclera.
B. conjunctiva.
C. macula.
D. canaliculus.

___ 8. In surgery to repair a retinal detachment, an
intraocular gas bubble may be placed to
_____ the retina.
A. extract
B. examine
C. tamponade
D. completely remove

___ 9. Whitish deposits of inflammatory cells on
the posterior surface of the cornea are called
_____
A. flare and cells.
B. keratic precipitates.
C. conjunctival injection.
D. stepping of the vessels.

___ 10. Physiologic cupping is _____
A. a normal finding.
B. evidence of a choked disc.
C. a sign of papilledema.
D. a sign of glaucoma.

___ 11. A retinal detachment arising from a tear is said to be a _____ detachment.
A. rhegmatogenous
B. intraocular
C. hyaloid
D. injected

___ 12. On physical examination, a patient with conjunctivitis might be said to have conjunctival _____, or hyperemia.
A. tearing
B. injection
C. hyphema
D. hemorrhage

___ 13. Sustained increase in intraocular pressure is _____
A. glaucoma.
B. hyperemia.
C. mydriasis.
D. retinitis.

___ 14. _____ may be a sign of hyperthyroidism.
A. Blepharospasm
B. Exophthalmos
C. Cupping of the disc
D. Arteriovenous nicking

___ 15. Which of the following is NOT an imaging technique to examine the eye?
A. Electroretinography.
B. Optical coherence tomography.
C. Fluorescein arteriography.
D. Slit lamp biomicrography.

Pharmacology

Instructions: Choose the best answer.

___ 1. Which of the following drugs is used to treat the inflammation that results from trauma, surgery, contact with chemicals, or allergies?
A. Gantrisin (sulfisoxazole).
B. Alomide (lodoxamide).
C. Chloroptic (chloramphenicol).
D. Pred Forte (prednisolone).

___ 2. Which of the following drugs does NOT belong in the group with the others?
A. Vistide (cidofovir).
B. Valcyte (valganciclovir).
C. Foscavir (foscarnet).
D. Vira-A (vidarabine).

___ 3. Which of the following drugs is NOT used to treat glaucoma?
A. Timoptic (timolol).
B. Carboptic (carbachol).
C. Humorsol (demecarium).
D. Cyclogyl (cyclopentolate).

___ 4. If a patient had allergic conjunctivitis, which drug would the physician prescribe?
A. Sulamyd (sulfacetamide).
B. Patanol (olopatadine).
C. Ocuflox (ofloxacin).
D. Vistide (cidofovir).

___ 5. Patients might need to be concerned about photophobia after administration of _____
A. Trusopt (dorzolamide).
B. Betaxon (levobetaxolol).
C. Mydriacyl (tropicamide).
D. Epifrin (epinephrine).

Dissecting Medical Terms

Instructions: As you learned in your medical language course, words are formed from prefixes, combining forms (root word plus combining vowel), and suffixes. Combining vowels (usually **o** but not always) are used to connect two root words or a root and a suffix. By analyzing these word parts, you can often determine the definition of a term without even looking it up (if you know the definition of the parts, of course!).

Being able to divide and analyze the words you hear into their component parts will also improve your auditory deciphering ability and spelling and help you research those words that you cannot easily spell or define.

For the following terms, draw a slash (/) between the components and then write a short definition based on the meaning of the parts. Remember that to define a word based on its parts, you start at the end, usually with the suffix. If there's a prefix, that is defined next, and finally the combining form is defined.

Example: achondroplasia

Divide & Analyze:
achondroplasia = ophthalmo/logy = study of + the eyes

Define: something that acts to prevent blood clot formation

1. akinesia
   Divide _____
   _____
   Define _____

2. blepharochalasis
   Divide _____
   Define _____

3. capsulorrhexis
   Divide _____
   Define _____

4. cryopexy
   Divide _____
   Define _____

5. dacryorhinocystitis
   Divide _____
   _____
   Define _____

6. endodiathermy
   Divide _____
   _____
   Define _____

7. hydrodelineation
   Divide _____
   Define _____

8. hydrodissection
   Divide _____
   Define _____

9. keratome
   Divide _____
   Define _____

10. neuroleptic
    Divide _____
    Define _____

11. panretinal
    Divide _____
    Define _____

12. paracentesis
    Divide _____
    Define _____

13. periocular

Divide _____

_____

Define _____

14. retrobulbar

Divide _____

_____

Define _____

15. sclerostomy

Divide _____

_____

Define _____

16. subretinal

Divide _____

_____

Define _____

17. superotemporal

Divide _____

_____

Define _____

18. tenotomy

Divide _____

_____

Define _____

19. trabeculectomy

Divide _____

_____

Define _____

20. vitrectomy

Divide _____

_____

Define _____

Spelling Exercise

Instructions: Review the adjective suffixes in your medical language textbook. Test your knowledge of adjectives by writing the adjectival form of the following ophthalmology words. Consult a medical dictionary to verify your spelling.

Noun	Adjective
1. aqua	_____
2. bulb	_____
3. cilia	_____
4. cortex	_____
5. macula	_____
6. nucleus	_____
7. oculus	_____
8. orbit	_____
9. sclera	_____
10. smoke	_____
11. trabecula	_____
12. vitreum	_____

Forming Plurals

Instructions: Review the rules for forming plurals. Test your knowledge of plurals by writing the plural form of the following terms. Consult a medical dictionary to confirm your spelling.

Singular	Plural
1. canaliculus	_____
2. canthus	_____
3. conjunctiva	_____
4. cortex	_____
5. fornix	_____
6. iris	_____
7. oculus	_____
8. paracentesis	_____
9. punctum	_____
10. sclera	_____

Abbreviations Exercise

Instructions: Expand the following common abbreviations and brief forms. Then memorize both abbreviations and definitions to increase your speed and accuracy in transcribing dictation

Abbreviation	Expansion
1. AV (nicking)	_____
2. BSS	_____
3. CMV	_____
4. D	_____
5. ECCE	_____
6. ERG	_____
7. I&A	_____
8. ICCE	_____
9. IOL	_____
10. LASIK	_____
11. LPI	_____
12. mmHg	_____
13. OCT	_____
14. OD	_____
15. OS	_____
16. OU	_____
17. PRK	_____
18. T-PRK	_____

Transcript Forensics

Instructions: This section presents snippets of transcribed dictations from clinic notes; history and physical examinations and consultations; operative reports and procedure notes; and discharge summaries. Explain the passage so that a nonmedical person can understand it.

Example: Best corrected visual acuities were 20/50 in the right eye and 20/40 in the left eye.

Explanation: On a vision test with the Snellen chart, the patient could see at 50 feet what individuals with "normal" vision could see at 20 feet in the right eye, and in the left eye, the patient could see at 40 feet what others with normal vision could see at 20 feet.

1. On examination, the patient has significant **conjunctival injection** with what looks like a subconjunctival **hemorrhage** on the medial aspect of the left eye. With **slit lamp examination**, there appears to be a threadlike object in the anterior chamber, and there is an obvious conjunctival hemorrhage on the left side. Her **visual acuity is 20/25** in both the right and left eye.

Explanation: _____
_____
_____
_____
_____
_____

2. History of uncontrolled primary **open angle glaucoma OU**. She had prior history of a **trabeculectomy** in the right eye with persistent **elevated IOP**.

Explanation: _____
_____
_____
_____
_____
_____

3. The **extraocular movements appear full**, although he still has **diplopia** in both lateral directions.

Explanation: _____
_____
_____
_____
_____
_____
_____

4. Eyes: The left **palpebral and bulbar conjunctivae**
are **erythematous. PERRLA. EOMI. Funduscopy**
without **hemorrhages, exudates,** lesions, or masses
bilaterally. **Gross** visual acuity intact.

Explanation: _____

_____

_____

_____

_____

5. PREOPERATIVE DIAGNOSES
Advanced chronic open angle glaucoma, left eye,
on **maximum tolerated medical therapy.** Dense
nuclear sclerotic and cortical cataract, left eye,
affecting activities of daily living.

Explanation: _____

_____

_____

_____

_____

_____

6. OPERATION
Trabeculectomy with **mitomycin. Phacoemulsification** and **posterior chamber IOL, OS.**

Explanation: _____

_____

_____

_____

_____

_____

7. Evaluation of the **discs** of her eyes was hampered
by **constriction** of the pupils; however, some mild
AV nicking could be detected. Funduscopy was
inadequate because of the **brisk pupillary
constriction.**

Explanation: _____

_____

_____

_____

_____

_____

_____

8. A clear **corneal temporal incision** was made using
a diamond knife. A continuous **curvilinear
capsulorrhexis** was then performed using a
cystitome. (*Note: This excerpt is from an operative
report/cataract extraction.*)

Explanation: _____

_____

_____

_____

_____

_____

9. Examination OD reveals **cup-to-disc ratio** 0.15.
Mild **venous dilation** and **vascular tortuosity** is
noted. Blurred macular detail consistent with
media **opacity** and **vitreous hemorrhage** is noted.

Explanation: _____

_____

_____

_____

_____

_____

10. IMPRESSION
Examination consistent with vitreous hemorrhage
OD secondary to **neovascularization** OD in an
area proximal to **poor perfusion** consistent with
previous branch **retinal vein occlusion** OD. (*Note:
This excerpt is from a fluorescein angiogram study.*)

Explanation: _____

_____

_____

_____

_____

Sample Reports

Sample ophthalmology reports appear on the following pages, illustrating a variety of reports. Fictional names are provided for illustration of proper format, and no resemblance to actual persons is intended. Sample transcripts were prepared according to *The Book of Style for Medical Transcription* (AHDI).

Operative Report

CLAY, NEIL
#797266

DATE OF SURGERY
April 2, [add year]

PREOPERATIVE DIAGNOSIS
Visually significant cataract of the right eye.

POSTOPERATIVE DIAGNOSIS
Visually significant cataract of the right eye.

SURGEON
Nathan Perry, MD

ANESTHESIA
Local with monitored anesthesia care.

PROCEDURE
Phacoemulsification with intraocular lens implant in the right eye.

DESCRIPTION OF PROCEDURE
The patient was taken from the preoperative holding area to the operating room, placed in the supine position, after which a retrobulbar block was given for local anesthesia. Local agents used were 2% lidocaine, 0.75% Marcaine in a 1:1 mix. Digital pressure was placed over the eye for approximately 5 minutes after which good anesthesia and akinesia were achieved. The patient was then prepped and draped in the usual sterile fashion. A lid speculum was then placed, after which a 75 blade was used to make a paracentesis tract at the 11:30 o'clock position. Healon was used to fill the anterior chamber, after which a clear corneal temporal incision was made using a diamond knife. A continuous curvilinear capsulorrhexis was then performed, first using a cystitome and then finished using Utrata forceps. Hydrodissection of the nucleus was then performed in all 4 quadrants. The lens nucleus was freely mobile after this procedure. Phacoemulsification of the nucleus was then performed in a 4-quadrant cracking method without difficulty. The remaining cortex was removed using irrigation-aspiration. Healon was used to fill the capsular bag after which the wound was opened 3 mm using a diamond knife. An Alcon

(continued)

Operative Report *(continued)*

CLAY, NEIL
#797266
Page 2

Laboratories intraocular lens (IOL), Model SN60WF, 14.5 diopters in power, serial # _____, was readied for insertion by placing the lens in the inserter, then placing the inserter in the Monarch delivery system. The inserter was then placed through the corneal incision, where the lens was delivered to the capsular bag. The trailing haptic was placed using a Kuglen hook. The remaining Healon was removed using irrigation-aspiration. Miochol was then placed through the paracentesis tract to promote miosis and fill the chamber. This was then irrigated using balanced salt solution (BSS). The wound had good integrity. There was no leakage noted. No suture was needed. The lid speculum was removed after Quixin drops were placed on the eye. The drapes were then removed from the patient, and a shield was placed over the eye. The patient tolerated the procedure well. There were no complications. He was taken to the recovery room in good condition.

NATHAN PERRY, MD

NP:hpi

d: 4/2/[add year]
t: 4/3/[add year]

Letter

May 17, [add year]

Thomas Oliphant, MD
2020 Lupus Way, Suite 20
Sewell, NY 12840

Re: Anna Lokotui

Dear Dr. Oliphant:

The patient was seen in February of this year and followed with a diagnosis of aphakia, left eye, and early nuclear cataract, right eye, as well as narrow angle glaucoma suspected in the right eye. She was placed on Pilocar 1% q.i.d., right eye. Gonioscopy showed a grade III angle superiorly using Scheie classification, with a grade II pigmentation. Her intraocular pressures were slightly elevated, and she was placed on Pilocar 1% b.i.d. In April she underwent YAG laser peripheral iridotomy, right eye, for narrow angle glaucoma, with subsequent widening of the peripheral iridotomy.

Her cataract progressed, and her visual acuity more recently has been 20/50 in the right eye. She has always had visual acuity in the left eye of counting fingers on the basis of the aphakia and a pupillary membrane with updrawn pupil. Her optic discs have had a cup-to-disc ratio of 0.34 in each eye, and the peripheral retinas have been within normal limits.

Recently she complained of redness and discomfort in both eyes on the basis of a moderate degree of superficial punctate keratitis and was placed on Lacri-Lube ointment at frequent intervals. Her intraocular pressure was 28 mmHg in the right eye and 20 mmHg in the left eye. Therefore, she was begun on Betoptic b.i.d. and epinephrine at bedtime to the right eye. Because of her superficial punctate and some allergic conjunctivitis, she was switched to Celluvisc q. 2 hours and cold compresses and was continued on her glaucoma drops.

IMPRESSION
1. Cataract, right eye.
2. Status post YAG peripheral iridotomy, right eye (OD), for narrow angle glaucoma.
3. Glaucoma suspected, each eye (OU).
4. Aphakia with pupillary membrane and updrawn pupil, left eye (OS).
5. Keratitis with ocular surface disease.

Thank you for the consultation on this patient. If I can be of any further help, please do not hesitate to contact me.

Best regards,

Bruce Seymour, MD

BS:hpi d: 5/17/[add year] 5/18/[add year]

Comic Relief

Dictation and transcription mistakes are common occurrences in ophthalmology transcripts.

Dictated	**Transcribed**
The patient had convergent strabismus at age 7.	The patient had convergence to business at age 7.
Eyes: Examination of the fundi revealed . . .	Examination of the fungi revealed . . .
The pupils and fundi were clear.	The pupils and front eye were clear.
The patient has a congenital cataract.	The patient has a genital cataract.
Bausch & Lomb Company	Boston Loan Company
AV nicking	AV necking
The eye was patched and the patient sent to her room.	The eye was patched and sent to her room.

Misdictations:

The eye was prepped in the usual manner for pelvic surgery.

Funduscopic exam is grade I mild arteriolar narrowing. No AV nicking, exudates, or hemorrhoids.

The patient has had cataract surgery and wears Cadillac glasses.

Cardiology

Learning Objectives

▶ Describe the structure and function of the cardiovascular system.

▶ Spell and define common cardiovascular terms.

▶ Identify cardiovascular vocabulary that might be used in the review of systems.

▶ Describe the negative and positive findings a physician looks for on examination of the cardiovascular system.

▶ List and describe the anatomic structures involved in the conduction system of the heart.

▶ List the 12 EKG leads and the names for the different points referenced on an EKG tracing.

▶ Describe the typical cause, course, and treatment options for common diseases of the cardiovascular system.

▶ Identify and define common diagnostic and surgical procedures of the cardiovascular system.

▶ List common cardiovascular laboratory tests and procedures.

▶ Identify and describe common cardiovascular drugs and their uses.

▶ Demonstrate knowledge of anatomical, medical, pharmacological, adjectival, and soundalike terms by accurately completing the exercises in this chapter.

Transcribing Cardiology Dictation

Introduction

Cardiology and cardiovascular surgery are both concerned with the diagnosis and treatment of diseases of the heart, great vessels, and peripheral circulation. The difference between cardiologists and cardiovascular surgeons lies in the methods used to treat these diseases.

The **cardiologist** is, by training, an internist who specializes in the diagnosis and medical treatment of cardiovascular disease. The cardiac surgeon specializes in the surgical treatment of cardiovascular disease. In no other area of medicine does an internist work so closely with a surgeon as in the management of cardiovascular disease.

Cardiologists must rely on their **cardiovascular surgeon** colleagues when surgical intervention is needed in the treatment of their patients. Similarly, cardiovascular surgeons rely on their cardiologist colleagues for the majority of their case referrals. The cardiologist and cardiovascular surgeon collaborate during a surgical procedure if the patient develops hemodynamic instability or refractory cardiac arrhythmia, and also during the postoperative period in the routine management of the cardiac surgery patient. Thus there is considerable overlap between the two specialties.

The **cardiovascular** or **circulatory system** (see ■ Figure 12-1) consists of the heart and the blood vessels

THE HEART

Broken heart, heavy heart, sacred heart—these phrases describe very deep human emotions. Do they really affect the heart?

Even in ancient times it was understood that the beating heart was at the core of the body. Of all the internal organs, only the heart makes a consistent pattern of noise that can be felt and heard through the skin and ex vivo (outside the body). Thus, it is not surprising that ancients attributed their physical existence to their "cores." In fact, the Latin word for heart is *cor*. From that simple Latin word has evolved a list of "emotional" words: cordial (hearty), core (the heart of, as in "It struck me to the core"), courage (bravery), discord (disagreement).

(arteries, capillaries, veins). The purpose of the system is to provide rapid delivery to the tissues of oxygen from the lungs; nutrients, minerals, vitamins, and water from the digestive system; hormones from glands; and white blood cells from bone marrow and lymphoid tissue, while removing waste products and delivering them to the lungs (carbon dioxide), liver (broken-down red blood cells), and kidney (surplus water, nitrogenous wastes) for excretion.

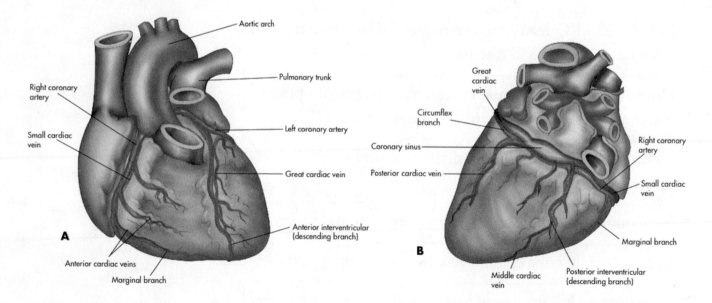

FIGURE 12-1. Coronary circulation. (A) Coronary arteries and veins of the anterior surface of the heart. (B) Coronary vessels of the posterior surface of the heart.

Anatomy Review

The heart is a pump—actually two synchronized **pumps**, each handling a different segment of the circulating blood at any given moment. The **right atrium** (antechamber) and the **right ventricle** receive venous blood from the systemic circulation and pump it into the lungs for gas exchange. The **left atrium** and **left ventricle** receive freshly oxygenated blood from the lungs and pump it through the arteries into the systemic circulation.

The contraction of a heart chamber is called **systole**; relaxation and refilling is called **diastole**. Valves in the heart (one for each of the four chambers) prevent backflow of blood from a chamber during systole. The heart is encased in a protective sac called the **pericardium**.

The names of the **coronary arteries and branches** are frequently mentioned in angiographic and surgical reports. The **major vessels** are the left main coronary artery, the left anterior descending (LAD) coronary artery, the right coronary artery (RCA), and the circumflex coronary artery. Names of **branches** of these take on additional terms, such as the left anterior descending diagonal (LADD). Other vessels to remember are the circumflex marginal, distal branches, and the posterior descendings. The major **conduits** are the aorta and pulmonary artery. The **valves** are aortic, mitral, pulmonary, and tricuspid.

Conduction System of the Heart

The conduction system of the heart (see ■ Figure 12-2) consists of highly specialized tissue capable of initiating and transmitting the electrical impulses that cause the heart to beat. The pacemaker of the heart is the **sinoatrial (SA) node**, a small nubbin of tissue in the upper part of the right atrium. Although nerves of the autonomic nervous system and circulating substances such as epinephrine and certain drugs can affect the rate and rhythm of the heart, the SA node continues to function as a **pacemaker**, stimulating regular cardiac contractions, even if all nerves to the heart are severed. In medical jargon, the SA node is almost universally called simply the **sinus**. Each electrical impulse generated by the SA node triggers a wave of depolarization that spreads over both atria, causing them to contract.

Located low in the right atrium is another mass of specialized tissue, the **atrioventricular (AV) node** (usually called simply the **node**). When the wave of depolarization set off by the SA node reaches the AV node, it is picked up and transmitted down the **bundle of His** ("hiss") to the septum between the two ventricles. In the septum the bundle of His divides into right and left bundle branches, of which the left further divides into anterior and posterior fascicles. All of these tracts of conducting tissue eventually break up into a network of **Purkinje fibers**, which penetrate the walls of the ventri-

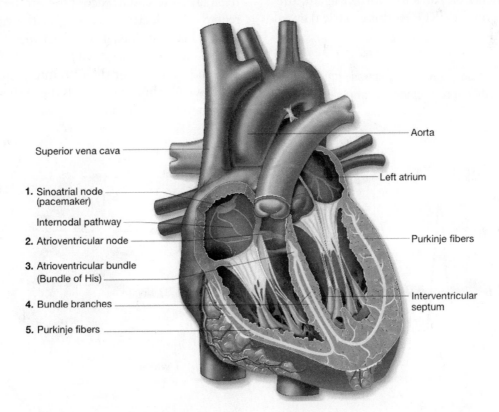

Superior vena cava

1. Sinoatrial node (pacemaker)

Internodal pathway

2. Atrioventricular node

3. Atrioventricular bundle (Bundle of His)

4. Bundle branches

5. Purkinje fibers

Aorta

Left atrium

Purkinje fibers

Interventricular septum

FIGURE 12-2. Conduction system of the heart

SLANG TERMS TO EXPAND IN TRANSCRIPTION	
a fib	atrial fibrillation
alk phos	alkaline phosphatase
cath	catheterization
cath'd	catheterized
crit	hematocrit
dig ("didge")	digoxin
fem-pop	femoral-popliteal
H&H	hemoglobin and hematocrit
lytes	electrolytes
nitro	nitroglycerin
V fib	ventricular fibrillation
V tach ("tack")	ventricular tachycardia

cles. The outward passage of the wave of depolarization through the muscular ventricular walls causes them to contract.

Electrocardiogram (ECG, EKG). A tracing of the electrical activity of the heart (see ■ **Figure 12-3**). An EKG traces the conduction of the electrical impulse generated by the SA node as it travels through the atria (P wave on the EKG) and through the ventricles (QRS complex on the EKG). Then, during the recovery period as the heart prepares to contract again, the T wave is evident on the EKG. As this electrical impulse

The monitor strip shows one brief episode of AV block for 3 beats and then a resumption of sinus rhythm with bradycardia.

travels through the heart, it can be detected on the skin by EKG electrodes.

The basic EKG records 12 leads. Three peripheral electrodes are placed on the right arm, left arm, and left leg. Six other electrodes are placed at precise locations on the chest around the heart area. The EKG technician can change from one lead to the next by using a dial on the EKG machine.

Leads I, II, and III (the so-called limb or bipolar leads) are obtained by simultaneously recording the electrical activity from the extremities. By combining the input from two of these three electrodes, the EKG machine generates a tracing for lead I (right arm and left arm,), lead II (right arm and left leg), and lead III (left arm and left leg).

The next three leads are called augmented leads because they increase or augment the amplitude or size of the tracing by 50%. The augmented leads are aVR (augmented voltage, right arm), aVL (augmented voltage, left arm), and aVF (augmented voltage, left foot).

The remaining six leads necessary to complete the 12-lead EKG are known as the precordial or chest leads. These electrodes are placed on the chest and are designated by a "V."

Lead V1 is positioned over the fourth intercostal space at the right sternal border and records the electrical activity of the right ventricle. Lead V2 is positioned over the fourth intercostal space at the left sternal border and records the electrical activity of the right ventricle. Lead V3 is positioned midway between V2 and V4 and records the electrical activity of the left ventricle. Lead V4 is positioned over the fifth intercostal space at the midclavicular line and records the electrical activity of the left ventricle. Lead V5 is positioned over the fifth

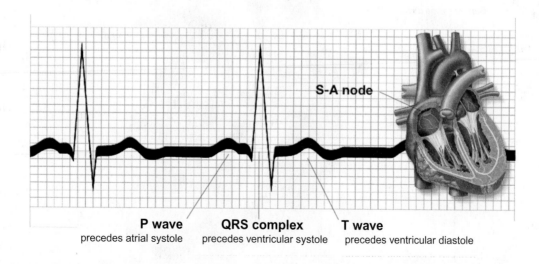

S-A node

P wave
precedes atrial systole

QRS complex
precedes ventricular systole

T wave
precedes ventricular diastole

FIGURE 12-3. Electriocardiogram (EKG) tracing

intercostal space at the anterior axillary line and records the electrical activity of the left ventricle. Lead V6 is positioned over the fifth intercostal space at the mid-axillary line and records the electrical activity of the left ventricle. Each of the 12 leads gives a different picture of the electrical condition of the heart.

An EKG showed atrial fibrillation with a fast ventricular response and nonspecific ST-T wave changes. A portable chest x-ray showed no evidence of cardiomegaly or acute infiltrates.

EKG revealed 3rd degree heart block with inferolateral ST-T wave changes consistent with ischemia.

Pause for Reflection

1. The heart is actually two synchronized _____.
2. Oxygenated blood is pumped into the arteries by the _____ side of the heart.
3. The _____ atrium and ventricle receive deoxygenated blood from the venous system and pump it to the lungs to be reoxygenated.
4. _____ is contraction of a heart chamber and _____ is relaxation.
5. The protective sac surrounding the heart is called the _____.
6. Name the four major arteries of the heart.
7. Name the four valves in the heart.
8. The major conduits of the circulatory system are the _____ and _____.
9. The pacemaker of the heart is the _____, commonly referred to simply as _____.
10. List the 12 EKG leads.
11. The _____ picks up the depolarization wave set off by the SA node and sends it to the _____.
12. The network of conducting fibers in the ventricles that represents the end-point of conduction is called the _____ fibers.
13. The electrical impulse generated by the SA node as it travels through the atria is represented on an EKG by the _____ and by the _____ _____ as it travels through the ventricles.
14. The _____ is evident on the EKG during the recovery period as the heart prepares to contract again.

LAY AND MEDICAL TERMS

chest pain (of cardiac origin)	angina pectoris
hardening of the arteries	arteriosclerosis atherosclerosis
heart attack	myocardial infarction
high blood pressure	hypertension

Vocabulary Review

akinesis Impairment of motion or loss of mobility; in cardiology the terms refers to a reduction of ventricular wall movement as detected by echocardiography.

arrhythmia Irregular rhythm of the heartbeat, with or without an abnormally slow or fast rate.

atrial fibrillation, atrial flutter (AF) Abnormal heartbeat in which the heart rhythm is fast and irregular.

atrioventricular block (AV block) Impairment of the conduction between the atria and ventricles of the heart.

bradyarrhythmia A pulse that is both irregular and abnormally slow.

bradycardia Abnormal slowness of the heartbeat (pulse less than 60/min).

bruit ("broo-ee") A rough vascular sound, synchronous with the heartbeat, heard on auscultation over a narrowing in an artery.

cardiomegaly Enlargement of the heart.

clubbing Club-shaped deformity of fingertips, seen in chronic pulmonary disease.

cor pulmonale Dilatation, hypertrophy, or failure of the right ventricle due to acute or chronic pulmonary disease.

crepitant rale A fine crackling rale.

dependent edema Swelling of the lower extremities, aggravated by the downward hanging position.

diaphoresis Sweating.

dyslipidemia Any of various disorders characterized by abnormally high levels of lipids (cholesterol, triglycerides) in the blood.

dyspnea Shortness of breath.

ABBREVIATION TRAPS IN CARDIOLOGY

ASHD (arteriosclerotic or atheroscerotic heart disease). Unless either term has been dictated in full elsewhere in the report, the abbreviation must be transcribed as dictated, even in a final diagnosis, because there is no way of knowing which of the disease processes is meant.

AV (arteriovenous)—may modify the words *access, anastomosis, aneurysm, depolarization, fistula, graft, malformation, shunt.*

AV (atrioventricular)—may modify the words *beat, block, complex, conduction, interval, node, rhythm, valve.*

BMP (basic metabolic profile)—a panel of 8 blood tests that includes electrolytes (sodium, potassium, CO_2 or bicarbonate, and chloride) plus glucose, calcium, BUN, and creatinine. It is a screening procedure that can detect a wide range of common metabolic disorders and imbalances

BNP (B-type natriuretic peptide)—a lab test for a hormone stored mainly in the ventricular myocardium; it is elevated in congestive heart failure and hypertension.

CK (creatine kinase)—a serum enzyme that can be chemically distinguished into three isoenzymes or fractions: the BB (CK-BB) isoenzyme is elevated in cerebral infarction, the MM (CK-MM) in muscular dystrophy and muscle crush injury, and MB (CK-MB) in myocardial infarction. When separated in the laboratory by electrophoresis, these isoenzymes appear as distinct bands in a visual display. Hence the expression MB band is roughly synonymous with MB isoenzyme. Do not confuse *creatine* with *creatinine.*

JVD (jugular venous distention)—Do not combine as jugulovenous.

PDA (patent ductus arteriosus)—a heart defect usually found in children and repaired by surgery.

PDA (posterior descending artery)—one of the main arteries supplying blood to the heart muscle and used in cardiac catheterization reports.

PND (paroxysmal nocturnal dyspnea)—sudden attacks of labored breathing, awakening the patient from sleep. Do not confuse with *postnasal drainage.*

edema Swelling due to the presence of fluid in tissue spaces.

effusion An abnormal accumulation of fluid in a body cavity, such as the pericardium.

embolism Obstruction of a blood vessel by a detached blood clot, air, fat, or injected material. An **embolus** is the material that causes the obstruction.

exudate Protein-rich fluid, inflammatory cells, and tissue debris deposited in or on tissues as a result of inflammation or degeneration.

fibrosis Excess fibrous connective tissue in an organ or tissue formed as a reparative or reactive process, as opposed to formation of fibrous tissue as a normal constituent of an organ or tissue.

gallop rhythm A cardiac rhythm that simulates the sound of a galloping horse on auscultation, usually due to the presence of a third or fourth heart sound, or both.

hepatojugular reflux Bulging of jugular veins when the liver is compressed because of increased pressure in the venous system. *Note*: Not reflex.

intervals On EKGs, AH or A-H, PA or P-A, PR or P-R, ST or S-T, and QT or Q-T when coupled with interval are all acceptable. By convention, QRS interval is transcribed without hyphens, and AV (atrioventricular) interval is not hyphenated.

irregularly irregular pulse An arrhythmia associated with atrial fibrillation; the pulse rate is irregular and the pulse amplitude varies.

CARDIOVASCULAR: *Irregularly irregular rate without murmur or gallop; tachycardic.*

ischemia Inadequate blood supply.

isorhythmic dissociation A type of atrioventricular dissociation characterized by atria and ventricles beating at similar rates, although independently.

joule (J) SI unit of electric power.

lumen The hollow interior of a vessel or other tubular structure.

orthostatic hypotension Low blood pressure brought on by a sudden change in body position, most often when shifting from lying down to standing.

palpitation(s) Various abnormal sensations accompanying heartbeat: unduly rapid heartbeat; noticeably irregular beat; a feeling that some or all heartbeats are unusually strong; a sense of missed beats; or intermittent flip-flop sensations in the heart. Do not confuse with **palpation**.

paroxysmal Occurring in sudden attacks or seizures (paroxysms).

pericarditis Inflammation of the pericardium, the membranous sac surrounding the heart.

peripheral edema Edema of the extremities.

pitting edema Edema that retains the mark of the examiner's fingers after release of pressure.

pleuritic Chest pain or discomfort from inflammation of the pleura caused by pneumonia and other diseases of the chest.

point of maximal intensity (PMI) The point on the chest wall where the impulse of the beating heart is most distinctly felt by the examiner's fingers.

precordial In front of the heart.

pulse The heartbeat, and by extension the rate of heartbeat, as measured at the wrist (radial pulse), the cardiac apex (apical pulse), or elsewhere.

rale (rhymes with "mail") A crackling or bubbling sound heard on auscultation of the breath sounds, usually due to fluid in small respiratory passages.

rhonchus (pl., **rhonchi**) A whistling or humming sound caused by passage of air through narrowed parts of the respiratory tract.

shock (precordial) An abnormally strong thrust applied to the chest wall by the beating heart, as detected by the examiner's fingers.

splitting Separation of the first or second heart sound, or both, into two distinctly audible components.

stenosis An abnormal narrowing in a blood vessel or other tubular organ or structure. The term **coarctation** is synonymous, but is commonly used only in the context of **aortic coarctation**.

ST-T wave changes A customary abridgment of the phrase "ST segment and T-wave changes." The ST segment is the part of the EKG tracing extending from the S wave to the T wave. There is no "ST wave."

syncope Sudden loss of consciousness; fainting.

CONFUSING PAIRS

atopic—related to hypersensitivity or allergy.

ectopic—located away from normal position or arising in an abnormal site or tissue.

Buerger disease (pronounced "bare-ZHAY")—a disease of the blood vessels.

Berger disease—a kidney disorder.

concentric—extending out from a common center.

eccentric—situated away from a center.

cor—heart   core—center

corps—organized group of individuals; silent *p* and *s*.

ejection—the discharge of blood from the heart, as in ejection fraction.

injection—infusion, or forcing liquid into a vessel, tissue, or organ.

hypertension—high blood pressure.

hypotension—low blood pressure.

loop—a curved structure or a low-voltage circular electrical wire used for cutting or cautery.

loupe—a magnification lens.

ostial—pertaining to an opening.

osteal—pertaining to bone, osseous.

palpitation—sensation caused by irregular heart beats.

palpation—use of the hands to examine body surfaces.

perfuse—to pour over or through.

profuse—abundant.

perfusion—delivery of oxygen and nutrients to tissues, and removal of carbon dioxide and other wastes by sufficient blood flow to the area.

profusion—abundance.

pericardial—pertaining to the sac surrounding the heart.

precordial—pertaining to the area in front of the heart and stomach; usually modifies lead ("leed") or area.

pericardium—the sac surrounding the heart.

precordium—the area of the body in front of the heart and stomach.

recanalization—restoration of blood flow by the creation of new canals.

recannulation—the reinsertion of a tube, cannula, into a vessel, duct, or cavity.

tachyarrhythmia   A pulse that is both irregular and abnormally rapid.

tachycardia   Rapid heart rate (over 100/min).

thrill   An abnormal sensation felt by the examiner over the heart when blood jets through an anomalous or narrowed orifice.

TIMI score   (Thrombolysis In Myocardial Infarction) A risk-scoring system developed to categorize a patient's risk of death and ischemic events and provide a basis for therapeutic decision making. The lower the number (from 0 to 3), the more serious the flow limitation.

(tunica) intima   The innermost layer or lining of an artery.

ventricular ectopy   Ventricular ectopic beats (VEB) are also called **premature ventricular contractions (PVCs)** as they may occur just before the normal beat of the ventricle. VEBs are easily seen on an electrocardiogram.

Medical Readings

History and Physical Examination

by John H. Dirckx, MD

Review of Systems.   The cardiovascular history begins with a review of past diagnoses of congenital or acquired heart murmurs, rheumatic fever, enlarged heart, coronary artery disease, heart attack, high blood pressure, varicose veins, thrombophlebitis, and treatments, past or present, prescribed for any of these. Note is made of the results of past diagnostic studies such as electrocardiograms, echocardiograms, stress testing, cardiac catheterization, and angiography, and of any surgical procedures, such as pacemaker implantation, valve repair or replacement, and coronary artery bypass graft.

Because **coronary artery disease** is a major cause of disability and death, any complaint of chest pain must be carefully evaluated to determine whether it represents **angina pectoris**, the cardinal symptom of coronary disease. A full description of chest pain includes its character, intensity, location, extent, radiation, duration, and frequency of occurrence; the effect of position, movement, breathing, and swallowing; associated symptoms such as shortness of breath, sweating, and palpitations; the effect of resting or taking medicines such as antacids or nitroglycerin; and triggering factors such as physical exertion, smoking, eating, strong emotion, or exposure to cold.

When shortness of breath is due to **cardiac failure**, it is typically less oppressive in the upright position (orthopnea) and may occur in attacks that awaken the patient during the night (**paroxysmal nocturnal dyspnea, PND**). **Orthopnea** is graded by the number of pillows needed to avoid respiratory distress (e.g., three-pillow orthopnea). Wheezing, coughing, and exertional dyspnea are common to cardiac and noncardiac disorders.

Physical Examination.   Auscultation provides more information about the heart than any other procedure. Stethoscopes used for cardiac auscultation have two chest pieces, a narrow, cone-shaped "bell" for lower pitched sounds and a wide, flat diaphragm for higher pitched sounds. The examiner changes back and forth from one to the other as needed during the examination. The stethoscope is applied to the chest in specific areas according to a basic routine, which may be varied as circumstances dictate.

Auscultation reveals a systolic murmur with a crescendo-decrescendo configuration beginning after S1, loudest in the right second intercostal space parasternally, which radiates to the neck, left sternal border, and apex.

Examination of the heart is ideally carried out with the patient seated and undressed from the waist up. Hence it logically follows the examination of the thorax, breasts, and axillae. The examiner has already noted such findings as pallor, flushing, cyanosis, respiratory distress, and dilated jugular veins. The anterior chest wall is inspected for pulsations and the point at which the cardiac impulse is strongest (**point of maximal intensity, PMI**) is found by **palpation**. The examiner's fingers not only locate this point but also detect any abnormalities associated with the heartbeat, such as a heaving of the chest wall due to unduly intense cardiac contractions, thrills due to passage of blood through abnormally narrowed valves or other orifices, and shocks from abnormally abrupt closure of valves in hypertension. **Percussion** can also be used to assess cardiac size and shape.

Four areas of the anterior chest are designated according to the **valves** whose sounds are best heard there: the **mitral** area, the **pulmonic** area, the **aortic** area, and the **tricuspid** area. The subject may need to change position, such as by leaning forward or lying on the left side, to enable the examiner to evaluate heart sounds adequately. The physician also listens for abnormal sounds: **murmurs** caused by abnormal flow of blood through a valve or other orifice; **clicks or snaps**, caused by abnormal valve function; **rubs**, creaking or grating sounds caused by friction between the beating heart and an inflamed pericardium; **bruits**, caused by passage of blood through a narrowed artery; and others.

The normally beating heart produces two **sounds** in alternation, traditionally represented as *lup-dup*. The first heart sound, or **S1**, which is louder, deeper in pitch, and longer, results from contraction of the ventricles and closure of the mitral and tricuspid valves. For practical purposes it is considered synchronous with the beginning of systole, or ventricular contraction. The second heart sound, **S2**, results from closure of the aortic and pulmonic valves just after systole ends. S2 is taken as the beginning of diastole, or ventricular relaxation and refilling.

The first and second **heart sounds** heard at specific valve areas are sometimes so designated: **A1**, the first heart sound at the aortic valve area; **P2**, the second heart sound heard at the pulmonic valve area; and so on.

> *The A2 was greater than P2, with a widely split second sound and no murmurs.*

Cardiac **murmurs** are produced by turbulence in the flow of blood passing forward through a stenotic valve, leaking back through an incompetent valve, or crossing from a place of higher pressure to a place of lower pressure through an abnormal orifice, such as an **interventricular septal defect**.

Murmurs are distinguished as to **sound quality** (harsh, blowing, high-pitched); **timing** (systolic, mid-systolic, late diastolic); **loudness** (grade 1 to 6 in one system, 1 to 4 in another; l/6 ["dictated as one over six"] = grade 1 on a scale of 1 to 6, a barely audible murmur); **radiation** (to apex, carotids, left axilla); **where best heard** (left sternal border, aortic valve area); **effect of position** (squatting, standing, recumbency); and **effect of respiratory movements** (inspiration, expiration, breath-holding).

> *Chest: Heart was regular rate and rhythm with a 3/6 systolic ejection murmur which radiates along the right sternal border and through the precordium to the carotids.*

Pause for Reflection

1. Listening to the heart with a stethoscope is called _____, and tapping the chest to discern structural alterations within the thorax is called _____.
2. A _____ is a creaking or grating sounds caused by friction between the beating heart and an inflamed pericardium, and a _____ is caused by passage of blood through a narrowed artery.
3. Contraction of the ventricles and closure of the mitral and tricuspid valves results in a sound that is louder, deeper in pitch, and longer; this sound is referred to as _____, and the sound associated with closure of the aortic and pulmonic valves just after systole ends is _____.
4. The first heart sound is referred to as A1 when it is heard at the _____, and the second heart sound as P2 when it is heard at the _____.
5. The diagnostician characterizes a heart murmur by the location where it is best heard, its radiation or transmission, its character, and its _____, which is generally graded on a scale of 1 to 6.

A Cardiovascular Surgeon's View
by Michael J. O'Donnell, MD

Cardiac catheterization was invented in 1929 by a physician named Werner Forssmann, who first tested the procedure by catheterizing his own circulatory system. Over the years it has progressed from a simple investigative technique to a powerful diagnostic procedure (see ■ **Figure 12-4**). The patient is premedicated and taken to the catheterization laboratory. A puncture is made in the groin and a catheter is fed under fluoroscopic guidance up through the vessel and into the chambers of the heart. If the blood supply to the legs is poor, the catheter is inserted through a brachial cutdown in the arm, a small incision in the upper part of the arm which is later sutured closed. A specialized pressure catheter allows the pressure in the heart chambers to be recorded.

Placement of the catheter in the coronary ostia (openings) and injection of contrast medium permits

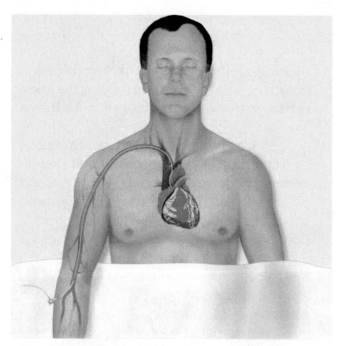

FIGURE 12-4. Cardiac catheterization using the brachial artery

radiographic visualization and recording of the coronary blood flow which is displayed on a computer monitor and a permanent recording made. The images are analyzed for narrowing or blockages in the arteries, wall motion abnormalities, and valve function.

The purpose of all of these cardiac diagnostic studies is to strive to treat the patient medically. In about half of the patients, however, an invasive therapy will be indicated. This may include coronary artery angioplasty, balloon valvuloplasty, or cardiac surgery either with coronary artery bypass grafting or repair or replacement of a valve.

Carotid Endarterectomy. The simplest cardiovascular surgical procedure is carotid endarterectomy. This involves opening up a segment of the internal carotid artery that has become obstructed by atherosclerotic disease, causing intermittent neurologic problems. In this procedure, the diseased portion of the artery is exposed via a surgical incision in the lateral aspect of the neck. Once the carotid artery is exposed, it is clamped above and below the obstruction. Then an incision is made into the vessel and the atherosclerotic material is peeled away. The incision in the vessel is sutured, the clamps are removed, and the skin is sewn closed. During this procedure, the patient is under general anesthesia but does not require the use of a heart-lung bypass machine.

Angioplasty. A blocked coronary artery may be treated with a minimally invasive procedure known as

a **PTCA (percutaneous transluminal coronary angioplasty)** (see ■ Figures 12-5 and 12-16). This procedure is often done immediately following the injection of a drug such as streptokinase or urokinase to lyse (break up) the clot. It can, however, be scheduled electively. A catheter with a tiny balloon on the 4 or 5 mm tip is placed at the site of the narrowing of the artery, and the balloon is inflated by means of a hand pump, to compress or squeeze the plaque back against the artery wall and open the blood flow through the vessel. A **stent**, often a stent coated with a drug to prevent clotting, may be inserted to keep the artery open. The advantage of this procedure is that it does not involve open heart surgery. The disadvantage is that this narrowing can recur, especially in those carrying inherited (familial) diseases. An angioplasty must be done in a hospital setting that provides surgery. If an artery tears open (dissects), the patient is taken to surgery for repair of the artery.

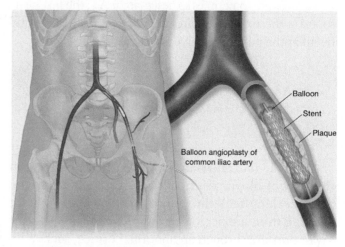

FIGURE 12-5. Balloon angioplasty of common iliac artery

Cardiopulmonary bypass. A patient with multiple occlusions may opt for open heart surgery, or **coronary artery bypass graft (CABG**, pronounced "cabbage") (see ■ Figure 12-6). Open heart procedures occur in two ways—opening the chest down the middle (median sternotomy), or, less usual, spreading the ribs and entering through this area (thoracotomy). A section of a large vein such as the saphenous vein from a lower extremity is harvested to use for the bypass. One end is attached to the aorta and the other end grafted in beyond the obstruction on a coronary artery. The **left internal mammary artery (LIMA)** may be detached from the chest wall and used to bypass an obstruction in the left anterior descending artery (LAD) or one of its major branches. LIMA grafts tend to remain open longer than venous grafts. Bypasses are named for the number of vessels reconnected—single, double, triple, or whatever number.

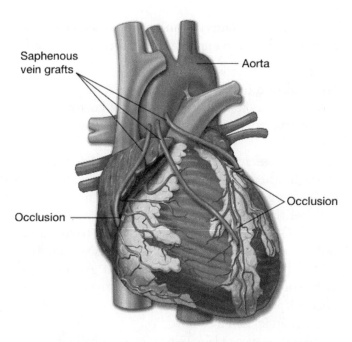

FIGURE 12-6. Coronary artery bypass graft (CABG)

A **heart-lung bypass machine** is used to take over the patient's cardiac and pulmonary function while surgery is being performed on the heart. The machine includes a pumping mechanism to maintain blood pressure and circulation to vital organs. In addition, the machine functions as an oxygenator since the lungs are bypassed once the patient's heart is placed in cardiac arrest. Thus the surgeon can perform an intricate procedure on a **nonbeating heart** without jeopardizing the patient's vital organs.

Although some endoscopic coronary artery bypass procedures are being performed, with robotic assistance, on a **beating heart**, these procedures have yet to become common or prove superior to the traditional bypass.

Pacemakers. New developments are occurring almost daily in the refinement of cardiac pacemakers (see ■ Figure 12-7). Pacemakers that can respond to the patient's metabolic work demands, as a normal heart would, are currently being evaluated. These ingenious devices are able to maintain variable heart rates depending on the body's demands in skeletal muscle activity, changes in core temperature, and changes in overall blood flow.

Pacemakers are identified by a three-letter code system, such as **DDD** or **VVI**, which need not be translated. The first letter indicates the chamber that is **paced**; the second letter denotes the chamber that is **sensed**; the third letter indicates whether the pacemaker is **inhibited** or **triggered** by the heart's own elec-

trical activity. For example, a **DDD pacemaker** serves the electrical activity of both the atrium and ventricle, paces (stimulates) both the atrium and ventricle to beat, and may cause (trigger) the atrium to contract while sending no signal (inhibited) to the ventricle, depending on what natural electrical activity is occurring in the heart at that time.

Defibrillators. Patients who have ventricular arrhythmias that do not respond to medical treatment are now given new hope with the development of **automatic implantable cardiac defibrillators (AICDs or ICDs)**.

In an AICD operation, electric pads that are secured to the surface of the heart with leads extending to a box (in the stomach area) which, like some types of pacemakers, can monitor the rhythm of the heart. When a sustained ventricular arrhythmia is detected, the device delivers a low-voltage shock directly to the

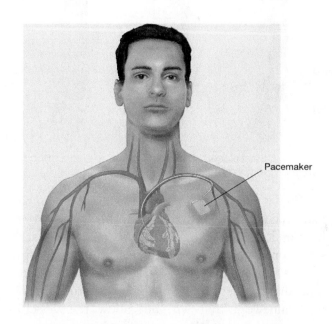

FIGURE 12-7. Permanent epicardial pacemaker

heart to restore a normal rhythm (**cardioversion**). Although the patient is able to sense this small electrical discharge, this is a small price to pay in view of the fact that the odds are against surviving a **cardiac arrest** occurring outside the hospital.

An **automated external defibrillator (AED)** is a device that provides a quick response and early defibrillation to victims of sudden cardiac arrest. It is used by fire departments, corporations, airlines and businesses that train employees in its use.

Catheters. In the treatment of intracardiac arterial disease, there has been rapid development in the technology of catheters, balloons, and guidewires. Research has been primarily directed toward newer materials to provide increased strength, decreased bulk, and smoother tracking over the guidewire. These changes allow more complex coronary angioplasty to be undertaken with a decreased risk of complications and restenosis.

Stents. A stent is a permanent intravascular device that can be inserted at the time of coronary angioplasty when acute closure of a vessel occurs. Introduced into the occluded area and then expanded, the stent provides a framework to support and keep the vessel open (see ■ Figure 12-8).

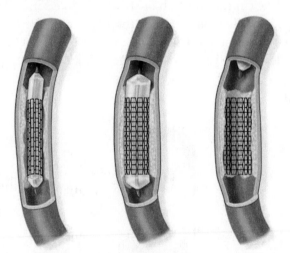

Figure 12-8 Stent placed in a coronary artery to relieve myocardial ischemia due to atherosclerosis

Stents may also be employed in patients who have had what is termed a chronic restenosis. These patients have undergone repeated angioplasty procedures for the same coronary artery lesion that continues to reappear despite multiple dilatations. The stent may be inserted immediately after balloon dilatation to form a supporting framework that will not allow the vessel to

restenose. New materials and coatings are constantly being developed to improve the performance of stents.

Lasers. There is continuing research in the area of **laser ablation** (eradication and removal with a laser) of coronary artery lesions. Various kinds of laser systems are under development. These include laser catheters that have a metal cap tip in which laser energy is used to heat the cap to extremely high temperatures so that it can melt through atheromatous lesions. Other catheter systems have what is termed direct laser energy emerging from the catheter tip to cut a channel through the atheromatous lesion. These catheters are currently able to reestablish only a small channel through an otherwise totally or subtotally occluded **atheromatous lesion**. After this procedure, a balloon catheter is advanced through the new channel, and **balloon angioplasty** is performed to make a larger channel for blood flow.

Another type of laser system is a **laser balloon**, which is essentially an angioplasty dilatation catheter with the capability of diffusing laser energy through the internal balloon surface outward to the endothelium of the coronary artery in contact with the balloon.

Other Devices. Mechanical **ablation** devices consist of either drill bits or coring tools that are placed into an artery with an atheromatous lesion. The drill, spinning at rates as high as 200,000 rpm, pulverizes the atheromatous lesion (**rotational atherectomy**). The other device cores or shaves the lesion with a blade. These devices are expected to prove more effective than balloon angioplasty in the treatment of atheromatous lesions, since they remove the lesion instead of just splitting or breaking it apart as in balloon angioplasty.

Pause for Reflection

1. Name 4 aspects of heart function that can be diagnosed or assessed by means of a cardiac catheterization.
2. The peeling away of atherosclerotic material in a carotid artery is called an _____.
3. Balloon dilatation of an atheromatous plaque in a coronary artery is called _____.
4. Using a saphenous vein graft or other vessel to create a new route around an obstruction in a coronary artery is called a _____.
5. A _____ is used to maintain circulation and oxygenation to the body during coronary artery bypass surgery.

Pause for Reflection *(continued)*

6. _____ maintain variable heart rates depending on the body's demands in skeletal muscle activity, changes in core temperature, and changes in overall blood flow.
7. Restoration of normal ventricular rhythm using a low-voltage shock directly to the heart is called _____.
8. A permanent intravascular device inserted at the time of coronary angioplasty to keep an artery open is called a _____.
9. An _____ procedure uses a mechanical ablation device to pulverize, core, or shave an atheromatous lesion causing artery blockage.

Common Diseases

Mitral Valve Prolapse

Abnormal bulging of mitral valve leaflets into the left atrium during left ventricular systole, due to structurally abnormal (floppy or billowing) valve leaflets.

Causes: May be inherited as an autosomal dominant trait. Often occurs in conjunction with other connective tissue abnormalities, particularly Marfan syndrome. Occurs in 1–5% of the general population, and is seen principally in women.

History: Usually there are no symptoms. A few patients experience nonspecific chest pain, palpitations with or without actual arrhythmia, dyspnea on exertion, fatigue, and syncope.

Physical Examination: Variable murmurs: usually midsystolic click and late systolic murmur. The patient may present other stigmata of connective tissue abnormality: thin body habitus, high palate, deformities of the chest wall (pectus excavatum, scoliosis).

Diagnostic Studies: Echocardiography confirms **valve prolapse** and indicates whether actual **regurgitation** occurs.

Course: Most patients have no symptoms and no complications. Rarely, regurgitation may have serious hemodynamic consequences. Endocarditis may develop on the mitral valve. Atrial fibrillation may occur. Sudden death may result from ectopic ventricular rhythms (**ventricular tachycardia**).

Treatment: Antibiotic prophylaxis of endocarditis before dental work and surgery. Beta-blockers usually control chest pain and arrhythmias. Rarely, surgical valve replacement.

Aortic Stenosis

Abnormal narrowing of the aortic valve opening, with reduction of left ventricular ejection volume during systole.

Causes: May be a consequence of acute rheumatic fever, but usually results from calcification of the valve with aging. Most patients are men over 50.

History: Weakness, dyspnea, chest pain, palpitations, syncope.

Physical Examination: Carotid pulsations are reduced. A precordial thrill may be noted. The second heart sound is reduced or absent. A harsh **"diamond-shaped" (crescendo-decrescendo) murmur** is heard at the base of the heart and transmitted to the carotids and cardiac apex.

Diagnostic Tests: Chest x-ray may show left ventricular dilatation and calcification of the aortic valve. Electrocardiogram, Doppler echocardiogram, and cardiac catheterization provide more precise and quantitative information.

Course: Left ventricular failure, arrhythmias, angina, syncope.

Treatment: Surgical replacement of the valve. Balloon dilatation of the valve may be successful.

Infective Endocarditis (Acute and Subacute Bacterial Endocarditis)

Bacterial infection of one or more heart valves (see ■ Figure 12-9).

Cause: Usually, the combination of preexisting congenital or acquired valvular disease or abnormal communications (septal defects) and bacteremia (after

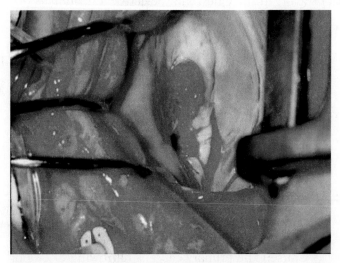

Figure 12-9. Endocarditis. Surgical procedure repairing a heart valve that has been scarred by bacterial endocarditis. The valve is the white tissue; the red area on the valve is a lesion. Source: Michael English, MD, Custom Medical Stock Photo.

HEART SOUNDS

Heart sounds are transcribed with a capital letter followed by a subscript number or a numeral on the baseline. Special characters such as subscripts do not transmit well electronically; hence, the common use of numerals on the baseline.

S1 or S_1 (first heart sound)

S2 or S_2 (second heart sound)

S3 or S_3 (third heart sound)

S4 or S_4 (fourth heart sound)

A2 or A_2 (aortic second sound, closure of the aortic valve)

P2 or P_2 (pulmonic second sound, closure of the pulmonary valve)

dental or surgical procedures or in systemic infection or septicemia).

History: Fever, chills, dyspnea, cough, abdominal pain, muscle or joint pain.

Physical Examination: Fever, pallor. Audible cardiac murmur, or change in quality or loudness of a pre-existing murmur. Signs of peripheral embolization of infective material (vegetations) from heart valves: petechiae of the palate and conjunctivae, splinter hemorrhages under fingernails, **Osler nodes** (tender purplish lumps in fingers, toes), **Janeway spots** (painless red spots of palms and soles), **Roth spots** (retinal exudates). Splenomegaly.

Diagnostic Tests: Anemia, leukocytosis, hematuria, proteinuria. Blood cultures may permit identification of the organism. Chest x-ray, electrocardiogram, echocardiogram supply diagnostic information.

Course: Valve leaflets may ulcerate and slough, with severe impairment of cardiac function. Fragments of infectious material (septic emboli) may be carried to brain, heart, kidney, and other tissues, or to the lung, causing local infective vascular lesions (mycotic aneurysms).

Treatment: Intravenous antibiotics for several weeks. Surgery may be undertaken in very severe cases.

Angina Pectoris

Paroxysmal chest pain due to myocardial ischemia, without permanent damage to heart muscle.

Cause: The primary cause is narrowing of one or more coronary arteries by arteriosclerosis. Arteritis, congenital vascular anomalies, emboli, severe anemia, cardiac **hypertrophy** (enlargement of a heart chamber due to increase in the thickness of its muscular wall), and cocaine intoxication can also lead to signs and symptoms of inadequate coronary blood flow. Risk factors for development of coronary arteriosclerosis include a family history of the disease, male gender, hypertension, cigarette smoking, diabetes mellitus, overweight, a sedentary lifestyle, and elevation of total cholesterol, LDL cholesterol, homocysteine, lipoprotein (a), or C-reactive protein.

History: Angina pectoris is a syndrome of anterior chest pain coming on abruptly and resolving spontaneously in less than 30 minutes. Pain is typically precipitated by physical exertion, strong emotion, exposure to cold, or eating a meal, and is relieved by rest or by taking nitroglycerin. The pain is described as a tightness, squeezing, or pressure; the patient often expresses this by holding a clenched fist in front of the chest. The pain may radiate into the neck, jaw, or arm, particularly the left. A variant, Prinzmetal angina, occurs at rest and is more common in women and younger patients than typical angina.

Physical Examination: There may be no abnormal findings, but the blood pressure is often elevated by pain and anxiety. Examination may disclose signs of underlying cardiovascular or systemic disease.

Diagnostic Tests: The electrocardiogram may be normal during an attack, but usually shows **ST-segment depression** and **flattened or inverted T waves**, indicating myocardial ischemia. There may also be evidence of conduction defects or ventricular hypertrophy. **Holter monitoring** allows recording of the EKG continuously for 24 hours. Stress testing records the electrocardiogram during standardized and closely supervised physical exertion. Angiography demonstrates narrowing of coronary vessels. Other studies (myocardial perfusion scintigraphy, radionuclide angiography, and echocardiography) can supply further information about the location and extent of coronary disease.

Course: Gradual progression to more severe disease (myocardial infarction, congestive heart failure) usually occurs, even with treatment. Unstable angina, which worsens with time despite treatment, has a less favorable prognosis.

Treatment: The standard treatment for an anginal attack is sublingual (under the tongue) nitroglycerin, which promptly abolishes pain of coronary ischemia by producing dilatation in the coronary arteries. Nitroglycerin can also be taken prophylactically before physical exertion. Longer-acting nitrate preparations, beta-blocking agents, and calcium-channel blockers taken regularly can prevent or mitigate attacks. Most patients are advised to take aspirin daily for its effect in inhibiting platelet aggregation and reducing the risk of myocardial infarction.

Coronary artery bypass graft (CABG) (see ■ Figure 12-6) uses veins or other materials to conduct blood past narrowed places in coronary arteries. **Percutaneous transluminal coronary angioplasty (PTCA, balloon angioplasty)** (see ■ Figures 12-5, 12-16) dilates narrowed places with a balloon passed into the circulation through an arterial catheter. A **metal stent** implanted at the time of angioplasty may provide long-term freedom from restenosis.

Myocardial Infarction (Heart Attack, Coronary Thrombosis)

Damage to a segment of heart muscle by severe impairment of coronary blood flow (see ■ Figure 12-10).

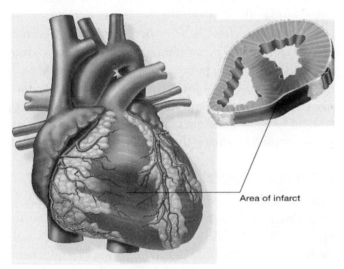

FIGURE 12-10. Myocardial infarction involving anterior wall of left ventricle and anterior portion of interventricular septum.

Causes: The underlying causes are the same as for angina pectoris. Myocardial infarction (MI) is usually due to **thrombosis** in a coronary artery already narrowed by arteriosclerosis. Arteritis, vasospasm, **embolism** (see ■ Figure 12-11), sudden hypotension, or cocaine can also precipitate infarction. Infarctions are typically designated by their location (apical infarction, inferior wall infarction).

History: Anterior chest pain, similar to angina but generally more severe and lasting more than 30 minutes. Pain often comes on at rest and is not relieved by nitroglycerin. Typically, men experience sweating, weakness, restlessness, shortness of breath, and nausea. Women may experience the same symptoms or may

perceive jaw or shoulder discomfort and/or chest tightness or discomfort without actual crushing pain. Rarely, infarction occurs without pain (**silent infarction**).

Physical Examination: The pulse and blood pressure may be increased, normal, or decreased. Mild fever often develops after the first 12 hours. The heart sounds may be soft or distant. An **atrial gallop** (fourth heart sound) is often heard. A **seagull murmur** of mitral regurgitation indicates rupture of a papillary muscle. The cardiac rhythm may be abnormal. A pericardial friction rub is often heard. Jugular venous distention and rales of pulmonary edema are seen in heart failure.

Diagnostic Tests: The electrocardiogram shows **ST-segment elevation** (changing later to depression) and inversion of **T waves** in leads pertaining to the area of infarction. **Q waves** indicate severe myocardial damage and a graver prognosis. The white blood cell count may be slightly elevated. Serial determination of the serum levels of the cardiac enzymes LDH (lactic dehydrogenase), CK-MB (the MB isoenzyme of creatine kinase), myoglobin, and troponins (C, I, and T) show characteristic rises. Fluoroscopy or other imaging techniques may show segmental wall motion at the site of infarction. Scintigraphy with technetium 99m pyrophosphate shows a hot spot at the site. **Doppler echocardiography** may also confirm the extent and location of infarction.

Course: About 20% of persons who sustain myocardial infarction die before reaching a hospital. With intensive therapy, the prognosis for the other 80% is good. During the acute phase, arrhythmia, shock, and congestive heart failure are serious possibilities. Other dangerous complications include **rupture of papillary muscle** (one of the muscles in the ventricles that control movements of the mitral and tricuspid valves) with

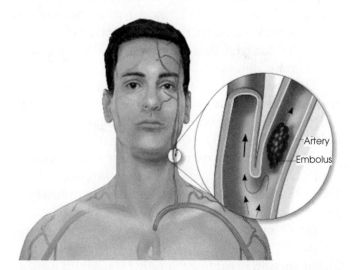

FIGURE 12-11. Embollus floating in an atery, resulting in occlusion

resulting serious valvular malfunction, **cardiorrhexis** (bursting of the ventricle), left **ventricular aneurysm** (extreme dilatation and thinning of the ventricle, with loss of contractile power), pericarditis, and formation of a **mural thrombus** (a localized clot adjacent to the infarcted area of ventricular wall).

Treatment: The standard treatment protocol includes hospitalization, administration of oxygen by inhalation and of narcotics for pain relief by injection, and continuous electrocardiographic monitoring. Thrombolytic agents (tPA [tissue plasminogen activator], streptokinase, or anistreplase) are administered intravenously to dissolve clots. Anticoagulants (aspirin, IV heparin) may also be administered. Beta-blocking agents are started early. In some centers, balloon angioplasty is performed during the acute phase of myocardial infarction.

Congestive Heart Failure (CHF)

A syndrome of impaired hemodynamics due to inability of the heart to maintain normal circulation.

Causes: Any condition that impairs the contractile force of the heart (ischemia due to coronary artery disease; myocarditis) or that overtaxes a normal heart (systemic or pulmonary hypertension, congenital or acquired valvular disease, hyperthyroidism). Right ventricular failure may be due to pulmonary hypertension or cor pulmonale.

A distinction is sometimes made between **forward failure** (inability of the heart to pump blood at a volume that is adequate for the needs of tissues) and **backward failure** (inability of the heart to distend adequately during diastole, with resulting increase of pressure in the venous system). Purely mechanical inadequacy of heart function is complicated by inappropriate hormonal and biochemical responses, including increase of peripheral vascular resistance due to sympathetic vasoconstriction and retention of sodium and water due to release of renin from kidneys whose blood flow is diminished.

History: Shortness of breath, particularly on exertion; orthopnea, paroxysmal nocturnal dyspnea, cough; fatigue, nocturia; anorexia and right upper quadrant fullness due to hepatic engorgement; ankle edema.

Physical Examination: Dyspnea, cyanosis, tachycardia, hypotension. Jugular venous distention. Left ventricular dilatation and hypertrophy. Diminished first heart sound. S3 gallop. Expiratory wheezes and rhonchi. Crepitant rales at bases; reduced breath sounds and dullness to percussion may indicate pleural effusion. Hepatomegaly, **hepatojugular reflux** (bulging of jugular veins when the liver is compressed because of increased pressure in the venous system). Pitting edema of the lower extremities, ascites.

Diagnostic Tests: The red blood cell count may be diminished. The electrocardiogram may indicate myocardial infarction, arrhythmia, or left ventricular hypertrophy. Echocardiography gives more precise information about ventricular size and function. Chest x-ray shows cardiomegaly, signs of pulmonary venous congestion (fine lines at the periphery of the lungs due to edema of pulmonary alveolar septa, called **Kerley B lines**), and sometimes pleural effusion. Radionuclide angiography shows that the **ventricular ejection fraction** (the fraction of the blood contained in the ventricle that is expelled during systole) is reduced.

Course: Congestive heart failure indicates a serious impairment of cardiovascular dynamics, and even with treatment the course is often steadily downhill. The prognosis for long-term survival is poor, and death often occurs suddenly.

Treatment: Rest, salt restriction, and early correction of identifiable precipitating factors. Diuretics (thiazides, loop diuretics, potassium-sparing diuretics), ACE inhibitors, and beta-blockers are used to reverse biochemical imbalances and hormonal effects that lead to sodium retention and circulatory volume overload. Digitalis glycosides increase the force of cardiac contraction.

Cardiomyopathy, Myocardiopathy

General terms for cardiac disorders that arise primarily from diseases of the heart muscle (myocardium) rather than from coronary artery disease, systemic or pulmonary hypertension, valvular disease, or congenital structural abnormality (see ■ Figure 12-12).

Cardiomyopathies vary widely in cause, pathophysiology, and clinical presentation and can accompany or

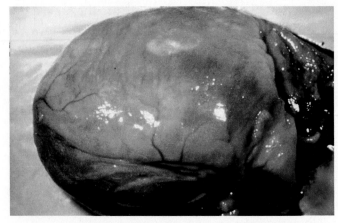

FIGURE 12-12. Enlarged heart resulting from cardiomyopathy.
Source: Pearson Education.

complicate other cardiac disorders. Cardiomyopathies are often categorized or classified by their presumed cause (alcoholic cardiomyopathy, infectious cardiomyopathy) or lack of a known cause (idiopathic cardiomyopathy), but the primary subdivisions are dilated (involving a dilated ventricle), hypertrophic (enlarged ventricle), and restrictive (rigid ventricular walls with poor filling).

The heart muscle is vulnerable to damage by a broad range of harmful influences, including infection (viral, parasitic, rickettsial), drugs and toxins (cancer chemotherapy agents, alcohol, cocaine, arsenic), radiation, metabolic disorders (amyloidosis, hemochromatosis, glycogen storage diseases), connective tissue disorders (systemic lupus erythematosus, scleroderma), generalized diseases of muscle (muscular dystrophy), and deficiency states (beriberi, due to lack of dietary thiamine). Most cases of cardiomyopathy are, however, idiopathic. Some types of hypertrophic cardiomyopathy are familial and are associated with the risk of sudden death at an early age.

Depending on its cause, cardiomyopathy can present as a dilated, flabby heart with poor contractility and diminished **ejection fraction (EF)** or as a thick-walled, hypertrophic heart with inadequate diastolic relaxation and filling. Most patients develop some degree of congestive heart failure, with dyspnea, tachycardia, and pulmonary or peripheral edema, and the typical physical findings outlined in the preceding section. Other symptoms may include chest pain, palpitation, and syncope.

Diagnosis is by EKG, echocardiography, and cardiac catheterization. Apart from standard measures to combat cardiac failure, drug therapy of myocardiopathies is of marginal effectiveness.

Treatment consists of either a heart transplant or making appropriate lifestyle changes, providing general support, and eliminating underlying disorders when possible. The prognosis for long-term survival in most forms of cardiomyopathy is poor.

Acute Pulmonary Edema

An extreme form of left ventricular failure in which respiratory symptoms predominate.

It can be precipitated by acute myocardial infarction or by any factors that increase the severity of existing cardiac failure. There are severe dyspnea, cough, and wheezing, with frothy pink sputum. The pulse is rapid and weak, the lips and nail beds cyanotic. Auscultation reveals rales and rhonchi in the lungs. The arterial oxygen is low. Chest x-ray shows cardiomegaly,

KILLER BLOOD CLOTS
Some people have a hormone that promotes exuberant clotting. If they sit or stand in one place for long periods of time, a blood clot can form in the legs, break loose, and travel to the lungs. David Bloom, an NBC network reporter who was assigned to Iraq to cover the Iraqi war, spent several days sitting and sleeping inside an artillery tank. He developed a blood clot in his leg that went into his lungs and killed him.

increased vascular markings, Kerley B lines, pleural effusion. Treatment includes oxygen by inhalation, morphine, and intravenous diuretics.

Shock

A condition in which the systemic blood pressure is too low to maintain adequate tissue perfusion.

Causes: **Hypovolemia** (reduced blood volume due to hemorrhage, dehydration, severe burns, ascites); cardiogenic (impairment of cardiac function by arrhythmia, myocardial infarction, myocarditis, acute valvular failure); vascular obstruction (**pericardial tamponade**, pulmonary embolism); dilatation of the circulatory system (septic shock, anaphylactic shock, toxic shock syndrome, neurogenic shock, drugs).

History: Weakness, palpitations, thirst, sweating, anxiety, loss of consciousness.

Physical Examination: The blood pressure is low and the pulse rapid. Peripheral pulses are weak or absent. The tilt test is positive (rise in pulse and drop in blood pressure when patient is moved from recumbent to erect position). In hypovolemic shock the skin is pale, cold, and clammy. In septic shock there may be high fever and flushing. Agitation, confusion, and deteriorating level of consciousness.

Diagnostic Tests: Procedures used during early treatment to assess the degree of shock include blood tests (complete blood count, electrolytes, arterial blood gases), urine flow, cardiac monitoring, and central venous pressure or pulmonary wedge pressure with Swan-Ganz catheter.

Course: Without treatment, shock may lead to irreversible damage: cerebral ischemia and infarction, myocardial infarction, renal failure.

Treatment: Vigorous treatment is required to maintain tissue perfusion and prevent irreversible consequences. The patient is placed in the **Trendelenburg**

IRREGULARITIES OF THE PULSE
Irregularities of the pulse are designated, some-what whimsically, as regular irregularities (having a pattern, albeit abnormal) and irregular irregu-larities (wholly random, without discernible pat-tern).

---

position (head lower than feet), and oxygen is admin-istered. Morphine sulfate is given for pain (unless there is respiratory depression or head injury). Volume replace-ment with blood, plasma, or artificial plasma expanders in hypovolemic shock. Treatment of underlying condi-tions. Compression of the arms, legs, and abdomen by an inflatable MAST (military antishock trousers) garment can maintain cerebral, coronary, and renal blood flow until bleeding or other underlying condition is controlled and blood volume restored. Dopamine, adrenal steroids, and other drugs may be administered.

Hypertension

Sustained elevation of arterial blood pressure above 140 mmHg systolic or 90 mmHg diastolic.

Cause: Unknown in more than 90% of cases, which are thus called **essential hypertension**. Essential hypertension shows a genetic pattern, running in fam-ilies and being much more common in African Amer-icans. Its development may depend on environmental factors, excessive dietary salt, sodium retention by the kidney, abnormalities of the renin-angiotensin system, obesity, alcohol abuse, and use of NSAIDs. **Secondary hypertension** is due to a demonstrable cause: renal parenchymal disease, renal ischemia, Cushing disease, primary aldosteronism, pheochromocytoma, or estrogen use in the form of oral contraceptives.

History: There may be no symptoms whatsoever until complications develop.

Physical Examination: Elevated blood pressure and accentuation of the second heart sound at the aortic valve area; otherwise there may be no findings. Retinopathy is indicated by detection of **Keith-Wagener-Barker changes** on ophthalmoscopic examination. Left ventricular hypertrophy may be indicated by precordial heave or by a systolic ejection murmur.

Diagnostic Tests: Laboratory studies may be nor-mal. The search for a cause of secondary hyperten-sion includes testing blood and urine for signs of renal disease.

Course: Some hypertensive patients experience a return of blood pressure to normal after a few weeks, months, or years. In most, however, elevation of blood pressure remains throughout life. Hypertension causes several forms of damage to the cardiovascular system (hypertensive cardiovascular disease), including left ven-tricular hypertrophy and dysfunction, arteriosclerosis, dilatation and dissecting aneurysm of the aorta, hyper-tensive encephalopathy, and hypertensive renal disease. In accelerated or malignant hypertension there is sus-tained high blood pressure responding poorly to treat-ment, and rapid progression of cardiovascular damage.

Treatment: Therapy of essential hypertension ide-ally includes lifestyle modification (reduction of alcohol intake, increased physical exercise), restriction of dietary salt, and control of overweight. Drug therapy is tailored to the severity of the disease, and typically starts with a single drug (a thiazide diuretic or a beta-blocker), others being added as needed: ACE inhibitors, angiotensin II receptor inhibitors, calcium channel blockers, methyldopa, alpha-receptor antagonists, guanethidine, and drugs of other classes.

Atherosclerosis

Hardening and even calcification of arterial walls, with narrowing of their lumens (see ■ Figures 12-13 and 12-14).

Cause: Inflammation and degeneration of arterial walls, with diffuse or plaquelike deposition of choles-terol crystals in the **tunica intima** (inner lining) of sys-temic arteries. Various inborn metabolic abnormalities in lipoproteins may predispose to abnormal elevation of serum cholesterol level and abnormal deposition of cholesterol in arterial alls. (Involvement of coronary

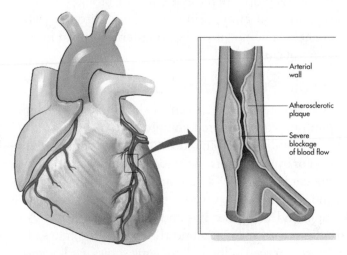

FIGURE 12-13. Atherosclerotic artery

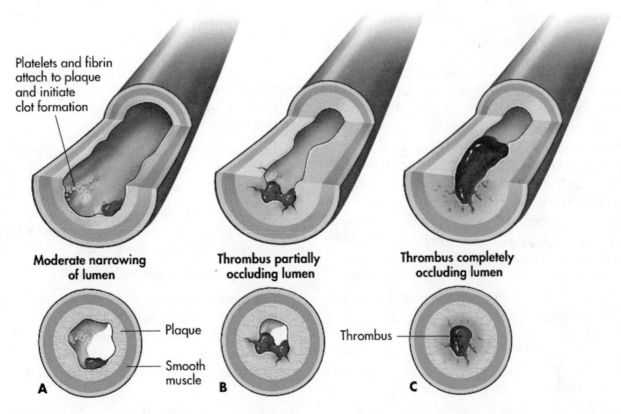

Platelets and fibrin attach to plaque and initiate clot formation

Moderate narrowing of lumen

Thrombus partially occluding lumen

Thrombus completely occluding lumen

Plaque

Smooth muscle

Thrombus

A

B

C

FIGURE 12-14. Thrombus formation in an atherosclerotic vessel depicting (A) the initial clot formation, and (B) and (C) the varying degrees of occlusion.

and cerebral arteries in the same process is a principal cause of coronary artery disease and cerebrovascular disease.)

History: Intermittent claudication: cramping muscle pain in calves, thighs, buttocks (depending on site of arterial obstruction) that is brought on by walking and relieved by rest. Erectile dysfunction.

Physical Examination: Weakness or absence of femoral, popliteal, or pedal pulses. Bruit over aorta, iliac or femoral arteries. Trophic changes (loss of hair, thinning of skin, pigmentation) in affected limb.

Diagnostic Tests: Evidence of reduced blood flow can be obtained by Doppler ultrasonography, transcutaneous oximetry, or other measures.

Treatment: Physical therapy and treatment with pentoxifylline or other agents may improve exercise tolerance slightly. Surgical treatment (endarterectomy or arterial grafting) yields much better results. Percutaneous transluminal angioplasty (balloon dilatation) is effective in selected cases.

Calf cramps come on after he has walked about one-half mile and require him to stop and rest.

Deep Vein Thrombophlebitis

Inflammation in the wall of a tributary of one of the common iliac veins in the pelvis or lower limb, associated with clotting of blood within the vein.

Causes: Congestive heart failure, sudden immobilization because of recent surgery or injury, oral contraceptives, malignancy. Cigarette smoking increases risk.

History: Pain or tightness in the calf or thigh, with edema distally. There may be no symptoms until **pulmonary embolism** occurs.

Diagnostic Tests: Doppler ultrasonography, impedance plethysmography, and venography confirm, localize, and quantify venous obstruction.

Course: There is considerable danger of **pulmonary embolism**. Healing may be followed by deep venous insufficiency, with chronic edema.

Treatment: Hospitalization. Intravenous or low-dose intramuscular heparin and oral anticoagulant.

Physical Examination: Distal edema may be the only objective sign. There may be pain or tenderness on calf rocking, or a positive **Homans sign** (calf pain or tightness on passive dorsiflexion of the foot).

Pause for Reflection

1. Sublingual nitroglycerin is used to treat _____, which may progress to more severe disease such as myocardial infarction or congestive heart failure, even with treatment.
2. An electrocardiogram showing ST-segment elevation (changing later to depression) and inversion of T waves, elevation of LDH, CK-MB and troponins is diagnostic of _____.
3. Physical findings including dyspnea, cyanosis, tachycardia, jugular venous distention, left ventricular dilatation and hypertrophy, diminished S1. S3 gallop, hepatojugular reflux, and pitting edema of the lower extremities suggest a diagnosis of _____.
4. _____ can present as a dilated, flabby heart with poor contractility and diminished ejection fraction (EF) or as a thick-walled, hypertrophic heart with inadequate diastolic relaxation and filling.
5. _____ is an extreme form of left ventricular failure with a chest x-ray showing cardiomegaly, increased vascular markings, Kerley B lines, pleural effusion.
6. _____ refers to high blood pressure of unknown cause, although it may run in families, but high blood pressure of demonstrable cause such as renal ischemia is known as _____.
7. Patients with atherosclerosis typically have a history of _____ or cramping muscle pain in calves, thighs, buttocks (depending on site of arterial obstruction) that is brought on by walking and relieved by rest.
8. Homans sign is indicative of _____.

Diagnostic and Surgical Procedures

aneurysm resection Surgical removal of a segment of vessel that has an abnormal ballooning and threatens to rupture.

arteriogram Injection of radiopaque dye directly into an artery to obtain x-rays of the vessel and its branches.

balloon angioplasty Stretching or breaking up atherosclerotic plaques in coronary arteries (see ■ Figures 12-5 and 12-16). See also **PTCA**.

bypass See *coronary artery bypass graft.*

cardiac catheterization A procedure that involves passing a flexible catheter through the femoral artery and into the heart to measure pressures within the heart's chambers. Dye is then injected to show patency or obstruction of the coronary arteries (see ■ Figure 12-4).

carotid endarterectomy Removal of hardened plaque from an obstructed carotid artery.

commissurotomy Surgical enlargement of the aperture of a stenotic heart valve, particularly the mitral, by stretching or cutting.

coronary artery bypass graft (CABG) Surgical procedure done to bypass one or more occluded coronary arteries by using a vein graft (often from the leg) (see ■ Figure 12-6).

CPR (cardiopulmonary resuscitation) The use of external compression of the heart coupled with breathing techniques to revive a victim whose heart and respirations have stopped.

ECG, EKG (electrocardiogram) A tracing of the electrical activity of the heart (see ■ Figure 12-3).

echocardiography A noninvasive diagnostic procedure in which an ultrasonic beam is directed at the heart and the returning echoes are recorded and analyzed; valuable for the measurement of cardiac chambers (wall thickness and cavity volume), assessment of ventricular function, and identification of valvular malfunction.

exercise stress test Test during which the patient exercises on a treadmill to stress the heart and reproduce symptoms of angina and EKG changes.

femoral-popliteal bypass Implantation of a vessel graft (real or artificial) into the femoral and popliteal arteries to bypass one or more blockages.

Holter monitoring A continuously recorded EKG as monitored by a portable EKG machine worn by the patient. This procedure is done on an outpatient basis for 24 hours to detect arrhythmias.

MUGA scan Radiologic procedure in which a radioactive isotope is injected into the arteries with a subsequent scan showing uptake of the isotope by the heart. These radioactive emissions are electronically collected and analyzed by computer, resulting in a series of successive images all taken at the same point in the cardiac cycle. This test is used to assess heart size, shape, and function. MUGA stands for multiple gated acquisition.

pacemaker implantation Placement of pacemaker electrodes to the heart to correct heart block or control persistent irregular rhythms (see ■ Figure 12-7).

percutaneous transluminal coronary angioplasty (PTCA) Procedure used to dilate an occluded artery, usually a coronary artery, by passing a catheter (with a deflated balloon section) to the site of the occlusion and inflating the balloon to compress the obstruction and enlarge the lumen of the vessel (see ■ Figure 12-16).

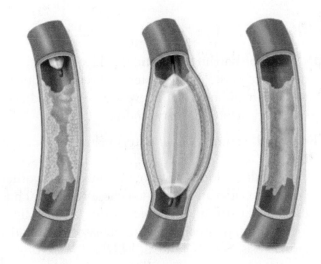

FIGURE 12-16. PTCA (percutaneous transluminal coronary angioplasty)

treadmill stress test See **exercise stress test**.

valve replacement Excision and replacement of a valve of the heart because of stenosis or insufficiency.

vein stripping Surgical removal of (usually) the saphenous leg vein and its branches to treat varicose veins (see ■ Figure 12-17).

venipuncture Insertion of a needle into a vein for the purpose of removing blood for testing, or to inject fluids, medicines, or diagnostic materials.

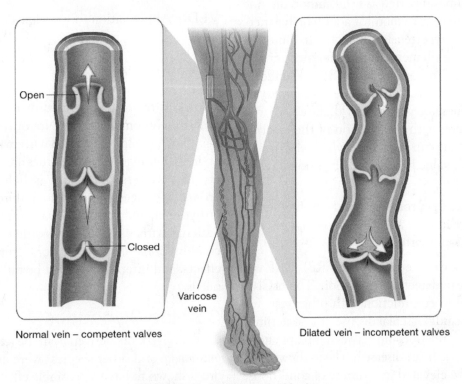

Open

Closed

Varicose vein

Normal vein – competent valves

Dilated vein – incompetent valves

FIGURE 12-17. Varicose vein stripping

Laboratory Procedures

BNP (B-type natriuretic peptide) A blood test used to detect, diagnose, and evaluate the severity of congestive heart failure; rising levels may also indicate worsening acute coronary syndrome (ACS).

cholesterol, serum A lipid (fatty) material formed in the liver and transported in the blood, which serves as a building block for various hormones and other substances. Elevation of serum cholesterol, which is usually due to an inherited disturbance of lipid metabolism, is associated with increased risk of atherosclerosis. See *HDL, LDL, VLDL.*

CK (creatine kinase) A serum enzyme that can be chemically distinguished into three isoenzymes or fractions: the BB (CK-BB) isoenzyme is elevated in cerebral infarction, the MM (CK-MM) in muscular dystrophy and muscle crush injury, and MB (CK-MB) in myocardial infarction. When separated in the laboratory by electrophoresis, these isoenzymes appear as distinct bands in a visual display. Hence the expression MB band is roughly synonymous with MB isoenzyme. Do not confuse *creatine* with *creatinine*. *CPK* (creatine phosphokinase) is an outdated term for *CK*.

electrolytes The electrolytes are sodium (Na), potassium (K), chloride (Cl), and bicarbonate (HCO_3) which is sometimes reported as total carbon dioxide (CO_2). They are used to monitor acid-base balance, kidney function, hypertension, response to diuretics, and potassium supplementation. Reference ranges: potassium 3.5–5.2 mEq/L; sodium 135–147 mEq/L; chloride 95–107 mEq/L; bicarbonate 19–25 mEq/L . Numerical values are sometimes dictated, in the order shown here, without mention of the electrolytes by name. One can determine which electrolyte goes with which value by knowing the normal reference ranges.

HDL (high-density lipoproteins) Lipid-carrying serum proteins associated with a relatively low risk of cholesterol deposition in arteries.

high sensitivity C-reactive protein (hsCRP) CRP is a nonspecific test to detect inflammation. The hsCRP is often ordered in conjunction with other tests for arteriosclerotic cardiovascular disease. It is sometimes ordered because a relationship between inflammation and arteriosclerotic heart disease has been shown, but because it can be elevated in a variety of conditions, it is not useful in diagnosing heart disease.

isoenzyme Any of a group of enzymes having similar chemical effects but differing in structure and often arising from different sources in the body. See *CK, LDH.*

LDH Abbreviation for lactic dehydrogenase, an isoenzyme. LDH1 is found in heart muscle; levels are increased after myocardial infarction. LDH2 is normally found in higher amounts in the serum than is LDH1. When the level of LDH1 surpasses that of LDH2, this is called a "flipped LDH." *LDH* need not be translated in reports.

lipoproteins, serum Serum proteins that bind and transport lipid materials including cholesterol.

LDL (low-density lipoproteins) Lipid-carrying serum proteins associated with a relatively high risk of cholesterol deposition in arteries.

MB bands See *CK (creatine kinase).*

troponins Troponins are the preferred tests for a suspected heart attack; they also help in evaluating the extent of heart injury and in distinguishing noncardiac chest pain. Troponin I and T are cardiac-specific whereas other tests such as the CK-MB or myoglobin are not. Reference ranges: troponin I 0–0.1 ng/mL (onset: 4–6 hrs, peak: 12–24 hrs, return to normal: 4–7 days); troponin T 0–0.2 ng/mL (onset: 3–4 hrs, peak: 10–24 hrs, return to normal: 10–14 days).

VLDL Abbreviation for *very low-density lipoproteins.*

Pharmacology

The drug treatment of cardiovascular disease is an exceedingly complex topic. Not only are diseases of the heart and circulation treated with many different kinds of drugs, but many of those drugs are effective in a variety of disorders, including ischemic coronary syndromes, congestive heart failure, hypertension, arrhythmia, and peripheral vascular disease. Nearly all patients with circulatory disorders receive balanced combinations of three or more drugs whose dosages, effects, and interactions must be tailored to individual needs.

Cardiac Glycosides

Cardiac glycosides derived from the foxglove plant (*Digitalis lanata* and other species) were among the earliest drugs shown to have a favorable effect in heart disease, strengthening and steadying the beat of the failing heart. *Digitalis* (often abridged to *dig,* which rhymes with *bridge*) is a general term for drugs of this class. Because of unpredictable dosage requirements and a considerable risk of toxicity (including nausea and potentially dangerous cardiac arrhythmias), blood levels of these agents may need frequent checking. Though largely supplanted nowadays by safer and more specific drugs, cardiac glycosides still have a role in the management of congestive heart failure.

> digoxin (Lanoxin, Lanoxicaps)

Beta-Blockers

Beta-blockers (beta-adrenergic blocking agents) reduce the stimulant effects of epinephrine and norepinephrine at various beta-adrenergic receptor sites in the circulatory system. They slow and stabilize the heart rate, diminish peripheral blood pressure, and reduce cardiac work and oxygen demand. They are widely used in the treatment of hypertension, angina pectoris, acute myocardial infarction, congestive heart failure, and some arrhythmias. The generic names of drugs in this class end in *-olol.*

> acebutolol (Sectral)
> atenolol (Tenormin)
> betaxolol (Kerlone)
> bisoprolol (Zebeta)
> esmolol (Brevibloc)
> metoprolol (Lopressor, Toprol-XL)
> nadolol (Corgard)
> nebivolol (Bystolic)
> peributolol (Levatol)
> pindolol (Visken)
> propranolol (Inderal, Innopran XL)
> sotalol (Betapace)
> timolol (Blocadren)

Alpha-Blockers

Alpha-blockers (alpha-adrenergic blocking agents) are used principally in the treatment of hypertension.

> clonidine (Catapres, Duraclon)
> doxazosin mesylate (Cardura)
> guanabenz (Wytensin)
> guanadrel (Hylorel)
> guanethidine (Ismelin)
> guanfacine (Tenex)
> methyldopa (Aldomet)
> phenoxybenzamine (Dibenzyline)
> prazosin (Minipress)

> "NITRO PASTE"
>
> Physicians often dictate "nitro paste" when the correct drug form is actually nitroglycerin ointment. The dosage of this coronary vasodilator is measured in inches of ointment (or fractions thereof) as it comes from the tube. The patient is supplied with disposable ruled applicators, with which the ointment is measured out and smeared over the skin in much the same way as one spreads mucilage or wallpaper paste—hence, probably, the popular misnomer "paste."
>
> When "nitro paste" is dictated, "nitro" should be expanded to "nitroglycerin," and "paste" should be translated "ointment"—unless departmental rules forbid using the right words when the dictator uses the wrong ones.
>
> Vera Pyle

> reserpine (Serpasil)
> terazosin (Hytrin)

A noncardioselective drug that blocks both alpha and beta adrenergic receptors is carvedilol (Coreg), used in the treatment of hypertension and congestive heart failure.

Calcium Channel Blockers

These drugs reduce heart rate and blood pressure and inhibit certain cardiac arrhythmias by blocking the passage of calcium ions across biologic membranes. They are used in the treatment of hypertension, angina pectoris, peripheral vascular disease, and some arrhythmias.

> amlodipine (Norvasc)
> diltiazem (Cardizem, Dilacor XR, Tiazac)
> felodipine (Plendil)
> israpidine (Dynacirc CR)
> nicardipine (Cardene)
> nifedipine (Adalat, Procardia)
> verapamil (Calan, Covera-HS, Isoptin, Verelan)

ACE Inhibitors

ACE (angiotensin-converting enzyme) inhibitors block the synthesis of angiotensin II, a hormone with vasoconstrictor and smooth muscle stimulant effects. Drugs in this class promote vasodilatation, decreasing pulmonary and peripheral vascular resistance and hence arterial pressure and cardiac work.

They are used in the treatment of hypertension and congestive heart failure. The generic names of drugs in this class end in *-pril*.

> benazepril (Lotensin)
> captopril (Capoten)
> enalapril (Vasotec)
> fosinopril (Monopril)
> lisinopril (Prinivil, Zestril)
> moexipril (Univasc)
> perindopril (Aceon)
> quinapril (Accupril)
> ramipril (Altace)
> trandolapril (Mavik)

Angiotensin II Blockers

Angiotensin II (two) receptor antagonists block the stimulant effect of angiotensin II on vascular smooth muscle. They are useful in the treatment of hypertension and left ventricular hypertrophy, particularly in patients intolerant to ACE inhibitors. The generic names of drugs in this class all end in *-sartan*.

> candesartan (Atacand)
> eprosartan (Teveten)
> irbesartan (Avapro)
> losartan (Cozaar)
> olmesartan (Benicar)
> telmisartan (Micardis)
> valsartan (Diovan)

Nitrates

Nitrates are vasodilators, chiefly used to relieve the pain of angina pectoris by increasing coronary artery flow. All of the following are trade names for nitroglycerin. Their routes of administration are indicated.

> Nitro-Bid (sustained-release capsule)
> Nitrodisc (transdermal patch)
> Nitro-Dur (transdermal patch)
> Nitrogard (transmucosal tablet)
> Nitrol (topical ointment)
> Nitrolingual (sublingual spray)
> Transderm-Nitro (transdermal patch)
> Tridil (IV)

Other nitrates given orally include:

> isosorbide dinitrate (Isordil, Sorbitrate)
> isosorbide mononitrate (Imdur)

Diuretics

Diuretics promote an increase in the renal excretion of water, sodium, and other ions, thus reducing peripheral and pulmonary edema in congestive heart failure. They are also first-line agents in the treatment of **essential hypertension**. These drugs vary widely in their mechanisms of action and particularly in the circulating ions whose excretion they favor.

> amiloride (Midamor)
> bumetanide (Bumex)
> chlorothiazide (CTZ) (Diuril)
> chlorthalidone (Thalitone)
> eplerenone (Inspra)
> furosemide (Lasix)
> hydrochlorothiazide (HCTZ) (Esidrix, HydroDIURIL, Microzide, Oretic)
> hydroflumethiazide (Diucardin)
> indapamide (Lozol)
> metolazone (Mykrox, Zaroxolyn)
> methyclothiazide (Enduron)
> spironolactone (Aldactone)
> torsemide (Demadex)
> triamterene (Dyrenium)

Each of the following antihypertensive drugs combines a diuretic with another antihypertensive agent. (Proprietary names are given first in this list.)

> Aldactazide (spironolactone + HCTZ)
> Aldoril (methyldopa + HCTZ)
> Apresazide (hydralazine + HCTZ)
> Combipres (clonidine + chlorthalidone)
> Dyazide (triamterene + HCTZ)
> Enduronyl (deserpidine + methyclothiazide)
> Hydropres (reserpine + HCTZ)
> Inderide (propranolol + HCTZ)
> Moduretic (amiloride + HCTZ)
> Renese-R (reserpine + polythiazide)
> Salutensin (reserpine + hydroflumethiazide)
> Tenoretic (atenolol + chlorthalidone)
> Zestoretic (lisinopril + HCTZ)

Antiarrhythmic Drugs

Cardiac arrhythmias can result from a variety of disturbances in the conduction system of the heart, and are treated with a correspondingly broad range of pharmacologic agents.

adenosine (Adenocard)
amiodarone (Cordarone)
bretylium (Bretylol)
disopyramide (Norpace)
flecainide (Tambocor)
ibutilide fumarate (Corvert)
lidocaine (Xylocaine)
mexiletine (Mexitil)
moricizine (Ethmozine)
procainamide (Procanbid, Pronestyl)
propafenone (Rythmol)
quinidine (Quinaglute Dura-Tabs, Quinidex)
tocainide (Tonocard)

Bile Acid Sequestrants

Bile acid sequestrants promote the intestinal excretion of cholesterol and are used in the treatment of hypercholesterolemia.

cholestyramine (Prevalite, Questran)
colesevelam (Welchol)
colestipol (Colestid)

HMG-CoA Reductase Inhibitors

HMG-CoA (3-hydroxy-3-methylglutaryl coenzyme A) reductase inhibitors block the synthesis of total cholesterol and LDL cholesterol. These drugs have been shown to delay progression of atherosclerosis and to decrease the risk of myocardial infarction and stroke in persons with hyperlipidemia. The generic names of drugs in this class end in -*statin*, and the drugs are collectively known as **statins**.

atorvastatin (Lipitor)
fluvastatin (Lescol)
lovastatin (Mevacor)
pravastatin (Pravachol)
simvastatin (Zocor)

Drugs that reduce serum triglyceride levels are used in selected hyperlipidemias.

clofibrate (Atromid-S)
fenofibrate (Tricor)
gemfibrozil (Lopid)

Vasopressors

Vasopressors used in medicine are potent selective stimulants of arterial smooth muscle, increasing the heart rate, raising systemic blood pressure by boosting peripheral vascular resistance, but maintaining coronary and renal blood flow. Administered by continuous IV infusion, they are often valuable in the management of severe cardiovascular collapse

dobutamine (Dobutrex)
dopamine (Intropin)
isoproterenol (Isuprel)
norepinephrine (Levophed)

Anticoagulants

Anticoagulants are used to prevent thrombosis of coronary and cerebral arteries in persons at risk of myocardial infarction or stroke and to prevent or treat deep venous thrombosis (DVT).

anisindione (Miradon)
ardeparin (Normiflo)
dalteparin (Fragmin)
danaparoid (Orgaran)
dicumarol
enoxaparin (Lovenox)
heparin
warfarin (Coumadin)

Tissue Plasminogen Activators (tPA)

Tissue plasminogen activators (tPA), synthesized by recombinant DNA technology, convert plasminogen in a blood clot to plasmin, which breaks down fibrin and dissolves the clot. When administered within the first 2–3 hours after myocardial infarction, thrombotic stroke, and peripheral vascular occlusion, these drugs can restore blood flow. They are given intravenously.

alteplase (Activase)
reteplase (Retavase)

Thrombolytic enzymes are used for the same indications and also act by dissolving clots. They are given intravenously.

anistreplase (Eminase)
streptokinase (Kabikinase, Streptase)
urokinase (Abbokinase)

Transcription Tips

Unless you transcribe exclusively in a physician specialist's office, the majority of the reports you encounter will be from the three main specialties of cardiology, gastroenterology, and orthopedics. Diseases of the cardiovascular system are quite prevalent, and the medical terminology is extensive. Even patients with noncardiac chief complaints may have chronic secondary cardiovascular disorders such as arrhythmia, hypertension, or elevated cholesterol level. This is particularly true of elderly patients.

1. Confusing terms related to the cardiovascular system (see box on page 381): Some of these terms sound alike; others are potential traps when researching. Memorize the terms and their meanings so that you can select the appropriate term for a correct transcript.

2. The spelling *anulus* is the official anatomical spelling, *not* annulus, although the latter is still found in references.

3. Watch out for spelling changes when forming derivatives.

   femoral-popliteal   or   femoropopliteal
   inferior-lateral   or   inferolateral

4. Note the challenging spellings of these common cardiology drugs:
   Cardizem (frequently mispronounced as "Cardiazem" or "Cardizyme")
   Catapres, Combipres (only one *s*)
   Inderal (*not* Inderol)
   Minipress and Lopressor (two *s's*)
   Rythmol (an antiarrhythmic drug, the spelling of which differs from the word *rhythm*)

5. Plurals. Generally, medical words derived from Latin or Greek are pluralized according to guidelines in the recommended references. However, some physicians prefer to pluralize Latin terms in the same way that English words are pluralized. Transcribe as dictated unless incorrect.

   cannulas   or   cannulae
   fistulas   or   fistulae
   lumens   or   lumina

6. Dictation Challenges

   anterior, inferior, interior—These directional terms can sound a lot alike, but if you are paying attention to context, you should not transcribe the wrong term in error. *Anterior* (in front of) and *inferior* (below, toward the bottom) can each modify myocardial infarction and be used to indicate location in a variety of contexts. If you think you hear "interior," stop and relisten because the only likely time it would be used, and very rarely at that, would be in a discussion of the inside of a hollow organ or structure, possibly by a pathologist or an endoscopist.

   "cabbage"—The dictator's pronunciation of CABG, acronym for coronary artery bypass graft.

   "irregularly irregular"—No, the doctor isn't stuttering. Heart rhythm may be said to be irregularly irregular or regularly irregular; listen closely and transcribe correctly.

   LIMA (left internal mammary artery) is pronounced "leema" and is used frequently as a conduit for coronary artery bypass.

   Triple A or AAA in a cardiology context stands for *abdominal aortic aneurysm*. It has a different meaning in orthopedics.

7. Abbreviation traps. Notice that many cardiac abbreviations contain the letters *V, P, B,* and *D;* these letters can all sound alike, so one must be extremely careful when transcribing abbreviations as well as expanding them. The abbreviations in the feature box earlier in the chapter have more than one translation and may even appear in the same report.

   Context will help you determine which to use. In addition, the appropriate modifiers will usually be apparent if you search a reputable medical dictionary or word book for the noun. Some references will give you a list of phrases beginning with the adjective. Try both types of searches if you cannot determine the correct translation from the context. If you're still unsure, transcribe the abbreviation. Be sure to translate the abbreviation correctly based on its meaning in the sentence.

Spotlight On

Transcribing Cardiology Dictation

by Kathleen Mors Woods

In literature and in life, the heart is always depicted as the soul of a person and is described in vivid terms. One may be called a heartbreaker, a heart throb, a sweetheart. One may be heartless, heartsick, brokenhearted, fainthearted, goodhearted, lighthearted, lionhearted, or have a big heart, a cold heart, a hard heart, or a heart as good as gold. These glossy descriptions take on a more meaningful tone when placed in a medical context and discussion of cardiology emerges.

In the medical field, we are concerned with cardiology as the study of the heart, its functions, and its diseases, the identification of these diseases by diagnostic tests, and ultimately the correction of defects.

When a newborn baby is diagnosed with a congenital heart defect, or a 16-year-old is stabbed in the chest, or a person's aorta is literally ripped out of the chest in an automobile accident (by hitting the steering wheel not wearing a seat belt), the cardiac surgeon is called upon to demonstrate a broad range of abilities in treating these patients. Transcribing reports on these procedures carries with it the excitement of a new technology, expanding every day through research and a commitment to life-saving techniques.

Cardiac Evaluation. Imagine the following scenario: Your neighbor has chest pain and goes to a cardiologist. The other factors for having this chest pain (for example, kidney stones or ulcers) have been ruled out. At the cardiologist's office, an electrocardiogram is performed. In electrocardiography, *lead* can mean either (1) an electrode attached to the patient or (2) a specific configuration of electrical signals fed to the galvanometer. There are 12 leads in the latter sense, but only five (right wrist, left wrist, right ankle, left ankle, chest) in the former sense.

If the patient's pain is caused by the decrease in blood flow due to a narrowing or obstruction of an artery carrying oxygen to the heart, and if damage has been done or is occurring, this will show up on the EKG. The pain, then, is caused by an obstruction (clot) in the vessel. If this clot remains in the vessel, the vessel is occluded and the muscle of the heart (myocardium) is damaged, for the area the vessel feeds dies.

If the patient is "evolving the infarction" (having a heart attack) and admitted to a hospital in a timely fashion, several other tests are performed, including measurement of blood levels of CK (creatine kinase) and troponins, which rise if heart cells are damaged during an infarction (but not during angina). New drugs are used to either dissolve the clot within the vessel or work with the body's own clotting factors to dissolve it. The patient may need to undergo a treadmill exercise stress test and be referred for a cardiac catheterization.

Abbreviations and Eponyms. In interpreting the dictation, the transcriptionist must become familiar with many abbreviations and eponyms. If a baby has a B-T shunt, it is the procedure named after the famous Blalock-Taussig blue baby operation first performed by those two physicians. Favaloro, Bovie, St. Jude, Carpentier-Edwards, and Björk-Shiley are all proper names (eponyms). If an eponym is the name of one person (Johns Hopkins, Austin Flint), it is not hyphenated.

Too often physicians dictate in abbreviations, and the transcriptionist should exercise discretion when transcribing them in medical reports. When you are required to type abbreviations, use only those abbreviations that will not be misinterpreted. If you drop one letter of an abbreviation, you change the medical meaning and location. The posterior descending artery is abbreviated *PDA*, which also stands for the congenital heart defect of *patent ductus arteriosus*. When you translate abbreviations, be sure to transcribe the correct meaning as indicated by the context of the report.

As a cardiology transcriptionist, you get to "know" a cardiology patient quite well through the medical history you transcribe, and you get a lot of satisfaction knowing that you are playing an essential role in a patient's return to good health.

Exercises

Medical Vocabulary Review

Instructions: Choose the best answer.

_____ 1. Which of the following terms indicates an arrhythmia that is abnormally slow and irregular?
A. Palpitations.
B. Bradyarrhythmia.
C. Tachyarrhythmia.
D. Irregularly irregular pulse.

_____ 2. Which of the following terms means swelling of the lower extremities, aggravated by the downward hanging position?
A. Edema.
B. Pitting edema.
C. Dependent edema.
D. Peripheral edema.

_____ 3. Which of the following terms means obstruction of a blood vessel by a detached blood clot, air, fat, or injected material?
A. Stenosis.
B. Fibrosis.
C. Exudate.
D. Embolism.

_____ 4. All of the following terms might be used to describe a murmur EXCEPT ___
A. bruit.
B. harsh.
C. gallop.
D. systolic.

_____ 5. The cardinal symptom of coronary disease is ____
A. hypertension.
B. cardiac murmurs.
C. angina pectoris.
D. paroxysmal nocturnal dyspnea.

_____ 6. An effusion is _____
A. swelling due to the presence of fluid in tissue spaces.
B. edema that retains the mark of the examiner's fingers after release of pressure.
C. an abnormal accumulation of fluid in a body cavity, such as the pericardium.
D. delivery of oxygen and nutrients to tissues, and removal of carbon dioxide and other wastes by sufficient blood flow to the area.

_____ 7. Patients with chronic pulmonary disease often exhibit _____ of the fingers.
A. cyanosis
B. clubbing
C. edema
D. fibrosis

_____ 8. Enlargement of a heart chamber due to increased thickness of its muscular wall is _____
A. akinesis.
B. ischemia.
C. hypertrophy.
D. cardiomegaly.

_____ 9. _____ hypotension is low blood pressure brought on by a sudden change in body position, most often when shifting from lying down to standing
A. Paroxysmal
B. Orthostatic
C. Isorhythmic
D. Pleuritic

_____ 10. Symptoms that occur in sudden attacks or seizures are said to be ____
A. pleuritic.
B. dependent.
C. paroxysmal.
D. orthostatic.

___ 11. A patient with right ventricular failure, hypertrophy, or dilatation due to acute or chronic pulmonary disease is said to have ____
A. cor pulmonale.
B. cardiomegaly.
C. hepatojugular reflux.
D. paroxysmal nocturnal dyspnea.

___ 12. Discharge of blood from the heart as determined by echocardiography or cardiac catheterization is referred to as the _____ fraction.
A. dilation
B. ejection
C. injection
D. conduction

___ 13. In the following sentence taken from a cardiac catheterization report, the correct translation of PDA is ____. Sentence: The right coronary proximally supplies the sinus nodal conus branch as well as the PDA and the postero-lateral ventricular system.
A. phased digital array.
B. patent ductus arteriosus.
C. posterior descending artery.
D. peripheral dependent angioedema.

___ 14. A lab test for a hormone stored mainly in the ventricular myocardium and elevated in congestive heart failure and hypertension is the _____
A. BNP (B-type natriuretic peptide).
B. CK-MB (creatine kinase, MB isoenzyme).
C. LDL (low-density lipoprotein).
D. hsCRP (high-sensitivity C-reactive protein).

___ 15. In a report of the physical examination of the neck, distention of the neck veins is called _____
A. jugular venous distention.
B. carotid artery distention.
C. carotid vascular distention.
D. hepatojugular reflux.

___ 16. Elevated _____, which are cardiac-specific proteins found in the blood, are more diagnostic of a myocardial infarction than other blood tests that might be performed.
A. troponins
B. myoglobins
C. creatine kinase
D. lactic dehydrogenase

___ 17. _____ is impairment of the conduction between the atria and ventricles of the heart.
A. Brady-tachycardia
B. Isorhythmic dissociation
C. Atrioventricular block
D. Irregularly irregular pulse

___ 18. Bulging of the neck veins when the liver is compressed because of increased pressure in the venous system is _____
A. jugular venous distention.
B. hepatojugular reflux.
C. point of maximal intensity.
D. paroxysmal nocturnal dyspnea.

___ 19. What is the meaning of the phrase "profuse diaphoresis" in this sentence? "The patient complained of profuse diaphoresis but no nausea or vomiting."
A. Excessive sweating.
B. Frequent, loose, watery stools.
C. A fluttering sensation caused by irregular heartbeat.
D. An abnormally strong thrust applied to the chest wall by the beating heart.

___ 20. A murmur heard at the base of the heart and transmitted to the carotids and cardiac apex in aortic stenosis may be described as a _____ murmur.
A. diamond-shaped
B. late diastolic
C. systolic ejection
D. harsh, blowing

Diagnostic and Surgical Procedures

Instructions: Match the following diagnostic and surgical procedures to their descriptions or definitions. Some answers may be used more than once.

_____ 1. cardiac catheterization

_____ 2. carotid endarterectomy

_____ 3. angioplasty

_____ 4. atherectomy

_____ 5. defibrillation

_____ 6. aneurysm resection

_____ 7. arteriogram

_____ 8. commissurotomy

_____ 9. echocardiography

_____ 10. exercise stress test

_____ 11. Holter monitoring

_____ 12. pacemaker implantation

_____ 13. venipuncture

_____ 14. coronary artery bypass graft

_____ 15. cardiopulmonary resuscitation

_____ 16. electrocardiogram

_____ 17. percutaneous transluminal coronary angioplasty

A. 24-hour EKG device worn by patient while going through usual daily activities

B. Cardioversion

C. EKG while patient is walking or running on a treadmill

D. A tracing of electrical activity of the heart

E. Injection of radiopaque dye directly into an artery to obtain x-rays of the vessel and its branches

F. Minimally invasive imaging procedure for assessing chamber pressures, wall motion abnormalities, coronary artery blood flow, valve function

G. Needle insertion into a vein to remove blood for testing, or to inject fluids, medicines, or diagnostic materials

H. Noninvasive ultrasound imaging to measure cardiac chamber wall thickness and cavity volume, assess ventricular function, and identify valvular malfunction

I. Dilation of an occluded artery using a balloon to compress the obstruction and enlarge the lumen of the vessel

J. Placement of electrodes to the heart to correct heart block or control irregular rhythms

K. Procedure to reduce narrowing in coronary artery by dilating the area of obstruction with a balloon or ablating the plaque with a laser

L. External compression of the heart coupled with breathing techniques to revive a victim whose heart and respirations have stopped

M. Procedure to remove atheromatous plaque in neck arteries

N. Surgical enlargement of the aperture of a stenotic heart valve, particularly the mitral, by stretching or cutting.

O. Surgical removal of a segment of vessel that has an abnormal ballooning and threatens to rupture

P. Using a mechanical device to remove atheromatous plaque from a coronary artery

Q. Anastomosing a vein segment from the aorta to a coronary artery to restore flow to an obstructed coronary artery

Dissecting Medical Terms

Instructions: As you learned in your medical language course, words are formed from prefixes, combining forms (root word plus combining vowel), and suffixes. Combining vowels (usually *o* but not always) are used to connect two root words or a root and a suffix. By analyzing these word parts, you can often determine the definition of a term without even looking it up (if you know the definition of the parts, of course!). Being able to divide and analyze the words you hear into their component parts will also improve your spelling and help you research those words that you cannot easily spell or define.

For the following terms, place a slash (/) between the components and then write a short definition based on the meaning of the parts. Remember that to define a word based on its parts, you start at the end, usually with the suffix. If there's a prefix, that is defined next, and finally the combining form is defined.

Example: biventricular
Divide & Analyze: biventricular = bi/ventricul/ar = pertaining to + two + lower chamber of heart
Define: pertaining to both lower chambers of the heart

1. Term bradyarrhythmia
   Divide _____

   Define _____

2. Term diaphoresis
   Divide _____

   Define _____

3. Term dyslipidemia
   Divide _____

   Define _____

4. Term echocardiogram
   Divide _____

   Define _____

5. Term endarterectomy
   Divide _____

   Define _____

6. Term endocarditis
   Divide _____

   Define _____

7. Term dysfunction
   Divide _____

   Define _____

8. Term hypokinesis
   Divide _____

   Define _____

9. Term hemodynamically
   Divide _____

   Define _____

10. Term hyperlipidemia
    Divide _____

    Define _____

11. Term infraclavicular
    Divide _____

    Define _____

12. Term interstitial
    Divide _____

    Define _____

13. Term ischemic
    Divide _____

    Define _____

14. Term isorhythmic
    Divide _____

    Define _____

15. Term thrombolytic
    Divide _____

    Define _____

16. Term regurgitation
    Divide _____

    Define _____

17. Term   nephrotoxicity
    Divide   _____
               _____
    Define   _____

18. Term   orthostatic
    Divide   _____
               _____
    Define   _____

19. Term   percutaneous
    Divide   _____
               _____
    Define   _____

20. Term   pneumothorax
    Divide   _____
               _____
    Define   _____

21. Term   revascularization
    Divide   _____
               _____
    Define   _____

22. Term   substernal
    Divide   _____
               _____
    Define   _____

23. Term   supraventricular
    Divide   _____
               _____
    Define   _____

24. Term   thrombocytopenia
    Divide   _____
               _____
    Define   _____

25. Term: transesophageal (echocardiogram)
    Divide   _____
               _____
    Define   _____

26. Term   unifocal
    Divide   _____
               _____
    Define   _____

Pharmacology

___ 1. Which of the following drugs is an anti-arrhythmic?
     A. Lasix.
     B. Tridil.
     C. Mexitil.
     D. Avapro.

___ 2. Which of the following generic drugs does not belong in the group with the others?
     A. diltiazem.
     B. quinapril.
     C. nifedipine.
     D. verapamil.

___ 3. Which of the following drugs is NOT included in the class of drugs known as angiotensin II antagonists?
     A. Isordil.
     B. Atacand.
     C. Cozaar.
     D. Avapro.

___ 4. If a patient had angina pectoris, you might expect the physician to prescribe which one of the following generic drugs?
     A. amiodarone.
     B. nitroglycerin.
     C. furosemide.
     D. gemfibrozil.

___ 5. Patients might need to be concerned about potassium loss when taking which of the following class of drugs?
     A. diuretics.
     B. digitalis.
     C. beta blockers.
     D. ACE inhibitors.

___ 6. Which of the following generic drugs is rarely used, except in the treatment of congestive heart failure, because of its unpredictable dosage requirements and risk of toxicity?
     A. captopril.
     B. digoxin.
     C. clonidine.
     D. metoprolol.

___ 7. Which of the following generic drugs is NOT used to treat patients with hyperlipidemia?
A. simvastatin.
B. fenofibrate.
C. atorvastatin.
D. hydrochlorothiazide.

___ 8. If a patient had essential hypertension, you might expect the physician to prescribe which one of the following generic drugs?
A. dopamine.
B. pravastatin.
C. spironolactone.
D. cholestyramine.

___ 9. Which of the following drugs is used to prevent thrombosis of coronary and cerebral arteries in persons at risk of myocardial infarction or stroke and to prevent or treat deep venous thrombosis?
A. Coumadin (warfarin).
B. Activase (alteplase).
C. Streptase (streptokinase).
D. Abbokinase (urokinase).

___ 10. Which of the following drugs is used in the treatment of hypertension and congestive heart failure because it promotes vasodilatation, decreasing pulmonary and peripheral vascular resistance, thus lowering arterial pressure and cardiac work load?
A. Norvasc (amlodipine).
B. Catapres (clonidine).
C. Sorbitrate (isosorbide dinitrate).
D. Capoten (captopril).

___ 11. Nitroglycerin ointment is measured in _____
A. inches.
B. grams.
C. milligrams.
D. units.

Spelling Exercise

Instructions: Review the adjective and adverb suffixes in your medical language textbook. Test your knowledge of **adjectives** by writing the adjectival form of the following cardiology words. Consult a medical dictionary to verify your spelling.

Noun	Adjective
1. angina	_____
2. angiographic	_____
3. anulus	_____
4. aorta	_____
5. apex	_____
6. atrium	_____
7. base	_____
8. cicatrix	_____
9. diastole	_____
10. diuresis	_____
11. dyslipidemia	_____
12. dyspnea	_____
13. ectopy	_____
14. hemodynamic	_____
15. implant	_____
16. ischemia	_____
17. myocardium	_____
18. obstruct	_____
19. sclera	_____
20. stenosis	_____
21. systole	_____
22. tachycardia	_____
23. thrombosis	_____
24. valve	_____
25. ventricle	_____

Abbreviations Exercise

Instructions: Expand the following common cardiology abbreviations and brief forms. Then memorize both abbreviations and definitions to increase your speed and accuracy in transcribing cardiology dictation.

Abbreviation   **Expansion**

1. APCs _____
   (inhibitor)
2. APCs _____
3. ARDS _____
4. AV (block) _____
5. AV _____
   (anastomosis)
6. BMP _____
7. BNP _____
8. BT _____
   (ligation, shunt)
9. CABG _____
10. cath _____
11. cath'd _____
12. circ _____
13. CK _____
14. coags _____
15. COPD _____
16. CVP _____
17. DNI/DNR _____
18. EOMI _____
19. EF _____
20. H&H _____
21. JVD _____
22. K _____
23. LAD _____
24. LIMA _____
25. LV _____
26. LVEF _____
27. lytes _____
28. lytics _____
29. MAP _____
30. mets _____
    (unit of measure)
31. MI _____
32. PACs _____
33. PDA _____
    (heart defect)
34. PDA _____
    (coronary artery)
35. PND _____
    (night-time shortness of breath)
36. PTCA _____
37. PVCs _____
38. PVR _____
39. RCA _____
40. RV _____
41. PA _____
42. SOB _____
43. SVT _____
44. TEE _____
45. vein _____
46. VSD _____

Transcript Forensics

This section presents snippets of transcribed dictations from clinic notes; history and physical examinations and consultations; operative reports and procedure notes; and discharge summaries. Explain the passage so that a nonmedical person can understand it. Pay particular attention to terms that are in bold type.

Example

Excerpt: On initial assessment, the patient was **hemodynamically stable** and complained of mild chest pain, **dyspnea, fatigue,** and diaphoresis.

Explanation: When the patient was first examined, blood pressure and pulse were normal but the patient complained of chest pain, shortness of breath, tiredness, and sweating.

1. **Excerpt:** A family history of intermittent **palpitations** and **syncope** in his brother raised suspicion for **ventricular tachycardia.**

Explanation: _____
_____
_____
_____
_____
_____
_____

2. **Excerpt:** At that point, 3 blood cultures came back positive for **enterococcus**. The patient, who has mitral valve disease, had no recent dental work and does use **antibiotic prophylaxis**.

Explanation: _____

_____

_____

_____

_____

3. **Excerpt:** Assessment: **Exertional dyspnea. Status post** aortic valve replacement with normal functioning **bioprosthetic aortic valve** by echocardiography. **Dyslipidemia.**

Explanation: _____

_____

_____

_____

_____

_____

4. **Excerpt:** CHEST: Examination revealed **diminished breath sounds** at the bases with mild **basilar crackles**. Otherwise clear to **percussion and auscultation**.

Explanation: _____

_____

_____

_____

_____

_____

5. **Excerpt:** The patient has also had a **biventricular pacemaker** and **defibrillator** placed. He currently complains of chest pain with any type of exertion. He states that with any walking he will develop **angina** and have to stop and rest. It is usually relieved with rest. He is on chronic **nitrate therapy**.

Explanation: _____

_____

_____

_____

6. **Excerpt:** This is a patient who, of course, given the history of **cardiomyopathy** with such **compromised ejection fraction,** is at risk for having not only atrial but also **ventricular arrhythmias**.

Explanation: _____

_____

_____

_____

_____

7. **Excerpt:** Left **ventriculography** revealed **akinesis** of the **anterior apical wall** with **global hypokinesis** and a **dilated left ventricle**. The catheterization report estimates an **ejection fraction** at 25%.

Explanation: _____

_____

_____

_____

_____

_____

8. **Excerpt:** This is a 9-month-old female presenting for repair of a severe **coarctation of her aorta** with arch hypoplasia. She underwent a Rastelli procedure including a Blalock-Taussig ligation, a **ventricular septal defect (VSD) repair,** and a **pulmonary homograft** right ventricle to pulmonary artery conduit.

Explanation: _____

_____

_____

_____

_____

9. **Excerpt:** He has an **ejection fraction** of about 25%, or probably lower, with **ischemic cardiomyopathy**. We would observe him and give him **supportive medical therapy** without any cardiac **invasive therapies**.

Explanation: _____

_____

_____

_____

Sample Reports

Sample cardiology reports appear on the following pages, illustrating a variety of reports. Fictional names are provided for illustration of proper format, and no resemblance to actual persons is intended. Sample transcripts were prepared according to *The Book of Style for Medical Transcription* (AHDI).

History and Physical Examination

OLSEN, NATALIE
Hospital #123456
Date of Admission: 11/17/[add year]
Attending Physician: Joseph Pieper, MD

CHIEF COMPLAINT
Chest pain.

HISTORY OF PRESENT ILLNESS
This 65-year-old white female was admitted to the hospital with chest pain on the night of admission. This lasted off and on for some time, for probably several hours. It was not relieved by nitroglycerin, and because of this she presented herself to the emergency department. She also has type 1 diabetes mellitus, and her sugars are sporadically in the 300–400 range. She has been unable to lose weight and is grossly obese.

PAST MEDICAL HISTORY
Please see old records for past medical history.

SOCIAL AND FAMILY HISTORY
See old records.

REVIEW OF SYSTEMS
GENERAL: System review is essentially unchanged from the last admission. She has occasional headaches.
HEENT: There is some decrease in her hearing.
Cardiorespiratory: She has cough and congestion but no pneumonia or tuberculosis (TB).
Gastrointestinal: Appetite and digestion have been good, and she has not had any GI bleeding.
Genitourinary: She has no urgency, frequency, or dysuria, but she has had urinary tract infections in the past.
Neuromuscular: Negative.
Musculoskeletal: Positive history for arthritis.

(continued)

History and Physical Examination *(continued)*

OLSEN, NATALIE
Hospital #123456
Date of Admission: 11/17/[add year]
Page 2

PHYSICAL EXAMINATION
VITAL SIGNS: Blood pressure is 140/80, pulse is 88 and regular, respirations 16 and regular.
GENERAL: This is a well-developed, obese female complaining of chest pain and shortness of breath.
HEENT: Head is normocephalic. She has bilateral arcus senilis and compensated edentulism
NECK: Neck is supple. No bruits noted.
BREASTS: Breasts are without masses.
LUNGS: Lungs reveal scattered wheezes and basilar rales.
HEART: Heart reveals a regular sinus rhythm. She has a soft apical murmur.
ABDOMEN: Abdomen is 4+ protuberant. No masses are felt.
EXTREMITIES: Unremarkable with the exception of 1+ edema. Peripheral pulses are diminished but present.
NEUROLOGIC: Reflexes are equal and active. Neurologic is physiologic.

IMPRESSION
1. Arteriosclerotic heart disease with chest pain and congestive heart failure. Rule out myocardial infarction.
2. Diabetes mellitus.
3. Exogenous obesity.
4. Degenerative osteoarthritis.

JOSEPH PIEPER, MD

JP:hpi
D&T: 11/17/[add year]

Emergency Department Note

PASQUALETTI, MARCUS
#9463452
12/17/[add year]

CHIEF COMPLAINT
Left-sided chest pain.

HISTORY OF PRESENT ILLNESS
This is a 62-year-old male who said that he fell yesterday afternoon. He said that he tripped while walking on the pavement and fell down onto his left side. This fall did not knock the wind out of him or cause a loss of consciousness, but he said it was a significant fall with pain in the left side of his chest. He was able to get up. There was no shortness of breath. He felt better, although he had some pain on the left side of his chest wall. He was able to sleep through the night, but this morning he continues to have pain in this area. It is worsened by any type of twisting or moving of his upper torso. He does not have shortness of breath or substernal chest pain, however. No abdominal pain, no nausea, no vomiting, no weakness or dizziness, and no other focal injuries. He comes into the emergency department for evaluation.

PAST MEDICAL HISTORY
Notable for diabetes, coronary artery disease, renal insufficiency, anemia, hypertension.

MEDICATIONS
Medications include Zaroxolyn, Lasix, Actos, spironolactone, and Lipitor.

ALLERGIES
No known drug allergies.

SOCIAL HISTORY
He lives at home, takes care of himself. No current smoking. He was a prior smoker.

REVIEW OF SYSTEMS
See my history of present illness and past medical history. Note the history of heart disease and diabetes. Note the recent fall. He has not had any similar pain. He does not have any weakness. No difficulty voiding, no nausea, no vomiting, no shortness of breath, no fevers, and no abdominal pain. All other systems are negative.

PHYSICAL EXAMINATION
VITAL SIGNS: On exam, pulse was 88, respiratory rate 18, blood pressure 132/97, pulse oximetry 98% on room air.
HEENT: Normocephalic, atraumatic. Mucous membranes pink and moist; oropharynx unremarkable.
NECK: Supple, nontender, no midline pain. Full range of motion.
LUNGS: Lungs reveal clear breath sounds bilaterally.

(continued)

Emergency Department Note *(continued)*

PASQUALETTI, MARCUS
#9463452
11/17/[add year]
Page 2

HEART: Regular rate and rhythm, normal S1 and S2, no murmurs, rubs, or gallops. He does have palpable chest wall pain on the left side of his chest in the midaxillary line, and this palpable pain extends around and under his left scapula. The pain seems to be aggravated when he tries to roll in bed. As long as he is sitting still, the pain is improved. There is no pain with deep inspiration.
ABDOMEN: Has bowel sounds, is soft and nontender and otherwise unremarkable. Specifically, there is no right or left upper quadrant pain.
PELVIS: Stable.
EXTREMITIES: Neurovascularly intact, 2+ radial pulses bilaterally, 2+ dorsalis pedis pulses bilaterally. Normal strength to flexion and extension in the lower and upper extremities. There is no pain with passive or active movement of the left arm.

HOSPITAL COURSE
I gave the patient a Lortab and we did a PA and lateral chest x-ray. This PA and lateral chest x-ray does not show any focal rib fractures, no effusions, no pneumothorax or other abnormalities. I have observed him now for over an hour. He is hemodynamically stable. He does have very focal reproducible pain on my exam, consistent with the mechanism of his fall. I think he has a chest wall contusion and may in fact have a rib fracture that we are not seeing on the x-ray. I discussed all this at length with the patient. I think he can be sent home with close followup. I gave him some Lortab to take for pain control. He will return immediately if he has worsening pain, shortness of breath, fever, weakness, or other symptoms of concern.

FRANKLIN TESSIER, MD

FT: hpi
d: 11/17/[add year]
t: 11/17/[add year]

Discharge Summary

PRING, ROBERT
#372941

DATE OF ADMISSION
6/21/[add year]

DATE OF DISCHARGE
6/26/[add year]

BRIEF HISTORY
This is a 60-year-old gentleman who underwent a stress test on June 6. He had several risk factors for coronary artery disease to include adult-onset diabetes mellitus, hypertension, obesity, and hyperlipidemia. He was only able to exercise for 4 minutes before demonstrating some significant ST-segment depressions. He eventually underwent a cardiac catheterization on June 12. This confirmed severe multivessel coronary artery disease. In view of these findings, surgical consultation was requested.

The patient was seen initially by Dr. _____ in his office, and after reviewing his situation and films, surgical myocardial revascularization was recommended, and he was admitted on this occasion for that purpose.

HOSPITAL COURSE
Following admission, he underwent a presurgical and preanesthetic evaluation. He was taken to the operating room on June 21. At that time, a coronary artery bypass graft operation x3 was performed. The left internal mammary artery was utilized as a conduit to bypass the 1.75 mm left anterior descending artery. Greater saphenous vein was also harvested and utilized to bypass the 2.5 mm mid obtuse marginal artery and a 1.75 mm right coronary artery.

Postoperatively, he was taken to CVICU in stable condition on no inotropic support. By the 1st postoperative morning, he was weaned from mechanical ventilation, extubated without any problems. Later, on the 1st postoperative day, the chest tubes and pacing wires were removed without any sequelae. On the 2nd postoperative day, we were able to transfer him to the PCU and monitor him on telemetry. The remainder of the hospital course was essentially unremarkable with the exception of requiring some aggressive pulmonary care secondary to his chronic obstructive pulmonary disease and probable chronic bronchitis. Despite this, he did progress well and was able to be discharged on postoperative day #5.

CONDITION ON DISCHARGE
Good.

(continued)

Discharge Summary *(continued)*

PRING, ROBERT
#372941
Page 2

DISCHARGE INSTRUCTIONS
He was appropriately instructed on wound incision care. He is not to lift any heavy objects over 5 pounds or drive a car for the next month. He will resume an American Heart Association diet. He will have a 2- to 3-week followup visit with both Dr. _____ and Dr. _____. He will take the following medications:
1. Darvocet-N 100, one to two tablets every 3 to 4 hours as needed for pain.
2. Lipitor 40 mg daily.
3. Zestril 10 mg daily.
4. Aspirin 81 mg daily.
5. He was also to continue taking his calcium supplements, vitamin D supplements and vitamin K supplements as he was taking at home.

FINAL DIAGNOSIS
Coronary artery disease.

PROCEDURES
Coronary artery bypass graft operation x3.

COMPLICATIONS
None.

HIEU PHAN, MD

HP: hpi

d: 6/27/[add year]
t: 6:28/[add year]

Comic Relief

She was seen at the emergency department last night for an episode of profound weakness and light-heartedness. (light-headedness).

The patient's blood pressure was enlarged to the left.

She is also taking quinine for leg cramps and high blood pressure which is pink.

The patient said she was too sick to be in the hospital and would return when she felt better.

d: The patient had a positive Homans sign.
t: The patient had a positive home inside.

d: Murmurs, gallops, and rubs
t: Memories, scallops, and rubs

d: The patient had a rapid heart beat.
t: The patient had a rabbit heart beat.

d: Heart and great vessels
t: Heart and engraved vessels

d: The patient had a syncopal episode.
t: The patient had a sink bowel episode.

Urology and Nephrology

Learning Objectives

▶ Describe the structure and function of the urinary tract and male reproductive system.

▶ Spell and define common genitourinary terms.

▶ Identify genitourinary vocabulary that might be used in the review of systems.

▶ Describe the negative and positive findings a physician looks for on examination of the external genitalia and male reproductive system.

▶ Describe the typical cause, course, and treatment options for common diseases of the excretory and male reproductive system.

▶ Identify and define common diagnostic and surgical procedures of the genitourinary system.

▶ List common genitourinary laboratory tests and procedures.

▶ Identify and describe common genitourinary drugs and their uses.

▶ Demonstrate knowledge of anatomical, medical, pharmacological, adjectival, and soundalike terms by accurately completing the exercises in this chapter.

Transcribing Urology and Nephrology Dictation

Introduction

Urology is a medical and surgical specialty concerned with the diagnosis and treatment of structural abnormalities, diseases, and injuries of the **genitourinary (GU) system**, which traditionally includes not only the kidneys and urinary tract but also the male reproductive organs. The female reproductive system and the relevant specialties of obstetrics and gynecology are discussed in Chapter 14. **Nephrology** is a branch of internal medicine devoted to the nonsurgical management of disorders of the kidney.

Anatomy Review

The **excretory system** includes the **kidneys**, the **ureters**, the **bladder**, and the **urethra** (see ■ Figures 13-1, 13-2, 13-3, 13-4).

The kidneys are paired, bean-shaped organs lying behind the abdominal cavity on either side of the aorta. The kidney is enclosed by a smooth connective tissue capsule somewhat like the skin of a sausage. The capsule can easily be peeled away from a normal kidney (although this does tear through a meshwork of

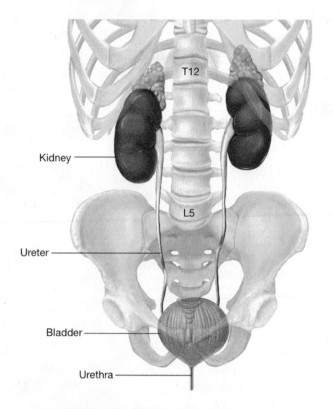

FIGURE 13-1. Position of the urinary organs

KIDNEYS, MORE THAN A FILTER

Everyone knows that the heart, the lungs, and the brain are vital organs—that is, that their absence or destruction is incompatible with life. But several other bodily structures, including the kidneys, are equally indispensable. The kidneys perform many highly selective excretory functions, reabsorbing most of the water that they filter and many of the substances dissolved in it, but also actively eliminating certain other substances from the blood.

The kidneys are paired structures whose shape is so familiar that expressions like *kidney beans* and *kidney-shaped swimming pool* are readily understood by all. They lie on either side of the midline just below the posterior attachments of the diaphragm, at the level of the twelfth rib and the first three lumbar vertebrae—much higher than lay persons usually seem to think. The right kidney is slightly lower than the left, probably because of the presence of the liver above it.

Each kidney is surrounded by a cushioning envelope of fat (perinephric fat) and lies deeply imbedded in the posterior abdominal wall. The kidneys are retroperitoneal, that is, they lie behind and outside the peritoneal cavity, which encloses most of the abdominal organs (stomach, small intestine, liver, spleen, and most of the large intestine).

Each kidney is about 12 cm in height, 6 cm in breadth, 3 cm in thickness, and weighs about 150 g. That's very close to the proportions, size, and weight of a standard computer mouse.

fine blood vessels), but not from one that has been scarred by chronic inflammation or infarction.

The principal functions of the kidney are the excretion of water and waste materials and the maintenance of water and electrolyte balance. Each kidney consists of an outer **cortex** (pl., **cortices**) and an inner **medulla** enclosing a funnel-shaped central cavity, the pelvis of the kidney. The cortex contains hundreds of

Kidneys: The kidneys have a thin capsule. The cortices show glomeruli of normal appearance. The tubules are not remarkable. The interstitial tissue shows no noteworthy change. The pelves are not remarkable.

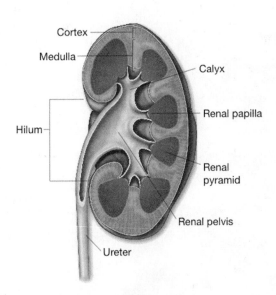

FIGURE 13-2. Kidney internal structures

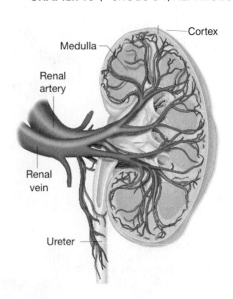

FIGURE 13-3. Kidney structure showing renal artery, vein, ureter

thousands of microscopic filtering units called renal corpuscles. In each of these a tangle of capillaries called a **glomerulus** (pl., **glomeruli**) is enveloped by a membranous cup, **Bowman capsule**, from which a renal tubule arises. The medulla is an intricate mesh-work of these tubules, where filtered water and other substances are selectively reabsorbed into the blood. The tubules empty their secretion into the pelvis (pl., **pelves**) of the kidney, from which it flows downward through the ureter and into the bladder. Each kidney has a pronounced **hilum** or notch at which an artery, a vein, and a ureter are attached.

The **urethra**, the outflow tract of the bladder, differs in the two sexes. The female urethra is short, emptying near the vestibule of the vagina but otherwise inde-pendent of the female reproductive system. The male urethra passes through the penis and in addition to its function in emptying the bladder, it serves as the chan-nel for the ejaculation of semen.

The **male reproductive system** (see ■ Figure 13-4) consists of the paired **testes (testicles)**, each with its collecting system (the **epididymis**, a coiled tubular structure attached to the testicle; and the **spermatic duct** or **vas deferens**, a tube that conducts sperm to the prostate), the **penis**, the **scrotum** (a cutaneous sac con-taining the testicles), the **prostate** (a gland surrounding the urethra just below the bladder), and the **seminal vesicles** (small pouchlike glands adjacent to the vas def-erens).

The **testicle** produces **spermatozoa** (sing., **sperma-tozoon**), each one of which is capable of fertilizing a female oocyte and carries the paternal contribution to the genetic makeup of the offspring. In addition, the testicles produce male hormones that are responsible for the development and maintenance of secondary sex-ual characteristics (facial and body hair, male body build, deep voice).

The **prostate** contains secretory cells that produce the fluid component of semen. It also contains smooth muscle, and under sexual stimulation it closes off the bladder from the urethra and brings about ejaculation of semen (prostatic fluid + spermatozoa) through the urethra.

Pause for Reflection

1. The renal artery, vein, and a ureter are attached to the kidney at a pronounced depression or pit in the kidney referred to as the _____.
2. What is the function of the testes? What is another name for the testes?
3. The _____ is a coiled tubular collecting system attached to the testicle; and the tube that conducts sperm to the prostate is called the _____.
4. Describe the location and list two functions of the prostate gland.

Vocabulary Review

acute tubular necrosis A generalized failure of the renal tubules to perform their excretory functions. Also referred to as *renal shutdown* or *shock kidney*.

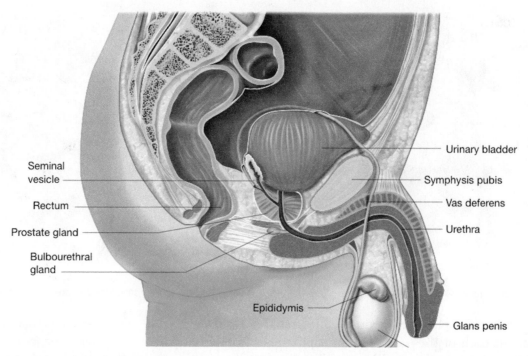

FIGURE 13-4. Male reproductive system, sagittal section, showing the organs of the pelvic cavity

adenocarcinoma of the prostate The most common malignancy of the prostate, it arises from glandular epithelium. Like benign prostatic hyperplasia (BPH), prostate cancer is an overgrowth of hormone-sensitive secretory cells.

albuminuria The presence of protein (proteinuria), not necessarily albumin, in the urine.

anuria Total cessation of urinary output.

azotemia See *uremia*.

bacteriuria The presence of bacteria in the urine.

benign prostatic hyperplasia (BPH) An overgrowth of androgen-sensitive glandular tissue that normally accompanies aging and causing varying degrees of urinary obstruction. It does not evolve into cancer.

bilirubinuria The presence of bilirubin in the urine resulting from liver disease or biliary duct obstruction.

calculus (pl., **calculi**) Stone; abnormal concretion, usually of mineral salts. May be found in the kidneys (renal calculi), bladder, and ureters. Can usually be successfully crushed in situ and the fragments flushed out by means of a cystoscope, but ESWL or an open procedure (generally laparoscopic) may sometimes be appropriate.

casts Plugs of material formed in renal tubules, detected on urinalysis. Casts are always abnormal.

condyloma (pl., **condylomata**) Genital wart.

cryptorchidism Failure of one or both of the testes to descend into the scrotum; also *cryptorchism* and *undescended testicle* (see ■ Figure 13-5).

crystals Detected on urinalysis.

Cushing syndrome Truncal obesity, moon facies, hypertension, impairment of glucose tolerance, osteoporosis, and other metabolic abnormalities caused by an excess of adrenocortical steroid, either from a tumor or hyperactivity of the adrenal gland or as a result of prolonged therapeutic administration of hormone.

dipstick A commercially produced strip of plastic or paper bearing a series of dots or squares of reagent, each designed to assess a specific chemical property of urine; often used to refer to the test itself.

diuresis An increase in the production of urine by the kidneys as a result of renal or systemic disease, toxic substances, or drugs administered to reduce body water, sodium, or both.

double-J stent A ureteral stent of flexible material with a J-shaped curl at each end, one to anchor the stent in the renal pelvis and the other to anchor it in the bladder.

dribbling Uncontrollable passage of drops of urine, particularly just after voiding.

dysuria Pain with urination.

enuresis Urinary incontinence. Do not confuse with *anuresis* (inability to urinate). See *anuria*.

E. (Escherichia) coli Gram-negative bacterium normally found in the intestine and responsible for many urinary tract infections.

Gleason score A numerical indicator of the malignant potential of prostatic carcinoma, determined by adding the grades of the two least differentiated biopsy specimens.

glycosuria The abnormal presence of glucose in the urine.

hematuria Blood in the urine.

hemoglobinuria Excretion of hemoglobin from broken-down red blood cells, as in transfusion reaction, sickle cell anemia, and malaria.

hesitancy Difficulty initiating the urinary flow.

holmium:YAG laser system Used with both percutaneous neophrolitholapaxy and ureteroscopic procedures.

hydrocele A circumscribed collection of fluid, especially a collection of fluid in the serous membrane covering the front and sides of the testis and epididymis (tunica vaginalis testis) or along the spermatic cord (see ■ Figure 13-6).

hydroureter Distention of the renal pelvis due to filling of the ureters and renal pelves with urine under pressure (see ■ Figure 13-9).

Patient is a 62-year-old white male with bladder outlet obstructive symptoms. These include hesitancy, a decrease in the force and strength of urinary stream, nocturia x0-3, urgency with some mild urge incontinence. Patient also makes note of terminal dribbling. Denies any stopping and starting of stream once stream has been established.

hydronephrosis Distention of the renal pelvis due to filling of the ureters and renal pelves with urine under pressure (see ■ Figure 13-9).

hyperbilirubinemia High concentrations of bilirubin in the blood causing yellowing of the skin and mucous membranes (jaundice).

hypovolemia A significantly decreased volume of circulating blood, usually due to excessive blood loss.

incontinence Involuntary passage of urine or stool.

ketonuria The abnormal presence of ketones in the urine.

KUB A plain radiograph of the kidneys, ureters, and urinary bladder. When dictated, it need not be expanded.

lues ("loo-eez") Syphilis.

micturition Voiding; urination.

nephritis Inflammation of the kidney.

nephron The anatomic and functional unit formed by a glomerulus and its renal tubule.

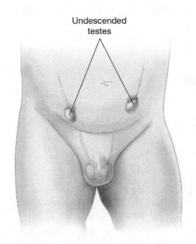

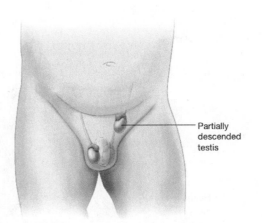

A   B

FIGURE 13-5. Cryptorchidism showing (A) undescended testes and (B) a partially descended testis..

LAY AND MEDICAL TERMS

the clap	gonorrhea
kidney stone	renal calculus
	nephrolithiasis
	renal lithiasis
pass water, pee, piss	urinate, micturate, void

---

nocturia Being awakened at night by the urge to void.

obstructive uropathy Disease or pathology of the urinary tract caused by obstruction.

occult blood Blood in the urine in such small amounts as to be undetected by the naked eye.

oliguria Marked reduction in the volume of urine excreted in 24 hours.

pH A measure of alkalinity or acidity.

pollakiuria Increased frequency of urination without increase in total volume excreted in 24 hours.

polyuria Increase in the 24-hour excretion of urine.

postvoiding dribbling Difficulty in stopping urination.

postvoiding residual Urine remaining in the bladder, as detected by catheterization after the patient has voided.

An intravenous pyelogram (IVP) showed a distended urinary bladder with a large postvoid residual.

proteinuria The abnormal presence of protein in the urine.

pyuria The presence of pus or pus cells (neutrophils) in voided urine.

radical In surgery, directed to the cause; directed to the root or source of a morbid process; it usually means removal of an entire organ or body part along with surrounding structures and sometimes lymph nodes.

reflux The backward flow of urine within any part of the urinary tract.

renal failure A severe decline in kidney function, with retention of urea, creatinine, potassium, and other substances normally excreted. Acute renal failure refers to abrupt onset.

renal hypertension The type of high blood pressure resulting directly from compromise of the circulation in at least one kidney.

rhabdomyolysis Rapid destruction of skeletal muscle tissue, associated with excretion of myoglobin in the urine. Myoglobin is harmful to the kidney and often causes kidney damage. Causes include excessive exercise, dehydration, severe burns, electrolyte imbalance, and medications.

seminal vesicles Small sac-like glands adjacent to the spermatic duct.

The testis showed a pink, fleshy, well-circumscribed mass consistent with seminoma.

spermatocele An abnormal sac (cyst) filled with milky or clear fluid that may contain sperm that develops in the epididymis. Generally painless and noncancerous but if a spermatocele grows large enough to cause discomfort, surgery can be performed (see ■ Figure 13-6).

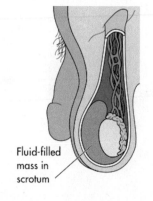
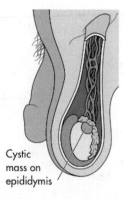
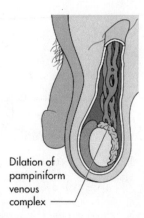

Fluid-filled mass in scrotum

Cystic mass on epididymis

Dilation of pampiniform venous complex

FIGURE 13-6. Hydrocele, spermatocele, and varicocele

stress incontinence Loss of urine when mechanical stress is placed on the bladder, as by coughing, laughing, sneezing, straining, or change in position.

TNTC (too numerous to count). This usually refers to a very large number of red blood cells or white blood cells seen on microscopic examination of urine. Because any number higher than 15–20 cells per high-power field indicates significant hematuria or pyuria, an exact count of 50 or more cells would provide no additional useful information. Doctors frequently dictate simply *TNTC*.

trabeculation Strands or bands of connective tissue sometimes extending from the capsule into the substance of an organ. Trabeculation of the bladder may be a secondary result of a bladder outlet obstruction due to hypertrophy and hyperplasia of the bladder muscle and the infiltration of the connective tissue.

uremia The buildup of urea and other nitrogenous wastes in the blood as a result of renal failure.

ureteral stent A flexible tube placed within a ureter to maintain its patency .

ureteropelvic junction (UPJ) The origin of the ureter from the renal pelvis.

ureterovesical junction (UVJ) The point at which a ureter enters the urinary bladder.

urinary tract infection (UTI) Infection of the bladder or of one or both ureters or kidneys (see ■ Figure 13-11).

varicocele Varicosities of the veins of the epididymis and testis accompanied by a constant pulling, dragging, or dull pain in the scrotum and a bluish appearance of the skin of the scrotum (see ■ Figure 13-6).

Medical Readings

History and Physical Examination
by John H. Dirckx, MD

Review of Systems: Kidneys and Urinary Tract. The kidneys and urinary tract (ureters, bladder, and urethra) and the reproductive system are considered together because of their close anatomic association and the frequency with which one disease affects both organ systems.

A thorough review of genitourinary history includes past diagnoses of congenital anomalies of the urinary or

There is a golf ball-sized left scrotal mass which is exquisitely tender. The mass is indistinguishable from the testicle and appears to lie in a horizontal position. The inferior portion of the scrotum transilluminates. The superior portion does not. The cord structures are palpable. There is no evidence of hernia. The right testicle is within normal limits.

genital tract; urinary tract infections; stone in a kidney, ureter, or bladder; sexually transmitted diseases; genitourinary surgery; and, for women, menstrual and reproductive history.

Symptoms suggesting renal or urinary tract disease are pain in one or both flanks, increase in frequency of urination (as opposed to increase in urine volume), **nocturia** (being awakened at night by the urge to void), burning or pain on voiding, difficulty voiding, diminution in the urinary stream, incontinence of urine, bedwetting in an older child or adult, blood in the urine, and any other marked change in the appearance of the urine.

Men are questioned about **urethral discharge** or burning; itching, rash, ulcers, or other lesions of the genitals; pain or swelling in the testicles; scrotal masses; and infertility.

Most persons are reticent about sexual matters, and not much is gained by determined probing unless the chief complaint involves the reproductive system in some way. When necessary, the interviewer may ask about the subject's sexual preference, frequency of sexual activity, number of different partners, participation in oral or anal sex, masturbation, and satisfaction with sexual activity. In addition, men are asked about difficulty in achieving or maintaining erections and premature or delayed ejaculation, women about pain during intercourse and any difficulty in attaining orgasm.

Physical Examination. With the patient standing, the physician inspects the **penis** and **scrotum** for dermatitis, ulcers, scars, and other skin lesions. The penis is assessed for developmental abnormalities, and the foreskin, if present, is retracted for inspection of the **glans**. The **urethra** may be milked to express any discharge. The scrotal contents are palpated, and any masses, testicular enlargement or deformity, or tenderness is noted. If one or both testicles are not felt in the scrotum, an attempt is made to locate them in the inguinal canals (**undescended testis, cryptorchidism**) (see ■ Figure 13-5).

Scrotal masses are assessed by **transillumination**. A bright focal light is placed behind and in contact with the scrotum, and the room lights extinguished. A cyst or hydrocele will transmit light; a solid tumor or hernia will not.

In a **digital rectal examination (DRE)** a gloved and lubricated finger is inserted into the rectum and gently rotated 360º to assess the internal surface of the rectum and the surrounding pelvic structures. The prostate is palpated for size, consistency, symmetry, and tenderness (see ■ Figure 13-7). The female genitourinary examination is discussed in Chapter 14, Obstetrics and Gynecology.

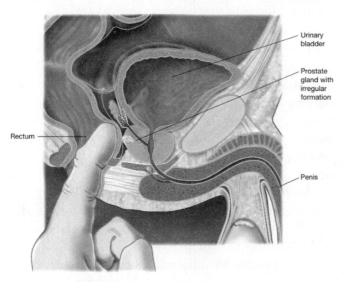

FIGURE 13-7. Digital rectal examination

Digital rectal exam showed a 45 g diffusely firm, non-suspicious prostate.

Pause for Reflection

1. List four symptoms that suggest renal or urinary tract disease.
2. The medical term for being awakened at night by the urge to void is _____.
3. On physical exam, inspection of the penis and scrotum is carried out to identify _____.
4. If one or both testicles are not felt in the scrotum, the patient may have a condition referred to as _____ or _____.
5. How is transillumination used to assess scrotal masses?

Urolithiasis

by John H. Dirckx, MD

Urolithiasis, the formation of stonelike concretions (calculi) in the urinary tract, is a common disorder and a significant cause of human suffering (see ■ Figure 13-8). Approximately 5% of the U.S. population will experience symptoms due to urinary calculi at some time during their lives. **Ureteral colic**, the pain that occurs when a stone that has formed in a kidney moves down and becomes lodged in the ureter, has been likened in severity to the pangs of childbirth. Persistent obstruction to the flow of urine by a stone often results in infection and may eventually cause kidney damage or destruction. Procedures to remove urinary calculi, including shock-wave lithotripsy, are among those most commonly performed by urologists.

The peak incidence of symptomatic urinary tract stones is between 20 and 60 years of age. Stone formation is 3–4 times as common in men as in women. Because calculi in the urinary tract may cause no symptoms, and because most stones that become lodged in a ureter eventually pass without treatment, the overall prevalence of urolithiasis is difficult to estimate.

Kidney stones. Stones form in the urinary tract for a variety of reasons. Most calculi that develop in the renal pelvis result from crystallization of salts that are present in abnormally high concentration in the urine. Such variations in the composition of the urine are usually due to metabolic or genetic factors. The great majority of renal calculi prove on analysis to be one of five types: calcium oxalate, calcium phosphate, ammoniomagnesium phosphate (struvite), uric acid, or cystine. A renal calculus may also form because of the presence of local disease (infection or necrosis of kidney tissue) or of urinary stasis due to an anatomic anomaly in the upper urinary tract.

In most instances, **urolithiasis** is first made manifest by the signal event of a stone slipping down from the renal pelvis into the ureter and getting stuck there. The typical clinical presentation of a stone in a ureter is the sudden onset of severe cramplike unilateral flank or abdominal pain radiating to the groin. This pain, which results from spasm in the muscle layer of the ureter triggered by the presence of an obstructing stone in its lumen, is often accompanied by nausea, vomiting, restlessness, and the passage of blood in the urine.

Physical examination may elicit only nonspecific tenderness at the site of pain. While laboratory detection of blood in the urine is strongly suggestive, a defin-

This is a 37-year-old white male, C4-5 quadriplegic secondary to motor vehicle accident, who has bilateral staghorn calculi filling the whole left renal pelvis. On the right there is a smaller amount of stone within the pelvis.

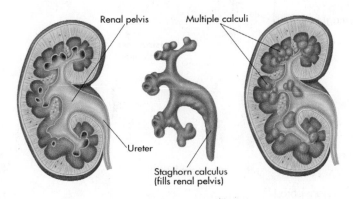

FIGURE 13-8. Staghorn calculus

itive diagnosis of urolithiasis requires either the demonstration of the **stone** by an imaging study or its retrieval after spontaneous passage or surgical extraction. An x-ray of the abdomen including the kidneys, ureters, and bladder (**KUB film**) is often the first diagnostic choice because it is inexpensive and requires no preparation.

Such studies, however, often miss small stones and cannot detect the 15% that are not radiopaque, such as uric acid stones. **Ultrasonography**, an attractive option because it involves no radiation, is disappointing in its ability to identify ureteral stones. Currently the imaging study of choice for the evaluation of acute flank pain is **non-enhanced, thin-cut helical computed tomography (CT)**, which can detect stones as small as 1 mm in diameter, regardless of their chemical composition.

Because about 95% of stones causing **ureteral colic** will pass spontaneously within 1–3 days, initial management consists of pain control and watchful waiting. Fluid intake is increased on the (unproved) assumption that a higher rate of urine flow will help flush out the obstructing stone. Ideally, all urine is strained so that if the stone is passed it can be identified and analyzed.

Indications for surgical extraction of a stone from the ureter include failure to pass spontaneously, ureteral obstruction with damming of urine above the obstruction to create **hydroureter** (distention of the ureter with urine) and **hydronephrosis** (distention of the renal pelvis) (see ■ Figure 13-9), and infection. The presence of a very large stone in a renal pelvis is also an indication for surgical intervention.

Currently the most frequently used mechanical treatment for urolithiasis is **ESWL (extracorporeal shock wave lithotripsy)**. First introduced in the 1980s, ESWL is a method of shattering stones in the urinary tract (also in the biliary tract) by means of ultrasound waves generated outside the body. This noninvasive procedure can break up more than 90% of urinary tract stones in adults, permitting passage of the fragments in the urine. The underlying physical principle is that, while soft tissues resist the impact of sound waves, rigid stones do not and are thus mechanically disrupted. At higher frequencies, some tissue injury may occur. The procedure is contraindicated in pregnancy, bleeding disorders, uncontrolled urinary tract infection, and some other conditions.

Hydration, analgesia, observation, and if stone does not pass within 72 hours or less, will probably recommend patient for ureteroscopy and stone basketing and, if needed, ultrasonic lithotripsy. If the stone cannot be mobilized downward, push-back and ESWL might be considered.

Earlier methods of ESWL required that the patient be immersed in a water bath. Nowadays the treatment head (**external lithotripter**) is applied directly to the patient's skin over the site of the stone and acoustic coupling is achieved by use of a topical gel. The procedure may be performed under general anesthesia or with analgesia and sedation. Fluoroscopic or ultrasonographic monitoring is maintained throughout. The most frequent adverse consequence of ESWL is *steinstrasse* (German, "stone street"), the impaction of fragments from a shattered stone in the lower ureter. Other postprocedure complications (ureteral pain, bleeding, infection) are uncommon. When ESWL fails to fragment a stone adequately, and in those patients for whom it is contraindicated, invasive procedures become necessary.

Ureteroscopy is the passage of an endoscope from outside the body through the urethra and the bladder into a ureter. The availability of flexible and increasingly sophisticated instruments (with digital camera chips and light-emitting diodes at their tips) has gained wide acceptance for ureteroscopy in the treatment not only of ureteral stones but also of those within the renal pelvis. Ureteroscopic procedures may be performed under intravenous sedation rather than general anesthesia.

Percutaneous nephrolitholapaxy is an alternative, minimally invasive surgical procedure for the extraction of stones from the renal pelvis by means of a rigid or flex-

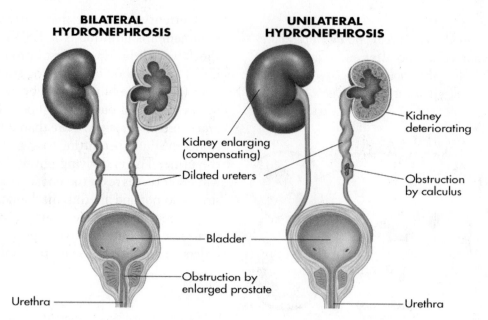

BILATERAL HYDRONEPHROSIS

UNILATERAL HYDRONEPHROSIS

Kidney enlarging (compensating)

Dilated ureters

Kidney deteriorating

Obstruction by calculus

Bladder

Obstruction by enlarged prostate

Urethra

Urethra

FIGURE 13-9. Hydronephrosis

ible endoscope (nephroscope) inserted through an incision in the skin overlying the kidney. This procedure is more feasible than a ureteral approach in children, and may be needed to manage very large renal stones.

Having gained endoscopic access to a stone, the urologist may remove it with forceps or a basket. A single-use **stone retrieval basket** consists of an open helical mesh formed by four strands of very fine nitinol wire, an alloy of nickel and titanium. Once a stone is snared between the wires, they are drawn tight around it. A tipless basket design permits grasping a stone wedged in a renal calyx with minimal risk of tissue injury.

The location, size, or physical characteristics of a stone may prevent successful use of either forceps or a basket. **Intracorporeal lithotripsy** involves the application of a shattering force directly to a stone by means of a device inserted endoscopically into the urinary tract. Electrohydraulic and pneumatic lithotripters function exactly like miniature jackhammers. Ultrasound systems are also available. The most widely used intracorporeal lithotripters at present employ laser technology. The **holmium:YAG system**, considered more efficient and safer than the neodymium:YAG, is currently preferred for use with both percutaneous nephrolitholapaxy and ureteroscopic procedures.

A **ureteral stent** is a flexible tube of biologically inert material that is placed within a ureter to maintain its patency despite the presence or continued formation of renal calculi. The stent is usually inserted from below through a cystoscope, and occupies the entire length of the ureter from the renal pelvis to the bladder. Each end

has a curl or pigtail (hence "**double-J stent**") to keep it from migrating out of its respective cavity. The presence of a stent may cause bladder pain, urinary frequency, or hematuria.

Depending on its purpose, a stent may be removed after a few days or left in place for 6–12 months. Stenting for 1-2 weeks may facilitate subsequent ureteroscopy by dilating the ureter. A stent that is intended to be removed after such a short period may have a string attached to its lower end, which protrudes from the urethra and is taped to the patient's leg. Removal is easily accomplished by traction on the string.

Bladder stones. The formation of a stone in the bladder nearly always reflects either local inflammation, such as that due to infection or radiation therapy, or **urinary stasis**, such as occurs with prostatic disease or after damage to bladder nerves (**neurogenic bladder**). Bladder stones generally consist of either calcium phosphate or uric acid. Occasionally a kidney stone may become arrested on its passage out of the body in the bladder, where it can serve as a nucleus for further stone formation.

Although frequently asymptomatic, a stone in the bladder can cause abdominal pain, pain or difficulty in urinating, urinary frequency, and hematuria. A large stone may be palpable on rectal examination, and imaging studies with or without intravenous injection of contrast material (**IVP, intravenous pyelogram**) are typically diagnostic. Lithotomy, the surgical removal of a bladder stone through an incision in either the lower abdomen or the perineum, was practiced in remote antiquity. Nowadays bladder stones can usually be successfully crushed in situ and the fragments flushed out by means of a cystoscope, but ESWL or an open procedure (generally laparoscopic) may sometimes be appropriate.

Pause for Reflection

1. Define urolithiasis and identify some of its causes.
2. The pain that occurs when a stone that has formed in a kidney moves down and becomes lodged in the ureter is called _____ and has been likened in severity to the pangs of childbirth.
3. Describe the typical clinical presentation of a ureteral stone.
4. How is definitive diagnosis of a ureteral stone made?
5. What are the indications for surgical intervention in the management of urolithiasis?
6. List the surgical treatment methods for urolithiasis.

Laboratory Examination of Urine

by John H. Dirckx, MD

In the modern clinical laboratory, microscopic examination and chemical analysis of urine can yield information not only about the urinary tract but also about other body systems, water and acid-base balance, nutrition, and the presence of toxic substances. A major advantage of urine examinations is that, under ordinary circumstances, specimens are readily available, without the need for invasive procedures or elaborate equipment.

For most of the tests done in the urinology laboratory, the preferred specimen is 60–90 mL of freshly voided urine. Although a random specimen is usually suitable, a **first-voided specimen** (the first urine passed after arising in the morning) may be more satisfactory in testing for trace substances because it is usually more concentrated.

A **clean-voided specimen (clean catch)** is one obtained after cleansing of the area around the urethral meatus (usually with liquid soap and cotton balls) to prevent contamination of the specimen with material from outside the urinary tract.

A **midstream specimen** is one that contains neither the first nor the last portion of urine passed. It is obtained by introducing a specimen container into the urine stream after voiding has begun and removing it

A clean-voided urine shows 15-20 white blood cells per high-power field, 8-10 red cells, 4+ occult blood, 1+ protein, negative for sugar, pH 5.5.

ASSESSMENT: *Acute cystitis.*

before voiding ceases. The purpose of this procedure is to obtain as pure as possible a sample of bladder urine, with minimal admixture of cells or other material from the urethra.

A **catheterized specimen** is obtained by urethral catheter (less often by suprapubic needle puncture of the bladder), either because the patient cannot void or to prevent contamination of the specimen. A **24-hour urine specimen** consists of all the urine passed by the patient during a 24-hour period.

A urine specimen is usually collected in a clean, dry bottle or cup of glass, plastic, or waxed or plasticized paper. The container need not be sterile except for bacteriologic work. Examination of urine is carried out as soon as possible after the specimen is obtained because blood cells in urine rupture early and bacterial growth in a standing specimen may alter its chemical composition. When a delay is expected, the specimen is refrigerated. A 1- or 2-gallon jug is used to collect a 24-hour urine specimen. The jug may be kept on ice during the collection period, and one of several preservatives may be placed in the jug before collection begins to inhibit the growth of bacteria in the specimen.

The principal diagnostic procedure in urinology is the **urinalysis**, a set of routine physical and chemical examinations. In most laboratories, the urinalysis includes direct observation of the specimen for color, turbidity, and other obvious characteristics; determination of specific gravity; microscopic examination of sediment for cells, crystals, and other formed elements; determination of pH; and chemical testing for glucose, protein, occult blood, and perhaps bilirubin and acetone.

Variations in color and clarity of urine usually reflect variations in concentration of solutes, including pigment. Because the daily solute load is fairly constant, changes in concentration are nearly always due to changes in volume of water excreted. Turbidity (cloudiness) may be due to the presence of phosphates, which are insoluble in alkaline urine. A smoky brown color ("**Coca-Cola urine**") often indicates the presence of hemolyzed blood. Color changes may be due to abnormal waste products (bilirubin, porphyrins), drugs (methylene blue, phenazopyridine), or pigments from foods (beets, blackberries). Mucus shreds, fragments of tissue, or calcareous material may be grossly evident in the specimen.

Microscopic examination of the urine is usually preceded by centrifugation of the specimen to concentrate any cells or other formed elements present. A polychrome stain such as the Sternheimer-Malbin stain (crystal violet and safranin in ethanol) may be added to the sediment to enhance the distinctive features of various cells, but is not essential. Microscopic examination is carried out on a small volume of fluid urine placed on a slide and covered with a cover slip. Dried smears of urine are not ordinarily suitable for examination.

Formed elements frequently found in urine are red blood cells, white blood cells, casts, crystals, bacteria, epithelial cells, and amorphous sediment. Cell counts are recorded as cells per high-power field, obtained as an average after examination and counting of several fields. A small number of red and white blood cells are present in normal urine.

A finding of more than 1 or 2 **red blood cells per high-power field (RBC/hpf),** called **microscopic hematuria**, indicates either bleeding in some part of the excretory system or contamination of the specimen with blood, possibly menstrual. **Hematuria** (see ■ Figure 13-10) occurs in acute glomerulonephritis, urolithiasis, hemorrhagic diseases, infarction of the kidney, tuberculosis of the kidney, benign or malignant tumors of any part of the urinary tract, and many cases of simple cystitis. The presence of more than 1 or 2 **white blood cells per high-power field (WBC/hpf),** known as **pyuria**, usually indicates infection in some part of the urinary tract.

Casts are microscopic cylindrical bodies that have been formed by concretion of cells or insoluble material within renal tubules and subsequently excreted in the urine. **Casts are always abnormal**. They are reported as the number counted per low-power field. Hyaline and waxy casts are homogeneous casts varying in refractivity. They consist of coagulated protein and are found in conditions associated with leakage of protein through glomeruli: nephritis, nephrotic syndrome (including lupus nephrosis and Kimmelstiel-Wilson disease), toxemia, and congestive heart failure. Granular casts are formed by aggregation of red or white blood cells or both in renal tubules and occur in many of the same conditions as hyaline and waxy casts.

A variety of **crystals** may be found on microscopic examination of the urine. Their chemical composition can usually be deduced from their shape. Crystals of uric acid, cystine, calcium oxalate, and triple phosphate may appear in the urine of persons who excrete abnormal quantities of these materials and are subject to stone formation. **Bacteria** in significant numbers in a freshly voided specimen (bacteriuria, bacilluria) suggest **urinary tract infection** (see ■ Figure 13-11). Some squamous **epithelial cells** (squames) are often found in urine and have little significance. **Amorphous sediment** is a general term for ill-defined solid material seen on microscopic examination of urine. It consists of chemical and cellular debris and is of no diagnostic importance.

Routine chemical testing of urine is usually performed with a dipstick, a commercially produced strip of plastic or paper bearing a series of dots or squares of reagent, each designed to assess a specific chemical property of urine. The **dipstick** is immersed briefly in the urine, and the test squares are observed for color changes. These tests are semiquantitative and are read by comparing the degree of color change in each square with an appropriate color chart. Results of dipstick tests other than pH and specific gravity are reported as either positive on a scale of 1 to 4 (1+, 2+, 3+, 4+) or negative.

The dipstick was negative except trace for protein.

The **pH** of urine (sometimes called simply the "reaction") is normally about 5.5. The urine may be alkaline (pH 8) in vegetarians and in persons with **urinary tract infection** due to urease-producing organisms such as *Proteus*, which split urinary urea to ammonia in the bladder.

The **specific gravity** of urine varies in direct proportion to the concentration of dissolved materials. It is ordinarily measured by means of a color change in the relevant square on a dipstick. A more precise measurement can be made by noting the depth to which a

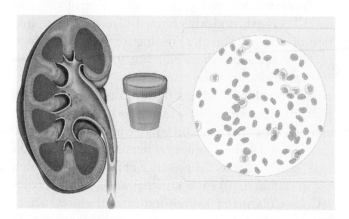

FIGURE 13-10. Hematuria, with red urine in the specimen container, and the microscopic view with red blood cells (red) and white blood cells (purple nuclei).

Urine Exam

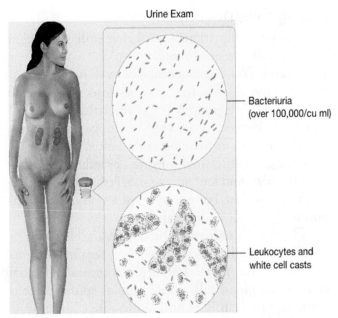

Bacteriuria
(over 100,000/cu ml)

Leukocytes and
white cell casts

FIGURE 13-11. Urinary tract infection

hydrometer, a precisely weighted float, sinks in the specimen. The normal specific gravity is 1.001 to 1.030 (which a dictator may pronounce "ten oh one" and "ten thirty"). The specific gravity is increased in dehydration (with normal renal function), toxemia, congestive heart failure, acute glomerulonephritis, and diabetes mellitus with glycosuria. The specific gravity is decreased (hyposthenuria) after ingestion or infusion of fluid (with normal renal function), in **diabetes insipidus**, and in renal failure with loss of concentrating ability.

The presence of **protein in the urine (proteinuria)** is usually due to leakage of albumin from the glomeruli. Hence it is often termed **albuminuria**, even though routine tests for protein in urine do not distinguish which proteins are present. Protein loss from the kidney occurs in glomerulonephritis, nephrotic syndrome, renal infarction, fever, and toxemia. In addition, most chemical tests for protein are positive in the presence of hematuria or pyuria.

Normally all of the plasma glucose that appears in glomerular filtrate is reabsorbed in the renal tubules. The detection of **glucose in the urine** (glycosuria) generally indicates an abnormal elevation of plasma glucose. The renal threshold for glucose is about 180 mg/dL. That means that at plasma levels above 180 mg/dL, more glucose appears in glomerular filtrate than can be reabsorbed by the tubules. **Glycosuria** is a cardinal finding in diabetes mellitus. It also occurs after rapid absorption of dietary glucose (alimentary glycosuria) and in some persons with abnormally low renal thresholds for glucose (renal glycosuria).

Occult blood refers to blood present in insufficient quantity to alter the color of the urine. A positive test for occult blood has generally the same significance as the finding of red blood cells in urine. **Acetone and other ketones** appear in the urine in diabetes mellitus with acidosis, in starvation, thyrotoxicosis, and high fever. Only bilirubin that has been conjugated with glucuronic acid is soluble in water. Hence the appearance of **bilirubin in the urine (bilirubinuria, choluria)** is noted in obstructive jaundice, in which conjugated bilirubin enters the blood stream from bile, but not in jaundice due to hemolysis or liver disease, in which only unconjugated bilirubin is elevated in the plasma.

Pause for Reflection

1. Urine is produced by the filtering of blood through numerous microscopic units called _____ and the filtrate is processed further in the _____.
2. Urine passes into a funnel-shaped collecting cavity called the _____, from which it flows downward through the _____, into the bladder, and out of the body through the _____.
3. Distinguish among the following expressions: (a) first-voided specimen, (b) clean-voided specimen, (c) clean catch specimen, (d) midstream specimen, (e) catheterized specimen, and (f) 24-hour specimen.
4. List the physical and chemical exams that are typically included in a standard urinalysis.
5. Describe three changes in color or clarity of the urine and their possible significance.
6. What is the purpose of microscopic exam of the urine?
7. Define the following terms and their significance: microscopic hematuria, pyuria, bacteriuria, proteinuria, albuminuria, glycosuria.

Common Diseases

Acute Renal Failure

An abrupt, severe decline in kidney function, with retention of nitrogenous waste products of protein metabolism (**azotemia, uremia**).

Cause: The abnormality may be **prerenal** (impaired blood supply to kidney), **renal** (also called parenchymal or intrinsic; disease of the kidney proper), or **postrenal**

MORE BEER, PLEASE!

"Why does beer go through you so fast? Because it doesn't have to stop and change color." So goes the old joke, but is there any truth to it?

In fact, it is not the color but the alcohol content in beer (and other alcoholic drinks) that stimulates the kidneys to produce more urine at a faster rate—the diuretic effect. We can see why in Australia the colloquial term for getting drunk is "to get pissed."

(obstruction of the outflow of urine from the kidney). Prerenal azotemia can result from renal artery stenosis, hypotension, or the effects of certain drugs (NSAIDs, ACE inhibitors) on renal blood flow. Renal azotemia can result from any severe disease of kidney tissue, including **acute glomerulonephritis**, **vasculitis** affecting the intrinsic renal circulation, and **acute tubular necrosis**.

History: Malaise, weakness, anorexia, nausea, reduced urine volume (**oliguria**). In advanced disease, vomiting, hematemesis, diarrhea, drowsiness, seizures, pruritus, cardiac arrhythmias, peripheral edema, dyspnea.

Physical Examination: Essentially negative. A pericardial friction rub may be heard in uremic pericarditis. In advanced disease, pallor, peripheral edema, pulmonary edema, congestive heart failure, coma.

Diagnostic Tests: The levels of BUN and creatinine are markedly increased in the blood. The serum pH is low (**metabolic acidosis**). Serum potassium and phosphorus levels are elevated and calcium is depressed. Anemia may be severe.

Course: The case mortality rate is 20% to 50% depending on the cause and underlying diseases. If the inciting cause is reversible, the renal failure itself may completely resolve. Most patients with reversible disease recover completely within six weeks. Typically there is an oliguric acute phase, followed by copious diuresis as renal function improves, and at length a return to normal urine volume. Infection is a common complication.

Treatment: Largely supportive. Restriction of water, protein, and potassium intake, with high carbohydrate diet and vitamin supplementation. Close monitoring of water and electrolyte balance. Renal dialysis or intravenous administration of glucose, insulin, and sodium bicarbonate, and oral sodium polystyrene sulfonate, to reduce serum potassium.

Acute Glomerulonephritis

Acute inflammation of renal glomeruli, with failure to excrete nitrogenous wastes.

Causes: Poststreptococcal glomerulonephritis is an autoimmune disease that follows infection (usually pharyngitis) with group A beta-hemolytic streptococci, type 12. In **Berger disease** (IgA nephropathy), immune complexes form in the glomerulus, often after a respiratory or gastrointestinal infection or a flulike illness.

History: Sudden appearance of tea-colored or Coca-Cola-colored urine, with reduction in urine volume and possibly peripheral edema.

Physical Examination: Blood pressure elevation (in poststreptococcal glomerulonephritis); peripheral edema.

Diagnostic Tests: The urine contains red blood cells, white blood cells, renal tubular epithelial cells, casts, and protein. Creatinine clearance and urinary sodium are reduced, and the 24-hour urinary excretion of protein is increased. In poststreptococcal disease, the ASO titer is elevated. Serum protein electrophoresis and antibody studies may indicate the presence of antibody to glomerular protein. Renal biopsy allows precise identification of tissue changes.

Course: Most patients with poststreptococcal glomerulonephritis recover without sequelae, but in a few the renal damage is rapidly progressive. About half of patients with Berger disease suffer progressive loss of kidney function.

Treatment: Largely supportive. Antibiotic to eradicate streptococci. Fluid restriction. Diuretics to reverse fluid retention. Attention to nutrition and control of hypertension. Renal dialysis if renal failure becomes severe.

Nephrotic Syndrome

A disorder of kidney function in which a large amount of protein is lost in the urine from damaged glomeruli.

Causes: Various abnormalities of glomeruli due to systemic disease (diabetes, systemic lupus erythematosus, amyloidosis); other forms: minimal change disease (lipoid nephrosis), focal glomerular sclerosis, membranous nephropathy, membranoproliferative glomerulonephritis.

History: Gradual onset of peripheral edema, with weight gain, dyspnea.

Physical Examination: Edema, ascites (excess fluid in abdominal cavity), anasarca (generalized edema); pulmonary edema, pleural effusion.

Diagnostic Tests: Marked increase in 24-hour urinary excretion of protein. Reduction of total protein and albumin in the serum. Increase in serum cholesterol level. There may be no cellular elements in the urine and no evidence of nitrogen retention. Renal biopsy provides histologic identification of the underlying disease process.

Treatment: Limitation of protein and salt intake; diuretics, cholesterol-lowering agents.

Diabetic Nephropathy

Progressive renal insufficiency with albuminuria and hypertension, occurring in persons with diabetes mellitus.

Cause: Thickening and degeneration of glomerular basement membrane and other pathologic changes that eventually occur in most patients with type 1 diabetes mellitus and in some patients with type 2. The incidence is higher in males, African Americans, Hispanics, and Native Americans. Most patients also have hypertension, which hastens the advance of renal damage.

History: Symptoms, which do not occur until damage is far advanced, are those of nephrotic syndrome (see above), chronic renal failure, or both.

Physical Examination: Edema, ascites. Hypertension.

Diagnostic Tests: Periodic determination of 24-hour urinary protein excretion (part of the routine surveillance of patients with diabetes mellitus) can detect microalbuminuria, a reliable marker of renal damage, early in the course of disease. With further progression, larger amounts of albumin are excreted, and measures of renal function show decline in glomerular filtration and in clearance of nitrogenous wastes. Serum levels of BUN, creatinine, and potassium are elevated. Metabolic acidosis may occur as a result of renal tubular dysfunction.

Course: Continual deterioration of renal function is usual. Use of certain drugs and injection of radiographic contrast media can precipitate acute renal failure. Diabetic nephropathy is currently the chief cause of end-stage renal failure requiring renal dialysis.

Treatment: Rigorous control of diabetes, with maintenance of plasma glucose as near normal as possible, can delay onset or progression of disease, but no treatment has been shown to reverse renal damage. Limitation of dietary protein and aggressive treatment of hypertension with ACE inhibitors or angiotensin II receptor blockers can delay progression of nephropathy. Urinary tract infections are promptly treated, and radiographic contrast media and drugs known to be toxic to the kidney are avoided. **End-stage renal failure** is treated with kidney transplantation, hemodialysis, or peritoneal dialysis.

Acute Pyelonephritis

Acute inflammation of kidney tissue and the renal pelvis due to infection (see ■ **Figure 13-12**).

Cause: Bacterial infection with *Escherichia coli*, *Proteus*, *Pseudomonas*, *Klebsiella*, *Enterobacter*, or *Staphylococcus aureus*. Infection usually ascends from the lower urinary tract (bladder and urethra), but may be spread through the circulation from a remote focus. Obstruction to urine flow caused by prostatic enlargement, a ureteral stone, or pregnancy may be the underlying cause. **Vesicoureteral reflux** of urine or anomalies of the urinary tract (tortuous or duplicated ureter) are also risk factors.

History: Fever, chills, nausea, vomiting, flank pain, urinary urgency, pollakiuria, dysuria.

Physical Examination: The temperature and pulse are elevated. Tenderness at one or both costovertebral angles is usually noted on palpation.

Diagnostic Tests: The white blood cell count is elevated. Examination of the urine shows white blood cells, red blood cells, and bacteria. Urine culture identifies the infecting organism.

Course: Pyelonephritis resolves promptly with antibiotic treatment unless an underlying problem of septicemia or urinary obstruction remains unresolved.

Treatment: Antibiotics (trimethoprim-sulfamethoxazole, ciprofloxacin) are administered orally or intravenously. Urinary obstruction must be relieved by catheterization, **nephrostomy** (draining urine from the renal pelvis), or other procedure.

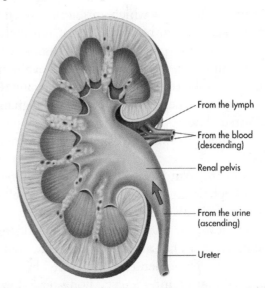

From the lymph

From the blood (descending)

Renal pelvis

From the urine (ascending)

Ureter

FIGURE 13-12. Pyelonephritis, showing various sources of infection

Urine culture obtained on admission came back growing greater than 100,000 E coli resistant to ampicillin, however, sensitive to gentamicin and first-generation cephalosporins.

Acute Cystitis

Acute inflammation of the bladder, usually due to bacterial infection.

Cause: Usually infection is due to *Escherichia coli* or other organisms ascending from the urethra. Cystitis is much commoner in women, in whom the urethra is short and straight, with its orifice in the vaginal vestibule where it is exposed to fecal contamination and trauma from sexual intercourse. Less commonly, cystitis may be due to urethral obstruction (principally in males), viral infection, bladder trauma, or spread of infection from adjacent pelvic organs. Pregnancy, diabetes mellitus, presence of an indwelling catheter, and advanced age are risk factors.

History: Fairly sudden onset of pollakiuria, urgency, urinary burning, and bladder spasms after voiding. Hematuria may occur. Often there is suprapubic or low back discomfort.

Physical Examination: Essentially unremarkable. Fever is absent. There may be suprapubic tenderness.

Diagnostic Examination: Laboratory studies of urine show white blood cells (sometimes clumped), red blood cells or occult blood, and bacteria. Tests for **leukocyte esterase** (an enzyme released by white blood cells in urine) and **nitrites** (formed by reduction of urinary nitrates by certain bacteria) are often positive. Urine culture identifies the causative organism, and sensitivity studies show which antibiotics are effective against it. Culturing, however, is not routinely performed except in atypical or recurrent disease. Cystitis is so uncommon in men that aggressive evaluation is usually undertaken in the male to identify any serious underlying cause such as obstruction or malignancy.

Course: The response to treatment is rapid, but many sexually active women experience frequent recurrences.

Treatment: Antibiotics (trimethoprim-sulfamethoxazole, cephalexin, ciprofloxacin) are often effective in courses of just two or three days. Urinary symptoms may be relieved by phenazopyridine (a bladder anesthetic taken orally) or antispasmodics. The frequency of recurrences in women can be reduced by regularly voiding just after intercourse. Long-term low-dose antibiotic prophylaxis also helps to prevent recurrences.

Bladder Cancer

Cancer of the urinary bladder is the fourth most common malignancy in men and the ninth most common in women in the United States. About 90% of bladder cancers arise from transitional cells, that is, epithelial cells in the bladder lining that appear cuboidal in the relaxed state but that assume a flatter, more squamous configuration when stretched by filling of the bladder with urine. Transitional epithelium, also called **urothelium**, is found in the renal pelvis, the ureters, and the urethra as well as the bladder.

His pathology report for bladder tumor showed high-grade urothelial carcinoma, extensive smooth muscle invasion, lymphatic invasion present.

Cause: Malignant changes in the lining of the bladder are triggered in most cases by chemical residues excreted by the kidneys and contained in the urine. By far the most common risk factor is tobacco smoking. Workers in many trades, including the manufacture of rubber and leather and occupations involving exposure to smoke and engine exhaust, are also at risk. Genetic factors are implicated by the difference in gender incidence. In addition, several oncogenes associated with increased risk of bladder cancer have been identified.

History: The most common presenting symptom is painless **hematuria**. Pain on urination, urinary frequency, and strangury suggest more advanced disease.

Diagnostic Tests: Urinalysis typically confirms the presence of red blood cells in urine. Cytologic study ("cell block") of urine or of bladder washings may yield a pathologic diagnosis of malignancy, but **cystoscopy with biopsy** of an observed lesion is far more sensitive, especially when the bladder lining is examined with fluorescent light (see ■ **Figure 13-13**). Biochemical detection of various protein markers in urine can identify specific types of cancer.

Course: Untreated **transitional cell carcinoma (TCC)** spreads to the muscular layer of the bladder and

ADMISSION DIAGNOSIS
Transitional cell carcinoma of the bladder invading the prostate.

DISCHARGE DIAGNOSES
Status post dilation of bladder neck contracture, transurethral resection of bladder tumor, transurethral resection of the prostate.

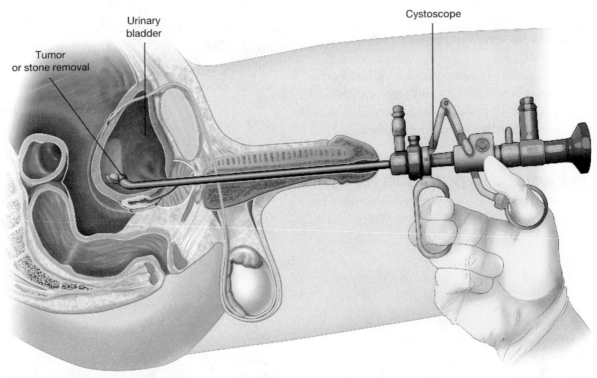

FIGURE 13-13. Cystoscopy

then invades surrounding tissues. Metastasis to pelvic lymph nodes, lungs, liver, and bone may occur.

Treatment: A tumor confined to the bladder mucosa (**papillary urothelial carcinoma**, **carcinoma in situ**) may be treated with electrocautery applied through a cystoscope. Any of several chemotherapeutic agents may then be instilled into the bladder to reduce the risk of recurrence. Cancer that has invaded the muscular layer of the bladder is treated with **cystectomy**, often with prophylactic removal of surrounding tissues or organs such as prostate or ovaries. Such surgery requires diversion of the urinary stream to the bowel or creation of an **artificial bladder** from a loop of bowel. Radiation, chemotherapy, or both may be used adjunctively after cystectomy for cancer.

Urinary Incontinence

Four distinct types of involuntary leakage of urine from the bladder are recognized. **Urge incontinence**, which occurs after a sudden, intense, irresistible urge to void, is the commonest type of incontinence in elderly persons. It is due to overactivity of the detrusor muscle of the bladder and often responds to treatment with an antispasmodic of the antimuscarinic class (darifenacin, oxybutynin, solifenacin, tolterodine).

Stress incontinence, which is seen almost exclusively in women, occurs when mechanical stress is placed on the bladder, as by coughing, laughing, or changing position. It may result from structural damage to the bladder as in childbirth. Treatment with pelvic muscle exercises (**Kegel exercises**) or estrogens may help. Surgical correction of anatomic abnormalities is often necessary and is highly successful.

Overflow incontinence is leakage of urine from an over-distended bladder, occurring almost exclusively in men with urinary obstruction due to prostatic disease. Treatment is correction of the obstruction.

Total incontinence is complete lack of control over voiding, usually due to neurologic disease, spinal cord injury, or radical prostatectomy. Continuous or intermittent catheterization may be the only effective means of controlling this type of incontinence. Incontinence is primarily a disorder of the elderly; besides the causes mentioned above, it may be due to dementia, urinary tract infection, diuresis, drugs, diminished mobility, and, in women, atrophic vaginitis.

Prostatitis

Inflammation of the prostate, typically due to bacterial infection, which may be acute or chronic. In acute prostatitis the presenting complaints are fever, urinary frequency and burning, occasionally urinary retention, and pain in the perineum or back. On digital rectal examination the prostate is found to be enlarged, warm, and exquisitely tender. The white blood count is elevated, and the urine contains white blood cells, red blood cells, and bacteria. Treatment is with oral or intravenous antibiotics.

In chronic prostatitis, symptoms are milder but of longer duration. Fever is absent and prostatic tenderness not so marked. Urinalysis yields normal results. Treatment is with antibiotics and must often be continued for a long time.

Benign Prostatic Hyperplasia (BPH)

Enlargement of the prostate accompanying aging, with varying degrees of urinary obstruction (see ■ Figure 13-14).

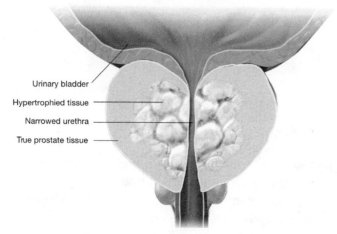

FIGURE 13-14. Benign prostatic hyperplasia

Cause: Some prostatic enlargement due to overgrowth of androgen-sensitive glandular elements occurs naturally with aging. Causes of severely symptomatic enlargement are unknown.

History: Gradual onset of urinary symptoms, which may be **obstructive** (decreased force and caliber of urinary stream, hesitancy, intermittency) or irritative (frequency, urgency, nocturia).

Physical Examination: The prostate is symmetrically enlarged on digital rectal examination, firm but not hard. Abdominal examination may indicate distention of the bladder. Catheterization after voiding may indicate residual urine.

Diagnostic Tests: Urinalysis may indicate evidence of infection (white blood cells) or of bladder irritation (red blood cells). The blood urea nitrogen (BUN) may be elevated if obstruction is advanced (**obstructive uropathy**). Intravenous pyelography may show bladder distention and bilateral ureteral dilatation. Urinary flowmetry gives an objective measure of the rate of flow from the bladder. Cystoscopy and urethroscopy may be of value in confirming the benign nature of the disorder.

PROSTATE CANCER

Prostate cancer is more common, occurs at an earlier age, and spreads more aggressively in African American men. Because malignant changes usually begin near the periphery of the gland, urinary symptoms occur late, if at all. In more than one third of patients, cancer has spread beyond the gland by the time the diagnosis is made. Prostate cancer can invade the bladder, rectum, and other pelvic structures by direct extension and can spread to more remote sites by metastasis. The bones of the spine and pelvis are the most frequent sites of metastasis.

Course: Symptoms may remain relatively mild for years, even decades. Obstruction may lead to infection and even to kidney failure. Benign prostatic hyperplasia does not evolve into carcinoma.

Treatment: Medical treatment with finasteride (an alpha-reductase inhibitor) or terazosin or doxazosin (alpha-adrenergic blocking agents) can reduce obstructive symptoms. In more severe cases, surgical excision of prostate tissue is indicated. **Transurethral resection (TUR)** is the usual procedure, but in some cases suprapubic (open) resection is preferred. Balloon dilatation of the prostate and transurethral laser excision are alternative procedures.

Adenocarcinoma of the Prostate

A malignant tumor arising from glandular epithelium of the prostate gland (see ■ Figure 13-15).

Cause: Adenocarcinoma of the prostate is the most common cancer in men (31% of all cancers diagnosed). The incidence of prostatic cancer found at autopsy in men over 50 is about 40%. However, prostate cancer causes only 11% of all cancer deaths in men. The risk of developing prostatic carcinoma is higher in men with a family history of it and in those who have undergone vasectomy. The tumor is testosterone-dependent (that is, it does not occur in men who have undergone **orchidectomy**). Adenocarcinoma of the prostate does not arise from benign prostatic hyperplasia.

History: There may be no symptoms. Diminished urine flow, urinary frequency, nocturia, and dribbling of urine may occur as in benign prostatic hyperplasia. The first symptom may be bone pain due to metastasis.

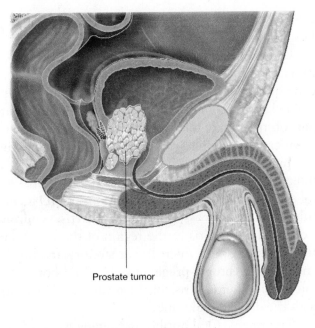

FIGURE 13-15. Prostate cancer

Physical Examination: The prostate, as palpated on digital rectal examination, may be unusually firm, nodular, or asymmetric.

Diagnostic Tests. The level of prostate-specific antigen (PSA), or acid phosphatase, or both in the serum is elevated in many cases of prostate carcinoma, particularly when metastasis has occurred. Transrectal ultrasound may detect abnormally dense areas within the prostate gland, representing tumor. Transrectal biopsy discloses zones of malignant tissue. The **Gleason grading system** gives a histopathologic estimate of malignancy and likely future behavior. X-ray studies and radionuclide bone scans may show metastases to bones of the spine or pelvis.

Course. Progression of disease is typically slow, and most patients die of other causes before the prostatic cancer has reached a lethal stage. Metastasis to lymph nodes and to the spine or pelvis eventually occurs. Urinary obstruction may lead to urinary tract infection and even renal failure.

Treatment. Surgical excision (usually **radical prostatectomy**), radiation by external beam or implanted radioactive needles; in advanced (metastatic) disease, castration or administration of estrogen (or an anti-androgen such as flutamide) to suppress tumor growth.

Gonorrhea

Infection of the genital tract by the gonococcus.

Cause: *Neisseria gonorrhoeae* (gonococcus), a gram-negative diplococcus that is transmitted almost

---

SEXUALLY TRANSMITTED DISEASES (STDs)

STDs are statistically more likely to occur in persons under 25 years of age, in members of ethnic minorities, in persons of low socioeconomic status, in persons with many sexual partners (especially prostitutes), and in sexually active gay men (but not in sexually active lesbians). Their incidence is also higher in urban areas. The only absolute protection against acquiring an infection through sexual contact is lifelong celibacy or maintenance of a permanently and mutually monogamous sexual relationship.

The diagnosis and treatment of STDs are rendered more difficult by the reluctance of most people to discuss their sexual behavior with health professionals and by the refusal of many patients to believe that a sexual partner has become infected by some third person. Diagnosis often demands alertness and a high degree of suspicion on the part of the healthcare worker. History-taking must be searching but nonthreatening and nonjudgmental.

---

exclusively by sexual contact. It attacks genitourinary mucous membranes, producing a purulent inflammation that may spread to adjacent organs or the peritoneum, and may progress to scarring. Infection of the pharynx or rectum can be acquired through oral or anal sex.

History: Men: After an incubation period of three to five days, severe pain on urination and a thick green urethral discharge. Women: Similar symptoms sometimes occur, along with vaginal or vulvar inflammation. Often, however, there are no symptoms unless **pelvic inflammatory disease (PID)** (spread of infection to the uterus and uterine tubes) occurs. PID causes pelvic pain and fever, with variable other symptoms.

Physical Examination: In men, evident purulent urethral discharge, with inflammation of the meatus. In women, acute disease may be manifested by urethritis, cervicitis, vaginitis, inflammation of **Bartholin glands** (secretory glands lateral to the vaginal vestibule), or proctitis. If PID ensues, fever, abdominal tenderness, extreme tenderness on manipulation of cervix.

Diagnostic Tests: DNA amplification tests performed on material obtained by cervical or urethral smear and on urine are valuable for diagnosis as well as for screening asymptomatic persons of either sex.

Stained smear of pus or secretions shows gram-negative diplococci inside WBCs. Culture on appropriate medium grows gonococci. Oral and anal specimens are positive when infection is in those areas.

Course: Acute urethral infection may resolve spontaneously, but in men it often spreads to the epididymis or prostate, or progresses to a stage of scarring, with resultant infertility. In women, spread to the vagina, cervix, uterus, tubes, and rectum often occurs. Tubal infection (**salpingitis**, PID) with scarring causes infertility and a heightened risk of ectopic pregnancy. In either sex, infection occasionally involves the skin, conjunctivae, joints, tendon sheaths, cardiac valves, or meninges. Spread of infection from mother to newborn can cause conjunctivitis with ensuing blindness.

Treatment: Antibiotic treatment with a single dose of intramuscular ceftriaxone is usually curative. It is standard practice to administer treatment for **chlamydial infection** at the same time since the infections so often occur together.

Chlamydial Infection

Urogenital infection with *Chlamydia trachomatis*.

Cause: Sexually transmitted infection of genital mucous membranes and related tissues with *Chlamydia trachomatis*, an intracellular gram-negative bacterium. Genital chlamydial infection (urethritis and cervicitis) is the commonest bacterial STD. Screening tests are positive in 10% of asymptomatic sexually active women.

History: Men: Urethral itching or burning, dysuria, thin serous discharge, one to four weeks after exposure. Anorectal pain and bleeding with rectal infection, common in gay men. Women: Dysuria and pollakiuria due to **acute urethral syndrome; dyspareunia** (pain with intercourse), vaginal bleeding, and vaginal discharge due to cervicitis; abdominal pain and fever due to pelvic inflammatory disease. Most women with chlamydial infection are asymptomatic.

Physical Examination: May be unremarkable. Thin, watery urethral discharge may be noted in males. In women, cervical erythema with mucopurulent discharge indicates cervicitis. With development of PID, fever, abdominal pain, and cervical tenderness become evident.

Diagnostic Tests: DNA amplification testing of urine is used for both diagnosis and for screening of asymptomatic persons. A urethral or cervical smear may show organisms with direct fluorescence antibody examination, enzyme-linked immunosorbent assay, or DNA probe.

Course: Spontaneous resolution often occurs, but in many patients chlamydial infection has long-term consequences. In men, infection can spread to the epididymis, produce urethral stricture with resulting urinary obstruction or infertility, or trigger an autoimmune disorder called **Reiter syndrome** (arthritis, conjunctivitis, mucocutaneous lesions). In about one fifth of infected women, infection spreads to the uterus and tubes (salpingitis, PID). Complications of PID include **tubo-ovarian abscess, Fitz-Hugh–Curtis syndrome** (localized peritonitis in the region of the liver), and **tubal scarring** with infertility or sterility and heightened risk of **ectopic pregnancy**. A child born to an infected mother is at risk of chlamydial conjunctivitis, with the danger of blindness.

Treatment: Oral antibiotic therapy with tetracycline, erythromycin, or a single dose of azithromycin is ordinarily curative. Treatment is often instituted on suspicion (urethritis or cervicitis with negative cultures of urine and discharge) because of the high probability of chlamydial infection in such cases. Persons treated for gonorrhea are also routinely treated for chlamydial infection as well.

Erectile Dysfunction (Impotence)

Failure of the penis to become erect after sexual stimulation, or to maintain sufficient rigidity for intercourse. Among many possible causes are atherosclerosis, neurologic disease or spinal cord injury, hormonal deficiency, side effects of medicines, anxiety, and depression. Diabetes mellitus, obesity, and cigarette smoking are risk factors. Most patients respond to oral phosphodiesterase inhibitors (sildenafil, tadalafil, vardenafil). Other methods of treatment include local injection of a vasodilator, induction of erection by means of a vacuum device, and implantation of a penile prosthesis.

This is a 31-year-old male in to discuss erectile dysfunction. Patient has noticed symptoms of a decrease in libido for the last 3 months. He has difficulty sustaining an erection and performing sexual intercourse. He has noted a decrease in desire over the past several years. He also does complain of some right testicular irritation.

ASSESSMENT
A 31-year-old male with complaints of erectile dysfunction, probably related to depressive symptoms.

Pause for Reflection

1. Discuss the causes of acute renal failure.
2. Distinguish between acute glomerulonephritis, nephrotic syndrome, acute pyelonephritis, and acute cystitis.
3. A disease caused by thickening and degeneration of glomerular basement membrane and other pathologic changes that eventually occur in most patients with type 1 diabetes mellitus and in some patients with type 2 is _____.
4. How is bladder cancer treated?
5. Distinguish among stress incontinence, overflow incontinence, and total incontinence.
6. List and briefly define three common diseases affecting the prostate.
7. Identify two common sexually transmitted diseases in men.
8. List modes of treatment for men with erectile dysfunction.

Diagnostic and Surgical Procedures

biopsy, prostatic Prostatic biopsy is usually performed in conjunction with a transrectal ultrasound (TRUS) examination to assess the size and configuration of the gland.

brachytherapy A form of cancer treatment in which radioactive material is inserted into the body close to the tissues to be treated.

cystolitholapaxy An endoscopic procedure in which bladder stones are crushed with a lithotrite and the resulting fragments are flushed out by irrigation.

cystoscopy Endoscopic examination of the interior of the urinary bladder.

cystourethroscopy A combination procedure consisting of urethroscopy and cystoscopy.

digital rectal examination (DRE) Examination of the interior of the rectum and adjacent structures, especially the prostate gland, with a finger inserted through the anus (see ■ Figure 13-7).

extracorporeal shock wave lithotripsy (ESWL) A method of shattering stones in the urinary tract (also in the biliary tract) by means of ultrasound waves generated outside the body. This noninvasive procedure can break up more than 90% of urinary tract stones in adults, permitting passage of the fragments in the urine.

holmium laser ablation of the prostate (HoLAP) Surplus prostatic tissue is vaporized rather than trimmed away.

holmium laser enucleation of the prostate (HoLEP) Uses a holmium laser to resect hyperplastic prostatic tissue instead of the electrical loop of traditional TURP.

hydrocelectomy Excision of a hydrocele.

intracorporeal lithotripsy The application of a shattering force directly to a stone by means of a device inserted endoscopically into the urinary tract. Electrohydraulic and pneumatic lithotripters function exactly like miniature jackhammers.

intravenous pyelogram (IVP) Radiograph of the urinary tract after intravenous injection of contrast material that is quickly excreted in the urine.

intravesical immunotherapy Instillation of an immunologic agent, often BCG, into the bladder for the treatment of superficial transitional cell carcinoma.

KUB A plain radiograph of the kidneys, ureters, and urinary bladder. It need not be expanded when dictated.

nephroscopy A ureteroscope that is of sufficient length and maneuverability to reach the renal pelvis is called a nephroscope. Direct examination of the renal pelvis can provide information about hematuria, calculous disease, tumors, and other disorders of the kidney.

orchiectomy Removal of a testicle.

panendoscopy Cystoscopy performed with an instrument that permits wide-angle viewing of the urinary bladder and urethra.

percutaneous nephrolithotomy Procedure in which a lodged stone in the renal pelvis or proximal ureter is surgically removed through the skin.

percutaneous nephrolitholapaxy An alternative, minimally invasive surgical procedure for the extraction of stones from the renal pelvis by means of a rigid or flexible endoscope (nephroscope) inserted through an incision in the skin overlying the kidney.

SLANG TERMS

Expand these slang brief forms when encountered in dictation.

cath	catheterization
cath'd	catheterized
cysto	cystoscopy
cysto'd	underwent cystoscopy

Exception: The term *prepped* (prepared) has become acceptable in its brief form through usage.

The patient was prepped and draped.

The skin was prepped prior to injection.

prostatectomy Removal of the entire prostate gland.

retrograde pyelography Radiography of the kidneys, ureters, and bladder following the injection of a contrast medium backward through a urinary catheter into the ureters and the calyces of the pelves of the kidneys. Useful in locating urinary stones and obstructions.

transperineal implantation of radioactive isotopes Treatment for prostate cancer.

transrectal ultrasound (TRUS) An ultrasound procedure to examine the prostate gland for tumors that cannot be felt by a digital rectal exam, and to estimate the size of the prostate gland. In a prostate needle biopsy, it is used to guide the needle to the right part of the prostate gland.

transurethral incision of the prostate (TUIP) Longitudinal incisions are made in the prostatic urethra without removal of any tissue.

transurethral resection of bladder tumor (TURB, TURBT) A resectoscope is inserted through the urethra into the bladder, and tumors are resected by means of an electrical loop; usually performed in conjunction with a cystoscopy.

transurethral resection of the prostate (TUR, TURP) A resectoscope is inserted through the urethra and advanced to the level of the hyperplastic prostate. The surgeon then shaves away surplus prostatic tissue encroaching on the lumen of the urethra by means of an electrical loop, which also seals severed blood vessels. The instrument is equipped with an irrigating system that flushes away blood and tissue.

transurethral ultrasound-guided laser incision of the prostate (TULIP) Resembles TUIP, but the incisions are made with a laser.

TUR Transurethral resection.

ureteroscopy The passage of an endoscope from outside the body through the urethra and the bladder into a ureter. Used in the treatment of ureteral stones but also of those within the renal pelvis.

urethroscopy A rigid urethroscope is a short tubular instrument designed to provide a view of the interior of the urethra. Used principally in examining the male urethra for prostatic enlargement or infection, urethral stricture (local narrowing due to scarring), varices, infectious lesions, and foreign bodies.

vasectomy Surgical division of the vas deferens in the male to effect sterility.

voiding cystourethrography (VCUG) A radiographic study of the bladder and urethra during voiding after injection of contrast medium through a catheter.

Laboratory Procedures

acid phosphatase Enzyme whose level in the serum is often increased in prostatic carcinoma.

amorphous sediment Unformed and generally insignificant debris seen in a urine specimen under microscopic examination.

antistreptolysin O (ASO) titer A blood test to measure antibodies against streptolysin O, a substance produced by group A streptococcus bacteria.

bilirubin A product of the breakdown of red blood cells, excreted in water-soluble form by the liver. In obstructive jaundice, excessive water-soluble (also called direct-reacting) bilirubin in the blood spills into the urine, giving it a greenish brown hue.

blood urea nitrogen (BUN) The serum level of urea nitrogen, a waste product of protein metabolism. Elevation indicates an impairment of kidney function.

catheterized urine specimen Specimen of urine obtained by passing a sterile catheter into the bladder.

clean-voided specimen (clean catch) Obtained after cleansing of the area around the urethral meatus to prevent contamination of the specimen with material from outside the urinary tract.

creatinine clearance A measure of kidney function, calculated from the serum creatinine level and the amount of creatinine excreted in the urine in 24 hours.

electrolytes, urinary Sodium, potassium, and chloride ions in the urine. Abnormal concentrations could indicate kidney disease.

first-voided specimen The first urine passed after arising in the morning.

midstream specimen One that contains neither the first nor the last portion of urine passed.

FTA-ABS Fluorescent treponemal antibody absorption test, to detect syphilis.

prostate-specific antigen (PSA) Blood test to screen for prostatic carcinoma.

RPR (rapid plasma reagin) Test for syphilis.

specific gravity The weight of a substance per unit of volume compared to pure water, which by definition has a specific gravity of 1.000. The specific gravity of urine (normally 1.001 to 1.030) is a rough measure of the amount of material dissolved in it.

24-hour urine specimen Consists of all the urine passed by the patient in a 24-hour period.

urinalysis (UA) A group of standard laboratory examinations of the urine, including determination of pH and specific gravity, chemical testing for sugar, albumin, occult blood, leukocyte esterase, nitrite, acetone, and bilirubin, and microscopic examination for red and white blood cells, bacteria, casts, crystals, and other formed elements.

urine culture Usually with colony count and sensitivity studies, to identify urinary pathogens.

VDRL Venereal Disease Research Laboratory test for syphilis. Abbreviation does not need to be expanded.

Pharmacology

Urinary tract drugs include antibiotics and other anti-infection agents, urinary tract analgesics, and urinary antispasmodics.

Antibiotics

The choice of an antibiotic for a urinary tract infection (UTI) depends not only on the causative organism but on the physiology of the excretory system. Because most UTIs are due to *E. coli* or other gram-negative pathogens, the drug selected must have proven effectiveness against such organisms. In addition, the drug chosen must be able to establish an effective tissue level despite the tendency of the kidneys to flush foreign chemicals out of the body as rapidly as possible.

> cinoxacin (Cinobac)
> ciprofloxacin (Cipro)
> fosfomycin (Monurol)
> nitrofurantoin (Furadantin, Macrobid, Macrodantin)
> norfloxacin (Noroxin)
> ofloxacin (Floxin)

Sulfonamides

Urinary tract infections can also be treated with sulfonamides (often called **sulfa drugs**). These drugs are not true antibiotics because they only inhibit the growth of bacteria, rather than killing bacteria as antibiotics do.

> sulfadiazine
> sulfamethoxazole (Gantanol, SMX)
> sulfisoxazole (Gantrisin Pediatric)

The combination of sulfamethoxazole with the folic acid inhibitor trimethoprim (Bactrim, Septra) is widely used in the treatment of upper and lower urinary tract infections, although strains of *E. coli* resistant to it are increasingly isolated.

Urinary Tract Analgesics and Antispasmodics

Oral medicines may be used to provide symptomatic relief of urinary burning, urgency, and frequency while more specific treatment is directed at the cause. Phenazopyridine (AZO, Azo-Tabs, Pyridium), absorbed into the circulation and excreted in the urine, acts on bladder and urethral mucous membranes as a topical anesthetic.

Much urinary tract pain is due to smooth muscle spasm triggered by infection, urinary retention, catheterization, or calculi. The long-established anti-cholinergic drug hyoscyamine (Anaspaz, Cystospaz, Dolsed, Urogesic Blue) is widely used to treat urinary tract spasm. Urge incontinence, which results from spasticity of the detrusor muscle of the bladder, responds particularly to drugs of a newer class, the antimuscarinics.

darifenacin (Enablex)
flavoxate (Urispas)
oxybutynin (Ditropan)
solifenacin (VESIcare)
tolterodine (Detrol LA)
trospium (Sanctura)

Drugs for Treatment of Benign Prostatic Hyperplasia (BPH)

alfuzosin (Uroxatral)
dutasteride (Avodart)
finasteride (Proscar)
tamsulosin (Flomax)
terazosin (Hytrin)

Drugs Used to Treat Male Erectile Dysfunction (ED)

alprostadil (Caverject, Muse)
sildenafil (Viagra)
tadalafil (Cialis)
vardenafil (Levitra)

Transcription Tips

1. Confusing terms related to the genitourinary system and the male reproductive system: Some of these terms sound alike; others are potential traps when researching. Memorize the terms and their meanings so that you can select the appropriate term for a correct transcript.

   anuresis—suppression of urine formation and excretion, anuria

   enuresis—urinary incontinence

   effected—carried out, made something happen (hemostasis was effected …)

   affected—acted upon, influenced (… apply to affected region …)

   efflux—the process of flowing out (e.g., outflow of urine; an English, not a medical term)

   reflux—backward flow (e.g. urine from bladder flowing back up the ureters)

   irritated—painful, red, swollen, inflamed (irritated lesion)

   irritative—dependent on or caused by irritation (irritative symptoms)

   obstructed—closed off, impeded (obstructed ureter)

   obstructive—causing obstruction (obstructive uropathy)

   prostate (noun)—a gland of the male reproductive system through which the urethra passes (frequently mispronounced by patients and a few clinicians)

   prostrate (adj.)—describes a posture of submission or a state of exhaustion or extreme grief

   radical (adj.)—directed at the root source (radical prostatectomy)

   radicle (noun)—the smallest branch of a vessel or nerve

   stent—a thin, flexible tube placed in the ureters to keep them open in cases of obstruction

   stint—a period of time spent doing something

   Uracid—a trademarked urinary acidifier to control ammonia production

   Urised—a discontinued urinary antibiotic still found in some resources

   ureter—the tube that conveys urine from the kidneys to the bladder (Mnemonic: There are two ureters, one from each kidney and there are two e's.)

   urethra—the canal that conveys urine from the bladder to outside the body (Mnemonic: There is only one, and there is just one e.)

   vesical (adj.)—pertaining to the urinary bladder (vesical neck)

   vesicle (noun)—small fluid-filled sac (seminal vesicles)

2. Spelling. Memorize the spelling of these urology terms. Note silent letters, doubled letters, and unexpected pronunciation.

   aggregate (double *g*'s)
   asymmetry (two *m*'s)
   bacteriuria (the first *i* is often inaudible)
   brachytherapy ("brake-ee-THER-a-pee")
   cystolitholapaxy (the –*la*- syllable may be inaudible)
   fluoroscopy (*not* floro-)
   glans penis (*not* glands)
   hypovolemia (*not* hyper-; the *v* is often difficult to hear)
   lues ("loo-eez")
   occult (two *c*'s)
   pollakiuria (two *l*'s, note *i* after the *k*)
   status post (two words)
   postvoiding (one word)
   verumontanum (one word)

3. Watch out for spelling changes when forming derivatives.

Noun	Adjective
diuresis	diuretic
penis	penile
testicle	testicular
vesicle	vesicular

Singular	Plural
calculus	calculi
condyloma	condylomata
testis	testes

Transcription Tips

4. Be careful when expanding these abbreviations.

    UPJ   ureteropelvic junction
    UVJ   ureterovesical junction

    It is unnecessary to expand these abbreviations:

    KUB   kidneys, ureters, and bladder (refers to a plain x-ray of the abdomen)
    pH   a measure of alkalinity or acidity; note lowercase p.
    PSA   prostate specific antigen
    UA   urinalysis

5. Dictation Challenges

    Urinalysis, not *urine analysis* even if urine analysis is dictated.

    Urine specific gravity is always written as the number 1 followed by a decimal point and three other numbers. Normal values range from 1.001 to 1.030. If you hear "ten ten," transcribe 1.010.

    The element *potassium* is abbreviated as K. Some brand name drugs containing potassium use K as part of the brand name (K-Dur), and these should be transcribed as indicated in a reputable reference. *KCl,* when it refers to the generic medication potassium chloride, should be expanded. When *K* is dictated referring to potassium as an electrolyte, as in laboratory data, it should be transcribed as potassium.

    The term *dartos* is often used alone when *tunica dartos* is meant; it may be transcribed as dictated.

6. Challenging drug spellings

    Note the challenging spellings or unusual capitalization of these common drugs.

    Anaspaz
    Caverject
    Cialis
    Cystospaz
    Detrol LA
    OxyContin
    Pyridium
    Urispas
    Urogesic Blue
    VESIcare
    Viagra

Spotlight On

Surviving Bladder Cancer

by John Starkey

Three years ago I was experiencing pain in my lower abdomen. Like most men I was hesitant about going to the doctor. My wife Joan convinced me to go to the Navy Hospital. The doctor pushed on my abdomen and I almost jumped off the table. He sent me for a CT scan and I returned to the doctor's office. The head surgeon of the hospital came and told me I had dodged a bullet. I had a ruptured appendix but it had walled itself off.

He then told me I had a mass either on my prostate or my bladder. I had had a weak stream but never thought of it as anything important; all men get enlarged prostates as they get older, so it didn't worry me. Although I had an appointment the next month with my urologist, the surgeon said I should call him now and tell him of the results of the CT scan. As for the walled-off appendix, I followed his advice and opted not to have surgery.

When I called Dr G, he told me to come in the next day. Dr G inserted a scope through my urethra and performed a cystoscopy. He found a large tumor. In two days I was in surgery at the hospital; the tumor was excised and sent to pathology. Dr. G was certain that it was cancer, and in several days the pathology report came back as transitional cell carcinoma, but it had not gone through the bladder wall.

I waited three months for the bladder to heal from the surgery before I started chemotherapy. I went through one treatment weekly for six weeks with chemotherapy BCG, which stands for Bacillus Calmette-Guérin. During cystoscopy, the surgeon instilled BCG into my bladder. The pain would have been unbearable if the scope had been inserted into the urethra without the use of a numbing gel (lidocaine jelly).

As a man over 74, I had an enlarged prostate which impeded the insertion of the scope and the catheter used to instill the BCG. For me, Dr. G used a coudè catheter which has a curved tip that bypasses the enlarged prostate. I had to remain on the table for a couple of hours, being turned this way and that so that the solution would bathe my entire bladder. Dr. G. told me not to be alarmed about severe burning during urination after the treatment with BCG (this usually ceases after the sixth or seventh urination, but the first is the worst because the lidocaine has worn off.)

I have had followup exams with a scope every six months. Since the first occurrence, I have had two more surgeries, one to remove two tumors which were less aggressive than the first, and one to remove a third tumor which showed no signs of cancer. The last three cystoscopies have shown no tumors. After each I received three weeks of BCG, one treatment each week.

In summary, it's cystoscopy, three months later BCG, three months later cystoscopy, three months llater BCG, and so on. This has been my routine now for three years. I am scheduled for three weeks of BCG to be done this fall as prophylaxis. Hopefully, it will be the last. After that, there will be exams probably every six months for a while and then annually.

I asked Dr G what caused bladder cancer, and without hesitation he said that, in men, smoking is the primary cause. (Why does the American Cancer Society not publicize this fact like they do lung cancer?)

Bladder cancer is the fourth most diagnosed cancer in men. In 2009, the most recent year for which there is data and the year that I was diagnosed, the American Cancer Society said there were 73,510 new cases of bladder cancer diagnosed (about 55,600 in men and 17,910 in women) and 14,880 deaths (about 10,510 in men and 4,370 in women). About 500,000 people in the United States are survivors of this cancer. Nine in ten people with bladder cancer are over age 55 with the average age of diagnosis being 73, so I guess I fit right in there with the average.

Advice to men: Don't smoke. I smoked for 50+ years and regret it. Get regular checkups. You're not invincible, no matter what you think. Men are taught they're supposed to tough it out, but the older you get, the more you realize how vulnerable you are.

Advice to wives: You need to hound your husbands. They may hate it, but it's for their own good.

Exercises

Medical Vocabulary Review

_____ 1. The capsule that covers the kidneys is called the _____
A. cortex.
B. hilum.
C. renal pelvis.
D. glomerulus.

_____ 2. Urine is formed in the _____
A. ureters.
B. urethra.
C. renal pelvis.
D. glomeruli and tubules.

_____ 3. Which of the following is NOT a part of the male reproductive system?
A. Testes.
B. Urethra.
C. Vas deferens.
D. Seminal vesicles.

_____ 4. The epididymis and vas deferens comprise the collecting system of the _____
A. kidneys.
B. testicles.
C. prostate.
D. seminal vesicles.

_____ 5. Spermatozoa and the male hormones responsible for development of secondary sexual characteristics are produced in the _____
A. scrotum.
B. prostate.
C. testicles.
D. adrenals.

_____ 6. What structure, under sexual stimulation, closes off the bladder from the urethra and brings about ejaculation of semen?
A. Prostate.
B. Epididymis.
C. Spermatic duct.
D. Seminal vesicals.

_____ 7. Which of the following best fits this definition? An overgrowth of androgen-sensitive glandular tissue that normally accompanies aging and causes varying degrees of urinary obstruction.
A. Prostatitis.
B. Urethral stricture.
C. Benign prostatic hyperplasia.
D. Adenocarcinoma of the prostate.

_____ 8. Calculi (renal stones) may be found in all of the following structures EXCEPT the _____
A. testes.
B. bladder.
C. ureters.
D. kidneys.

_____ 9. Which is the term that best fits this definition? Failure of one or both of the testes to descend into the scrotum.
A. Hydrocele.
B. Spermatocele.
C. Cryptorchidism.
D. Cushing syndrome.

_____ 10. Increased production of urine resulting from renal or systemic disease, toxic substances, or drugs administered to reduce body water and/or sodium is a condition known as _____
A. dribbling.
B. diuresis.
C. dysuria.
D. incontinence.

___ 11. Which of the following refers to pain on urination?
A. Dysuria.
B. Oliguria.
C. Anuresis.
D. Azotemia.

___ 12. Another term for hydronephrosis is _____
A. hydrocele.
B. hydrocalyx.
C. hydrorrhea.
D. hydroureter.

___ 13. In a patient with yellowing of the skin and mucous membranes (jaundice), the workup might include a urinalysis, the results of which are likely to show what substance in the urine?
A. Ketones.
B. Glucose.
C. Bilirubin.
D. Acid phosphatase.

___ 14. Being awakened at night by the urge to void is referred to as _____
A. anuria.
B. oliguria.
C. polyuria.
D. nocturia.

___ 15. Another word for urinary incontinence is

_____
A. anuresis.
B. enuresis.
C. diuresis.
D. kaliuesis.

___ 16. Which of the following refers to excessive distention of the veins of the epididymis and testis?
A. Hydrocele.
B. Cystocele.
C. Varicocele.
D. Spermatocele.

___ 17. Backward flow of urine within any part of the urinary tract is _____
A. reflux.
B. efflux.
C. hydroureter.
D. hydronephrosis.

___ 18. Disorders of kidney function include all of the following EXCEPT _____
A. Cushing syndrome.
B. glomerulonephritis.
C. acute renal failure.
D. renal tubular necrosis.

___ 19. A general term for ill-defined solid material seen on microscopic examination of urine is

_____
A. casts.
B. crystals.
C. turbidity.
D. amorphous sediment.

___ 20. On a urinalysis, cell counts are recorded as number of cells per _____
A. deciliter of urine ([cells]/dL).
B. high power field ([cells]/hpf).
C. milliliter of urine ([cells]/mL).
D. cubic centimeters of urine ([cells]/cc).

Diagnostic and Surgical Procedures

Instructions: Match the following diagnostic and surgical procedures to their descriptions or definitions. Some answers may be used more than once or not at all.

____ 1. brachytherapy

____ 2. cystolitholapaxy

____ 3. cystoscopy

____ 4. cystourethroscopy

____ 5. extracorporeal shock wave lithotripsy

____ 6. hydrocelectomy

____ 7. intravesical immunotherapy

____ 8. panendoscopy

____ 9. retrograde pyelography

____10. transurethral resection of the prostate

A. Endoscopic treatment by which bladder stones are crushed using a lithotrite, with the fragments being subsequently washed out

B. Endoscopy of the urinary bladder via the urethra

C. Examination of the GU system in which a contrast medium is injected backward through a urinary catheter into the ureters and calyces of the pelves of the kidneys with the flow observed radiographically

D. Examination using an instrument that permits wide-angle viewing of the urinary bladder and urethra

E. Excision of a fluid-filled sac in the scrotum

F. Form of radiotherapy in which sealed sources of radioactive material are inserted temporarily into body cavities or directly into tumors

G. Instillation of a drug such as BCG into the bladder for the treatment of bladder cancer

H. Noninvasive method of shattering urinary tract stones using ultrasound

I. Surplus prostatic tissue encroaching on the lumen of the urethra is shaved away using an electrical loop

J. Use of a urethroscope to examine the male urethra for prostate enlargement

Laboratory Procedures

Instructions: Match the following laboratory procedures to their descriptions or definitions. Some answers may be used more than once, some not at all.

____ 1. acid phosphatase

____ 2. ASO titer

____ 3. bilirubin

____ 4. BUN

____ 5. creatinine

____ 6. creatinine clearance

____ 7. FTA-ABS

____ 8. PSA

____ 9. RPR (rapid plasma reagin

____ 10. urinalysis

A. A measure of kidney function based on the amount of a specific nitrogenous waste excreted by the kidneys in the volume of urine collected over a 24-hours period

B. Blood test to screen for prostatic carcinoma

C. Its appearance in the urine is indicative of obstructive jaundice

D. Nitrogenous waste excreted by the kidneys, serum levels of which are elevated in renal failure and other conditions of impaired renal function

E. Panel of tests including pH and specific gravity, glucose, albumin, leukocyte esterase, nitrite, acetone, bilirubin, red and white blood cells, crystals, casts, etc.

F. Serum blood test to measure antibodies against a substance produced by group A Streptococcus bacteria

G. Serum level of a nitrogenous waste product of protein metabolism, elevated in impaired kidney function

H. Test for syphilis

I. Urine specimen obtained after cleansing of the area around the urethral meatus to prevent contamination

Pharmacology

Instructions: Choose the best answer.

___ 1. Factors affecting the choice of therapy for urinary tract infections include all of the following EXCEPT _____
    A. the causative organism.
    B. whether the drug is a true antibiotic.
    C. proven effectiveness against the organism.
    D. the ability to establish an effective tissue level.

___ 2. Which of the following drugs does not belong in the group with the others?
    A. Cipro (ciprofloxacin).
    B. Floxin (ofloxacin).
    C. Macrodantin (nitrofurantoin).
    D. Gantanol (sulfamethoxazole).

___ 3. Which of the following drugs is NOT an antispasmodic?
    A. Pyridium (phenazopyridine).
    B. Detrol LA (tolterodine).
    C. Ditropan (oxybutynin).
    D. Urispas (flavoxate).

___ 4. If a patient had urge incontinence, you might expect the physician to prescribe which one of the following drugs?
    A. Noroxin (norfloxacin).
    B. Avodart (dutasteride).
    C. VESIcare (solifenacin).
    D. Pyridium (phenazopyridine).

___ 5. A generic drug used in combination with the folic acid inhibitor trimethoprim for the treatment of upper and lower urinary tract infections is _____
    A. sulfamethoxazole.
    B. ciprofloxacin.
    C. nitrofurantoin.
    D. ofloxacin.

___ 6. Which of the following drugs is used for treatment of benign prostatic hyperplasia?
    A. Levitra (vardenafil).
    B. Proscar (finasteride).
    C. Detrol LA (tolterodine).
    D. Dolsed (methenamine).

___ 7. Which of the following drugs is NOT used to treatment erectile dysfunction?
    A. Caverject, Muse (alprostadil).
    B. Viagra (sildenafil).
    C. Cialis (tadalafil).
    D. Hytrin (terazosin).

Dissecting Medical Terms

Instructions: As you learned in your medical language course, words are formed from prefixes, combining forms (root word plus combining vowel), and suffixes. Combining vowels (usually *o* but not always) are used to connect two root words or a root and a suffix. By analyzing these word parts, you can often determine the definition of a term without even looking it up (if you know the definition of the parts, of course!). Being able to divide and analyze the words you hear into their component parts will also improve your auditory deciphering ability and spelling and help you research those words that you cannot easily spell or define. It will also help you decipher, define, and spell coined words that may not appear in reliable resources.

For the following terms, draw a slash (/) between the components and then write a short definition based on the meaning of the parts. Remember that to define a word based on its parts, you start at the end, usually with the suffix. If there's a prefix, that is defined next and finally the combining form is defined. The actual definition of medical words does not always equal the sum of their parts because of changes in meaning over time; when this is the case, adjust your final definition to fit today's use.

Example: adenocarcinoma
Divide & Analyze: adenocarcinoma = adeno/carcin/oma = tumor + gland + malignant cancer
Define: a malignant cancerous tumor of a gland

1. Term   prophylaxis
   Divide _____
    _____
   Define _____

2. Term   hyperplasia
   Divide _____
    _____
   Define _____

3. Term   brachytherapy
   Divide _____
    _____
   Define _____

4. Term   fluoroscopy
   Divide _____
    _____
   Define _____

5. Term   cystolitholapaxy
   Divide _____
    _____
   Define _____

6. Term   dyssynergia
   Divide _____
    _____
   Define _____

7. Term   dysfunctional
   Divide _____
    _____
   Define _____

8. Term   hemiscrotal
   Divide _____
    _____
   Define _____

9. Term   hydronephrosis
   Divide _____
    _____
   Define _____

10. Term   hyperbilirubinemia
    Divide _____
     _____
    Define _____

11. Term   hypovolemia
    Divide _____
     _____
    Define _____

12. Term   intravesical
    Divide _____
     _____
    Define _____

13. Term   nephropathy
    Divide _____
     _____
    Define _____

14. Term   organomegaly
    Divide _____
     _____
    Define _____

15. Term   panendoscopy

Divide _____

_____

Define _____

16. Term   radiopaque

Divide _____

_____

Define _____

17. Term   retrograde

Divide _____

_____

Define _____

18. Term   rhabdomyolysis

Divide _____

_____

Define _____

19. Term   pyelography

Divide _____

_____

Define _____

20. Term   urodynamic

Divide _____

_____

Define _____

Spelling Exercise

Instructions: Review the adjective suffixes in your medical language textbook. Test your knowledge of adjectives by writing the adjectival form of the following urology or nephrology words. Consult a medical dictionary to verify your spelling.

Noun	Adjective
1. diuresis	_____
2. diverticulum	_____
3. elect	_____
4. erection	_____
5. erythema	_____
6. gland	_____
7. pertaining to the kidneys (2 adjectives)	
	_____
	_____
8. papilla	_____

9. penis _____

10. prostrate _____

11. scrotum _____

12. testicle _____

13. trabecula _____

14. trabeculate _____

15. urine _____

16. vesica (bladder) _____

17. vesicle (sac) _____

Abbreviations Exercise

Instructions: Expand the following common urology and nephrology abbreviations and brief forms. Then memorize both abbreviations and definitions to increase your speed and accuracy in transcribing urology and nephrology dictation. Although some abbreviations do not need to be translated in healthcare documents, you do need to know the translation in order to be sure that you are hearing the abbreviation correctly.

Abbreviation	Expansion
1. BPH	_____
2. BMP	_____
3. BUN	_____
4. CBC	_____
5. CHF	_____
6. CNS	_____
7. CK	_____
8. CVA	_____
9. DVT	_____
10. EBL	_____
11. ECF	_____
12. PSA	_____
13. TCC	_____
14. TCF	_____
15. TNTC	_____
16. TURP	_____
17. TSH	_____
18. UTI	_____

Transcript Forensics

This section presents snippets of transcribed dictations from clinic notes; history and physical examinations and consultations; operative reports and procedure notes; and discharge summaries. Explain the passage so that a nonmedical person can understand it. Pay particular attention to terms that are in bold type.

1. **Excerpt**: GU examination revealed a normal penis. His testes were both descended. There was a probable right **spermatocele** present superior to the testis. His rectal examination revealed a 20 g non-nodular prostate. IMPRESSION: The overall impression is urethral stricture disease

Explanation: _____

_____

_____

_____

_____

_____

_____

2. **Excerpt**: Patient is a 62-year-old white male with **bladder outlet obstructive** symptoms, including hesitancy, a decrease in the force and strength of urinary stream, **nocturia** x0-3, urgency with some mild urge incontinence. Patient also makes note of terminal dribbling. Denies any stopping and starting of stream once stream has been established.

Explanation: _____

_____

_____

_____

_____

_____

_____

3. **Excerpt**: **Cystoscopy** was performed, which revealed a deep **diverticulum** of the bladder with inflammatory or **neoplastic lesion** within the diverticulum. This area was biopsied, and biopsy showed ulceration and chronic inflammation of the bladder but no **malignancy**.

Explanation: _____

_____

_____

_____

_____

_____

_____

_____

4. **Excerpt**: An IVP showed a distended urinary bladder with a large **postvoid residual**. Upper tracts were unremarkable except for some **cortical** scarring and small cortical renal cysts.

Explanation: _____

_____

_____

_____

_____

_____

5. **Excerpt**: DIAGNOSIS: Left **ureterolithiasis** with partial ureteral obstruction and **hydronephrosis**.

Explanation: _____

_____

_____

_____

_____

_____

_____

6. **Excerpt:** The patient was admitted for pain control. **Serum creatinine was 1.7.** He underwent cystoscopy and left **retrograde pyelogram**, which revealed a possible left **ureteral stricture**. This was dilated; there were no stones apparent, and a double-J stent was left in place.

Explanation: _____

_____

_____

_____

_____

_____

_____

7. **Excerpt:** Patient had an **IVP** in the emergency room earlier today, which shows partial to complete obstruction of the left ureter at the **UVJ** with a large stone approximately 8 x 5 mm lodged at the UVJ. Patient has no other **calcifications** visible. IMPRESSION: Left lower **ureteral stone** with obstruction.

Explanation: _____

_____

_____

_____

_____

_____

_____

8. **Excerpt: Hydration, analgesia,** observation, and if stone does not pass within 72 hours or less, will probably recommend patient for **ureteroscopy** and **stone basketing** and, if needed, **ultrasonic lithotripsy.** If the stone cannot be mobilized downward, push-back and **ESWL** might be considered.

Explanation: _____

_____

_____

_____

_____

_____

_____

_____

9. **Excerpt:** The patient preoperatively had a **creatinine of 0.6,** his white count 6500. Coagulation studies were normal. Urinalysis showed greater than **200 white cells, 15 red cells, and calcium phosphate crystals.** Culture of the bacteria grew out **klebsiella and pseudomonas.**

Explanation: _____

_____

_____

_____

_____

_____

_____

_____

10. **Excerpt:** The patient has a heavily **trabeculated** bladder with an enlarged occlusive prostate. **Transrectal ultrasonography** showed a volume of 31.9 mL with poor bladder emptying. Transrectal biopsy revealed a pathologic diagnosis of chronic **prostatitis** and **benign prostatic hyperplasia.**

Explanation: _____

_____

_____

_____

_____

_____

_____

Sample Reports

Sample urology and nephrology reports appear on the following pages, illustrating a variety of reports. Fictional names are provided for illustration of proper format, and no resemblance to actual persons is intended. Sample transcripts were prepared according to *The Book of Style for Medical Transcription* (AHDI).

Chart Note

CHESSON, ELIZABETH
June 20, [add year]

SUBJECTIVE
This is a 24-year-old white married female who complains of urinary burning and frequency beginning approximately 5 days ago. She denies any prior urinary problems. She has had no chills, fever, flank pain, or hematuria. She has noted nocturia x3 since the onset of her symptoms. She has had no nausea or abdominal pain. She denies vaginal discharge or itching. Last menstrual period began 17 days ago. She is on Demulen 1/35-28 for birth control but has taken no other medicines. She is sexually active in a stable and apparently exclusive marital relationship. Her general health is good, and she denies recent upper respiratory infection (URI). She has never been pregnant.

OBJECTIVE
Temperature 98.6, pulse 72 and regular, blood pressure 116/80. The patient is alert and in no distress. Her skin is pale, warm, and dry. There is no costovertebral angle tenderness, and palpation of the abdomen indicates no masses or organomegaly. The bladder is not palpable or tender. On pelvic exam there is no evidence of vulvar edema or erythema and no discharge. The cervix is clean, and only scant mucoid material is seen in the vault. She had a negative (class 1) Pap smear about 8 months ago. Bimanual exam reveals a normal-sized uterus which is slightly retroflexed. The adnexal areas are normal. There are no masses or abdominal tenderness, and the rectal examination is negative.

A clean-voided urine shows 15-20 wbc/hpf, 8-10 red cells, 4+ occult blood, 1+ protein, negative for sugar, pH 5.5.

ASSESSMENT
Acute cystitis.

PLAN
1. Cipro 250 mg q.12 h. x3 days.
2. Pyridium 200 mg q.4-6 h. p.r.n. burning.
3. Increase oral fluids.
4. I discussed the probable origin of her condition with the patient and advised her to make a practice of voiding immediately after intercourse in the future.
5. The patient is to call in the day after tomorrow if she has any persisting symptoms.

JF:hpi

History and Physical Examination

SALDATE, DAVID
#987123456
Admitted 6/1/[add year]

HISTORY
This 43-year-old male was admitted through the emergency department with a history of less than 1 day of acute ureteral colic on the left side. The patient had an IVP in the emergency department earlier today which shows partial to complete obstruction of the left ureter at the ureterovesical (UV) junction, with a large stone approximately 8 x 5 mm lodged at the UV junction. The patient has no other calcifications visible. The patient denies any previous history of urinary tract stones or other GU problems except for prostatitis a couple of years ago. The patient has no other significant medical problems.

PAST MEDICAL HISTORY
Otherwise negative.

ALLERGIES
None.

MEDICATIONS
None. Follows usual diet.

FAMILY HISTORY
No familial history of kidney stones or other significant hereditary disease.

PHYSICAL EXAMINATION
GENERAL: A well-nourished, well-developed male in no acute distress.
HEAD AND NECK: Eyes: Pupils equal, round, react to light. Ears, nose, and throat clear. Neck supple; no JV distention or bruit.
CHEST: Lungs clear to percussion and auscultation.
HEART: Regular rhythm, no murmur.
ABDOMEN: Soft. Slight left CVA tenderness; slight left lower quadrant tenderness. No rebound.
GENITALIA: Within normal limits. Penis: Normal male.
EXTREMITIES: No cyanosis, clubbing, or edema.
NEUROLOGIC: Oriented x3 with no gross deficits.

IMPRESSION
Left lower ureteral stone with obstruction.

RECOMMENDATION
Hydration, analgesia, observation, and if the stone does not pass within 72 hours or less, will probably recommend patient for ureteroscopy and stone basketing, and if needed, ultrasonic lithotripsy. If the stone cannot be mobilized downward, push back and ESWL might be considered.

LEO PEREZ, MD
LP:hpi
d: 6/1/[add year]   t: 6/1/[add year]

Consultation

PARK, MARCO
#9872435
June 1, [add year]
Medical 701B

HISTORY

Apparently this patient presented to the emergency department last night about midnight with excruciating left flank pain radiating down into the left groin and testicle, chills, nausea, vomiting, and slight urinary burning, all of about 2 hours' duration, and a stat urine showed 60-80 red cells. Apparently he was given Stadol 2 mg IM for analgesia and some IV fluids, and he had an emergency IVP run which showed a radiopaque stone measuring about 0.5 cm partially blocking the left ureter at a point about 2 cm above the ureterovesical junction. There was moderate hydronephrosis without appreciable dilatation of the caliceal system, and some dye was getting past the block. I have reviewed these films, and they show normal urinary tract anatomy on the right and on the left, except as noted.

When I examined him about 10 a.m., he was still in considerable distress although noticeably obtunded by a dose of Demerol given about one-half hour prior to my visit. He was sufficiently alert, however, to give a good clear history. Apparently this man has had two previous episodes of left-sided ureteral colic followed by spontaneous passage of stones, once while on military service in Turkey and once since then, but on neither occasion were the stones preserved for analysis.

His general health is good, and he takes no medicine. He has never had a urinary tract infection. There is no known family history of renal lithiasis, gout, or bone or joint disease; however, he is adopted. He is 41 years of age, married, with two daughters, and is employed as a manager of a recreation center.

EXAMINATION

Temperature is 99.2, pulse 100, blood pressure 150/80. Physical exam is quite benign except that he is pale, sweating, restless, and in considerable distress and tender at the left costovertebral angle and in the left upper quadrant over the kidney and ureter. External genital exam is unremarkable. I did not attempt to do a rectal exam. He has an IV running, even though he is now taking oral fluids and he is not nauseated. He is voiding painlessly, and his urine is being strained. I did not see his urine, but according to the patient and the attendant, it is not grossly bloody.

DIAGNOSIS

Left ureterolithiasis with partial ureteral obstruction and hydronephrosis.

RECOMMENDATIONS

1. Continue analgesia and hydration.
2. Continue straining urine and preserve any solid material passed for chemical analysis.
3. Clean-voided midstream urine for culture and sensitivity.
4. After this has been obtained, start Cipro 500 mg q.12 h. orally.

(continued)

Consultation *(continued)*

PARK, MARCO
#9872435
June 1, [add year]
Medical 701B
Page 2

RECOMMENDATIONS (continued)

5. He is now about 12 hours post onset of symptoms, but there is still a good statistical chance that he will pass his stone spontaneously. We are going to get another IVP at 4 p.m., and if he is still obstructed, I think we had better attempt to bring this stone down with a snare before he gets enough local edema to obstruct completely or gets into trouble with a red-hot ascending pyelonephritis.
6. In any event, he needs a biochemical analysis of his problem, and depending on that, he may need dietary or drug prophylaxis against further calculus disease.

Thank you for the privilege of collaborating in the care of this patient.

MARC GIOVANNI, MD

MG:hpi

D:6/1/[add year]
T: 6/2/[add year]

Operative Report

KEVORKIAN, LUKE
#25624134
SURGERY 400-C

DATE OF SURGERY
June 4, [add year]

PREOPERATIVE DIAGNOSIS
Recurrent bladder neck obstruction.

POSTOPERATIVE DIAGNOSIS
Recurrent bladder neck obstruction.

TITLE OF OPERATION
Cystoscopy and transurethral resection of the prostate.

TECHNIQUE
Upon administration of satisfactory spinal anesthesia, the patient was placed on the cystoscopy table in the lithotomy position. The external genitalia were prepped and draped in the usual manner for endoscopy. The #24 Wappler instrument was passed under direct vision, revealing a normal distal urethra. There is no evidence of stricture or other localized lesion. As one enters into the prostatic urethra, he has a normal-appearing verumontanum. There is a small apical growth on the patient's left side, but this is not impressive. He has a very large obstructing-appearing lobe coming in from the right side, mainly superiorly, with only a relatively small amount near the floor. As one enters the prostatic urethra, there is a slightly scarred bladder neck contracture apparent; however, it is of wide caliber and would not be considered significant. The instrument was then irrigated, and cystoscopy was done with both right-angle and Foroblique lens systems. The main thing one sees here is a heavily trabeculated bladder, multiple bands and ridges, no true diverticulum. No stones are identified. There is no evidence of inflammation or tumor.

At this point, the McCarthy-Storz Foroblique resectoscope sheath was introduced, size 28 in character, after accepting comfortably 28 and 30 van Buren sounds. A standard transurethral resection of the prostate was done. The ureteral orifices sat nicely back from the bladder neck, and I instilled indigo carmine just for security. Once the bladder neck was cut down on the bladder side, I then started at 11 o'clock and subsequently 1 o'clock cutting lateral lobe tissue out bilaterally and then cut the tissue as it fell in. Because of his decompensating bladder, I did a fairly radical and deep transurethral resection of the capsule throughout. I did stay within the verumontanum but took out apical lobes as safely as I could. At the end of the resection, there was some venous bleeding but no evidence of arterial bleeding. The prostatic urethra was wide open. All chips were then irrigated from the bladder and a #26 three-way Foley inserted. It was inflated to 55 mL. We observed him for venous bleeding; this stopped almost immediately and remained clear. At that point he was transferred to the recovery room with vital signs stable, in good general condition.

SEAN LARKIN, MD

SL:hpi   d: 6/5/[add year]   t: 6/6/[add year]

Operative Report

PASMA, DANIEL
#618758

DATE
October 22, [add year]

PREOPERATIVE DIAGNOSIS
Hematuria, right lower quadrant pain.

POSTOPERATIVE DIAGNOSIS
Hematuria, right lower quadrant pain.

OPERATION PERFORMED
Cystoscopy and bilateral retrograde pyelograms.

SURGEON
MICHAEL COGGER, MD

INDICATIONS FOR PROCEDURE
This 49-year-old gentleman has been experiencing right lower quadrant pain radiating to his right leg and groin. He has had extensive x-rays and extensive GI workup, all negative. He presents at this time for urologic evaluation.

FINDINGS
The urethra was normal without strictures. The prostate was 2 cm in length, nonobstructing. The ureteral orifices effluxed clear urine. Bilateral bulb tip retrograde pyelograms revealed no filling defects, no stones seen.

PROCEDURE
Patient brought to the operating room where, under general anesthesia, he was prepped and draped in the usual fashion. Cystoscopy was carried out with the Olympus 21 French cystoscope utilizing the 12- and 70-degree lens, with the above findings. Bilateral bulb tip retrograde pyelograms were obtained with the above findings. Fluoroscopy was used to visualize peristalsis of the ureters, especially the right, and no hang-up of contrast was seen, and there was free flow from the kidney down to the bladder. The bladder was drained. Patient tolerated the procedure well.

MICHAEL COGGER, MD

MC:hpi

d: 10/1/[add date]
t: 10/2/[add date]

Operative Report

LAPIERRE, WAYNE
#256781

DATE OF OPERATION
April 11, [add year]

PREOPERATIVE DIAGNOSIS
Redundant foreskin.

POSTOPERATIVE DIAGNOSIS
Redundant foreskin.

PROCEDURE
Circumcision.

ANESTHESIA
Local with IV sedation. Local was approximately 12 mL of 1% lidocaine mixed with 0.5% Marcaine.
IV sedation included 100 mL of IV Demerol, 5 mg of IV Versed.

COMPLICATIONS
None apparent.

SPECIMENS
None.

DESCRIPTION OF PROCEDURE
Patient brought to the operating room and placed in the supine position. The penis, scrotum, and
perineum were prepped and draped in the usual sterile fashion. Initially, a penile block was performed
with lidocaine-Marcaine mix. This created adequate anesthesia of the distal penile foreskin. The foreskin
was then marked just proximal to the corona of the glans penis and on the inner foreskin 1 cm proximal
to the glans. Incisions were made over the marked area, and the foreskin was removed in a sleeve
technique. A 4-quadrant closure was done with 3-0 chromic interrupted suture using a horizontal
mattress at the frenulum. The 4-0 chromic interrupted suture was then used in between these quadrants.
Final inspection revealed excellent hemostasis and an excellent closure. Please note that prior to closing
the foreskin, the underlying dartos fascial layers were cauterized for hemostasis, which was excellent. At
the end of the procedure, Bacitracin was applied to the incision. A Telfa and a lightly compressive Coban
dressing were applied.

He tolerated the procedure well, was transferred to the recovery room in stable condition. There were no
apparent complications.

ROY TRAWICK, MD
RT:hpi d&t: 4/11/[add year]

Comic Relief

Correct	Incorrect
Correct	**Incorrect**
d: The urine showed pyuria.	t: The urine showed pyorrhea.
d: Examination of prostate, normal.	t: Exophthalmos of prostate, normal.
d: The testis was pulled up into the wound by stripping off the tunicus dartos.	t: Dermatitis was pulled up into the wound by sipping off the tourniquet.
d: Mayo clamps were used.	t: Male clamps were used.
d: The wound was treated with ice packs.	t: The wound was treated with ice picks.
d: The cystic duct was traced to its junction.	t: The cystic duct was chased to its junction.
d: A lazy S incision was made.	t: A lazy ass incision was made.
d: Venous filling time, 10 seconds bilaterally.	t: Penis filling time, 10 seconds bilaterally.
d: Broken stricture in the urethra.	t: Boa constrictor in the urethra.

Obstetrics and Gynecology

Learning Objectives

▶ Describe the structure and function of the female reproductive system.

▶ Spell and define common ObGyn terms.

▶ Identify ObGyn vocabulary that might be used in the review of systems.

▶ Describe the negative and positive findings a physician looks for on examination of the female reproductive system.

▶ Describe the course and care of a patient during pregnancy and delivery, including complications of pregnancy and delivery.

▶ Describe the typical cause, course, and treatment options for common diseases of the female reproductive system, including sexually transmitted diseases and infertility.

▶ Identify and define common diagnostic and surgical procedures of the female reproductive system.

▶ List common ObGyn laboratory tests and procedures.

▶ Identify and describe common ObGyn drugs and their uses.

▶ Demonstrate knowledge of anatomical, medical, pharmacological, adjectival, and soundalike terms by accurately completing the exercises in this chapter.

Transcribing Obstetrics and Gynecology Dictation

Introduction

Gynecology is the branch of medicine that is concerned with diseases peculiar to women, chiefly diseases of the reproductive system. **Obstetrics** is the medical specialty devoted to the management of pregnancy and childbirth. Although many physicians work in both fields and are referred to as obstetrician-gynecologists (ObGyn), some prefer to limit their practice to one specialty or the other.

Obstetricians care for patients who are pregnant or planning to becoming pregnant. They handle a patient's prenatal care, follow the pregnancy, supervise labor and deliver the baby, and provide postpartum care. Some obstetricians specialize in genetic counseling and prenatal diagnosis, others in assisted reproduction and infertility.

Gynecologists often function as primary care physicians for women, caring for their general health as well as their reproductive organs, breasts, and sexual function. Gynecologists manage hormonal disorders and treat gynecologic infections including sexually transmitted diseases.

Anatomy Review

The **female reproductive system including the breasts** (see ■ Figures 14-1, 14-2, 14-3) is concerned exclusively with procreation. Unlike that of the male, it does not share structures with the urinary tract to any significant extent. The female reproductive organs are divided into **internal genitalia (ovaries, uterus,** and **vagina)** and **external genitalia** (labia majora, labia minora, clitoris, and vaginal vestibule, collectively forming the **vulva**).

The nonpregnant adult **uterus** is roughly the size and shape of a pear. It rests on the floor of the pelvis with its conical narrower portion, the **cervix** (Latin, 'neck'), pointing downward. The body or **corpus** (the remainder of the uterus) lies in the pelvic cavity. The domelike top, or **fundus**, of the uterus lies between the rectum posteriorly and the urinary bladder anteriorly. Normally the uterus tilts forward, resting on the top of the bladder and making a considerable angle with the axis of the vagina.

From either side of the uterine fundus, a hornlike projection gives rise to one of the two **uterine tubes** (fallopian tubes). Each of these sweeps laterally to form a funnel-shaped expansion (**fimbria**) near one of the ovaries. Approximately the lower one-half of the cervix, the portio vaginalis (i.e., 'vaginal portion'), extends

down through the anterosuperior part of the **vaginal vault** to lie within the vagina. The upper half or portio supravaginalis, as its name implies, is above the vagina. Many physicians, evidently believing that portio means something like 'porch' or 'portico', omit the qualifying adjective and refer to the portio vaginalis simply as "the portio."

A narrow passage (about 0.75 cm in diameter), the **endocervical canal**, runs through the cervix to connect

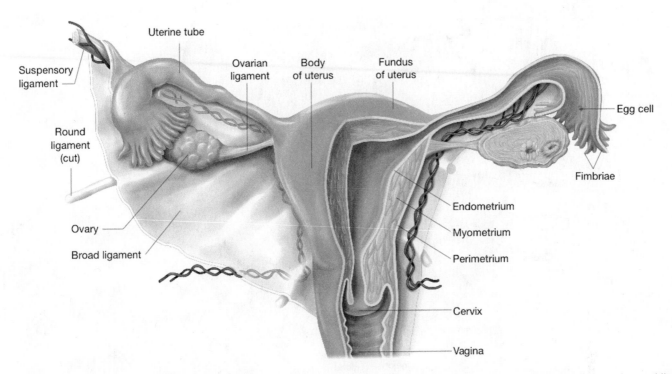

FIGURE 14-1. Female reproductive system, internal organs. Cutaway view shows the uterus and its relationship to the ovaries and the vagina.

the cavity of the uterus with the vagina. The upper end of this canal, opening into the uterine cavity, is called the **internal os** (Latin, 'mouth'), and the lower end is the **external os**.

The body or corpus of the uterus consists largely of muscle (**myometrium**), whose contractions expel the fetus during childbirth. In contrast, the cervix contains mostly fibrous connective tissue rather than muscle. A mucosal membrane (**endometrium**) lines the interior of the uterus. The endometrium varies in thickness and structure with the phases of the menstrual cycle. It is shed during menstruation.

The female reproductive system also includes the **breasts** (mammary glands), which provide nourishment to the newborn child (see ■ Figure 14-2). The mature nonpregnant breast consists principally of fibrous connective tissue and fat, in which glandular elements are radially disposed and communicate by ducts with the nipple. Like the endometrium, the glandular tissue of the breast responds to cyclical variation in the levels of ovarian and pituitary hormones.

Pelvic examination reveals essentially healthy vagina with blood in the vault and cervical os. The uterus is anteverted, 6 weeks' size, and mobile. Adnexa are grossly normal. No palpable masses. Rectal examination was negative.

This 45-year-old married mother of 3 children first noted a 2.5 x 2.5 cm hard, irregular, nontender mass in the upper outer quadrant of the left breast about 6 weeks ago.

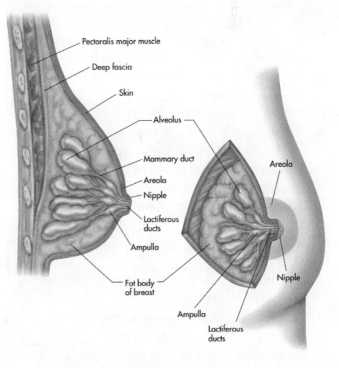

FIGURE 14-2. Breast.

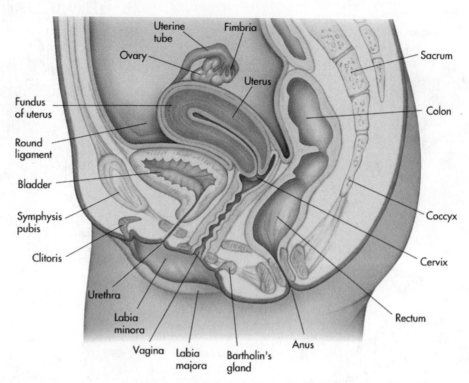

FIGURE 14-3. The female reproductive organs, sagittal section

Pause for Reflection

1. The ovaries, uterus, and vagina constitute the _____ and the labia majora, labia minora, clitoris, and vaginal vestibule are referred to as the _____ or _____.
2. The three principal parts of the uterus are the _____ ("neck"), the _____ ("body") and the _____ (domelike top).
3. The hornlike projections on either side of the fundus give rise to the _____ tubes, which may also be referred to as _____ tubes.
4. The ends of these tubes are called _____.
5. The lower half of the cervix extends down into the upper anterior portion of the _____.
6. The narrow passage that runs through the cervix to connect the uterus to the vagina is called the _____; its upper opening is called the _____ and the lower opening is the _____.
7. The membrane that lines the interior of the uterus is called the _____.
8. The muscular structure of the uterus is the ____.
9. Both the _____ and the _____ respond to cyclical variation in the levels of ovarian and pituitary hormones.

Vocabulary Review

adnexa (plural only; takes a plural verb) Organs adjacent to the uterus—ovaries, tubes, broad ligaments, round ligaments, and associated blood vessels.

amenorrhea Absence of menstruation.

anovulation Failure of ovulation to occur at the expected times.

antepartum Before childbirth.

Apgar score The sum of points assigned on assessment of a newborn's heart rate, respiratory effort, muscle tone, reflex irritability, and color, usually calculated at 1 and 5 minutes after birth.

Bartholin glands A pair of glands located on either side of the vaginal orifice that secrete mucus for lubrication during intercourse.

boggy uterus More spongy or elastic than expected.

Braxton Hicks contractions Weak and irregular contractions of the uterus occurring during mid to late pregnancy.

BUS Bartholin glands, urethra, and Skene glands.

cephalopelvic disproportion (CPD) The fetal head is too large to pass through the maternal pelvis.

cervical incompetence A medical condition in which a pregnant woman's cervix begins to dilate (widen) and efface (thin) before her pregnancy has reached term. It may cause miscarriage or preterm birth during the second and third trimesters.

cervical intraepithelial neoplasia (CIN) Dysplasia that is seen on a biopsy of the cervix and classified as follows: CIN I—mild dysplasia; CIN II—moderate to marked dysplasia; CIN III—severe dysplasia to carcinoma in situ.

cesarean delivery (cesarean section, C-section) Birth of the fetus through a surgical incision into the uterus through the abdominal wall.

Chadwick sign Purplish discoloration of the cervix and vagina in early pregnancy.

choriocarcinoma A malignant tumor that can develop from either the chorion of a normal pregnancy or a hydatidiform mole. It grows rapidly and metastasizes early, often before an abnormal pregnancy is suspected. Quantitative assay of hCG plays a role in the detection and management of both of these placental neoplasms.

cystocele Bulging of the urinary bladder through the anterior vaginal wall.

cystourethrocele Prolapse of the urethra and bladder into the vagina.

dilatation The expansion of the uterine ring to a size (about 10 cm) through which the fetal head can pass.

dysmenorrhea Pain occurring with menstruation and often severe. The lay term for dysmenorrhea is "(menstrual) cramps."

dyspareunia Pain in the vulva, vagina, or pelvis with sexual intercourse.

dysplasia Cell abnormalities heralding eventual development of malignancy.

dystocia Abnormal slowing or arrest of the progress of labor.

dysuria Pain in the urethra or vulva with urination.

ectopic pregnancy Pregnancy in which implantation has occurred somewhere other than the endometrium—in the uterine tube, on the pelvic peritoneum, or even on an ovary.

effacement The flattening of the cervix from a tubular structure to a ring during labor.

LAY AND MEDICAL TERMS	
afterbirth	placenta
bag of waters	amniotic membranes and fluid
birth control	contraception
change of life	menopause
clap	gonorrhea
cramps	dysmenorrhea
periods	menses
tubal pregnancy	ectopic pregnancy
water breaking	gush of fluid from vagina
womb	uterus

endometrial stripe On an ultrasound, refers to the thickness of the endometrium; an endometrial stripe of more than 4 or 5 mm is an indication for an endometrial biopsy in a postmenopausal woman.

estimated date of confinement (EDC). Calculated by going back 3 months and then forward 7 days from the first day of the last menstrual period. May also be called **EDD (estimated date of delivery).**

failure of descent, failure to descend A delay in the progression of labor in which the baby fails to descend into the birth canal.

fetal hypoxemia Reduction in fetal plasma oxygen tension.

fetal macrosomia Excessive body size and weight.

fetal pyelectasis Dilatation of a renal pelvis observed in a fetus.

fourchette A fold of skin crossing the posterior commissure of the labia minora. Episiotomy may be performed during delivery to avoid irregular tearing of the fourchette.

funic souffle A whistling sound due to the flow of blood in the umbilical cord, heard on auscultation of the pregnant abdomen.

gestational diabetes Carbohydrate intolerance first occurring or first noted during pregnancy. This is a risk factor for polyhydramnios (excessive volume of amniotic fluid) and fetal macrosomia.

gravid Pregnant.

gravida Pregnant woman.

Hegar sign Softening of the cervix in early pregnancy, as palpated on pelvic examination.

hydatidiform mole A benign neoplasm developing from the chorion of a pregnancy that is abnormal because of a certain type of chromosomal aberration. The tumor, which consists of fluid-filled vesicles clumped somewhat like grapes, may enlarge and stretch the uterus just like a normal pregnancy. A fetus may or may not be present along with the tumor.

hypermenorrhea Abnormally high volume of menstrual discharge.

hypomenorrhea Abnormally low volume of menstrual discharge.

intrauterine device (IUD) A device placed in the uterus to prevent conception. Two types available in the U.S. are the copper Paragard and the hormonal Mirena.

intrauterine pregnancy (IUP) A normal pregnancy that develops within the uterus.

introitus The vestibule of the vagina, at the level of the labia minora, urethral meatus, and Bartholin glands.

lactation Producing milk from the breasts.

last menstrual period (LMP) Used in calculating EDC in pregnancy and also pertinent in menstrual disorders.

longitudinal lie The relation of the long axis of the fetus to that of the mother. In the longitudinal lie the fetal axis is parallel to mother's.

Lugol solution An iodine-based staining solution. During a colposcopy, Lugol's is applied to the vagina and cervix. Normal tissue will stain, but tissue suspicious for cancer will not. Also called a *Schiller test*, so *Schiller-positive* indicates that the tissue did not stain, a seeming paradox.

meconium Stool formed in the fetal intestine before birth.

menarche The onset of the first menstrual period.

menometrorrhagia Excessive menstrual bleeding occurring both during menses and at irregular intervals.

menopause The cessation of regular menstrual periods.

menorrhagia Regularly occurring menstrual flow that is excessive in volume and lasts longer than a normal menstrual period.

metrorrhagia Menstrual bleeding occurring at irregular but frequent intervals.

miscarriage Spontaneous abortion.

mittelschmerz Intermenstrual pain due to peritoneal irritation by a small volume of blood escaping from the ovary at the time of ovulation.

multigravida A woman who has been pregnant more than once.

multipara A woman who has given birth more than once.

nuchal cord Occurs when the umbilical cord becomes wrapped around the fetal neck 360 degrees. Half of nuchal cords resolve before delivery.

nulligravida A woman who has never been pregnant.

nullipara A woman who has never given birth.

oligohydramnios Less than the normal amount of amniotic fluid, defined as 500 mL or less at term and smaller amounts at earlier gestational ages. Too little amniotic fluid can cause severe fetal abnormalities, and the mortality rate is high.

oligomenorrhea Infrequent or scanty menstrual bleeding.

para Live birth.

parturient A woman in labor.

parturition Childbirth.

pelvic relaxation Weakening of the pelvic floor muscles and ligaments, often a result of childbirth or aging and resulting in prolapse of the uterus or bladder.

polyhydramnios Excessive volume of amnionic fluid.

polymenorrhea Menstrual bleeding that occurs with abnormal frequency.

position The relation of the presenting part to the right or left side of the birth canal. In right occiput anterior (ROA) the fetal occiput is anterior and directed toward the right side of the mother.

postcoital Occurring after sexual intercourse.

postpartum Following childbirth.

postvoiding residual The amount of urine left in the bladder after urination.

preeclampsia Abnormal development of high blood pressure that may be accompanied by proteinuria and edema, all due to toxemia during pregnancy.

premature rupture of membranes (PROM) Rupture of the amniotic sac (bag of waters) prior to the onset of labor.

presenting part The part of the fetus that is nearest to, or has entered, the birth canal. With a longitudinal lie this is either the head or the breech (buttocks).

primary amenorrhea Failure of menses to start at puberty (by age 14–16).

primigravida A woman who is pregnant for the first time.

primipara A woman who has given birth once.

puerperal Pertaining to the puerperium.

puerperium The period between the birth of the child and the return of the uterus to its normal size, with regeneration of endometrium.

rectocele Bulging of the rectum through the posterior vaginal wall.

secondary amenorrhea Cessation of menses that have been normal in the past.

serous cystadenoma A benign cystic tumor of the ovary.

spirochete A spiral-shaped bacterium. The organisms that cause syphilis and Lyme disease are spirochetes.

spontaneous abortion Miscarriage.

station The position of the fetal presenting part with respect to the maternal ischial spines as labor progresses. **Station minus two** means that the presenting part lies 2 cm above the spines.

tubo-ovarian abscess An abscess formed between a uterine tube (fallopian tube) and its adjacent ovary.

uterine descensus Prolapse of the uterus. Also called *descensus uteri*. In first-degree descensus, the cervix of the uterus is within the vaginal orifice; second-degree, the cervix is outside the orifice; and third-degree, the entire uterus is outside the orifice.

uterine sound A long flexible instrument with graduated measurements used for exploring the length and direction of the cervix and uterus. May be used as a verb, as in "The uterus was sounded to a depth of 8 cm."

vulva The group of structures that make up the female external genitalia (labia majora, labia minora, clitoris, the vaginal orifice, and the urinary meatus).

yeast A one-celled fungus; often used interchangeably with *Candida albicans*.

Medical Readings
History and Physical Examination
by John H. Dirckx, MD

Review of Systems. The menstrual history includes age at onset of menses (**menarche**), regularity of cycles, interval between periods, duration of periods, and the date of the last normal menstrual period. In addition, the interviewer inquires about menstrual cramps (**dysmenorrhea**), heaviness of flow, and intermenstrual or postmenopausal bleeding.

This patient is a 16-year-old gravida 1, para 0, menarche at age 13, whose last menstrual period was March 11, who had a positive beta hCG; previous to that, normal menstrual cycles every 28 days.

The **female reproductive history** covers pregnancies, miscarriages, abortions, stillbirths, normal deliveries, and cesarean births; any complications of pregnancy such as hemorrhage or toxemia. The salient points of the reproductive history are customarily noted according to one of two formulas. In one of these, pregnancies, term deliveries, and miscarriages are recorded respectively as gravida, para, and abortus (or G, P, and Ab) with a numeral. Thus, G 3, P 2, Ab 1 refers to a woman who has been pregnant three times, has delivered two children at term, and has had one miscarriage. The other formula consists of a set of four numerals (for example, 2–0–1–2) representing respectively deliveries at term, premature deliveries, miscarriages, and children currently living. Either of these systems can prove ambiguous with respect to multiple pregnancies and their outcome.

The patient is also questioned about the use of condoms, diaphragms, oral contraceptives, or other contra-

The patient is a 28-year-old white female, gravida 2 para 1–0–0–1 who has elected to have a vaginal birth after cesarean section (VBAC), having undergone a primary C-section in 2004.

ceptive methods; pelvic pain, vaginal discharge, vulvar itching, sores, or rash; and any **breast complaints** (pain, swelling, masses, bleeding or discharge from the nipple).

Physical Examination. In women the examination of the external and internal genitourinary organs and the rectum and anus is normally performed with the patient in the lithotomy position. The patient lies on her back on a specially equipped examining table with her feet in stirrups, her thighs flexed sharply on her abdomen, and her knees spread wide apart. If she cannot assume the lithotomy position, the left lateral (Sims) position may be used instead.

The physician inspects the pubes and vulva for hair distribution (**escutcheon**), developmental anomalies, cutaneous lesions, swellings, and signs of inflammation. The urethral meatus and Bartholin and Skene glands are inspected and palpated. The integrity of the pelvic floor is assessed by having the patient bear down while the examiner observes for **cystocele** (bulging of the urinary bladder through the anterior vaginal wall), **rectocele** (bulging of the rectum through the posterior vaginal wall), or **uterine prolapse** (fallen uterus causing the cervix to protrude through the vaginal opening). Any vaginal discharge is also observed, and the perineum and anus are examined.

The patient is a 64-year-old woman who is gravida 4, para 4, referred because of a large cystocele and uterine prolapse.

Visual inspection of the cervix is an integral part of every gynecologic examination. The physician inserts a warmed and lubricated bivalve speculum into the vagina and by spreading its blades and adjusting its position obtains a view of the cervix, fornices, and vaginal walls. Vaginal specula are manufactured in various sizes and shapes to meet most needs. However, adequate visualization of the cervix may not be possible in prepubertal children, extremely obese women, or those with abnormal pelvic architecture.

Specimens may be taken for cultures or cytologic study (**Pap smear**). A gynecologist may use a colposcope, which provides bright light and strong magnification, to inspect the cervix for signs of dysplasia.

After removing the speculum, the examiner inserts one or two fingers of the dominant hand, gloved and lubricated, into the vagina and places the other hand on the patient's abdomen (**bimanual pelvic examination**). In this manner the size, shape, and position of

the uterus can be assessed, and any masses or tenderness in the pelvic cavity can be detected. Normal uterine adnexa (ovaries, tubes, broad ligaments, round ligaments, and associated blood vessels) can seldom be felt. The physician concludes the examination of the female subject by performing a digital rectal examination. With the patient in the lithotomy position, the examiner inserts one finger in the vagina and another in the rectum at the same time (**rectovaginal exam**).

The **breast examination** (see ■ Figure 14-2) consists of the following steps:

Inspection of the breasts with the subject in the upright position, first with arms at sides, then with arms raised, and finally with hands pressed against hips to render underlying muscles taut.

Palpation of each breast in both the upright and supine positions, with attention to the axillae.

Assessment of nipples for inflammation, bleeding, or discharge.

Pause for Reflection

1. The ObGyn review of systems focuses primarily on the menstrual history, including _____ and whether the patient has experienced any _____ with her periods.

2. The term _____ refers to the number of pregnancies a woman has had, _____ to the number of deliveries, and _____ to the number of abortions or miscarriages.

3. The physical exam is performed with the patient in the _____ position or in the left lateral, _____, position if she cannot assume the usual position.

4. Physical signs of loss of pelvic floor support for the uterus include _____ (bulging of the urinary bladder through the anterior vaginal wall), or _____ (bulging of the rectum through the posterior vaginal wall), or _____ (downward displacement of the cervix or entire uterus into the vagina).

5. The size, shape, and position of the uterus and any masses or tenderness in the pelvic cavity is assessed on _____ examination.

6. A _____ exam concludes the exam of the internal and external genitalia.

7. _____ and _____ of the breasts concludes the ObGyn physical exam.

Common Diseases

Premenstrual Syndrome (PMS)

A group of distressing physical and psychologic symptoms experienced in varying degrees and proportions by many women during the week preceding onset of menstruation: swelling of breasts, waist, and ankles, breast soreness, weight gain, irritability, drowsiness, depression, changes in appetite and libido. **Premenstrual dysphoric disorder (PMDD)**, a severe form of PMS associated with extreme anxiety, depression, anger, sleep and appetite disorders, and impairment of occupational and social functioning, is recognized by some authorities as a distinct condition.

The cause is unknown, but genetic predisposition, heightened sensitivity to cyclical changes in hormone levels, and dysregulation of serotonin metabolism are believed to play a part. Treatment with selective serotonin reuptake inhibitors (SSRIs) such as fluoxetine, sertraline, and paroxetine is often effective. Other measures that may help are counseling, a regular program of exercise, and restriction of sodium, caffeine, alcohol, and sugar.

Dysmenorrhea

Pelvic pain occurring with menstruation.

Causes: *Primary:* "Normal" menstrual cramps, occurring in 50–75% of all women, and due to uterine vasoconstriction and spasm resulting from withdrawal of progesterone effect. *Secondary:* Endometriosis, **pelvic inflammatory disease (PID)**, use of an IUD (intrauterine device), tumor of the uterus, cervical stenosis (due, for example, to scarring after induced abortion).

History: Cramping pain felt low in the pelvis, often radiating to the back or inner thighs, often accompanied by nausea, diarrhea, headache, or prostration. Pain begins usually on the first day of the menstrual period and lasts 1–2 days. In secondary dysmenorrhea, symptoms are more variable.

Physical Examination: Generally unremarkable in primary dysmenorrhea. Endometriosis, salpingitis, or uterine neoplasm may be detected as a cause of secondary dysmenorrhea.

Diagnostic Tests: In secondary dysmenorrhea, pelvic ultrasound or MRI may identify the underlying cause. Diagnostic D&C may disclose a cause within the uterine cavity. Laparoscopy identifies endometriosis or PID.

Course: Primary dysmenorrhea tends to diminish in severity after age 25, and particularly after childbirth.

Without treatment, secondary dysmenorrhea may continue throughout the reproductive years.

Treatment: Nonsteroidal anti-inflammatory drugs (ibuprofen, naproxen, mefenamic acid) usually provide good symptomatic relief. Oral contraceptives may be prescribed for more sustained control. Endometriosis is treated with drugs or surgery.

Dysfunctional Uterine Bleeding (DUB)

Unusually heavy or light bleeding from the uterus, typically unpredictable, or amenorrhea, in the absence of pregnancy or any demonstrable abnormality (neoplasm, infection) of the uterus.

Causes: Most cases are due to **anovulation** (failure to ovulate). This is a common occurrence and can result from physical or emotional stress, marked weight loss (as in anorexia nervosa or stringent dieting), strenuous exercise (running, gymnastics), excess or deficiency of thyroid hormone, polycystic ovary disease, recent discontinuance of oral contraceptives, lactation, and other causes. About one-third of patients with amenorrhea have elevated levels of **prolactin**; in rare cases, this is due to overproduction of prolactin by a pituitary tumor.

History: Unusually heavy or light bleeding, typically irregular; often amenorrhea lasting for three or more cycles. Symptoms of underlying disease may also be present.

Physical Examination: Generally unremarkable. May show obesity or emaciation, stigmata of thyroid or ovarian disease (goiter, exophthalmos, hirsutism), or other evidence of an underlying disorder. Cysts may be palpable in the ovaries. Presence of normal breast development and axillary and pubic hair confirms normal estrogen effect. A palpable, nontender uterus of normal size and shape rules out congenital absence of the uterus (in primary amenorrhea) and helps to exclude uterine tumors or infection.

Diagnostic Tests: A pregnancy test is always done to rule out normal or ectopic pregnancy or recent miscarriage or abortion. Determination of blood levels of estrogen, LH, FSH, T_4, TSH, and prolactin is standard. In amenorrhea in which pregnancy has been ruled out, oral administration of a progesterone (medroxyprogesterone acetate) for five days is normally followed within 10 days by a discharge of blood from the uterus if the endometrium is healthy and the estrogen level adequate. Absence of a response suggests a severe uterine disorder (**endometrial scarring**) or estrogen deficiency due to pituitary or ovarian disease.

Pelvic ultrasound may help to confirm the presence or absence of uterine or ovarian disease. Laparoscopy may be needed for definitive diagnosis. CT or MRI of the head may be performed if a pituitary tumor is suspected.

Course: Depends on the underlying condition. Extremely heavy bleeding can lead to shock or anemia.

Treatment: Depends on the underlying condition. For many patients, a course of oral contraceptive provides cyclical hormone levels sufficient to induce what seem like normal menstrual cycles and flow. Clomiphene may be given to an anovulatory woman who wants to conceive. **Hyperprolactinemia** (abnormal elevation of prolactin) in the absence of a pituitary neoplasm is treated with bromocriptine. Thyroid, ovarian, or pituitary disease, or abnormalities of pelvic anatomy and physiology, may require other specific treatment.

Uterine Myoma (Fibromyoma, Fibroid)

A benign neoplasm of uterine muscle (see ■ **Figure 14-4**).

Cause: Unknown.

History: There may be no symptoms. Abdominal or pelvic pain or pressure, heavy vaginal bleeding, dysmenorrhea, urinary frequency, infertility.

Physical Examination: Pelvic examination shows one or more discrete, firm masses in the uterine wall. With heavy bleeding there may be tachycardia, pallor, or even shock.

Diagnostic Tests: With heavy bleeding the hemoglobin level may be low. Ultrasound or MRI studies can clearly delineate the nature of the problem.

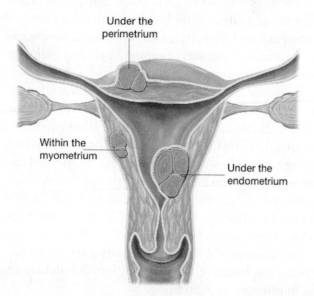

FIGURE 14-4. Fibroid tumors of uterus

Course: Uterine myomas tend to grow larger and more numerous with time. With significant bleeding there is a risk of chronic anemia or sudden onset of shock. Myomas in the pregnant uterus can lead to fetal loss, premature or difficult labor, or severe postpartum hemorrhage.

Treatment: Small or solitary myomas can be removed surgically (**myomectomy**). If tumors are large or numerous, **hysterectomy** (removal of the uterus) may be indicated. Before surgery, leuprolide or nafarelin is administered to reduce the size and vascularity of tumors.

Endometriosis

Growth of endometrial tissue outside of the uterus, particularly in the ovaries and on the pelvic walls.

Cause: Unknown. The problem affects about 2% of American women. Implants of endometrial tissue can occur in a wide variety of locations, including any peritoneal surface, the rectal mucosa, and the ovaries (causing **endometrial** or **"chocolate" cysts**, so-called because of their color).

History: Onset is usually during the middle to late 20s. Severe dysmenorrhea, often beginning days before the onset of menstruation and continuing for a week or more. Pain is constant and may be diffuse, with rectal pain and dyspareunia. Many patients are infertile (unable to conceive). Rectal bleeding may occur from implants in the rectum.

Physical Examination: Tender nodules of endometrial tissue may be palpated in the pelvis, particularly **Douglas's cul-de-sac** (lowermost part of pelvic cavity, between uterus and rectum), the ovaries, or the rectum.

Diagnostic Tests: Ultrasound, MRI, or barium enema may identify **endometrial implants**. Often laparoscopy is required to arrive at a definitive diagnosis. At laparoscopy, endometrial implants often appear as hemorrhagic cysts or **"powder burn" lesions** on peritoneal surfaces.

Course: Pain (including dyspareunia) and infertility tend to persist throughout the reproductive years. Medical or surgical treatment may diminish pain, but most treatment methods may further impair fertility.

Treatment: Analgesics and various hormone analogues (leuprolide, nafarelin, oral contraceptives) or hormone inhibitors (danazol) may help. Focal endometriosis may be ablated laparoscopically with a laser. For severe or generalized disease, **hysterectomy** (removal of uterus), **oophorectomy** (removal of ovaries), or both may be indicated.

Carcinoma of the Cervix

A slowly growing, invasive carcinoma of the uterine cervix, predominantly of squamous cell origin.

Causes: Squamous cell carcinoma of the cervix develops as a consequence of **cervical dysplasia**, which in turn is caused in a majority of cases by cervical infection with **human papillomavirus** (HPV, genital wart virus), particularly types 16, 18, and 31. The progression from dysplasia to invasive carcinoma typically takes 5–10 years. Peak incidence of cervical carcinoma occurs in the late 30s. Risk factors for cervical carcinoma are smoking, prolonged use of oral contraceptives, sexual contact with many partners, and HIV infection.

History: Irregular vaginal bleeding or spotting, particularly after intercourse; abnormal vaginal discharge; bowel or bladder pain or dysfunction.

Physical Examination: Cervical ulceration. With advanced disease, evidence of pelvic invasion or metastasis; a **fistula** (abnormal passage or communication) between the vagina and the bladder or rectum may occur.

Diagnostic Tests: Premalignant cellular changes can be detected early by routine Pap smear. HPV typing, performed either simultaneously with a routine Pap smear or as a followup to an abnormal smear, can confirm the presence of the virus and identify its type. About 20% of women with **ASCUS** (abnormal squamous cells of undetermined significance) eventually develop squamous intraepithelial lesions or invasive carcinoma. Detection of cellular dysplasia (low-grade squamous intraepithelial lesion, **LGSIL**, or high-grade squamous intraepithelial lesion, **HGSIL**) calls for followup in the form of colposcopy, cervical biopsy, and possibly surgical or laser excision of a cone of cervical tissue including the entire squamocolumnar junction. These provide precise information about the type and stage of disease.

Course: Severe bleeding may occur from ulceration and erosion of the cervix and surrounding tissues. Extension can lead to bilateral ureteral obstruction, with resultant kidney failure, or to rectovaginal or vesicovaginal fistula. The five-year survival rate with treatment is about 60%.

Treatment: Early removal of localized disease by conization or, preferably, hysterectomy. In advanced disease, radiation is an alternative to radical surgery. A vaccine now available against HPV, which is particularly active against viral types associated with a high risk of malignant change, can be expected to reduce the

HUMAN PAPILLOMAVIRUS (HPV)

Almost all cervical cancers begin with cellular changes induced by infection with human papillomavirus (HPV), a sexually transmitted disease. Genital HPV infection is the most common viral sexually transmitted disease in the Western world. Because the risk of contracting this infection through a single unprotected contact with an infected person is a staggering 50%, it isn't surprising that at least 50% of all sexually active women have been infected with HPV.

incidence of cervical cancer markedly during the coming decades.

Fibrocystic Disease (or Condition) of the Breast (Cystic Mastitis, Mammary Dysplasia)

Formation of benign but painful cysts in the breasts (see ■ Figure 14-5).

Cause: Probably inappropriate response of breast tissue to ovarian hormones. The condition affects as many as one third of all women between the ages of 25 and 50. The theory that caffeine (from coffee, tea, and chocolate) exacerbates symptoms remains unproven.

History: One or more lumps in the breast, typically painful and tender, and more so just before the onset of menses. Lumps are frequently multiple and may change markedly in size within 2–3 days. Lumps typically disappear eventually, but meanwhile others often develop.

Physical Examination: One or more fluctuant, usually tender masses in one or both breasts. Occasionally nipple discharge is noted.

Diagnostic Tests: Needle aspiration of a cyst usually leads to its disappearance. Biopsy material obtained by fine-needle aspiration or other method from a solid or cystic mass helps to rule out malignant change. Biopsy may show **hyperplasia** of epithelial tissues, associated

There was evidence of fibrocystic process and a fairly well-circumscribed lump in the upper quadrant region of her right breast at approximately the 12 o'clock position. The lump measured about 3 cm in width by about 2 cm in length.

with an increased risk of malignant tumor of the breast. Mammography and ultrasound examinations may help to distinguish cysts from solid tumors.

Course: Fibrocystic disease tends to persist, with remissions and exacerbations, until menopause, and then to resolve completely and permanently. Forms of fibrocystic disease associated with proliferation of epithelial elements carry a slightly higher risk of progression to carcinoma of the breast.

Treatment: Analgesics, education, close observation for persisting or dominant lump, which may prove to be a solid tumor requiring further observation. For severe disease, danazol and, rarely, mastectomy may be advised.

Breast Cancer

A malignant tumor of the female breast, arising most frequently from ductal epithelium. The commonest cancer in women, and the second commonest cause of cancer death (after lung cancer) in women. One in eight or nine women will develop breast cancer (see ■ Figure 14-5).

Cause: Women who have no children, or whose first pregnancy occurs late in the childbearing years, are at increased risk of breast cancer. So are women who have a family history of breast cancer, particularly cancer occurring at an early age in one or more female relatives, which may be associated with the BRCA1 or BRCA2 oncogene. The risk of breast cancer is increased by estrogen replacement therapy after menopause.

History: A solitary, firm, nontender mass in the breast, usually discovered by the patient accidentally or during breast self-examination. Sixty percent occur in the upper outer quadrant of the breast. Occasionally nipple discharge is the presenting symptom. With advancing disease, swelling and local pain. Bone pain, weight loss, and jaundice are symptoms of systemic spread through metastasis.

Physical Examination: There may be enlargement or abnormal contour of one breast on inspection. The tumor is felt as a hard, ill-defined, nontender solitary mass. There may be skin or nipple retraction, fixation of the tumor to the underlying chest wall or the overlying skin, and signs of local inflammation (swelling, redness, ulceration). Axillary lymph nodes may be found enlarged if cancer cells have spread to them.

Diagnostic Tests: Mammography (a specialized x-ray procedure) can identify changes indicative of breast cancer (calcification, mass, or both) as much as two years before a tumor becomes palpable, and is therefore a valuable screening procedure for asymptomatic women over 40, and for younger women believed to be at increased risk because of a family history of early-onset breast cancer or presence of BRCA1 or BRCA2 as detected by genetic testing. **Ultrasound examination** can supply valuable additional information.

Biopsy is required for confirmation of malignancy and precise identification of tumor type. A biopsy can be obtained through the skin by either a large-needle or fine-needle technique. **Excisional biopsy** (removal of the tumor followed by frozen-section examination

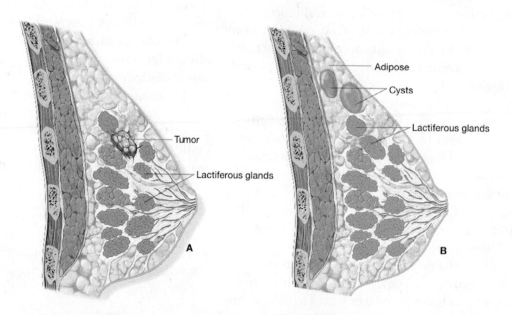

FIGURE 14-5. A. Carcinoma of breast. B. Fibrocystic disorder of breasts.

This is a 62-year-old female with biopsy-proven breast cancer of the lateral portion of the left breast. She was scheduled for lumpectomy with lymph node dissection.

before closure of the surgical site) is the method usually chosen when clinical and mammographic evidence supports a diagnosis of cancer.

Course: An untreated breast cancer typically enlarges, invades surrounding and underlying tissues, and causes extensive cutaneous ulceration. Breast cancers spread to axillary and mediastinal lymph nodes, liver, bone, and brain. For a solitary localized tumor, the five-year survival rate is 95% and the 10-year survival rate is 90%. The figures for disease that has become systemic before treatment is instituted are 5% and 2%, respectively. Five-year and even 10-year rates do not adequately reflect the long-term mortality of breast cancer, which is eventually the cause of death in most patients except when cancer is discovered very early by screening procedures.

Treatment: The basic treatment of breast cancer is **surgical removal of the tumor**. Various further procedures, including **radical mastectomy** (removal of the entire breast as well as surrounding and underlying tissues and axillary lymph nodes) may be appropriate with certain types and stages of cancer.

Both radiation treatments and chemotherapy are usually administered after surgery. Radiation is not usually needed after radical mastectomy, but the procedure is mutilating and psychologically devastating. In metastatic disease, elimination of estrogen stimulation through either oophorectomy (removal of the ovaries) or administration of tamoxifen, a chemical anti-estrogen, delays progression of disease and mitigates symptoms.

Pause for Reflection

1. List 3 causes of dysmenorrhea not due to "normal menstrual cramping."
2. _____ is unpredictable, unusually heavy or light bleeding from the uterus or cessation of menses in the absence of pregnancy or any demonstrable abnormality of the uterus.
3. Endometrial implants may appear as _____ on the ovaries or as hemorrhagic cysts or _____ on peritoneal surfaces.

(continued)

Pause for Reflection *(continued)*

4. A benign neoplasm of the uterine muscle is called _____.
5. A majority of cases of cervical dysplasia are caused by _____; cervical dysplasia may ultimately develop into _____.
6. Screening diagnostic procedures for breast cancer include _____ and _____; however, _____ is required for confirmation of malignancy and precise identification of tumor type.

Sexually Transmitted Diseases

A **sexually transmitted disease (STD)** is any infectious disease that is transmitted from one person to another through sexual contact. The only thing all STDs have in common is their mode of transmission. In other respects they vary widely among themselves. Changes in national sexual mores have led to the emergence of sexually transmitted infections that were not previously known or recognized, such as **chlamydia** and **AIDS**, and to marked increases in the incidence of some formerly rare infections such as **genital herpes** and **genital warts**. Some of the viruses that cause genital warts induce cervical cancer.

All of the classically recognized STDs can be transmitted through vaginal intercourse. Most of them can also be transmitted through oral-genital contact and anal intercourse with resulting oropharyngeal, anorectal, or systemic infection. STDs affecting the skin (genital warts, pubic lice) or transmitted through the skin (syphilis, AIDS) can be acquired during intimate contact even though genital exposure is avoided or a condom is used.

The only absolute protection against acquiring an infection through sexual contact is lifelong celibacy or maintenance of a permanently and mutually monogamous sexual relationship. Some degree of protection against STDs is afforded by practicing "safe (or safer) sex"—which basically means using condoms and avoiding high-risk behaviors such as anal intercourse—and by limiting the number of sex partners.

The diagnosis and treatment of STDs are rendered more difficult by the reluctance of most people to discuss their sexual behavior with health professionals and by the refusal of many patients to believe that a sexual partner has become infected by some third person. Diagnosis often demands alertness and a high degree of suspicion on the part of the healthcare worker. History-taking must be searching but nonthreatening and non-judgmental. Often the most suggestive point in the history is exposure to a new sexual partner within two months before the appearance of symptoms.

In treating any patient with an STD, the physician must reckon with two epidemiologic realities: the fact that at least one of the patient's sexual partners (and possibly all of them) is also infected, and the statistical probability that a person with one STD has other STDs. Failure to treat sexual partners prophylactically will lead to eventual reinfection of most patients. More-over, unless both partners in a relationship are treated at the same time, they may keep reinfecting each other, a phenomenon known as "ping-ponging." STD screening tests are a standard part of prenatal care as well.

Urethritis and Pelvic Inflammatory Disease

Genital infections due to **chlamydia** are currently the most common of all bacterial STDs.

Cause: Although, strictly speaking, chlamydia is the name of the causative organism, in clinical parlance genital infections due to this organism are often called simply "chlamydia." *Chlamydia trachomatis* is highly contagious; at least 50% of sexual partners of persons with chlamydia are also infected. Moreover, 20% of men and 80% of women with the disease have no symptoms and do not know that they are infected (and infectious).

In women the most frequent form of chlamydial infection is **mucopurulent cervicitis**, which may cause slight bleeding or pain with intercourse but is often discovered only on routine pelvic examination. Chlamydia also causes **acute urethral syndrome** in women, in which symptoms of increased urinary frequency and urinary burning mimic cystitis, but urine cultures are sterile.

Diagnosis: Chlamydial DNA can be detected in cervical, vaginal, or urethral specimens and in urine by various nucleic acid amplification tests. Urine tests are standard for screening asymptomatic women.

Patient presents with a history of having been evaluated for complaints of increasing central pelvic pain, increasing vaginal discharge and symptoms of cystitis, deep dyspareunia, sacral backache. When evaluated the patient was felt most likely to have a chlamydia pelvic inflammatory disease.

Course: As many as 20% of women with untreated chlamydia will eventually develop **acute salpingitis**, also called **pelvic inflammatory disease (PID)**, due to spread of infection to one or both uterine tubes. PID is more likely to occur in a woman with an **intrauterine device (IUD)**, and acute attacks are more common during menstruation. The symptoms of pelvic pain and fever are fairly nonspecific, but severe tenderness on manipulation of the cervix and on palpation of the uterine adnexa during pelvic examination is highly suggestive of the diagnosis.

PID may progress to **tubo-ovarian** abscess or to peri-hepatitis (**Fitz-Hugh–Curtis syndrome**). A more common consequence of PID is scarring of the uterine tubes with resulting infertility or sterility and heightened risk of **ectopic pregnancy**.

Treatment: Chlamydia responds to treatment with various antibiotics. Currently recommended drugs are doxycycline (Doryx, Vibramycin, Vibra-Tabs), tetracycline (Panmycin, Sumycin, Tetracyn, Tetralan), or azithromycin (Zithromax, Zmax). All of the patient's sexual partners must be treated prophylactically, regardless of symptoms or laboratory test results. Tubo-ovarian abscess and salpingitis that do not respond to antibiotics may require surgical treatment.

Gonorrhea

Infection of the genital tract of either sex by *Neisseria gonorrhoeae*, a gram-negative diplococcus. This disease has been known for centuries and goes by the colloquial name of "**the clap**." Physicians often refer to the causative organism as the **gonococcus, GC** for short, and this abbreviation frequently stands for the disease itself in medical slang.

Cause: Like chlamydia, gonorrhea is an infection of the genital mucous membranes, causing urethritis in men but frequently asymptomatic in women; it too is capable of progressing to PID with its complications of tubo-ovarian abscess and Fitz-Hugh–Curtis syndrome and its aftermath of tubal scarring with resultant infertility or sterility and increased risk of tubal pregnancy. Also like chlamydia, gonorrhea can cause severe eye infection, resulting in blindness, in an infant born to an infected mother.

Diagnosis: The diagnosis of gonorrhea can be made by examination of a gram-stained smear of urethral discharge for the typical intracellular diplococci or by culture of urethral, cervical, or other material on special media such as Thayer-Martin agar, which is designed to favor the growth of gonococci. Highly sensitive rapid tests based on detection of gonococcal DNA in urethral, cervical, or vaginal specimens or in urine have largely supplanted smear and culture. Urine testing is widely used to screen high-risk subjects.

Treatment: Increasing problems of resistance to penicillin have led to the abandonment of this drug for the treatment of gonorrhea. A single intramuscular injection of ceftriaxone is highly effective in eradicating gonococcal infection. Several cephalosporins (cefixime, cefuroxime, cefpodoxime) are effective in a single oral dose.

All patients treated for gonorrhea are also treated prophylactically for chlamydia because of the high frequency with which these diseases occur together. In addition, all sexual contacts of patients with gonorrhea are treated prophylactically against both diseases, regardless of symptoms or results of tests.

Genital Herpes

Herpes simplex is a viral infection of skin or mucous membranes characterized by painful localized blistering and ulceration, with a tendency to periodic recurrences. Type 1 herpes simplex virus (HSV-1) was formerly associated almost exclusively with lesions of the lips and face (**orofacial herpes, herpes labialis, cold sore, fever blister**), while type 2 (HSV-2) caused most lesions of the genitals (**genital herpes, herpes progenitalis**). Currently, however, as many as one half of first-episode cases of genital herpes are caused by type 1. Recurrences of cutaneous lesions, and viral shedding in the absence of overt symptoms, are much less frequent with type 1 infection.

Transmission is by direct contact with an infected person. The incubation period may be as short as one week, but sometimes the virus remains dormant for months or years before causing symptoms. Apparently persons with latent infection (no active lesions) can spread the disease to others, at least in certain circumstances. Genital herpes is always spread through sexual contact.

Physical Examination: Regardless of its location, herpes simplex appears as a small cluster of vesicles surrounded by a reddened zone of skin or mucous membrane. Itching or burning is often intense and may precede the appearance of lesions. Within a day or two the vesicles slough and become shallow, painful ulcers. A first attack of herpes simplex may be accompanied by swelling and inflammation of regional lymph nodes and fever. The lesions heal spontaneously after 1–2 weeks; however, the virus remains in the body for the life of the patient, lying dormant in spinal cord ganglia.

Course: A recurrence of herpes simplex at the same site as the original eruption can be triggered at any time by various physical or emotional stresses, including fever, sunburn, menses, and fatigue. Recurrent herpes simplex is usually milder than the primary attack and of shorter duration, and fever and lymph gland involvement seldom occur. Recurrences may come at intervals of days, weeks, months, or years; many patients never experience any recurrences at all.

In women with genital herpes, severely painful vulvar lesions are the rule, but when the cervix is the site of the eruption, it may go unnoticed. Anorectal lesions result from anal intercourse. Neonatal infection, acquired at birth by a child born to a mother with active genital herpes, often leads to disseminated disease with a high mortality rate.

Diagnosis of herpes simplex is usually obvious on direct examination. Confirmation may be obtained by means of a **Tzanck smear**, a stained preparation of material scraped or expressed from a lesion, which shows abnormal balloon cells with viral inclusion bodies. A **Pap smear** may also show these changes, but culture of the virus is much more specific and is the diagnostic procedure of choice. These tests are relatively insensitive, however, and cannot distinguish between herpes and other viral eruptions (chickenpox, herpes zoster).

Detection of antibody to viral glycoprotein in serum not only identifies persons who have been infected and are therefore infectious but also distinguishes between types 1 and 2, refining prognosis and guiding treatment, including prophylaxis against recurrences.

Treatment of genital herpes with acyclovir, famciclovir, or valacyclovir shortens the period of clinical symptoms and of viral shedding, but does not eradicate the virus. Long-term prophylaxis with these agents has been helpful for some patients with frequent recurrences. Because genital herpes is a risk factor for cervical cancer, women with a history of this disease are advised to have regular Pap smears throughout life. A woman who goes into labor with active genital herpes is delivered by cesarean section to prevent transmission of infection to the newborn.

Genital Warts

A **wart** is a benign skin tumor induced by infection with the **human papillomavirus (HPV)**. Genital warts (venereal warts), occurring on the skin and mucous membranes of the genitals and anus, are spread almost exclusively through sexual contact. Perianal spread may result from anal intercourse but is often due to migration of virus from the patient's own genital lesions.

History: Genital warts are highly contagious: 60–90% of sexual partners of persons with genital warts also have genital warts. They are the most common viral STD, and their incidence is increasing. Genital warts are more likely to develop during pregnancy and in persons with impaired immunity.

Physical Examination. In men genital warts usually appear on the penis, occasionally within the urethra or about the anus. In women genital warts typically affect the labia and perianal skin but may involve the vaginal lining and cervix. The principal symptom of genital warts is their visible presence. Itching and vaginal discharge may occur, and warts sometimes ulcerate or become infected with skin bacteria.

Cause: HPV types 6 and 11 cause the classical genital wart known as **condyloma acuminatum** (plural, **condylomata acuminata**). This is a slender, often finger-shaped growth with a narrow attachment to the skin, a tapered tip, and a somewhat rough texture. HPV types 16 and 18 cause flat warts rather than classical condylomata acuminata. These latter viral types are associated with a high risk of dysplasia or cancer in affected genital skin or mucous membranes, which may progress to invasive carcinoma of the cervix.

Examination revealed perianal condylomata and vulvar intraepithelial neoplasia (VIN) around the posterior fourchette as well as the right anterior vulvar lesion (measuring 1 cm). Comes in today for treatment of biopsy-proven perianal condylomata.

Diagnosis: Genital warts can usually be diagnosed by simple inspection, but many cases of latent infection are only recognized on Pap smear or cervical biopsy. A standard procedure for identifying genital warts and other lesions of the cervix is **colposcopy**, an inspection of the cervix with a low-power binocular microscope. In both sexes, visualization of small, flat, or atypical warts is enhanced by prior application of 5% acetic acid (white vinegar) for a few minutes to the area of skin or mucous membrane to be examined. Acetic acid causes blanching (**acetowhitening**) in typical HPV lesions. This procedure is not highly specific, but at least it helps the examiner to decide which lesions should be biop-

sied. Screening tests based on molecular biology can confirm the presence of HPV and identify its type. HPV screening is often performed at the same time as a routine Pap smear to enhance the diagnostic value of the smear.

Treatment: A wide variety of methods are used to treat genital warts, including surgical excision, electrodesiccation, cryosurgery, and laser ablation; application of liquid nitrogen, corrosive chemicals (trichloroacetic acid, dichloroacetic acid), or antimitotics (podophyllin, 5-FU); and intralesional injection of interferon. The choice of treatment depends on the site, character, and extent of involvement. Currently liquid nitrogen is favored for most lesions. Regardless of the method used, several treatments are usually needed to eliminate all warts, and rates of recurrence or treatment failure with all methods are substantial. A vaccine against types of HPV known to be associated with genital warts (6 and 11) and cervical cancer (16 and 18) is currently recommended for all young women.

Pelvic Inflammatory Disease (PID), Salpingitis, Endometritis

Acute or chronic bacterial infection of the uterus and tubes.

Causes: Sexually transmitted infection with *Neisseria gonorrhoeae* or *Chlamydia trachomatis* ascending from the lower genital tract; infection with other organisms (streptococci, *Haemophilus influenzae*) may be blood borne. Risk factors include **nulliparity** (never having borne a viable child), nonwhite race, smoking, and sexual contact with many partners.

History: Pelvic pain, chills, fever, menstrual irregularities, purulent vaginal discharge, dyspareunia. Acute symptoms are more likely to occur during menses. With **Fitz-Hugh–Curtis syndrome**, right upper quadrant pain.

Physical Examination: Fever, abdominal tenderness; marked tenderness on manipulation of cervix and palpation of adnexa. Right upper quadrant tenderness in Fitz-Hugh–Curtis syndrome.

Diagnostic Tests: The white blood cell count is variably elevated. Smear and culture of material obtained from the cervix (or from Douglas's cul-de-sac by **culdoscopy**) (see ■ Figure 14-6) may identify the infecting organism. Pelvic ultrasound and laparoscopy are used to refine the diagnosis.

Course: In about 25% of patients, the condition becomes recurrent or chronic even after treatment, with pelvic pain, infertility, and increased risk of

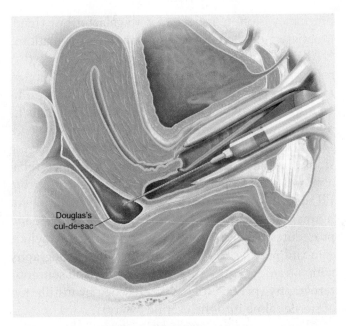

FIGURE 14-6. Culdoscopy

ectopic pregnancy. Complications of PID include tubo-ovarian abscess with danger of rupture into the peritoneal cavity, and Fitz-Hugh–Curtis syndrome, a localized peritonitis in the right upper quadrant.

Treatment: Hospitalization, intravenous antibiotics (cefoxitin, clindamycin). For milder disease, outpatient treatment with oral antibiotics may suffice. Surgical drainage of abscesses; for severe disease, hysterectomy with bilateral salpingo-oophorectomy.

Vaginitis, Vulvovaginitis

Inflammation of the vagina and vulva, generally due to infection and manifested by vaginal discharge and vulvar itching or pain. Most cases are due to one of three organisms:

Vaginal candidosis: *Candida albicans*, a yeastlike fungus, frequently causes vulvar pruritus and a thick white curdy discharge. Infection is more common in diabetes mellitus and pregnancy and in women taking oral contraceptives or broad-spectrum antibiotics.

Examination shows intense erythema of the vulva and curdy white material in the vaginal vault. A wet preparation of this material in potassium hydroxide examined microscopically identifies the causative organism. Culture may also be performed. Treatment is with topical antifungal medicines (miconazole, terconazole, clotrimazole) in vaginal suppositories, creams, or ointments, or with oral fluconazole in a single dose. Recurrences are common.

Trichomonas vaginitis: *Trichomonas vaginalis* is a sexually transmitted protozoan parasite that causes vul-var itching and vaginal discharge. Vaginal examination shows erythema, particularly of the cervix (**"strawberry cervix"**), and a watery, frothy, malodorous yellowish-brown discharge. Wet preparation of vaginal discharge shows motile protozoa. Treatment is with oral metronidazole for the patient and all sexual partners. (Symptoms in men are usually absent; dysuria and urethral discharge may occur.)

Bacterial vaginosis: *Gardnerella vaginalis* is at least one of the organisms involved in **bacterial vaginosis**, a mixed vaginal infection that causes a thin grayish discharge with a foul fishy odor but not much vulvar irritation or itching. Microscopic examination of discharge material shows **clue cells** (epithelial cells heavily studded with bacteria). This condition is associated with increased risk of premature labor and preterm birth. Treatment is with oral or vaginal metronidazole or clindamycin.

Pause for Reflection

1. Name 2 STD infections that can lead to pelvic inflammatory disease.
2. Genital herpes is treated with _____.
3. Genital warts are caused by infection with _____.
4. Classical genital warts known as _____ are not associated with cervical dysplasia or carcinoma.
5. The viral types that are associated with a high risk of dysplasia or cancer in affected genital skin or mucous membranes, which may progress to invasive carcinoma of the cervix, are _____.
6. Complications of PID include _____ with danger of rupture into the peritoneal cavity, and _____, a localized peritonitis in the right upper quadrant.
7. Name 3 organisms that may cause vaginitis, vulvovaginitis, or vaginosis.

Infertility

The diagnosis of fertility problems in women and the application of various techniques of reproductive assistance make up a substantial part of modern gynecologic practice. **Infertility** (also called **subfertility**) is defined as the inability of a couple to achieve conception after 12 months of frequent, unprotected intercourse. It is currently estimated that 10–15% of couples are infertile. In at least one third of cases, the male is the infertile member of the couple.

The absence of ovaries or of anatomic structures essential for the reception of sperm and its union with an oocyte obviously renders conception impossible, a condition known as **sterility**. Chromosomal aberrations can induce sterility by preventing the fertilization or normal development of oocytes. An infertility workup seeks to rule out sterility and to identify disorders that make conception less likely but not impossible. In as many as one fourth of cases, no cause is found.

Diagnostic Evaluation of Infertility

Diagnostic evaluation begins with medical and sexual history and general physical examination. A history of menstrual irregularity or of pelvic inflammatory disease (PID), tubal pregnancy, or tubal or pelvic surgery may point to causes of inability to conceive, as may signs of endocrine dysfunction (hirsutism, galactorrhea). Occupational or medical exposure to toxic chemicals or radiation can offer a clue to reproductive failure. Chronic disease, debility, malnutrition, drug or alcohol abuse, and other constitutional factors can impair the efficiency of an otherwise normal reproductive system.

When the initial assessment provides no conclusive explanation for failure to conceive, laboratory testing and imaging studies may provide the answer. The first question to be answered is whether the woman is ovulating. Ovulation can be confirmed by various procedures, including serial determination of basal body temperature and measurement of LH, FSH, or progesterone (the latter produced by the corpus luteum, the part of a mature ovarian follicle remaining after release of its oocyte).

Any severe physical or emotional stress can inhibit ovulation for one or two cycles by upsetting the equilibrium of the hypothalamic-pituitary-gonadal axis. Among numerous causes of persistent failure to ovulate are primary ovarian failure (premature menopause), endometriosis, polycystic ovary syndrome, abrupt or marked weight loss (as in anorexia nervosa), strenuous exercise (female athlete syndrome), chronic emotional stress, and endocrine abnormalities due to thyroid, pituitary, or gonadal dysfunction.

In about one third of women with chronic ovulatory failure, the serum level of the anterior pituitary hormone prolactin is elevated above the maximum normal limit of 580 milliunits/L. The chief role of this hormone is regulating breast development and lactation in pregnancy. Elevation (hyperprolactinemia) outside of pregnancy is often associated with galactorrhea (inappropriate milk secretion) and inhibition of ovulation.

Known causes of hyperprolactinemia include thyroid and renal disease, prescription drugs (hormones, phenothiazines, dopamine antagonists, and many others), and (often with elevation above 5000 milliunits/L) a functioning adenoma of the anterior pituitary gland.

When ovulation is found to be normal, imaging studies or laparoscopy may be used to detect tubal abnormalities (congenital deformities, scarring from PID or excision of a tubal pregnancy) or deviations from normal uterine anatomy (fibroids, polyps). Ultrasound procedures useful in assessing uterine anatomy include standard **pelvic sonography**, **transvaginal sonography** with a transducer inserted in the vagina, and **sonohysterography** (pelvic ultrasound preceded by instillation of sterile saline into the uterine cavity).

These procedures assess uterine anatomy but provide no information about tubal patency. **Hysterosalpingography** (see ■ Figure 14-7) is a radiologic procedure in which x-ray images are obtained after injection of a radiopaque contrast medium through the cervix and into the uterine cavity. If the uterine tubes are patent, contrast material can be seen passing through them and spilling into the pelvic cavity. In a few cases this technique proves to be therapeutic by reestablishing patency in tubes narrowed by minor scarring or anatomic malformation.

Chromosomal abnormalities associated with sterility are detectable by karyotyping and molecular biology studies.

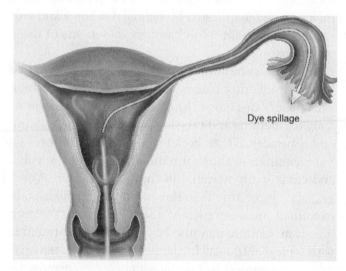

Radiopaque dye injected into
uterus; tubal filling and spillage
monitored with fluoroscopy

FIGURE 14-7. Hysterosalpingography

Some forms of infertility, such as stenosis of the uterine tubes, respond to surgical correction. Drugs used to enhance fertility in women are agents that promote the development of ovarian follicles by various mechanisms. Levels of the gonadotropins FSH and LH or of gonadotropin-releasing hormone, all produced by the pituitary, can be boosted with injections of natural or synthetic hormones. Clomiphene citrate, a selective estrogen receptor modulator (SERM), and letrozole, an aromatase inhibitor, can be given orally to stimulate the ovaries by inhibiting the negative feedback effect of estrogen. The use of fertility drugs is associated with risks of birth defects and multiple pregnancy.

Assisted Reproductive Technology (ART)

Assisted reproductive technology (ART) includes a range of mechanical and surgical methods by which the likelihood of conception by infertile couples can be increased.

Artificial Insemination

Artificial insemination is the implantation of semen from the male partner in the female genital tract by mechanical means (syringe and cannula) rather than through sexual intercourse. This technique may be useful in cases of **oligospermia** (low concentration of sperm in semen) or low concentration of motile, structurally normal sperm, or in various circumstances that render vaginal intercourse difficult or impossible. It is also frequently tried when thorough evaluation of both partners provides no explanation for failure to conceive.

The wife of a man who is sterile may be artificially inseminated with the sperm of a donor who is matched as closely as possible to the husband in physical traits such as height, weight, physique, and color of skin, eyes, and hair. This technique may also be used when genetic studies of both partners indicate a high risk of abnormal offspring or when only one partner has AIDS.

In Vitro Fertilization (IVF)

In vitro fertilization (IVF) is the process of incubating an oocyte and sperm together in the laboratory under conditions that favor fertilization. Once fertilization occurs and cell division has begun, one or more embryos are suspended in a transfer medium and injected into the uterus with a cannula inserted into the cervix. In an alternative procedure called **zygote intrafallopian transfer (ZIFT)**, the fertilized oocyte is placed in a uterine tube by a laparoscopic procedure rather than in the uterine cavity.

In preparation for IVF, hormones are administered to control the maturation of ovarian follicles and to increase the chances that several will mature at once. Oocytes are then harvested from the ovary with an ultrasonically guided needle inserted through the abdominal wall. Sperm are obtained by ejaculation or by needle aspiration from a testicle. Oocytes, sperm, or both may be provided by donors rather than derived from the infertile couple.

In cases where fertilization is considered unlikely to occur in vitro, a single sperm may be injected mechanically into an oocyte by a technique called **intracytoplasmic sperm injection (ICSI). Gamete intrafallopian transfer (GIFT)** is the laparoscopic placement of oocytes and sperm together in a uterine tube instead of their combination in a laboratory vessel.

The live birth rate after a single ART procedure varies from 10% to 30%, depending on the procedure and the reasons for its use. As with fertility drugs, all methods of ART are associated with some risk of birth defects and multiple pregnancy.

Pause for Reflection

1. Distinguish between infertility and sterility.
2. Identify at least one gynecologic, one occupational, and one nongynecological medical reason as a possible cause for infertility.
3. List the procedures that can confirm that the patient is ovulating.
4. List 3 causes of persistent failure to ovulate.
5. Name and describe the radiologic procedure used to assess tubal patency.
6. Distinguish among the different forms of assisted reproductive technology.

Obstetrics

Physiology of Pregnancy

Fertilization usually occurs in a uterine (fallopian) tube, and considerable embryonic development has already occurred before implantation in the uterine lining takes place. At the site of implantation, the fertilized **oocyte** (now called an **embryo**) forms a specialized plate of tissue, the **chorion**, through which it draws nourishment

PREGNANCY TERMS

nulligravida—a woman who has never been pregnant.

nullipara—a woman who has never given birth.

primigravida—a woman who is pregnant for the first time.

primipara—a woman who has given birth once.

multigravida—a woman who has been pregnant more than once.

multipara—a woman who has given birth more than once.

parturition—childbirth.

parturient—a woman in labor.

antepartum—before childbirth.

postpartum—after childbirth.

puerperium—the time between the birth of the child and the return of the uterus to its normal size, with regeneration of endometrium.

puerperal—pertaining to the puerperium.

from the underlying endometrium by way of fingerlike projections (**villi**). During the third week after conception, the embryo differentiates into three primitive cell layers: **ectoderm**, from which epidermis, the nervous system, the eye, the ear, and dental enamel develop; **mesoderm**, the source of muscle, bone, connective tissue, the circulatory system, and the genitourinary system; and **endoderm**, which gives rise to the liver, the pancreas, and the epithelial linings of the respiratory, digestive, and genitourinary systems.

Further development consists of a complex series of divisions, foldings, and fusions as the basic framework of the body is laid down and the formation of organ systems (organogenesis) proceeds. By the end of the eighth week, organogenesis is largely complete. After the ninth week of gestation, the embryo is called a **fetus**. Its further development is largely a matter of growth and maturation.

The chorion evolves into the **placenta**, a round flat disk of tissue to which the blood vessels in the umbilical cord are attached. Although interchange of oxygen, carbon dioxide, nutrients, and wastes takes place in the placenta by diffusion between maternal and fetal circulations, the circulations do not mix. The placenta produces **(human) chorionic gonadotropin (hCG)**, the basis of virtually all current pregnancy tests.

The fetus develops within a fluid-filled membranous sac, the **amnion**. Amnionic (also amniotic) fluid serves as a shock-absorber and also participates in nutrient and excretory functions. During pregnancy the lining of the uterus undergoes structural change and is called the **decidua**. Chorion, amnion, and decidua are known collectively as fetal membranes.

Multiple pregnancy (twins, triplets) can occur as a result of either fertilization of a single oocyte by more than one spermatozoon (identical twins) or fertilization of more than one oocyte, each by a different spermatozoon (fraternal twins). The average duration of a normal pregnancy from conception to delivery is 280 days (40 weeks). This period is divided into three trimesters of three months each.

Symptoms and Signs of Pregnancy

Amenorrhea (cessation of menses).

Nausea and vomiting. Typically confined to the earlier part of the day, or worse then ("morning sickness"), and often aggravated by the smell, sight, or even the thought of food. About 50% of pregnant women experience some nausea between the sixth and the sixteenth weeks of pregnancy.

Swelling and soreness of the breasts due to edema (milk secretion does not occur until after childbirth).

Enlargement of the uterus. Enlargement can be detected on pelvic examination by about the sixth week of pregnancy. After the twelfth week, the **fundus** (curved upper surface or dome) of the uterus rises above the pubic bone and the uterus becomes an abdominal organ. Uterine enlargement may be responsible for symptoms occurring at various stages of pregnancy such as urinary frequency, varicosities of the vulva and lower limbs, constipation, hemorrhoids, and heartburn.

Weak and irregular contractions of the uterus (**Braxton Hicks contractions**) begin early in pregnancy

Purplish discoloration of the cervix and vagina (**Chadwick sign**) is due to increased vascularity.

Softening of the cervix (**Hegar sign**) can sometimes be observed on palpation during pelvic examination.

Presence of a fetus can be detected by ultrasound examination at and after six weeks' gestation. X-ray examination (avoided during early pregnancy because of the risk of fetal damage) shows fetal development somewhat later.

Fetal heart action can be detected by echocardiography by the sixth week and by Doppler ultrasonography by the eighth week. Fetal heartbeat can be heard with a special stethoscope (fetoscope) by about 18 weeks' gestation. The rate is normally 120–160 beats per minute, and the heart tones sound like the ticking of a watch.

Other circulatory sounds that can occasionally be heard are a **funic souffle** (rhymes with "truffle"; a whistling sound synchronous with fetal heartbeat, due to flow of blood in the umbilical cord) and a **uterine souffle** (rhymes with "truffle"; a softer rushing sound synchronous with maternal heartbeat, due to increased flow of blood in uterine arteries).

Fetal movement (quickening) is first appreciable around 16–20 weeks' gestation.

Skin changes: Increased pigmentation of areolae (darker zones around nipples); chloasma (brownish patches on the face and elsewhere).

Positive pregnancy test: Chemical tests for the beta fraction of human chorionic gonadotropin in blood or urine become positive between 6 and 10 days after implantation.

Prenatal Care

At the first prenatal visit, pregnancy is confirmed and the probable date of delivery is estimated. According to the time-honored Naegele Rule, the EDC (expected date of confinement; "confinement" is an old euphemism for childbirth) is found by going back three months and then forward seven days from the first day of the last menstrual period (LMP). Thus, if the LMP began on August 8 the EDC would be May 15.

The mother's history is carefully reviewed, with particular attention to prior reproductive history (stillbirths, miscarriages, abortions, premature labor or other complications of pregnancy, previous cesarean delivery).

Other elements of the history that may have an impact on the course and outcome of pregnancy are the mother's use of tobacco, alcohol, coffee, prescription and nonprescription medicines, or drugs of abuse; history of sexually transmitted diseases such as chlamydia, genital herpes, or AIDS; personal or family history of genetically transmitted disorders; presence of systemic disease such as diabetes mellitus, hypertension, thyroid disease, or heart disease; and occupational exposures, such as lead or radiation, that could cause fetal harm.

The initial prenatal examination includes determination of maternal height, weight, and blood pressure; assessment of general health and nutritional status; and a search for significant disorders. Naturally the examination focuses on the reproductive system and the

GRAVIDA AND PARA

The terms *gravida* and *para* are used to describe a woman's reproductive history. The pregnant uterus is said to be a *gravid uterus*. Gravida, followed by a number, refers to the number of pregnancies the patient has had, including ectopics, hydatidiform moles, abortions (either spontaneous or surgical), and normal pregnancies.

Para, followed by a number, refers to the number of deliveries after the 20th week of gestation (live or stillbirth, single or multiple, vaginal cesarean) and does not correspond to the number of infants. A woman who has had only one pregnancy—even if she delivers twins or quintuplets—is still gravida 1, para 1. If she has had one delivery, an ectopic pregnancy, and an abortion (less than 20 weeks' gestation) prior to a delivery, she will be gravida 3, para 1.

Para may also be expressed as a four-digit number, with each digit representing a particular type of birth in this order: term infants, premature infants, abortions or miscarriages, living children.

Both of the following examples refer to the same patient.

The patient is gravida 6, para 3
  (6 pregnancies, 3 live births).
The patient is gravida 6, para 2–1–0–3
  (6 pregnancies, 2 term infants, 1 premature infant, 0 miscarriages, 3 living children).

A woman who is para 0–3–0–2 could have had three separate pregnancies resulting in premature deliveries, of which two children are now living, or she could have had triplets in one delivery with two living children, or even one premature and one twin premature delivery with two living children. Clearly, this system isn't exactly precise. Confused? Remember TPAL: Term deliveries, Premature infants, Abortions, and Living children.

Another method of documenting obstetrical history is an index called GPMAL. The letters refer to Gravida, Para, Multiple births, Abortions, and Live births, and are expressed in numbers separated by hyphens to represent the specific information. Some physicians dictate para 3–2–0–1–2, which may be transcribed as gravida 3, para 2–0–1–2, or para 3, 2–0–1–2.

developing fetus. **Pelvimetry** refers to certain standard measurements of the bones of the pelvis to assure an adequate birth passage for the fetus.

Laboratory studies carried out as part of routine prenatal care include a complete blood count, urinalysis, blood type, Rh antibody screen, rubella titer (to confirm maternal immunity to rubella, a potential cause of fetal damage), serologic test for syphilis, and Pap smear. Other tests that may be performed depending on risk factors include screening for sexually transmitted diseases (chlamydia, gonorrhea, HIV, syphilis) and for genetic diseases (sickle cell anemia).

Attention to **maternal nutrition** includes assuring adequate intake of protein, iron, calcium, and vitamins including folic acid. A weight gain of 20–30 pounds is considered most compatible with good maternal and fetal health. The patient is advised to avoid alcohol and tobacco and to limit caffeine intake. Maternal use of alcohol, caffeine, or nicotine is associated with lower birth weight, a sensitive indicator of suboptimal fetal development.

Prescription and nonprescription medicines are avoided if possible, and taken only when the expected benefit outweighs the risk of fetal harm. Nearly any drug administered to a pregnant woman will reach the fetal circulation in some concentration. Drugs that are capable of causing developmental anomalies are called teratogens. The risk of teratogenesis is limited almost exclusively to the period from the third through the eighth week of development, but a few drugs (ACE inhibitors, sulfonamides, tetracyclines) can cause fetal harm later in pregnancy. Drugs that are absolutely contraindicated during pregnancy because of unacceptably high risk include sex hormones (estrogens, androgens, progesterones), certain antibiotics (fluoroquinolones, tetracyclines, vancomycin), isotretinoin, radionuclides, valproic acid, and warfarin.

Certain maternal infections are also associated with a risk of **fetal malformation**. These include rubella in the first trimester and toxoplasmosis, cytomegalovirus, and herpes simplex later in pregnancy.

Standard prenatal care consists of regular visits every four weeks through the seventh month of gestation. During the eighth month visits are every two weeks, and after the 36th week they are weekly. At each visit the patient's weight and blood pressure are recorded, the urine is tested for protein and sugar, and the height of the uterine fundus above the pubic symphysis is measured. The examiner palpates the uterus and listens for fetal heart tones, normally audible by the fifth month. As pregnancy progresses, more and more information about the fetus can be gained by palpation.

Fetal ultrasound is routinely performed at 18–20 weeks to confirm fetal size and assess development. The examination may be repeated later to resolve any doubts. Repetition at four-week intervals is standard in multiple pregnancy. If needed for prenatal diagnosis of suspected anomalies, chorionic villus sampling is done at 10–12 weeks, amniocentesis at 12–18 weeks.

At 26–28 weeks the patient is screened for gestational diabetes (discussed later in this chapter) by determination of plasma glucose one hour after a standard oral glucose load. An Rh-negative mother is given a prophylactic dose of an immune globulin to suppress possible immune response to blood from an Rh-positive fetus.

Normal Labor and Delivery

Childbirth is a natural process that only occasionally requires skilled medical or surgical intervention. The role of the obstetrician or midwife is to observe the progress of labor while attending to the comfort of the mother and monitoring fetal and maternal well-being, prepared to render assistance as needed but generally allowing events to proceed naturally.

The **stages of labor** are as follows (see ■ Figure 14-8):

1st stage: from the onset of labor to full dilatation of the cervix.
2nd stage: from full dilatation of the cervix to delivery of the fetus.
3rd stage: from delivery of the fetus to delivery of the placenta.

The **onset of labor** is usually signaled by intermittent pelvic and back pains due to uterine contractions, at first mild and random but eventually growing stronger and coming at shorter and more regular intervals. Once labor has begun, the parturient may experience a bloody show—passage of a small amount of bloody material from the vagina, representing a plug of mucus that has been expelled from the cervix by uterine contractions. Eventually the amnionic sac ruptures, releasing a gush of fluid ("breaking of the waters") from the vagina.

The birth canal consists of two concentric passages—an inner soft-tissue tube made up of the cervix, vagina, and vulva and an outer rigid channel formed by the pelvic bones—through which the fetus must pass. The force that propels the fetus through this canal is

A

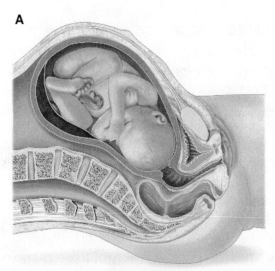

DILATION STAGE:
Uterine contractions dilate cervix

B

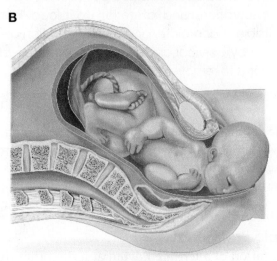

EXPULSION STAGE:
Birth of baby or expulsion

C

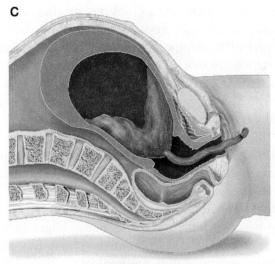

PLACENTAL STAGE:
Delivery of placenta

FIGURE 14-8. Stages of labor

supplied chiefly by uterine contractions, augmented by voluntary or involuntary contractions of the abdominal muscles including the diaphragm ("bearing down").

The principal soft-tissue obstacle to the advancement of the fetus is the cervix. Near the end of pregnancy the cervix undergoes a process of softening ("ripening") so that when labor begins it can stretch to accommodate the presenting part. Cervical stretching consists of two more or less simultaneous processes. **Effacement** is the flattening of the cervix from a tubular structure to a ring, and **dilatation** is the expansion of that ring to a size (about 10 cm) through which the fetal head can pass.

A lesser soft-tissue obstacle to delivery is the **vulva**. Encirclement of the largest diameter of the fetal head by the vulva is called **crowning**. Delivery typically ensues shortly after crowning has occurred, unless the passage of the fetus through the bony pelvis is delayed or arrested.

The bony birth canal is not only rigid and barely large enough to accommodate passage of the fetal head, but also tortuous. The pelvic inlet, or superior pelvic strait, is formed by the pubic bones, the ilia, and the promontory of the sacrum. In entering the pelvic inlet, the greatest diameter of the **presenting part** (the anteroposterior diameter of the fetal head) must rotate into an oblique position. The pelvic outlet, or inferior pelvic strait, is formed by the inferior rami of the ischia and pubic bones and the sacrotuberous and sacrospinous ligaments. In passing through the pelvic outlet the presenting part must rotate back to an anteroposterior orientation.

The obstetrician follows the progress of the first stage of labor by performing periodic rectal examinations to note the extent of **cervical effacement** and **dilatation** and the **station of the presenting part**, that is, its position with respect to the ischial spines. ("Station minus two" means that the presenting part is 2 cm above the spines.)

When the cervix is fully dilated ("complete") the parturient is positioned on a delivery table or birthing bed, obstetrical anesthesia (if any) is administered, continuous fetal monitoring is begun (usually by electronic pulse detector applied to the maternal abdomen), and the attendant dons sterile gown and gloves.

Failure of the second stage of labor to progress at the expected rate, evidence of fetal distress, inability of the mother to assist or cooperate (heart disease, mental illness), or certain complications (maternal hemorrhage, prolapse of the umbilical cord) may dictate one or more forms of obstetrical intervention: **episiotomy** (an incision in the posterior midline to enlarge the soft tissue passage), application of forceps or a vacuum cup extractor to the fetal head, or **cesarean delivery** (birth of the fetus through a surgical incision into the uterus through the abdominal wall).

During and immediately after the birth process the upper respiratory passages of the newborn are cleared of mucus and amnionic fluid, resuscitation measures are undertaken if spontaneous respirations do not begin immediately, and the umbilical cord is clamped and cut. The placenta is spontaneously expelled from the uterus within the next few minutes by further uterine contractions. The birth canal is carefully inspected for injuries or unexpected bleeding. Any laceration found (or an episiotomy, if one was performed) is surgically repaired. Hormones are administered by injection to hasten contraction of the uterus so as to arrest postpartum bleeding.

Pause for Reflection

1. Distinguish between an embryo and a fetus.
2. Name the hormone that is the basis of virtually all pregnancy tests; what is the stage of pregnancy at which this test becomes positive?
3. Define the following: (A) Braxton Hicks contractions, (B) Chadwick sign, (C) Hegar sign.
4. How is the expected date of confinement calculated?
5. List 4 laboratory tests that may be carried out during pregnancy.
6. Explain the statement, "The patient is 4 cm dilated, 50% effaced, -2 station."
7. What is an episiotomy?

Disorders of Pregnancy and Childbirth

Spontaneous Abortion (Miscarriage)

Spontaneous termination of pregnancy before the fetus is sufficiently developed to survive. The dividing line between abortion and premature delivery (with at least the possibility of survival of the infant) is arbitrarily placed at 20 weeks' gestation or a birth weight of 500 g.

At least 10% of pregnancies are believed to end in miscarriage, usually during the first trimester. More than 60% of these early miscarriages occur after embryonic or fetal death due to developmental abnormality. Inherited

---

SPONTANEOUS ABORTIONS

Threatened abortion: Any vaginal bleeding, with or without uterine cramping, during the first half of pregnancy.

Inevitable abortion: Rupture of membranes before the period of fetal viability.

Incomplete abortion: Expulsion of a nonviable fetus with retention of part or all of the placenta in the uterus.

Missed abortion: Retention of a dead fetus in the uterus for an extended period (often several weeks) before diagnosis is made.

Habitual abortion: A history of three or more consecutive spontaneous abortions.

Threatened abortion is treated with rest, careful observation, and attention to blood loss. Inevitable, incomplete, and missed abortion are treated by cervical dilatation and curettage of the uterus to remove all products of conception.

---

genetic disorders account for very few of these abnormalities. Miscarriage can also be due to a variety of maternal factors: severe illness or malnutrition, endocrine deficiency, uterine infection or trauma, cervical incompetence, and alcohol or nicotine use.

Ectopic Pregnancy

Implantation of a fertilized ovum at a site other than the endometrium, usually (95%) in a uterine tube (tubal pregnancy) (see ■ Figure 14-9). The risk of tubal implantation is increased by any factor that delays migration of the fertilized oocyte from the tube to the uterine cavity (developmental anomaly, neoplasm, scarring due to infection or surgery). Development of a fetus in a uterine tube eventually leads to rupture of the tube and life-threatening maternal hemorrhage. The classical triad of amenorrhea followed by scanty vaginal bleeding and severe abdominal pain occurs often but not always. An adnexal mass may be felt on pelvic examination. Serum pregnancy test is positive but progesterone level is low.

In tubal pregnancy, ultrasound shows an adnexal mass but no gestational sac in the uterus. Laparoscopy allows direct visualization of the dilated tube. Uncommonly, an ectopic pregnancy may implant on the abdominal or pelvic wall or on an ovary. Treatment is surgical control of hemorrhage and removal of the ectopic pregnancy with preservation of the tube if possible.

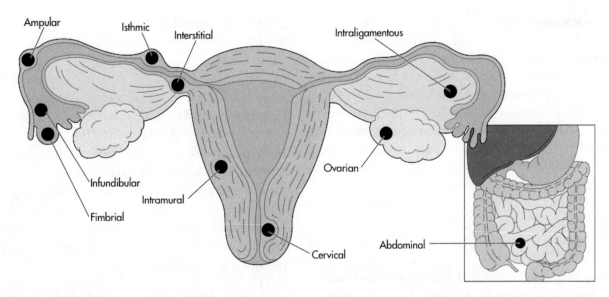

FIGURE 14-9. Various implantation sites in ectopic pregnancy, with the fallopian tube the most common (tubal pregnancy).

Abruptio Placentae

Separation of the placenta from the endometrium before onset of labor. Trauma is only occasionally the cause. The risk is increased by advanced maternal age, multiparity, hypertension, and cigarette smoking. Abdominal or pelvic pain resulting from stretching of the placenta and dissection of leaking blood into uterine muscle is accompanied by vaginal bleeding. Premature labor often begins within a few hours. The uterus is tender and may show asymmetric swelling. Ultrasound is not always helpful in demonstrating placental separation. Maternal hemorrhage can lead to loss of both mother and child. Treatment is by fluid or blood replacement as needed and cesarean delivery.

Placenta Previa

Implantation of the placenta partially or entirely over the internal cervical os (see ■ Figure 14-10). The risk is increased by advanced maternal age, multiparity, and multiple pregnancy. Uterine anomalies or previous uterine surgery may be contributory. Significant placenta previa occurs in about 0.5% of all pregnancies. Painless vaginal bleeding occurs in the third trimester as the malpositioned placenta separates from the endometrium with enlargement of the fetus. Ultrasound examination confirms placental position.

The finding of placenta previa on ultrasound in the second trimester is common (up to 40% of pregnancies), but most of these have resolved on repeat ultrasonography in the third trimester. Maternal hemorrhage can lead to loss of both mother and child. If labor begins, blockage of the internal cervical os by the placenta may interfere with the expulsion of the fetus. Treatment is with fluid replace-

ment and preterm delivery, usually cesarean, as needed to save the fetus and prevent life-threatening maternal hemorrhage.

Premature (Preterm) Labor

Premature labor is defined as onset of labor after attainment of fetal viability but before fetal maturity is reached, usually at 40 weeks' gestation. Premature labor is the most common third trimester complication of pregnancy. Causes include premature rupture of membranes (PROM), cervical incompetence, multiple pregnancy, polyhydramnios (excessive volume of amnionic fluid), placenta previa, and abruptio placentae. Management includes maternal and fetal monitoring, main-

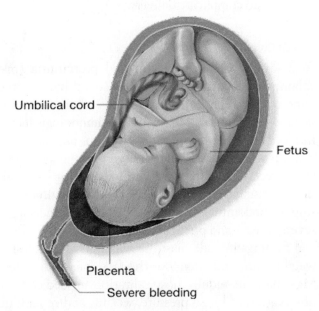

FIGURE 14-10. Placenta previa

tenance of maternal hydration, and avoidance of analgesics and anesthetics as much as possible because of their possible adverse effects on the premature infant. Labor is permitted to continue if the cervix is dilated to 4 cm or more, if membranes are ruptured, if there is evidence of fetal distress, and especially in the presence of preeclampsia or other complication of pregnancy for which prompt delivery would be beneficial. Otherwise labor is arrested by administration of a tocolytic drug: a beta-adrenergic agonist (isoxsuprine, ritodrine, terbutaline), calcium channel blocker (nifedipine), or magnesium sulfate.

Gestational Diabetes

Carbohydrate intolerance that begins, or is first recognized, during pregnancy. Gestational diabetes occurs in 3–6% of pregnancies. It may be due to hormonal and physiologic alterations of pregnancy, and hence fully reversible. However, at least half of women with this disorder eventually develop clinical diabetes mellitus. The one-hour postprandial glucose is elevated on routine testing at 24–28 weeks' gestation and the diagnosis is confirmed by abnormal results of a three-hour glucose tolerance test.

This condition may be associated with fetal macrosomia (excessive body size and weight), congenital anomalies, and **polyhydramnios** (excessive quantity of amniotic fluid); heightened risk of urinary tract infection (pyelonephritis) in the mother. Treatment is by strict attention to diet, with avoidance of concentrated sugar and fats. Insulin may be required for adequate control of blood sugar level. Labor may be induced early if fetal size threatens to complicate delivery.

Toxemia of Pregnancy

A syndrome of hypertension and proteinuria (**preeclampsia**) occurring during the second half of pregnancy, which can progress to a stage characterized by seizures (**eclampsia**). Metabolic or immunologic factors induced by the developing chorion appear to be causative. The risk is greater for very young mothers or those over 40, and for those with preexisting hypertension or vascular or renal disease. Headache, visual blurring, or abdominal pain due to hepatic edema suggest severe disease and predict progression to seizures. Physical findings include diastolic hypertension, excessive weight gain, and edema of the face, hands, and feet. Most patients require hospitalization for bed rest and observation of blood pressure, weight, and renal function, as well as fetal monitoring. Hypertension and

seizures are controlled pharmacologically. The severity of the condition may dictate early induction of labor.

Dystocia

Dystocia, defined as any abnormal slowing or arrest of the progress of labor once it has begun, can be due to maternal factors (uterine dysfunction, excessive anesthesia, pelvic deformity), fetal factors (large baby, hydrocephalus, breech presentation), or some combination of these. **Cephalopelvic disproportion** means that the fetal head is too large to pass through the maternal pelvis. Dystocia that cannot be readily corrected by pharmacologic measures or nonsurgical manipulation is a principal indication for cesarean delivery.

Nonreassuring Fetal Status (Fetal Distress)

A general term for findings on fetal cardiac monitoring that suggest **fetal hypoxemia** (reduction in plasma oxygen tension). Normally the fetal pulse slows during a uterine contraction because of compression of the fetal head and returns to a normal rate (120–160/minute) immediately afterwards. Prolonged or nonuniform deceleration of the pulse rate or tachycardia can indicate a significant threat to fetal welfare.

Serious causes include developmental abnormality of the placenta, prolapse (premature descent through the cervix) or compression of the umbilical cord, and uterine rupture. The pH of fetal blood obtained by scalp incision (in a cephalic presentation) is 7.2 or lower in the presence of significant fetal hypoxemia. Management includes administration of oxygen to the mother and diligent search for a correctible cause. Often no cause is found and labor and delivery proceed normally. Circumstances may dictate prompt vaginal or cesarean delivery.

Pause for Reflection

1. What distinguishes a spontaneous abortion from a premature delivery?
2. Implantation of a fertilized ovum at a site other than the endometrium, usually in a uterine tube, is referred to as a(n) _____.
3. Distinguish between the two types of disorders of pregnancy that involve the placenta.
4. Name the most common third trimester complication of labor and list 3 possible causes.

(continued)

Pause for Reflection *(continued)*

5. Describe toxemia of pregnancy.
6. List 2 maternal and 2 fetal factors contributing to dystocia.
7. What is the general term for findings on fetal cardiac monitoring that suggest fetal hypoxemia?

Diagnostic and Surgical Procedures

amniocentesis A procedure to withdraw amniotic fluid through a needle from the uterus of a pregnant woman. The fetal cells and chemicals in the fluid are studied to identify fetal abnormalities.

amniotic fluid index (AFI) An ultrasound procedure used to assess the amount of amniotic fluid that surrounds the baby. The uterus is divided into four quadrants and the deepest, unobstructed vertical pocket of fluid in each quadrant is measured in centimeters. The values for each quadrant are added up for the AFI. Too little fluid (oligohydramnios) could be detrimental to the baby; too much (polyhydramnios) could be associated with gestational diabetes mellitus or cause premature labor.

This is an 18-year-old G1, P0, at 41-6/7 weeks presented for postdates induction. In her evaluation she was noted to have a nonreactive nonstress test (NST). She had an ultrasound performed that showed an amniotic fluid index (AFI) of approximately 0 to 1, a nonreactive NST, minimal tone, no breathing, no movement. The decision was made in light of this to proceed towards primary low transverse cesarean section.

anterior colporrhaphy Plication of the vaginal muscularis fascia overlying the bladder (pubocervical fascia) to repair a cystocele. A midline incision is made in the vaginal mucosa and the vagina dissected sharply away from the pubocervical fascia lateral to the inferior pubic ramus. Absorbable mattress sutures are placed in layers on the pubocervical fascia, excess vaginal mucosa trimmed away, and remaining mucosa closed with running or interrupted sutures.

anterior and posterior (A&P) repair A combination of anterior and posterior colporrhaphy for the repair of cystocele, rectocele, and uterine prolapse.

basal body temperature Daily determination of oral temperature on arising is useful in confirming and dating ovulation. Daily graphing of basal body temperature will show a rise of 0.75 to 1.0°F (0.2 to 0.5°C) approximately one day after ovulation.

biopsy, cervical A colposcopically directed procedure that may involve removal of plugs of tissue with a punch-type instrument or removal of a cone of tissue including the entire squamocolumnar junction (see ■ Figure 14-11).

biopsy, endometrial Removal of tissue with a suction tube device from the endometrium for histologic examination to identify infection, neoplasm, or other abnormality. The procedure may be performed in a doctor's office with or without anesthesia (see ■ Figure 14-11).

biopsy, excisional Removal of a tumor followed by frozen-section examination before closure of the surgical site (see ■ Figure 14-11).

breech birth The delivery of a newborn buttocks first.

cervical cerclage A surgical treatment for cervical incompetence in which a ring of strong suture of special tape is placed around the cervix and tightened to prevent the cervix from thinning and stretching so as to avoid premature delivery.

cesarean delivery (cesarean section, C-section) Removal of the fetus (usually term or near-term) surgically though an incision in the abdomen and uterus.

Given that the baby was found to be large for gestational age and had an oblique lie, the decision was made to proceed with primary low transverse cesarean section.

chorionic villus sampling Removal of a biopsy specimen from the chorion, which carries a significant risk of causing miscarriage, for the purpose of genetic testing to see if the patient is at risk for having a baby with Down syndrome or other genetic defect.

colposcopy Examination of the cervix with an illuminated low-power microscope, which facilitates identification of suspicious cervical lesions requiring biopsy.

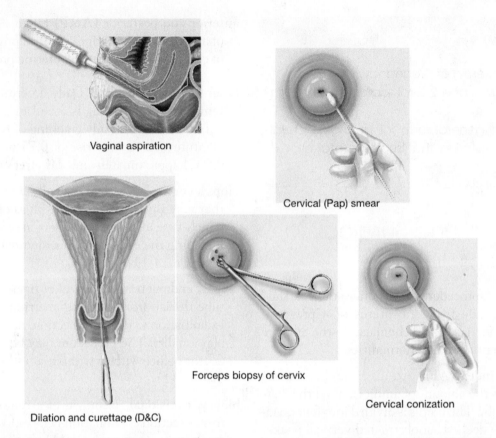

Vaginal aspiration

Cervical (Pap) smear

Forceps biopsy of cervix

Cervical conization

Dilation and curettage (D&C)

FIGURE 14-11. Biopsy to remove a tissue sample for microscopic exam: aspiration, endoscopic, excisional, or needle.

conization of the cervix Removal of a cone of tissue from the cervix for microscopic examination (see ■ Figure 14-11).

culdoscopy Endoscopic inspection of the cul-de-sac (pouch of Douglas), the lowermost part of the perito-

> *A 24-year-old G5 P2 diagnosed with a missed and an incomplete abortion by ultrasound as well as presenting to the emergency room with dilated cervix and vaginal bleeding, taken to the OR for suction D&C after consultation with the patient.*

neal cavity, which lies between the uterus and the rectum. The instrument is introduced vaginally under anesthesia (see ■ Figure 14-6).

dilatation and curettage (D&C) Scraping of the endometrium, after stretching of the cervix with graded dilators, to obtain specimen material for the diagnosis of endometrial disease. This procedure, performed under anesthesia (general, spinal, or intravenous), is also used therapeutically for various endometrial disorders (see ■ Figure 14-11).

endometrial ablation Surgical destruction (ablation) of the endometrium (uterine lining) for dysfunctional uterine bleeding. A variety of ablating modalities including laser, radiofrequency, thermal balloon (ThermaChoice), electricity, cryosurgery (freezing), and microwave may be used. The procedure may done under local or spinal anesthesia. A **hysteroscope** may be used for visualization.

episiotomy An incision in the posterior midline to enlarge the vulvar opening during childbirth.

Falope ring sterilization A small silastic band is placed around a loop of the uterine (fallopian) tube to close it off to prevent pregnancy. Although intended to be permanent, some women choose this method because it is sometimes reversible.

hysterectomy Surgical removal of the uterus.

hysterosalpingogram A test to assess infertility in which radiopaque dye is injected into the uterus and fallopian tubes, and x-rays are taken to show if the tubes are patent (clear) or obstructed (see ■ Figure 14-7).

laparoscopy Inspection of pelvic viscera through a laparoscope, a tubular instrument with illumination and magnification, inserted through a small incision in the abdominal wall. Minor surgical procedures can be performed through the instrument.

loop electrosurgical excision procedure (LEEP) Use of a thin low-voltage wire loop to remove cervical tissue for histological analysis as part of a colposcopy; it may be performed in a doctor's office or as an out-patient surgical procedure in a hospital or clinic.

mammogram A radiographic image of the breast produced with special equipment and techniques to screen for carcinoma in women without breast symptoms.

Marshall-Marchetti-Krantz (MMK) procedure An operation for urinary stress incontinence, performed retropubically.

marsupialization Surgical technique of cutting a slit into a cyst and suturing the edges of the slit to form a continuous surface from the exterior surface to the interior of the cyst. Sutured in this fashion, the cyst remains open and can drain freely. This technique is used to treat a cyst when a single draining would not be effective, and complete removal of the surrounding structure would not be desirable.

nonstress test (NST) A noninvasive (thus, nonstress) test to monitor the fetal heart rate during fetal movement and during contractions in labor by means of an external monitor placed around the mother's belly.

oophorectomy Surgical removal of an ovary.

Pap (Papanicolaou) smear A vaginal speculum is inserted and cells detached from the vaginal walls, the squamocolumnar junction, and the endocervical canal by gentle scraping. Disposable instruments used for this purpose include the Ayre spatula, the Cyto-brush, and the Cervex-Brush. Cell specimens are spread on a glass microscope slide and immediately sprayed with a fixative solution that arrests cellular metabolism and prevents distortion of cells due to drying. In liquid-based cytology the specimen is immersed in a fluid medium and spread on a slide after transfer to a cytology laboratory. Smears are stained by the Papanicolaou technique and screened, usually with computer assistance, for signs of cellular dysplasia or other abnormalities. Results are reported according to the Bethesda system (see page 496).

Pomeroy technique Used in tubal ligation.

posterior colporrhaphy Repair of a posterior vaginal defect (rectocele). Typically, a transvaginal approach is used and incorporates a posterior colpoperineorrhaphy with plication of the levator ani muscle. The rectovaginal fascia is plicated in the midline and excess vaginal mucosa excised and repaired with absorbable sutures.

robotically assisted laparoscopic surgery Widely used in gynecology to perform oophorectomy, myomectomy, and hysterectomy and to treat endometriosis and prolapse of the pelvic floor.

sacrocolpopexy A laparoscopic or open abdominal procedure for repair of apical vaginal prolapse. One end of a graft is sutured to the anterior and posterior vaginal wall with the other end attached high up in the pelvis to sacral ligaments or the sacral promontory. Variations in techniques and graft materials are many.

salpingectomy Surgical removal of a uterine (fallopian) tube.

sonogram See *ultrasound*.

TAH-BSO Total abdominal hysterectomy and bilateral salpingo-oophorectomy.

tubal ligation Surgical division of the uterine (fallopian) tubes to obtain sterility (see ■ Figure 14-12).

ultrasound The use of sound waves to assess tumors of the ovaries, uterus, breast, as well as the fetus in a pregnant woman.

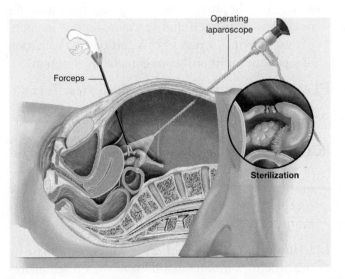

FIGURE 14-12. Tubal ligation

Laboratory Procedures

AFP (alpha fetoprotein) A test performed on maternal serum, usually around 16–18 weeks' gestation. Maternal AFP may be abnormally low when the fetus has Down syndrome and abnormally elevated when the fetus has a neural tube defect. AFP is also a marker for certain cancers. This test is included in a triple screen or quadruple screen.

beta-hCG See *hCG.*

chocolate agar A culture medium containing blood which, when autoclaved, turns chocolate brown. It is used to culture *Neisseria gonorrhoeae* and *Haemophilus influenza.*

Coombs test, direct A test to determine whether the patient's red blood cells have become coated with an antiglobulin. The test is positive in newborns with hemolytic disease due to Rh incompatibility and in other patients with acquired hemolytic disease.

Coombs test, indirect A test to determine whether the patient's serum contains antiglobulin to red blood cells. This test is positive in the mother of an infant with hemolytic disease due to Rh incompatibility and in other patients with acquired hemolytic disease.

dark-field microscopy A microscopic technique using special lighting that makes it easier to identify *Treponema pallidum,* the organism that causes syphilis.

estradiol The principal estrogen (female hormone) secreted by the ovary. Measurement of its level in serum gives an estimate of ovarian function.

FSH (follicle-stimulating hormone) A hormone secreted by the anterior pituitary gland that stimulates ovulation in women and spermatogenesis in men. Measurement of serum FSH is part of the evaluation of a patient for infertility or gonadal dysfunction.

FTA (fluorescent treponemal antibody) test An indirect immunofluorescence test, highly specific for syphilis.

hCG, HCG (human chorionic gonadotropin) A hormone produced by the placenta and detected in various blood and urine tests for pregnancy. A more specific test detects only the beta subunit of this hormone, hence the term beta-hCG.

LH (luteinizing hormone) A hormone produced by the anterior pituitary gland. In women it stimulates ovulation and formation of the corpus luteum, and in men it stimulates production of androgens in the testicle. Measurement of LH is part of the evaluation of a patient for infertility or gonadal dysfunction.

OraQuick In-Home HIV test The first over-the-counter in-home HIV test kit approved by the FDA that does not need to be sent to a laboratory for analysis. An oral fluid sample is taken by swabbing the upper and lower gums and placed into a developer vial, and results are obtained within 20 to 40 minutes.

pregnancy test See *HCG.*

quadruple screen A triple screen with the addition of inhibin A. May be dictated as *quad screen.*

RPR (rapid plasma reagin) Test for antibody to *Treponema pallidum.* Used in the diagnosis of syphilis.

semen analysis Examination of semen to determine the number, shape, and motility of spermatozoa as a part of an infertility evaluation.

smear and culture Microbiologic study of secretions or other materials from the cervix, vagina, urethra, rectum, or from superficial lesions, to identify causes of infection.

spinnbarkeit When the estrogen level is high but the progesterone level is low (the conditions existing just before and just after ovulation), a specimen of cervical mucus can be drawn out into strings or strands several centimeters in length. This property is called **spinnbarkeit** (German, "ability to be drawn out into a string"). When both estrogen and progesterone are present in large amounts, cervical mucus loses this property, and attempts to draw it out into a string fail.

STD screen Sexually transmitted disease screen.

STS (serologic test for syphilis) A general term referring to any test used to identify syphilis by a serologic method.

TPI (*Treponema pallidum* immobilization) A diagnostic test for syphilis.

triple screen A panel of tests that includes AFP (alphafetoprotein), hCG (human chorionic gonadotropin), and uE3 (unconjugated estriol) obtained during the second trimester to evaluate for certain fetal abnormalities such as trisomy 21 (Down syndrome), trisomy 18 (Edwards syndrome), neural tube defect, spina bifida, or anencephaly. May be dictated as *tri screen.*

Tzanck smear A stained smear of material from a cutaneous or mucosal lesion, intended to identify changes due to viral infection from herpes simplex or varicella.

VDRL (Venereal Disease Research Laboratory) A serologic test for syphilis. (It does not need expansion.)

Pharmacology

Drugs used to treat women with obstetrical and gynecologic problems include drugs for infertility and vaginal infections, drugs that stimulate or suppress labor contractions, drugs that correct menstrual disorders and endometriosis, estrogen replacement therapy, and prophylactically prescribed birth control agents. Few drugs are prescribed during pregnancy, particularly during the first trimester, due to the increased risk of birth defects; however, antibiotics for infections and drugs to maintain good health (such as insulin or heart medications), as well as prenatal vitamins, iron, and folic acid, are given.

Ovulation-Stimulating Drugs for Infertility

These drugs block estrogen receptors on the ovary so estrogen cannot enter. The ovary responds to the lack of estrogen by signaling the pituitary gland that estrogen levels are low, and then the pituitary gland secretes luteinizing hormone (LH) and follicle-stimulating hormone (FSH). These hormones stimulate a nonovulating ovary to develop an ovarian follicle and release mature eggs. These drugs also aid in the formation of the corpus luteum, which secretes progesterone to maintain the pregnancy if the egg is fertilized.

Ovulation-stimulating drugs are appropriate for patients with anovulation (failure to ovulate), but are not appropriate for patients with infertility due to blocked uterine tubes or other mechanical problems that require surgical intervention.

> choriogonadotropin alfa (Ovidrel)
> clomiphene (Clomid, Serophene)
> follitropin alfa (Gonal-F)
> follitropin beta (Follistim)
> human chorionic gonadotropin (HCG or hCG) (A.P.L., Pregnyl, Profasi)
> letrazole (Femara)
> lutotropin alfa (Luveris)
> menotropins (Humegon, Pergonal, Repronex)

> sermorelin (Geref)
> urofollitropin (Fertinex, Metrodin)

Note: Clomid can be used alone, but menotropins and urofollitropin must be given concurrently with hCG to achieve a complete therapeutic effect.

Uterine Relaxants

Premature or preterm labor and delivery greatly increase morbidity and mortality in infants. Premature labor contractions can be inhibited by using uterine-relaxing drugs that act on beta$_2$ receptors in the smooth muscle of the uterus. These drugs are known as **tocolytics** (from the Greek words *tokos* "childbirth," and *lysis* ("release, dissolution"). The relaxant ritodrine decreases both the frequency and strength of contractions.

Uterine Stimulants

Women in labor may be given a uterine stimulant if their uterine contractions are too weak to effect delivery (uterine inertia) or if complications such as preeclampsia or diabetes necessitate induction of labor. Normally, oxytocin (Pitocin), produced by the pituitary gland, stimulates the uterus by binding to special oxytocin receptors in the uterine muscle. Oxytocin as a drug increases both the frequency and strength of uterine contractions.

Oxytocin is not indicated when prolonged labor is due to cephalopelvic disproportion—the baby's skull is too large to fit through the mother's pelvic outlet.

> hexoprenaline (Delaprem)
> oxytocin (Pitocin)

Labor is composed of uterine contractions as well as cervical dilatation (widening) and effacement (thinning). When the cervix does not dilate and thin, dinoprostone (Cervidil, Prepidil) may be applied topically to the cervix to ripen it.

Postpartum Bleeding

Postpartum bleeding is due to uterine relaxation, which results in increased bleeding at the site of placental separation. Drugs used to treat postpartum bleeding include:

> carboprost (Hemabate)
> ergonovine (Ergotrate)
> methylergonovine (Methergine)
> oxytocin (Pitocin, Syntocinon)

Drugs Used to Treat Endometriosis

Endometriosis develops when tissue from the uterus implants within the pelvic cavity and on the ovaries and other organs. It remains sensitive to hormonal influences, shedding blood when the uterus begins menstruation. Endometriosis causes pelvic pain, inflammation, and cyst formation. After hormonal drugs suppress the menstrual cycle for several months, endometrial implants may atrophy. Hormonal drugs used to treat endometriosis include:

>danazol (Danocrine)
>goserelin (Zoladex)
>leuprolide (Lupron Depot)
>nafarelin (Synarel)
>norethindrone (Aygestin)

Oral Contraceptives

Birth control pills exert a hormonal influence to prevent pregnancy and are 95% effective if taken as directed. Most oral contraceptives contain a combination of estrogen and progestin that is taken for 21 days. During the final seven days of the 28-day menstrual cycle, the patient may take no tablets, seven sugar-filled tablets, and seven sugar tablets with iron (Fe). Other oral contraceptives contain only progestin.

Combination oral contraceptives that contain both estrogen and progestin are divided into three basic groups according to the relative amounts of progestin and estrogen provided during each day of the menstrual cycle. These three basic groups of combination oral contraceptives include monophasics, biphasics, and triphasics.

Monophasic oral contraceptives provide fixed amounts of progestin and estrogen in each tablet for each day of the 21-day period. The amounts of progestin and estrogen are designated by two numbers in the trade name of the drug. Example: Norinyl 1+50 contains 1 mg of progestin and 50 mg of estrogen in each tablet. Because an increased incidence of side effects (particularly thrombophlebitis) has been associated with higher estrogen dosages, a physician may elect to prescribe Norinyl 1+35, which contains 1 mg of progestin and just 35 mg of estrogen in each tablet.

Demulen 1/50	Demulen 1/35
Loestrin 1.5/30	Loestrin 1/20
Norinyl 1+50	Norinyl 1+35
Ortho-Novum 1/50	Ortho-Novum 1/35

Lunelle provides a fixed amount of progestin and estrogen in a once-monthly injection. Ortho Evra is a transdermal patch drug that provides a fixed amount of progestin and estrogen. NuvaRing provides a fixed amount of progestin and estrogen in a vaginal ring.

Biphasic oral contraceptives provide a fixed amount of estrogen in every tablet for each day of the 21-day period; the amount of progestin is fixed in the first half of the cycle but then increases in the second half of the cycle. This change is designated by two numbers following the trade name. Example: Ortho-Novum 10/11 provides 0.5 mg of progestin and 35 mg of estrogen in each tablet for the first 10 days; for the final 11 days, each tablet contains 1 mg of progestin and 35 mg of estrogen.

Triphasic oral contraceptives provide a fixed amount or slightly varying amount of estrogen for each day of the 21-day time period, while the amount of progestin increases or varies throughout that time. This is designated, at least in the case of Ortho-Novum, by the numbers 7/7/7 which show that the amount of progestin increases every 7 days. Other drugs in this category have the prefix *tri-* in their trade names to indicate the three phases of different dosages of progestin in the 21 days.

>Cyclessa
>Estrostep Fe, Estrostep 21
>Ortho-Novum 7/7/7
>Ortho-Tri-Cyclen
>Tri-Levlen
>Tri-Norinyl
>Triphasil
>Trivora-28

Contraceptives that contain only progestin are slightly less effective in preventing pregnancy than combination contraceptives, particularly if the patient forgets to take even one daily tablet. However, the risks (particularly thrombophlebitis) and other side effects of estrogen therapy due to combination oral contraceptives are avoided. Progestin-only contraceptives are taken orally, given by injection, implanted under the skin, or inserted into the uterus.

>medroxyprogesterone (Depo-Provera)
>Micronor
>Mirena
>Nor-QD
>Ovrette
>Progestasert

Plan B is a progestin-only drug that is taken in two doses after intercourse to prevent pregnancy, and Plan B One-Step is a single dose with the same effectiveness.

Drugs Used to Treat Irregular Menstruation

Primary hypothalamic amenorrhea, the absence of menstruation due to decreased levels of gonadotropin-releasing hormone (GnRH), may be treated with a drug that stimulates the release of luteinizing hormone (LH) and follicle-stimulating hormone (FSH) from the pituitary gland. A special pump is needed to administer the drug IV in pulses that mimic the natural release of GnRH from the pituitary gland. Example: gonadorelin (Lutrepulse).

Amenorrhea and abnormal uterine bleeding may also be treated with progesterone-like drugs that act directly on the tissues of the endometrium to restore a normal menstrual cycle.

hydroxyprogesterone (Hylutin)
medroxyprogesterone (Amen, Cycrin, Provera)
norethindrone (Aygestin)
progesterone (Crinone)

Combination estrogen/progestin drugs used to treat irregular menstruation include Premphase and Prempro.

INTRAVENOUS FLUIDS

Commonly used intravenous fluids include normal saline, dextrose, and Ringer injection; these fluids are sometimes referred to as crystalloids when referring to fluid replacement during surgery.

IV FLUIDS
1000 mL of crystalloid

Normal saline (NS) is the commonly used phrase for a solution of 0.9% NaCl. Less commonly, this solution is referred to as physiological saline or isotonic saline, neither of which is technically accurate. NS is used in IV therapy to supply extra water to a dehydrated patient, to supply daily water and salt needs (maintenance IV therapy) of a patient who is unable to take them by mouth, for the IV delivery of drugs, or to replenish circulating blood volume due to loss of blood through trauma or surgery. Intravenous solutions with reduced saline concentrations typically have dextrose (glucose) added to maintain a safe osmolality while providing less sodium chloride.

D5/0.45 normal saline
half normal saline in 5% dextrose
D5W and half normal saline

Dextrose is referred to by its percentage in water; thus D5W is 5% dextrose in water. Half normal saline is 0.45% saline because it is half of the 0.9% normal saline solution.

Ringer injection, lactated, is also used in combination with 5% dextrose for fluid resuscitation after a blood loss due to trauma, surgery, or a burn injury. It is isotonic with blood and administered intravenously. It is used because the byproducts of lactate metabolism in the liver counteract acidosis, which is a chemical imbalance that occurs with acute fluid loss or renal failure.

Although the "official name" is Ringer injection, lactated, you will more often hear *lactated Ringer's solution* or *Ringer's lactate solution* or the abbreviations *LR* (lactated Ringer's), *RL* (Ringer's lactate) or *LRS* (lactated Ringer's solution).

Transcription Tips

1. Confusing terms related to the female reproductive system: Some of these terms sound alike; others are potential traps when researching. Memorize the terms and their meanings so that you can select the appropriate term for a correct transcript.

   bimanual—performed with two hands

   by manual—by hand

   perineal—the area between the pubic arch and the anus

   peritoneal—the serous membrane lining the abdomen

   perianal—the area surrounding the anus

   peroneal—pertaining to the thigh and usually modifying nerves, vessels, muscles

   radical—directed at the root source (radical hysterectomy, radical mastectomy)

   radicle—the smallest branch of a vessel or nerve

   vesical—pertaining to the urinary bladder

   vesicle—small fluid-filled sac

2. Slang terms. Expand these slang brief forms when encountered in dictation.

   primip ("prime-ip")   primipara

   multip ("mul-tip)   multipara

3. Spelling. Memorize the spelling of these ObGyn terms.

   Note these terms beginning with *post-*

   postmenopausal

   postpartum   postvoiding

   Note these terms ending in *–rrhagia.*

   menometrorrhagia

   menorrhagia   metrorrhagia

   Note these terms ending in *-rrhea.*

   amenorrhea   dysmenorrhea

   oligomenorrhea   polymenorrhea

   Note these terms ending in *–rrhaphy*

   colporrhaphy   perineorrhaphy

   Note silent letters, doubled letters, and unexpected pronunciation.

   anovulation (*not* an ovulation or inovulation)

   chlamydia

   cul-de-sac (hyphens are mandatory)

   cystadenoma

cystosarcoma phyllodes	mittelschmerz
	oophorectomy
descensus uteri	Pfannenstiel incision
dyspareunia	pneumoperitoneum
dystocia	placenta previa
endometriosis	preeclampsia
fourchette	pyelectasis
gonococcus	salpingo-oophorectomy
menarche	single-tooth(ed) tenaculum
menstruation	souffle (rhymes with *truffle*)
mesosalpinx	Tzanck smear

4. Watch out for spelling changes when forming derivatives.

   The term *parous* (not "Paris"), a derivative of *para*, describes a woman who has given birth either vaginally or by cesarean section after the 20th week of gestation; however, a *parous introitus* means the patient has had a vaginal delivery. *Parity* is the number of such deliveries.

curet	surgical instrument
curettage	surgical procedure
curetting	process using a curet
curettings	material obtained during a curettage
salpinx	tube
salpingectomy	excision of tube
salpingitis	inflammation of tube

5. Note the challenging spellings of these common drugs. Memorize the spellings of these drugs with unusual internal capitalization.

   MetroGel-Vaginal   MICRhoGAM

   RhoGAM   WinRho SDF

6. Be careful when translating these abbreviations.

   A&P (anterior and posterior)

   A&P (auscultation and percussion)

   BUS (Bartholin gland, urethra, and Skene gland) (not Bartholin, urethral, and Skene glands)

7. Dictation Challenges

   The abbreviation *VBAC* (acronym for vaginal birth after cesarean section) is often pronounced "vee-back."

Spotlight On

Listening to Your Body

by Brenda Hurley

We have all heard the clichés about paying attention to our body; I am living proof how true that really is. I have enjoyed reasonably good health and have too often taken it for granted. My healthcare event did not start with a thunderstorm of pain or something ominous that would immediately grab my attention, but instead a small amount of red-tinged vaginal discharge. It was not painful, not enough to call outright bleeding, and it was intermittent instead of consistent in occurrence. Like any woman, I ignored it for months because I was sure it would just go away. It really did not get worse, but it did not go away either.

Finally I told my primary care doctor about it. My doctor immediately was concerned with any bleeding in a postmenopausal woman (me). Surely my doctor was overreacting, I thought. This was not bleeding, it was only blood-tinged discharge! Do you see how we rationalize things to make them seem less important when all we are doing is being stagnant in denial? I was.

So a referral to a GYN specialist was made. Okay, I accepted (before I saw the specialist) that I must have endometritis and an antibiotic would be needed to fix my little problem. The specialist did an exam and pelvic ultrasound. He was undecided himself since there was nothing really obvious found on either. He put me on a medication with my promise that if this blood-tinged discharge returned, I would make a followup appointment. I was back in his office in just a few months. I was now convinced that I would likely need a D&C or a different medication to clear this up.

After having transcribed a zillion D&C procedures in my long MT career, I knew this attitude was not uncommon. As an MT, we just love to make the diagnosis when we transcribe reports, and in real life as well. So I was diagnosing myself, and in this case I was wrong.

The specialist again did an exam and ultrasound because he wanted to see if there was any pronounced endometrial stripe. It was still inconclusive,

so he did an endometrial biopsy. That was no fun! He told me that the biopsy would be sent to pathology and they would call me with the results. I knew all of that, of course, because I worked as a transcriptionist in pathology for 12 years. I knew about the biopsies, the processing of the tissue specimens, and the macroscopic and microscopic reporting, all done to conclude with a final diagnosis.

I was so convinced that this was a persistent endometritis that I did not worry a moment from the time I left the doctor's office. I had a big birthday celebration quickly approaching and a 4th of July trip planned, as well as full-time work, so there was much to do over the next week.

On my 60th birthday the doctor called to tell me that I had been diagnosed with adenocarcinoma of the endometrium. Not the birthday present I expected. He referred me to a GYN oncologist who specializes in the da Vinci robotic-assisted laparoscopic hysterectomy. Of note, I had seen this procedure and this same surgeon on an online presentation to educate the community about this state-of-the-art procedure now available through their facility. I viewed the procedure because of my interest in new surgical techniques and terminology, believing it would be useful for me as an MT, but instead it was useful for me as a patient.

I quickly went to work on becoming my own healthcare advocate. I created a detailed document that included my past medical and surgical histories, significant family history, medications, allergies, and emergency contact information. Before my appointment I again reviewed the online video on the da Vinci procedure and took notes for questions that I would ask when I met with the GYN oncologist and his staff.

I also went online to research adenocarcinoma of the endometrium to better understand what it is and the risk factors for occurrence. I found that I was right on target for this cancer. In fact, if I had not been so deep in denial, I would have easily seen that the risk factors were perfectly aligned to me and my symptoms. These include (1) never having been pregnant; (2) my age group; (3) larger than normal abdominal fat (yes, that's me); and (4) post-menopausal bleeding.

I was armed with my health data sheet, my questions, and a much better understanding of what it is that I have when I met with the GYN oncologist and his staff. Immediately they were impressed with my health data sheet, of which I quickly announced that I am a medical transcriptionist and that all of the terms are spelled correctly. The doctor still dictates all of his office visits and procedures, so we immediately clicked. In fact, he joked that he probably didn't need to get out the anatomy chart to show me where the uterus is. I told him that if he got the anatomy chart out, I would show it to him instead. We skipped the anatomy chart.

We went through my questions. I made notes. When done, he said that if all of his new patients came as prepared as I was, he could see three times more patients.

Within a month I had the surgery and was on the road to a full recovery. The pathology from my uterus showed that the cancer had invaded the myometrial wall but not beyond it. No one knows how much longer it would have taken the cancer to get through the wall, but definitely my followup would have been very intensive if it had. Since my cancer was graded as a stage I, I did not require any chemotherapy or radiation. My story would be very different if I had stayed in denial and allowed the cancer to continue to grow.

Your story is still being written. Be proactive, not in denial. When your body is telling you something is wrong, see your doctor. Do it sooner rather than later because disease processes wait for no one.

THE BETHESDA SYSTEM OF CLASSIFICATION

The Bethesda system is now generally used to report Pap smear findings. In this system, a full cytologic report contains (1) a statement of the adequacy of the specimen (for example, whether columnar cells from the endocervix are present), (2) a general categorization (presence or absence of premalignant or malignant epithelial cell changes), and (3) a descriptive summary of all findings, including evidence of acute infection with *Trichomonas* or *Candida* and the patient's hormonal status.

Mild dysplasia of squamous cells, including cellular atypia characteristic of HPV infection, is designated a low-grade squamous intraepithelial lesion (LGSIL or LSIL).

Changes that suggest HPV infection are koilocytosis (unusually clear or vacuolated cytoplasm with a dense border, presence of a perinuclear halo) and nuclear pyknosis (shrinkage of the nucleus with condensation of stainable material). Squamous intraepithelial lesions that do not meet criteria for either of these categories may be called either atypical squamous cells of undetermined significance (ASCUS) or atypical squamous cells suggestive of high-grade lesions (ASC-H).

The finding of ASC-H, LGSIL, or HGSIL is an indication for colposcopically directed biopsy of the cervix. A woman with ASCUS or ambiguous Pap smear reports may undergo a repeat Pap smear after an interval, colposcopy and biopsy, or DNA testing for high-risk HPV types. Currently, viral typing is the preferred method.

Exercises

Medical Vocabulary Review

Instructions: Choose the best answer.

_____ 1. Which of the following means "excessive menstrual bleeding occurring both during menses and at irregular intervals"?
A. Menorrhagia.
B. Polymenorrhea.
C. Hypermenorrhea.
D. Menometrorrhagia.

_____ 2. Dysplasia seen on a specimen obtained by Pap smear is classified using which of the following methods?
A. Apgar score.
B. CIN I, II, III.
C. Naegele rule.
D. Bethesda system.

_____ 3. _____ is when the fetal head is too large to pass through the maternal pelvis.
A. Failure of descent
B. Fetal macrosomia
C. Cephalopelvic disproportion
D. Spontaneous abortion

_____ 4. A woman who has never been pregnant is a _____
A. multigravida.
B. nulligravida.
C. primipara.
D. multipara.

_____ 5. Onset of the first menstrual period is referred to as _____
A. menses.
B. menarche.
C. amenorrhea.
D. menstruation.

_____ 6. A term meaning "occurring after sexual intercourse" is _____
A. postcoital.
B. dyspareunia.
C. parturient.
D. dysmenorrhea.

_____ 7. The entrance to the vaginal vault is called the _____
A. os.
B. vulva.
C. introitus.
D. adnexa.

_____ 8. A surgical instrument for exploring the length and direction of the cervix and uterus is a _____
A. sound.
B. speculum.
C. tenaculum.
D. forceps.

_____ 9. The _____ refers to the distribution of pelvic hair.
A. fornix
B. menarche
C. escutcheon
D. Skene gland

_____ 10. Pain occurring with menstruation is _____
A. dyspareunia.
B. dysmenorrhea.
C. pelvic inflammatory disease.
D. dysfunctional uterine bleeding.

_____ 11. _____ are benign neoplasms of uterine muscle.
A. Fibroids
B. Papillomas
C. Cystadenomas
D. Endometriomas

___ 12. ____ may appear as "chocolate" cysts on the ovaries or powder burn lesions on the peritoneum.
A. Fibromyomas
B. Uterine myomas
C. Endometrial implants
D. Cervical intraepithelial neoplasia

___ 13. Cervical carcinoma develops from cervical dysplasia which, in a majority of cases, is caused by _____
A. chlamydia.
B. gonorrhea.
C. endometriotic implants.
D. human papillomavirus.

___ 14. All of the following can cause vaginitis EXCEPT _____
A. *Candida albicans*.
B. *Trichomonas vaginalis*.
C. *Gardnerella vaginalis*.
D. *Chlamydia trachomatis*.

___ 15. The fetus develops within a fluid-filled membranous sac called the _____
A. chorion.
B. uterus.
C. amnion.
D. placenta.

___ 16. _____ refers to the period of time before childbirth.
A. Antepartum
B. Postpartum
C. Parturition
D. Puerperium

___ 17. _____ is flattening of the cervix from a tubular structure to a ring.
A. Ripening
B. Crowning
C. Dilatation
D. Effacement

___ 18. Separation of the placenta from the endometrium before the onset of labor is ____
A. abruptio placentae.
B. placenta previa.
C. placental delivery.
D. threatened abortion.

Laboratory Procedures

Instructions: Match the following laboratory procedures to their descriptions or definitions. Some answers may be used more than once, others not at all.

___ 1. AFP
___ 2. Coombs test
___ 3. FSH
___ 4. hCG
___ 5. LH
___ 6. RPR
___ 7. STS
___ 8. triple screen
___ 9. Tzanck smear
___ 10. VDRL

A. Anterior pituitary gland hormone that stimulates ovulation in women
B. A panel of tests obtained during the second trimester to evaluate for certain fetal abnormalities
C. Test used in the diagnosis of syphilis
D. Test to identify changes due to viral infection from herpes simplex or varicella
E. Test performed on maternal serum at around 16–18 weeks' gestation for detection of fetal abnormalities
F. The principal female hormone secreted by the ovary; its level in serum gives an estimate of ovarian function
G. An indirect immunofluorescence test, highly specific for syphilis
H. Tests for Rh incompatibility between mother and infant
I. Pregnancy test
J. Used to detect *Neisseria gonorrhoeae* and *Haemophilus influenzae*

Diagnostic and Surgical Procedures

Instructions: Match the following diagnostic and surgical procedures to their descriptions or definitions. Some answers may be used more than once.

___ 1. amniocentesis

___ 2. anterior colporrhaphy

___ 3. A&P repair

___ 4. amniotic fluid index

___ 5. bilateral tubal ligation

___ 6. cervical cerclage

___ 7. chorionic villus sampling

___ 8. colposcopy

___ 9. endometrial ablation

___ 10. endometrial biopsy

___ 11. LEEP

___ 12. marsupialization

___ 13. nonstress test

___ 14. salpingectomy

___ 15. tubal ligation

A. Biopsy of the fetal membranes in which the fertilized oocyte is implanted

B. Colporrhaphy to repair both cystocele and rectocele

C. Examination of the cervix with an illuminated low-power microscope

D. Excision of a portion of a uterine tube and suturing the cut ends for sterilization

E. Excision of a uterine tube

F. Noninvasive test to monitor fetal heart rate

G. Procedure to prevent premature labor

H. Removal of a cone of tissue from the cervix for microscopic examination

I. Removal of cervical tissue with a low-voltage wire for histological analysis as part of a colposcopy

J. Removal of tissue from the uterine lining with a suction tube device for histologic examination

K. Repair of cystocele, rectocele, and uterine prolapse

L. Slitting open a cyst and suturing edges to create a continuous surface from the exterior to the interior for drainage

M. Sterilization procedure using a ring device to close off the uterine tubes

N. Surgical destruction of the uterine lining

O. Surgical procedure to repair cystocele

P. Ultrasound procedure in which the fluid in each of four quadrants of the uterus is measured

Q. Procedure to withdraw amniotic fluid for analysis

Pharmacology

Instructions: Choose the best answer.

_____ 1. Which of the following drugs is an ovulation-stimulating drug for infertility that can be used alone?
   A. Clomid (clomiphene).
   B. Delaprem (hexoprenaline).
   C. Fertinex, Metrodin (urofollitropin).
   D. Humegon, Pergonal (menotropins).

_____ 2. Which of the following drugs does not belong in the group with the others?
   A. Crinone (progesterone).
   B. Pitocin, Syntocinon (oxytocin).
   C. Hylutin (hydroxyprogesterone).
   D. Provera (medroxyprogesterone).

_____ 3. Which of the following drugs is NOT a monophasic oral contraceptive?
   A. Demulen 1/50.
   B. Loestrin 1/20.
   C. Ortho-Novum 7/7/7.
   D. Ortho-Novum 1/50.

_____ 4. Primary hypothalamic amenorrhea may be treated with _____, a drug that stimulates the release of LH and FSH from the pituitary gland by means of a special pump that delivers the drug IV in pulses that mimic the natural release of GnRH from the pituitary gland.
   A. Lutrepulse (gonadorelin).
   B. Crinone (progesterone).
   C. Aygestin (norethindrone).
   D. Hylutin (hydroxyprogesterone).

_____ 5. Which type of contraceptive may be taken orally, given by injection, implanted under the skin, or inserted into the uterus?
   A. Monophasic.
   B. Biphasic.
   C. Triphasic.
   D. Progestin-only.

_____ 6. Drugs that relax the uterus and inhibit uterine contractions to prevent premature labor are called _____
   A. stimulants.
   B. tocolytics.
   C. hormones.
   D. anxiolytics.

_____ 7. Patients with infertility due to reasons other than anovulation should be treated with _____
   A. hormones.
   B. uterine relaxants.
   C. surgical intervention.
   D. ovulation-stimulating drugs.

_____ 8. If uterine contractions are too weak to effect delivery or if complications such as pre-eclampsia or diabetes necessitate induction of labor, a patient may be given _____
   A. Pitocin (oxytocin).
   B. Cervidil (dinoprostone).
   C. Aygestin (norethindrone).
   D. Yutopar (ritodrine).

_____ 9. Oxytocin is contraindicated when prolonged labor is due to _____
   A. uterine inertia.
   B. preeclampsia or diabetes.
   C. cephalopelvic disproportion.
   D. nonreassuring fetal heart tones.

_____ 10. Postpartum bleeding due to uterine relaxation may be treated with all of the following EXCEPT _____
   A. Pitocin (oxytocin).
   B. Yutopar (ritodrine).
   C. Hemabate (carboprost).
   D. Ergotrate (ergonovine).

Dissecting Medical Terms

Instructions: As you learned in your medical language course, words are formed from prefixes, combining forms (root word plus combining vowel), and suffixes. Combining vowels (usually *o* but not always) are used to connect two root words or a root and a suffix. By analyzing these word parts, you can often determine the definition of a term without even looking it up (if you know the definition of the parts, of course!). Being able to divide and analyze the words you hear into their component parts will also improve your spelling and help you research those words that you cannot easily spell or define.

For the following terms, place a slash (/) between the components and then write a short definition based on the meaning of the parts. Remember that to define a word based on its parts, you start at the end, usually with the suffix. If there's a prefix, that is defined next, and finally the combining form is defined.

Example: anteverted
Divide & Analyze: anteverted = ante/vert/ed =
  *possessing or having characteristics of + turn + before
Define: Tipped or bent forward (e.g., anteverted uterus)

*-*ed* and *–ing* are participle verb endings that turn words into adjectives, so the meaning of the ending depends on how the word is used.

1. Term   antepartum
   Divide _____
   _____
   Define _____

2. Term   bimanual
   Divide _____
   _____
   Define _____

3. Term   colporrhaphy
   Divide _____
   _____
   Define _____

4. Term   cystadenoma
   Divide _____
   Define _____

5. Term   dysmenorrhea
   Divide _____
   _____
   Define _____

6. Term   dyspareunia
   Divide _____
   _____
   Define _____

7. Term   episiotomy
   Divide _____
   _____
   Define _____

8. Term   hydrodissection
   Divide _____
   _____
   Define _____

9. Term   hypotonic
   Divide _____
   _____
   Define _____

10. Term   hysterosalpingogram
    Divide _____
    _____
    Define _____

11. Term   intraepithelial
    Divide _____
    _____
    Define _____

12. Term   ipsilateral
    Divide _____
    _____
    Define _____

13. Term   leukorrhea
    Divide _____
    _____
    Define _____

14. Term   macrosomia
    Divide _____
    _____
    Define _____

15. Term   menometrorrhagia
    Divide _____
    _____
    Define _____

16. Term   mesosalpinx
    Divide   _____
              _____
    Define   _____

17. Term   oligohydramnios
    Divide   _____
              _____
    Define   _____

18. Term   perineorrhaphy
    Divide   _____
              _____
    Define   _____

19. Term   pyelectasis
    Divide   _____
              _____
    Define   _____

20. Term   salpingo-oophorectomy
    Divide   _____
              _____
    Define   _____

Spelling Exercise

Instructions: Review the adjective and adverb suffixes in your medical language textbook. Test your knowledge of **adjectives** by writing the adjectival form of the following ObGyn words. Consult a medical dictionary to verify your spelling.

Noun	Adjective
1. appendix	_____
2. areola	_____
3. cervix	_____
4. cornu	_____
5. endometriosis	_____
6. endometrium	_____
7. erythema	_____
8. fimbria	_____
9. fundus	_____
10. globule	_____
11. habit	_____

12. hemorrhage   _____
13. histopathology _____
14. hymen   _____
15. hyperplasia   _____
16. isthmus   _____
17. menses   _____
18. multipara   _____
19. sterile   _____
20. uterus   _____

Abbreviations Exercise

Instructions: Expand the following common ObGyn abbreviations and brief forms. Then memorize both abbreviations and definitions to increase your speed and accuracy in transcribing ObGyn dictation.

Abbreviation	Expansion
1. AFP	_____
2. AFI	_____
3. BSO	_____
4. BUS	_____
5. CIN	_____
6. CVA	_____
7. D&C	_____
8. DTRs	_____
9. ECC	_____
10. EDC	_____
11. I&D	_____
12. L&D	_____
13. LEEP	_____
14. LMA	_____
15. LMP	_____
16. MAC	_____
17. NST	_____
18. RL or LR	_____
19. TAH-BSO	_____
20. UTI	_____

Transcript Forensics

This section presents snippets of transcribed dictations from clinic notes; history and physical examinations and consultations; operative reports and procedure notes; and discharge summaries. Explain the passage so that a nonmedical person can understand it. Pay particular attention to terms that are in bold type.

Example

Excerpt: This patient is a 16-year-old **gravida** 1, **para** 0, **menarche** at age 13, whose last menstrual period was March 11, who had a positive **beta hCG**; previous to that, normal menstrual cycles every 28 days.

Explanation: This 16-year-old patient is pregnant as indicated by the use of gravida and a positive beta hCG, unknown status. Her first menstrual period was at age 13. Cycles are normal.

1. **Excerpt:** ASSESSMENT: Twin pregnancy, both **breech**, at 35 weeks and 4 days by reasonably good dates, with **proteinuria**, a couple of elevated blood pressures, **nonstress tests** that have not been truly **reactive** for some time.

   Explanation: _____
   _____
   _____
   _____
   _____
   _____
   _____

2. **Excerpt:** PREOPERATIVE DIAGNOSES: An 18-year-old **gravida 3, para 2-0-0-2**, at 32 weeks' gestation, late prenatal care. Severe **oligohydramnios**. **Fetal distress** noted by fetal tachycardia; baseline heart rate in the 230s.

   Explanation: _____
   _____
   _____
   _____
   _____
   _____
   _____
   _____

3. **Excerpt:** OBSTETRIC LABORATORY DATA: Blood type is A, **Rh is positive**, antibody negative. **Rubella immune**. Gonococcus (GC) negative, chlamydia negative. Hepatitis B surface antigen negative. HIV negative. Patient has had a **triple screen** done this pregnancy, which was also within normal limits. This patient is group B strep negative.

   Explanation: _____
   _____
   _____
   _____
   _____
   _____
   _____
   _____

4. **Excerpt:** The patient is a 62-year-old with **endometrial carcinoma** admitted for operative exploration. Final pathology report shows a deeply invasive, **high-grade papillary serous carcinoma** of the endometrium with **nodes negative**.

   Explanation: _____
   _____
   _____
   _____
   _____
   _____

5. **Excerpt:** PREOPERATIVE DIAGNOSIS
   1. Anemia.
   2. Menorrhagia.
   3. Uterine fibroids.

   Explanation: _____
   _____
   _____
   _____
   _____
   _____
   _____

6. **Excerpt**: After an adequate level of general anesthesia, the patient was changed to the **lithotomy position**. The patient was prepped and draped in a sterile manner. A single-toothed tenaculum was used to grasp the anterior lip of the cervix. The **uterus sounded** to 12 cm. The **cervix was then dilated** up to a 20 Hegar dilator. **Sharp curettings** were taken in all four quadrants. Findings on the frozen section were **hyperplastic polyp**.

Explanation: _____
_____
_____
_____
_____
_____
_____
_____

7. **Excerpt**: Patient presents with a history of having been evaluated for complaints of increasing central pelvic pain, increasing vaginal discharge and symptoms of **cystitis**, deep **dyspareunia**, sacral backache. When evaluated the patient was felt most likely to have a **chlamydia pelvic inflammatory disease**.

Explanation: _____
_____
_____
_____
_____
_____
_____
_____

8. **Excerpt**: There was a moderate amount of yellowish, **purulent-appearing leukorrhea**. The external genitalia appeared to have a mild amount of inflammation. **Bartholin and Skene glands and urethra** were not really remarkable. The cervix was 4+ tender to motion bilaterally. The **adnexal areas** on bimanual exam showed the uterus to be anteverted, anteflexed, normal size, **exquisitely tender** to palpation. **Rectovaginal exam** showed what was felt to be bilateral adnexal masses, 3-4 cm in size, with the right being more tender than the left. Rectal exam also showed some thickening of the **cul-de-sac of Douglas**, but no nodularity of the uterosacral ligaments noted.

Explanation: _____
_____
_____
_____
_____
_____
_____
_____
_____
_____
_____

9. **Excerpt**: A 5 mm **hysteroscope** was introduced into the uterine cavity, and the above-noted findings were confirmed. Both **tubal ostia** were visualized and found **patent**. The endocervical canal appeared clean with no lesions. A sharp curet was then introduced into the uterine cavity, and the **endometrial curettings** were obtained and sent for pathology.

Explanation: _____
_____
_____
_____
_____
_____
_____
_____

Sample Reports

Sample ObGyn reports appear on the following pages, illustrating a variety of reports. Fictional names are provided for illustration of proper format, and no resemblance to actual persons is intended. Sample transcripts were prepared according to *The Book of Style for Medical Transcription* (AHDI).

History and Physical Examination

CHAUVIN, LAURA
#253249
Admitted: 6/11/[add year]

HISTORY OF PRESENT ILLNESS
This patient is a 34-year-old female, gravida 0, last menstrual period November 20. Patient presents with a history of having been evaluated for complaints of increasing central pelvic pain, increasing vaginal discharge and symptoms of cystitis, deep dyspareunia, sacral backache. When evaluated the patient was felt most likely to have a chlamydia pelvic inflammatory disease. She was at that time treated with 2 g of Claforan IM and given a 3-week course of Vibramycin. She was instructed to return p.r.n. for worsening symptoms. She returned, states that several days after the completion of her menstrual cycle the pelvic pain returned, particularly severe in the left side over that ovary, and she also began having problems with cystitis symptoms, i.e., frequency, hesitancy, dysuria, as well as increasing secondary dyspareunia. Also relates history of night sweats, chills, fever elevation up to 102.

PAST MEDICAL HISTORY
Allergies: Past medical history includes drug allergy to aspirin.
Current Medications: Bactrim DS and Triphasil oral contraceptive pills.
Surgical: The patient had one prior admission, at which time diagnostic laparoscopy and laser laparoscopy were performed for endometriosis.

PHYSICAL EXAMINATION
GENERAL: On physical exam, she was a well-developed, well-nourished female in moderate distress.
HEENT, NECK, CHEST: Eyes, ears, nose, throat, neck, lungs, heart were not remarkable.
ABDOMEN: The CVA area was negative. Abdomen was soft. No organomegaly was noted. There was some diffuse lower abdominal tenderness to palpation, with the left being more severe than the right.
PELVIC: There was a moderate amount of yellowish, purulent-appearing leukorrhea. The external genitalia appeared to have a mild amount of inflammation. Bartholin and Skene glands and urethra were not really remarkable. The cervix was 4+ tender to motion bilaterally. The adnexal areas on bimanual exam showed the uterus to be anteverted, anteflexed, normal size, exquisitely tender to palpation. Both adnexal areas were thick and nodular, exquisitely tender to palpation. Rectovaginal exam showed what was felt to be bilateral adnexal masses, 3–4 cm in size, with the right being more tender than the left.

(continued)

History and Physical Examination

CHAUVIN, LAURA
#253249
Admitted: 6/11/[add year]
Page 2

Rectal exam also showed some thickening of the cul-de-sac of Douglas, but no nodularity of the uterosacral ligaments noted.

IMPRESSION
1. Probable pelvic inflammatory disease. Rule out tubo-ovarian abscess.
2. History of endometriosis. Rule out relapse of endometriosis.

DEBORAH BAERWALD, MD

DB:hpi

d: 6/11/[add year]
t: 6/12/[add year]

History & Physical Examination

CROSCILL, MARLENE
#092431
ADMITTED: 5/5/[add year]

CHIEF COMPLAINT
Uterine prolapse.

HISTORY OF PRESENT ILLNESS
This is a 64-year-old woman who is gravida 4, para 4, referred because of a large cystocele and uterine prolapse. The patient states that when she is on her feet, a bulge comes out of the vagina between her legs. She was found to have a large cystocele and a 2nd degree uterine prolapse, the cervix protruding through the os even with the patient lying down and when she strains. She does not have any significant problem with urinary tract control. She enters at this time for vaginal hysterectomy and anterior and posterior (A&P) repair.

PAST HISTORY
Her general health has been reasonably good. She is taking Lanoxin 0.25 mg, 1/2 tablet per day.

PHYSICAL EXAMINATION
GENERAL: A well-developed, well-nourished, slender white female at 131 pounds. Blood pressure was 130/70.
EARS: Negative.
EYES: Pupils small, react well to light. Sclerae clear.
MOUTH: I believe the patient has dentures. The throat is clear. The tonsils are absent.
NECK: Supple. No masses felt.
BREASTS: Quite good turgor for her age. No masses are felt.
LUNGS: Clear to percussion and auscultation (P&A).
HEART: Regular rhythm, no murmurs.
ABDOMEN: Soft and nontender.
GYN EXAM: There is relaxation. When the patient strains, the bladder bulges down and out and the cervix comes out through the introitus.
RECTAL: Negative. No intrinsic masses. Moderate rectocele.
EXTREMITIES: No significant deformities are noted. No edema. Reflexes are physiologic.

IMPRESSION
Second-degree uterine prolapse; cystocele with some rectocele.

PLAN
Vaginal hysterectomy, anterior repair, and possibly posterior repair at the same time.

JOSHUA VILLA, MD

JV:hpi d: 5/5/[add year] t: 5/5/[add year]

Operative Report

VOLONTE, NATALIE
#174259

DATE OF OPERATION
February 25, [add year]

PREOPERATIVE DIAGNOSIS
1. Missed abortion.
2. Habitual aborter.

POSTOPERATIVE DIAGNOSIS
1. Missed abortion.
2. Habitual aborter.

OPERATION PERFORMED
Dilatation and evacuation by suction.

SURGEON
Andrew Wildt, MD

ANESTHESIA
General by laryngeal mask airway (LMA).

COMPLICATIONS
None.

PATHOLOGY
Products of conception to Genetics.

ESTIMATED BLOOD LOSS
100 mL.

FLUIDS
500 mL of lactated Ringer's.

INDICATIONS FOR SURGERY
This 30-year-old female, gravida 4, para 3, presented at 12 weeks' gestation with fetal demise for evacuation.

(continued)

Operative Report

VOLONTE, NATALIE
#174259
Page 2

FINDINGS AND PROCEDURE
The patient was taken to the operating room at which point a general anesthetic was administered. She was placed in the lithotomy position, prepped and draped in the usual fashion. Examination under anesthesia showed the uterus to be of 8 weeks' size, anterior, mobile. No adnexal masses could be palpated. A speculum was placed in the vaginal vault, single-tooth tenaculum placed on the uterine cervix. The cervix was dilated. A #9 suction curet was passed. Multiple passes were made, with moderate to large return of tissue, which was collected and handed off for Genetics and for specimen processing. Sharp curet was passed. A good cry was noted in all quadrants with no further return of tissue. Pitocin was started. Good hemostasis was secure. One more single cleansing pass was made with no further return of tissue. All instruments were then removed from the vagina. Good hemostasis was noted. The patient tolerated the procedure well and went to the recovery room in a stable condition.

ANDREW WILDT, MD

AW:hpi

d: 02/25/[add year]
t: 02/26/[add year]

Comic Relief

Correct	Incorrect
d: Pap smear	t: Pabst beer
d: Missed conception	t: Misconception
d: Frank blood was present.	t: Fake blood was present.
d: No evidence of carcinoma in situ.	t: No evidence of carcinoma in sight too.
d: This baby boy was born to a primip, who is Rh positive.	t: This baby boy was born to a prime hip who is Rh positive.
d: The patient underwent a tubal ligation.	t: The patient underwent a two-ball ligation.
d: On curettage there was no evidence of a fetus.	t: On curettage there was no evidence of a penis.
d: This grand multiparous was given a sterile vaginal exam.	t: This Grandma Kipperus was given a sterno vascline exam.
d: Pfannenstiel incision	t: Fan and steal incision

Gastroenterology

Learning Objectives

▶ Describe the structure and function of the gastrointestinal system.

▶ Spell and define common gastrointestinal terms.

▶ Identify vocabulary that might be used during the gastrointestinal review of systems.

▶ Describe the negative and positive findings a physician looks for on examination of the abdomen.

▶ Describe the typical cause, course, and treatment options for common diseases of the gastrointestinal system.

▶ Identify and define diagnostic and surgical procedures of the gastrointestinal system.

▶ List common gastrointestinal laboratory tests and procedures.

▶ Identify and describe common gastrointestinal drugs and their uses.

▶ Demonstrate knowledge of anatomical, medical, pharmacological, adjectival, and soundalike terms by accurately completing the exercises in this chapter.

Transcribing Gastroenterology Dictation

Introduction

Four miserable-looking people, standing abreast of each other, chant and gesture in turn, "Nausea, heartburn, indigestion, upset stomach, diarrhea!" The television commercial is for Pepto-Bismol, a pink pepperminty potion for gastrointestinal distress. You relate to these people because you've experienced some of those symptoms; perhaps you've actually taken Pepto-Bismol. Hopefully, though, you haven't experienced all these symptoms at once!

> *If she eats spicy foods, she has heartburn and vomits. She has a poor appetite, difficulty swallowing solids or liquids, gas, and bloating. She also has alternating diarrhea and constipation.*

No one can truthfully claim they have been spared nausea, heartburn, indigestion, upset stomach, or diarrhea. Some of these symptoms are actually a sign that your body is working hard to rid itself of invading germs. "Throwing up" after ingesting or acquiring something harmful is nature's way of getting rid of the offending organism; so is diarrhea. These and other conditions fall under the medical specialty of **gastroenterology**, which is the study of the **gastrointestinal (GI)** or **digestive system**, also known as the **alimentary canal**.

> *Gastrointestinal system: No history of prior peptic ulcer disease, hematemesis, or melena. Appetite remains good. Bowels are working well. Stools of normal color.*

All physicians receive some specialized training in gastroenterology, even if they choose to practice in another specialty. For more complex conditions or diseases, however, they might refer a patient to a **gastroenterologist**, a medical doctor who specializes in treating patients with digestive system problems. A notable subspecialty is **proctology**, the study of the rectum and its related structures; practitioners are proctologists. While gastroenterologists generally carry out endoscopies themselves, surgery that involves cutting and suturing is usually performed by **general surgeons**. Pediatric gastroenterologists treat children with more complex gastrointestinal problems.

The **GI system** includes all those structures concerned with the ingestion of solids and liquids, their

> The world of gastroenterology is a fascinating one. I particularly enjoy being a gastrointestinal surgeon. It's like Christmas every day—I open a new package and I never know for sure what I am going to find!
>
> Thomas L. Largen, MD, FACS

mechanical and chemical breakdown into usable nutrients, the absorption of these into the circulation, and the excretion of solid wastes.

Anatomy Review

The **alimentary canal** is a coiled but unbranched tube extending from the lips to the anus and divided into mouth, oropharynx, esophagus, stomach, small intestine (duodenum, jejunum, ileum), and large intestine (colon, rectum).

> *On upper GI endoscopy, the esophagus and stomach appeared to produce a normal amount of mucus. The gastric antrum appeared to be normal. There was mild erythema in the pyloric channel and the prepyloric area with a minimal amount of bile reflux.*

Numerous microscopic glandular structures occur in the walls of the digestive tract (gastric glands, intestinal glands), and in addition larger secretory organs (salivary glands, liver, pancreas) pour their products through ducts into parts of the tract. These secretions serve to liquefy and lubricate food and to break down fats, proteins, and carbohydrates to fatty acids, amino acids, and simple sugars, respectively.

The **peritoneum** is a delicate serous membrane that lines the abdominal and pelvic cavities (**parietal peritoneum**) and also covers the stomach, small intestine, and colon (except for the distal part of the rectum), as well as the liver, spleen, uterus, ovaries, ureters, and dome of the bladder (**visceral peritoneum**). Structures such as the pancreas and kidneys that lie behind the peritoneal cavity are called retroperitoneal.

The **liver**, the largest gland in the body, lies in the right upper quadrant of the abdomen just below the **diaphragm** and is largely covered by peritoneum. The liver performs numerous vital functions and is intimately concerned with carbohydrate and nitrogen metabolism and with removal of certain waste products. **Bile**, the secretory product of the liver, passes through a duct into the duodenum. Bile contains **bile salts**, which help in the digestion of fats, and bilirubin, a breakdown product of hemoglobin. Bile does not flow steadily into the duodenum, but is stored in the **gallbladder**, a bulb or pouch connected by the cystic duct to the common bile duct. Ingestion of a fatty meal stimulates contraction of the gallbladder and increased flow of bile into the intestine.

The **pancreas** is a flat retroperitoneal organ lying behind and below the stomach, with its right end (head) embraced by the sweep of the duodenum. It is composed of two types of glandular tissue: groups of cells that secrete enzymes for the digestion of carbohydrate, protein, and fat, which are poured through a duct into the duodenum near the orifice of the common bile duct; and other groups of cells that secrete hormones (insulin, glucagon, somatostatin) and release them directly into the bloodstream.

Pause for Reflection

1. Perform a Google image search for anatomic terms to enhance your understanding of GI structures.
2. List the major structures of the GI tract, in order, starting with the mouth and finishing with the anus.
3. Which structures or organs are involved in the production, storage, and transport of bile? What function does bile perform?
4. What is the function of the pancreas?

Vocabulary Review

adenoma A benign tumor arising from glandular epithelium.

adynamic ileus Bowel obstruction caused by decreased bowel motility, often secondary to peritonitis.

ampulla of Vater. Also known as the **hepatopancreatic ampulla**. Formed by the union of the pancreatic duct and the common bile duct.

anal condyloma (pl., **condylomata**) Growths found on the skin around the anus (rectal opening) or in the lower rectum. Also called **anal warts**.

anal verge The distal end of the anal canal, forming a transitional zone between the skin of the anal canal and the perianal skin.

anorexia Loss of appetite.

The patient takes Beano before every meal because of bloating and gas after eating, especially after cruciferous vegetables. He recently began taking Lactaid to help with his intolerance to dairy.

biliary colic Pain in the gallbladder region due to passage of gallstones along the bile duct.

bloating An overly full, distended feeling, usually from excessive intestinal gas.

borborygmus (pl., **borborygmi**) Audible rumbling and gurgling sounds in the digestive tract.

bowel gas pattern On abdominal film, the normal radiographic appearance of gas in the intestine.

cardia The first of five portions of the stomach adjacent to and surrounding the cardiac opening where the esophagus connects to the stomach; it is not anatomically divided but used for reference.

colon Term that can mean part or all of the large intestine.

constipation Firm, difficult stools.

diarrhea Abnormal frequency, urgency, and looseness of stools.

diverticulum (pl., **diverticula**) An abnormal outpouching of a hollow organ such as the colon.

dysphagia Difficulty swallowing.

dysplasia Alteration in size, shape, and organization of adult cells.

endorectal Inside the rectum; said of diagnostic or therapeutic instruments or procedures.

enterocolitis Inflammatory disease of both the small and large intestines.

erosive gastritis Inflammatory condition characterized by multiple erosions of the mucous membrane lining the stomach.

esophageal stenosis Narrowing of the esophagus caused by the buildup of scar tissue or by a congenital defect.

esophagogastric (EG) junction (also, **cardioesophageal** or **gastroesophageal [GE] junction**) The transition site from the stratified squamous epithelium of the esophagus to the simple columnar epithelium of the cardia of the stomach.

fistula Abnormal passage or communication between organs, or from an organ through to the outside surface of the body.

fistulotomy A fistulotomy is surgery to open a fistula to allow it to heal.

The scope was eventually passed up to the splenic flexure, transverse colon, hepatic flexure, then dropped down into the ascending colon, where the cecum was encountered.

flatulence, flatus Excessive intestinal gas.

flexure A bend. The **hepatic flexure** and **splenic flexure** are bends in the large bowel where it bends first to the left and then downward respectively.

gastrostomy button, balloon-tipped A small skin level gastrostomy tube made of silicone. It has an inflatable balloon at one end (inside the body) and an external base (outside the body) at the other.

heartburn Burning pain in the epigastrium or chest due to digestive disorders. Also called **pyrosis**.

hematemesis Vomiting blood.

hematochezia Passage of blood from the rectum.

hemorrhoids Anal varicose veins.

hepatorrhaphy Suturing a ruptured or lacerated liver.

hepatomegaly Enlargement of the liver.

hepatopancreatic ampulla See *ampulla of Vater*.

hernia Protrusion of organ or tissue through an abnormal opening.

hyperplasia An increase in the number of cells in a tissue or organ.

ileus Intestinal obstruction. See *adynamic ileus*.

intussusception Prolapse of one part of the intestine into another.

jaundice Discoloration of skin and sclerae by excessive bile pigment.

melena Black stools (often due to the presence of blood).

mesentery The fan-shaped membrane on the posterior (back) wall of the abdominal cavity that supports the ileum and jejunum.

neoplasia The progressive multiplication of cells that results in the formation and growth of a tumor.

obstipation Total inability to pass stool.

palliative Directed to the relief of symptoms rather than the elimination of their cause.

perineal area The region between the thighs and containing the roots of the external genitalia; in males, it is the area between the scrotum and anus, in the female the area between the vulva and anus.

pilonidal cyst, sinus, abscess A cyst that develops along the tailbone (coccyx) near the cleft of the buttocks, approximately 5 cm from the anus. These cysts usually contain hair and skin debris.

polyps Massive overgrowths of chronically inflamed mucosa.

postprandial Following a meal.

prepyloric area The area just before the pylorus.

rebound tenderness Additional stab of pain when pressure on abdomen is released, often indicating peritoneal irritation.

rugae Deep accordion-type folds in the stomach that flatten out when food arrives.

sessile polyp A relatively flattened growth that is usually benign but can transform into a malignant growth.

seton A silk string or a rubber band used to help a fistula to drain.

shelving edge of Poupart ligament The shelflike edge of the inguinal ligament. Referred to in inguinal hernia repair dictation.

sphincter A muscular ring that constricts passage or closes an orifice, e.g., the **lower esophageal** sphincter (cardiac sphincter), the **pyloric** or **prepyloric** sphincter, **cricopharyngeal** sphincter, and **anal** sphincter.

splenomegaly Enlargement of the spleen.

squamocolumnar junction The point where the normal squamous epithelium of the esophagus meets the normal columnar epithelium of the stomach.

tenesmus Straining at stool, usually without result and often painful.

transrectal Said of a diagnostic or surgical procedure that is performed through the rectum.

Treitz, ligament of A fibromuscular band extending from the diaphragm to the small intestine at the site of transition from duodenum to jejunum.

volvulus Intestinal obstruction due to twisting of the bowel.

water brash Heartburn with regurgitation into the mouth of fluid that may be sour or almost tasteless.

Medical Readings
History and Physical Examination
by John H. Dirckx, MD

Review of Systems. The gastrointestinal history is concerned mainly with two types of symptoms: **abdominal pain** of any type or degree (though abdominal pain often results from nondigestive causes); and any disturbances of **digestive function**, including anorexia, nausea, vomiting, and diarrhea. Symptoms due to disorders of the liver or biliary tract, the pancreas, or the rectum or anus are also included here.

In reviewing the past **digestive tract history**, the examiner inquires about previous diagnoses of hiatal hernia, ulcer, gallstones or gallbladder disease, pancreatitis, colitis; any tumors of the alimentary canal or associated structures; results of gastrointestinal x-rays or other diagnostic studies (esophagoscopy, gastroscopy, colonoscopy); operations on the digestive organs, including appendectomy and hemorrhoid surgery; and use of antacids, laxatives, enemas, or prescription medicines for digestive symptoms.

Abdominal pain may be described as burning, crampy, or dull. It may be constant, intermittent, or of varying intensity. It may remain in one place or radiate or migrate to another, perhaps in the back or chest. It may be brought on, aggravated, or relieved by eating, not eating, drinking, having a bowel movement, or assuming certain positions. It may be provoked by taking certain

medicines or eating certain foods; a record of any food intolerances is an important part of the digestive history.

Symptoms besides abdominal pain that draw attention to the digestive system are anorexia, nausea, pain or difficulty in swallowing that seems to originate below the pharynx, vomiting, flatulence, constipation, diarrhea, abnormal appearance of the stools, weight loss, jaundice, and anorectal pain, swelling, or bleeding. A history of **vomiting** prompts inquiries about its frequency and the volume and character of emesis. Blood that is mixed with gastric contents often has a characteristic **coffee-grounds appearance**. **Jaundice** (a yellow color of the skin, mucous membranes, and ocular sclerae) indicates an excessive quantity of bile pigment in blood and tissues. It can result from intrinsic liver disease (hepatitis, hepatic failure) or from obstruction of the biliary tract by a gallstone or a tumor.

Because constipation and diarrhea mean different things to different people, the interviewer must carefully determine the frequency and consistency of the patient's stools. Even with normal bowel habits, an abnormal stool color can indicate disease. Clay-colored stools occur in obstruction of the biliary tract because bile does not reach the intestine. Blood that has passed through much of the intestine before appearing in the stool may look tarry black (**melena**) because of chemical changes in blood pigment.

Inguinal hernia may also be considered with the gastrointestinal history because most hernias contain loops of bowel and eventually affect digestive or eliminative function. The patient is asked about swelling or bulging in the groin or scrotum that is accentuated by coughing or straining and diminishes or disappears in the recumbent position.

Physical Examination of the abdomen is performed to assess skin turgor and muscle tone, to determine the size, shape, and position of the abdominal and pelvic organs, and to detect any masses or tenderness. The physician starts with light **palpation**, which provides information about the abdominal wall and any zones of tenderness, and then progresses to deep palpation to study the internal organs and search for masses. An area of pain or tenderness known to the physician is examined last.

Throughout the examination, the physician closely observes the patient's face for signs of distress. **Rebound tenderness**, a transient stab of pain when the abdomen is pressed and then suddenly released, denotes local or generalized peritoneal irritation. The physician may look for tenderness in the liver or gallbladder by gentle fist **percussion** over the right lower ribs or by hooking the fingers of the examining hand under the right costal margin and asking the patient to inhale deeply. **Costo-vertebral angle tenderness** occurs in inflammation or infection of the kidney or ureter.

Most normal intra-abdominal structures cannot be distinctly felt through the abdominal wall. By vigorous palpation of a very thin patient, one can feel parts of the normal liver, spleen, and kidneys, but ordinarily these organs must be enlarged before they can be palpated. No part of the digestive tract can normally be felt, nor can the pancreas, gallbladder, or ureters. In an obese patient, even gross abnormalities can escape detection by palpation.

Percussion can be used to measure the **liver span** (the width of liver dullness between lung and bowel resonances) and to distinguish between a solid organ or tumor, which yields a dull or flat note, and bowel distended by gas, which yields a hollow or resonant note. It can also confirm the presence of **ascites** (free fluid in the peritoneal cavity) by detecting a change in the percussion note as the patient rolls from the supine position to the right or left side (shifting dullness).

Pause for Reflection

1. Another word for vomiting is _____.
2. An excessive amount of bile pigment in the blood and tissues resulting in yellowing of the skin, mucous membranes, and ocular sclerae is a condition known as _____.
3. Black, tarry stools indicate that blood has passed through much of the intestine before appearing in the stool; black, tarry stools are referred to as _____.
4. A transient stab of pain when the abdomen is pressed and then suddenly released denotes local or generalized peritoneal irritation and is referred to as _____.
5. On exam of the abdomen, to distinguish between a solid organ and bowel gas, the physician uses a method called _____.
6. A change in the percussion note as the patient rolls from the supine position to the right or left side may be referred to as _____ ; this finding is indicative of free fluid in the peritoneal cavity or a condition known as _____.

Common Diseases

Gastroesophageal Reflux Disease (GERD)

Backflow of gastric juice into the esophagus.

Cause: Structural or functional incompetence of the **lower esophageal sphincter (LES)**, associated with disordered gastric motility and prolonged gastric emptying time. In a few cases, reflux of gastric juice may be facilitated by **esophageal hiatus hernia** (weakness or dilatation of the opening in the diaphragm where the esophagus passes through, with herniation of part or all of the stomach into the thorax; often asymptomatic). Reflux of acid gastric juice into the esophagus causes inflammation because the esophageal mucosa is not adapted to resist acid and digestive enzymes (see ■ **Figure 15-1**).

History: Recurrent epigastric and retrosternal distress, usually described as heartburn; belching, nausea, gagging, cough, hoarseness in varying proportions. There is a strong association with asthma, obesity, and diabetes mellitus. Symptoms are triggered or aggravated by recumbency (especially after a meal), vigorous exercise, smoking, overeating, caffeine, chocolate, alcohol, and certain drugs.

Physical Examination: Unremarkable.

Diagnostic Tests: Imaging studies confirm reflux of swallowed barium from the stomach and may identify ulceration or stricture. The 24-hour monitoring of esophageal pH with a swallowed electrode proves a sustained abnormal acid state in the esophagus. Endoscopy gives direct visual proof of inflammation and may identify a zone of **Barrett esophagus** (cellular change due to chronic inflammation).

Course: The underlying disorder of the LES and of gastric motility is irreversible. Severe reflux disease can lead to peptic ulceration of the esophagus, with eventual stricture due to scarring. Another possible complication is Barrett esophagus, a metaplasia (transformation) of normal squamous esophageal epithelium into columnar epithelium; some cases of Barrett esophagus progress to adenocarcinoma.

Treatment: Avoidance of smoking, alcohol, caffeine, and large meals. Over-the-counter antacids may suffice to control symptoms. Otherwise, acid production may require suppression by H_2 antagonists (cimetidine, ranitidine, famotidine, nizatidine) or proton pump inhibitors (omeprazole, lansoprazole). Prokinetic drugs (bethanechol, metoclopramide, cisapride) may improve sphincter function and gastric motility.

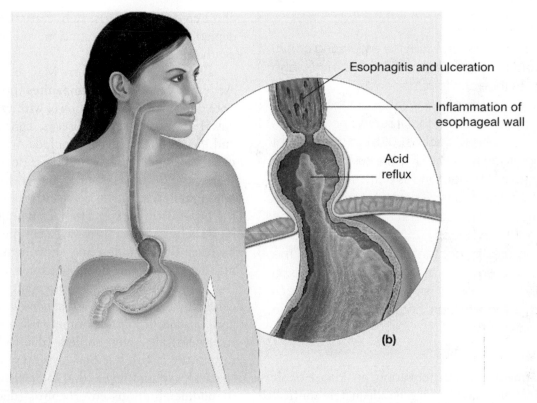

FIGURE 15-1. Acid reflux. (a) A hiatal hernia or diaphragmatocele. (b) A portion of the stomach protrudes through the diaphragm into the thoracic cavity.

Peptic Ulcer Disease (PUD) and Gastritis

Inflammation and ulceration of the stomach, duodenum, or both by acid gastric juice (see ■ Figure 15-1).

Cause: Most commonly, infection of the gastric mucosa by *Helicobacter pylori*, a motile bacterium that survives in the acid environment of the stomach by secreting urease, an enzyme that converts urea to ammonia and bicarbonate, thus providing a protective alkaline medium for itself. *H. pylori* infection, which is spread from person to person by the fecal-oral route, results ultimately in a marked increase of acid production.

Peptic ulceration can also result from regular use of prostaglandin-inhibiting drugs—adrenal corticosteroids and nonsteroidal anti-inflammatory agents such as ibuprofen and aspirin. In rare cases it is part of Zollinger-Ellison syndrome, in which a tumor of the pancreas produces excessive amounts of the hormone gastrin and thus causes hypersecretion of gastric acid. Severe stress, head injuries, and burns are sometimes complicated by peptic ulcer. Most peptic ulcers occur in the duodenum, but the stomach may be involved as well or instead.

History: Burning epigastric pain that comes on within an hour after meals and is relieved by taking antacids or food. Night pain is common. Tobacco, alcohol, caffeine, and certain foods aggravate symptoms, apparently by stimulating acid production. With complications—hematemesis, melena, **early satiety** (feeling that the stomach is full after only one or two mouthfuls of food), weight loss, severe abdominal pain, collapse.

Physical Examination: Unremarkable. Abdominal tenderness is variable and may be absent. With hemorrhage: pallor and tachycardia. With perforation—boardlike rigidity of the abdomen due to chemical peritonitis.

Diagnostic Tests: Upper GI studies with contrast can show ulceration, scarring, obstruction, or perforation. Endoscopy visualizes ulcers, bleeding sites, and scarring, and it is important to rule out carcinoma in gastric lesions. Infection by *H. pylori* can be confirmed by culture, biopsy, serologic testing, or breath-testing for evidence of urease activity on orally administered isotopically tagged urea.

Course: Without treatment, peptic ulcer disease tends to persist, with remissions and exacerbations, for many years. The most serious complications are hemorrhage (the principal cause of ulcer mortality), obstruction due to scarring, perforation of the digestive tract with release of gastric juice into the peritoneal cavity, and penetration into the retroperitoneal space.

APPENDIX

The cecum is a short sac in the ascending colon. Dangling from the cecum is the appendix, also known as the vermiform appendix.

The appendix was once thought to be a vestigial organ, meaning that it served no purpose. However, there is a school of medical thought that no organ in the body is useless and that we simply do not understand its purpose.

In fact, the appendix contains lymphoid tissue and may be important in immune function. The appendix can become inflamed (appendicitis) and rupture, its contents leaking out into the abdominal cavity and leading to peritonitis, a deadly condition. A small, hard bit of feces called a fecalith can also develop inside the appendix.

Treatment: Smoking cessation, avoidance of alcohol and caffeine. Acidity may be adequately controlled by over-the-counter antacids, H_2 antagonists (cimetidine, ranitidine, famotidine, nizatidine) in over-the-counter or prescription strength, or proton pump inhibitors (omeprazole, lansoprazole). Proven *H. pylori* infection is treated with a course of therapy including bismuth subsalicylate and two antibiotics, tetracycline or amoxicillin, and metronidazole or clarithromycin.

Gastroenteritis

Inflammation of the stomach and intestine, manifested by abdominal pain, vomiting, and diarrhea; usually acute, infectious, and self-limited.

Causes: Infection with viruses (adenovirus, echovirus, coxsackievirus, rotavirus), bacteria (*Escherichia coli* H157:O7 and other virulent strains, *Campylobacter, Yersinia, Salmonella, Shigella, Clostridium*), protozoa (*Entamoeba histolytica, Giardia lamblia*), fungi (*Candida albicans*). Most of these infections are acquired by the fecal-oral route. Some are much more likely to occur in immunocompromised persons. Outbreaks are usually due to contaminated food or water. "Food poisoning" is due to toxins produced by staphylococci, *Salmonella, Clostridium*, or other organisms. Gastroenteritis can also be a reaction to medicines, foods, poisonous plants, toxic chemicals.

History: Usually abrupt onset of abdominal distress or cramping, anorexia, nausea, vomiting, and diarrhea. Chills, fever, malaise. Hematemesis and bloody diarrhea are ominous signs. In severe or protracted disease, or in children or the elderly, dehydration and electrolyte depletion can lead to prostration, vascular collapse, and death.

Physical Examination: May be unremarkable. Abdominal tenderness, **tympanites** (hollow percussion note due to distention of bowel with gas), hyperactive bowel sounds. In severe disease, signs of dehydration and electrolyte depletion include dryness of mucous membranes, **decreased skin turgor** (loss of normal consistency and fullness), tachycardia, hypoactive deep tendon reflexes, and decreased urine output.

Diagnostic Tests: Stool examination for white blood cells and organisms, with culture for pathogenic bacteria. Blood studies may show hematologic abnormalities or fluid and electrolyte imbalance.

Course: Most cases of gastroenteritis, even those caused by bacteria such as *Salmonella, Campylobacter*, and *Yersinia*, resolve spontaneously without specific treatment. However, cholera (due to *Vibrio cholerae*, rare in the U.S.), bacillary dysentery (due to *Shigella* species), typhoid fever (due to *Salmonella typhi*), and **pseudomembranous enterocolitis** (due to toxin-producing *Clostridium difficile*, often following treatment with antibiotics that kill normal intestinal flora) are all severe and potentially fatal infections requiring prompt, aggressive antimicrobial treatment. Gastroenteritis in small children or in elderly or debilitated persons can lead to dangerous electrolyte and water depletion and vascular collapse.

Treatment: Largely symptomatic and supportive. Over-the-counter products may suffice to control nausea, cramping, and diarrhea. Water and electrolytes may be replaced orally or intravenously as indicated. Antibiotic treatment is indicated only in certain specific infections. Trimethoprim-sulfamethoxazole or ciprofloxacin are effective in bacillary dysentery (shigellosis), typhoid fever, and cholera; pseudomembranous enterocolitis is treated with metronidazole or vancomycin.

Appendicitis

Acute inflammation of the appendix.

Cause: Obstruction of the appendiceal lumen by a **fecalith** (stonelike mass of hardened feces), seed, or parasite, or by swelling due to infection or neoplasm. Obstruction is followed by inflammation, impairment of blood supply, necrosis, and rupture.

History: Gradual onset of generalized abdominal distress gradually becoming more severe and steady and localizing in the right lower quadrant. Anorexia, nausea, vomiting, fever, chills, constipation. Sudden spontaneous relief of pain suggests perforation.

Physical Examination: Slight fever and tachycardia, tenderness and rebound tenderness over **McBurney point** (about one third of the distance from the right anterior superior iliac spine to the umbilicus), tenderness and rebound tenderness in the same area on rectal or pelvic examination. Diminished bowel sounds. After perforation, boardlike rigidity of the abdomen indicating peritonitis, signs of toxicity, vascular collapse. In infants, the elderly, and pregnant women, the findings may be atypical or deceptively mild.

Diagnostic Tests: Moderate elevation of the white blood cell count, with left shift (increase of band or immature forms). Focused CT may show a mass, ileus, or other signs of peritonitis, or an opacity in the appendiceal lumen; barium injected by rectum fails to fill the appendix.

Course: Without treatment the condition has a mortality rate over 90%. Most cases progress to perforation within 12–36 hours, followed by generalized peritonitis, septicemia, and collapse.

Treatment: Surgical removal of the appendix (by open procedure or laparoscopy) is the only effective treatment. Perforation requires surgical repair, intravenous fluids, and antibiotics.

Irritable Bowel Syndrome (IBS)

Intermittent or chronic abdominal distress and bowel dysfunction without any demonstrable organic lesion.

Cause: Unknown. A derangement of the normal interaction between the brain and the bowel is postulated. IBS is more likely to occur with emotional stress, dietary irregularities, and heavy intake of caffeine. Lactose intolerance and abuse of antacids or laxatives may be partly responsible. The disorder is more common in women and in persons under 65. As many as 50% of patients report a history of verbal or sexual abuse.

History: Intermittent lower abdominal pain, often relieved by having a bowel movement; alternating diarrhea and constipation; a sense of inadequate evacuation after bowel movement; excessive mucus in stools; flatulence.

Physical Examination: Essentially negative.

Diagnostic Tests: Stool examinations, barium enema, colonoscopy, and blood studies are all negative.

Course: Symptoms tend to wax and wane for many years, with intervals of complete remission.

Treatment: Regular eating habits, avoidance of coffee and other triggering factors. Antispasmodics may be prescribed to reduce bowel motility and cramping. Alosetron and tegaserod usually provide control of severe symptoms, but only in women.

> ### BUTTERFLIES IN THE STOMACH
>
> The **vagus nerve** (pronounced like "Vegas") runs from the brain to the intestines; thus, there is a definite connection between what you think and what you feel "in your gut." If you've ever had butterflies in your stomach during anticipation of an exciting or scary event, it's a very real feeling.
>
> The **enteric nervous system** (ENS) contains muscles, nerves, and neurotransmitters which help with digestion. During stressful situations, an abnormal number of signals can fire, leading to abdominal discomfort.

Crohn Disease (Regional Enteritis, Regional Ileitis)

A chronic inflammatory disease of the bowel that can lead to intestinal obstruction, abscess and fistula formation, and systemic complications (see ■Figure 15-2).

Cause: Unknown. The disease shows a familial pattern of incidence.

History: Recurrent crampy or steady abdominal pain, nausea, diarrhea, **steatorrhea** (excessive fat in stool), hematochezia, weakness, weight loss, and fever.

Physical Examination: Abdominal tenderness, signs of complications.

Diagnostic Tests: The white blood count and erythrocyte sedimentation rate are elevated. There may be mild anemia and reduction of serum levels of potassium, calcium, magnesium, and other substances.

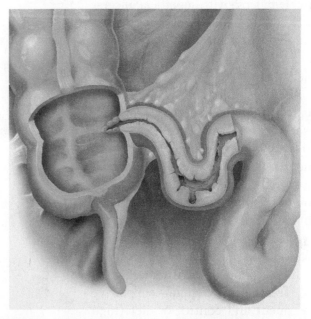

FIGURE 15-2 Crohn disease in the ileum of the small intestine

Barium enema shows regional narrowing of the lumen ("**string sign**") alternating with areas of normal caliber. Sigmoidoscopy and colonoscopy show local inflammation with **skip areas** (intervening zones of normal mucosa). On biopsy, all layers of the bowel are seen to be involved, not just the mucosa as in ulcerative colitis.

Course: Complications include intestinal obstruction, formation of abscesses and fistulas, perforation of the bowel.

Treatment: Low-fiber diet, drugs to reduce intestinal motility, aminosalicylates (sulfasalazine, mesalamine), corticosteroids (prednisone, budesonide), immunomodulators (azathioprine, mercaptopurine), and monoclonal antibodies (infliximab, adalimumab).

Ulcerative Colitis

A chronic inflammatory disease of the colon, chiefly the left colon, causing superficial ulceration.

Cause: Unknown.

History: Bloody diarrhea, abdominal cramps, tenesmus, anorexia, malaise, weakness, hemorrhoids or anal fissures. Bowel movements may occur more than 20 times a day and may awaken the patient at night.

Physical Examination: Fever, abdominal tenderness, signs of complications.

Diagnostic Tests: The white blood count and erythrocyte sedimentation rate are elevated. Anemia may be present. Stool examination reveals mucus, blood, and pus, but no bacteria or parasites. Serum electrolytes and protein may be depleted. Sigmoidoscopy and colonoscopy show erythematous, friable mucosa with superficial ulceration, and sometimes **polyp** formation. Biopsy shows chronic inflammation and microabscesses of the crypts of Lieberkühn.

Course: The course is intermittent, with spontaneous remissions and exacerbations. Physical and emotional stress and dietary irregularities may increase symptoms. Possible complications include colonic hemorrhage, perforation, **toxic dilatation** (extreme dilatation of the colon, compounded by effect of bacterial toxins); polyp formation with progression to carcinoma; arthritis, spondylitis; iritis; oral ulcers.

Treatment: General supportive treatment and control of diet (high protein, low milk) are crucial to long-term management of the disease. Aminosalicylates and corticosteroids suppress colonic inflammation and reduce symptoms. When these fail, immunosuppressants and monoclonal antibodies may provide satisfactory control. Severe or intractable disease may require hospitalization with intravenous alimentation and fluid replacement and antibiotic treatment to combat sepsis. About 25% of persons with ulcerative colitis eventually undergo surgery (colectomy and ileostomy).

Diverticulosis and Diverticulitis

A **diverticulum** (plural, **diverticula**) is a blister- or bubble-like outpouching of a hollow or tubular organ. **Diverticulosis** of the colon is the formation of one or more such outpouchings of the colon. **Diverticulitis** (see ■ Figure 15-3) means inflammation and infection of colonic diverticula.

Cause: Unknown; more common in middle-aged and elderly.

History: Most patients with diverticulosis have no symptoms. The diverticula may be discovered incidentally on routine examination (barium enema, colonoscopy). A few patients may experience irregular bowel habits or abdominal pain. Patients in whom diverticulitis develops experience acute abdominal pain, nausea, vomiting, constipation, and sometimes fever or blood in the stools.

Physical Examination: With the development of diverticulitis, there may be mild fever, abdominal tenderness, and even the sensation of a mass, most often

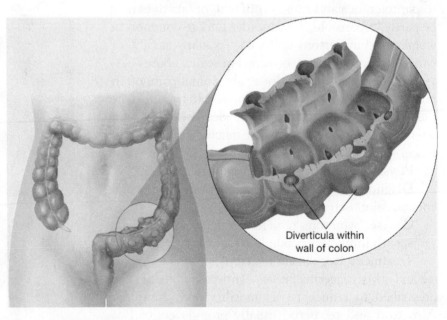

Diverticula within wall of colon

Figure 15-3. Diverticulitis.

in the region of the sigmoid colon (left lower quadrant of the abdomen).

Diagnostic Tests: The white blood count and sedimentation rate may be slightly elevated. The stool may be positive for occult blood. Barium enema, sigmoidoscopy, or colonoscopy may be performed to identify and localize the lesion, but are contraindicated in the presence of acute inflammation because of the danger of perforation of the bowel. X-ray studies may be used to identify free air in the peritoneal cavity due to perforation, and CT scan may be done to detect abscess formation. Diagnostic evaluation needs to be particularly thorough to rule out malignancy.

Course: Diverticulitis may lead to hemorrhage, perforation of the bowel, obstruction due to fibrous scarring, fistula formation, abscess formation.

Treatment: Patients with mild or no symptoms may require no treatment but are often advised to follow a high-fiber diet. During the acute phase of diverticulitis, patients are kept at bed rest, with nothing by mouth (n.p.o.), intravenous fluids and nutrition, and, if necessary, a nasogastric tube. Usually antibiotic treatment is used because of the risk of peritonitis and abscess formation. Metronidazole, ciprofloxacin, and trimethoprim-sulfamethoxazole are the drugs usually used. As many as one third of patients with diverticulitis will need surgery to drain an abscess or to resect a segment of badly diseased colon.

Intestinal Obstruction

Blockage of the flow of digestive fluids through the small or large intestine.

Causes: Surgical adhesions, hernia, neoplasms, gallstones, **volvulus** (twisting of a loop of intestine) (see ■ Figure 15-4), **intussusception** (passage of a segment of intestine into the segment distal to it), foreign body, fecal impaction. Obstruction due to causes outside the bowel (volvulus, hernia) are often complicated by **strangulation** (ischemia of the involved portion of bowel).

History: Crampy abdominal pain, nausea, vomiting, obstipation. Obstruction of the small intestine causes more severe and rapidly progressing symptoms than obstruction of the colon.

Physical Examination: Abdominal distention, **borborygmi** (gurgling sounds due to intestinal activity); increased bowel sounds, often high-pitched or in peristaltic **rushes** (urgent-sounding series of squeaking or gurgling sounds occurring with overactive peristaltic

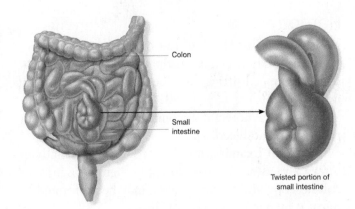

FIGURE 15-4. Volvulus

movements). A fullness or mass may be palpated at the site of obstruction. Tenderness in the presence of strangulation. The rectum is empty of stool unless fecal impaction is the cause of obstruction.

Diagnostic Tests: The white blood count is elevated, particularly in the presence of strangulation. Blood chemistries may show electrolyte imbalance and dehydration due to vomiting and sequestration of fluid above the obstruction. Abdominal x-rays show dilated loops of bowel containing fluid levels, and may demonstrate the cause (volvulus, gallstone). Barium enema may be necessary to identify an obstruction in the colon.

Treatment: A nasogastric tube with suction to decompress the bowel proximal to the obstruction. Intravenous fluids to correct dehydration and electrolyte imbalance. Surgery is often necessary to relieve obstruction and to resect infarcted areas of bowel in cases of strangulation.

Adynamic Ileus

Failure of normal flow of materials through the digestive tract because of atony or paralysis of the bowel.

Causes: Recent abdominal surgery, peritonitis, mesenteric ischemia or infarction, medicines (opiates, anticholinergics).

History: Nausea, vomiting, obstipation, abdominal distention. Pain mild or absent.

Physical Examination: Abdominal distention, little or no tenderness, bowel sounds diminished or absent.

Diagnostic Tests: X-ray of the abdomen shows distended loops of small intestine with fluid levels.

Treatment: Nasogastric tube and suction, intravenous fluids, correction of the underlying cause if possible.

Hemorrhoids

Dilated veins just above or just below the anus.

Cause: Unknown. Constipation with straining at stool, prolonged sitting, and local infection have been implicated.

History: Anorectal discomfort or pain, swelling or protrusion, and bleeding.

Physical Examination: Dilated veins externally or internally, as seen by endoscopy. Sigmoidoscopy or colonoscopy and barium enema may be performed to rule out malignancy.

Course: Symptoms are typically mild and intermittent. Bleeding is occasionally significant. Thrombosis of stagnant blood within a hemorrhoid results in acute pain and swelling, but the problem resolves spontaneously in a few weeks.

Treatment: High-fiber diet, stool softeners, hot sitz baths, soothing applications or suppositories. With severe pain or bleeding, surgery is indicated. Band ligation is used for internal hemorrhoids; external hemorrhoids are treated by excision or cryosurgery.

Acute Peritonitis

Acute inflammation of the peritoneum.

Causes: Infection (penetrating abdominal wounds, surgery, peritoneal dialysis for renal failure, spread from digestive or urinary tract or from a systemic site); chemical irritation (leakage of gastric or intestinal contents, bile, pancreatic secretions from injured, diseased, or perforated structure); systemic disease; neoplasm.

History: Fairly abrupt onset of severe local or generalized abdominal pain, nausea, vomiting, fever.

Physical Examination: Elevated temperature and pulse. Boardlike rigidity of abdomen, tenderness and rebound tenderness. Diminished or absent bowel sounds and abdominal distention due to ileus.

Diagnostic Tests: The white blood count is elevated. Blood studies may also show electrolyte imbalances due to peritoneal effusion, vomiting, and dehydration. Anemia may occur. Fluid obtained by abdominal paracentesis may show amylase or lipase (indicating leak of intestinal contents or pancreatic juice), significant cellular abnormalities, or infecting microorganisms. Various types of imaging may be of use in confirming and identifying intra-abdominal catastrophe.

Course: Without treatment the outlook is poor. Septicemia and vascular collapse often occur within a few hours of onset. In some patients, peritonitis becomes localized, with **abscess** formation, particularly

subphrenic (just below diaphragm) or pelvic. Peritonitis often results in eventual formation of fibrous adhesions that may produce intestinal obstruction.

Treatment: Hospitalization, nothing by mouth (n.p.o.), gastrointestinal suction to decompress the bowel and draw off secretions, intravenous fluids, narcotics for pain, antibiotics for infection, surgery to repair underlying abnormality.

Abdominal Hernia

A localized weakness in the musculoaponeurotic wall of the abdomen, with protrusion of abdominal contents. Abdominal hernias are classified according to position as:

umbilical (at the navel): often congenital, seldom requiring surgical repair because they resolve during infancy.

inguinal (in the groin) (see ■Figure 15-5):

 direct inguinal: due to thinning and stretching of the lower abdominal wall, often with aging.

 indirect inguinal: (usually congenital) weakness and bulging in the inguinal canal, the passage through which, in the male fetus, the testicle descends from the abdominal cavity to the scrotum; a similar potential passage exists in women.

femoral: herniation into the femoral canal, through which the femoral artery and vein pass from the pelvis into the thigh.

Cause: Congenital weakness or malformation; thinning of the abdominal musculature by aging. Herniation may be precipitated or aggravated by vigorous or repeated straining of the abdominal wall (chronic con-

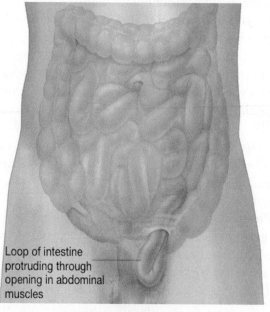

Loop of intestine protruding through opening in abdominal muscles

FIGURE 15-5. Inguinal hernia

stipation, urinary obstruction, heavy lifting, chronic cough).

History: A tender bulge in the abdominal wall that enlarges with straining. Intestinal obstruction may occur with severe abdominal pain, nausea, vomiting, weakness, shock, and collapse.

Physical Examination: A fluctuant bulge in the abdominal wall that enlarges with straining and can be reduced with manipulation or recumbency unless **incarceration** has occurred. A defect in the abdominal wall at the site of the hernia can be palpated. Visible or palpable mass, tenderness. Evidence of strangulation or bowel obstruction.

Diagnostic Tests: Barium enema and other studies may be done to rule out obstructive disease of the bowel or urinary tract.

Complications: Strangulation (compromise of blood supply), **incarceration** (inability to reduce hernia), bowel obstruction.

Treatment: Surgical repair of the defect, sometimes with implantation of reinforcing mesh.

Hepatitis A

Hepatitis is a general term referring to inflammation of the liver. Hepatitis can be caused by various drugs, toxic chemicals, and infections. Viral infections are the most important causes of hepatitis.

Cause: Hepatitis A virus. Transmission is by the fecal-oral route. Contaminated food and water are important means of infection.

History: Anorexia, nausea, vomiting, malaise, upper respiratory or flulike symptoms, fever, joint pain, aversion to tobacco, abdominal discomfort, diarrhea or constipation. Infection may be asymptomatic in children.

Physical Examination: Fever, jaundice, enlargement and tenderness of the liver, splenomegaly, cervical lymphadenopathy.

Diagnostic Tests: The serum bilirubin is elevated, and liver function tests are abnormal. Atypical lymphocytes may appear in the blood. Anti-HAV (IgM) antibody appears early in the course of the disease and disappears after recovery. IgG antibody develops later and persists indefinitely, indicating past history of, and immunity to, the disease.

Course: Symptoms characteristically resolve within 2–3 weeks. The mortality is very low.

Treatment: Supportive and symptomatic.

Hepatitis B

Cause: Hepatitis B virus. Transmission is by blood (shared needles, needle stick injury in healthcare workers) or sexual contact. Maternal transmission to neonates occurs also.

History: Fever, anorexia, nausea, vomiting, malaise, joint pain and swelling, rash, aversion to tobacco, abdominal pain, bowel irregularities.

Physical Examination: Fever, jaundice, enlargement and tenderness of liver. Splenomegaly, cervical lymphadenopathy.

Diagnostic Tests: The serum bilirubin is elevated, and liver function tests are abnormal. Atypical lymphocytes may appear in the blood. Hepatitis B surface antigen (HB_SAg) appears early in the disease and indicates presence of infection and infectivity of the patient. Antibody to surface antigen ($AntiHB_S$) indicates recovery, immunity to future infection, and lack of infectivity. Presence of HB_SAg after the acute phase suggests chronic infection.

Course: The incubation period may be 6–12 weeks or longer, and acute illness may persist for as long as 16 weeks. The mortality rate is somewhat higher than that of hepatitis A. Some patients become carriers of the disease, able to transmit infection months or years after recovery. In some, a chronic phase occurs. **Chronic persistent hepatitis** is mild and generally asymptomatic, while **chronic active hepatitis** leads to gradual deterioration of liver function, cirrhosis, and an appreciable risk of hepatocellular carcinoma.

Treatment: Chiefly supportive. Chronic hepatitis is treated with interferon alfa-2b and lamivudine.

Hepatitis C (HCV)

A mild or asymptomatic viral hepatitis usually transmitted by sharing needles or by blood transfusion. In about 85% of cases it becomes chronic, with risk of cirrhosis and hepatocellular carcinoma. Carriers can be identified by serologic testing. Treatment is with interferon alfa or ribavirin. Liver transplantation.

Cirrhosis (Portal Cirrhosis, Cirrhosis, Laënnec Cirrhosis)

A chronic disorder of the liver characterized by inflammation of secretory cells followed by nodular regeneration and fibrosis.

Causes: The principal cause of cirrhosis (see ■ **Figure 15-6**) is chronic alcohol abuse. About 20% of persons with hepatitis C eventually develop cirrhosis. Other toxic, metabolic, nutritional, and infectious fac-

ESOPHAGEAL VARICES

Today there are new treatments and medications to treat diseases that once eluded the medical community. In *Intern* by Alan E. Nourse, a patient in 1965 dies a gruesome death from a condition for which there was no effective treatment at the time: esophageal varices. Esophageal varices are varicose veins in the lower esophagus. This condition, often the result of alcohol abuse, is caused by portal hypertension, where bloodflow through the liver is diminished due to cirrhosis (liver degeneration often accompanied by scarring or fibrosis). The pressure from the limited bloodflow to the liver causes backup pressure in veins of the esophagus, which can then balloon from a few millimeters to over one centimeter in circumference and leak or burst. Bleeding is profuse and profound.

About 1988 a relatively simple treatment to control esophageal varices was developed: injection of saline solution into the varices, resulting in shrinkage of the dilated vessels. Today beta-blockers and/or radiofrequency ablation are used to shrink dilated blood vessels and prevent bleeding. The condition can still be dire if a dilated vessel begins to leak or burst, however.

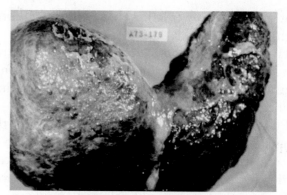

FIGURE 15-6. Cirrhosis of the liver from chronic alcoholism. Source: Pearson Education.

tors may play a part in the genesis of cirrhosis. The cirrhotic liver contains various combinations of fatty change and fibrosis forming small and large nodules.

History: Usually gradual onset of anorexia, nausea, weakness, weight loss, abdominal swelling due to **ascites** (accumulation of fluid in the abdominal cavity), and often jaundice. Disturbance of sex steroid hormone metabolism causes impotence in men and amenorrhea in women.

Physical Examination: Fever, muscle wasting, pleural effusion, **ascites**, peripheral edema. The liver is usually enlarged and may be firm or even hard. The spleen may also be enlarged. Jaundice appears relatively late. Elevation of estrogen level causes gynecomastia in men, spider angiomas (**spider nevi**) on the face and upper trunk, and palmar erythema. The tongue may appear smooth, shiny, and inflamed. With advanced disease there may be coarse, flapping tremors (**asterixis**) and delirium due to hepatic failure, which may progress to hepatic coma.

Diagnostic Tests: Laboratory tests show elevation of bilirubin and enzymes such as aminotransferases, lactic dehydrogenase (LDH), and alkaline phosphatase, which rise in the presence of liver cell damage. Anemia may be present, and coagulation studies may yield abnormal results. Liver biopsy confirms presence of typical histologic changes. Imaging studies including radioactive liver scans provide further information. Esophagoscopy may show **esophageal varices**.

Course: Symptoms may wax and wane over a period of years, often in response to varying levels of alcohol consumption. Progressive hepatic failure often occurs. Fibrosis within the liver typically shuts off branches of the portal circulation and increases the pressure in the portal vein (**portal hypertension**). In consequence, other vessels (particularly the lower esophageal venous plexus) dilate and become varicose (bulging) or tortuous (coiled, twisted). Hemorrhage from bleeding esophageal varices is often life-threatening, particularly when hepatic disease causes a coagulation disorder. There is an increased incidence of hepatocellular carcinoma in persons with cirrhosis.

Treatment: Abstinence from alcohol, attention to nutrition, particularly carbohydrate, protein, vitamins. Rest, sodium restriction, and diuretics for edema and ascites. Severe ascites may require abdominal **paracentesis** (removal of peritoneal fluid with a needle passed through the abdominal wall). Patients with portal hypertension and bleeding esophageal varices may need a **portacaval shunt** (surgical procedure allowing portal vein blood to bypass the liver and empty directly into the inferior vena cava).

Cholelithiasis (Gallstones)

The formation of gallstones is a common disorder, generally due to some disturbance in the flow of bile from the gallbladder or in the composition of bile (see ■ Figure 15-7). Gallstones are more common in women and in elderly persons. Risk factors include pregnancy, diabetes mellitus, high serum cholesterol, Crohn disease, and sickle cell anemia. In the latter condition, stones consist primarily of bilirubin from hemolyzed red blood cells. In the other conditions, gallstones are composed primarily of cholesterol.

Gallstones are often asymptomatic ("**silent**"), but about 90% of persons with **cholecystitis** (inflammation of the gallbladder) have preexisting **cholelithiasis**. Stones may be demonstrated on plain abdominal films, but ultrasound and imaging after injection of opaque medium are more sensitive and specific. Potential serious complications are blockage of the **common bile duct** by a stone with ensuing obstructive jaundice, blockage of the **cystic duct** with ensuing cholecystitis, and passage of a stone into the intestine with the potential for causing bowel obstruction (**gallstone ileus**).

Treatment of symptomatic gallstones is surgical removal (along with the gallbladder), usually through a **laparoscope**. Stones can also be crushed and flushed out with instruments passed through an endoscope inserted through the mouth and threaded into the common bile duct. Oral bile salts (chenodeoxycholic acid, ursodeoxycholic acid) and extracorporeal shock wave lithotripsy (ESWL) sometimes dissolve stones.

Acute Cholecystitis

Acute inflammation of the gallbladder.

Causes: Most patients with cholecystitis have preexisting cholelithiasis (see ■ Figure 15-7). Impaction

> **FEMALE, FAT, AND FORTY**
> Cholelithiasis refers to stones (calculi) that have formed in the gallbladder. Overweight women aged 40 or older are more likely than men to develop gallstones, hence an old diagnostic medical phrase "female, fat, and forty." People who experience relatively fast weight loss or are yo-yo dieters are also at increased risk.
>
> *This 25-year-old Caucasian female is admitted for cholecystectomy. She developed gallstones after weight-loss surgery. A gallbladder ultrasound was taken routinely prior to her gastric bypass, and at that time the gallbladder appeared normal.*

of a stone in the cystic duct leads to obstruction of the flow of bile from the gallbladder, with ischemia, acute inflammation, and sometimes abscess formation or perforation.

History: Fairly acute onset of severe epigastric and right upper quadrant pain, nausea, and vomiting.

Physical Examination: Fever and jaundice may be present. In the right upper quadrant of the abdomen there are tenderness, rebound tenderness, and **involuntary guarding** (spasm of abdominal muscles on palpation). Bowel sounds are reduced or absent. Occasionally a mass can be felt below the liver edge, representing a distended gallbladder.

Diagnostic Tests: The white blood cell count, bilirubin, and levels of serum enzymes reflecting hepatic damage may all be elevated. Imaging studies (plain abdominal x-ray, ultrasound, scans with radiotagged media) may precisely identify the problem.

Course: Acute cholecystitis may resolve spontaneously. Often relapses occur with gradual development of chronic cholecystitis. Inflammation may culminate in **gangrene** (tissue death due to compromise of blood supply) or perforation of the gallbladder, or may ascend into the liver via the biliary tract (ascending cholangitis).

Treatment: Chiefly supportive, with narcotics for pain, intravenous fluids, and close observation. Impending or actual perforation is treated by surgical (laparoscopic) decompression (drainage) of the gallbladder or, preferably, by removal of the gallbladder (cholecystectomy).

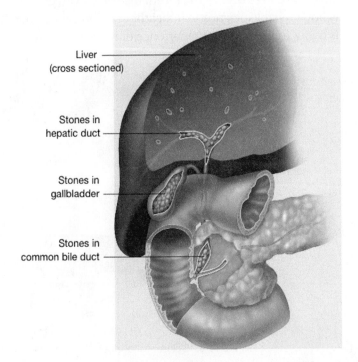

Liver (cross sectioned)

Stones in hepatic duct

Stones in gallbladder

Stones in common bile duct

FIGURE 15-7. Cholelithiasis

Acute Pancreatitis

Acute inflammation of the pancreas.

Causes: Most cases occur in alcoholics or in persons with chronic biliary tract disease (cholelithiasis, cholecystitis). In these instances, obstruction of the pancreatic duct by edema, or backflow of bile from the duodenum into the pancreatic duct, causes release of pancreatic enzymes into the substance of the gland, with resulting intense inflammation, necrosis, and often hemorrhage. Other causes are **hypercalcemia** (abnormally high level of calcium in the blood), **hypertriglyceridemia** (abnormally high level of triglycerides in the blood), abdominal trauma or surgery, certain medicines, and viral infection including mumps. An acute attack of pancreatitis is often precipitated by excessive alcohol consumption or by eating a large meal.

History: Abrupt onset of severe, persisting epigastric pain, worse on lying flat, and radiating to the flanks and back. Nausea, vomiting, sweating, prostration, restlessness.

Physical Examination: Pallor, tachycardia, fever, epigastric tenderness, reduced or absent bowel sounds. Jaundice or hypotension may occur. In the presence of severe pancreatic hemorrhage, a bluish discoloration of the skin may appear over the left flank (**Turner** or **Grey Turner sign**). There may be evidence of ascites or a left **pleural effusion** (inflammatory fluid in pleural cavity).

Diagnostic Tests: Blood studies may show leukocytosis, hyperglycemia, anemia, and **hypocalcemia** (drop in serum calcium). Blood levels of pancreatic enzymes (amylase, lipase) are typically elevated. Imaging studies may show gallstones, a mass representing the swollen pancreas, left **atelectasis** (collapse of part of left lung caused by shallow breathing at site of pain), or left pleural effusion (inflammatory fluid in pleural cavity).

Course: Acute pancreatitis has a high mortality rate and, among survivors, a high recurrence rate. Possible outcomes include abscess formation, splenic vein thrombosis, ileus, shock, renal failure, adult respiratory distress syndrome, severe hypocalcemia with tetany, formation of **pseudocysts** (pockets of inflammatory fluid and debris between the pancreas and surrounding tissues), and progression to chronic disease.

Treatment: Hospitalization, narcotics for pain relief, nasogastric suction, intravenous fluids with attention to water balance, nutritional needs, and replacement of calcium. Surgery may be required to control hemorrhage, correct underlying disease, or drain pseudocysts.

Adenocarcinoma of the Colon and Rectum

A malignant neoplasm arising from glandular epithelium in the large intestine (see ■ Figure 15-8). In both men and women, colon cancer ranks second as a cause of cancer deaths in the U.S. One half of all colon cancers are situated in the sigmoid colon or rectum. These tumors tend to grow slowly but may eventually become bulky; they may encircle and constrict the bowel.

Causes: Most colon cancers arise by malignant transformation of benign **polyps** (adenomas). Several oncogenes are associated with heightened risk of developing primary cancer in the colon; some of these predispose to formation of multiple malignant tumors, which may involve organs other than the bowel. Risk factors for developing colon cancer include age over 40, a history of adenomas (benign polyps) of the colon, a family history of colon cancer, and a history of ulcerative colitis.

History: Depending on the location of the tumor, crampy abdominal pain, change of bowel habits, bloody stools, weakness, fatigue.

Physical Examination: A mass may be felt on abdominal or digital rectal examination. The liver may be enlarged or irregular in contour if hepatic metastases are present.

Diagnostic Tests: The red blood count may be low as a result of hemorrhage. Chemical examination of the stool may detect occult blood. The carcinoembryonic antigen (CEA) titer in the serum may be elevated. This is not a reliable diagnostic indicator of colon cancer but is useful in watching for recurrence or metastatic disease

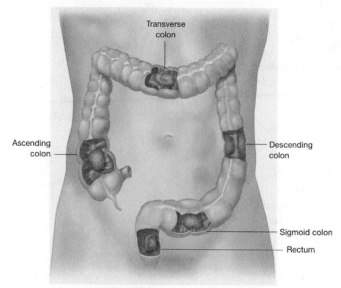

FIGURE 15-8. Colorectal cancer

after surgery. With extensive hepatic metastases, liver function tests become abnormal. Barium enema demonstrates mucosal defects, a space-occupying lesion, or an encircling obstruction. Abdominal CT scan may provide additional information. Endorectal ultrasound is valuable in distal lesions. Chest x-ray may show pulmonary metastases. Colonoscopy with biopsy provides definitive diagnosis.

Course: The overall survival rate in treated colon cancer is about 35%. If complete resection of primary tumor can be carried out, the survival rate is about 55%.

Treatment: The procedure of choice is surgical resection. **Rectal carcinoma** may require **abdominoperineal resection** (removal of the entire lower bowel, including the anus) with sigmoid **colostomy.** Tumors higher in the colon may be able to be resected with simple anastomosis of normal bowel above and below the surgical site. Chemotherapy and radiation therapy are valuable adjuncts to surgery in colon carcinoma.

Abdominal Injury

Blunt injury can cause bruising, laceration, or severe hemorrhage of internal organs (liver, spleen, kidney, digestive tract, urinary bladder). In penetrating abdominal injuries, the risk of damage and particularly of hemorrhage is much increased. Puncture of the stomach or intestine releases digestive fluids into the peritoneal cavity and causes chemical peritonitis. Hemorrhage into the abdominal cavity is called **hemoperitoneum**.

The diagnosis of abdominal injury depends on careful physical examination, x-ray studies and scans, and **peritoneal lavage** (injection of fluid through a needle passed through the abdominal wall, followed by its withdrawal and laboratory examination). This procedure can detect blood, digestive fluids, urine, or other substances not normally present.

Management includes supportive care and prompt surgical intervention to repair leaking blood vessels or punctured organs.

Pause for Reflection

1. Chronic GERD may lead to a precancerous condition known as _____.
2. The most common cause of peptic ulcer disease is _____.
3. Gastroenteritis can be a reaction to medicines, foods, poisonous plants, toxic chemicals, or due to toxins produced by _____.
4. On physical exam, slight fever and tachycardia, tenderness and rebound tenderness over _____, tenderness and rebound tenderness in the same area on rectal or pelvic examination suggest that the patient has appendicitis.
5. Intermittent or chronic abdominal distress and bowel dysfunction without any demonstrable organic lesion is known as _____.
6. ____ disease is suggested when a barium enema shows regional narrowing of the lumen (referred to as a _____ sign), alternating with areas of normal caliber. Sigmoidoscopy and colonoscopy show local inflammation with ____.
7. Distinguish between the terms *diverticulum*, *diverticulosis*, and *diverticulitis*.
8. Distinguish between the following causes of intestinal obstruction: *volvulus, intussusception,* and *strangulation of the colon.*
9. Atony or paralysis of the bowel results in a condition known as _____.
10. When it becomes necessary to treat hemorrhoids with surgery, the patient may undergo _____ for internal hemorrhoids or _____ or _____ for external hemorrhoids.
11. Elevated temperature and pulse; boardlike rigidity of abdomen, tenderness and rebound tenderness; and diminished or absent bowel sounds and abdominal distention due to ileus are distinguishing features of _____.
12. Distinguish among the 4 types of abdominal hernia.
13. The form of hepatitis that often leads to the need for a liver transplant is _____.
14. A chronic disorder of the liver characterized by inflammation of secretory cells followed by nodular regeneration and fibrosis is _____.
15. Distinguish between *cholelithiasis* and *cholecystitis.*
16. Most adenocarcinomas of the colon and rectum arise by malignant transformation of _____.
17. Hemorrhage into the abdominal cavity is called _____.
18. Injection of fluid through a needle passed through the abdominal wall, followed by its withdrawal and laboratory exam, is a procedure called _____.

Diagnostic and Surgical Procedures

anastomosis Surgical joining of two organs or vessels.

appendectomy Surgical excision of the vermiform appendix.

barium enema (BE) A radiological imaging study that uses barium given rectally to outline the colon and rectum.

capsule endoscopy A relatively new procedure in which a tiny camera is swallowed in the form of a capsule. As it moves through the digestive tract over a period of about eight hours, pictures of the internal structures are taken and transmitted to a recording device worn about the patient's waist. Doctors can then review the full-color images to detect abnormalities. Also called **wireless capsule endoscopy**.

cholecystectomy Surgical removal of the gallbladder. It can be done either through an open incision or through minimally invasive laparoscopy.

colectomy Surgical excision of part or all of the colon.

colonoscopy Endoscopic procedure to view the colon using a flexible (fiberoptic) endoscope (see ■ Figure 15-9).

colostomy A surgically created opening from the colon to the abdominal wall, through which feces are passed rather than by the rectum; may be temporary or permanent.

endoscopy Insertion of a tube with a light source into a body cavity to view and often to biopsy the structures. Common types of endoscopies are esophagoscopy, gastroscopy, gastroduodenoscopy, anoscopy, sigmoidoscopy, and colonoscopy.

esophagogastroduodenoscopy (EGD) Endoscopic procedure to view the esophagus, stomach, and duodenum.

exploratory laparotomy Inspection of the abdominal and pelvic cavities through an incision in the abdominal wall.

gastrectomy Excision of a portion or all of the stomach.

gastroscopy Endoscopic procedure to view the stomach.

hemicolectomy Surgical excision of approximately half the colon.

hemorrhoidectomy Surgical excision of hemorrhoids (anal varicose veins).

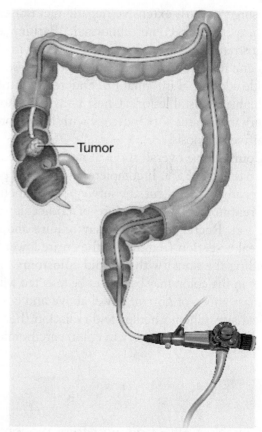

FIGURE 15-9. Colonoscope.
Source: CNRI, Photo Researchers, Inc.

herniorrhaphy Surgical repair of a hernia (protrusion of organ or tissue through an abnormal opening).

imaging studies Flat, upright, and (usually left) lateral decubitus films of the abdomen; fluoroscopic studies with swallowed or injected barium or other contrast medium (barium swallow, upper GI series, small bowel series, barium enema); CT or MRI for specific indications (for example, to assess gallbladder, masses); and ultrasound studies.

KUB x-ray Plain x-ray to image the kidneys, ureters, and bladder (hence KUB).

laparoscopy Inspection of abdominal cavity through an endoscope inserted through an incision in the abdominal wall.

polypectomy The surgical removal of outgrowths (polyps).

portacaval shunt Surgical procedure allowing portal vein blood to bypass the liver and empty directly into the inferior vena cava.

pyloroplasty Incision of the pylorus and reconstruction of the pyloric channel to relieve pyloric obstruction.

resection Surgical removal.

splenectomy Surgical removal of the spleen, usually precipitated by splenic injury.

upper GI series (UGI) with small bowel follow through An x-ray series that uses barium taken orally to outline the esophagus, stomach, and small intestine.

Laboratory Procedures

absorption tests Based on determination of blood or stool levels of substances that have been ingested in measured amounts.

alkaline phosphatase An enzyme whose level in the serum is often increased in bone disease and obstructive liver disease.

ALT (alanine aminotransferase) An enzyme whose level in the serum is elevated in hepatitis, cirrhosis, and other liver diseases.

ammonia, serum A breakdown product of protein metabolism, increased in hepatic failure.

amylase, serum An enzyme whose level is increased in pancreatitis and mumps.

AST (aspartate aminotransferase) An enzyme whose level in the serum is elevated in myocardial infarction, liver disease, and other conditions.

bilirubin, conjugated Bilirubin that has been conjugated (combined with glucuronic acid) by the liver so that it is water-soluble.

bilirubin, direct Bilirubin that reacts directly with testing chemicals because it has been rendered water-soluble (combined with glucuronic acid) in the liver. Its level is increased in biliary obstruction.

bilirubin, indirect Bilirubin in the serum that does not react directly with testing chemicals because it has not yet been conjugated (combined with glucuronic acid) in the liver. Its level is increased in disorders that impair the function of liver cells.

bilirubin, unconjugated Fat-soluble bilirubin that has not been conjugated (combined with glucuronic acid) by the liver.

bilirubin, urinary Bilirubin in the urine; it can be measured with a dipstick. Any amount is considered abnormal; usually it indicates obstructive liver disease or hepatitis.

carcinoembryonic antigen (CEA) A glycoprotein occurring in the normal embryo and also detectable in the serum of some adults with cancer of the colon.

CLO (Campylobacter-like organism) test To detect *H. pylori* in acid peptic disease. Also, *rapid urease test.*

examination of stool For occult blood, fat, pathogens (bacteria, fungi, parasites), abnormal constituents.

5'-nucleotidase (pronounced "five prime nucleotidase") A serum enzyme whose level increases in biliary obstruction. Testing for this enzyme helps to distinguish liver disease from bone disease as possible causes of elevated serum alkaline phosphatase.

Helicobacter pylori **(H. pylori)** A gram-negative organism which is the cause of many peptic ulcers.

Hemoccult test For occult blood in the stool.

LFTs (liver function tests).

Meckel scan Imaging procedure in which radioactive material is injected into a vein to outline a small abnormal outpouched area of the ileum.

occult blood Blood present in quantities too small to be detected by naked-eye observation but detected by microscopic or chemical examination.

stool for ova and parasites (O&P) Examination of stool for parasites or their ova (eggs).

Pharmacology

Drugs for Peptic Ulcers and GERD

Several types of drugs are used to treat peptic ulcers, including antacids, H_2 blockers, antispasmodics, and others.

Antacids

Antacids were the original, and for many years the only, treatment for peptic ulcers. They are weak bases that exert a therapeutic effect by neutralizing hydrochloric acid. This raises the pH of the stomach contents, which decreases mucous membrane irritation and also inhibits the action of pepsin.

Antacids contain aluminum, magnesium, calcium, sodium, or a combination of these as the active ingredients. Some antacids contain simethicone to relieve flatulence and gas; simethicone acts by changing the surface tension of air bubbles trapped in the GI tract to allow them to be expelled. Others contain aspirin or acetaminophen for pain relief. Antacids are available without a prescription and include Bromo Seltzer, Di-Gel, Gaviscon, Maalox, Mylanta, Phillips' Milk of Magnesia, Riopan, Rolaids, and Tums.

H_2 Blockers

The release of gastric acid is triggered by histamine, which acts on special histamine receptors (known as H_2 receptors) in the gastric parietal cells lining the stomach. Drugs that block these receptors and prevent release of acid are known as H_2 blockers and are used to treat ulcers and gastroesophageal reflux disease (GERD). Examples include cimetidine (Tagamet), famotidine (Pepcid), nizatidine (Axid AR), and ranitidine (Zantac).

Proton Pump Inhibitors

Unrelated to H_2 blockers, proton pump inhibitors decrease gastric acid by blocking the final step of acid production within the gastric parietal cell. This final step involves an enzyme system known as the proton pump, hence the name of this drug category.

> esomeprazole (Nexium)
> lansoprazole (Prevacid)
> omeprazole (Prilosec)
> pantoprazole (Protonix, Protonix IV)
> rabeprazole (AcipHex)

Drugs Used to Treat *H. pylori* infections

Successful eradication of *H. pylori* requires the use of two antimicrobial agents combined with bismuth (such as Pepto-Bismol) and either an H_2 blocker or a proton pump inhibitor such as lansoprazole (Prevacid) or omeprazole (Prilosec). Antimicrobials and bismuth disrupt the cell walls surrounding bacteria, causing cell death. Antimicrobials for *H. pylori* infections include:

> amoxicillin (Amoxil, Trimox, Wymox)
> clarithromycin (Biaxin)
> metronidazole (Flagyl, Protostat)
> tetracycline (Achromycin V, Panmycin, Sumycin)

GI Stimulants for GERD

GI stimulants increase the rate of gastric emptying in order to keep excess acid from accumulating in the stomach. An example is metoclopramide (Maxolon, Reglan).

Drugs Affecting GI Muscle Tone and Motility

Drugs Relieving GI Spasm

Spasm of the smooth muscle layer of the GI tract is responsible for much of the pain caused by a wide variety of digestive disorders. GI spasms can be relieved by antispasmodic drugs, which are also known as **anticholinergic drugs**. Anticholinergic drugs exert their therapeutic action in the following way. Muscle contraction and peristalsis in the GI tract are controlled by the parasympathetic nervous system through the release of the neurotransmitter acetylcholine. Acetylcholine acts on cholinergic receptors to stimulate muscular contractions and begin peristalsis to move food through the GI tract. If peristalsis is too strong and causes spasms, anticholinergic drugs can be given to block the effects of acetylcholine to stop the spasms and slow peristalsis.

> dicyclomine (Bentyl, Di-Spaz)
> L-hyoscyamine (Anaspaz, Levbid, Levsin,
> Levsin Drops, Levsin/SL, Levsinex Timecaps)
> methantheline (Banthine)
> propantheline (Pro-Banthine)

These drugs combine an antispasmodic drug with the central nervous system sedative phenobarbital or the antianxiety drug Librium.

> Bellergal-S (belladonna, phenobarbital)
> Donnatal, Donnatal Extentabs (L-hyoscyamine,
> scopolamine, phenobarbital)
> Librax (clidinium, Librium)

Antidiarrheal Drugs

Antidiarrheal drugs produce a therapeutic effect by slowing peristalsis in the intestinal tract or by absorbing extra water in diarrheal stools. Some antidiarrheal drugs exert their effect because they contain opium or related narcotic drugs. Although these drugs have pain-relieving properties, a common side effect is constipation. This side effect then becomes the therapeutic effect in treating diarrhea.

Drugs for diarrhea which contain opium or related substances are classified as narcotics and may be controlled substances, depending on the actual addictive properties of the particular drug. Examples include difenoxin (Motofen), diphenoxylate (Lomotil), and paregoric (Pantopon). Non-narcotics include loperamide (Imodium).

ULCER THERAPY

Not long ago, medical professionals were taught that peptic ulcer disease was brought on by high levels of stress in some individuals—an emotional disease, of sorts. The condition was treated with a bland diet (no spicy or irritating foods), antacids, and stress reduction. In refractory cases (unresponsive to treatment), radical surgery was performed to cut the vagus nerves (vagotomy), reconstruct the pylorus (pyloroplasty), and even remove part of the stomach (partial gastrectomy).

In 1983 a new bacterial organism, now known as *Helicobacter pylori*, or *H. pylori*, was discovered to thrive in the stomachs of patients with stomach ulcers. This organism is sensitive to antibiotics, and patients who were given courses of antibiotics often experienced great relief. Further medical research proved that *H. pylori* exists in the digestive tracts of much of the population as well; thus, it was unclear why some people were more susceptible to its adverse effects.

Ulcer treatment today is quite different than in the past. While antacids are still prescribed, newer drugs such as Prevacid and Nexium inhibit the production of stomach juices, making the stomach less "environmentally friendly" to *H. pylori* and reducing the corrosive effects of acid.

Probiotic therapy has also proven useful in some individuals. These are substances containing normal intestinal flora (good bacteria) that line the digestive tract. When antibiotics kill off pathogens, they also decimate the protective intestinal flora. Probiotics (notice how the word is the opposite of antibiotics) such as *Lactobacillus acidophilus* supplements can be found in acidophilus milk, in pill or in capsule form.

A healthy diet, adequate exercise, and stress reduction, however, are still good modes of therapy for everyone!

Nonprescription drugs for diarrhea contain non-opiate substances such as kaolin and pectin which absorb water. Examples include Donnagel, Kaolin, and Kaopectate. Drugs used to treat bacterial or protozoal diarrhea or traveler's diarrhea include ciprofloxacin (Cipro) and doxycycline (Doryx, Vibramycin, Vibra-Tabs).

Laxatives

Laxatives are used for the short-term treatment of constipation, along with dietary and other measures to promote regularity. They are also used to empty the colon in preparation for imaging studies, endoscopy, or surgery. Laxatives are classified according to their mode of action. Some OTC products contain representatives of more than one class.

Stimulant or irritant laxatives act on the intestinal mucosa to induce peristalsis. Examples include castor oil, bisacodyl (Correctol, Dulcolax), and senna derivatives (Ex-Lax, Fletcher's Castoria, Senokot). Overuse of laxatives of this type can result in dependency as well as nutritional and electrolyte imbalance.

Most laxatives work by augmenting the bulk of the stool, increasing its water content, or both. Bulk-producing laxatives promote bowel regularity by modifying the volume and consistency of the stool with nonabsorbable and chemically inert fiber or cellulose. Their action is the most natural and safest. Examples include psyllium husk (Metamucil), methylcellulose (Citrucel), and polycarbophil (Equalactin, Konsyl Fiber).

Stool softeners (Colace, Dialose, Surfak) contain docusate, a surfactant that renders stool more plastic by enhancing the incorporation of bowel fluid. Mineral oil, a highly refined, non-absorbable petroleum derivative, prevents the absorption of water from the colon and exerts a lubricant action as well.

Osmotic laxatives promote bowel action by increasing the water content of stool through osmotic activity on secretory membranes, including those of the small intestine. The osmotic agents in saline laxatives are mineral salts: magnesium sulfate (Epsom salt), magnesium hydroxide (milk of magnesia, MOM), and magnesium citrate (Citromag). Hyperosmotic laxatives contain poorly absorbed organic compounds of high molecular weight: polyethylene glycol (MiraLax, GlycoLax), lactulose (Cephulac, Chronulac, Kristalose).

Suppositories containing glycerin stimulate defecation by their presence in the rectum. Enemas of plain warm water also stimulate bowel activity mechanically besides producing a cleansing effect. Stimulant and osmotic agents may also be given rectally.

Drugs for Specific GI Disorders

Drugs Used to Treat IBS

The traditional treatment of inflammatory bowel syndrome includes modification of diet and lifestyle and the use of antispasmodics, antidiarrheals, and laxatives as appropriate. More specific agents that alter the response of the bowel to hormones of the serotonin family are effective in women but not in men. In patients whose predominant symptom is diarrhea, the 5-HT$_3$ receptor antagonist alosetron (Lotronex) reduces stool frequency and cramping. In patients with constipation, the 5-HT$_4$ partial agonist tegaserod (Zelnorm) increases stool frequency and reduces bloating and discomfort.

Ulcerative Colitis Drugs

Antispasmodic and anti-inflammatory drugs used to treat ulcerative colitis include 4-ASA (Pamisyl, Rezipas), mesalazine (Dipentum), sulfasalazine (Azulfidine), and topical corticosteroids such as hydrocortisone (Cortenema, Cortifoam).

Antiemetics

Antiemetics are used to control nausea and vomiting arising from illnesses of the GI tract, as a side effect of drugs, surgery, radiation or chemotherapy, or from vertigo or motion sickness. Vomiting patients may be given medication in rectal suppository form because they are unable to keep oral medications down.

For severe nausea and vomiting, chlorpromazine (Thorazine) and prochlorperazine (Compazine) are prescribed. Medications such as promethazine (Phenergan), thiethylperazine (Torecan), and trimethobenzamide (Tigan) are prescribed for moderate nausea and vomiting.

Vertigo is caused by irritation to the inner ear which upsets balance and stimulates the vomiting center. Motion sickness arises from repeated motion, such as in a car, which also overstimulates the inner ear. Drugs to treat these problems seem to act by either reducing the sensitivity of the inner ear to motion or inhibiting the increased inner ear stimuli from reaching the chemoreceptor trigger zone and the vomiting center in the brain.

> dimenhydrinate (Dramamine)
> diphenhydramine (Benadryl)
> meclizine (Antivert, Bonine)
> promethazine (Phenergan)
> scopolamine (Transderm-Scop)

Note: All of these drugs are given orally, with the exception of scopolamine (Transderm-Scop), which is manufactured as a small transdermal patch worn behind the ear.

Antiemetics for Patients Undergoing Chemotherapy

Chemotherapy drugs directly stimulate the vomiting center in the brain. In addition, some cause release of serotonin in the small intestine; this stimulates the vomiting reflex. Because the nausea and vomiting in response to chemotherapy can be severe and prolonged, antiemetic drugs are often given prophylactically prior to beginning chemotherapy.

> chlorpromazine (Thorazine)
> dronabinol (Marinol)
> granisetron (Kytril)
> metoclopramide (Reglan)
> ondansetron (Zofran)
> prochlorperazine (Compazine)
> promethazine (Phenergan)
> trimethobenzamide (Tigan)

Immunosuppressants

The following are immunosuppressant drugs given to liver transplant patients to prevent rejection of donor organs.

> cyclosporine (Neoral, Sandimmune)
> muromonab-CD3 (Orthoclone OKT3)
>   (monoclonal antibody)
> tacrolimus (Prograf)
> Xomazyme-H65

Transcription Tips

1. Confusing terms: Some of these terms sound alike; others are potential traps when researching.

   acidic—presence of acid

   ascitic—abnormal accumulation of abdominal fluid (noun, ascites)

   dysphagia—difficulty swallowing

   dysplasia—alteration in size, shape, and organization of adult cells

   dysphasia—speech impairment, usually as a result of cerebrovascular accident or brain trauma

   ileum—a portion of the small intestine

   ilium—a pelvic bone

   mucus (noun)—a slimy substance produced by the mucous membranes

   mucous (adjective)—pertaining to mucus; it will precede a noun like membranes or discharge

   perineal—pertaining to the area between the genitalia and the anus

   peritoneal—pertaining to the serous membrane lining the abdomen

   perianal—pertaining to the area surrounding the anus

   peroneal—pertaining to the tibia; usually referring to nerves, vessels, muscles

   tortuous—twisted (colon)

   torturous—of, relating to, or causing torture

   tract—an anatomical term, a collection of organs that work together as in digestive tract or GI tract, or a passage, as in fistulous tract.

   track—a path or marks that look like a path, as in needle tracks

2. The following slang terms should be expanded when dictated:

alk phos	alkaline phosphatase
appy	appendectomy
bili	bilirubin
C diff	*C difficile*
H&H	hemoglobin and hematocrit
procto	proctoscopy
sig	sigmoidoscopy
tic	diverticulum

3. Spelling tips:

inflamed	but	inflammation
spleen	but	splenectomy

   The spelling *distention* is preferred; *distension* is an acceptable alternative.

   Although *antacids* have an anti-acid effect, the "i" is omitted from *anti-* in the correct spelling although it is sometimes pronounced.

   In contrast, *antiemetic* is correct even though the first "i" is often not clearly pronounced.

4. Memorize the spelling of these difficult gastrointestinal terms:

borborygmus	cirrhosis
guaiac	hemorrhoid
hepatorrhaphy	intussusception

5. Note the challenging spellings of these common gastrointestinal drugs:

   AlternaGEL

   CoLyte

   Dulcolax (the first *L* is often not pronounced)

   Evac-Q-Kit

   Fleet enema (often dictated incorrectly as Fleet's)

   GoLYTELY

   Maalox (double *a*)

   Mylanta (*y*, not *i*)

   Mylicon (*y*, not *i*)

   Phillips' Milk of Magnesia

   Zantac (not to be confused with Xanax, an antianxiety drug)

6. Dictation Challenges

   A typical dictation error is the plural of *diverticulum*, which is always *diverticula*, not *diverticulae*, *diverticuli*, *diverticulee*, or *diverticulas*, regardless of how pronounced.

   Physicians often dictate *melanotic* when they mean *melenic*. *Melenic* refers to the presence of melena, the passage of dark, bloody stools. *Melanotic* refers to melanosis, the presence of excessive melanin (pigment), usually in the skin, and is not related to the stool.

Transcription Tips

7. Dictation Challenges

Although you will often hear "coffee-ground emesis" dictated, common sense demands the plural, "coffee-grounds emesis," in this phrase.

When listening to dictation, do not confuse the anatomical term *colon* with the punctuation mark. Sometimes dictators say "colon mark" when they are dictating the punctuation mark.

Certain accents may cause the words *bile* and *bowel* to sound alike in dictation. Being "in the zone" and aware of the context and meaning of the words you are transcribing will prevent a transcription error like confusing *bile* and *bowel*.

8. *Dilation* and *dilatation* are often used interchangeably. They refer to the action of stretching or enlarging an organ or part of the body, e.g., dilation or dilatation of the stomach or esophagus.

9. The esophagus is the long "swallowing tube" that courses from the back pharynx to the stomach, while the trachea is the "breathing tube" that carries air into the lungs. Do not confuse the two!

Spotlight On

Transcribing Gastroenterology Dictation

by Bron Taylor

One of the satisfactions of this work is the degree to which you can teach yourself about medicine. You don't have to major in anatomy or become a pharmacy student, if you keep your ears and eyes open and soak up all the medical information you can, all the time.

The amount of anatomy to be learned is finite—there are a certain number of muscles and bones and nerves to learn, and anatomy can be learned so well that using it becomes automatic. New drugs and procedures are being constantly introduced, but once one knows the bulk of them, most of the work is done.

We don't want to give the impression that there is so much new information to be learned with every report that the transcriptionist must spend every day in a time-consuming search for new information. There are patterns that underlie what the dictators are saying, and it all makes good sense, and it's a great satisfaction to learn these—by any means. The reports themselves will teach you a great deal.

It's especially important in the beginning stages to resist pressure to guess and thus avoid leaving blanks in reports. Unfortunately, there are supervisors who encourage guessing and who will not allow blanks in reports, who think that pages without gaps are "good enough." You have to resist this pressure because it is just not safe to guess when you're working on a patient's permanent medical record.

Too many words sound alike. One of the best tools you can develop is a little bell of doubt that rings for you when you're really not sure what you're transcribing. When this little bell goes off, trust it—if you have a hunch that it might be wrong, it probably IS wrong. Look it up, ask someone, and, if you have to leave a blank, do that—and attach a note to the dictator.

With study and experience, one acquires a picture of what's happening behind the dictation, and everything starts to make sense. Mumbles become clear, your questions to the doctors become more astute and generate more interesting answers, you catch more mistakes, and you begin to see the bigger picture and realize how it all fits together. Some days you'll have the satisfaction of having a new procedure or drug already in mind before it's dictated, which is a nice "a-ha" feeling and brightens your day.

Not every day will be fascinating, for much of the dictation will be repetitive, but there are many rewards hidden in the dictation.

Exercises

Medical Vocabulary Review

Instructions: Choose the best answer.

___ 1. The first part of the small intestine is the ___
A. stomach.
B. esophagus.
C. duodenum.
D. sigmoid.

___ 2. The membranous sac that lines the abdominal and pelvic cavities, covering most of the organs, is the ___
A. omentum.
B. peritoneum.
C. jejunum.
D. diverticulum.

___ 3. _____ is produced in the liver, passes through a duct into the duodenum, and helps in the digestion of fats.
A. Bile
B. Acid
C. Salt
D. Bowel

___ 4. The _____, a retroperitoneal organ, produces enzymes passed through a duct into the duodenum for the digestion of carbohydrates, protein, and fat and insulin and other hormones which are released directly into the bloodstream.
A. liver
B. pylorus
C. pancreas
D. gallbladder

___ 5. A common cause of peptic ulcer disease is ___
A. *Helicobacter pylori.*
B. *Clostridium difficile.*
C. *Escherichia coli.*
D. *Giardia lamblia.*

___ 6. Which of the following tests might have been reported as revealing guaiac-positive stool?
A. Barium enema.
B. Hemoccult test.
C. IgM antibody.
D. Colonoscopy.

___ 7. The endoscopic procedure done to view the entire upper gastrointestinal tract is the ____
A. gastroscopy.
B. esophagoscopy.
C. small bowel follow-through.
D. esophagogastroduodenoscopy.

___ 8. Which of the following is NOT a localized weakness in the musculoaponeurotic wall of the abdomen, with protrusion of abdominal contents?
A. Umbilical hernia.
B. Femoral hernia.
C. Hiatus hernia.
D. Indirect inguinal hernia.

___ 9. A surgical procedure undertaken for purely diagnostic reasons is the _____
A. exploratory laparotomy.
B. diagnostic ultrasound.
C. magnetic resonance imaging.
D. laparoscopic cholecystectomy.

___10. Which of the following drugs is used in the treatment of *Helicobacter pylori* infections?
A. Flagyl.
B. gemfibrozil.
C. Pepcid.
D. Zofran.

___11. Which of the following is the generic drug name for Flagyl?
A. amoxicillin.
B. tetracycline.
C. metronidazole.
D. clarithromycin.

___ 12. Which of the following best describes the drug Pepcid?
A. It is an antispasmodic, anticholinergic drug used to slow peristalsis.
B. It is an antimicrobial used in combination with an antacid to treat *Helicobacter pylori* infection.
C. It is a proton pump inhibitor used to treat ulcers and gastroesophageal reflux disease.
D. It is an H$_2$ blocker antacid used to treat ulcers and gastroesophageal reflux disease.

___ 13. Ulcers and gastroesophageal reflux disease response to the drug Prilosec because it ___
A. neutralizes hydrochloric acid and raises the pH of the stomach contents.
B. is a combination of an antispasmodic drug with the a central nervous system sedative.
C. controls muscle contraction and peristalsis in the GI tract through the release of the neurotransmitter acetylcholine.
D. is a proton pump inhibitor that decreases gastric acid by blocking the final step of acid production to treat peptic ulcers.

___ 14. If you were suffering with irritable bowel syndrome, you might want to do all of the following EXCEPT ___
A. use a Fleet enema or GoLYTELY.
B. take an antispasmodic medication.
C. take alosetron or tegaserod, if you're a woman.
D. avoid foods and beverages that trigger a flareup.

___ 15. Proven *H pylori* infection is treated with a course of therapy including bismuth subsalicylate and two antibiotics, either ___
A. tetracycline or amoxicillin and metronidazole or clarithromycin.
B. esomeprazole or lansoprazole and omeprazole or pantoprazole.
C. cimetidine or famotidine and nizatidine or ranitidine.
D. scopolamine or phenobarbital and clidinium or chlordiazepoxide HCl.

___ 16. Which of the following statements best describes Zantac?
A. It is an H$_2$ blocker and the generic name is ranitidine.
B. It is a proton pump inhibitor and the generic name is omeprazole.
C. It is an H$_2$ blocker and the generic name is cimetidine.
D. It is a proton pump inhibitor and the generic name is ranitidine.

___ 17. Antiemetic drugs are often given prophylactically prior to beginning chemotherapy; this class of drugs includes which of the following?
A. Zofran (ondansetron).
B. Sandimmune (cyclosporine).
C. Duragesic (fentanyl).
D. Versed (midazolam HCl).

Spelling Exercise

Instructions: Review the adjective suffixes in your medical language textbook. Test your knowledge of **adjectives** by writing the adjectival form of the following gastroenterology words. Consult a medical dictionary to verify your spelling.

Noun	Adjective
1. abdomen	
2. antrum	
3. axilla	
4. bile (2 adj.)	
5. cecum	
6. colon	
7. cyst	
8. diaphragm	
9. diverticulum	
10. duodenum	
11. edema	
12. erosion	
13. esophagus	
14. fascia	
15. fiber	
16. fibril	
17. gluteus	
18. icterus	
19. pancreas	
20. umbilicus	

Forming Plurals

Instructions: Test your knowledge of plurals by writing the plural form of the following gastroenterology words. Consult a medical dictionary to confirm your spelling.

Singular	Plural
1. adenoma	_____
2. condyloma	_____
3. diverticulum	_____
4. borborygmus	_____

Abbreviations Exercise

Instructions: Expand the following common GI abbreviations and brief forms. Then memorize both abbreviations and definitions to increase your speed and accuracy in transcribing GI dictation.

Abbreviation	Expansion
1. appy	_____
2. AVM	_____
3. BE	_____
4. bili	_____
5. CEA	_____
6. EGD	_____
7. GE	_____
8. GERD	_____
9. GI	_____
10. IBS	_____
11. KUB	_____
12. lap chole	_____
13. LES	_____
14. LFTs	_____
15. LLQ	_____
16. LUQ	_____
17. NG (tube)	_____
18. n.p.o.	_____
19. p.o.	_____
20. procto	_____
21. PUD	_____
22. RLQ	_____
23. RUQ	_____
24. tic	_____
25. UGI series	_____

Dissecting Medical Terms

Instructions: As you learned in your medical language course, words are formed from prefixes, combining forms (root word plus combining vowel), and suffixes. Combining vowels (usually *o* but not always) are used to connect two root words or a root and a suffix. By analyzing these word parts, you can often determine the definition of a term without even looking it up (if you know the definition of the parts, of course!). Being able to divide and analyze the words you hear into their component parts will also improve your spelling and help you research those words that you cannot easily spell or define.

For the following terms, draw a slash (/) between the components and then write a short definition based on the meaning of the parts. Remember that to define a word based on its parts, you start at the end, usually with the suffix. If there's a prefix, that is defined next, and finally the combining form is defined.

Example: prepyloric

Divide & Analyze: pre/pyloro/ic
pertaining to (-ic)

Define: before (pre-) the pylorus (pylor)

1. appendectomy
   Divide _____
   _____
   Define _____

2. arthralgia
   Divide _____
   _____
   Define _____

3. bronchoscope
   Divide _____
   _____
   Define _____

4. colonoscopy
   Divide _____
   _____
   Define _____

5. epigastric
   Divide _____
   _____
   Define _____

6. fistulotomy
   Divide _____

   _____
   Define _____

7. gastrostomy
   Divide _____

   _____
   Define _____

8. hepatorrhaphy
   Divide _____

   _____
   Define _____

9. hypopharynx
   Divide _____

   _____
   Define _____

10. infraumbilical
    Divide _____

    _____
    Define _____

11. intra-abdominal
    Divide _____

    _____
    Define _____

12. intradermally
    Divide _____

    _____
    Define _____

13. laparoscopic
    Divide _____

    _____
    Define _____

14. laparotomy
    Divide _____

    _____
    Define _____

15. laryngectomy
    Divide _____

    _____
    Define _____

16. nasogastric
    Divide _____

    _____
    Define _____

17. paracolic
    Divide _____

    _____
    Define _____

18. perianal
    Divide _____

    _____
    Define _____

19. periumbilical
    Divide _____

    _____
    Define _____

20. polypectomy
    Divide _____

    _____
    Define _____

21. subcuticular
    Divide _____

    _____
    Define _____

22. subglottic
    Divide _____

    _____
    Define _____

Sample Reports

Sample gastroenterology reports appear on the following pages, illustrating a variety of reports. Fictional names are provided for illustration of proper format, and no resemblance to actual persons is intended. Sample transcripts were prepared according to *The Book of Style for Medical Transcription* (AHDI).

Chart Note

LACOURSIERE, SUZANNE
February 5, [add year]

The patient has primary biliary cirrhosis. I refilled the patient's colchicine. Articles were sent to the patient on primary biliary cirrhosis. The patient should have LFTs and a serum cholesterol drawn every 8 months, and I ordered a chem-25, CBC, iron, and TIBC. The results of these tests were within normal limits with the following important exceptions: serum iron was 45, which is low; TIBC was 433, which is high; and percent iron saturation was 10, which is low. Her ferritin was 10, which is also low. These results taken together indicate that the patient was iron deficient, and so I started her on Feosol 1 p.o. b.i.d. Her GGT was 105, which is elevated, and alkaline phosphatase was 209, which is also elevated. A CT scan of the abdomen has been done and was negative.

She continued to have abdominal pain. I gave her a trial of Reglan 10 mg p.o. q.i.d. and also scheduled an upper GI with small bowel follow through. The upper GI showed hesitancy in opening of the duodenal bulb, but the bulb was intrinsically normal and the duodenum was normal as well. The remainder of the upper GI series and small bowel series was normal. I don't believe the hesitancy in the opening of the duodenal bulb to be significant.

I saw the patient again with continued complaints of abdominal pain. At that time her friend had just died of colon cancer. She complained of fatigue and malaise, as well as new symptoms of reflux and heartburn.

My impression is that she has irritable bowel syndrome as well as esophageal reflux. I gave her a prescription for Sinequan 25 mg q.d. and a sample supply of Tagamet 400 mg b.i.d. The Tagamet improved her symptoms, as she called in for a refill.

HIEU NGUYEN, MD

HN:hpi
d: 2/25/[add year]
t: 2/26/[add year]

Consultation

KIM, YOONSUN
#9463452
July 24, [add year]
Referring physician: Mark Blank, MD

CHIEF COMPLAINT
Diarrhea and abdominal discomfort.

HISTORY OF PRESENT ILLNESS
This 31-year-old Korean female presented to the office today, having been referred by Dr. Blank for evaluation. She states she has been having problems with watery diarrhea. She admitted to nausea and vomiting on one occasion. These symptoms have been going on for approximately 1-1/2 months now. She said that her bowel movements had been regular. She denied any blood or mucus in her stools, although she added that she has some hemorrhoidal tags, and she did have a little bit of blood at times.

The patient claimed that she tried Donnagel and Pepto-Bismol without much help. It appeared that she also had diarrhea at night, and she may have 10 to 12 bowel movements a day. The patient's appetite has been depressed. She has lost approximately 18 pounds in the last 1-1/2 months.

PAST MEDICAL HISTORY
The patient claimed that she has perennial vasomotor rhinitis for which she receives treatment from Dr. Blank. There was no history of any other significant illnesses in the past.

SOCIAL HISTORY
The patient works as a medical transcriptionist. She denied smoking or the intake of any alcoholic beverages. She denied the intake of any coffee.

ALLERGIES
The patient claimed that she is allergic to penicillin and erythromycin.

FAMILY HISTORY
The patient has no knowledge of diabetes mellitus in her family. She claimed that her paternal grandparents suffer from hypertension. There was no history of cancer. The patient says that her father is an alcoholic, and he had gastrointestinal bleeding, question from gastritis or ulcer.

REVIEW OF SYSTEMS
Respiratory: Cough secondary to allergies and sinus problems.
Cardiovascular: The patient stated that she has palpitations at times experienced over the last 1-1/2 months.
Gastrointestinal: See History of Present Illness. The patient denied any esophageal symptoms but occasionally has indigestion.
Musculoskeletal: She gets slight discomfort in her right hip but takes no medication for that. This discomfort was only experienced in the last few months.

(continued)

Consultation

KIM, YOONSUN
#9463452
July 24, [add year]
Page 2

Genitourinary: Denied any flank pain, burning with micturition, change in the color or stream of urine.
Neurological: The patient claimed that in the last 1-1/2 months, she has experienced diplopia on 3 occasions lasting for less than 30 seconds. She had severe frontal headaches recently which lasted for half a day, which have subsided. She thinks this is because of her sinuses and allergies. She has a history of migraine headaches but only 3 to 4 times yearly. Denies any dizzy spells, blackouts, seizure disorder, paresthesia, or focal weakness.

PHYSICAL EXAMINATION
VITAL SIGNS: Height 5 feet 5-1/2 inches, weight 261 pounds. Blood pressure 168/92, pulse 100 per minute and regular with good volume. Respirations 18 to 20.
GENERAL: The patient is a well-developed slightly obese 31-year-old Caucasian female in no acute distress, alert, very well oriented, pleasant, and a good historian.
HEAD AND NECK: Examination of the head and neck was essentially unremarkable. There was no conjunctival pallor or scleral icterus. Funduscopic examination was normal.
CARDIOVASCULAR: Jugular venous pressure was not elevated. Carotid pulses were good and equal on both sides. Heart sounds were normal with no murmurs or gallops.
LUNGS: Trachea was central. Expansion was good and equal on both sides. Breath sounds were normal with no adventitious sounds.
ABDOMEN: The abdomen was soft and obese. There was slight tenderness on deep palpation in the epigastrium without any guarding or rebound. There were no palpable masses and no palpable organomegaly.
RECTAL: Examination revealed no external skin tags, no external anal fissures, and normal sphincter tone. There were no palpable masses or tenderness in the rectal ampulla, which was empty of stool.
EXTREMITIES: No finger or toe clubbing. No cyanosis or pedal edema.
NEUROLOGIC: Motor power, tone, and coordination were intact. Deep tendon reflexes were 1+ and equal on both sides. Sensation was not tested.

IMPRESSION
Abdominal pain and diarrhea, question of inflammatory bowel disease; differential diagnoses below.

DENISE LOEWEN, MD

DL:hpi
d: 7/24/[add year]
t: 7/25/[add year]

History and Physical Examination

CHICHESTER, MARK
#90438
Admitted: 6/1/[add year]
Medical 302C

ADMISSION DIAGNOSIS
Metastatic colon cancer.

HISTORY OF PRESENT ILLNESS
A 61-year-old white male who is status post sigmoid resection and segmentectomy of the liver for colon cancer, who presents because of liver metastasis on CT scan despite one year of 5-FU therapy. He is without complaint of loss of appetite, weight loss, nausea, vomiting, jaundice, melena, or hematochezia. He denies change in bowel habits since the operation but does chronically have bulky stools.

PAST MEDICAL HISTORY
Resection of the sigmoid with segmentectomy of the left lobe of the liver, secondary to metastases, and a primary colocolostomy. Metastases were also noted to the regional and retroperitoneal lymph nodes, which were also resected. Therapy with 5-FU was given as above.

MEDICATIONS ON ADMISSION
None.

ALLERGIES
None.

FAMILY HISTORY
There is no family history of cancer.

SOCIAL HISTORY
The patient does not smoke or drink.

PHYSICAL EXAMINATION
VITAL SIGNS: Blood pressure 110/70, pulse of 60, respiratory rate 18, temperature 36.
GENERAL: This is a well-developed, well-nourished white male in no acute distress.
HEAD & NECK: HEENT unremarkable. Neck is supple without jugular venous distention (JVD), adenopathy, or bruit.
CHEST: Lungs are clear.
HEART: Regular rate and rhythm.

(continued)

History and Physical Examination

CHICHESTER, MARK
#90438
Admitted: 6/1/[add year]
Medical 302C
Page 2

ABDOMEN: Soft, nondistended, and nontender. Liver is approximately 8-10 cm in span and does not descend below the right costal margin. There is no splenomegaly or masses.
LYMPH NODES: There is no palpable adenopathy throughout.
RECTAL: Normal anal sphincter tone. No masses. Stool was Hemoccult-negative.
NEUROLOGIC: Neurologically the patient is intact.

ADMISSION LABORATORY
Hemoglobin 14.4. White blood cells 6.9 with 66 segs, 19 lymphs, 5 monos, 9 eos, and 1 baso. Platelets 295,000. Astra was within normal limits. The profile showed an alkaline phosphatase of 141, AST of 29, total bilirubin of 0.5, total protein 7.5, albumin 3.9. PT is 11.5 and PTT is 28.1. Chest x-ray showed a small, approximately 1 cm nodule in the right lower lung and was otherwise normal.

PRINCIPAL DIAGNOSIS
Metastatic colon cancer.

KAREN ZEMPOLICH, MD

KZ:hpi
d: 6/1/[add year]
t: 6/1/[add year]

Comic Relief

Crude terms for passing gas usually elicit a snicker; so do euphemisms such as, "I have no idea what you're talking about." The same goes for other audible bodily functions. Gastroenterology reports often contain inadvertently funny passages, too, especially when it comes to "unmentionable" topics.

She complains of passing flatus at inopportune moments—not that there are many opportune moments.

Rectal exam revealed hyperplasia of the thyroid gland.

The patient eats lunch before every meal.

This GI is seen for GI complaints.

The patient stated she has problems swallowing but managed to down a wad of French fries during the interview.

She experiences nausea just before she goes to bed with her husband on an empty stomach.

Her weight loss surgery was canceled this morning because she ate a Whopper last night.

PEARSON
myhealthprofessionskit™

To access the online exercises and transcription practice, go to **www.myhealthprofessionskit.com**. Select "Medical Transcription," then click on the title of this book, ***Healthcare Documentation: Fundamentals & Practice***. Then click on the Gastroenterology chapter.

Orthopedics

16

Learning Objectives

▶ Describe the structure and function of the musculoskeletal system.

▶ Spell and define common orthopedic terms.

▶ Identify musculoskeletal vocabulary that might be used in the review of systems.

▶ Describe the negative and positive findings a physician looks for on examination of the back and extremities.

▶ Identify and define common fractures of the extremities.

▶ Describe the typical cause, course, and treatment options for common diseases of the musculoskeletal system.

▶ Identify and define common diagnostic and surgical procedures of the musculoskeletal system.

▶ List common orthopedic laboratory tests and procedures.

▶ Identify and describe common orthopedic drugs and their uses.

▶ Demonstrate knowledge of anatomical, medical, pharmacological, adjectival, and soundalike terms by accurately completing the exercises in this chapter.

Transcribing Orthopedic Dictation

Introduction

Have you ever had a broken bone or sprained an ankle? If so, you're in good company. Nearly everyone has experienced some kind of musculoskeletal problem at one time or another. In fact, orthopedic complaints are the number-one reason Americans seek medical care. According to the National Center for Health Statistics, orthopedic conditions (injuries, diseases, disorders) account for over half of physician office visits. Clearly, the person responsible for transcribing medical dictation must possess more than a casual acquaintance with orthopedics.

This is a 14-year-old gentleman who was playing football earlier today. He sustained a Salter-Harris II fracture of the distal tibia. There was displacement of over 1 cm. We did a reduction maneuver and were able to reduce the fracture relatively well. Under fluoroscopic guidance, we held it in an anatomically reduced position. We made a small percutaneous incision medially, and then using a guidewire pinned it across the fracture site, avoiding the growth plate. This held the fracture nicely reduced. We measured the guidewire and chose a 46 mm length screw, reamed, and then placed a 4.0 cannulated screw across the fracture site.

A medical doctor (MD) who specializes in treating injuries, diseases, and disorders of the musculoskeletal system is known as an **orthopedist** or **orthopedic surgeon.** Orthopedists usually train an additional three years in the diagnosis and treatment of bones, joints, muscles, and their corresponding tendons and ligaments.

Sports medicine physicians specialize in treating athletic injuries. Nonphysicians involved in musculoskeletal system care include physical therapists, massage therapists, personal trainers, and athletic trainers. Many revolutionary treatments have come from sports medicine.

A **neurologist** is a medical doctor who has had additional training in the study of the nervous system (neurology). A **neurosurgeon** performs surgery on the brain, spinal cord, and peripheral nervous system. A neurosurgeon is a neurologist, but a neurologist is not necessarily a neurosurgeon. How are these two disciplines related to orthopedics? The spinal column. Both orthopedic surgeons and neurosurgeons perform back surgery to correct conditions such as slipped disk, bulging disk, narrowing of the space between two vertebrae, and similar surgeries (see Chapter 17, Neurology).

He was found to have disk space degeneration at L1-2, L2-3, L3-4, L4-5, and L5-S1, with posterior bulging at L4-5 and L5-S1.

The **musculoskeletal system** comprises those structures that lend support and mobility to the body and that enable us to perform voluntary actions: bones, cartilage, muscles, and associated connective tissue structures (tendons, ligaments).

BONES

You may be one of the millions of students who moaned audibly when discovering that there are 206 bones in the human body. The good news is that it is not necessary to memorize all the individual bones. Excellent reference book skills are absolutely essential. You must be able to locate an anatomic structure in a medical dictionary, verify that it is the correct choice, and spell it perfectly. You and your medical dictionaries (print or electronic) will become best friends.

The smart approach is to memorize the approximate location of major bones. Every human being—male or female—has the same bones as you or me, with rare exceptions. There are a finite number of bones, and they don't change. Many structures related to bones have a similar name, and once you know where a bone is located, you can find its related structure in your references easier and faster.

"A both-bone fracture of the lower leg was present" will make sense when you understand that the tibia and fibula are two leg bones. If you know that the calcaneus is in the heel, it's much easier to locate the calcaneal (Achilles) tendon.

Learning the bones of the body is easier when you approach the task in small steps. Begin with the bones of the head and neck and work down as you learn where they are located and how they are spelled.

Dictators are much more likely to use the English term for a bone rather than its Latin equivalent "os"—for example, "occipital bone" rather than "os occipitale"; "head of the femur" rather than "caput femoris."

Anatomy Review

Bone is a type of tissue in which a framework or matrix of organic (protein) fibers is reinforced by deposits of calcium and phosphorus salts, which provide strength and rigidity. Bone is not inert material. It has a rich blood supply, it can heal after severe injury, and its calcium content is in equilibrium with the calcium level of the blood. Most bones are covered by a dense sheet of connective tissue called **periosteum**.

Each of the **long bones** of the extremities (see ■ Figure 16-1) is divided into a **diaphysis** (shaft), an **epiphysis** (enlarged, knobby end) and a **metaphysis** (between the diaphysis and the epiphysis). **Long bones**, and some others, are hollow and contain bone marrow in their cavities. **Bone marrow** is the site of production of red blood cells, white blood cells, and platelets.

Cartilage is a noncalcified connective tissue similar to bone. In most joints, the contacting surfaces of the bones are covered by protective layers of cartilage. Some weight-bearing joints (intervertebral joints, knees) contain thick cushions of tougher cartilage (**fibrocartilage**). Cartilage also provides semirigid support for the nose, the external ear, the larynx, and the trachea and bronchi.

Muscle is a unique type of tissue that has the property of contracting (shortening) under appropriate stimulation, usually neural. The respiratory, digestive, and urinary tracts contain **smooth muscle**, which is **innervated** by (receives its nerve supply from) the autonomic nervous system and is not subject to voluntary control. The muscle of the heart is also not subject to voluntary control.

The anatomic description of each **voluntary muscle** includes mention of its shape and position, its origin (bone or other structure that serves to anchor it), insertion (bone or other structure that is moved or stabilized by the muscle), action, blood supply, and innervation. Each muscle is supplied by a nerve containing **motor fibers** (to transmit impulses from the brain and spinal cord) and **sensory fibers** (for **proprioception**, that is, perception of position and movement). Each motor nerve is attached to its muscle at a motor end-plate, where nerve impulses trigger contraction of muscle fibers.

While some muscles are attached directly to the periosteum of the bones that serve as their origin and insertion, most muscles are modified at one or both ends and equipped with **connective tissue** bands that serve for attachment to muscle. A narrow cordlike band is called a **tendon**; a broad sheetlike connection is called an **aponeurosis**. Some tendons (for example, those at the wrist and ankle) pass through tubular sheaths that act somewhat like pulleys to control direction of pull and reduce local friction.

A **joint** is the site at which two bones **articulate** (connect, generally in an arrangement whereby one or both can move with respect to the other). The ends of bones forming a joint are usually protected by **articular cartilage** and sometimes by heavier fibrocartilage cushions (intervertebral disks, menisci of knees). The entire joint

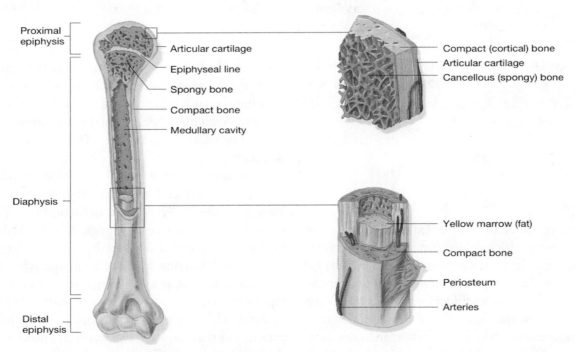

Proximal epiphysis
Articular cartilage
Epiphyseal line
Spongy bone
Compact bone
Medullary cavity

Compact (cortical) bone
Articular cartilage
Cancellous (spongy) bone

Diaphysis

Yellow marrow (fat)
Compact bone
Periosteum
Arteries

Distal epiphysis

FIGURE 16-1. Long bone components

is surrounded by a capsule of **synovial membrane**, a delicate, highly vascular connective tissue that secretes a lubricating fluid in small amounts.

A **ligament** is a band of inelastic connective tissue extending across the joint from one bone to the other to limit both the direction and the extent of motion at the joint. Most joints have several ligaments (the knee has 12).

Pause for Reflection

1. The dense sheet of connective tissue covering most bones is called the _____.
2. The shaft of a long bone is called the _____.
3. The contacting surfaces of the bones of the knee are covered by protective layers of thick _____.
4. While some muscles are attached directly to the periosteum of the bones that serve as their origin and insertion, most muscles are connected by narrow cordlike bands called _____ or a flat, sheetlike connection called an _____.
5. The subcutaneous tissue overlying some bony prominences contains one or more purselike cushions containing a little fluid to protect underlying surfaces and reduce friction; these cushions are called _____.
6. The site at which two bones connect or _____, generally in an arrangement whereby one or both can move with respect to the other, is called a _____.
7. A band of inelastic connective tissue extending across the joint from one bone to the other to limit both the direction and the extent of motion at the joint is called a _____.

Joint Movements

Joint movements of the upper extremities. Normal **wrist** movements include flexion, extension, radial deviation, ulnar deviation, supination, and pronation. The **elbow** can be put into flexion, extension, pronation, or supination. The **shoulder** (which has two major joints) can be put through internal rotation, external rotation, adduction, abduction, flexion, and extension (see ■ Figure 16-2).

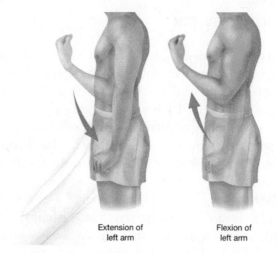

Extension of left arm · Flexion of left arm

FIGURE 16-2. Extension of left arm (left). Flexion of left arm (right).

Joint movements of the lower extremities. The **ankle** can be put through dorsiflexion, plantar flexion, eversion and inversion, and limited rotation. Normal **knee** movements include flexion and extension, but to some degree there are also rotation and sliding movements. Normal **hip** movements consist of abduction, adduction, internal rotation, and external rotation.

The **neck** can rotate on its axis, bend forward (flex) and backward (extend). Some flexible people can also move their neck from side to side on its axis.

> *The paramedics reported that at the accident site, the patient was moving the upper and lower extremities as well as the neck before he was immobilized on the gurney.*

Recall that **flexion** is to move a body part in toward the body. To flex your biceps muscle in the arm, bend your elbow. **Extension** is to move away from the body. To extend your arm, straighten it and lock the elbow. The physician may check for ability to extend and flex muscles by asking the patient to move joints in a certain direction.

The examiner may test for limitation of abduction and adduction of certain joints. **Abduction** is to draw away from the midline, while **adduction** is to draw in toward the body (see ■ Figure 16-3). Abduction increases the angle; adduction decreases the angle.

Internal rotation involves a circular-type of joint movement inward, just as **external rotation** is a similar type of movement outward. To test for internal rotation of the shoulder, for example, the doctor might have the patient put the arm back and move the hand as far up the back as possible. To check external rotation of the

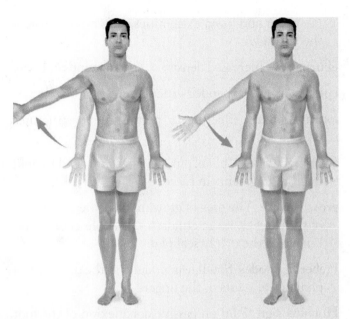

FIGURE 16-3. Abduction (left). Adduction (right).

shoulder, the examiner might ask the patient to put the arm out to the side with the elbow bent slightly and palm up, then move the elbow so that the palms rotates backward with the thumb pointing as far down as possible.

Dorsiflexion of the foot is with ankle bent upward and toes pointed toward the head (a **cephalad** direction). In **plantar flexion**, the ankle is bent downward with toes pointed toward the sole of the foot (see ■ Figure 16-4).

Volar means "palmar," and thus **volar flexion** is when the fingers are bent in toward the palm. **Ulnar deviation** or **drift** results when the fingers are shifted toward the pinkie finger, as might be seen in rheumatoid arthritis.

Inversion means to turn a body part inward, while **eversion** is turning outward. Eversion of the feet is the

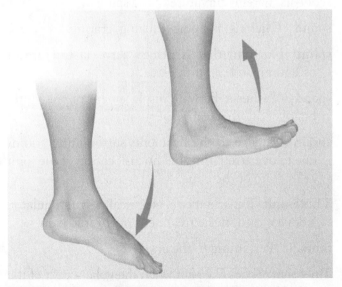

FIGURE 16-4. Plantar flexion of foot (left). Dorsiflexion of foot.

Tapping Out

When casino card dealers finish a shift, they "tap out." This involves one clap of the hands, then putting the hands in supination and pronation, respectively, to show they are not leaving the casino with unauthorized chips.

required position for a ballet dancer. **Pronation** indicates a downward or face-down position. When the palms of the hands are facing downward, they are in pronation. If they are facing upward, they are in **supination**.

There was 2/5 strength with dorsiflexion and plantar flexion of the feet bilaterally.

The elbow is limited to 160 degrees of extension and 75 degrees of flexion.

There was no evidence of tendinous involvement, and full flexion was observed as well as extension.

Her arm shows forward flexion of about 90 degrees, abduction 60 degrees, external rotation 20 degrees, and internal rotation 50 degrees.

Pause for Reflection

1. Bending the neck forward, bending the arm at the elbow to form an angle, or bending the leg at the knee is called _____.
2. Straightening the arm at the elbow or the leg at the knee is a movement called _____.
3. When the patient is asked to put the arm back and move the hand as far up the back as possible, the examiner is testing for _____ _____.
4. When the foot is bent upward at the ankle with the toes pointing toward the head, the foot is said to be in _____ and in _____ when bent in the opposite direction.
5. When the palms are facing downward, they are in _____ and in _____ when they are facing upward.
6. The site at which two bones connect is called _____.

Vocabulary Review

AK amputation Above-the-knee amputation.

ankylosis Immobility and consolidation of a joint due to disease, injury, or surgical procedure.

avascular necrosis Death of bone tissue with destruction of adjacent joint due to obstruction of blood supply as a result of trauma; long-term systemic treatment with corticosteroids in patients with lupus, rheumatoid arthritis, or vasculitis; chronic alcohol abuse; blood disorders; and other diseases.

BK amputation Below-knee amputation.

bone wax Gel-like material that is exactly like wax used in the kitchen. It has the ability to seal little pores in the bone that are exuding blood.

bony crepitus The crackling sound produced by the rubbing together of fragments of fractured bone.

bony process A component of bone, not bone itself. The greater and lesser trochanters are processes of the femur (thigh) bone.

bridging Formation of a bridge from one bone to another by abnormal calcium deposition, as in osteoarthritis.

bursa Purselike cushion containing a little fluid to protect underlying surfaces and reduce friction.

callus formation An unorganized meshwork of woven bone, which is formed following fracture of a bone and is normally replaced by hard adult bone.

cast Application of a solid material to immobilize an extremity or position of the body in the treatment of a fracture, dislocation, or severe injury. It may be made of plaster of Paris or fiberglass.

cervical Pertaining to the neck.

condyle A rounded projection on a bone. It usually serves as an articulation site at which two anatomical structures meet.

cortex, cortical bone. Compact bone which is dense and hard on the bone surface, like the bark of a tree.

crepitus See *bony crepitus* and *joint crepitus*.

deep tendon reflexes (DTRs) Occur in response to sudden stretching of a muscle, usually induced by tapping a tendon with a rubber-headed reflex hammer. Tendon reflexes are tested in several muscles of the upper and lower extremities, with comparison of the two sides.

eburnation Increased density of articular ends of bone.

epiphysis The expanded articular end of a long bone.

extraarticular Affecting or pertaining to structures other than joints.

fixation device A plate, pin, nail, or screw used to hold fracture fragments in place.

growth plate The area of growing tissue near the ends of the long bones in children and adolescents. Also known as the epiphyseal plate.

Heberden nodes Small firm nodules at the distal interphalangeal joints of the fingers.

Homans sign Pain on passive dorsiflexion of the foot indicative of deep venous thrombosis.

joint crepitus A grating sensation caused by the rubbing together of the dry synovial surfaces of joints.

kyphosis Forward hunching of the upper spine.

lumbar Pertaining to the midback.

osteophytes, osteophyte formation Outgrowths of bone from the surface.

rasp, raspatory A surgical file.

sacral Pertaining to the sacrum, a wedge-shaped mass of bone at the lower end of the spine that represents the fusion of five vertebrae and articulates with the pelvic bones.

saucerization Radical surgical excision of infected bone.

scoliosis Lateral curvature of the spine.

sounds Clicking, popping, rubbing, grating.

splint Flat nail that is placed across a fracture or osteotomy to hold it in place.

spondylolisthesis Forward displacement of one vertebra over another.

sprain Damage to the ligaments surrounding a joint due to overstretching, but no dislocation of the joint or fracture of the bone.

TENS unit Transcutaneous electrical nerve stimulator, a device used in the treatment of chronic pain.

thoracic Pertaining to the chest.

Tinel sign Shocklike pain when the volar aspect of the wrist is tapped; indicative of carpal tunnel syndrome.

Medical Readings

History and Physical Examination

by John H. Dirckx, MD

Review of Systems. The subject is questioned about prior diagnosis of, and treatment for, any fractures or dislocations, severe sprains, bursitis, tendinitis, or arthritis.

Most painful inflammatory conditions of the back and extremities are due to injury—either a single violent event or repeated straining or overuse. Hence the interviewer will attempt to elicit a history of trauma or unusual activities (moving furniture, sudden excessive athletic activity, change of job). Less likely possibilities are local infection and systemic disorders such as rheumatoid arthritis and gout.

As with pain anywhere, an effort is made to establish a complete profile of back or extremity pain by learning its exact location, radiation, severity, intermittency, aggravating or mitigating factors, and effect on normal function. A patient complaining of muscle or joint pain will be asked about concomitant heat, swelling, stiffness, or spasm, and the effects of rest, exercise, and medicines.

Physical Examination. A full orthopedic examination requires considerable cooperation from the patient in assuming various positions and performing various movements. In performing the orthopedic examination, the physician looks for any developmental or traumatic deformities not previously noted and any evidence of generalized conditions such as muscle wasting or weakness, stiffness, or tremors. The terms **varus** and **valgus** refer to abnormal deviations in joints of the extremities. In a **varus** deformity, the bone distal to the affected joint is deviated inward; hence **genu varum** means **bowleg**. **Valgus** is outward deviation of the distal bone; hence **genu valgum** means **knock-knee**.

The physician puts joints through a **passive range of motion (ROM)** and has the patient put them through an **active range of motion**, with or without resistance by the examiner. Muscles are assessed for development, bilateral symmetry, strength, tone, and spasm or tenderness. Bones are assessed for deformity, masses, or tenderness.

A **joint** is not simply the place where two bones are hooked together but a complex structure with highly specialized tissues, subject to many injuries and diseases. The physician examines joints for swelling, stiffness, thickening of synovial membranes, fluid, tenderness,

LAY AND MEDICAL TERMS	
ankle bone	talus
collar bone	clavicle
breast bone	sternum
elbow	olecranon process
finger or toe bone	phalanx
heel	calcaneus
kneecap	patella
seat bone	ischium
shin bone	tibia
shoulder blade	scapula
slipped disk	herniated nucleus pulposus
tail bone	coccyx
thigh bone	femur

and instability. The range of motion in a joint can be quantified with a **goniometer**, a simple device consisting of two arms connected at a movable joint, with a scale that reads in degrees of rotation.

In examining an injured extremity, the physician notes any swelling, deformity, cutaneous trauma, ecchymosis, or hematoma formation. The age of subcutaneous hemorrhage can be judged by its color. Muscular and skeletal structures are palpated for tenderness, spasm, deformity, or discontinuity, and active and passive ranges of motion are checked. Joints are palpated for crepitus or effusion and tested by manipulation for **ligamentous laxity**. The circulation and sensation of the part are also carefully evaluated.

The **back** is examined first with the subject standing and facing away from the examiner. Any spinal curvature or developmental deformities are noted, as well as any surgical scars. The heights of the iliac crests are compared as a rough test of leg length equality. The spinous processes of the vertebrae, the sacroiliac joints, and the sciatic notches are assessed by palpation for tenderness, the muscles for tenderness and spasm. The examiner notes the range of spinal movements as the subject bends forward, backward, and to the sides. The subject then lies supine (face up) on the examining table, and the physician tests for disorders of the sacroiliac and hip joints and for sciatic nerve irritation by manipulation of the lower extremities.

The **neck** is not simply a column for supporting the head. Through it pass all nerve connections between brain and body, all inspired oxygen and exhaled carbon dioxide, all swallowed food and drink, and all blood supply to the brain, which consumes 25% of the body's oxygen intake. Because subtle abnormalities of the neck can herald life-threatening developments, the region is carefully assessed.

The **neck** is subject to many musculoskeletal injuries and disorders, some of which can affect its configuration and mobility in obvious ways. The examiner tests neck mobility by gently grasping the subject's head and putting it through a range of movements, noting any restrictions due to joint stiffness, muscle spasm, or pain.

Pause for Reflection

1. In the Review of Systems, if the patient is complaining of painful inflammatory conditions of the back and extremities, the interviewer will attempt to elicit a history of _____.
2. On physical examination, when the examiner observes abnormal deviations in joints of the extremities, if the bone distal to the affected joint is deviated inward, the patient is said to have a _____ deformity; if there is outward deviation of the distal bone, the patient has a _____ deformity.
3. When the physician puts a joint through a range of motion, it is said to be _____; when the patient moves the joint through range of motion, it is said to be _____.
4. Palpation of the joints allows the examiner to assess the presence or absence of _____ characterized by a rubbing or grating sound and _____ evidenced by swelling due to the presence of fluid in the joint.
5. Manipulation of the patient's joint by the examiner is a test for _____.

Trauma

You might remember from grade school that there are 206 bones in the human body. We are actually born with over 300 bones, but many of these fuse together to form one larger bone. That's a lot of bones to break!

Our bodies continue to weave new bone as long as we live. In neonates (newborns), bone growth is greatly accelerated such that a fractured bone will heal in a matter of days. Fractures are common in children. A fracture at the **epiphyseal plate**, or **growth plate**, in a child is serious, however, because it can cause stunting of bone growth.

This 8-year-old gymnast fell off the uneven parallel bars, landing on her right side, and sustained a radio-humeral fracture perilously near the epiphyseal plate.

The older we get, the slower our bone growth and ability to form **callus**, the bony substance responsible for knitting broken bones together properly. Our bones become more brittle as we age, and a fall is more likely to result in a fracture than it would have were we younger. A fractured bone in an elderly person may take months to heal, may form a cartilaginous repair instead of bony, or may not heal at all. Sometimes, **osteophyte** formation occurs around the healed fracture site. The **periosteum**, which covers the surface of all bones except at the joints, has nerve endings, unlike the rest of the bone, and is responsible for feeling pain on manipulation of a fractured bone.

Generally, fractures may be classified as **open**, **closed**, **displaced**, or **nondisplaced** (see below), but additional distinctions are numerous. Fractures are generally identified by the **name of the bone** involved (metacarpal fracture, phalangeal fracture, calcaneal fracture), **appearance** (bucket-handle, comminuted, angulated), an **eponym** (Colles), or **classification** system (Salter-Harris) (see ■ Figure 16-5).

angulated fracture Fracture in which the fragments are at an angle to one another.

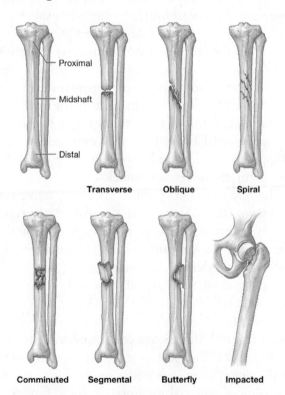

FIGURE 16-5. Classification of fractures

avulsion fracture Forcible separation of a fragment of bone at a site of tendon or ligament attachment.

bimalleolar fracture Fracture of the medial and lateral malleoli, the bony prominences on the sides of the ankle.

both-bone fracture Fracture of two adjacent bones in a limb, either radius and ulna (forearm) or tibia and fibula (leg).

bucket-handle fracture Microfractures through the immature part of the bone edge of the metaphysis in infants, caused by shearing, often seen in rapid acceleration and deceleration forces to the extremity.

buckle fracture A type of **impaction** fracture that generally occurs at the transition from diaphysis to metaphysis.

butterfly fracture A long-bone fracture in which the central fragment is triangular-shaped.

closed fracture Fracture with no open skin wound (see ■ Figure 16-6). Also called *simple fracture*.

Colles fracture Fracture of the distal radius with dorsal displacement, with or without involvement of the ulna.

comminuted fracture Fracture in which the bone is shattered, splintered, or crushed into many small pieces or fragments.

complex fracture Closed fracture with extensive injury to adjacent tissues.

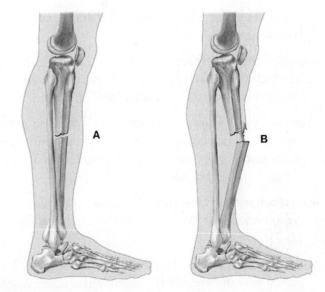

FIGURE 16-6. (A) Closed (or simple) and (B) open (or compound) fractures

compound fracture Also called *open fracture*.

compression fracture Fracture caused by longitudinal force. Usually refers to fracture of the vertebrae.

displaced fracture Fracture in which the fragments are not in anatomic alignment.

femoral neck fracture Fracture through the neck of the femur, proximal to the greater and lesser trochanter (see ■ Figure 16-7).

greenstick fracture Fracture in which there is an incomplete break; one side of bone is broken and the other side is bent. This type of fracture is commonly

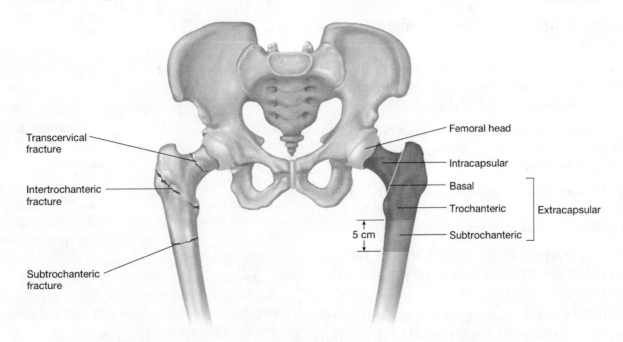

Transcervical fracture

Intertrochanteric fracture

Subtrochanteric fracture

Femoral head

Intracapsular

Basal

Trochanteric

Subtrochanteric

Extracapsular

5 cm

FIGURE 16-7 Intracapsular and extracapsular areas of the hip and types of hip fractures

found in children due to their softer and more pliable bone structure.

impacted fracture Fracture commonly seen in children in which the broken ends of the bone are driven into each other. May also be called *buckle fracture*.

intercondylar fracture Fracture of the humerus between its two condyles, the rounded prominences at the end of the humerus, in the shape of a T. Also called *T-shaped fracture*.

intertrochanteric fracture Fracture between the greater and lesser trochanters of the hip (see ■ Figure 16-7).

nondisplaced fracture Fracture in which the break is partial or complete, but the alignment is maintained.

nonunion fracture Fracture in which the realigned bone fragments have failed to heal.

oblique fracture Fracture that is curved or slanting, neither transverse nor at an acute angle, caused by a rotational force.

open fracture Fracture in which the broken end of a bone pierces through the skin. It may recede back and be hidden, but leaves an open wound. This type of fracture is particularly ominous because of the risk of a deep bone infection (see ■ Figure 16-6). Also called *compound fracture*.

pathological fracture Fracture of a bone weakened due to disease such as osteomyelitis or other disease, not due to injury.

Salter-Harris fracture Fracture of the epiphyseal plate in children.

spiral fracture Also called a **torsion fracture** in which the bones have been twisted apart by a rotational force. Often seen in cases of physical abuse.

stress fracture A crack in the cortex of a bone caused by repetitive stress, as in running, rather than by a single violent event.

torus fracture Fracture in which there is a bulging or swelling of the cortex of the bone with little or no displacement. Not the same as a *torsion fracture*.

transverse fracture of the radius Complete fracture that is straight across the bone at right angles to the long axis of the bone.

trimalleolar fracture Fracture of the medial and lateral malleoli and the posterior process of the tibia.

He sustained an open, highly comminuted right tibiofibular fracture, and there is an external fixation device on the right leg.

Treatment of fractures varies depending on severity and may include a **cast**, **brace**, **splint**, **reduction** (aligning displaced fragments), or surgery (**open reduction**). **Pins, nails, rods,** or **screws** are often be used to stabilize the fragments (**internal fixation**).

Occasionally an **external fixation device** may be required. This involves drilling holes through the skin and into the bone, inserting hardware into the bone, and securing it with a device on the outside of the body.

To regain mobility (use) after the cast or splint comes off, physical therapy may be ordered with active or passive range of motion exercises, ultrasound, whirlpool, and/or application of dry or moist heat.

Moist heat, ultrasound, and range-of-motion exercises were prescribed for her shoulder injury.

Pause for Reflection

1. Stunted bone growth in a child may result from a fracture of the _____ or _____ plate.
2. A sign that a fracture is healing is the presence of _____.
3. A patient feels pain on manipulation of a broken bone because of nerve endings in the _____.
4. The risk of a deep bone infection is particularly associated with a(n) _____ fracture.
5. A serious fracture in which the bone fragments are not aligned is a(n) _____ fracture.
6. A(n) _____ fracture is a fracture of the hip.
7. _____ or _____ fractures involve the bones of the ankle.
8. A(n) _____ fracture is a fracture of the humerus.
9. _____ and _____ is an operative procedure in which pins, rods, screws, or nails are used to secure fracture fragments in alignment.
10. _____ involves drilling holes through the skin and into the bone, inserting hardware into the bone, and securing it with a device on the outside of the body.

Common Diseases

Muscular Dystrophy

This term includes a number of inherited disorders of voluntary muscle tissue having various clinical features. Some begin in infancy and others in middle age; some cause death within a few years and others progress slowly and have little impact on lifestyle or life expectancy.

Progressive muscular weakness and wasting of muscle tissue are features of most types of muscular dystrophy. In some types, enlargement of affected muscles (**pseudohypertrophy**) occurs. Some are associated with mental retardation or other defects.

Diagnosis is made by history (including family history), physical examination, electromyography, muscle biopsy, and detection of elevated serum creatine kinase. Prenatal diagnosis is possible. Treatment is purely supportive and consists of physical therapy and regular exercise.

Scoliosis

Lateral curvature of the spine in the erect position, due to malalignment of vertebrae. Two types are recognized. **Structural scoliosis** affects the vertebrae primarily. It may be caused by bone, nerve, or muscle disease, but in 90% of cases the cause is unknown. In most of these cases a genetic cause is likely. This type of scoliosis is both more common and more severe in women. Onset is around the age of puberty.

Nonstructural scoliosis occurs as a result of abnormality or disease other than in the affected vertebrae. Many cases are due to significant discrepancy in leg length, which brings about a compensatory curve in the upper spine to keep the head and shoulders level.

In both types of scoliosis, there is usually some rotational deformity of the spine in addition to lateral curvature. Generally there are no symptoms at first, and detection is made on routine physical examination, chest x-ray, or school screening. Direct inspection of the back often fails to disclose mild scoliosis, especially in overweight patients. When a person with scoliosis bends forward from the waist, one side of the thorax appears more prominent than the other because of the rotatory component of the deformity. X-ray examination and measurement of the curvature is needed for precise diagnosis.

A curvature of more than 20 degrees is considered significant, particularly because it is likely to progress. When significant scoliosis is detected before the mid-teens, vigorous efforts are made to correct it before spinal growth ceases. Correction is by bracing or casting. In severe or neglected cases, surgical fusion of the spine may be indicated. Untreated scoliosis may lead to severe deformity and disability, even compromise of cardiac and pulmonary function.

Tendinitis (Tenosynovitis)

Inflammation of a **tendon** or, more precisely, of a **tendon sheat**h. The cause is usually repetitive or extreme strain on the tendon, as in an occupational or athletic setting. The symptoms are pain on active or passive movement of the part, localized tenderness over the tendon, and sometimes swelling and **crepitus** (grating, grinding, or crunching sounds) with movement. Disability may be severe, but spontaneous resolution usually occurs if the inciting activity can be stopped.

Treatment is with analgesics and anti-inflammatory agents, wrapping or splinting, and local heat. Injection of adrenal corticosteroid into the site of inflammation often yields prompt temporary relief, but repeated injections may lead to complications, including rupture of the tendon.

Carpal Tunnel Syndrome (CTS)

Pain, tingling, and hypesthesia or anesthesia in the thenar (the fleshy part of the palm proximal to the thumb and index finger), with weakness and eventual atrophy in muscles of the thenar supplied by the median nerve, as a result of compression of this nerve on the volar aspect of the wrist where it passes through the carpal tunnel, formed by wrist bones and the nonyielding carpal ligament (see ■ Figure 16-8).

Many cases are induced by repetitive wrist flexion, as in jobs or hobbies. The incidence is increased during pregnancy and among persons with certain systemic diseases (diabetes mellitus, hypothyroidism, rheumatoid arthritis).

Pain and tingling sometimes wake the patient at night and elicit the response of shaking the hand to restore normal feeling. **Tinel sign** (shocklike pain when the volar aspect of the wrist is tapped) and **Phalen sign** (reproduction of pain or paresthesia when both wrists are flexed with the hands firmly pressing one another back-to-back for 60 seconds) are positive. Electromyography and nerve conduction velocity studies can confirm the site of nerve compression.

Treatment: Removal of known underlying causes; splinting, at least at night; physical therapy; local injection of corticosteroid; and often surgical division of the carpal ligament.

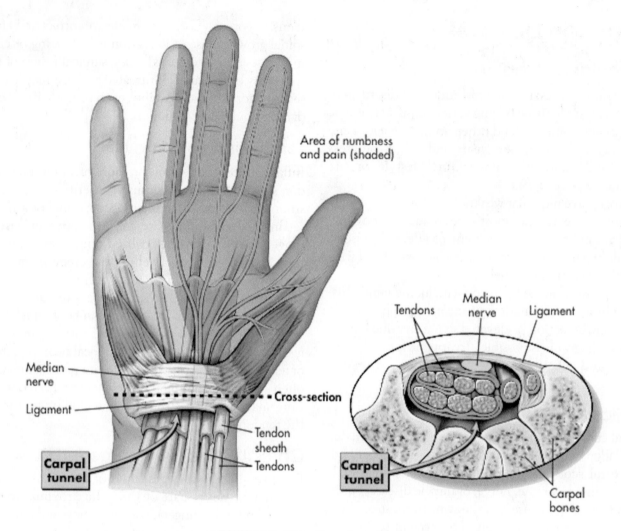

FIGURE 16-8. Carpal tunnel syndrome

Bursitis

Inflammation of a **bursa** (see ■ Figure 16-9), usually due to local trauma, often repetitive (kneeling on concrete, working overhead). Inflammation can also result from local infection or as an extension from an inflamed joint. Onset is typically sudden; initial symptoms are sharply localized pain and tenderness and often pronounced swelling, with **fluctuancy** (the sensation of contained fluid on palpation) due to accumulation of inflammatory fluid within the affected bursa. The diagnosis is usually evident from the history and physical examination.

If infection is suspected, the bursa must be aspirated and the fluid examined by smear and culture for pathogenic microorganisms. Treatment options include rest, immobilization if necessary, local heat, nonsteroidal anti-inflammatory drugs, local corticosteroid injections, and antibiotics for infection if present.

Common sites of bursitis are subdeltoid (near the point of the shoulder), olecranon (near the point of the elbow), prepatellar (overlying the patella; housemaid's knee), popliteal (**Baker cyst**; fluctuant swelling of the bursa behind the knee joint, which communicates with the joint space, as a result of local trauma or disease), and calcaneal (near the point of the heel).

Fibromyalgia Syndrome

A syndrome of chronic musculoskeletal pain accompanied by weakness, fatigue, and sleep disorders.

Cause: Unknown. The condition occurs almost exclusively in adult women with onset before age 50. Depression and viral infection have been proposed as underlying causes in some cases. The disorder sometimes occurs in hypothyroidism.

History: Chronic widespread aching and stiffness, typically bilaterally symmetrical and involving particularly the neck, shoulders, back, and hips, which is aggravated by use of affected muscles. Usually there are associated fatigue, a sense of weakness or inability to perform certain movements, paresthesia, difficulty sleeping, and headaches.

Physical Examination: Trigger points: sharply localized and extremely tender points, particularly in the neck and back, and often bilaterally symmetric. Some of these points may correspond to sites of pain and others may be painless until palpated. Otherwise examination is normal. There is no fever or local swelling or redness, and joints are not involved.

Diagnostic Tests: Complete blood count, erythrocyte sedimentation rate, and imaging studies yield uniformly normal results.

Course: The condition tends to be chronic, with moderate to severe disability, but symptoms can usually be mitigated by treatment. Symptoms do not progress, and objective signs of disease never develop.

Treatment: Education, exercise, physical therapy. Duloxetine, milnacipran, and pregabalin relieve pain and related symptoms in many patients.

Torn Meniscus

The menisci are crescent- or C-shaped pads of fibrocartilage within the **knee joint** (see ■ Figure 16-9), one medial and one lateral, that cushion shocks between the femur and the tibia. Injury to a meniscus is common and usually results from twisting the knee joint with the foot planted, often in an athletic setting. The patient hears a **pop** and feels sudden severe pain. Swelling develops soon, and the knee may lock or buckle with weightbearing. The **medial meniscus** is torn 10 times as often as the **lateral meniscus**. Meniscal tears do not heal. A piece broken off a meniscus remains in the joint as a **loose body** and may impair mobility.

Exam shows effusion of fluid into the joint space, crepitus, and a positive **McMurray test**—extension of the knee from full flexion with the leg and foot externally rotated causes an audible or palpable snap in medial meniscus tear; extension with the leg and foot internally rotated causes a snap in lateral meniscus tear. Treatment is with ice, elevation, a bulky compression dressing, and crutches, with attention to maintaining mobility and muscle strength and tone in the **quadriceps muscle** (the large four-headed muscle on the front of the thigh that extends the knee joint). Mild tears may eventually become asymptomatic. For persistent symptoms, **arthroscopic** (but occasionally open) **surgery**

A bucket-handle lesion of the medial meniscus was identified on MRI scanning of the right knee.

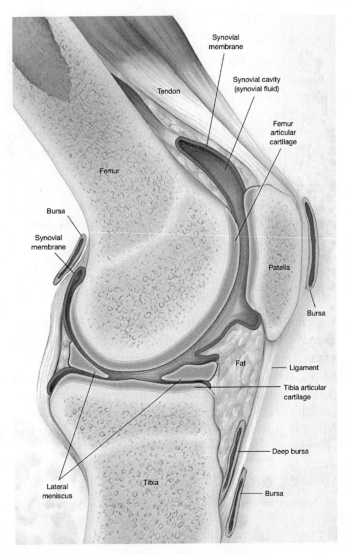

FIGURE 16-9. Knee joint

is required, with removal of loose fragments and reshaping of remaining cartilage.

Patellofemoral Syndrome

Pain in the **knee** (see ■ Figure 16-9), occurring most often in active teenagers or young adults, due to abnormal friction between the patella (kneecap) and the groove on the femur in which it slides. Any disturbance in the normal alignment or tracking of the patella in its groove, such as may result from uneven pull by the four heads of the **quadriceps muscle**, can cause chronic trauma to the back of the patella, with resultant **degenerative changes** (roughening, fraying, even complete loss of cartilage), known collectively as **chondromalacia patellae**. The principal symptom is pain with walking, especially on stairs, and with squatting.

Physical examination shows tenderness on manipulation of the patella and sometimes swelling and crepitus. X-rays are negative. Some cases resolve spontaneously

TORN MENISCUS

Cartilage is vital to freedom of movement. In fact, loss of cartilage (degeneration) affects the shape and makeup of a joint so it doesn't function smoothly. It can cause fragments of bone and cartilage to float in joint fluid, resulting in pain and dysfunction.

The menisci in the knees are made up of fibro-cartilage. You may have heard someone say they "tore" the cartilage in their knee, meaning the meniscus. Degeneration of cartilage is also linked to loss of synovial fluid, often resulting in osteo-arthritis.

with rest and anti-inflammatory medicines. **Quadriceps exercises** (repeatedly bringing the knee into full extension, with tensing of the muscles of the front of the thigh) often help to correct muscle imbalances. Shaving the roughened posterior surface of the patella arthroscopically may relieve pain. If tracking of the patella in its groove on the anterior femur is grossly deviant, surgical transplantation of the patellar tendon may be needed.

Osteoporosis

A disorder in which the density of bone is inadequate for its normal supporting function (see ■ Figure 16-10).

Causes: Resorption of calcium from bone to maintain serum calcium level, a complex phenomenon involving parathyroid hormone, intestinal and renal function, activity level, and dietary intake of calcium, phosphorus, and vitamin D. Postmenopausal deficiency of estrogen increases sensitivity of bone to factors that promote calcium loss; 80% of patients are post-menopausal women. Other causes include genetic disorders (cystic fibrosis, Marfan syndrome, osteogenesis

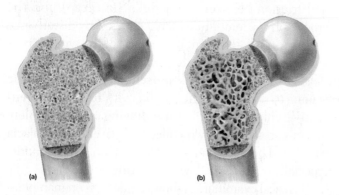

FIGURE 16-10. Osteoporosis: (a) Normal spongy bone. (b) Spongy bone with osteoporosis.

imperfecta), endocrine disorders (diabetes mellitus, Cushing syndrome, thyrotoxicosis, hyperparathy-roidism), prolonged amenorrhea in female athletes, and reduced level of mobility and physical activity because of illness, injury, or lifestyle. Asian or Caucasian race, underweight, dietary calcium deficiency, alcohol use, and cigarette smoking are all risk factors.

History: Backache, reduction of stature, **kyphosis** (forward hunching of the upper spine) (see ■ Figure 16-11), **pathologic fractures** (fractures for which under-lying abnormality of bone are partly responsible).

Physical Examination: Unremarkable except for features noted above.

Diagnostic Tests: X-ray examination shows bone deformity or fractures but does not reliably demonstrate minor degrees of demineralization. Bone density is more accurately assessed by CT scan, single-photon absorp-tiometry (SPA), dual-energy x-ray absorptiometry (DEXA), or ultrasound.

Course: Osteoporosis is responsible for 50% of frac-tures occurring in women over age 50. Compression fractures of the vertebrae and traumatic fractures of the wrist and femoral neck are most common. Gradual col-lapse of vertebrae causes loss of body height and senile kyphosis. The one-year mortality after hip fracture is about 20%.

Treatment: Administration of calcium along with vitamin D and calcitonin (orally or nasally). Bisphos-phonates (alendronate, etidronate) improve resistance of bone to enzymatic breakdown. Raloxifene (a selec-tive estrogen receptor modulator), strontium ranelate, and teriparatide (synthetic parathyroid hormone) reduce fracture risk in postmenopausal osteoporosis. Men with reduced androgen levels are treated with testosterone. Physical therapy, increased mobility.

Osteomyelitis

Bacterial infection of bone.

Cause: Infection with staphylococci, streptococci, or other organisms. Bacteria may be introduced directly into bone tissue (gunshot wound, surgery, compound fracture) or migrate there from adjacent soft tissue infection (sinusitis, deep abscess) or a remote source (systemic infections such as typhoid or tuberculosis, bacteremia in IV drug abusers). Osteomyelitis due to *Salmonella* frequently occurs as a complication of sickle cell disease and other inherited hemoglobin abnormal-ities.

History: Gradual or sudden onset of bone pain, fever, and chills.

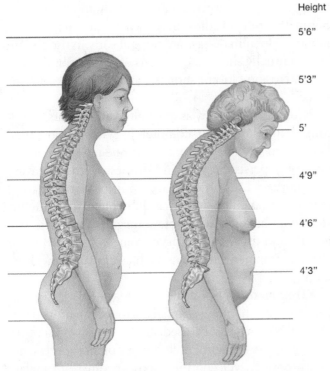

Height
5'6"
5'3"
5'
4'9"
4'6"
4'3"

FIGURE 16-11. Spinal changes caused by osteoporosis. Kyphosis shown at 50 and 70 years old.

Physical Examination: Fever, tenderness of site of infection. In severe infection there may be signs of toxemia.

Diagnostic Tests: The erythrocyte sedimentation rate is elevated. Causative organisms can be cultured from material aspirated from infected bone or from the blood. Serologic studies can identify infection due to *Salmonella*. X-ray or, preferably, CT and MRI studies show local swelling, decalcification, and eventually erosive destruction of bone.

Course: Without prompt treatment, infection may become chronic. Bone destruction can lead to severe deformity and disability.

Treatment: Rest, immobilization, analgesics. Antibiotics based on culture findings. Surgical drainage of the infection site. Severe or advanced disease may require radical surgical excision of infected bone (**saucerization**). Physical therapy as needed.

Arthritis

Inflammation of one or more joints. Arthritis is not just one disease but a group of many (perhaps over 200) that have joint inflammation as a common feature.

Degenerative Joint Disease (DJD; Osteoarthritis)

A joint disorder characterized by degeneration of articular cartilage.

Cause: Unknown. Familial factors may be involved. Cartilage protecting articular surfaces of bones degenerates, allowing bony surfaces to touch and erode each other. Hypertrophy of bone at the affected site adds to symptoms. Onset of symptoms is typically in early middle-age. Trauma, overweight, and the presence of other orthopedic disorders in the area of the affected joint may precipitate or accelerate symptoms.

History: Gradual onset of pain and stiffness in joints, particularly the intervertebral joints, hips, and knees; pain is aggravated by activity and relieved by rest.

Physical Examination: Stiffness, crepitus, and occasional swelling of affected joints. **Heberden nodes** (small firm nodules at the distal interphalangeal joints of the fingers) may be present.

Diagnostic Tests: X-rays show narrowing of joint spaces due to destruction and wearing away of cartilage; increased density (**eburnation**) of articular ends of bone due to mutual compaction after loss of protective cartilage; and hypertrophy of bone near the joint, with formation of **osteophytes** (outgrowths of bone from the surface) variously described as beaking, lipping, and bridging (forming a bridge from one bone to the other).

Course: Progressive pain and stiffening of joints, with eventual deformity and disability, may occur.

Treatment: Rest, physical therapy, prescribed exercise programs, correction of underlying causes if possible, weight reduction in overweight patients, mild analgesics (acetaminophen). Surgical replacement of the hip or knee joint reduces pain and improves mobility.

Rheumatoid Arthritis

A chronic systemic disease causing inflammatory changes in many tissues, particularly joint membranes (see ■ Figure 16-12).

Cause: Formation of antibody to one's own tissues, particularly **synovial membranes**. About 1–2% of the population are affected, and the disease is three times more common in women. It tends to run in families. Onset is typically between 20 and 40 and may be triggered by emotional or physical stress, surgery, or childbirth.

History: Gradual onset of pain, stiffness, and warmth in joints, particularly **smaller joints** (proximal

RHEUMATOID ARTHRITIS

Rheumatologists specialize in the field of rheumatology, the branch of medicine that deals with rheumatic disorders. A rheumatologist is not usually an orthopedist, but rather a pediatrician or internal medicine physician who devotes an additional two to three years to specialized rheumatology training.

Rheumatic diseases are thought to be caused by an autoimmune disorder, perhaps triggered by a virus, in which the body's own defenses begin to attack its own structures. The body's defenses do not seem to recognize the synovial membrane surrounding a joint and attack it as an invader.

interphalangeal and metacarpophalangeal joints, wrists, knees, ankles, and toes). Stiffness is worse in the morning (**"jelling"**). Malaise, fever, and weight loss may accompany the onset of the disease.

Physical Examination: Tenderness, warmth, stiffness of affected joints. Enlargement and deformity of joints, including ulnar deviation of finger joints, may occur late. About 20% of patients have subcutaneous nodules over bony prominences on extremities.

Diagnostic Tests: The erythrocyte sedimentation rate is elevated. A mild anemia is common, and platelets may be increased. Testing for rheumatoid arthritis (RA) factor is positive in about 75% of patients, and for antinuclear antibody in about 20%. Serum protein studies may detect an increase in immune globulin. X-rays are normal early in the disease but eventually show osteoporosis of bone near affected joints, erosion of joint surfaces, and narrowing of joint spaces.

Course: In as many as one half of all patients, symptoms remit largely or completely within two years. Patients in whom symptoms continue may have intermittent or persistent pain and stiffness, with increasing deformity and fusion of affected joints. Extraarticular manifestations include pericarditis, pleurisy with effusion, lymphadenopathy, splenomegaly, vasculitis, dry mouth and eyes (Sjögren syndrome), and peripheral nerve entrapment problems such as carpal tunnel syndrome.

Treatment: The standard treatment is aspirin (ASA), but other nonsteroidal anti-inflammatory drugs (NSAIDs) may also be used. In refractory cases other drugs may prove useful, including immunosuppressants (azathioprine, cyclosporine, methotrexate), antimalarials, gold salts, and adrenal corticosteroids. All of these drugs have problematic side effects or toxicities. Physical therapy is important in maintaining mobility. Surgery may be needed to correct severe deformity.

Gout

A systemic disease with joint symptoms due to deposition of urate crystals.

Causes: Elevation of serum uric acid due to overproduction, impaired excretion, or both. Some forms of gout are hereditary. Signs and symptoms of gout can be

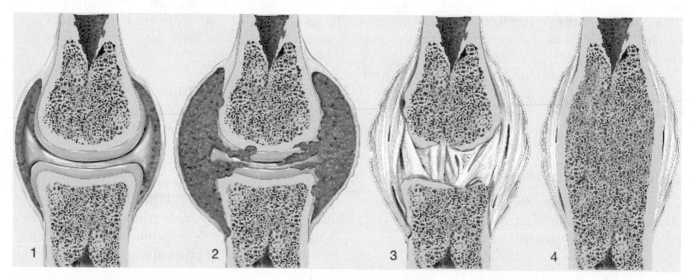

FIGURE 16-12. Rheumatoid arthritis: 1. Inflammation of synovial membrane and beginning changes. 2. Progression of inflammation and beginning of cartilage destruction. 3. Complete loss of synovial membrane, which leads to fibrous tissue. 4. Advanced stage of complete joint loss and osteoporosis.

precipitated by certain drugs (thiazide diuretics, nicotinic acid, low-dose aspirin), malignancies of blood-forming tissues and other disorders characterized by rapid breakdown of cellular nucleic acid, renal disease, hypothyroidism, and lead poisoning (saturnine gout). Nearly all patients are men over 40.

History: Recurrent acute episodes of severe pain, tenderness, and swelling, usually affecting a single joint, often occurring at night, and separated by symptom-free intervals. The first metatarsophalangeal joint is most often affected. After the acute episode, itching and scaling of the skin overlying the affected joint. Eventual development of nodules in soft tissues.

Physical Examination: Redness, swelling, and exquisite tenderness of the affected joint. **Tophi** (nodular deposits of urate crystals with local inflammation) may appear in cartilage (the outer ear), in tissues around joints (subcutaneous tissue, tendons), or at other sites.

> *The patient presented with pain in the great toe of the right foot and had a significantly elevated uric acid level.*

Diagnostic Tests: The serum **uric acid level** is generally elevated, as well as the erythrocyte sedimentation rate. Microscopic examination of material aspirated from affected joints or tophi shows urate crystals. In chronic disease, x-rays may show tophi in bone as punched out (radiolucent) areas.

Course: Without treatment an acute attack can last for days or weeks. Chronic disease may lead to joint destruction, deformity, and disability. Uric acid kidney stones are a common complication. With advanced disease, renal failure may occur.

Treatment: An acute attack of gout is promptly aborted by nonsteroidal anti-inflammatory agents or corticosteroid. Rest and immobilization may also be important in shortening the attack. Options for prophylactic treatment between attacks include drugs that inhibit uric acid production (allopurinol) or increase its excretion (probenecid). Colchicine can also be used. Abstinence from certain foods (liver, sweetbreads, anchovies) and alcohol is usually recommended, but the impact of dietary restrictions is minimal in a patient taking adequate doses of prophylactic medicine.

Lupus Erythematosus (LE)

A chronic inflammatory disorder of connective tissue due to formation of antibody to nucleoprotein. In this autoimmune disorder the body attacks its own connective tissue.

Cause: Unknown. Ninety percent of patients are young women. Antinuclear antibody and anti-DNA antibody are found in the serum.

History: Gradual or abrupt onset of widely varying symptoms: joint pain, butterfly rash over the cheeks, discoid lesions and other skin changes (purpura, alopecia), fever, chest pain, mood changes and other psychiatric symptoms.

Physical Examination: Fever, signs of swelling and inflammation in joints, malar "butterfly" eruption, lymphadenopathy, splenomegaly, pericardial or pleural friction rub heard on auscultation.

Diagnostic Tests: The erythrocyte sedimentation rate is elevated, white blood cells (particularly lymphocytes) and platelets are decreased. Tests based on detection of abnormal antibodies (LE cell preparation, antinuclear antibody, anti-DNA antibody) are often positive. Serologic test for syphilis may be falsely positive. Urinalysis may show proteinuria, red blood cells, and casts.

Course: The disease is chronic and relapsing, with spontaneous remissions and exacerbations. With treatment the 10-year survival rate is about 95%. Most patients eventually develop kidney disease (lupus nephritis), and death is usually due to renal failure.

Treatment: NSAIDs and general supportive measures may suffice to control symptoms. Antimalarial drugs (hydroxychloroquine and others), adrenal corticosteroids, and immunosuppressive drugs (azathioprine, cyclophosphamide) are useful in more severe cases.

OUCH!

Have you ever wondered why some shots (injections, immunizations) are given in the "backside"? It's because the gluteus maximus—the main muscle in the buttocks—is the largest muscle in the body and is capable of absorbing more of the drug with less trauma.

Some drugs like penicillin must be administered intramuscularly (IM) into a deep muscle, such as the outer (lateral) gluteal area or the ventrogluteal area (over the hip). The gluteal muscles of infants and small children are not well developed until they have been walking for a few years.

Pause for Reflection

1. _____ refers to a number of inherited disorders characterized by progressive muscular weakness and wasting of muscle tissue.
2. _____ is a lateral curvature of the spine in the erect position, due to malalignment of vertebrae.
3. Inflammation of a tendon sheath usually caused by repetitive or extreme strain on the tendon is a condition known as _____ or _____.
4. Carpal tunnel syndrome is diagnosed by a positive _____ sign, which is a shocklike pain when the volar aspect of the wrist is tapped, and a positive _____ sign, reproduction of pain or paresthesia when both wrists are flexed with the hands firmly pressing one another back-to-back for 60 seconds.
5. Fluctuant swelling of the bursa behind the knee joint, which communicates with the joint space, as a result of local trauma or disease, denotes a _____.
6. When inflammatory fluid accumulates in the purselike cushions overlying some bony prominences, it results in a condition known as _____.
7. Sharply localized and extremely tender points, particularly in the neck and back and often bilaterally symmetric, on physical exam are a key feature of _____; these points of extreme tenderness are called _____ points.
8. A _____ is a piece broken off a meniscus that remains in the joint.
9. A _____ is evidenced on physical exam by effusion of fluid into the joint space, crepitus, and an audible or palpable snap on extension of the knee from full flexion with the leg and foot externally rotated.
10. A _____ consists of extending the knee from full flexion with the leg and foot externally rotated when testing for a medial meniscus tear or extending the knee with the leg and foot internally rotated when testing for a lateral meniscus tear.
11. A disorder in which the density of bone is inadequate for its normal supporting function is _____.
12. Bone density is assessed by CT scan, single-photon absorptiometry (SPA), _____,

Diagnostic and Surgical Procedures

anterior drawer test With the patient supine, the injured knee is bent to 90 degrees. The physician then grasps the upper end of the tibia and pulls it anteriorly. Excessive movement means the **anterior cruciate ligament (ACL)** within the knee joint is damaged or torn.

arthrocentesis Insertion of a needle into the joint cavity in order to remove or aspirate fluid. May be done to remove excess fluid from a joint or to obtain fluid for examination.

arthroscopy A surgical procedure which involves an incision into a joint and the insertion of an arthroscope to view the structures inside the joint.

arthroplasty The surgical replacement of all or part of a joint, such as the hip, knee, or shoulder.

bone mineral density (BMD) test Measures the amount of calcium in regions of the bones.

bone scan A nuclear imaging test which, following the intravenous administration of radioisotope, uses a scanning device to detect areas of abnormal uptake in the bones to identify fractures.

carpal tunnel release Surgical cutting of the ligament in the wrist to relieve nerve pressure caused by carpal tunnel syndrome, which can result from repetitive motion such as typing (see ■ Figure 16-8).

closed reduction of fracture Correcting a fracture by realigning the bone fragments by manipulation without entering the body

crossed (or contralateral) straight leg raising With the patient supine, the unaffected leg is held straight and flexed at the hip. If sciatica is present, the patient will experience pain in the opposite, affected side.

cubital tunnel syndrome A type of entrapment neuropathy with a complex of symptoms resulting from injury or compression of the ulnar nerve at the elbow, including pain and numbness along the ulnar aspect of the hand and forearm, and weakness of the hand.

deep tendon reflexes (DTRs) Occur in response to sudden stretching of a muscle, usually induced by tapping a tendon with a rubber-headed reflex hammer. Tendon reflexes are tested in several muscles of the upper and lower extremities, with comparison of the two sides.

densitometry Determination of variations in density (for example, bone density) by comparison with that of another material or with a certain standard. See *dual photon densitometry*.

DEXA (dual-energy x-ray absorptiometry) Enhanced form of x-ray technology that is used to measure bone loss. Stationary devices usually check the spine and hips. Portable devices, some utilizing ultrasound as well, are used on wrists and hands.

dual photon densitometry A quantitative assessment of a patient's bone density, and comparison with normal ranges for persons of the same age and sex.

electrophysiologic studies Measurement of electrical activity in nerves and muscles. See *EMG* and *NCV*.

EMG (electromyogram) Test to determine the response pattern of muscles when stimulated by an electrical impulse from a needle electrode inserted into the muscle.

fixation Procedure to stabilize a fractured bone while it heals. **External fixation** includes casts, splints, and pins inserted through the skin. **Internal fixation** includes pins, plates, rods, screws, and wires that are applied during an open reduction (see ■ Figures 16-13 and 16-14).

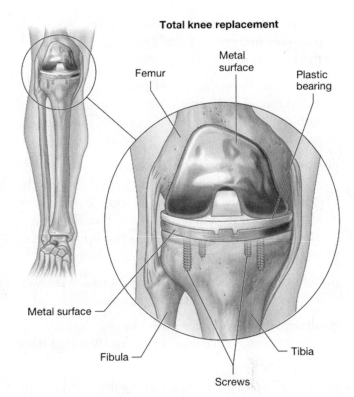

Total knee replacement

FIGURE 16-14. Total knee replacement

imaging studies Including x-ray, the most common and least expensive diagnostic tool for assessing bone structure and integrity. Also called *radiograph*, *film*, *roentgenogram*, and *roentgenograph*. MRI, CT scan, and *nuclear medicine studies* are also used for diagnostic purposes.

Lachman test Similar to the **anterior drawer test**, but performed with the patient's knee flexed only to 15–20°. Also used to evaluate **anterior cruciate ligament** stability.

laminectomy Surgical cutting through the posterior arch of one or more vertebrae and removal of herniated disk material.

Lasègue sign or test See *straight leg raising*.

McMurray test or sign Extension of the knee from full flexion with the leg and foot externally rotated causes an audible or palpable snap in **medial meniscus tear**; extension with the leg and foot internally rotated causes a snap in **lateral meniscus tear**.

NCV (nerve conduction velocity) Measured by timing the passage of nerve impulses between a stimulating and a recording electrode, which are a precisely measured distance apart.

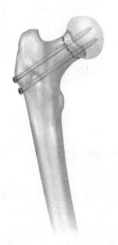
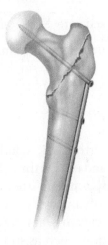

FIGURE 16-13. Hip repair of subcapital fracture (left) and intertrochanteric fracture (right)

open reduction, internal fixation (ORIF) A surgical procedure to correct a fracture that requires alignment and fixation with a plate, pin, or screw.

Phalen sign Reproduction of pain or paresthesia in **carpal tunnel syndrome** when both wrists are flexed with the hands firmly pressing one another back-to-back for 60 seconds.

pivot-shift test With the patient supine, the foot is held in the physician's hand. The physician then turns the foot inward while pushing on the outside of the knee with the opposite hand, at the same time flexing and extending the patient's leg. This test is also used to evaluate anterior cruciate ligament stability.

posterior drawer sign A test designed to detect instability of the **posterior cruciate ligament**.

quadriceps exercises Repeatedly bringing the knee into full extension, with tensing of the muscles of the front of the thigh.

rotator cuff tear repair Re-attaching the tendon to the head of humerus (upper arm bone). A partial tear may need only a trimming or smoothing procedure called a debridement. A complete tear within the thickest part of the tendon is repaired by stitching the two sides back together (see ■ Figure 16-15).

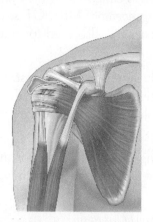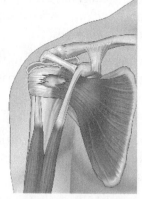

FIGURE 16-15. Partial and full-thickness tears of the rotator cuff

straight leg raising With the patient supine, the leg is elevated with the knee straight to the point where pain is experienced in the back or leg itself, or dorsiflexion of the foot causes an increase in pain. This test is done to determine if **nerve root irritation** such as **sciatic nerve root compression** is present. Also called *Lasègue sign* or *test*.

Tinel sign Shocklike pain when the volar aspect of the wrist is tapped; indicative of **carpal tunnel syndrome**.

traction Applying a pulling force on a fractured or dislocated limb or the vertebral column in order to restore normal alignment. Example, Buck's traction.

Laboratory Procedures

aldolase Elevated levels are indicative of muscle disease, such as muscular dystrophy.

alkaline phosphatase An enzyme whose level in the serum is often increased in bone disease and obstructive liver disease. The slang "alk phos" should be expanded.

ANA (antinuclear antibody) An antibody detected by immunofluorescence in patients with rheumatoid arthritis, lupus erythematosus, and other autoimmune diseases.

C-reactive protein (CRP) A test used to detect rheumatoid arthritis.

erythrocyte sedimentation rate (ESR, sed rate) The rate at which red blood cells settle to the bottom of a specimen of whole blood that has been treated with anticoagulant. The rate is expressed in millimeters per hour (mm/h), as measured in a standard glass column. Elevation of the sedimentation rate occurs in various inflammatory and malignant diseases but is diagnostic of none. An acceptable brief form is *sed rate*.

LE cell prep Lupus erythematosus cell test.

RA test Rheumatoid arthritis test. See *rheumatoid factor*.

rheumatoid factor (RF) An antibody present in the serum of patients with rheumatoid arthritis and other autoimmune disorders.

sed rate See *erythrocyte sedimentation rate*.

uric acid, serum A breakdown product of purine metabolism, increased in gout and other disorders.

Pharmacology

Orthopedic conditions such as arthritis (rheumatoid and osteoarthritis), bursitis, tendinitis, gout, and muscle spasms are treated with aspirin, nonsteroidal anti-inflammatory drugs (NSAIDs), gold salts, and muscle relaxants, among others. Acute musculoskeletal conditions such as strains, sprains, and "pulled muscles" are treated with analgesics and anti-inflammatory drugs.

The physician may also elect to prescribe a skeletal muscle relaxant.

Drugs used to treat osteoarthritis reduce pain and inflammation. These drugs include salicylates (such as aspirin), nonsteroidal anti-inflammatory drugs (NSAIDs), and COX-2 inhibitors. In addition, corticosteroids may be used. None of these drugs, however, can reverse the cartilage and bone damage that has already occurred in the joint.

Salicylic Acid Compounds

The oldest drug used to treat arthritis is **aspirin**. Aspirin is also known as *acetylsalicylic acid*, abbreviated ASA. It has anti-inflammatory, analgesic, and antipyretic actions. Salicylates (salicylic acid compounds) include:

aspirin (Arthritis Foundation Pain Reliever, Ecotrin, Empirin, Extended Release Bayer 8-Hour Caplets, Norwich Extra-Strength)
choline salicylate (Arthropan)
choline salicylate/magnesium salicylate (Trilisate)
diflunisal (Dolobid)
salsalate (Disalcid)

Because salicylate drugs such as aspirin are irritating to the stomach, and long-term therapy with such drugs has been shown to cause peptic ulcers, some manufacturers have taken precautions to reduce this irritation. Ecotrin is manufactured as an enteric-coated tablet that does not dissolve in stomach acid; it dissolves only when it comes in contact with the higher pH environment of the duodenum.

Aspirin is often combined with an antacid to raise the pH of the stomach, inhibit the action of pepsin, and neutralize stomach acid, all of which prevent the formation of peptic ulcers during aspirin therapy.

Arthritis Pain Formula
Ascriptin, Ascriptin A/D, Ascriptin Extra Strength
Bayer Buffered Aspirin, Bayer Plus Extra Strength
Bufferin, Tri-Buffered Bufferin
Cama Arthritis Pain Reliever

Acetaminophen

Although acetaminophen is an analgesic like aspirin, it lacks the ability to inhibit the production of prostaglandins and has no anti-inflammatory action. The American College of Rheumatology recommends using acetaminophen to treat osteoarthritis because it has fewer side effects than NSAIDs.

acetaminophen
Aspirin Free Anacin Maximum Strength
Panadol
Tylenol
Tylenol Arthritis
Tylenol Arthritis Extended Relief
Tylenol Extra Strength
Tylenol Regular Strength

NSAIDs (Nonsteroidal Anti-inflammatory Drugs)

NSAIDs ("en sayds" or "en seds") inhibit the production of prostaglandins for an anti-inflammatory effect, and they also relieve pain directly (analgesic effect). NSAIDs have less of a tendency than aspirin to cause stomach irritation or peptic ulcers. Their structure is similar enough to aspirin that patients allergic to aspirin should not take NSAIDs. NSAIDs include:

diclofenac (Cataflam, Voltaren, Voltaren-XR)
etodolac (Lodine, Lodine XL)
fenoprofen (Nalfon Pulvules)
flurbiprofen (Ansaid)
ibuprofen (Advil, Advil Liqui-Gels, Haltran, Motrin, Motrin IB)
indomethacin (Indocin, Indocin SR)
ketoprofen (Orudis, Orudis KT, Oruvail)
meclofenamate (Meclomen)
meloxicam (Mobic)
nabumetone (Relafen)
naproxen (Aleve, Anaprox, Anaprox DS, Naprelan, EC-Naprosyn, Naprosyn)
oxaprozin (Daypro)
piroxicam (Feldene)
sulindac (Clinoril)

Arthrotec contains an NSAID (diclofenac) combined with a synthetic prostaglandin (misoprostol) that protects the gastric mucosa and prevents the formation of peptic ulcers.

COX-2 inhibitors, which also belong to the larger category of NSAIDs, selectively inhibit the enzyme cyclooxygenase-2 (COX-2) to decrease the production of prostaglandins and relieve pain.

celecoxib (Celebrex)

Corticosteroids

Corticosteroids, which are produced naturally in the adrenal cortex, have a powerful anti-inflammatory effect and are given orally to treat acute episodes of osteoarthritis associated with inflammation of the synovial membrane. Because of the side effects associated with prolonged oral use, corticosteroid drugs are used only to treat acute exacerbations.

> betamethasone (Celestone Soluspan)
> dexamethasone (Dalalone, Dalalone D.P., Dalalone L.A., Decadron, Decadron-LA, Hexadrol)
> hydrocortisone (Hydrocortone)
> methylprednisolone (Depo-Medrol, Depopred-40, Depopred-80)
> prednisolone (Hydeltrasol, Key-Pred 25, Key-Pred 50, Key-Pred-SP, Predalone 50, Prednisol TBA)
> triamcinolone (Aristocort Forte, Aristospan Intra-articular, Kenalog-40)

Hyaluronic acid is secreted by the synovial membrane of a joint and helps to maintain the lubricating quality of the synovial fluid. These drugs, derivatives of hyaluronic acid, are injected into the joints of patients with osteoarthritis:

> hyaluronic acid derivative (Hyalgan, Synvisc)
> sodium hyaluronate (Supartz)

Gold Salts

Gold salts contain actual gold (from 29% to 50% of the total drug) in capsules or in solution for injection; they are used to treat active rheumatoid arthritis. Rheumatoid arthritis is an autoimmune disease in which the patient's own macrophages attack and damage cartilage. Gold salts inhibit the activity of macrophages but cannot reverse past damage.

> auranofin (Ridaura)
> aurothioglucose (Solganal)
> gold sodium thiomalate (Myochrysine)

Unlike other antiarthritis drugs, gold salts are never prescribed for osteoarthritis, as this disease is caused by degenerative wear and tear, not by an immune response. NSAIDs are the first line of treatment for rheumatoid arthritis, but if these fail, gold salts may be added to the treatment regimen. Plaquenil (hydroxychloroquine) is also effective in treating rheumatoid arthritis, as well as anakinra (Kineret), which is human interleukin-1 produced through recombinant DNA technology.

Osteoporosis Drugs

Osteoporosis is a thinning of the bone due to demineralization.

Osteoporosis is much more common in women than in men, and most common in postmenopausal women. As estrogen levels decrease in menopause, the rate of bone formation decreases but the rate of bone breakdown remains constant, causing the bones to slowly and progressively thin. Additional risk factors for osteoporosis include Caucasian or Asian race, slender build, smoking, and alcohol abuse.

Osteoporosis is prevented or treated by supplementing calcium, and increasing exercise (to stimulate bone growth). Estrogen taken orally or administered through a transdermal patch reverses postmenopausal bone loss but increases the risk of cardiovascular disease, thromboembolism, and certain cancers.

The hormone **calcitonin** is normally produced by the thyroid gland and regulates calcium and the rate of bone resorption (breakdown). Miacalcin, an analog of human calcitonin derived from salmon, is given by injection or nasal spray to inhibit calcium loss in osteoporosis.

These drugs decrease the rate of bone resorption by inhibiting osteoclasts (cells that break down bone).

> alendronate (Fosamax)
> etidronate (Didronel)
> pamidronate (Aredia)
> risedronate (Actonel)

Evista (raloxifene) belongs to the class of drugs known as selective estrogen receptor modulators (SERMs) and activates estrogen receptors to decrease the rate of bone resorption.

Skeletal Muscle Relaxants

These drugs relieve muscle spasm through action on the central nervous system. Most also have a sedative effect.

> carisoprodol (Soma)
> chlorphenesin (Maolate)
> chlorzoxazone (Paraflex, Parafon Forte DSC)
> cyclobenzaprine (Flexeril)
> diazepam (Valium)
> metaxalone (Skelaxin)
> methocarbamol (Robaxin, Robaxin-750)
> orphenadrine (Norflex)

These skeletal muscle relaxants are used to treat severe muscle spasticity in patients with multiple sclerosis, cerebral palsy, stroke, or spinal cord injury.

baclofen (Lioresal)
dantrolene (Dantrium)
tizanidine (Zanaflex)

Combination skeletal muscle relaxants include Norgesic (orphenadrine and aspirin), Robaxisal (methocarbamol and aspirin), Soma Compound (carisoprodol and aspirin), and Soma Compound with Codeine (carisoprodol, aspirin, codeine).

Drugs Used to Treat Gout

Gout is caused by a metabolic defect that allows uric acid to accumulate in the blood. The kidneys are unable to excrete the excess uric acid, and it crystallizes within the joints, causing pain and inflammation.

Drugs used to treat gout act either by increasing the excretion of uric acid in the urine or by inhibiting enzymes that produce uric acid in the blood.

allopurinol (Zyloprim)
colchicine
potassium citrate/sodium citrate (Polycitra, Polycitra-LC)
probenecid (Benemid)
sulfinpyrazone (Anturane)

In addition, certain NSAIDs have been found to be of particular benefit in treating gout.

indomethacin (Indocin, Indocin SR)
naproxen (Aleve, Anaprox, Anaprox DS, EC-Naprosyn, Naprosyn)
sulindac (Clinoril)

Drugs Used to Treat Phantom Limb Pain

After amputation many patients experience pain that seems to come from the absent limb. Nerve impulses coming from just above the area of amputation are interpreted by the brain as being from the missing limb. This pain diminishes over time but is treated with tricyclic antidepressants that have been found to be effective in treating different types of pain.

amitriptyline (Elavil)
amoxapine (Asendin)
desipramine (Norpramin)
doxepin (Sinequan, Sinequan Concentrate)
imipramine (Tofranil, Tofranil-PM)
nortriptyline (Aventyl, Aventyl Pulvules, Pamelor)
protriptyline (Vivactil)

Transcription Tips

1. Confusing terms related to the musculoskeletal system: Some of these terms sound alike; others are potential traps when researching. Memorize the terms and their meanings so that you can select the appropriate term for a correct transcript.

   adduct (draw away from); abduct (draw closer to)

   apophyseal (pertaining to a bony projection or outgrowth); epiphyseal (pertaining to the expanded articular end of a long bone)

   apposition (near each other); opposition (opposite each other)

   aseptic (without microorganisms); septic (pertaining to the presence of microorganisms)

   break (fracture); brake (stop)

   buckle (collapse); buccal (inside of cheek)

   callus (n., tissue that forms at a fracture site, a sign of healing); callous (adj., relating to a callus or callosity, a hardened thickening of the epidermal keratin layer due to repeated friction or pressure, nothing to do with a bone)

   cervical (relating to the neck, in any sense); surgical (as in surgical neck of humerus; the narrow portion below the head and tuberosities)

   dens (small bone); dense (thick); dents (indentations)

   device (n., instrument); devise (v., develop)

   effusion (fluid build-up); fusion (growing together of two parts); infusion (put in)

   eminence (bony prominence); imminence (something about to occur)

   flexor (a muscle which flexes a joint); flexure (a bend in an organ or structure)

   gait (manner of walk); gate (barrier)

   graft (join or combine); graph (diagram)

   grate (scraping noise); great (ample)

   Hohmann retractor (used for hip surgery); Hoen retractor (discontinued small bone retractor but still in references and on the Internet)

   humeral (pertaining to the humerus, an arm bone); humoral (pertaining to immunity from antibodies in the blood)

   humerus (arm bone); humorous (funny)

   ilium (hip bone); ileum (part of the small intestine)

   malleolus (bony prominence on either side of ankle); malleus (bone of middle ear)

   metacarpal (small bones of the hand) metatarsal (small bones of the feet)

   knuckle (of fingers); nuchal (adjective for neck)

   malalignment (out of whack); malignment (talk bad about)

   osteal (pertaining to bone, syn. osseous); ostial (pertaining to an opening)

   osteophyte (outgrowths of bone from the surface); osteocyte (mature bone cell)

   overdo (do too much); overdue (late)

   peroneal (pertaining to the fibula); perineal (pertaining to the area between the genitalia and anus)

   phalanges (bones); flanges (rims)

   rays (fingers or toes); raise (lift); raze (tear down)

   realign (to return to a condition of straightness); reline (to put in another liner)

   rent (n., a tear); rend (past tense of rent, torn)

   sac (fluid-filled area, like a cyst); sack (bag)

   shear (to cut or break off); sheer (see-through)

   shears (breaks off OR scissors); sheers (see-through curtains)

   site (a place); cite (to say or reference); sight (vision)

   straight (aligned); strait (narrow)

2. Watch out for spelling changes when forming derivatives.

femur	but	femoral
tendon	but	tendinitis
bone	but	bony

3. Difficult to spell terms:

   psoas muscle (silent p)

   Flexeril (a muscle relaxant), *not* Flexoril

   Weightbearing, weight bearing, weight-bearing—which is the correct spelling? Consulting a dictionary will not provide the answer. We have *followed the rationale of Vera Pyle's Current Medical Terminology:* "The trend in language is to combine words without hyphens after compound nouns become common. . . . It seems

Transcription Tips

simpler and cleaner to make weightbearing and nonweightbearing single words."

Although you will find the spellings *orthopaedics* and *orthopaedist* in dictionaries and on the Internet, these spellings are not used in healthcare documentation in the United States except in the official names of some organizations, orthopedic groups, and hospitals.

4. Expand these slang brief forms when dictated.

tib-fib   tibia-fibula (n.) or tibiofibular (adj.)
fem-pop   femoral-popliteal or femoropopliteal

5. Dictation Challenges

abduction and adduction. Because "adduction" and "abduction" sound so similar, especially in dictation, the dictator may try to clarify by saying "a-d-duction" or "a-b-duction." Sometimes this is helpful, sometimes not; the pronunciation of "b" is a lot like that of "d." To summarize, *abduction* increases the angle; *adduction* decreases the angle.

ORIF. The abbreviation is often mistranslated. It is *open reduction and internal fixation*, two different procedures done during the same surgery. It may be transcribed with the conjunction or as *open reduction-internal fixation* or even *open reduction, internal fixation* but not open reduction internal fixation or open reduction/internal fixation.

crepitus (defined in the Vocabulary Review). Often pronounced as "crepitance" or "crepitants"; the dictator means *crepitus*. *Crepitant* (an adjective, no "s") may be used to describe rales in the lung examination.

Physicians frequently mispronounce *tensor fasciae latae* as if it were spelled "tensor fascia lata" and chondromalacia patellae as if it were spelled "chondromalacia patella." Note the correct spellings.

Some structures have two (or more) names that may be used interchangeably, even in the same dictation:

calcaneus = os calcis
navicular bone = scaphoid bone
(bony) pelvis = innominate bone = os coxae
xiphoid cartilage = ensiform cartilage

6. Research Challenges: Doctors often mix English and Latin anatomic terms. If you cannot find the adjective you're hearing under the English noun, try the Latin noun. You also need to look under the singular noun, even if you're hearing the plural noun.

English, Latin Singular	*English, Latin Plural*
articulation, articulatio	articulations, articulationes
joint, articulatio	joints, articulationes
bone, os	bones, ossa
condyle, condylus	condyles, condyli
ligament, ligamentum	ligaments, ligamenta
muscle, musculus	muscles, musculi
nerve, nervus	nerves, nervi
tendon, tendo	tendons, tendines

For many English nouns, references may not include the adjective you're hearing with the noun you're hearing, but you can often find the adjective listed under other nouns with similar meanings.

When The Dictator Says, Also Check

device	apparatus, component, bandage, prosthesis, splint
dressing	bandage, splint, cast, boot
maneuver	technique, method
operation	procedure, technique, method
phenomenon	sign, test
procedure	amputation, approach, flap, graft, maneuver, method, operation, technique
syndrome	disease, disorder, condition, sign
sign	test, phenomenon, reflex
technique	maneuver, method, procedure, operation
test	reflex, sign

Spotlight On

Totally Hip

by Judith Marshall

"You are too old, too fat, too poor, and too crippled. No one will ever go out with you. Besides, your husband just died. Shame on you."

Nothing like an old girlfriend to point me in the wrong direction. I hopped on the Internet anyway. Perhaps hop is too strong a word. I limped onto the Internet. The dotcoms were loaded with men seeking women. I met a few of them for coffee but no planets collided or stars exploded.

Then I found David and from his first words on the telephone, I just knew he was delicious. We spoke on the phone for a week and met for dinner in a restaurant parking lot. He slid into my car because I had two things to tell him. I told him that later that month I was scheduled for a serious biopsy. It could be cancer. He gazed at me quietly and said he would be there and what else? I told him the total hip replacement (THR) was scheduled soon. In the trunk I had a walker and a cane but that day I held his hand and walked into the restaurant.

He simply said he would be there. And he was. Nothing fazed David. He liked me and I liked him. He loaded my walker into his car and for the next couple of months, we went to museums and zoos, wineries, movies, and shopping, sightseeing on the Maine and Rhode Island coasts. He was with me from 5 a.m. the day of the first surgery and brought me home and took care of me. The biopsies were negative.

Nothing really prepared me for the hip surgery. Not even the excellent classes the hospital offered or the Internet web sites. In on Monday, out on Thursday, maybe even home, no rehab—that is what they told me. The idea of a foreign body in my body was not uncomfortable, since I already had metal, mesh, and plastic. Why not titanium and ceramic? The best surgeon, the best hospital, the best anesthesiologist—what was there to fear? The worsening pain over seven years made the decision for me. Either buy a wheelchair or have the hip replaced. The surgery was booked nine months ahead. So I had time to lose over 100 pounds, join a gym, get a nutritionist, and join a weight loss support group. And chase men.

Except for David I was virtually alone but strangely calm as September 22 dawned. After surgery, medication dulled the initial pain, and that first evening I was surprised at how ravenously hungry I was. A superb supper was served by lovely people in long white-sleeved shirts, black vests, and bow ties. If it were not for the catheter and the IV running, I would have thought I was in a Las Vegas bistro. Then David appeared next to my bed wearing a black suit and a Roman collar. For a moment I thought I was dead. He called me Sister Mary Catherine and asked if I would like to make a confession of my sins. Since he could not find a rosary, he used Mardi Gras beads. In retrospect I wonder how much I confessed in that Dilaudid dream. We still play Sister Mary Catherine and Father Dave and there usually is some penance involved. But that is another story.

Yes, they really do get the patients out of bed the second day. I told the physical therapists who looked about 12 years old that I really did not care too much about how soon I would be walking but more importantly when I could have sex. They blushed and giggled. I had to ask the surgeon, who raised his eyebrows and said "in about a month." He was absolutely correct about that.

David arrived the second night as Uncle Moishe, a character he developed with a voice which took me back to my childhood in the old neighborhood. Uncle Moishe soothed me. Medical personnel hovered near the door listening intently as they heard a heavily accented man tell jokes and stories, wondrously peppered with Yiddish phrases. Uncle Moishe knew I loved herring in sour cream so he brought along an eight-foot stuffed fish-shaped pillow with brilliant speckles and red and black coloring. When I was sitting in a chair, I put Solomon (the fish had to have a name) with his head on the pillow and his huge tail partially covered by bedclothes, then I would wait for various personnel to come in and do a double-take or laugh, and it amused me through that difficult day. I had such great fun with that fish.

Hospital day three was a hundred years long. A petite female aide tried to prop me up so that I could sit and stand. The hip prosthetic weighed more than she did, and as both of us were about to

Spotlight On Totally Hip *(continued)*

topple to the floor, I saw a bulbous red nose under an enormous multi-colored wig and a clown with balloons walked into the room. David entertained me and the astonished aide while the hospital room doorway filled with delighted nurses. He knew I had a fear of clowns (*fearus clownus* in medical terms). I find them sinister but not that clown, not that night.

Day four brought the ambulance drivers and they strapped me into the stretcher and Solomon the Fish lay on top of me. We paraded out of the hospital and the two wise-cracking attendants enjoyed every minute. "Waddya gawkin' at, never seen a fish before?" "Look what we caught in the Charles River!" "This mermaid is going to rehab!"

The rehab was paradise compared to the hospital. A huge private room with a shower big enough to accommodate a horse in a hoist and a grand window with a view of autumn foliage. Whatever I asked for, David brought to me, including gallons of coffee. The worst problems for me were filth and constipation. The nursing staff said they were too busy to give me a bath. David, always unfailingly polite, ordered them to find a chair with wheels and he and an aide rolled me into the shower room. I clung to the safety rails while David hosed me down like a pig at a county fair. Then he washed my hair and rinsed it. He patted me dry, blow dried my hair, and powdered my bottom. If that is not love, what is?

When I went for physical therapy, he became a Marine drill instructor, a coach, a personal trainer, and a general pain in the neck. He forced me to go farther and faster. He walked backwards while I walked towards him with the walker, cursing him and whining. We went to occupational therapy together and he did the exercises with me, shouting encouragement for me to walk stairs. I had enough gas to fly to Chicago but he never complained.

On discharge, he loaded my belongings into the car and took me home. He fed the cat, went food shopping, made supper, and then sat by the bed until I fell asleep and he went home. The next day I went back to work in my home office. We visited several zoos in the autumn, went mall-walking and sightseeing in museums all winter. He booked New Year's weekend in a Cape Cod hotel with a heated pool and hot tub. The surgeon said to walk

in the pool and so I did, with David wearing goggles, swimming around like Jaws and yelling, "One, two, three, four, march." By month six I was dancing at Bavarian night, stepping tentatively and clinging to David. A month after that I was wearing my new ballerina flats, doing the twist, the foxtrot, and jitterbugging. I sold my walker and threw out the cane.

Each major surgery is a journey for the patient. In the age 65–70 range, approximately 120,000 are performed in the U.S. annually at a cost of $43,000 to $63,000. Patients with THR report satisfaction rates of over 90 percent while knee replacement surgery satisfaction runs about 70 percent.

If a person is contemplating total hip replacement, some hints and caveats.

1. If the hospital holds a class for patients, take it.

2. Do not make yourself crazy reading Internet stories and blogs. The same people writing them are the ones who terrorized you decades ago with horror stories of childbirth or gallbladder operations.

3. Choose your spouse and your children wisely because you will need them. Not everyone can find a David. Cultivate many friends, especially younger people.

4. Try to have an efficacious bowel regimen early on in your postoperative phase. One Colace a day is not going to suffice. Do not wait until the situation becomes a matter of explode or die. Be vocal, be assertive and totally without shame as you perch upon your throne euphemistically called the bedside commode. Discontinue pain medication as soon as possible; it's constipating. And try to familiarize yourself with the proper medical terminology used on the road to recovery. "Did we poop and pee today?" chirped the morning aide every single morning.

5. Appreciate that any form of bathing which does not include a shower in the postoperative period is not enough. Line up friends and relatives to help or hire strangers in advance. Maintain your dignity even though stark naked and soaking wet.

6. Send thank-you notes and letters to the people who helped you through this process, especially the physical therapy and food service folks.

The surgery was a miracle for me after years of dreaming of walking and dancing.

Exercises

Medical Vocabulary Review

Instructions: Choose the best answer.

_____ 1. The enlarged knobby area at each end of a long bone is called the _____
A. diaphysis.
B. epiphysis.
C. metaphysis.
D. apophysis.

_____ 2. Narrow, cordlike connective tissue that attaches muscle to bone is called _____
A. callus.
B. tendon.
C. ligament.
D. aponeurosis.

_____ 3. Articulation is another word for _____
A. joint.
B. cartilage.
C. synovium.
D. bone marrow.

_____ 4. Healing of a bone fracture is evidenced by the formation of _____
A. callus.
B. calcium.
C. callosity.
D. crepitus.

_____ 5. A childhood fracture may result in stunted bone growth if it involves the _____
A. periosteum.
B. cortical bone.
C. cancellous bone.
D. epiphyseal plate.

_____ 6. Outgrowths of bone from the surface may occur in diseases such as osteomyelitis and as a result of fracture or other trauma; these outgrowths are _____
A. eburnation.
B. osteoarthritis.
C. Heberden nodes.
D. osteophyte formation.

_____ 7. A grating sensation caused by the rubbing together of the dry synovial surfaces is a sign of _____
A. eburnation.
B. joint crepitus.
C. saucerization.
D. spondylolisthesis.

_____ 8. Positive Tinel and Phalen signs are diagnostic of _____
A. fibromyalgia.
B. tenosynovitis.
C. muscular dystrophy.
D. carpal tunnel syndrome.

_____ 9. A fluctuant swelling of the bursa behind the knee joint is _____
A. bursitis.
B. a meniscal tear.
C. a Baker's cyst.
D. avascular necrosis.

_____ 10. Crescent- or C-shaped pads of fibrocartilage within the knee joint that cushion shocks between the femur and the tibia are the _____
A. deep tendon reflexes.
B. tendons and ligaments.
C. motor and sensory fibers.
D. medial and lateral menisci.

___ 11. The _____ consists of extension of the knee from full flexion with the leg and foot externally rotated.
A. Lachman test
B. McMurray test
C. anterior drawer test
D. straight leg raising test

___ 12. Disturbance in the normal alignment or tracking of the patella in its groove causing chronic trauma to the back of the patella with roughening, fraying, and even complete loss of cartilage is characteristic of a condition called ____
A. chondromalacia patellae.
B. osteogenesis imperfecta.
C. fibromyalgia syndrome.
D. avascular necrosis.

___ 13. The large four-headed muscle on the front of the thigh that extends the knee joint is the ____
A. adductor magnus.
B. quadriceps muscle.
C. gluteus medius muscle.
D. gluteus maximus muscle.

___ 14. Compression fractures of the vertebrae and traumatic fractures of the wrist and femoral neck are common in women with a bone density disorder called ____
A. necrosis.
B. osteogenesis.
C. osteoporosis.
D. spinal stenosis.

___ 15. Positive Tinel and Phalen signs and nerve compression documented by EMG and nerve conduction studies are diagnostic of ____
A. carpal tunnel syndrome.
B. fibromyalgia syndrome.
C. patellofemoral syndrome.
D. avascular necrosis syndrome.

___ 16. Sharply localized pain and tenderness, swelling, and fluctuancy due to accumulation of inflammatory fluid within the purselike cushions that protect underlying surfaces and reduce friction in the joint is indicative of ____
A. arthritis.
B. tendinitis.
C. synovitis.
D. bursitis.

___ 17. Bacterial infection of the bone is a condition known as ____
A. osteoarthritis.
B. tenosynovitis.
C. osteomyelitis.
D. rheumatoid arthritis.

___ 18. _____ is a chronic systemic disease caused by the formation of antibodies to one's own tissues, particularly the synovial membranes.
A. Avascular necrosis
B. Fibromyalgia syndrome
C. Lupus erythematosus
D. Rheumatoid arthritis

___ 19. _____ is caused by the elevation of serum uric acid due to overproduction, impaired excretion, or both.
A. Gout
B. Arthritis
C. Tendinitis
D. Baker cyst

___ 20. Elevated erythrocyte sedimentation rate, decreased white blood cells and plates, and often positive antinuclear antibody, anti-DNA antibody are diagnostic for ____
A. tenosynovitis.
B. avascular necrosis.
C. lupus erythematosus.
D. rheumatoid arthritis.

Diagnostic and Surgical Procedures

Instructions: Match the following diagnostic and surgical procedures to their descriptions or definitions. Some answers may be used more than once, or not at all.

_____ 1. anterior drawer test

_____ 2. arthroscopy

_____ 3. dual-energy x-ray absorptiometry

_____ 4. electromyogram

_____ 5. Lachman test

_____ 6. McMurray test

_____ 7. open reduction, internal fixation

_____ 8. pivot-shift test

_____ 9. straight leg raising

A. Test to determine response pattern of muscles when stimulated by electrical impulse from a needle electrode inserted into the muscle.

B. Surgical procedure to align and fixate a fracture with a plate, pin, or screw

C. A surgical procedure using a device to view the structures inside the joint

D. Test to determine if nerve root irritation such as sciatic nerve root compression is present

E. Test to evaluate anterior cruciate ligament stability

F. Enhanced form of x-ray technology used to measure bone loss

G. Test to evaluate for medial or lateral meniscus tear

Dissecting Medical Terms

Instructions: As you learned in your medical language course, words are formed from prefixes, combining forms (root word plus combining vowel), and suffixes. Combining vowels (usually **o** but not always) are used to connect two root words or a root and a suffix. By analyzing these word parts, you can often determine the definition of a term without even looking it up (if you know the definition of the parts, of course!).

Being able to divide and analyze the words you hear into their component parts will also improve your auditory deciphering ability and spelling and help you research those words that you cannot easily spell or define.

For the following terms, draw a slash (/) between the components and then write a short definition based on the meaning of the parts. Remember that to define a word based on its parts, you start at the end, usually with the suffix. If there's a prefix, that is defined next, and finally the combining form is defined.

Example: achondroplasia

Divide & Analyze:
 achondroplasia = a/chondr/o/plasia
 = without + cartilage + development
Define: lack of development of cartilage

1. dysarthria
 Divide _____

 Define _____

2. myotomy
 Divide _____

 Define _____

3. supination
 Divide _____

 Define _____

4. fibrotic
 Divide _____

 Define _____

5. interphalangeal
Divide
_____
_____
Define
_____

6. articulation
Divide
_____
_____
Define
_____

7. intramedullary
Divide
_____
_____
Define
_____

8. subluxated
Divide
_____
_____
Define
_____

9. paramedial
Divide
_____
_____
Define
_____

10. meniscectomy
Divide
_____
_____
Define
_____

11. fasciotomy
Divide
_____
_____
Define
_____

12. ankylosing
Divide
_____
_____
Define
_____

13. patellofemoral
Divide
_____
_____
Define
_____

14. chondromalacia
Divide
_____
_____
Define
_____

15. transfixation
Divide
_____
_____
Define
_____

16. tenodesis
Divide
_____
_____
Define
_____

17. osteotome
Divide
_____
_____
Define
_____

18. myoplasty
Divide
_____
_____
Define
_____

19. supraclavicular
Divide
_____
_____
Define
_____

20. antebrachial
Divide
_____
_____
Define
_____

Spelling Exercise

Instructions: Review the adjective suffixes your medical language textbook. Test your knowledge of **adjectives** by writing the adjectival form of the following words. Note that for some suffixes, the vowel may change when adding the adjective suffix. For some, the adjective form is the past participle of the verb. Consult a medical dictionary to verify spelling.

Example: apophysis apophyseal

Noun or Verb	Adjective
1. cartilage	
2. clavicle	
3. epithelium	
4. necrosis	
5. diaphysis	
6. distend	
7. epiphysis	
8. interdigitate	
9. femur	
10. fibula	
11. humerus	
12. ilium	
13. patella	
14. malleolus	
15. radius	
16. spondylolisthesis	
17. tendon	
18. ligament	
19. ulna	
20. avulse	
21. purulence	
22. periosteum	
23. trauma	
24. trochlea	
25. vola	

Forming Plurals

Instructions: Test your knowledge of plurals by writing the plural form of the following terms. Consult a medical dictionary to confirm your spelling.

Singular	Plural
1. fibula	
2. thorax	
3. apex	
4. epiphysis	
5. arthritis	
6. phalanx	
7. chondroma	
8. ganglion	
9. retinaculum	
10. callosity	
11. raphe	
12. ecchymosis	
13. exostosis	
14. meniscus	
15. malleolus	

Combining Words

Instructions: Test your knowledge of combined words by hyphenating where appropriate or forming a single word from the following pairs. Consult a dictionary to verify your spelling and the definition.

Example: anterior and inferior anterior-inferior

Phrase	Combined Form
1. posterior and lateral	
2. tibial and fibular	
3. talar and fibula	
4. clavicular and pectoral	
5. coracoid and acromial	
6. curved and linear	
7. cerebral and vascular	
8. costal and vertebral	
9. deltoid and pectoral	
10. dorsal and medial	
11. dorsal and radial	
12. femoral and popliteal	
13. glenoid and humeral	
14. metacarpal and phalangeal	
15. patellar and femoral	

Abbreviations Exercise

Instructions: Expand the following common abbreviations and brief forms. Then memorize both abbreviations and definitions to increase your speed and accuracy in transcribing dictation

Abbreviation	Expansion
1. ACL	_____
2. AK, AKA	_____
3. AP	_____
4. ATFL	_____
5. BMP	_____
6. BNP	_____
7. CABG	_____
8. CRP	_____
9. CVA	_____
10. CVA	_____
11. DIP	_____
12. DP	_____
13. DVT	_____
14. EBL	_____
15. EHL	_____
16. EIP	_____
17. EMG	_____
18. EOMI	_____
19. EPL	_____
20. I&D	_____
21. I&D	_____
22. IM	_____
23. IP	_____
24. IT	_____
25. LCL	_____
26. LMA	_____
27. MAC	_____
28. MCP	_____
29. ML	_____
30. MP	_____
31. ORIF	_____
32. PCL	_____
33. PERRLA	_____
34. PIP	_____
35. PT	_____

Transcript Forensics

Instructions: This section presents snippets of transcribed dictations from clinic notes; history and physical examinations and consultations; operative reports and procedure notes; and discharge summaries. Explain the passage so that a nonmedical person can understand it.

Example

Knee pain: He had a **bucket-handle tear** of his right **medial meniscus** removed about 5 years ago.

Explanation: The knee cartilage in the right knee (the medial, or inner side of the knee) was torn in the shape of a bucket handle, and it was surgically cut away.

1. She had **avascular necrosis** of the left hip and underwent **surgical intervention**. At the time of that surgery she was found to have **arthritic osteoporotic cavity defects** in the acetabulum.

Explanation: _____
_____
_____
_____

2. Examination revealed a **genu valgum** of 9 degrees, **Q angle** of 16 to 17 degrees with a slight **patellar tilt**, but **positive patellar inhibition** with lateral movement of the patella.

Explanation: _____
_____
_____
_____

3. There was tenderness and **fullness** along the tibial tendon and **peroneal tendons** behind the medial and lateral **malleoli**.

Explanation: _____
_____
_____
_____

4. There is severe **hallux valgus deformity** of the left great toe with **pronation** of her left foot.

Explanation: _____

_____

_____

_____

5. There is a **bony exostosis** of the calcaneus causing **impingement** of the Achilles tendon, resulting in **tendon shortening** and **gait impairment**.

Explanation: _____

_____

_____

_____

6. **Bone densitometry studies** were done at the Osteoporosis Center, and diagnosis of osteoporosis of the spine without evidence of compression fracture was made.

Explanation: _____

_____

_____

_____

_____

7. There is **recurrent tendinitis** in the left arm which has been successfully injected in the past with **cortisone**. A **tennis elbow armband** was placed on the left arm, and he was begun on **Anaprox**.

Explanation: _____

_____

_____

_____

8. It was determined that an **external fixation device** would be required.

Explanation: _____

_____

_____

_____

9. The patient stepped on a nail several weeks ago, resulting in possible **osteomyelitis** of the calcaneus. He is scheduled for **calcaneal biopsy**.

Explanation: _____

_____

_____

_____

10. A **Rush rod** was inserted to stabilize the two ends of the fracture.

Explanation: _____

_____

_____

_____

11. Our attention was directed to the femur. The **neck** was further debrided of its soft tissue.

Explanation: _____

_____

_____

_____

12. An **orthopedic cutting block** was used to make an oblique cut through the bone.

Explanation: _____

_____

_____

_____

13. Three **portals** were made and the **outflow cannula** attached.

Explanation: _____

_____

_____

_____

Sample Reports

Sample orthopedic reports appear on the following pages, illustrating a variety of reports. Fictional names are provided for illustration of proper format, and no resemblance to actual persons is intended. Sample transcripts were prepared according to *The Book of Style for Medical Transcription* (AHDI).

Progress Note

KRATZ, NEIL
#942136
July 10, [add year]

PROBLEM LIST
1. Diabetic right foot ulcer.
2. Uncontrolled type 2 diabetes.

INTERVAL HISTORY
The patient is applying Promogran with dressing changes. He has ordered orthotics, which he will have in about 3 weeks.

PHYSICAL EXAMINATION
He is afebrile. Examination of the right plantar foot wound measures 0.4 x 0.3 x 0.3 cm which is a reduction in size of a wound that is granulating well. There is no drainage or odor.

ASSESSMENT
Healing wound to the right plantar foot.

PLAN
Wound will be dressed with Promogran today. He will be seen back in 2 weeks' time.

EMILY MORGAN, MD

EM:hpi

d: 7/10/[add date]
t: 7/10/[add date]

Operative Report

APPLEBAUM, SARAH
#89810

DATE OF OPERATION
August 6, [add year]

PREOPERATIVE DIAGNOSIS
Failed hardware, right hip, status post open reduction and internal fixation (ORIF) with nonunion.

POSTOPERATIVE DIAGNOSIS
Failed hardware, right hip, status post open reduction and internal fixation (ORIF) with nonunion.

OPERATION PERFORMED
Hardware removal of right hip nonunion and femur nonunion with open reduction and internal fixation of right hip and femur nonunion, with addition of Norian bone filler.

SURGEON
RICHARD HOWARD, MD

ASSISTANT
LEON FAIRBORN, MD

ANESTHESIA
General.

ESTIMATED BLOOD LOSS
3000 mL.

INDICATIONS
A 69-year-old female who sustained a very comminuted and displaced fracture that extended from her hip down to near her knee. There were spiral and butterfly fragments, and it was a very unstable, complex fracture. She underwent intramedullary (IM) nailing in March and has actually been doing reasonably well up until recently. This week she developed significant pain. X-rays taken demonstrated that the nail had broken. She presents now for the revision of the hardware with bone grafting and re-reduction.

DESCRIPTION OF PROCEDURE
After successful induction of anesthesia, she was placed on the fracture table, and her right lower extremity was prepped and draped in the normal sterile fashion. A longitudinal incision was made on the lateral aspect of the leg, from the proximal aspect of the hip down to about 10 cm proximal to the knee. We dissected down to the iliotibial (IT) band. The IT band was split, and then the vastus lateralis was elevated off the bone. We identified the greater trochanter and were able to remove the proximal portion of the nail. We then removed the screw that had been advanced into the femoral neck and head. We then removed the locking screw distally.

(continued)

Operative Report

APPLEBAUM, SARAH
#89810
August 6, [add year]
Page 2

series of trials, we were able to remove the distal portion of the nail using 2 different guidewires. This, after much struggle, worked rather nicely. We then subsequently removed a great deal of scar tissue from the proximal nonunion site. This was accomplished after meticulous dissection and reestablishment of the anatomy. We subsequently, after we removed a great deal of scar tissue, aligned the bones up, held them reduced with clamps, and then placed cerclage wires around the fracture to help keep it aligned. A guidewire was advanced across the fracture. We subsequently reamed up to a size 13 reamer and then advanced a 12 mm x 36 mm nail across the fracture sites. The reconstruction screw was placed through the nail up into the femoral head under guidance. We elected to leave this nail without distal fixation in hopes that this would compress at the fracture site. We then irrigated thoroughly and then squirted some Norian bone graft filler from Synthes into the defects in the bone. We subsequently irrigated it and repaired the wounds over Hemovac drains in normal fashion. The skin was approximated with staples. Sterile dressings were applied. The patient went to the recovery room in stable condition.

RICHARD KING, MD

RK:hpi

d: 8/6/[add year]
t: 8/7/[add year]

Comic Relief

Dictation and transcription mistakes are common occurrences in orthopedic documents. Here are some favorites.

His left arm was fractured when his car was jacked.

The patient was referred to our car for physical therapy.

The patient was able to bear weight on the knee after meniscectomy, and by discharge it had completely disappeared.

The patient claims that he is numb from the toes down.

When she slipped on the ice, her right leg went east and her left leg went west.

PEARSON
myhealthprofessionskit™

To access the online exercises and transcription practice, go to **www.myhealthprofessionskit.com**. Select "Medical Transcription," then click on the title of this book, ***Healthcare Documentation: Fundamentals & Practice***. Then click on the Orthopedics chapter.

Neurology

Chapter Outline

Learning Objectives

▶ Describe the structure and function of the nervous system.

▶ Spell and define common neurology terms.

▶ Identify neurology vocabulary that might be used in the review of systems.

▶ Describe the negative and positive findings a physician looks for on neurologic examination.

▶ Describe the typical cause, course, and treatment options for common diseases of the nervous system.

▶ Identify and define common diagnostic and surgical procedures of the nervous system.

▶ List common neurologic laboratory tests and procedures.

▶ Identify and describe common neurologic drugs and their uses.

▶ Demonstrate knowledge of medical, pharmacological, adjectival, and soundalike terms by accurately completing the exercises in this chapter.

Transcribing Neurology Dictation

Introduction

Neurology is a branch of medicine that focuses on disorders of the nervous system, particularly the central nervous system (CNS). A **neurologist** is a physician with three years of postdoctoral training and specialty board certification in the diagnosis and non-surgical management of developmental anomalies, injuries, infections, and degenerative and neoplastic diseases of the brain, spinal cord, and peripheral nerves.

Neurosurgery is a surgical subspecialty devoted to the operative treatment of nervous system disorders, particularly head wounds and intracranial neoplasms. A **neurosurgeon** is a physician with six to seven years of postdoctoral training and board certification in surgery of the central nervous system.

Neuropsychiatry is a medical specialty combining features of neurology and psychiatry. A **neuropsychiatrist** is a physician with both psychiatric and neurologic training who treats patients with emotional or behavioral disorders related to organic disease affecting higher brain centers (cerebral cortex, limbic system), such as epilepsy, attention deficit disorder, and dementia.

Anatomy Review

The **nervous system** (see ■ Figure 17-1) is an exceedingly complex arrangement of nerve cells and their fibers that extends throughout the body and receives, processes, and interprets sensory stimuli; initiates and coordinates voluntary muscular movement; regulates autonomic processes such as heartbeat, vascular constriction and dilatation, bronchiolar caliber, sweating, and gastrointestinal secretion and motility; carries out complex mental functions and operations including memory and recall of past events, recognition of persons and objects, abstract reasoning and practical problem solving, judgment, and language production and comprehension; and is the seat of mood and emotions.

All nerve tissue is made up of **nerve cells** and their processes. Although nerve cells vary widely in structure and function, all conform to a basic pattern. Each nerve cell (**neuron**) consists of a cell body containing a nucleus; one or more short treelike processes called **dendrites**; and a single long straight process, the **axon**. Dendrites conduct nerve impulses toward the cell body, and are therefore called **afferent processes**; axons conduct impulses away from the cell and are therefore called

efferent processes. The point of contact between processes of two different cells is called a **synapse**. Chemical substances called neurotransmitters are produced in infinitesimal quantities at nerve endings and serve to transmit nerve impulses, either stimulating or inhibiting, across the synapse.

The axons of some nerve cells are enveloped in a thin layer of fatty white material called **myelin**. The **myelin sheath** serves as an electrical insulator. Nerve tissue consisting of many myelinated fibers is called **white matter**; tissue consisting chiefly of nerve cell bodies is called **gray matter**.

The nervous system is divided into two major sections: the **central nervous system**, consisting of the brain and spinal cord; and the **peripheral nervous system**, consisting of the peripheral motor and sensory nerves and the **autonomic nervous system**. The **brain** (see ■ Figure 17-2), which entirely fills the cranial cavity, is traditionally broken down into major parts on the basis of gross anatomic features:

The **cerebrum**, made up of two symmetric hemispheres and concerned with the higher mental processes; its surface, the **cerebral cortex**, is thrown into deep convolutions like the kernel of a walnut. The convexities (raised areas) are called **gyri**, and the grooves between them are called **sulci**. Deeper grooves (**fissures**) divide each hemisphere into four lobes: **frontal**, **temporal**, **parietal**, and **occipital**.

The **cerebellum** lies behind the cerebrum and looks like a smaller version of it, as its name implies. Its principal function is coordination of voluntary motor activity.

Four structures—diencephalon, mesencephalon or midbrain, pons, and medulla oblongata—compose, from front to back, the **ventral surface of the brain**; the last three make up the **brain stem**. The medulla continues below the skull as the **spinal cord**.

The brain and spinal cord are covered by three protective membranes called **meninges**. The outer membrane, the **dura mater**, is in contact with the bony interior of the skull and spinal column. Within the dura is the delicate **arachnoid membrane**, and within that is the **pia mater**, which lies on the surface of the brain and spinal cord.

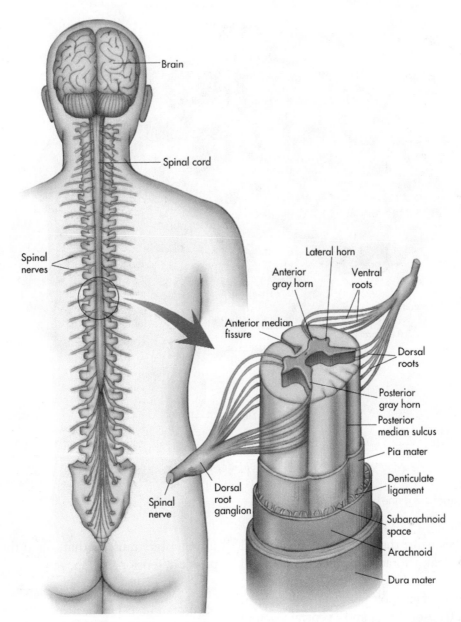

FIGURE 17-1. The nervous system including the brain, spinal cord, and spinal nerves with an expanded view of a spinal nerve

Within the cerebrum and the diencephalon is a system of communicating hollow chambers (the two **lateral ventricles**, the **third ventricle**, and the **fourth ventricle**). **Cerebrospinal fluid** (CSF) is a watery medium that is both formed and reabsorbed within the skull and serves primarily as a shock absorber. It surrounds the brain and spinal cord in the subarachnoid space and also fills the ventricular system and the hollow central canal of the spinal cord.

Twelve pairs of cranial nerves (traditionally represented by Roman numerals) emerge from the ventral surface of the brain and brain stem and serve important sensory and motor functions, chiefly within the head.

The **spinal cord** is made up largely of axons of nerve cells, some with cell bodies in the brain (carrying motor impulses to various spinal segments) and others with cell bodies in the cord itself (carrying sensory impulses from spinal segments to various brain centers). Whereas the visible surface of the cerebral cortex is made up of gray matter (cell bodies), with white matter inside, in the spinal cord the white matter, consisting of ascending and descending myelinated nerve fibers, is on the outside, and the gray matter is within.

The **peripheral nervous system** comprises all nerve tissue outside the brain and spinal cord. Its two major divisions are the **spinal nerves** and the **autonomic nervous system**. Spinal nerves are those that originate in the spinal cord and pass between pairs of vertebrae to supply the body with sensation and voluntary motor power. There are 31 sets of spinal nerves, one arising

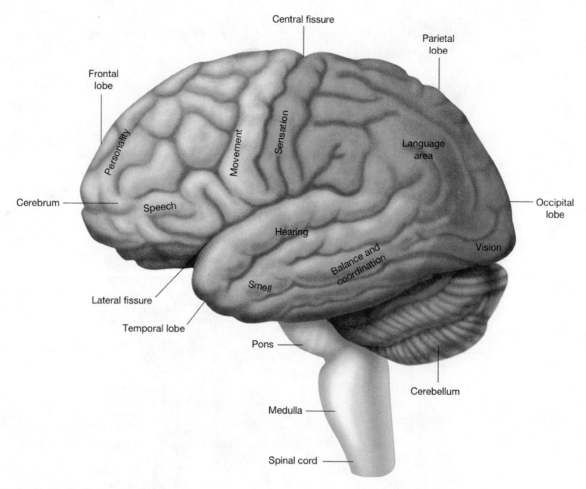

FIGURE 17-2. Major structures of the brain

from each spinal segment; these segments correspond closely to the cervical, thoracic, lumbar, and (fused) sacral vertebrae.

Each spinal segment gives off a pair of nerve roots on each side: a **dorsal (sensory) root** and a **ventral (motor) root**. Each dorsal root has a visible node or swelling (**ganglion**) containing cell bodies of sensory nerves. The dorsal and ventral roots fuse to form **segmental nerves**, which pass forward around the body and give off branches to all external surfaces and internal structures, particularly muscles of the trunk and extremities.

Each visible and named peripheral nerve is a bundle of thousands of myelinated axons of motor neurons whose cell bodies lie in the brain and spinal cord, and of dendrites of sensory nerves, whose cell bodies are located in the dorsal root ganglia. **Motor nerves** send signals to voluntary muscles throughout the body. **Sensory nerves** carry impulses from sensory structures in the skin that respond to pain, pressure, light touch, hot, and cold; from visceral sensors that respond to pressure or stretching and pain; and from proprioceptive sensors

in voluntary muscles that signal the brain as to their position, tension, and movement.

Sensory exam: Has decreased pin sensation, stocking-glove fashion, up to about the wrists and the hands, to just about the knees and the legs. This was for pain sensation. Joint position sense appears to be intact.

The **autonomic nervous system** is a purely motor system concerned with automatic or involuntary activities or processes, such as heart rate and digestion. The bodily effects of emotion (tachycardia, sweating, pallor, sense of constriction in the chest) largely result from the actions of the autonomic nervous system.

Nerves of the sympathetic or thoracolumbar division arise from a series of ganglia lying along each side of the thoracic and lumbar segments of the spinal cord, but outside the spinal column. These communicate with the spinal cord and with one another by both myelinated and nonmyelinated fibers. The **sympathetic**

Neurologically there are no focal signs, but the patient is very confused. She is not oriented to person, place, time, or situation. Her memory is extremely poor.

nervous system is concerned with the so-called fight or flight response mediated by **epinephrine** and **norepinephrine**. Nerves of the sympathetic division are distributed to the eye, where they cause pupillary dilatation; the heart, where they increase the pulse rate; the lungs, where they cause bronchodilation; and the skin, where they constrict blood vessels, stimulate secretion of sweat, and cause erection of hairs.

The **parasympathetic** or **craniosacral** division of the autonomic nervous system provides motor innervation to cranial, thoracic, abdominal, and pelvic viscera, generally of an opposite nature to sympathetic innervation. That is, parasympathetic activity occurs chiefly during periods of rest or quiet, and is associated with cardiac rate and with such physiologic processes as gastrointestinal secretion and motility and sexual activity.

Parasympathetic nerves arise only from the brain and from sacral segments of the spinal cord. Three cranial nerves (III, VII, and IX) send parasympathetic fibers to structures in the head (iris, ciliary body, salivary glands); a fourth (X) sends fibers to thoracic, abdominal, and pelvic viscera (heart, lungs, digestive system). Parasympathetic nerves from sacral segments of the spinal cord supply the urinary tract and reproductive system.

Pause for Reflection

1. Describe the key components of a nerve cell.
2. What is the myelin sheath?
3. Name and describe the major sections of the nervous system.
4. Name the main divisions of the brain and describe their principal functions.
5. Name the meninges and describe their location.
6. What are the ventricles of the brain?
7. Distinguish between the cranial nerves and the spinal cord.
8. Describe the 2 major components of the peripheral nervous system.
9. Describe the function and main components of the autonomic nervous system.

Vocabulary Review

altered level of consciousness Varying from slight drowsiness or inattentiveness, to confusion and disorientation, to deep coma from which the subject cannot be aroused by any stimulus.

absence ("ab sáhnce") **seizure** (petit mal) Brief loss of attention and perception.

amnesia Loss of memory, recent, remote, or total.

anesthesia Total loss of sensation on one or more parts of the body surface.

aphasia Impairment of the ability to communicate through spoken or written language, or to understand spoken or written language, or both.

ataxia Impairment of complex movements due to loss of proprioceptive impulses from the muscles of the trunk or limbs.

athetosis Slow, writhing, involuntary movements of the face or limbs.

Babinski reflex Consists of dorsiflexion of the great toe and flaring of the other toes in response to stroking the sole of the foot toward the toes; an indication of disease or injury affecting a corticospinal tract. A normal reflex is downgoing, except in newborns and infants, in which the normal Babinski reflex is upgoing.

causalgia Burning or stinging due to irritation or inflammation of nerves.

cephalgia, cephalalgia Headache. Local or generalized, intermittent or constant; can result from infection, neoplasm, or hemorrhage within the cranium, obstruction to the flow of cerebrospinal fluid, trauma, or migraine.

Chaddock reflex Extension of the great toe elicited by tapping the ankle behind the lateral malleolus, a sign of disease or injury of a corticospinal tract.

chorea Rapid, jerky, purposeless involuntary movements of one or several muscle groups.

complex seizure Impaired alertness or unconsciousness; sometimes with psychic symptoms or automatisms.

deep tendon reflexes Occur in response to sudden stretching of a muscle, usually induced by tapping a tendon with a rubber-headed reflex hammer. Tendon reflexes are tested in several muscles of the upper and

LAY AND MEDICAL TERMS

fainting	syncope
fit, convulsion	seizure; epileptic seizure
numbness	hypesthesia, anesthesia, or paresthesia
pins and needles	parathesias
spinal tap	lumbar puncture
stroke	cerebrovascular accident (CVA)
water on the brain	hydrocephalus

lower extremities, with comparison of the two sides. Also called *muscle stretch reflexes*.

dementia Deterioration of mental function.

Glasgow coma scale Used to assess a patient's level of consciousness after a head injury. Verbal, motor, and sensory responses to stimuli are graded on a scale of 1 through 5. The values for each are added together for a total score. A score of 7 or less indicates coma; a score of 3 or less indicates brain death.

dorsiflexion Bending upward of the hand or foot.

dysequilibrium Loss of balance sense; tendency to fall without support.

flaccidity Absence of muscle tone and absence of reflexes.

generalized seizure A seizure in which the entire cerebral cortex is involved.

grand mal seizure See *tonic-clonic*.

graphesthesia The ability to recognize letters or numbers traced on the skin.

headache See *cephalgia, cephalalgia*.

hydrocephalus An increase in the volume of cerebrospinal fluid in the ventricular system of the brain, usually accompanied by an increase of pressure and eventually by reduction of brain substance.

hypesthesia Partial loss of sensation on one or more parts of the body surface.

incoordination Jerkiness and awkwardness in activities requiring smooth coordination of several muscles.

intention tremor Tremor occurring only during voluntary movement.

lamina of vertebral arch (L., *lamina arcus vertebrae*. Either of the pair of broad plates of bone flaring out from the pedicles of the vertebral arches and fusing together at the midline to complete the dorsal part of the arch and provide a base for the spinous process.

myoclonic seizures Repeated shocklike, often violent contractions in one or more muscle groups.

neuropathy A general term for pathological change in any part of the peripheral nervous system.

nuchal rigidity Marked stiffness of the neck, a cardinal finding in meningitis.

paralysis Complete loss of muscular function.

paresis Muscle weakness.

paresthesia A sense of tingling or prickling ("pins and needles") on a part of the body surface. The lay term "numbness" is applied indiscriminately to hypesthesia, anesthesia, and paresthesia.

partial seizure Seizure in which only part of one cerebral cortex is involved.

pathologic reflexes Present only in neurological disorders, such as Babinski reflex or Chaddock reflex.

petit mal seizure (absence seizure) Characterized by brief loss of attention and perception.

Phalen sign Reproduction of pain or paresthesia in carpal tunnel syndrome when both wrists are flexed with the hands firmly pressing one another back-to-back for 60 seconds.

plantar flexion Bending downward of the hand or foot.

porencephaly One or more cysts or cavities in a cerebral hemisphere communicating with the ventricular system. There may be little or no neurologic impairment.

postictal state After awakening from seizure, subject is drowsy and amnesic for a variable period.

proprioception Position sense.

radiculopathy A general term for disease of the nerve roots.

reflex A muscular contraction occurring in response to a sensory stimulus.

resting tremor Tremor occurring only when the affected muscles are not being used for purposeful activity.

seizures Sudden, transitory impairment of central nervous system function, with or without loss of consciousness, and with or without local or generalized tonic and clonic contractions of voluntary muscles.

simple seizure No unconsciousness; local twitching or jerking; perception of flashing lights or other abnormal sensory phenomena.

spasm Sustained contraction, usually painful, of a muscle.

spasmodic torticollis Twisting of the neck and unnatural position of the head caused by spasms of neck muscles, particularly the sternocleidomastoid and trapezius muscles.

spasticity Tight muscles with resistance to manipulation and hyperactive reflexes.

spina bifida A failure of closure of one or more vertebrae in the posterior midline, which may be associated with bulging of meninges (**meningocele**) or of spinal cord and meninges (**meningomyelocele**) (see ■ Figure 17-3).

spondylosis (1) Ankylosis—immobility and consolidation of a joint due to disease, injury, or surgical procedure, or (2) degenerative spinal changes of the vertebrae, intervertebral disks, and surrounding ligaments and connective tissue due to osteoarthritis, sometimes accompanied by pain and paresthesias.

status epilepticus Series of grand mal seizures without waking intervals.

stereognosis The ability to identify objects solely by feeling them.

superficial reflexes Muscle contractions in response to stroking the skin; those of the abdominal wall are tested as part of a complete neurologic examination.

syncope (fainting) Sudden loss of consciousness, usually transitory, due to circulatory or neurologic abnormality, including central nervous system intoxication or injury, but frequently the result of strong emotion in the absence of organic disease.

tic A rapid involuntary muscle twitch, typically recurrent and stereotyped, affecting one or several body areas.

Tinel sign Shocklike pain when the volar aspect of the wrist is tapped; indicative of carpal tunnel syndrome.

tonic-clonic seizure In the tonic phase the victim becomes rigid, often cries out, loses consciousness, falls, stops breathing. In the clonic phase there is generalized muscular jerking; may bite tongue or lips, may be incontinent of urine or stool.

The patient is a very pleasant 79-year-old gentleman who presented to the emergency room with acute onset of tonic-clonic seizure activity with loss of consciousness, which lasted about 30 minutes.

tremor(s) Shaking of parts of the body supplied by voluntary muscles, principally the arms, forearms, and hands.

two-point discrimination The ability to distinguish two adjacent, simultaneous pinpricks.

vertigo A subjective sense of spinning. Dysequilibrium and vertigo sometimes occur together, and both are indiscriminately referred to as dizziness by the laity.

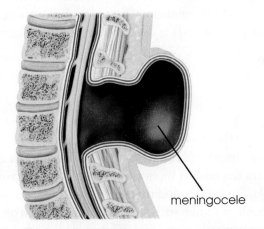

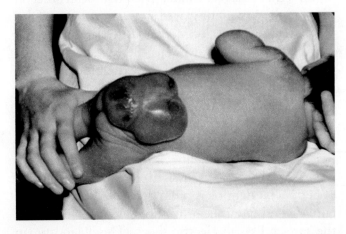

meningocele

FIGURE 17-3. (Left) Cross-sectional view of a meningocele of the spinal cord. (Right) Photograph of a child born with spina bifida, with a large meningocele. Source: Biophoto Associates, Photo Researchers, Inc.

Medical Readings

History and Physical Examination

by John H. Dirckx, MD

Review of Systems. This broad category includes disorders of the central and peripheral nervous systems and injuries and diseases that affect not only skeletal muscle but also bones, joints, ligaments, and associated structures. The patient is questioned about prior diagnosis of, and treatment for, seizures, brain concussion, brain tumor, stroke, paralysis, neuritis, any fractures or dislocations, severe sprains, bursitis, tendinitis, or arthritis.

Neurologic: The patient denies any syncope, vertigo, hemiparalysis, or paresthesias except for the feeling of numbness in his feet.

Symptoms suggestive of **central nervous system disease** are severe or unusual headache; unexplained drowsiness or dysequilibrium; confusion; disorientation; sudden deterioration of memory, judgment, or emotional stability; tremors; incoordination; disorders of speech; weakness, clumsiness, paralysis, or spasticity of the extremities; and seizures. Often, detailed information on these points must be obtained from someone other than the patient. In obtaining a full picture of any of these symptoms, the interviewer asks whether it is constant, intermittent, or progressive; to what extent it impairs normal function; and whether any cause can be suggested for the symptom, such as a recent or remote injury or use of alcohol or drugs.

In gathering data about **syncopal episodes** or seizures, the physician will try to learn from an observer whether the patient displayed any warning signs of distress, cried out, fell, lost consciousness completely or only became confused; whether there was local or general twitching or writhing of the extremities; whether the patient was incontinent of urine during the seizure; and how long after the seizure any weakness, drowsiness, or confusion remained.

Peripheral nerve disorders are suggested by numbness, paresthesia (a tingling or "pins and needles" sensation), weakness, or paralysis in an extremity. The pain of peripheral neuritis is often described as stinging or burning and often seems to shoot along or just under the surface like an electric shock. The diagnostician inquires whether symptoms are brought on or aggravated by fatigue, certain activities or positions, or a cold or damp environment, and whether there has been exposure to toxic drugs or chemicals.

The Neurologic Examination. The examination of the central and peripheral nervous systems, like that of the heart, consists almost exclusively of tests of function. Many of these tests require the cooperation of the patient. However, the more urgent the need for a neurologic exam, the less capable the patient may be to cooperate. The extreme example is the **comatose patient**, whose life may depend on prompt and accurate diagnosis but who cannot cooperate at all. The basic neurologic examination is augmented by special procedures as history and findings direct.

Most parts of the neurologic examination are carried out on a regional basis and interspersed with examinations of other systems. In analyzing and recording findings, however, the physician classifies them according to anatomic and functional divisions of the nervous system. The **central nervous system (CNS)** comprises the brain and spinal cord; the peripheral nervous system, the cranial and spinal nerves. Peripheral nerve fibers are either motor (efferent) fibers carrying impulses to muscles, or sensory (afferent) fibers carrying impulses to the spinal cord or brain stem. Both kinds of fibers are often combined in a single nerve trunk.

The physician tests **sensory functions** by stimulating appropriate receptors and noting the patient's responses. **Motor functions** are tested by observing the patient's ability to perform certain actions. Even in an unconscious patient, testing the **deep tendon reflexes** enables the examiner to assess the integrity of the spinal reflex arcs, which consist of both sensory (stretch receptor) and motor nerve fibers. But evaluation of complex voluntary movements and muscle coordination requires the conscious collaboration of the patient. Assessment of cerebral functions (memory, orientation, thinking capacity, mood) is described in the psychiatry chapter.

Neurologic exam reveals no gross sensory or motor deficients.

If the patient is stuporous or unconscious, the physician tries to determine the degree of central nervous system depression by noting the size and reactivity of the pupils, the rate and rhythm of breathing, the response to noxious stimuli such as loud noises and firm pressure over bony prominences, and the presence of certain primitive reflexes such as the corneal and gag reflex. In the **doll's**

eye maneuver, the examiner rotates the patient's head from side to side and notes the effect on eye position. Normally the eyes rotate in a direction opposite to that in which the head is moved, tending to maintain the same direction of gaze (**oculocephalic reflex**). Failure of the eyes to rotate around their own vertical axes during this maneuver indicates **brain stem damage**.

Pause for Reflection

1. Describe an observer's role in the examiner's attempt to obtain a full picture of the patient's neurological review of systems.
2. What symptoms might a patient report if there is a peripheral nerve disorder present?
3. In general, how does the examiner test for sensory and motor function?
4. What does the examiner do if the patient is stuporous or unconscious?
5. Describe the doll's eye maneuver.

Cranial Nerves

The twelve pairs of cranial nerves (traditionally represented by Roman numerals) emanate from the brain stem and pass to structures in the head and neck. They serve important sensory and motor functions, chiefly within the head. The cranial nerves are assessed individually by the following maneuvers:

I. **Olfactory**: Testing sense of smell. This assessment is often omitted, hence the frequent expression, "Cranial nerves II through XII are intact." It can be evaluated by asking the patient to identify common substances (soap, tobacco) by their odors.

II. **Optic**: Testing the patient's vision with standard eye charts. Checking peripheral vision and visual fields by simple techniques. Examination of the ocular fundi with an ophthalmoscope.

III. **Oculomotor**: Testing ocular movements; observing for strabismus, nystagmus, and drooping of eyelids. Testing the ability of the pupil to constrict when stimulated by light and when focused on a near object. The oculomotor nerve innervates four of the six extraocular muscles. The fourth nerve (trochlear) innervates only the superior oblique, the sixth (abducens) only the lateral rectus. In examining the eyes the physician doesn't assess each muscle separately, but rather observes whether both eyes follow the movements of a fingertip or light carried through a random

sequence of movements. Once that procedure has been carried out, all extraocular muscles (and movements) have been assessed.

IV. **Trochlear**: Assessed with cranial nerve III.

V. **Trigeminal**: Sensitivity to light touch (wisp of cotton or fine brush) and pain (sterile needle) are tested over the skin of the face. The **blink reflex** to touching the cornea with cotton is also tested. The integrity of motor branches to the muscles of mastication is tested by having the patient open the mouth wide and then clench the teeth together.

VI. **Abducens**: Assessed with cranial nerve III.

VII. **Facial**: Testing muscles of facial expression by having the patient wrinkle the forehead, close the eyes tightly, retract the lips so as to show the teeth, and purse the lips as for whistling. Taste on the anterior two thirds (front part) of the tongue may be tested by touching the tongue with a drop of salt or sugar solution or vinegar.

VIII. **Vestibulocochlear**: Hearing and equilibrium. Cold caloric test: when ice water is poured into the ear canal, a normal vestibular apparatus causes nystagmus with the quick component to the opposite side. Hearing is tested in each ear separately.

IX. **Glossopharyngeal**: With impairment of innervation to one side of the palate, the uvula deviates to the normal side, particularly during the **gag reflex**. Swallowing is affected by impairment of either the ninth or the tenth cranial nerve.

X. **Vagus**: The patient's ability to speak and to swallow is observed.

XI. **Accessory**: The patient's ability to push against the examiner's hand with each side of the chin indicates integrity of the nerve supply to the sternocleidomastoid and trapezius muscles.

XII. **Hypoglossal**: The examiner notes the symmetry of development of the tongue muscles at rest and the symmetry of movement when the tongue is protruded. Impairment of a hypoglossal nerve causes deviation of the tongue to the affected side.

Pause for Reflection

1. List each cranial nerve and the sensory or motor function associated with it.
2. Describe the manner in which each cranial nerve is tested.
3. Explain the expression "Cranial nerves II through XII are intact."

Spinal Nerves

The **spinal nerves** emerge from the spinal cord in pairs, one right and one left, and supply the body from the occiput downward with sensory and motor fibers (see ■ Figure 17-4). A pair of spinal nerves is named from the vertebra above which (cervical region) or below which (other regions) it emerges. Thus the L2 pair emerge below the second lumbar vertebra.

Sensory innervation of the skin is assessed by the subject's ability to recognize **light touch** (wisp of cotton), **pain** (sterile needle), **hot and cold** (test tubes of hot and cold water) on various parts of the body surface. Examination may include tests of **stereognosis** (ability to recognize an object by handling it), **vibratory sense** (ability to sense the vibration of a tuning fork when the stem is placed on a bone near the surface, such as the elbow or the shin), **two-point discrimination** (ability to distinguish two points close together on the skin).

Proprioception is tested by having the subject report whether a toe or finger is moved up or down by the examiner, and by observation of stance and gait. The **Romberg test** (having the subject stand with feet together and eyes open, then eyes closed) assesses position sense in the trunk and legs.

Motor innervation is tested by observation of muscle development, tone, and voluntary movement in the trunk and limbs, with comparison of the two sides. The examiner notes any wasting, paralysis, spasm or rigidity, or involuntary movements (tremors, tics, chorea, athetosis). Coordination is tested by having the subject perform **rapid alternating movements** with the hands or feet. The **finger-to-nose** and **heel-to-shin tests** and **tandem walking** are other ways of judging coordination.

Reflexes: A reflex is a muscular contraction occurring in response to a sensory stimulus, such as tapping the patellar tendon. All the nerve cells and fibers involved in a reflex are located in a spinal cord segment, and its sensory and motor roots form a so-called **reflex arc**; the brain is not involved.

Muscle stretch (deep tendon) reflexes occur in response to sudden stretching of a muscle, usually induced by tapping a tendon with a rubber-headed reflex hammer. Tendon reflexes are tested in several muscles of the upper and lower extremities, with comparison of the two sides.

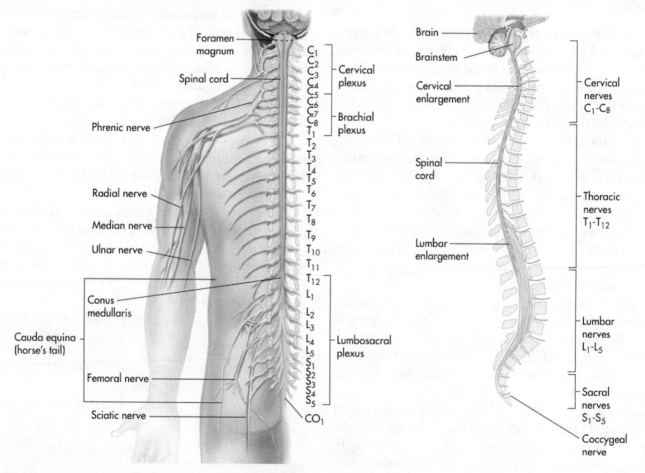

FIGURE 17-4. The 31 pairs of spinal nerves

Superficial (cutaneous) reflexes are muscle contractions in response to stroking the skin; those of the abdominal wall are tested as part of a complete neurologic examination.

Pathologic reflexes are present only in neurologic disorders. The **Babinski reflex** consists of dorsiflexion of the great toe and flaring of the other toes in response to stroking of the sole of the foot toward the toes. The **Chaddock reflex** is the same response to tapping the lateral aspect of the ankle. These and similar pathologic reflexes, along with spastic paralysis and rigidity, indicate an **upper motor neuron lesion**—interruption of motor tracts from the cerebral cortex to the spinal segment involved, without impairment of the reflex arc. Flaccid paralysis, absence of normal and abnormal reflexes, and muscle wasting indicate a **lower motor neuron lesion**—interruption of motor tracts from spinal cord to muscle.

Pause for Reflection

1. How is sensory innervation of the skin tested?
2. How is proprioception tested?
3. How are motor innervation and coordination tested?
4. Define *reflex*. Distinguish among deep tendon reflexes, superficial reflexes, and pathologic reflexes.
5. Define upper motor neuron lesion and how such a disorder is determined.
6. Define lower motor neuron lesion and how it is diagnosed.

Common Diseases

Multiple Sclerosis (MS)

A chronic sensory and motor disorder of variable presentation, due to loss of myelin from nerve cells in the central nervous system.

Cause: Patchy deterioration of the myelin sheaths of nerve tracts in the brain and spinal cord and in the optic nerve leads to deterioration of nerve function. The cause is unknown; genetic, infectious, and autoimmune factors have been suggested. Onset is usually between the ages of 20 and 40. The incidence is higher in women and in cooler latitudes. Disease is sometimes apparently precipitated by fatigue, emotional stress, pregnancy, or viral respiratory infection.

History: Irregular, intermittent or progressive impairment of sensory or motor function: hypesthesia, paresthesia, visual disturbances, disorders of equilibrium; muscular weakness, spasticity, or unsteadiness; tremors, nystagmus, diplopia, disturbances of swallowing or bladder function.

Physical Examination: Findings on neurologic examination are typically diffuse and highly variable: hypesthesia or anesthesia, irregularly distributed muscle weakness with spasticity and hyperactive deep tendon reflexes, Babinski reflex, impaired superficial abdominal reflexes, ataxia, uncoordinated (scanning) speech, tremors, nystagmus, temporal pallor of the optic disks followed by optic atrophy, visual field defects, emotional lability.

Diagnostic Tests: The spinal fluid may show moderate lymphocytosis and elevation of the immune globulins, including oligoclonal IgG globulins (antibody to myelin) not found in serum. The electroencephalogram may show nonspecific abnormalities. MRI of the brain and spinal cord shows multiple patchy lesions. Visual evoked potential testing may corroborate the diagnosis.

Course: The disease is highly unpredictable. Four **patterns** are distinguished: relapsing remitting, primary progressive, secondary progressive, and progressive relapsing. Presenting symptoms often remit for months or years. Typically the disease progresses gradually, with remissions and exacerbations, and eventually produces some disability. Relapses may be triggered by excessive fatigue.

Treatment: Increased rest, particularly during periods of heightened symptoms. Adrenocortical steroids often mitigate neurologic impairment, particularly during acute relapses. Physical therapy and muscle relaxants are helpful in dealing with muscle weakness and spasm. Immunotherapy, plasmapheresis, and synthetic myelin protein are among treatments currently being evaluated. Psychotherapy or counseling may be necessary.

Guillain-Barré Syndrome

A chronic inflammation of peripheral nerves, causing muscle weakness or paralysis.

Cause: Formation of autoantibody to myelin, with resultant segmental demyelination of peripheral nerve fibers, usually reversible. Precipitating causes: acute infection (influenza, infectious mononucleosis, varicella-zoster), myocardial infarction, certain vaccines, surgery.

History: Progressive, symmetric muscle weakness in both arms and legs, paresthesia, hypesthesia, and pain, coming on 1–4 weeks after the precipitating event. The cranial nerves may be involved. Loss of bladder control and respiratory paralysis may occur.

Physical Examination: Peripheral sensation is impaired, and deep tendon reflexes are diminished or absent. The pulse and blood pressure may be elevated.

Diagnostic Tests: The spinal fluid contains elevated protein but normal cell counts.

Course: The case fatality rate is about 5%. About 65% of patients who recover have minor neurologic impairment and 10% remain severely disabled.

Treatment: Physical therapy; cardiac monitoring and pulse oximetry, with mechanical ventilation as needed. Intravenous immune globulin. Plasmapheresis to remove antibody from serum.

Amyotrophic Lateral Sclerosis (ALS, Lou Gehrig Disease)

Progressive paralysis and wasting of muscles due to degeneration of motor neurons.

Cause: Unknown. There is a genetic predisposition, and men are affected more than women by a ratio of 3:1. Viral or autoimmune factors cannot be excluded. Possible precipitating factors include trauma, extreme stress or fatigue, viral respiratory infection, and myocardial infarction.

History: Onset, between the ages of 30 and 50, of weakness and wasting of voluntary muscles, particularly those in the hands and feet. **Fasciculations** (repeated twitching of small groups of voluntary muscle fibers) may precede any other symptoms. Eventually, with brain stem involvement, difficulty in speaking, eating, and even breathing. Depression commonly occurs with progressive deterioration.

Physical Examination: Muscle weakness and atrophy, visible fasciculations, evidence of cranial and spinal motor nerve malfunction without sensory impairment. Hyperactive deep tendon reflexes, spasticity, and rigidity indicate upper motor neuron degeneration.

Diagnostic Tests: Electromyography and muscle biopsy confirm loss of motor nerve supply to affected areas.

Course: Usually the disease is steadily progressive and death occurs in 2–5 years.

Treatment: Purely supportive; physical therapy, muscle relaxants; nasogastric tube or gastrostomy feedings, tracheotomy and respirator as needed.

Parkinsonism (Parkinson Disease, Paralysis Agitans)

A chronic, progressive neurologic disorder causing muscle tremor and rigidity.

The patient was diagnosed with Parkinson disease. His gait progressively became worse over the last 5 years, and he started falling more consistently. Over the last 6 months, his balance worsened and he felt light-headed, especially with walking. . . . He was referred for a ventriculoperitoneal (VP) shunt.

Cause: Unknown. Neurologic symptoms are due to deterioration and dopamine depletion in certain brain nuclei (corpus striatum, globus pallidus, substantia nigra). It is more common in men and onset is usually between 45 and 65. Certain toxic chemicals (carbon disulfide, carbon monoxide), drugs (chlorpromazine, haloperidol, and other neuroleptic drugs), and a history of encephalitis can induce parkinsonian symptoms.

History: Resting tremor, initially in one extremity, that is exacerbated by emotional stress and reduced during voluntary motion. Stiffness, rigidity, and **bradykinesia** (slowness of movement) commonly occur, with postural instability and gait disorders.

Physical Examination: Immobile, masklike face (**parkinsonian facies**), with infrequent blinking. Reduced automatic movements such as swinging the arms while walking. Hyperactive deep tendon reflexes and resistance to passive movement of joints, often with **"cogwheel" rigidity**. A flexed posture, a shuffling and seemingly hurried (festinating) gait, and difficulty in standing from a sitting position are typical. Seborrhea (excessive secretion of sebum) on the scalp and face and excessive drooling are also often seen. The handwriting becomes smaller (**micrographia**). There may be mild deterioration of mental function.

Course: Typically progressive, with death in about 10 years.

Treatment: Drug treatment is helpful in advanced disease: amantadine, anticholinergics (trihexyphenidyl, ethopropazine), levodopa and carbidopa, bromocriptine, and selegiline. Surgical removal of degenerating brain tissue may be a good choice in younger patients. Physical and speech therapy and counseling are important for most patients.

Encephalitis

Inflammation of the brain due to viral infection.

Cause: Most cases of encephalitis are due to viruses transmitted by mosquitoes (Eastern and Western equine encephalitis, Japanese B encephalitis) or ticks. Numerous other viruses (coxsackievirus, herpes simplex virus, mumps virus, HIV) can cause encephalitis.

History: Abrupt onset of fever and headache, with muscle weakness or paralysis, restlessness, personality or behavioral changes, delirium, seizures, and lethargy perhaps progressing to coma.

Physical Examination: Fever, depressed level of consciousness, signs of meningeal irritation, evidence of focal or diffuse neurologic damage including tremors, paralysis, hyperreactive reflexes, and pathologic reflexes.

Diagnostic Tests: Serologic studies can identify the causative virus. The CSF shows increase of pressure, protein, and cells. Abnormal findings on electroencephalogram (EEG) are nonspecific.

Course: Most cases resolve without sequelae after a few weeks, but many are followed by residual paralysis, seizures, and parkinsonism.

Treatment: Largely supportive. Physical therapy; attention to nutrition and hydration. Drug therapy as needed to provide sedation, relieve fever and headache, and control convulsions. Herpes simplex encephalitis responds to acyclovir. In severe disease, adrenal corticosteroids may reduce cerebral edema and inflammation.

Meningitis

Infection of the meninges, with neurologic and systemic effects.

Causes: Infection with bacteria (*Staphylococcus*, pneumococcus, meningococcus, *Haemophilus influenzae*, *Escherichia coli*, *Mycobacterium tuberculosis*), viruses (mumps virus, coxsackievirus, herpes simplex virus), fungi, or protozoans. Causative organisms may be introduced by a penetrating head wound, spread locally from infections of the ears or sinuses, or reach the meninges through the bloodstream from remote sites (pneumonia, endocarditis). Symptoms vary considerably with the etiologic agent; signs and symptoms are milder in viral than in bacterial meningitis and the prognosis more favorable. Meningitis due to meningococcus (*Neisseria meningitidis*) is a rapidly progressive and highly lethal disease, particularly because the meningococcus causes a severe toxemia that can lead to shock and death, even in the absence of signs of meningitis.

HEENT revealed marked stiffness of the neck with nuchal rigidity. Positive Brudzinski, Kernig signs.

PROVISIONAL DIAGNOSIS
Acute bacterial meningitis.

This child was born with cystic hydromas secondary to meningitis and has a permanent shunt in place. The child has had increasing frequency of seizures over the past few months and has been treated in the emergency room and hospitalized on several occasions for these. Today the patient requested that his mother pump his shunt and then began having left-sided seizures without vomiting or dyspnea.

History: Abrupt onset of fever, headache, and vomiting. Painful stiffness of the neck and back muscles, visual disturbances, and irritability, twitching, or seizures. Clouding of the sensorium, delirium, and coma may follow rapidly.

Physical Examination: Fever, depressed level of consciousness. Signs of meningeal irritation include **nuchal rigidity** (stiffness of the neck, with inability to touch the chin to the chest), painful stiffness of other muscles, hyperreflexia, **Kernig sign** (inability to extend the knee when the thigh is flexed), **Brudzinski sign** (passive flexion of the neck causes active flexion of the hip and knee). In an infant, bulging of the fontanelles.

Diagnostic Tests: Lumbar puncture shows elevated pressure. The CSF may be purulent. White blood cells and protein are elevated. In bacterial meningitis, CSF glucose is low. Smear and culture of the fluid identify bacterial agents. In viral (aseptic) meningitis the fluid is clear and the glucose is normal; viral culture may identify the cause.

Course: Without treatment, viral meningitis nearly always resolves without sequelae, and bacterial meningitis nearly always proves fatal, particularly in children and the elderly. **Meningococcemia**, which may occur with or without meningitis, causes a petechial rash and profound and fulminant systemic abnormalities, including widespread hemorrhages and vascular collapse, sometimes due to adrenal hemorrhage (**Waterhouse-Friderichsen syndrome**). Patients who have recovered from meningitis may have residual mental retardation, paralysis, or seizures.

Treatment: Meningitis is an emergency. Hospitalization and administration of intravenous antibiotics are routine. Antibiotics are started even before reports of CSF studies are available, and discontinued or changed on the basis of these studies. Antibiotics are usually continued for three weeks or longer. Supportive care, including physical therapy, attention to nutrition and hydration, artificial ventilation, and measures to control fever, reverse shock, and reduce intracranial pressure, is vitally important. Asymptomatic persons who have been closely exposed to a patient with meningococcal meningitis receive prophylactic rifampin or ciprofloxacin to terminate the carrier state. A vaccine active against some strains of meningococcus is available.

West Nile Virus Disease

An infection of wild crows and jays transmitted by several species of mosquito. Human infection, first recognized in the U.S. as recently as 1999, has now spread throughout all of the contiguous states.

Although human infection is usually subclinical, encephalitis, meningitis, and paralytic syndromes may occur, especially in the elderly, in whom the mortality rate is significant. Adults who recover from the disease often have residual neurologic, muscular, or psychiatric impairment.

Transmission by blood transfusion and organ transplantation has occurred, but person-to-person transmission by mosquitoes is not recognized. The highest incidence of human infections occurs during the mosquito season (late spring, summer, and early fall).

Treatment is strictly symptomatic and supportive. Elimination of mosquito breeding places and use of insect repellent are strongly recommended as preventive measures.

Migraine Headache

Recurring severe unilateral headache with neurologic concomitants.

Cause: Unknown. Head pain is apparently related to constriction, dilatation, and throbbing of meningeal and other vessels. Chemical factors (release of vasodilator substances, depletion of plasma serotonin) probably play a part. The disease runs in families and is more common in young women, affecting about 15% of adult women in the U.S. Oral contraceptives may bring on headaches in susceptible women.

History: Recurring episodes of severe unilateral throbbing headache accompanied by nausea, vomiting, photophobia, intolerance to noise, and sometimes neurologic symptoms (diplopia, transient local anesthesia or paralysis). In **migraine with aura**, the patient experiences a warning symptom (aura) before the headache begins. Most often this consists of seeing flashes or zigzags of light in both eyes, usually with transitory visual field defects (**scintillating scotomas** and **fortification spectrum**).

In **migraine without aura**, the headache may be less severe and more generalized. Headaches typically last for many hours and may be severely incapacitating. Often complete relief is not obtained until after sleep. In susceptible persons, a migraine headache may be triggered by emotional stress, fatigue, menstruation, skipping a meal, certain foods (chocolate, prepared foods containing nitrates), or alcohol.

Physical Examination: Essentially normal during attacks, and entirely so between attacks.

Diagnostic Tests: Chiefly of use in ruling out more serious disorders; no specific findings.

Course: The disorder often begins in childhood and continues for many years. Depending on the presence of triggering factors, headaches may occur daily or at intervals of months or years.

Treatment: Mild analgesics sometimes help; nonsteroidal anti-inflammatory drugs (aspirin, ibuprofen, naproxen), especially when combined with caffeine, provide adequate relief for many patients. Selective serotonin receptor agonists (sumatriptan, rizatriptan, zolmitriptan) orally or by injection can abort a headache at any stage of its development. For patients who have extremely frequent headaches (one or more a week), prophylactic treatment usually provides good control. Prophylactic drugs include beta-adrenergic blocking agents (propranolol, atenolol) and others (amitriptyline).

Epilepsy

A neurologic disorder in which the patient experiences recurrent seizures consisting of transient disturbances of cerebral function due to paroxysmal neuronal discharge.

Causes: Seizure disorders, especially those first causing symptoms in childhood, are often idiopathic (without demonstrable cause). Seizures can be induced by cerebral trauma, infection, vascular disease, neoplasms, degenerative diseases (Alzheimer disease), drugs and

He was noted at times to have some jerking myoclonic-type of movements in his upper extremities, particularly the left.

chemical poisons, metabolic disorders (renal failure, hypoglycemia), and, in children, high fever. In persons with idiopathic epilepsy, seizures may be triggered by physical or emotional stress, lack of sleep, fever, drugs, alcohol, alcohol withdrawal, menstruation, or flashing lights.

Symptoms: Seizures are classified on the basis of overt presentation:

Partial (only part of one cerebral cortex is involved).

> **Simple** (no unconsciousness): Local twitching or jerking; perception of flashing lights or other abnormal sensory phenomena.
>
> **Complex** (impaired alertness or unconsciousness): Sometimes with psychic symptoms or automatisms.

Generalized (entire cerebral cortex involved).

> **Absence** (petit mal): Brief loss of attention and perception.
>
> **Tonic-clonic (grand mal)**: Tonic phase: victim becomes rigid, often cries out, loses consciousness, falls, stops breathing. Clonic phase: generalized muscular jerking, may bite tongue or lips, may be incontinent of urine or stool. Postictal state: after awakening, patient is drowsy and amnesic for a variable period.

Myoclonic: Repeated shocklike, often violent contractions in one or more muscle groups.

Status epilepticus: One or a series of grand mal seizures lasting more than 30 minutes without waking intervals.

Physical Examination: Between seizures there is no detectable abnormality. Signs of neurologic disease may be found in secondary epilepsy.

Diagnostic Tests: The electroencephalogram generally shows focal abnormalities in the rate, rhythm, or relative intensity of cerebral cortical rhythms, allowing diagnosis and classification of epilepsy. Laboratory studies and CT scan or MRI may be performed to rule out treatable causes of epilepsy.

Treatment: In idiopathic epilepsy, long-term treatment with anticonvulsant medicine (phenytoin, carbamazepine, valproic acid, phenobarbital, ethosuximide, and others) provides excellent control for most patients. Blood levels of medicine may require monitoring to ensure optimum dosage. Avoidance of triggering factors is important. For intractable cases, surgical treatment is sometimes successful.

Bell Palsy

Weakness or paralysis of muscles on one side of the face caused by inflammation or compression of the seventh cranial nerve (facial nerve) as it passes through the bony facial canal and emerges at the stylomastoid foramen behind the ear. The cause is unknown, but exposure to cold and herpes simplex virus infection have been suggested. Onset of symptoms is often accompanied by pain below or behind the ear.

Onset of facial weakness is usually abrupt, producing a characteristic asymmetry of the face and diminished ability or inability to close the eyes, smile, or purse the lips. Speech and eating may be slightly disturbed. There may be impairment of hearing and taste on the tip of the tongue.

The diagnosis is clinically evident, but electromyography and nerve conduction velocity studies may give indications of prognosis. More than half of cases resolve spontaneously in a few days to a few weeks, but residual weakness and asymmetry of the face, occasionally severe, may be permanent. A systemic corticosteroid is usually prescribed.

Transient Ischemic Attack (TIA)

Sudden onset of neurologic symptoms that resolve completely within 24 hours.

Cause: Transient interruption of blood supply to some part of the brain. Common causes include blockage by an **embolus** (from an infected heart valve, mural thrombus, or sloughed arteriosclerotic plaque) and reduction in blood supply due to the combined effects of arterial disease (arteritis, systemic lupus erythematosus) and reduced flow (hypotension; subclavian steal syndrome, in which blockage of a subclavian artery near its origin leads to reversal of blood flow in a vertebral artery to provide collateral flow beyond the obstruction, at the expense of brain tissue normally supplied by the vertebral artery).

History: Sudden onset of focal neurologic symptoms (weakness, numbness, unilateral loss of vision, diplopia, speech disturbances, vertigo, ataxia, falling) depending on site of circulatory impairment, resolving in less than 24 hours (usually in less than four hours).

Physical Examination: Flaccid weakness or paralysis, hyperreflexia, Babinski reflex, hypesthesia or anesthesia, depending on site of lesion. All neurologic signs resolve within 24 hours.

Diagnostic Tests: CT scan may be done to rule out hemorrhage. Arteriography, MR angiography, or carotid duplex ultrasonography may be used to assess the cerebral circulation. X-ray, laboratory, and electrocardiography or echocardiography may trace the underlying cause.

Course: By definition a TIA has no complications. Many patients, however, will eventually have one or more strokes.

Treatment: No treatment is needed for the acute episode, which has often resolved before the patient is seen by a physician. Depending on the reason for the attacks, treatment directed against future attacks may include carotid endarterectomy, control of cardiac or systemic disease, and use of anticoagulant medicines. Long-term prophylactic administration of drugs that inhibit platelet aggregation (aspirin, ticlopidine) reduces the risk of further attacks. Heparin and Coumadin may be needed if there is a major problem with thrombotic disease.

Stroke (Brain Attack, Cerebrovascular Accident, CVA)

Sudden onset of neurologic symptoms due to interruption of blood supply to some part of the brain. Stroke ranks third as a cause of death in the U.S. (see ■ Figure 17-5).

Cause: Blockage of a cerebral artery by a clot (thrombosis) or **embolus**, or local hemorrhage from a cerebral vessel (see ■ Figure 17-6).

Most cases are due to underlying vascular disease (arteriosclerosis, cerebral aneurysm, hypertension, diabetes mellitus, valvular heart disease).

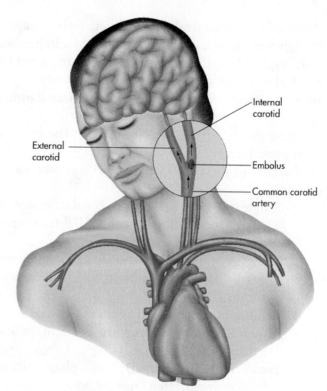

FIGURE 17-6. Embolus traveling to the brain

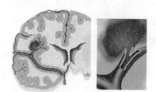

Cerebral hemorrhage: Cerebral artery ruptures and bleeds into brain tissue.

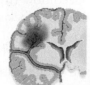

Cerebral embolism: Embolus from another area lodges in cerebral artery and blocks blood flow.

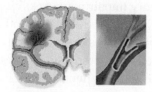

Cerebral thrombosis: Blood clot forms in cerebral artery and blocks blood flow.

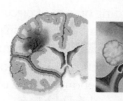

Compression: Pressure from tumor squeezes adjacent blood vessel and blocks blood flow.

FIGURE 17-5. Four common causes for cerebrovascular accidents

History: Sudden onset of weakness, numbness or paralysis, usually on one side of the body, or other neurologic deficit (loss of vision, dizziness, difficulty speaking, confusion, loss of consciousness), depending on part of brain affected. Severe headache, vomiting, or seizures may also occur. Usually there is a history of cardiovascular disease, sometimes of preceding TIAs. Neurologic deficit may progress to coma and death.

Physical Examination: Evidence of neurologic deficit, depending on location and extent of brain tissue involved, and duration of circulatory impairment. Muscle weakness or paralysis, which may initially be flaccid but eventually becomes spastic, with rigidity, hyperreflexia, Babinski and other pathologic reflexes. Aphasia, confusion, delirium, coma.

Diagnostic Tests: CT scan of the head can show areas of hemorrhage or infarction. Magnetic resonance imaging may also be used, without contrast material. Lumbar puncture helps to distinguish hemorrhage (blood in fluid, elevated opening pressure) from thrombosis. Blood studies, electrocardiography, and other diagnostic procedures may be used to identify underlying disease.

Course: Many cases of stroke resolve without any residual symptoms. Paralysis, weakness, or dementia may worsen. Stroke may progress rapidly to a fatal termination when the damage is extensive.

Treatment: If neurologic impairment is progressive and hemorrhage has been ruled out, anticoagulants (IV heparin followed by oral Coumadin) are used during the acute phase. In selected cases, tissue plasminogen activator (tPA) is administered to dissolve a freshly formed thrombus. Vigorous supportive treatment (oxygen, parenteral nutrition, prevention of respiratory and urinary tract infection, prevention of bedsores) must be instituted early. Physical therapy is important to maintain mobility and achieve maximum rehabilitation as neurologic function returns. Braces or splints may be necessary to promote mobility despite weakness of certain muscle groups.

Hydrocephalus

An increase in the volume of cerebrospinal fluid (CSF) in the ventricular system of the brain, with concomitant reduction of brain tissue (see ■ Figure 17-7).

Congenital Hydrocephalus

Enlargement of the head by excessive fluid pressure within the ventricular system, evident at birth or within the first few weeks of life.

Causes: Obstruction to the normal outflow of cerebrospinal fluid from the ventricular system due to a congenital defect, often the result of maternal infection (toxoplasmosis, rubella, cytomegalovirus, syphilis).

Physical Examination: Abnormally large circumference of the head at birth, or disproportionate increase in head size during early infancy, and bulging fontanels. Paralysis of upward gaze (setting sun sign).

Diagnostic Tests: CT, MRI, and ultrasonography confirm ventricular enlargement and may indicate the site of obstruction. **Cisternography** (radiographic studies after injection of radiopaque medium into the ventricular system) can provide more precise data.

Course: Without treatment, progressive enlargement of the ventricular system, with damage to the

The assessment is acute focal seizure secondary to underlying seizure disorder. Ventricular-peritoneal shunt appears to be functioning adequately.

cerebral hemispheres and other intracranial structures resulting in developmental retardation, feeding problems, seizures, coma, and early death.

Treatment: Surgical insertion of a **shunt** from the obstructed ventricular system to the right atrium of the heart or to the peritoneal cavity. As the child grows, increasingly longer shunts must be inserted. **Third ventriculostomy** (surgical creation of an aperture in the floor of the third ventricle) can correct hydrocephalus due to obstruction of the sylvian aqueduct by allowing drainage of CSF to the subarachnoid space,

Acquired Hydrocephalus

Causes: Obstruction of CSF circulation by a neoplasm or by scarring from intracranial infection, head trauma, or hemorrhage.

History: Headache, lethargy, nausea, blurred or double vision, dysequilibrium, memory loss.

Physical Examination: In infants with open fontanels, enlargement of the head and bulging of fontanels. Paralysis of upward gaze, other focal or nonfocal neurologic signs, cognitive impairment, papilledema.

Diagnostic Tests: **Lumbar puncture** shows CSF pressure to be elevated but laboratory studies of the fluid indicate no chemical or hematologic abnormalities. CT, MRI, and ultrasonography confirm ventricular enlargement and may indicate the site of obstruction. Cisternography can provide more precise information.

Treatment: Standard shunting procedures are generally successful in correcting acquired hydrocephalus.

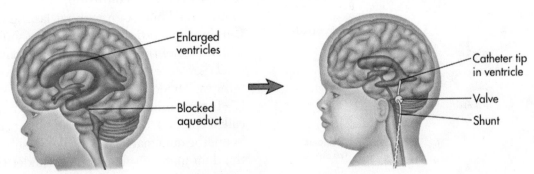

FIGURE 17-7. Hydrocephalus

Note these two important variants. In **normal pressure hydrocephalus (NPH)**, elevation of CSF pressure occurs only intermittently and may not be detected on lumbar puncture. Continuous intraventricular pressure recordings over a period of several hours may confirm periodic elevation of pressure. **Brain atrophy**, which occurs in some cases of dementia and schizophrenia, can lead to enlargement of the ventricular system with compensatory increase in the volume of CSF, but no increase in pressure.

Polyneuritis

A disease process involving a number of peripheral nerves.

Causes: Hereditary (Charcot-Marie-Tooth disease, Dejerine-Sottas disease, Friedreich ataxia), metabolic (diabetes mellitus, uremia), vitamin deficiency, alcoholism, drugs (INH, phenytoin), chemical poisons (lead, arsenic), autoimmunity (Guillain-Barré syndrome).

History: Hypesthesia, anesthesia, paresthesia, causalgia, weakness, muscle wasting involving various areas often in an irregular and shifting pattern.

Physical Examination: Reflexes diminished or absent; muscular atrophy.

Diagnostic Tests: Electromyography and nerve conduction velocity tests confirm neural malfunction. Emphasis is on finding a systemic cause (diabetes mellitus, other metabolic diseases, lead poisoning).

Treatment: Removal or treatment of underlying cause, if possible.

Herniated Disk (Herniated Nucleus Pulposus, HNP; Slipped Disk)

Extrusion of the soft center of an **intervertebral disk**, with symptoms due to pressure on adjacent spinal nerves (see ■ Figure 17-8).

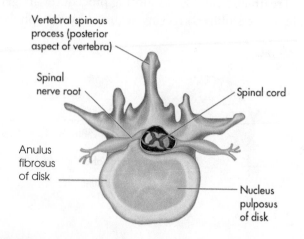

Vertebral spinous process (posterior aspect of vertebra)

Spinal nerve root

Spinal cord

Anulus fibrosus of disk

Nucleus pulposus of disk

FIGURE 17-8. Herniated intervertebral disk

Cause: *Predisposing cause*: Degeneration of the intervertebral disk due to aging or other pathologic process. *Precipitating cause*: Lifting or straining that puts unusual force on the disk.

History: Pain in the back or extremities, often of sudden onset and associated with lifting or straining. The pain may radiate along the course of an extremity like an electric shock and may be associated with paresthesia and hypesthesia. Movement or coughing may aggravate pain. Bowel or bladder function may be affected.

Physical Examination: There may be tenderness at the site of herniation. Neurologic examination may show impairment of deep tendon reflexes due to compression of dorsal nerve roots.

Diagnostic Tests: CT and myelography (x-ray of spine with contrast medium injected into the subarachnoid space) may show bulging or displacement of a disk. MRI is a more sensitive technique for showing herniation.

Course: Prolonged disability may occur if the condition is left untreated, although milder cases may often be asymptomatic.

Treatment: Bed rest, analgesics, and muscle relaxants usually provide symptomatic relief. With radiologic evidence of severe or progressive disease or significant neurologic impairment, **laminectomy** (cutting through the posterior arch of one or more vertebrae) and removal of herniated disk material are indicated.

Head Injuries

Blunt or penetrating wounds of the head can cause irreversible damage to the brain, and hemorrhage within the brain or between the brain and the skull (see ■ Figure 17-9). Such injuries are frequently lethal or result in permanent impairment of mental function.

Cerebral concussion is defined as a violent blow to the skull that causes brief unconsciousness but does no permanent damage to the brain or its supporting structures. In **cerebral contusion**, there is local injury to brain tissue, but again without lasting consequences. **Cerebral laceration** is a still more violent injury in which part of the brain is torn. The outcome is often death or severe permanent impairment (paralysis, seizures, dementia).

Intracranial hemorrhage can be extradural (also called epidural, between the outermost covering of the brain, the dura mater, and the skull), subdural (beneath the dura mater), subarachnoid (under the arachnoid membrane covering the brain), or intracerebral (within

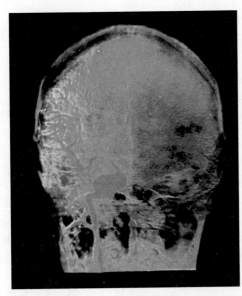

FIGURE 17-9. Cerebral angiography. The pink area on top of the brain indicates the location of a hemorrhage. Source: CNRI, Photo Researchers, Inc.

the substance of the brain). **Extradural hemorrhage** usually results from arterial bleeding and often proves rapidly fatal. **Subdural hemorrhage** is often venous, with chronic signs and symptoms (gradually progressing headache, stupor, personality change, or neurologic impairment). **Subarachnoid hemorrhage** is less often due to trauma than to rupture of a congenital aneurysm (abnormal bulge or weakness in a cerebral artery, present from birth). Any intracranial hemorrhage is life-threatening because of the danger of irreversible damage from compression of brain tissue within the rigid, nonexpanding skull. The treatment of head injury demands prompt and decisive action to conserve brain tissue and arrest hemorrhage.

Intracranial Neoplasms

Most tumors occurring within the cranial cavity, whether benign and malignant, arise from supporting tissues and cells (meninges, neuroglia) rather than from nerve tissue. Intracranial neoplasms cause symptoms by compressing or invading brain centers or tracts, by blocking the circulation of CSF and so increasing intracranial pressure, or by causing local hemorrhage.

Symptoms include headache (steady, increasing in severity, and often localized), nausea and vomiting, and focal or general neurologic impairment (dysequilibrium,

hearing loss, visual field defects, paralysis) depending on the site of the tumor.

Physical examination may show papilledema due to increased intracranial pressure and various neurologic deficits, which may help to localize the lesion.

Diagnosis of a space-occupying lesion is confirmed by various imaging techniques, including CT and MRI with injected contrast materials. In some cases angiography, electroencephalography, lumbar puncture, or brain biopsy may provide important diagnostic and prognostic information. Brain tumors are treated by surgical excision, guided by stereotactic localization. Chemotherapy and radiation are employed in the treatment of malignant tumors.

Benign Brain Tumors

Meningioma is a relatively common benign tumor, derived from meningeal cells, that grows slowly and causes symptoms by compressing adjacent structures. On CT scan it has a homogeneous appearance, and because of its rich blood supply its image is greatly enhanced after injection of contrast material ("tumor blush"). Prognosis after surgical removal is highly favorable. **Craniopharyngioma** arises in the area of the optic chiasm (the crossing of the right and left optic nerves on the undersurface of brain) and the pituitary gland. Hence the presenting symptoms are usually visual field defects and evidence of pituitary functional impairment. **Vestibular schwannoma** (formerly called acoustic neurinoma) develops from nerve sheath cells of the eighth cranial nerve, and by compressing the nerve causes hearing loss, tinnitus, and vertigo.

Malignant Brain Tumors

Most primary malignancies of the brain arise from neuroglia. **Astrocytoma** and **astroblastoma** are gliomas displaying moderate anaplasia. The most malignant brain tumor is **glioblastoma multiforme**, a highly undifferentiated and rapidly growing neoplasm that invades locally, spreads within the brain via the cerebrospinal fluid, and may even metastasize to sites outside the skull, particularly the cervical lymph nodes and the lungs. Despite surgery and radiation therapy, the lesion is uniformly lethal.

Pause for Reflection

1. What is the treatment for hydrocephalus?
2. Describe the symptoms and physical exam findings in patients with multiple sclerosis.
3. What are the precipitating events and what is the treatment for Guillain-Barré Syndrome?
4. How is amyotrophic lateral sclerosis diagnosed?
5. Describe the symptoms and physical findings in patients with Parkinson disease.
6. Distinguish among the 3 infectious diseases of the brain and spinal cord: encephalitis, meningitis, West Nile virus.
7. How does migraine with aura differ from other migraine headaches?
8. Distinguish among the different symptoms used to classify seizures on the basis of their presentation.
9. Distinguish between a transient ischemic attack and a stroke.
10. How is polyneuritis diagnosed?
11. What condition is defined as "Extrusion of the soft center of an intervertebral disk, with symptoms due to pressure on adjacent spinal nerves"? How is severe or progressive disease or significant neurologic impairment treated?
12. Distinguish among cerebral concussion, cerebral contusion, and cerebral laceration.
13. Distinguish among extradural, subdural, and subarachnoid hemorrhage.
14. Distinguish among benign and malignant brain tumors.

Diagnostic and Surgical Procedures

brain scan A diagnostic imaging procedure that can be performed using CT, MRI, or PET imaging. These neuroimaging procedures use a scintillator or scanner to trace and record the accumulation of a radioisotope injected intravenously. The nature and rate of accumulation in brain tissue can identify intracranial masses, lesions, tumors, or infarcts.

cerebral angiography An imaging study that uses an injected contrast medium to show cranial vasculature (see ■ Figure 17-9).

corpectomy Excision of all or part of a vertebral body for decompression of the spinal cord with the removed bone being replaced by a graft

craniotomy Surgical incision into the cranium, which necessitates drilling or sawing through the bone of the skull.

craniectomy Surgical removal of part of the bone of the skull.

digital subtraction angiography X-ray images of the head with and without contrast medium are processed by a computer, which deletes all shadows common to both films (skull bones, soft tissue profiles and interfaces), leaving only the vascular system visible.

diskectomy Excision of an intervertebral disk.

electroencephalography (EEG) Measurement and recording of electrical activity in the brain from several sites simultaneously (see ■ Figure 17-10). Electrodes are attached with fine needles to standard sites on the scalp, and the record is made on a strip of moving paper. Tracings are usually made after administration of a short-acting sedative (with the subject asleep, if possible). The effects of hyperventilation and of photic stimulation (exposure to a flashing light) are recorded also. The EEG is particularly useful in identifying and classifying seizure disorders.

electrophysiologic studies Measurement of electrical activity in nerves and muscles. Electromyography (EMG) involves insertion of fine needle electrodes into voluntary muscles. Nerve conduction velocity (NCV) is measured by timing the passage of nerve impulses between a stimulating and a recording electrode, which are a precisely measured distance apart.

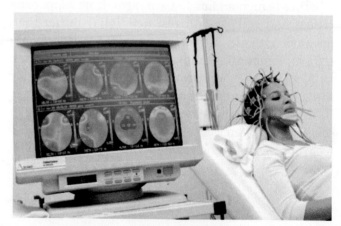

FIGURE 17-10. Electroencephalography.
Source: AJ Photo, Photo Researchers, Inc.

finger-to-nose test The patient extends the arms outward laterally, closes the eyes, and tries to touch the finger to the nose. Tests coordination.

Gamma Knife stereotactic radiosurgery A form of radiation therapy using specialized equipment that focuses hundreds of tiny beams of radiation on a tumor in the brain delivering a strong dose of gamma radiation to the site where the beams meet but having little effect on the brain tissue as the individual beams pass through. Gamma Knife is a trademarked device.

heel-to-shin test With the patient standing straight, the heel of one foot is placed against the shin of the opposing leg. Tests coordination.

hemilaminectomy Excision of one side of the vertebral lamina.

laminectomy Excision of the posterior arch of a vertebra.

laminotomy Division of the lamina of a vertebra.

lumbar puncture (LP) Withdrawal of a specimen of cerebrospinal fluid from the subarachnoid space by inserting a needle between two vertebrae (usually L4 and L5) at the lower end of the spinal column (see ■ Figure 17-11). A **manometer** (graduated glass tube) is used to measure the pressure of the fluid at the beginning of the procedure (**opening pressure**) and the end (**closing pressure**). Specimens of fluid are examined microscopically (stained smear) for cells (neutrophils and lymphocytes) and pathogenic microorganisms; chemically for glucose, protein, and other substances; by culture for bacterial pathogens; and, if indicated, serologically for evidence of syphilis, Lyme disease, or other infections, and by cytologic techniques for malignant cells. Normal CSF is water clear. **Xanthochromia** (yellowness) of the fluid suggests recent but not current hemorrhage. Frank blood in the specimen may indicate subarachnoid hemorrhage but may also be due to local injury by the needle (**traumatic tap**).

microdiskectomy Debulking of a herniated nucleus pulposus using an operating microscope or loupe for magnification. This procedure may be performed as a minimally invasive procedure using an arthroscope to access the site of herniation.

MRI of the spine An imaging procedure that uses an external magnetic field to evaluate the spinal cord and nerve roots. MRI has largely replaced myelography except in cases where it is contraindicated because the patient has a medical device, such as a cardiac pacemaker. In such cases, myelography and/or a CT scan may be performed.

myelography Visualization of the spinal canal (the tubular enclosure of the spinal cord formed collectively by the vertebrae) with real-time fluoroscopy with contrast medium introduced into the subarachnoid space by lumbar puncture. The procedure may be followed by a CT scan to better define the anatomy and any abnormalities.

somatosensory evoked potential Waves recorded from the spinal cord or cerebral hemisphere after electrical stimulation or physiological activation of peripheral sensory fibers; analysis of deviations in latency or amplitude can detect or characterize lesions of the peripheral or sensory conduction pathways.

spinal tap See *lumbar puncture*.

tandem walking test Tests the subject's ability to walk with one foot in front of the other in a straight line. A coordination test, often used by police officers to assess drivers for substance abuse.

Laboratory Procedure

CSF (cerebrospinal fluid) The fluid medium of the central nervous system (brain and spinal cord), which can be sampled by lumbar puncture (spinal tap) for chemical testing, cell counts, and culture.

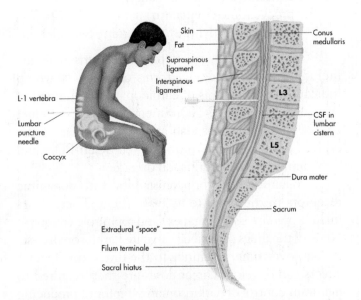

Skin
Fat
Supraspinous ligament
Interspinous ligament
L-1 vertebra
Lumbar puncture needle
Coccyx
Conus medullaris
L3
CSF in lumbar cistern
L5
Dura mater
Sacrum
Extradural "space"
Filum terminale
Sacral hiatus

FIGURE 17-11. Lumbar puncture (spinal tap)

Pharmacology

Epilepsy Drugs

Drugs used to treat epilepsy are known as anticonvulsants because epilepsy is characterized by seizures or convulsions. Barbiturates are sedative drugs, some of which also possess an anticonvulsant action. Barbiturates are controlled substance drugs (Schedule IV) that inhibit conduction of nerve impulses coming into the cortex of the brain and depress motor areas of the brain.

> mephobarbital (Mebaral)
> phenobarbital (Luminal, Solfoton)

Hydantoins act on the cell membrane of neurons in the cortex of the brain. These drugs affect the flow of sodium in and out of the cell, thereby preventing the neuron from depolarizing and repolarizing (sending out an impulse) too rapidly or repeatedly.

> ethotoin (Peganone)
> mephenytoin (Mesantoin)
> phenytoin (Dilantin Infatabs, Dilantin Kapseals, Dilantin-125)

Succinimides depress the cortex and raise the seizure threshold.

> ethosuximide (Zarontin)
> fosphenytoin (Cerebyx)
> methsuximide (Celontin Kapseals)
> phensuximide (Milontin Kapseals)

Benzodiazepine drugs act on several different types of receptors throughout the body to affect memory, emotion, and muscles. They exert an anticonvulsant effect on receptors in the brainstem.

These are controlled substance drugs (Schedule IV).

> clonazepam (Klonopin)
> clorazepate (Tranxene, Tranxene-SD, Tranxene-SD Half Strength, Tranxene-T)
> diazepam (Diazepam Intensol, Valium)

The mechanism of action of these antiepileptic drugs varies.

> acetazolamide (Diamox)
> carbamazepine (Atretol, Carbatrol, Epitol, Tegretol, Tegretol-XR)
> clobazam (Frisium)
> felbamate (Felbatol)
> gabapentin (Neurontin)

> lamotrigine (Lamictal, Lamictal Chewable Dispersible Tablet)
> primidone (Mysoline)
> valproic acid (Depacon, Depakene, Depakote ER)

No one drug has therapeutic effects against all types of seizures. Some drugs that are effective for controlling one type of seizure may actually provoke another type.

Parkinson Disease Drugs

Drug therapy for Parkinson disease is divided into two main categories: drugs that increase or enhance the action of dopamine in the brain, and drugs that inhibit the action of acetylcholine. All of these drugs act to restore the natural balance between dopamine and acetylcholine. Drugs that increase the amount of dopamine, enhance its action in the brain, or directly stimulate dopamine receptors include:

> amantadine (Symmetrel)
> bromocriptine (Parlodel, Parlodel Snap Tabs)
> carbidopa (Lodosyn)
> levodopa (L-dopa, Larodopa)
> pergolide mesylate (Permax)
> pramipexole (Mirapex)
> ropinirole (Requip)
> selegiline (Carbex, Eldepryl)

Drugs that inhibit the action of acetylcholine in the brain are called anticholinergic drugs and include:

> benztropine (Cogentin)
> biperiden (Akineton)
> diphenhydramine (Benadryl)
> procyclidine (Kemadrin)
> trihexyphenidyl (Artane, Artane Sequels)

Combination drugs used to treat Parkinson disease include the various dosage forms of Sinemet, which indicate the milligrams of carbidopa per milligram of levodopa: Sinemet 10-100, Sinemet 25-100, Sinemet 25-250. The FDA has also approved the use of the orphan drugs apomorphine, NeuroCell-PD, and Spheramine to treat Parkinson disease.

Dopamine-receptor agonists bind with dopamine receptors in the brain to activate them. These drugs include pramipexole (Mirapex) and ropinirole (Requip). None of the drugs prescribed can cure Parkinson disease. In fact, over time, tolerance to the drugs' therapeutic effects can develop. Larger doses are then required to maintain control of parkinsonian symptoms, producing more side effects. When doses can no longer be increased or side effects become intolerable, the physician will gradually withdraw all medication, placing the patient on a "drug holiday" for a few days. When therapy is again initiated, the patient will respond to lower doses of antiparkinsonian drugs.

Insomnia Drugs

Drugs used to induce sleep are termed hypnotics after *hypnos*, the Greek word for *sleep*.

acecarbromal (Paxarel)
chloral hydrate (Aquachloral Supprettes)
estazolam (ProSom)
eszopiclone (Lunesta)
flurazepam (Dalmane)
glutethimide (Doriden)
lorazepam (Ativan)
quazepam (Doral)
temazepam (Restoril)
triazolam (Halcion)
zaleplon (Sonata)
zolpidem (Ambien, Ambien CR)

Over-the-counter (OTC) sleep aids commonly contain the antihistamine diphenhydramine, phenyltoloxamine citrate, doxylamine succinate, or pyrilamine maleate. These sleep aids use the antihistamine's side effects of drowsiness as the therapeutic effect to treat insomnia.

Bufferin AF Nite Time
Compoz Nighttime Sleep Aid
Excedrin P.M., Excedrin P.M. Liquigels
Nytol
Sominex
Extra Strength Tylenol PM
Sominex, Sominex Pain Relief

Transcription Tips

1. Confusing terms related to the neurology system: Some of these terms sound alike; others are potential traps when researching. Memorize the terms and their meanings so that you can select the appropriate term for a correct transcript.

   abductor—a muscle that draws an extremity away from the body (dictated "a-b-duc-tor")
   adductor—a muscle that draws an extremity toward the body (dictated "a-d-ductor")
   conscious—aware of oneself and surroundings
   conscience—moral convictions
   cistern—a closed space or reservoir for fluid, as cerebellopontine angle cistern
   system—a series of interconnected or interdependent parts that function together
   aura—a motor or sensory phenomenon associated with the onset of a seizure or migraine
   ora (1) the plural of *os*, (2) an edge or margin
   concussion—the condition that results from a violent jar or shock
   convulsion—a seizure
   contusion—a bruise or subcutaneous hemorrhage
   dysphasia—speech impairment
   dysphagia—difficulty swallowing
   dysplasia—abnormal development
   dura mater (one *t*) (rhymes with "later")
   white matter (two *t*'s) (rhymes with "fatter")
   faucial—palatine (tonsil)
   facial—pertaining to the face
   fascial—pertaining to fascia, a sheet or band of fibrous tissue
   gait—manner of walking
   gate—a break in a fence
   nuchal—pertaining to the neck
   knuckle—a knob or the upper part of a finger joint
   noxious—harmful, damaging to tissue
   nocuous—harmful (not used in medicine)
   peak—highest point
   peek—look quickly or briefly
   radical—extreme
   radicle—smallest branch of vessel or nerve
   sheath—covering of an organ, nerve, muscle
   sheet—a bed covering or tissue resembling a sheet
   sellar—pertaining to the sella turcica
   cellar—an underground room below a house
   thecal—In neurology, pertaining to the dura mater of the spinal cord
   fecal—pertaining to stool
   cecal—pertaining to the cecum of the colon
   coma—unconsciousness
   comma—a punctuation mark

2. Slang Terms. Expand these slang brief forms when encountered in dictation.

gastroc	gastrocnemius
tib	tibia or tibial

3. Spelling. Memorize the spelling of these difficult-to-spell terms. Note silent letters, doubled letters, and unexpected pronunciation.

anxiety	fluoroscopy
anxious	meralgia paresthetica
anulus	wallerian
ectopy	

   Note: *Disk* is the preferred spelling in all instances except ophthalmology. The term *diskectomy* is spelled only with a *k*.

4. Watch out for spelling changes when forming derivatives.

   neural foramen (sing.), foramina (pl.)
   foraminotomy, not foramenotomy

5. Note the challenging spellings or unusual capitalization of these common neurology drugs.

diphenhydramine	phenobarbital
eszopiclone	phensuximide
fentanyl	phenytoin
fosphenytoin	ProSom
Halcion	Restoril
mephenytoin	selegiline
mephobarbital	trihexyphenidyl

6. Dictation Challenges

   The French term *absence* ("ab sáhnce") describes seizures that used to be called "petit mal" ("petty mahl").

Spotlight On

My Husband's Journey

by Jody Bogdanovich

The human brain is an amazing, vital, and resilient organ, but I did not fully understand or appreciate that fact until my husband was involved in a motorcycle accident in which he suffered a traumatic brain injury (TBI), classified as severe, with three skull fractures and a shear injury. He was airlifted and intubated en route to a level 1 trauma center where he spent the next two months recovering, slowly but surely, until he was well enough to travel 600 miles back home to continue treatment as an outpatient.

We were traveling in another state when my husband crashed. I was able to spend the entire time at his bedside and witness the daily progress as his brain and other injuries healed, first in the emergency room, then in the intensive care unit, the neurology unit, and finally in the neurologic inpatient rehabilitation wing of the hospital.

We will never know what caused my husband to lose control of his motorcycle, since the initial part of the accident was not witnessed. I was riding my own motorcycle ahead of him and did not see what happened, but hearing the crash from behind, I pulled off the road and witnessed first his motorcycle tumble past me, and then my husband. It was captured in my mind in slow motion, as he repeatedly rolled, his arms instinctively crossed over his chest, his bare head hitting the pavement multiple times, causing closed coup-contrecoup injuries.

Apparently his novelty-type helmet came off after the initial impact. The doctors said later that if not for the protection of his helmet, albeit minimal, the first blow to his head would have been fatal. The helmet, though not ideal, did save his life. We were riding in a state with no helmet law, and I was grateful he was wearing one. I, however, was not, but this traumatic experience has made me a firm believer in wearing the proper safety gear at all times.

The initial head CT scan showed a dramatic midline shift caused by subdural hematoma as well as edema. The doctors monitored his brain closely. He did not need a craniotomy to relieve pressure or to evacuate the blood. Although it was a long slow process, the swelling eventually resolved and the old blood was absorbed. Periodic CT scans and an MRI showed the two hemispheres of the brain equalizing in size.

The TBI patient goes through several stages of recovery, and from what I observed during the weeks I spent on the neurology rehab floor, watching not only my husband's progress but also the progress of other patients, no matter what age, gender, or mode of traumatic brain injury, they all seemed to go through the same transitions.

In the early phase, after they emerge from a coma, TBI patients become very agitated and combative, requiring restraints and in some cases netting over the bed that allows the patient to move around but not escape. Then I noticed the patients sporting a vacant stare, a disturbing glassy-eyed, almost zombie-like appearance, which eventually clears. It was a tremendous relief to finally see a twinkle in my husband's eyes as the fog gradually lifted from his psyche.

Speech therapy, physical therapy, occupational therapy, and eventually recreational therapy were all important elements in my husband's recovery.

He was fortunate in that he did not lose his ability to speak, but he did have aphasia. One of the doctors compared a brain injury to a computer shutting down and the recovery process is like the computer rebooting (in technical terms, the brain is rebuilding synapses). As my husband's brain was healing and rewiring, he would oftentimes say the wrong word—close to what he meant to say, but not quite.

Eight days after his accident, he was asked by a nurse, "How are you feeling today?" My husband replied, "Oh, somewhere between a C and a D." Good answer coming from the school teacher that he was, and probably a fair assessment. He also complained that he was tired of being in "quarantine" and kept referring to his proposed discharge date as his date of "extradition." He referred to his students back home (grades K-12) as "little creatures," "critters," or "animals." And when he became frustrated with being told that he was not allowed to do certain things, like leave the hospital, chew tobacco, or watch certain television shows that would overstimulate him, he complained that there were "too many big bosses around here."

Spotlight On My Husband's Journey *(page 2)*

During the hospitalization, my husband started fabricating a story. Although he had no memory of the accident, he told the doctors that several other "bikes" were chasing me, so he rode towards them so I could get away, and they ran him off the road. The truth was, there were no other vehicles of any kind on that remote stretch of highway at the time of his accident. The doctors explained that this is called confabulation; he (his brain) was trying to make sense of something that he could not remember or understand, so he was filling in the blanks and thus making up a story, or confabulating.

Another thing he did during the hospitalization was perseverate, where he would focus on or obsess about one thing. For instance, one of the early phases of TBI recovery is extreme agitation and even aggressiveness, to the point where patients need to be restrained. My husband persistently asked to be removed from the restraints, and then started demanding that I or nursing staff give him a knife or scissors so he could cut the bands from his wrists. Several times we caught him very slyly trying to unfasten the restraints while keeping his hands hidden under the bed covers. Even an injured brain can be very resourceful.

The doctors were focusing on the most serious of my husband's multiple injuries, which in this case was the brain trauma. They had ruled out any internal organ injuries, spinal injuries, or broken long bones, but he did have broken ribs, a broken clavicle, scalp and forehead lacerations, and various contusions, as well as a serious road rash to his forearms.

My husband was upset that his back hurt and the doctors weren't doing anything about it. He complained that his back was out of alignment and repeatedly asked me to walk on his back or get a chiropractor to come in to "pop" his back. The doctors and nurses assured him his back was fine and it was probably the broken ribs causing pain, but he continued to demand to see a chiropractor. He also was obsessed about seeing his motorcycle (eventually the recreational therapist took him to the bike shop where his bike was being stored).

The activity he repeated that really wore me out started after he progressed through physical therapy to the point where he was ambulating without assistance. He decided he was ready to be discharged and would continually pace around the room, rounding up all our belongings, and piling them in a wheelchair. I gave up trying to keep the room organized while he was going through this phase of perseveration.

Complications arose during my husband's hospitalization, such as seizures, and he suffered through a severe case of singultus (or hiccups) which lasted several days. He developed problems with his digestive system which required insertion of a nasogastric tube to relieve pressure in his stomach and through which he was temporarily fed. Not surprisingly, he had a constant headache. He also was treated for hypertension and hyperglycemia, neither of which he had prior to his accident, and he developed deep venous thromboses (DVTs) in both his arms. All but the DVTs were directly attributable to the insult to his brain.

Finally, the day of "extradition" arrived when my husband was released from "quarantine," and he was discharged from inpatient care. He underwent several months of outpatient treatment back home with physical, speech, and occupational therapists.

He also required followup with a neurologist, who performed an EEG and weaned him off seizure medication. He developed a neurogenic bladder, a sequela of his TBI, and was referred to a urologist. He also has had ongoing issues with anger management and has been counseled by a psychologist.

He established care with a neuropsychologist for executive functioning difficulties. He learned new ways to help with time management, organization, problem-solving, memory—cognitive processes. He will always have trouble with short-term memory.

After complaining of knee pain, an MRI revealed he had a complex tear of the meniscus and ligament in his left knee attributable to the accident, for which he underwent surgery.

Despite the dramatic recovery from his severe TBI, my husband was not able to resume his teaching and coaching career and had to take a disability retirement. Thanks to the expert care from medical professionals, family, and friends, my husband is a living testament to the extraordinary capacity of the brain to recover from trauma.

Exercises

Medical Vocabulary Review

Instructions: Choose the best answer.

___ 1. The expression "altered level of consciousness" refers to ____
A. deep coma, unarousable.
B. confusion and disorientation.
C. drowsiness or inattentiveness.
D. all of the above.

___ 2. A patient who has suffered a stroke with impaired ability to understand spoken or written language, or both is said to have ___
A. amnesia.
B. aphasia.
C. dementia.
D. absence.

___ 3. Rapid, jerky purposeless involuntary movements of one or several muscle groups is ___
A. paresis.
B. chorea.
C. a simple seizure.
D. myoclonic seizure.

___ 4. A grand mal seizure is a(n) _____ type of seizure.
A. absence
B. simple
C. complex
D. tonic-clonic

___ 5. Marked stiffness of the neck, a cardinal finding in meningitis, is ____
A. paresthesia.
B. hypesthesia.
C. partial paralysis.
D. nuchal rigidity.

___ 6. Bending upward of the foot is ____
A. dorsiflexion.
B. plantar flexion.
C. a Babinski reflex.
D. a Chaddock reflex.

___ 7. Loss of balance sense or tendency to fall without support is ____
A. ataxia.
B. athetosis.
C. dysequilibrium.
D. graphesthesia.

___ 8. An intention tremor ____
A. occurs only during voluntary movement.
B. occurs only during involuntary movement.
C. occurs during both voluntary and involuntary movement.
D. is done on purpose to confuse the examiner.

___ 9. Twisting of the neck and unnatural position of the head caused by spasms of neck muscles is ____
A. partial paralysis.
B. porencephaly.
C. torticollis.
D. nuchal rigidity.

___ 10. Disease of the nerve roots is ____
A. neuropathy.
B. radiculopathy.
C. idiopathic.
D. a pathological reflex.

___ 11. Impaired alertness or unconsciousness, sometimes with psychic symptoms or automatisms, is ____
A. a complex seizure.
B. a petit mal seizure.
C. a generalized seizure.
D. a myoclonic seizure.

___12. Reflexes that occur in response to sudden stretching of a muscle, usually induced by tapping a tendon with a rubber-headed hammer, are called ____
A. pathologic reflexes.
B. superficial reflexes.
C. hyperactive reflexes.
D. deep tendon reflexes.

___ 13. Degenerative spinal changes of the vertebrae, disks, and spinal ligaments and connective tissue due to osteoarthritis, is called ____
A. ankylosis.
B. athetosis.
C. spondylosis.
D. stereognosis.

___ 14. Paralysis is ____
A. muscle weakness.
B. complete loss of muscle function.
C. loss of function on one side of the body.
D. loss of function in all extremities.

___ 15. A Glasgow coma scale of 15 means that the patient is ____
A. conscious.
B. in a coma.
C. brain dead.
D. confused and disoriented.

___ 16. Partial loss of sensation on one or more parts of the body surface is ____
A. anesthesia.
B. dysesthesia.
C. hypesthesia.
D. paresthesia.

___ 17. Pain or tingling when both wrists are flexed with the hands firmly pressing one another back-to-back for 60 seconds is called a ____
A. Tinel sign.
B. postictal state.
C. paresthesia.
D. Phalen sign.

___ 18. Sudden, usually transitory, loss of consciousness due to circulatory or neurologic abnormality is ____
A. paralysis.
B. syncope.
C. presyncope.
D. a postictal state.

___ 19. The cranial nerves that relate to ocular movements are ____
A. cranial nerves I, III, and VI.
B. cranial nerves III, IV, and VI.
C. cranial nerves I, V, and VIII.
D. cranial nerves IX, X, and XII.

___ 20. On physical examination of the spinal nerves, tests of coordination include all of the following EXCEPT ____
A. two-point discrimination.
B. rapid alternating movements.
C. finger-to-nose testing.
D. tandem walking.

Diagnostic and Surgical Procedures

Instructions: Match the following diagnostic and surgical procedures to their descriptions or definitions. Some answers may be used more than once or not at all.

____ 1. corpectomy

____ 2. craniotomy

____ 3. diskectomy

____ 4. electroencephalography

____ 5. electromyography

____ 6. finger-to-nose test

____ 7. Gamma Knife radiosurgery

____ 8. heel-to-shin test

____ 9. hemilaminectomy

____ 10. laminectomy

____ 11. laminotomy

____ 12. lumbar puncture

____ 13. microdiskectomy

____ 14. myelography

____ 15. nerve conduction study

A. Excision of the posterior arch of a vertebra

B. Test of coordination

C. Excision of one side of the posterior arch of a vertebra

D. A form of radiation therapy that delivers a strong dose of radiation to a tumor but has little effect on intervening normal brain tissue

E. Insertion of fine needle electrodes into voluntary muscles to measure electrical activity

F. Division of the posterior arch of a vertebra

G. Excision of all or part of a vertebral body

H. Drilling or sawing through the bone of the skull.

I. Timing of the passage of nerve impulses between a stimulating and a recording electrode

J. A test or coordination performed as part of a physical examination

K. Intervertebral disk excision

L. Fluoroscopy of the spinal canal using contrast introduced into the subarachnoid space by lumbar puncture

M. Recording of electrical activity from several sites of the brain simultaneously to identify or classify seizure disorders

N. Removal of cerebrospinal fluid from the subarachnoid space using a needle inserted between two vertebrae at the lower end of the spinal column

O. Debulking of a herniated nucleus pulposus using an operating microscope or loupe for magnification

Pharmacology

Instructions: Choose the best answer.

____ 1. Which of the following drugs is a treatment for epilepsy?
A. Ativan (lorazepam).
B. Symmetrel (amantadine).
C. Luminal (phenobarbital).
D. Paxarel (acecarbromal).

____ 2. Which of the following drugs does not belong in the group with the others?
A. Requip (ropinirole).
B. Symmetrel (amantadine).
C. L-dopa, Larodopa (levodopa).
D. Doriden (glutethimide).

____ 3. Which of the following drugs is NOT a benzodiazepine?
A. clonazepam.
B. estazolam.
C. diazepam.
D. clorazepate.

____ 4. If a patient had insomnia, you might expect the physician to prescribe which one of the following drugs?
A. Mirapex (pramipexole).
B. Neurontin (gabapentin).
C. Lunesta (eszopiclone).
D. Symmetrel (amantadine).

____ 5. Patients might need to be concerned about habituation or addiction when taking which of the following?
A. barbiturates and benzodiazepines.
B. hydantoin and succinimides.
C. hypnotics and antihistamines.
D. dopaminergics and anticholinergics.

____ 6. Which drug might be prescribed for a patient with Parkinson disease?
A. Cogentin (benztropine)
B. Halcion (triazolam)
C. Neurontin (gabapentin)
D. Mysoline (primidone)

____ 7. Which category of epilepsy drugs acts on the cell membrane of neurons in the cortex of the brain, affecting the flow of sodium in and out of the cell, thereby preventing the neuron from sending out an impulse too rapidly or repeatedly?
A. benzodiazepines.
B. hydantoins.
C. succinimides.
D. barbiturates.

____ 8. Which of the following statements is NOT true?
A. No one drug has therapeutic effects against all types of seizures.
B. Barbiturates and benzodiazepines are Schedule IV drugs.
C. Drugs used to treat epilepsy are stimulants and act to control seizures by confusing the motor neurons in the brain.
D. Some drugs that are effective for controlling one type of seizure may actually provoke another type.

____ 9. An orphan drug approved by the FDA to treat Parkinson disease is ____
A. apomorphine.
B. amantadine.
C. ropinirole.
D. pramipexole.

____ 10. Which of the following statements is NOT true?
A. Parkinson disease cannot be cured with drugs.
B. Tolerance to Parkinson drugs' therapeutic effects can develop.
C. Patients often require larger and larger doses to maintain control of symptoms.
D. When therapy becomes ineffective with one Parkinson drug, patients are switched to a different type of drug for continued treatment.

Dissecting Medical Terms

Instructions: As you learned in your medical language course, words are formed from prefixes, combining forms (root word plus combining vowel), and suffixes. Combining vowels (usually **o** but not always) are used to connect two root words or a root and a suffix. By analyzing these word parts, you can often determine the definition of a term without even looking it up (if you know the definition of the parts, of course!).

Being able to divide and analyze the words you hear into their component parts will also improve your auditory deciphering ability and spelling and help you research those words that you cannot easily spell or define.

For the following terms, draw a slash (/) between the components and then write a short definition based on the meaning of the parts. Remember that to define a word based on its parts, you start at the end, usually with the suffix. If there's a prefix, that is defined next, and finally the combining form is defined.

Example: atrophic
Divide & Analyze:
    atrophic = a/troph/ic = pertaining to + nourishment + away
Define: pertaining to wasting away

1. abductor
   Divide _____

   Define _____

2. ankylosis
   Divide _____

   Define _____

3. corpectomy
   Divide _____

   Define _____

4. dorsiflexion
   Divide _____

   Define _____

5. dysphasia
   Divide _____

   Define _____

6. electromyogram
   Divide _____

   Define _____

7. fluoroscopy
   Divide _____

   Define _____

8. hemorrhage
   Divide _____

   Define _____

9. iatrogenic
   Divide _____

   Define _____

10. lumbodorsal
   Divide _____

   Define _____

11. microsurgical
   Divide _____

   Define _____

12. myoclonic
   Divide _____

   Define _____

13. neuropathy
   Divide _____

   Define _____
   _____

14. neurovascularly
   Divide _____

   Define _____
   _____

15. paraspinal
   Divide _____

   Define _____
   _____

16. percutaneous
   Divide _____

   Define _____
   _____

17. periventricular
   Divide _____

   Define _____
   _____

18. pseudomeningocele
   Divide _____

   Define _____
   _____

19. radiculopathy
   Divide _____

   Define _____
   _____

20. subperiosteal
   Divide _____

   Define _____
   _____

Spelling Exercise

Instructions: Review the adjective suffixes in your medical language textbook. Test your knowledge of adjectives by writing the adjectival form of the following neurology terms. Consult a medical dictionary to verify your spelling.

Noun	Adjective
1. anxiety	_____
2. apex	_____
3. atrophy	_____
4. axilla	_____
5. cadaver	_____
6. diabetes	_____
7. ectopy	_____
8. epilepsy	_____
9. fascia	_____
10. fluctuancy	_____
11. foramen	_____
12. kyphosis	_____
13. lamina	_____
14. Parkinson	_____
15. perineum	_____
16. periosteum	_____
17. perone	_____
18. radicle	_____
19. spine	_____
20. spondylosis	_____

Abbreviations Exercise

Instructions: Expand the following common abbreviations and brief forms. Then memorize both abbreviations and definitions to increase your speed and accuracy in transcribing dictation

Abbreviation	Expansion
1. C5–C6	_____
2. CNS	_____
3. CN II–XII	_____
4. CPR	_____
5. CSF	_____
6. CVA	_____
7. DC	_____
8. DC	_____
9. DVT	_____
10. EDB	_____
11. EEG	_____
12. EHL	_____
13. EMG	_____
14. L5–S1	_____
15. m/sec	_____
16. msec	_____
17. mV	_____
18. MRI	_____
19. NCS	_____
20. NCV	_____

Transcript Forensics

Instructions: This section presents snippets of transcribed dictations from clinic notes; history and physical examinations and consultations; operative reports and procedure notes; and discharge summaries. Explain the passage so that a nonmedical person can understand it.

Example:

NEUROLOGICAL: His reflexes are slightly hyperactive on the right side.

Explanation: The patient's muscular response in the right leg was more active than normal when the examiner tapped below the knee with a mallet.

1. He has very slow **mentation** and his attention span is not long. There is slurring of speech but there's no **unilateral paralysis**.

Explanation: _____
_____
_____
_____
_____

2. ADMITTING DIAGNOSIS
Cervical **spondylytic radiculopathy** and cervical **ankylosis**.

Explanation: _____
_____
_____
_____
_____
_____

3. There has been no evidence of **DVT**, and the patient has remained **neurovascularly intact**.

Explanation: _____
_____
_____
_____
_____

4. Medications include **Lortab** 7.5 mg 1 to 2 p.o. q.4-6 hours p.r.n., **Decadron** 2 mg today and 1 mg tomorrow, and the **resumption** of all previous medications. He is also advised to continue home exercise program and **progressive ambulation**. [Note: Be sure to explain what the medications are for.]

Explanation: _____
_____
_____
_____
_____

5. A 58-year-old female with history of diabetes and thigh pain more prominent on the left side. Question of **lumbosacral radiculopathy** or **meralgia paresthetica**. [Note: Include in your explanation the significance of the history of diabetes.]

Explanation: _____

_____

_____

_____

_____

_____

6. CHIEF COMPLAINT
The patient presented to the emergency room with **acute onset** of **tonic-clonic seizure activity** with **loss of consciousness**, which lasted about 30 minutes. There was no associated **urinary or bowel incontinence**.

Explanation: _____

_____

_____

_____

_____

_____

_____

7. HEENT EXAMINATION: **Normocephalic, atraumatic**. Extraocular muscles intact. Both tympanic membranes were intact. Pharynx was without **erythema**, without **exudate**.

Explanation: _____

_____

_____

_____

_____

_____

8. INR was 0.9, PTT 25.9. AST 22, ALT 41, alkaline phosphatase 117. Cardiac enzymes: CK 8, troponin less than 0.04, BNP 12.8. [Note: Explain the purpose of each test and whether the value is normal or abnormal.]

Explanation: _____

_____

_____

_____

_____

_____

9. ASSESSMENT AND PLAN
New-onset seizure disorder. The patient was **loaded** with **fosphenytoin** 1 g in the emergency room. We will admit for observation to **telemetry** with **seizure precautions**.

Explanation: _____

_____

_____

_____

_____

_____

10. **Subperiosteal dissection** was used along the **paraspinal muscles** on the left side, exposing the **lamina** of L4 as well as L5. [This is an excerpt from an operative report for excision of a herniated disk.]

Explanation: _____

_____

_____

_____

_____

_____

Sample Reports

Sample neurology reports appear on the following pages, illustrating a variety of reports. Fictional names are provided for illustration of proper format, and no resemblance to actual persons is intended. Sample transcripts were prepared according to *The Book of Style for Medical Transcription* (AHDI).

Chart Note

MILLER, JULIE
Age 74
June 20, [add year]

This very pleasant 74-year-old woman has rather advanced parkinsonism, present for many years. It is affecting her daily living to a great degree. She has difficulty dressing, has frequent falls occasionally related to freezing or to festination, but also occurring without any apparent cause. She has marked hesitancy on changing direction and unsteadiness with fatigue. She has a minor problem with sialorrhea, eating, and swallowing. She is able to maintain her personal hygiene without any difficulty. She has had some symptoms of depression along with her Parkinson disease.

On neurologic exam she did have mild to moderate impairment in cognition and short-term memory, although she is oriented x3. She has a mild tremor, worse in the left arm than the right. She has rigidity in the upper extremities. She has marked poverty of movement, with long delays in initiating movement and frequent freezing. She has a moderately flexed posture and cannot straighten to command. She has postural instability. Her speech is mildly dysarthric. She has paucity of spontaneous facial expression. Her gait is characterized by shuffling strides with festination in propulsion. She does not need assistance with gait. She can arise from a chair with difficulty only after multiple attempts. She has micrographia. Deep tendon reflexes are symmetrical, and toes are downgoing. Cranial nerves are unremarkable.

She has been on Sinemet 25/100 t.i.d. for the last 6 years or so. She will be going on vacation soon, and I would not attempt to add a second antiparkinsonian medication. However, I have asked her to increase her Sinemet dose to q.i.d. We will see how she does with Sinemet and plan to add bromocriptine 1 mg per day when she returns.

PW:hpi

Operative Report

HERBEL, KAREN
Hospital #746272

DATE OF OPERATION
November 1, [add year]

PREOPERATIVE DIAGNOSIS
Pseudoarthrosis, C6-7, recurrent radiculopathy.

POSTOPERATIVE DIAGNOSIS
Pseudoarthrosis, C6-7, recurrent radiculopathy.

OPERATIVE PROCEDURE
1. C6 laminectomy with bilateral decompression, dictated separately by Dr. _____.
2. Two-level posterior spinal fusion, C5 to C7.
3. Application of bilateral lateral mass plate, C5 to C7.

SURGEON
JEFF PETERSON, MD

ANESTHESIA
General.

COMPLICATIONS
None.

OPERATIVE NOTE
Patient identified, brought to the operating room. General endotracheal anesthesia was induced, followed by placement of Mayfield tongs and turning the patient prone onto padded rolls. The neck area was thoroughly prepped with a razor, Betadine scrub, and Betadine solution and draped in sterile fashion. The left posterior iliac crest was also sterilely prepped with a razor, Betadine gel, and draped in a sterile fashion. A midline skin incision was made followed by exposure of the posterior elements of C5, C6, and C7 bilaterally. Intraoperative x-ray proved quite difficult despite preoperative positioning, due to the patient's extremely large body habitus. Successful identification of levels was performed from counting from the x-ray landmarks available, and from direct examination, which demonstrated evidence of solid fusion at C5-6 and minimal motion at C6-7, normal motion C4-5. Subsequent to localization, a complete C6 laminectomy was performed with bilateral decompression. Stabilization was then performed using bilateral lateral mass plates. A high-speed bur was used to decorticate the C6-7 facet joints bilaterally. The C5-6 facet joints appeared to be fused. Bilateral unicortical screws were placed through the lateral mass plates at C5, C6, and C7.

(continued)

Operative Report *(continued)*

HERBEL, KAREN
Hospital #746272
Page 2

An oblique incision was made over the left posterior iliac crest followed by exposure of the posterior superior iliac spine, harvesting of cancellous bone graft from between the tables of the ilium. This was placed in the decorticated lateral surfaces and at the joints. Intraoperative x-ray was not repeated due to the difficulty of visualizing. The wound was copiously irrigated with antibiotic solution.

Both wounds were then closed in layers. Dry Gelfoam was placed in the iliac crest for hemostasis. A Hemovac drain was placed in the cervical wound. Layered closure was performed with 0 Vicryl suture in the muscle and fascia, interrupted 2-0 Vicryl sutures subcutaneously, and staples on the skin. The patient was returned to the supine position and extubated. Mayfield tongs were removed. The patient was placed in a Miami J collar. There were no complications. Sponge and needle counts were correct x2.

JEFF PETERSON, MD

JP:hpi

d: 11/1/[add year]
t: 11/2/[add year]

Comic Relief

Correct	Incorrect
d: There were no localizing neurological signs.	t: There were no localizing neurological sins.
d: Tactile stimulation	t: Tackle stimulation
d: Finger-to-nose testing was done well.	t: Finger in the nose testing was done well.
d: The patient was followed by the Neurology Service.	t: The patient was fouled up by the Neurology Service.
d: Patient does point testing and rapid alternating movements well.	t: Patient does pint testing and rapid alternating movements well.

PEARSON
myhealthprofessionskit™

To access the online exercises and transcription practice, go to **www.myhealthprofessionskit.com**. Select "Medical Transcription," then click on the title of this book, ***Healthcare Documentation: Fundamentals & Practice***. Then click on the Neurology chapter.

Diagnostic Imaging

18

Learning Objectives

▶ Spell and define common vocabulary related to diagnostic imaging.

▶ Define various diagnostic imaging procedures.

▶ Identify and describe imaging techniques that do not involve x-rays.

▶ Explain selected techniques and views used in diagnostic imaging.

▶ Correlate selected contrast agents and radionuclides to the studies in which they are used.

▶ Demonstrate knowledge of diagnostic imaging terms and procedures by accurately completing the exercises in this chapter.

Transcribing Diagnostic Imaging Dictation

Introduction

Diagnostic Imaging is the use of physical principles and technology to visualize parts of the body that cannot be seen directly and to assess their function. Images can be created by penetrating tissues with ionizing radiation (x-ray, fluoroscopy), by testing their ability to absorb or reflect nonionizing radiation (ultrasound), by observing the response of their hydrogen ions to shifts in a magnetic field (magnetic resonance imaging, MRI) (see ■ Figure 18-1), or by detecting and recording the absorption and distribution of radioactive materials introduced into the body (nuclear medicine).

Radiology is the branch of medicine that employs x-rays in diagnosis and therapy. By extension, the term often includes ultrasound, MRI, and some aspects of nuclear medicine. A radiologist is a physician with advanced training and board certification in radiology. Most radiologists limit their practice to a specialized branch of the field, such as diagnostic x-ray studies, CT scans, ultrasonography, or x-ray therapy (the treatment of cancer and certain other lesions with external beam radiation or with implanted nuclear material). An **interventional radiologist** uses fluoroscopic imaging to guide catheters, balloons, stents, filters, and other instruments introduced into the cardiovascular and other systems through the skin.

A **radiographic technician** is a nonphysician with practical training in the operation of diagnostic equipment and the performance of x-ray examinations. Technicians often specialize too, limiting their activities to employment with a particular radiologist or practice group.

Some diagnostic procedures (fluoroscopy, angiography) are conducted by a radiologist, others (chest x-ray, IVP, obstetrical ultrasound examination) by a technician working independently of a radiologist. In either event, the interpretation of the images produced is the province of the radiologist.

Most imaging studies are performed according to established routines that specify patient preparation, patient positioning and placement of film, selection of equipment (film type and size, grids, filters) and equipment settings (voltage, exposure time, distance from x-ray source to patient).

An imaging study, or group of studies, is ordinarily ordered by a physician to aid in the diagnostic evaluation of symptoms or abnormal findings. Before ordering an examination the physician may consult with a radiologist to determine the most appropriate studies for the intended purpose. In some settings (for routine health evaluations, before certain types of surgery, or in workers exposed to certain hazardous airborne substances), a chest x-ray or other radiologic study may be performed as a screening procedure in a person without symptoms or suspected abnormalities.

Orders for imaging studies are transmitted in writing to the radiologic department or laboratory. Ordinarily an imaging requisition contains information for the radiographic technician and radiologist about significant medical history and physical findings. Any history of allergy, particularly to radiographic contrast media, is noted. When previous imaging studies have been performed, they are made available to the radiologist for comparison with current studies and perhaps to guide the choice of further examinations.

Many examinations require special preparation of the patient, such as fasting, laxatives, enemas, withholding of regular medicines, administration of premedication, local or general anesthesia, and placement of endoscopes or catheters.

A radiologist dictates a report of findings observed during an examination and after review of films, with conclusions or radiographic diagnoses as appropriate, and the report is then sent to the ordering physician.

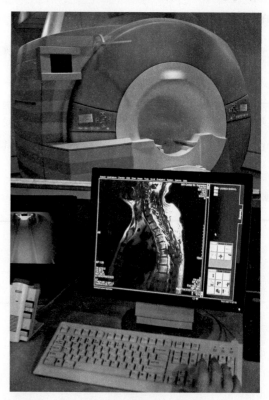

FIGURE 18-1. Magnetic resonance imaging (MRI).
(Source: smart.art / Fotolia)

For mammography, federal law requires that a report in nontechnical language also be transmitted to the patient.

Radiologic diagnoses may be quite specific ("Left pneumothorax with 30% collapse of the lung and no mediastinal shift," "Solitary Lincoln cent in the ascending colon with no evidence of bowel obstruction"). Often, however, only very general observations or conclusions can be recorded, with a note recommending **clinical correlation** (interpretation of radiographic findings, or the lack thereof, in the light of the patient's history and findings on physical examination and other diagnostic testing).

The radiologist's report may include comments about the quality of images obtained by a technician (improper patient positioning, faulty developing technique), patient preparation (necklace left in place for chest x-ray, stool in the colon during barium enema examination), or other factors that may adversely affect the diagnostic accuracy of the study (poor patient cooperation or movement during exposure of films).

The **modern imaging laboratory**, whether a freestanding operation or a department in a hospital, may employ dozens of radiologists and technicians, perform thousands of procedures each month, and have a capital investment of many millions of dollars in equipment.

Besides devices used to perform imaging studies, the furnishings of an x-ray department include apparatus for the administration of contrast agents, supplies for the medical support of patients including emergency resuscitation equipment, and specialized examining tables capable of being adjusted to any desired position and equipped with necessary supports, restraints, and padding. A diagnostic suite and its equipment may be adaptable for a broad variety of examinations, or may be "dedicated"—that is, designed specifically, or used exclusively, for a single type of procedure such as mammography or cerebral angiography.

Vocabulary Review

acoustical shadowing The inability of ultrasound to reach and delineate structures located in the "shadow" of an organ or tissue that reflects a large amount of ultrasound.

air bronchogram A radiographic shadow of an air-filled bronchus passing through an airless segment of lung.

air-fluid level A line representing the level of a collection of fluid seen in profile, with air or gas above it.

air-space disease As seen on chest x-ray, disease or abnormality of lung tissue that encroaches on space normally filled by air.

anterolisthesis Spondylolisthesis, a forward displacement of one vertebra over another resulting from congenital deformity of or damage to vertebral articular processes.

artifact Something present in an image which isn't natural to the structure or tissue. An **aliasing artifact** in ultrasonography is due to a sampling error. In MRI, an aliasing artifact is due to the appearance of a structure outside the field of view within the image. A **summation artifact** in mammography is the appearance of harmless shadows photographically superimposed to resemble cancerous lesions that disappear when the breast is viewed from another angle.

atelectasis Incomplete expansion of the lung or part of a lung.

blood pool The circulating blood, into which radionuclides are injected for various types of circulatory scans.

blunted costophrenic angle On chest x-ray, a costophrenic angle that is flattened or distorted by scarring or pleural fluid.

bony island Benign developmental abnormality consisting of a localized zone of increased density in a long bone.

bowel gas pattern On abdominal film, the normal radiographic appearance of gas in the intestine.

bridging osteophytes Osteophytes (bony outgrowths) on adjacent vertebrae that meet and fuse, forming a "bridge" across the joint space.

clinical correlation (advised or recommended) Interpreting an imaging study in light of the patient's medical history and objective findings on physical examination and laboratory testing.

collateral vessels Vascular channels newly formed from existing ones to maintain the circulation of a tissue or organ whose normal blood supply has been impaired by disease or injury.

collecting system The nonexcretory portions of the kidney, which collect newly formed urine and conduct it to the ureter; the minor and major calices and the renal pelvis.

confluent Merged, not discrete or distinct.

consolidative process An abnormal process that increases the density of a tissue or region. Also called *consolidation*.

contiguous images A series of scans without intervals of unexamined tissue between them. Also called *stacked scans*.

costophrenic angle The angle at the junction of the ribs and diaphragmatic pleura.

cut A CT section or image; a scan.

demineralization Reduction in the amount of calcium present in bone, due to disease or immobilization.

echo characteristics The frequency, intensity, and distribution of echoes produced by a structure or region on ultrasound examination.

echo pattern The ultrasonographic appearance of a structure as seen on a visual display.

ectasia (-ectasis) Dilatation or distention of a tubular structure, as in the bronchi or intestines.

ectopy, ectopia The appearance of a structure or organ outside its normal location.

effacement Abnormal flattening of the contour of a structure.

extraaxial Outside the brain or external to the pia mater, the meningeal membrane that covers the brain, spinal cord, and the proximal portions of the nerve root. Extraaxial masses are more likely to be meningiomas, fluid, or hemorrhage. Compare *intraaxial*.

extravasation of contrast Leakage of contrast medium from the structure into which it is injected through a perforation or other abnormal orifice.

filling defect A zone within a tubular structure that is not filled by injected contrast medium (usually a tumor or abnormal mass).

free air Air or gas in a body cavity where it does not belong, usually after escape from the GI tract.

gas density line A linear band of maximal radiolucency, representing or appearing to represent a narrow zone of air or gas.

granuloma A small nodular collection of cells as an inflammatory response to infectious or noninfectious agents.

great vessels The major vascular trunks entering and leaving the heart: the superior and inferior venae cavae, the pulmonary arteries and veins, and the aorta.

high field strength scanner An MRI device using a static magnetic field of maximal intensity.

hypoaeration Abnormal reduction in the amount of air in lung tissue.

hypokinesis Abnormal reduction of mobility or motility; reduced contractile movement in one or both cardiac ventricles.

ileus Small bowel obstruction due to failure of peristalsis.

impingement Contact or pressure, generally abnormal, between two structures.

internal fixation device Any appliance placed surgically in or on a bone to stabilize a fracture during healing.

interstitial markings The radiographic appearance of lung tissue, as opposed to the appearance of air contained in the lung.

interval change Change in the radiographic appearance of a structure or lesion in the interval between two examinations.

intraaxial Inside the brain. Intraaxial tumors are more likely to be gliomas, astrocytomas, or metastatic disease. Compare *extraaxial*.

isthmus A narrow connection between two larger bodies or parts.

label To render a substance radioactive by incorporating a radionuclide in it; also, to cause a tissue or organ to take up radioactive material. Also called *sensitize* or *tag*.

leukomalacia Softening of the white matter of the brain.

loculated effusion A collection of fluid in a body cavity whose distribution is limited by adjacent normal or abnormal structures.

lucent defect An abnormal zone of decreased resistance to x-rays.

lytic (osteolytic) lesion A disease or abnormality resulting from or consisting of focal breakdown of bone, with reduction in density.

mass effect The radiographic appearance created by an abnormal mass in or adjacent to the area of study.

mass lesion Anything that occupies space within the body and is not normal tissue.

midline shift Displacement of a structure that is normally seen at or near the midline of the body, such as the pineal gland or the trachea.

opacification An increase in the density of a tissue or region, with increased resistance to x-rays.

origin of a vessel The commencement of a vessel as it branches off from a larger vessel.

parenchyma The physiologically active tissue of an organ, as opposed to fat and connective tissue.

peribronchial cuffing Thickening of bronchial walls by edema or fibrosis, as seen in asthma, emphysema, cardiac failure, and other acute and chronic respiratory and circulatory disorders.

peristaltic wave A wave of muscular contractions passing along a tubular organ (such as the intestine), by which its contents are advanced.

pleural effusion An abnormal accumulation of fluid in the pleural cavity.

pole of kidney The upper or lower extremity of a kidney.

posterior sulcus The groove formed by the intersection of the diaphragm and the posterior thoracic wall, as seen in a lateral chest x-ray.

probe Ultrasound transducer.

pulmonary vascular markings As seen on chest x-ray, the normal radiographic appearance of the branches of the pulmonary arteries and veins about the hila of the lungs.

pulmonary vascular redistribution Increased prominence of upper pulmonary vessels and reduced prominence of lower pulmonary vessels at the lung hila in left ventricular failure and other disturbances of circulatory dynamics.

radiolucent Offering relatively little resistance to x-rays (by analogy with *translucent*).

radionuclide Radioactive isotope; a species of atom that spontaneously emits radioactivity.

radiopaque Resisting penetration by x-rays.

reconstitution Maintenance of flow in an artery beyond an area of narrowing or obstruction by establishment of collateral circulation.

resolution The ability of an optical, radiographic, or other image-forming device to distinguish or separate two closely adjacent points in the patient. In CT, resolution is measured in lines per millimeter. The higher the resolution, the sharper and more faithful the image.

runoff The flow of blood and contrast medium through the branches of an artery into which the medium has been injected.

sacralization Abnormal bony fusion between the fifth lumbar vertebra and the sacrum.

sensitize To introduce radioactive material into a fluid, tissue, or space for purposes of performing a radioactive scan; essentially the same as *label*. Also called *label* and *tag*.

serial scans A series of scans made at regular intervals along one dimension of a body region.

signal intensity The strength of the signal or stream of radiofrequency energy emitted by tissue after an MRI excitation pulse.

small bowel transit time The time required for swallowed contrast medium to pass through the small bowel and appear in the colon.

sonolucent Offering relatively little resistance to ultrasound waves (as air or fluid) and hence generating few or no echoes.

spiculated Spiked, thorny.

spurring Formation of one or more jagged osteophytes, as in osteoarthritis.

stacked scans Also called *contiguous images*.

strandy infiltrate A pulmonic infiltrate that appears as strands or streaks of increased density in a chest film.

subcutaneous emphysema Air or gas in subcutaneous tissue.

suboptimal Not as good as might have been expected; usually referring to technical factors in an x-ray study, such as positioning, film quality, and patient cooperation.

surface coil In MRI, a simple flat coil placed on the surface of the body and used as a receiver.

tag Also called *label* and *sensitize*.

tail of breast A wedge-shaped mass of normal breast tissue extending toward the axilla.

takeoff of a vessel The origin of a branch from a larger vessel, as demonstrated radiographically with injected contrast medium.

TE (echo time) The interval between the first pulse in a spin echo examination and the appearance of the resulting echo.

tenting of hemidiaphragm On PA chest x-ray, a distortion of the diaphragm by scarring, in which an up-pointing angular configuration (like a tent) replaces all or part of the normal curved contour of a hemidiaphragm.

tertiary contractions Aberrant contractions of the esophagus, occurring after the primary and secondary waves of normal swallowing.

tibial plateau The flattened surface at the upper end of the anterior aspect of the tibia.

T1 On MRI, the time it takes for protons to return to their orientation to a static magnetic field after an excitation pulse.

TR (repetition time) On MRI, the interval between one spin echo pulse sequence and the next.

T2 On MRI, the time it takes for protons to go out of phase after having been shifted in their orientation by an excitation pulse.

uptake Absorption or concentration of a radionuclide by an organ or tissue.

ventricular ejection fraction That portion of the total volume of blood in a ventricle that is ejected during ventricular contraction (systole); usually expressed as a percent rather than a fraction.

volvulus Intestinal obstruction due to twisting of the bowel.

washout phase Scintiscanning of the lungs at the conclusion of the inhalation phase of a lung scan, after an interval during which all inhaled radionuclide would be expected to have been exhaled.

Medical Readings
Diagnostic Radiology
by John H. Dirckx, MD

X-rays are a form of electromagnetic radiation having a wavelength between that of gamma rays and that of ultraviolet rays. Their importance in medicine arises from their ability to penetrate most of the tissues of the human body and to expose photographic film in a manner similar to light. Diagnostic x-rays are produced by a high-voltage electron tube (Coolidge tube) with equipment that controls the intensity of the beam, its direction and shape, and the duration of emission.

X-rays pass through the part of the body under study and create an image on a sheet of film that is protected from light in a film holder or cassette. Since no lenses are used to focus x-rays, the image is about the same size as the patient, and correspondingly large sheets of film must be used. The standard film size for chest x-rays is 14 x 17 inches (35.5 x 43 cm).

Most x-ray equipment is permanently installed in a properly equipped and shielded radiographic suite. Portable x-ray machines are available to perform certain types of examination in an emergency department, at the bedside, in the patient's home, intraoperatively (during the course of a surgical procedure), or for mass screening in a nursing home, factory, or correctional facility.

X-ray film is developed in an automatic processing machine similar to those used in conventional photography. A developing solution reacts chemically with the silver-containing emulsion on the film in proportion to the amount of radiation that has reached each area of the film. After a timed exposure to the developer, the film passes through a fixative or "hypo" bath that arrests all further chemical reaction. Finally the film is rinsed with water and dried by a current of warm air. A film processor yields a dry, finished film ready for viewing less than five minutes after the exposure was made.

Not all radiographic studies produce permanent images. In **fluoroscopy**, a continuous stream of x-rays passing through a part of the body is made to create an image on a sensitive screen. The image is enhanced electronically so that the dose of radiation can be kept to a minimum. Fluoroscopic monitoring is used extensively in studies with contrast media (gastrointestinal series, angiography) and in invasive and interventional cardiology to track the position of catheters, stents, and other devices.

Although modern picture archiving and communicating systems make it possible to store and retrieve x-ray images digitally and to transmit them instantly anywhere in the world, much of the day-by-day diagnostic work in radiology (chest x-rays, examinations of injured limbs) involves the production of one or more negative images on sheets of film. By long-established convention, these negatives are not printed on paper, as is done in conventional photography. Instead, the negative itself serves as the picture. For examination or "reading," the film is placed on a **backlighted view box** that provides bright, even illumination.

Different tissues offer different amounts of resistance to the passage of x-rays and produce correspondingly lighter or darker images on film. A structure or body area that allows x-rays to pass freely, resulting in a darker or black area on the film, is said to be **radiolucent** (by analogy with *translucent*). A structure or object that blocks x-rays, resulting in less exposure of the film and a lighter or white area, is said to be **radiopaque**.

The radiologist can distinguish only four degrees of density in tissue: **metal density** (bone, gallstones, urinary calculi, metallic foreign bodies including orthopedic hardware); **water density** (body fluids and most soft tissues other than fat); **fat density**; and **air** or **gas density** (air in respiratory passages, gas in digestive passages, or either of these in inappropriate places). Shapes or outlines appear in an x-ray image only where two zones of contrasting density touch or overlap.

The radiologist can see the outline of a **bone** (which is of metal density) because it is silhouetted against surrounding soft tissues of water density. A bubble of air in the stomach is visible because it, too, is surrounded by, and contrasts with, water-density tissue. But where two structures of like density (e.g., two muscles, or the spleen and the pancreas) are contiguous, no silhouette is produced, and the border or interface between them is not represented in the image.

Unlike a photograph, an x-ray picture gives no information about the depth or contours of the structures shown. An x-ray picture is literally just a shadow or group of shadows. Everything is represented in an absolutely flat, **two-dimensional image**. An x-ray film of a right hand, when turned over, cannot be distinguished from an x-ray of a left hand. For that reason, an x-ray picture of any part of a limb is normally labeled R or L at the time of exposure. A metal letter clipped to the corner of the film holder becomes a part of the image.

Pause for Reflection

1. Briefly describe the manner in which an x-ray is obtained and produced.
2. How does fluoroscopy differ from standard x-ray imaging?
3. Distinguish between radiolucent and radiopaque.
4. Describe the 4 degrees of tissue density.
5. How is a radiograph alike or unlike a photograph?

Plain Radiography

The term **plain film** (not "plane film") refers to any radiographic study performed without the use of contrast material. For each part of the body and each diagnostic purpose, standard procedures (positioning of the patient, machine voltage setting, exposure time) have been developed to yield the desired information with maximum speed and efficiency and a minimum of exposure to harmful radiation.

The standard **PA (posteroanterior) chest film** is the most frequently performed of all plain radiographic examinations. For this study the patient stands facing the film holder and the x-ray tube is aimed horizontally at the patient's back. The backs of the wrists are placed on the hips and the elbows rotated forward so as to move the scapulae laterally as far as possible, and the breath is held in full inspiration.

This single study can provide a great deal of critical diagnostic information. Solid tumors and abnormal accumulations of fluid (**water density**) are readily apparent when they encroach on lung tissue, which is largely filled with air (**gas density**). The heart and great vessels appear sharply silhouetted against the background of air in lung tissue, so that abnormalities in their size and shape are also clearly evident.

In reading a **chest film**, the radiologist looks for changes in the density and contour of soft tissues (muscles of the neck and thorax, breasts); indications of deformity, disease, or trauma in bones (spine, ribs, scapulae, humeri); irregularities, thickening, or calcification of the pleural margins, or fluid in the pleural space; abnormalities of the diaphragmatic contour; and variations in the size, shape, and position of the heart, great vessels (aorta, pulmonary artery, superior and inferior venae cavae) and other structures in the mediastinum (the part of the thorax between the lungs).

The outline or contour of the heart, being a two-dimensional shadow, is aptly termed a silhouette (see ■ Figure 18-2). In a standard PA chest film the width of the cardiac silhouette at its widest is normally less than half the width of the thorax at its widest. The comparison of these two widths (heart width divided by thoracic width), called the **cardiothoracic ratio (CTR)**, is therefore normally less than 0.5.

The normal "lung markings"—radiopaque tubular structures at the hila of the lungs, which branch and taper as they spread toward the periphery—are not bronchi but branches of the right and left pulmonary arteries. Distortion or asymmetry of the pattern created by these vessels may indicate a space-occupying lesion

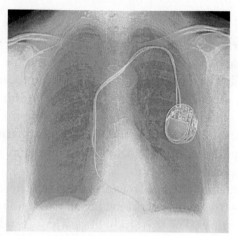

FIGURE 18-2. Color-enhanced x-ray of implanted pacemaker (Courtesy of UHB Trust/Getty Images)

within lung tissue, pneumothorax (air in the pleural space), or other abnormal condition.

A **lateral chest film** is often performed in conjunction with a PA film, or as a supplement to it when the initial study shows some abnormality. A left lateral film (with the left side of the chest nearest to the film holder) is usually preferred because it provides a sharper image of the heart. Right and left oblique views of the chest may be obtained to clarify the diagnosis.

Plain films of the abdomen are less valuable than chest films because most of the abdominal organs are of the same (water) density. Abdominal films are useful, however, in identifying disorders characterized by abnormal distribution of air or gas (distention of bowel due to obstruction, gas in the peritoneal cavity from a ruptured bowel), in confirming the presence and location of kidney stones and swallowed foreign bodies, and in identifying certain other disorders.

A plain film of the abdomen may be obtained as a screening examination, particularly in a patient with acute abdominal pain, to determine whether other studies are needed and to help in the selection of those studies. A plain film performed as a preliminary to contrast studies is called a **scout film**. Because such an examination is often done to screen for a stone in the urinary tract, it may also be called a **KUB** (kidneys, ureters, bladder) film.

A single abdominal film is ordinarily made with the patient lying supine (face up) and the film holder contained in a receptacle within the examining table. When there is concern about the possibility of a ruptured bowel, with leakage of gas into the peritoneal cavity, several plain films may be made with the patient in different positions, usually **flat, upright, and left lateral decubitus** (that is, lying on the left side). For the latter

examination, the film holder is placed vertically and the x-ray beam is directed horizontally across the table, hence the common term "**cross-table view.**" Such a combination of films may be called an **acute abdomen series** or a **free air study**.

X-ray studies of the **extremities** are performed to assess the effects of injury (fracture, dislocation), to locate foreign bodies, or to diagnose disorders of bones or joints (congenital deformities, metabolic or circulatory disorders, benign and malignant tumors, rheumatoid arthritis, degenerative joint disease). A single x-ray view of an extremity may be of limited usefulness. Because all structures are superimposed in one composite two-dimensional image, a small fracture or zone of bone disease may escape detection. A metallic foreign body will probably be visible, but its exact location in the three-dimensional extremity cannot be determined from a two-dimensional study. For most extremity studies, therefore, three exposures are made: anteroposterior (AP), lateral, and oblique.

A **stress film** is made while mechanical stress is applied to one or more joints. A stress film may show abnormal laxity of a joint, such as that due to a ligamentous tear, which would not be apparent on a standard view. In the examination of a shoulder to detect a tear of the acromioclavicular ligament, films may be taken both with and without the patient holding a weight in the hand on the affected side.

X-rays of the **axial skeleton** (skull, spinal column, ribs, and sternum) may be performed in cases of injury or to diagnose bone or joint disease. However, specialized examinations (CT, MRI, angiography) have largely supplanted plain skull films in the assessment of brain disorders (hemorrhage, neoplasms), and are also more valuable than plain films in evaluating injury or disease of the vertebrae.

Special studies of the **nasal bones**, the **bony orbit**, and other **facial bones** may be performed to evaluate acute injury. Radiographic studies of the **paranasal sinuses** may show thickening of mucous membranes and an air-fluid level due to accumulation of secretions in a sinus whose ostium is blocked by swelling. But computed tomography (CT) is more accurate in the diagnosis of acute and chronic sinusitis, and shows nasal polyps better.

Mammography (see ■ Figure 18-3) is the radiologic evaluation of the female breast, primarily to search for or evaluate abnormal masses that may be malignant.

The apparatus used to perform mammography includes, besides an adjustable x-ray source and a film

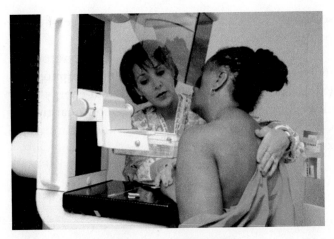

FIGURE 18-3. Mammography

holder, a compression paddle that serves to flatten out the breast during the examination. By thinning the layer of tissue to be examined, compression permits a lower dose of radiation. In addition, the compression paddle steadies the patient and reduces the risk of movement during the exposure.

A **screening mammogram** is performed according to a standard protocol to evaluate the breasts of a woman who has no breast complaints or abnormal findings. In contrast, **diagnostic mammography** refers to a more specific and individualized radiographic study that is done to evaluate local breast pain or abnormal findings such as a palpable lump or nipple discharge or to follow up on an abnormal screening mammogram.

In screening mammography, an x-ray of each breast is made in two projections. For the **mediolateral oblique (MLO)** view, the x-ray tube is positioned in front of the chest and aimed horizontally toward the breast to be examined, with the film holder placed laterally under the patient's raised arm. For the **craniocaudal** or **cranial-caudal (CC)** view, the film holder is placed horizontally under the breast and the x-ray beam is directed downward from above.

For diagnostic mammography, each breast is imaged separately in CC and MLO projections, with the addition of supplemental views tailored to the specific problem. These supplemental views can include lateromedial (LM) and mediolateral (ML) views.

For interpretation, a film of the right breast is displayed side by side on a viewbox with the corresponding view of the left breast, as if they were mirror images. This facilitates comparison of the two breasts and serves to emphasize minor differences in their radiographic appearance. **Digital mammography**, permitting review of digital images on a high-resolution monitor, improves the accuracy of mammographic screening.

Mammographic findings that suggest cancer are ill-defined densities within breast tissue and microcalcifications (very small deposits of calcium), particularly those that are irregularly clustered or spiculated (appearing like small spikes or thorns). These findings are nonspecific. It is estimated that a woman having screening mammograms regularly throughout life has a 50% chance of eventually having a false-positive report (suspicious for cancer in the absence of cancer). Reporting of mammographic findings has been standardized by **BIRADS** (see box, page 630).

Pause for Reflection

1. Define plain film.
2. List the different views that may be used in obtaining a chest x-ray; which is the most common?
3. What are the two names by which a plain film of the abdomen may be called? Explain the logic or rationale behind these names.
4. What positions may the patient be placed in when obtaining a plain film of the abdomen?
5. What are the three exposures or views used when obtaining x-rays of the extremities and why are they needed?
6. What is a stress film?
7. Describe the views used in screening mammography? What additional views are included in diagnostic mammography?
8. Explain the BIRADS categories for reporting diagnostic mammography findings.

Bone Densitometry

Osteoporosis, a common disorder of middle-aged and elderly women, is characterized by decreased mass and decreased mineral density of bone, with increased susceptibility to fractures. Bone mass declines with age and is influenced by sex, race, weight, and other factors. Osteoporosis is responsible for 50% of fractures occurring in women over age 50.

Compression fractures of vertebrae and fractures of the wrist and hip (neck of the femur) due to falls are the most common. Assessment of bone density is currently recommended for all women over 65 and for younger women who are at increased risk of osteoporosis.

Because mineral density must be decreased by about one-third before any reduction is apparent in an x-ray image, standard radiography is an insensitive test for osteoporosis. Bone densitometry is an application of radiographic technology to osteoporosis screening.

Most of the bone densitometry techniques in current use measure the extent to which a low dose of radiation is absorbed by bone. The patient sits or lies motionless with the body area under study placed between an x-ray source and a scanner. Skeletal areas examined include the wrist, lumbar spine, and hip. Besides producing an image of the area examined, the study yields a numerical score that can be used to measure the degree of osteoporosis and to quantify the risk of fracture.

The several methods used for bone densitometry include **single-photon** and **dual-photon absorptiometry** (SPA and DPA), **single-energy** and **dual-energy x-ray absorptiometry** (SXA and DEXA), and **quantitative CT**. An ultrasound procedure, which does not involve x-rays, is also available.

The interpretation of a bone densitometry study includes a comparison of the findings with established

MAMMOGRAM REPORTS—BIRADS

The American College of Radiology (ACR) has developed a standard way of describing mammogram findings. In this system, the results are sorted into categories numbered 0 through 6. This system is called the Breast Imaging Reporting and Data System (BIRADS). Having a standard way of reporting mammogram results lets doctors use the same words and terms and ensures better followup of suspicious findings.

Here is a brief review of what the categories mean:

X-ray assessment is incomplete.

Category 0: Additional imaging evaluation and/or comparison to prior mammograms is needed.

This means a possible abnormality may not be clearly seen or defined and more tests are needed, such as the use of spot compression (applying compression to a smaller area when doing the mammogram), magnified views, special mammogram views, or ultrasound.

This also suggests that the mammogram should be compared with older ones to see if there have been changes in the area over time.

X-ray assessment is complete.

Category 1: Negative

There is no significant abnormality to report. The breasts look the same (they are symmetrical) with no masses (lumps), distorted structures, or suspicious calcifications. In this case, negative means nothing bad was found.

Category 2: Benign (non-cancerous) finding

This is also a negative mammogram result (there is no sign of cancer), but the reporting doctor chooses to describe a finding known to be benign, such as benign calcifications, lymph nodes in the breast, or calcified fibroadenomas. This ensures that others who look at the mammogram will not misinterpret the benign finding as suspicious. This finding is recorded in the mammogram report to help when comparing to future mammograms.

Category 3: Probably benign finding. Followup in a short time frame is suggested.

The findings in this category have a very good chance (greater than 98%) of being benign (not cancer). The findings are not expected to change over time. But since it is not proven benign, it is helpful to see if an area of concern does change over time. Followup with repeat imaging is usually done in six months and regularly thereafter until the finding is known to be stable (usually at least two years). This approach helps avoid unnecessary biopsies, but if the area does change over time, it allows for early diagnosis.

Category 4: Suspicious abnormality. Biopsy should be considered.

Findings do not definitely look like cancer but could be cancer. The radiologist is concerned enough to recommend a biopsy. The findings in this category can have a wide range of suspicion levels. For this reason, some doctors may divide this category further:

4A: Finding with a low suspicion of being cancer

4B: Finding with an intermediate suspicion of being cancer

4C: Finding of moderate concern of being cancer, but not as high as Category 5.

Category 5: Malignancy highly probable.

norms. The result of this comparison is reported as a **T-score**, which is based on comparison of the patient's bone mineral density with that of a healthy woman in her 30s. A **Z-score**, based on comparison of the patient's measurements with those of a person of the same sex and age, may also be calculated.

Pause for Reflection

1. List the different methods for bone densitometry.
2. Why is bone densitometry performed?
3. What is the T-score?

Contrast Radiography

X-ray images of soft-tissue structures such as the brain and spinal cord and the circulatory, digestive, and genitourinary systems typically lack sufficient detail for diagnostic purposes because most of the structures represented in the image are of the same density. This deficiency has been very largely overcome by the use of contrast media in diagnostic radiography. A **contrast medium** (sometimes called a dye) is a liquid or semisolid material that appears with metal density in a radiographic image. Introduced into a hollow structure such as the colon or the aorta, it imparts to an x-ray picture a solid, opaque image of that structure.

A **myelogram** is a radiographic examination of the spinal cord after injection of a contrast agent into the subarachnoid space. The procedure is usually performed to identify abnormalities of the spinal cord and its nerve roots, particularly compression by a herniated disk, a tumor, arthritic osteophytes (spiky outgrowths of bone), or spinal stenosis (narrowing of the spinal canal). Myelography has been largely supplanted in clinical practice by MRI.

The standard contrast medium for gastrointestinal studies is **barium sulfate**. Various concentrations are used depending on the type of examination to be performed. Abnormalities that may be noted in a barium study are **filling defects** (areas where the barium fails to fill out the expected contour of the organ because of the presence of a tumor), **ulcerations** (breaks or erosions in the integrity of the mucosal lining), **strictures** (narrowing of the lumen due to scarring), **distortion** or **displacement** due to external factors (swelling, tumors, or hemorrhage outside the digestive tract), and disturbances

in **gastrointestinal motility** (undue rapidity or slowness of peristaltic movement of barium through the tract).

The sensitivity of a barium study can be enhanced by performing an **air-contrast (double-contrast)** examination. Air or gas is introduced into the digestive tract to distend its walls after most of the barium has passed through or, in the case of a barium enema, has been expelled from the colon.

In a **barium swallow** the patient drinks a sufficient volume of barium suspension to fill and outline the esophagus while the radiologist observes its passage fluoroscopically, taking spot films as appropriate. When the diagnostic focus is not limited to the esophagus, the barium swallow examination is followed by observation of the passage of contrast medium into the stomach and duodenum (**upper GI series**) with the patient lying face up on the x-ray table. Passage of barium through the small intestine normally takes 2–4 hours or longer.

For a full upper GI examination with **small-bowel follow-through**, further fluoroscopic assessment and spot films are performed at intervals, ideally until some barium appears in the cecum (first part of the colon).

A **barium enema** (see ■ Figure 18-4), the standard radiographic examination of the large intestine, involves introducing barium suspension into the rectum by means of an enema tube. In preparation for this examination, the colon must be emptied of stool with laxatives, suppositories, cleansing enemas, or some

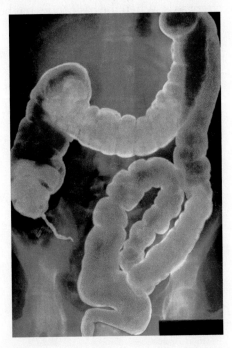

FIGURE 18-4. Color-enhanced x-ray of colon taken during barium enema examination. Note the thin stream of barium filling the appendix in the right lower quadrant. (CNRI/Science Photo Library/Photo Researchers, Inc.)

combination of these. The procedure is not considered complete until some barium is seen in the **distal ileum** (the part of the small intestine that empties into the colon), indicating that the entire colon has been visualized. If an upper GI study has recently been performed, examination of the colon is postponed until barium remaining from the earlier examination has passed out of the body.

Cholangiography is the study of the biliary tract after oral or intravenous administration of a radiopaque material that is concentrated by the liver and secreted in bile, or after injection of medium directly into the duct system. After the performance of a baseline cholangiogram, **cholecystokinin (CCK)** may be injected intravenously to stimulate contraction of the gallbladder. A followup study showing an **ejection fraction** of less than 35% (that is, retention of 65% or more of the radiopaque bile in the gallbladder) suggests obstruction of the cystic or common bile duct. **Cholescintigraphy**, a nuclear medicine procedure discussed later in this chapter, is often preferred now to contrast radiography of the biliary tract.

Intravenous pyelography (IVP) (see ■ Figure 18-5) is a radiographic study of the urinary tract (renal pelves, ureters, bladder, and urethra) after intravenous injection of a contrast agent that is rapidly excreted by the kidneys. Exposures of the lower abdomen and pelvis are made before administration of contrast medium and at standard intervals afterwards. When the basic series has been com-

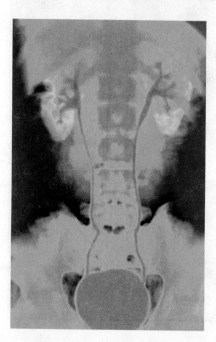

FIGURE 18-5. Intravenous pyelogram (IVP) showing normal renal collecting systems, ureters, and fully distended bladder. Source: CRNI, Photo Researchers, Inc.

pleted, the patient is asked to void and another film is taken to assess residual urine in the bladder.

In **retrograde pyelography**, the upper urinary tract is visualized with contrast medium that has been injected directly into it, one ureter at a time, from below. With a cystoscope, a ureteral catheter is threaded under direct vision into the opening between one ureter and the bladder. Contrast medium is injected in retrograde fashion under fluoroscopic monitoring and spot x-ray films are made.

A **voiding cystourethrogram (VCUG)** is performed to assess the anatomy of the bladder and urethra and, in particular, the function of the bladder during voiding. A contrast medium is instilled into the bladder by means of a urethral catheter. Spot films are recorded in various projections while the bladder is distended with medium. The catheter is then removed and further films are taken as the patient voids (empties the bladder).

In a **stress cystogram**, the patient is not instructed to void while imaging studies are performed. Instead, the patient coughs, strains, or bears down as for a bowel movement, while trying to hold back the flow of urine. This test is done to detect stress incontinence (involuntary leakage of urine with increase of pressure in the abdominopelvic cavity, as from coughing or laughing).

Hysterosalpingography is a radiographic examination of the uterine cavity and uterine tubes with contrast medium injected through the cervix. The principal indications for this procedure are infertility and habitual abortion (repeated miscarriage), but it may also be used to diagnose tumors and other disorders of the female genital tract. A contrast medium is injected through a catheter or cannula placed in the uterine cervix. Filling of the uterine cavity and uterine tubes is monitored fluoroscopically and spot films are taken. Occasionally the injection of contrast medium under pressure corrects infertility by dilating a narrowed uterine tube without the need for other intervention.

Angiography is the radiographic study of blood vessels (less often, lymph vessels) into which a radiopaque medium has been injected. The principal reason for performing an angiographic examination is to detect malformation, narrowing (stenosis), blockage (occlusion), or injury of a blood vessel. In addition, angiography often enhances the diagnostic value of plain radiography by showing displacement of blood vessels or other changes of vascular pattern due to tumors, swelling, hemorrhage, or trauma.

The injection of contrast medium may be made with the catheter so placed that an entire arterial system (for example, both renal arteries) is visualized (flush method), or the tip of the catheter may be directed into a specific vessel or branch for a more selective examination.

Angiography differs from other contrast studies in that the structures outlined (blood vessels) are already full of fluid, and that fluid is in motion. Because injected contrast medium immediately becomes diluted by the blood, it must be highly concentrated in order to retain its potency as an opacifying agent. And because the medium is immediately swept along through the vessels by the flow of blood, the study consists of a **series of images** made at split-second intervals after injection, as well as being recorded videographically on tape.

A major application of **arteriography** is in the evaluation of the chambers and valves of the heart, the coronary arteries, and the aorta and pulmonary arterial circulation. Arteriography is also extensively used to assess the circulation of the brain, the abdominal viscera, and the extremities.

Cerebral angiography (contrast examination of the vasculature of the brain) is performed to identify and localize obstruction to blood flow and also to detect vascular anomalies such as aneurysm (abnormal local dilatation of an artery) and arteriovenous malformations. Because displacement of normal vascular patterns can indicate an intracranial tumor or a hematoma (local accumulation of blood due to hemorrhage) or other consequence of head trauma, cerebral angiography is often used in cases of head injury or as an adjunct to other studies in patients with unexplained severe headache, seizures, or other clues to the possible presence of a tumor. In addition, cerebral angiography is performed to provide vascular mapping before certain types of surgery, and it may also be done postoperatively to assess beneficial results of surgery or to look for complications.

In **coronary angiography** a catheter is introduced into a peripheral artery and advanced toward the heart under fluoroscopic guidance. The tip of the catheter is then manipulated into the origin of one of the two coronary arteries and contrast medium is injected. Coronary angiography is currently the most precise diagnostic procedure available to confirm and localize narrowing of coronary arteries by disease and to estimate the extent to which blood flow is compromised.

This examination is performed routinely in the assessment of patients with known or suspected coronary artery disease. Modern techniques of coronary angiography have developed in parallel with the field of cardiac catheterization, and both types of procedure are often performed during the same diagnostic session. Moreover, therapeutic procedures pertaining to interventional cardiology (percutaneous transluminal angioplasty, stent placement) may be undertaken immediately after angiography if one or more sites of significant vascular narrowing are identified.

Aortography (contrast imaging of the thoracic and abdominal aorta, with medium injected through a catheter in a femoral or brachial artery) is indicated when other studies fail to provide adequate information about atherosclerotic lesions, aneurysms, or aortic dissection. By advancing the catheter under fluoroscopic monitoring, the radiologist can perform selective angiography of the liver, spleen, pancreas, or kidneys when indicated.

Renal angiography may be performed to identify renal artery stenosis (an important cause of secondary hypertension), thrombosis or embolism of a renal artery, or structural abnormality within a kidney due to congenital anomaly, trauma, or tumor. Renal angiography is also a standard part of the evaluation of a donor kidney for renal transplant.

Other contrast studies include **venography** (phlebography), examination of peripheral veins to diagnose deep vein thrombosis; **lymphangiography**, a radiographic examination of lymphatic channels, performed for the diagnosis of lymphomas (malignant tumors of lymphoid tissue) or of malignancies that have metastasized to lymph nodes; and **arthrography**, the radiographic examination of a joint into which a contrast medium has been injected.

Pause for Reflection

1. Define *contrast medium* or *dye*.
2. Briefly define the following studies: *myelography, cholangiography, hysterosalpingography, lymphangiography, arthrography.*
3. List and describe the contrast procedures on the gastrointestinal tract that incorporate the use of barium sulfate.
4. List and describe the contrast studies performed on the kidneys and bladder.
5. List and describe the angiographic studies done on the circulatory system (heart and brain).

Computed Tomography (CT)

Computed tomography (CT), also called **computed axial tomography (CAT)**, is an application of computer technology to diagnostic radiology. Instead of exposing a sheet of photographic film after passing through the patient, the x-rays are detected and recorded by one or more scintillation counters (devices that detect and measure radiation). The x-ray source and scintillation counter are mounted on a frame or gantry, allowing them to rotate 360° around the patient and "cut" across any selected plane. A series of exposures are made according to a predetermined protocol that has been programmed into the equipment. Data on the amount of x-ray that penetrates the patient at each exposure are collected, digitized, and analyzed by a computer that generates a cross-sectional image or profile corresponding to the plane cut by the x-ray beam.

A CT examination results in a series of images or slices showing the anatomy of the patient at right angles to the x-ray beam, exactly as if the body were actually being sliced into cross-sections. For viewing, CT images are oriented as if the patient were lying supine (face up) and the observer were looking at the sections from the patient's feet. The thickness of each slice and the distance between slices are determined by computer settings. An examination can result in sample slices at regular intervals or in a sequence of contiguous images without intervals of unexamined tissue between them.

In conventional CT, the x-ray source moves from one position to another in stepwise fashion around the patient and exposures are made individually. In **helical** (or **spiral**) **CT** the x-ray tube emits radiation continuously as it rotates through a predetermined arc while the table supporting the patient moves at a constant speed at a right angle to this arc to yield a series of cuts. Because helical CT produces a series of images more quickly, it reduces artifacts from breathing movements and allows an entire organ or body region to be scanned during a single session.

The information acquired during a CT examination is stored as raw digital data. By manipulating these data, the radiographer can enhance the visibility of certain tissues or structures as they appear in an image, while suppressing others. By more sophisticated programming of the CT computer, it is possible to perform multi-planar reconstructions (projections of anatomy in planes other than at a right angle to the viewer).

Computed tomography has replaced conventional x-ray studies for many applications because it permits finer discrimination between tissue densities. Contiguous soft-tissue structures whose borders or silhouettes are not represented in an x-ray image can often be clearly distinguished in a CT scan. Hence CT provides superior visualization of enlarged or displaced organs and of soft-tissue masses (cysts, neoplasms, hemorrhage), and is particularly valuable in diagnostic screening of the **head**, thorax, abdomen, and pelvis. In addition, it is more sensitive than conventional radiology in detecting variations in calcification and bone density and in identifying subtle **fractures**.

CT examinations of the head are useful in identifying and localizing hemorrhage both after acute trauma (to identify epidural or subdural hematoma) and in stroke (to rule out hemorrhage before administration of a thrombolytic agent). Studies of the respiratory tract with **helical CT** and **multiplanar imaging** have application in the diagnosis of bronchial disease and asthma and in screening high-risk populations (smokers over 60) for lung cancer. In acute abdominal pain, CT is valuable in diagnosing such disorders as ureteral calculus, bowel obstruction, and appendicitis. It can also detect deep vein thrombosis (DVT) in the pelvis or a lower limb.

As with conventional radiography, the sensitivity of some computed tomography studies can be enhanced by administration of a **contrast medium** during the examination. Barium may be given orally or rectally in studies of the gastrointestinal tract. In CT angiography, contrast medium is infused intravenously rather than being introduced into an artery by catheter. After making a circuit through the heart and lungs, the medium appears in the arterial supply of the structures being studied in sufficient concentration to render those vessels and structures visible.

Another contrast medium used with CT is **xenon**, a colorless, odorless, and chemically inert elemental gas. Inhalation of a mixture of xenon and oxygen results in excellent demarcation of respiratory passages on CT scanning. Inhaled xenon is absorbed into the circulation and rapidly diffused throughout the body, enhancing the visibility of soft tissues such as abdominal viscera. Because it readily passes the blood-brain barrier, xenon studies are valuable in the evaluation of regional cerebral blood flow.

Ultrasonography

Ultrasonography (or sonography) is a means of visualizing internal structures by observing the effects they have on a beam of sound waves. The sound waves used for this procedure have a higher frequency (pitch) than the human ear can detect. The upper limit of human hearing is about 20,000 Hz (hertz, or cycles per second); diagnostic ultrasonography uses frequencies between 1 and 10 MHz (megahertz, one million Hz).

Ultrasound waves pass through air, gas, and fluid without being reflected. However, they bounce back from rigid structures such as bone and gallstones, creating an echo that can be detected by a receiver. Solid organs such as the liver and kidney partially reflect ultrasound waves in predictable patterns. Waves are also reflected from the interface between two structures having different acoustic properties, such as fluid and the structure that contains it (e.g., cyst, urinary bladder).

Ultrasound waves for diagnostic sonography are generated by a transducer (a piezoelectric crystal or ceramic chip), which emits vibrations when stimulated by electricity. The same crystal acts as a receiver, detecting echoes and converting them back into electrical signals. The transducer used in ultrasonographic examinations is contained in a hand-held scanning head or probe, which the examiner places on the surface of the patient's body. A gel is applied to the skin surface to reduce friction and ensure even contact.

The echoes detected by the receiver and transformed by it into electrical data are processed by a computer and converted to an image on a television screen. In analyzing sonographic data, the computer uses the strength of each echo to determine the **acoustical impedance** (resistance to the passage of sound waves) of the structure that generated it, and the **echo time** (delay in return of echo after emission of the sound wave) to determine the distance between the transducer and the structure.

The images produced are in **gray-scale**. That is, each pixel ("picture element," smallest discrete component of the image) appears in a shade of gray whose darkness or lightness is in proportion to the intensity of the signal represented. A tissue or organ that reflects ultrasound strongly is said to be **hyperechoic**, or to display high **echogenicity**, while a tissue that reflects ultrasound weakly is said to be **hypoechoic** and to display low echogenicity.

Because water and other fluids do not reflect at all, they are said to be **anechoic** or **sonolucent** (by analogy with **translucent** and **radiolucent**). A highly echogenic structure, such as a bone, prevents sound waves from generating images of tissues behind it, a phenomenon known as acoustic shadowing.

A-mode sonography, using a solitary transducer, yields only information about the size or position of a given target, such as a mass or organ. In **B-mode** sonography, a scanner containing as many as 100 transducers, each "listening" to an echo from a slightly different angle, permits the generation of a two-dimensional image. Rapid processing of signals can convert a succession of B-mode scans into a sequence of images that flow together to give the observer an illusion of motion.

This is called **M-mode** (for "motion") or real-time scanning. By this technique, movement such as the beating of the heart is perceived as it occurs. By the application of technology similar to that used in computed tomography, two-dimensional B-mode sonographic images can also be combined to produce three-dimensional images.

Because it involves no harmful radiation, ultrasonography is particularly useful during **pregnancy** and in the examination of children. It is widely used in the diagnosis of acute or chronic pain, masses, and trauma of the abdomen or pelvis. Because it can determine the size of masses and distinguish between cysts and solid tumors, it is a standard procedure in evaluating masses or swellings in the thyroid gland, liver, pancreas, spleen, kidney, and prostate. Because it shows gallstones and urinary calculi clearly, it is particularly useful in obstructive disease of the biliary and urinary tracts. It can also be used to guide the performance of a biopsy, particularly of the prostate, or (during surgery) the placement of a needle in a cyst or other lesion.

The **Doppler phenomenon** is the familiar change in the pitch of sound waves as heard when their source is moving with respect to the hearer. Doppler sonography applies this effect to obtain information about flow through blood vessels. **Duplex Doppler sonography** combines standard ultrasound imaging with computer analysis of Doppler data to graph the speed and direction of **blood flow** through the vessels under study. A further refinement is the use of color to indicate the direction of blood flow. In **color Doppler** sonography, each pixel containing information on blood flow is color-coded according to the direction and velocity of blood flow, blue indicating flow away from the transducer and red indicating flow toward the transducer.

Ultrasonography is a routine part of prenatal care. Ordinarily an **obstetrical sonogram** is performed at 18 to 20 weeks' gestation (see ■ Figure 18-6). An examination may be performed earlier to confirm the presence of pregnancy or, in cases of vaginal bleeding, to assess fetal viability and rule out ectopic pregnancy. Other specific indications for **diagnostic sonography** during pregnancy include diagnosis of multiple pregnancy, fetal malformation, or polyhydramnios (excessive amniotic fluid) and localization of the placenta (in cases of placenta previa or before amniocentesis). **Transvaginal sonography**, with the scanning head placed inside the vagina, yields superior detail in certain circumstances.

Sonography permits accurate determination of fetal size and calculation of gestational age. Early in pregnancy the **crown-rump length** is most useful in calculating age. Later the **biparietal diameter** (transverse width of the skull) correlates most closely with age. In the third trimester, the circumference of the fetal abdomen may be measured as a means of estimating fetal size and weight.

Ultrasound is used to determine the **biophysical profile (BPP)** of a fetus (see ■ Figure 18-7). This is a precise assessment of fetal well-being that may be performed during the third trimester of a high-risk pregnancy or when there is suspicion of fetal distress. The profile is based on a set of five observations made during a 30- to 60-minute session of continuous ultrasound surveillance and monitoring of fetal heart rate. The components of the profile are:

1. **Body and limb movements**: Should occur at least three times during the observation period.

2. **"Breathing" movements**: At least one, lasting 30 seconds or more, should be observed.

3. **Stretching movements** of fetal limbs and spine should occur and should be followed by a return to a flexed posture.

4. **Amniotic fluid index (AFI)**: The space between the fetus and the wall of the amniotic sac is measured in all four quadrants. The sum of the measurements is normally between 6 and 25 cm.

5. **Spontaneous increases in fetal heart rate**, typically accompanied by fetal movements, should occur at least twice. (This observation is called, somewhat illogically, a **nonstress test** to distinguish it from a stress test, in which the fetal heart rate is monitored after administration of an agent to promote uterine contractions.)

A score of either 0 or 2 (never 1) is recorded for each of the five assessments. A total score of 8 or 10 is a satisfactory profile. A score of 6 or 8 indicates the

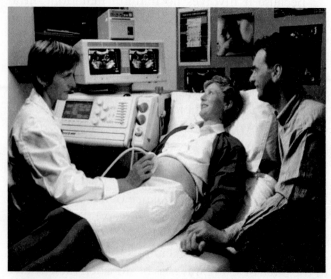

FIGURE 18-6. Obstetric ultrasound

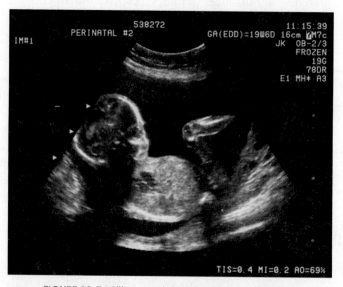

FIGURE 18-7. Ultrasound showing outline of a fetus

need for a repeat test in 12–24 hours. A score of 4 or less is presumptive evidence of fetal hypoxemia, demanding prompt investigation and, if the fetus is sufficiently mature, induction of labor.

Echocardiography is the application of ultrasonography to the examination of the heart. An echocardiogram, performed with a scanning head applied to the anterior and lateral chest wall, gives information about the size of the cardiac chambers (atria and ventricles), the thickness and motion of chamber walls, and the condition of the pericardium and great vessels. The addition of **Doppler imaging** shows the direction and velocity of blood flow, assesses valve function, and permits calculation of the **ventricular ejection fraction** (the proportion of the blood present in the left ventricle at the end of diastole that is ejected during systole, usually expressed as a percent rather than a fraction).

Echocardiography is a standard procedure in the evaluation of congenital and acquired valvular disease, including mitral valve prolapse, and in congestive heart failure and other disorders characterized by inadequate pumping action of the heart. A general reduction in ventricular wall motion is called **hypokinesis**; a more localized reduction of motion is called **asyneresis**. An ejection fraction less than 40% suggests cardiac failure.

Pause for Reflection

1. How does ultrasonography differ from conventional x-ray?
2. Define the following terms: hyperechoic, echogenicity, anechoic, sonolucent, hypoechoic, and acoustic shadowing.
3. Distinguish among A-mode, B-mode, and M-mode ultrasonography.
4. What is Doppler sonography and its applications?
5. What are the uses of ultrasonography in obstetrics?
6. What are the indications for echocardiography?

Magnetic Resonance Imaging (MRI)

Magnetic resonance imaging is a method of visualizing internal structures electronically rather than with x-rays. Although this technique yields cuts or cross-sectional images similar to those of computed tomography, it is based on entirely different physical principles. As with x-ray and ultrasound, MRI detects and records differences in the physical properties of contiguous or adjacent tissues—for example, bone as contrasted with muscle, or normal liver as contrasted with a cyst. But whereas an x-ray examination detects varying resistance of tissues to penetration by x-rays, and ultrasonography detects varying resistance to penetration by sound waves, MRI detects varying concentrations or densities of hydrogen atoms (protons) in tissues.

A magnet attracts not only iron atoms but also any other atoms that, like iron, have an unequal number of protons and neutrons in their nuclei. The degree to which such an atom responds to magnetic attraction depends on its nuclear structure and is expressed as a physical constant called **spin**.

The simplest of all atoms is that of hydrogen, which, with but a single proton in its nucleus, possesses spin and responds to magnetic attraction. If the human body is placed in a static magnetic field of sufficient strength, then a significant number of its hydrogen atoms align themselves with the field like trillions of infinitesimal compass needles.

In an MRI examination, the patient is placed inside a static magnetic field generated by a large, powerful magnet. A pulse of radio waves (excitation pulse) is then used to create, for a brief period, a second magnetic field at a right angle to the static field. While this second field is acting on the body, the hydrogen ions (protons) change their orientation, and when the second field is turned off, they go back to their previous orientation to the static magnetic field.

As the protons return to their previous orientation, they give off a stream of radiofrequency energy or "signal," which can be detected by a suitably placed receiving coil. The intensity of the signal given off by any tissue is proportional to the hydrogen ion concentration (or proton density) of that tissue. Muscle emits a very high signal, bone a very low one, air or gas almost none.

The time it takes for the protons to return to their former orientation after an excitation pulse is called the **spin-lattice relaxation time**, abbreviated as **T1**. This **time interval**, a fraction of a second, is directly proportional to the hydrogen ion density or **proton density (PD)** of the sample. The greater the proton density of the tissue examined, the greater the delay in returning to the previous orientation, and the longer the **T1**.

When the **excitation pulse** is applied, the protons in the sample respond together, or in phase, as they take up their new orientation. After the excitation pulse ceases, but before all the protons have come back to their former orientation to the static magnetic field, they tend to get out of phase with each other, as adjacent molecules collide. Once the protons go out of phase, a signal can no longer be detected by the receiving coil. The time it takes for the protons to go out of phase is called the **spin-spin relaxation time**, or **T2**.

Because both T1 and T2 vary in proportion to the proton density of the sample, they can be used by a computer to generate an image of the sample. In order to obtain cross-sectional images, it is necessary to modify the magnetic resonance system by adding yet a third magnetic field. This gradient magnetic field, created by a separate coil, introduces a positional element into the signals detected by the receiver. A computer decodes and analyzes the signals, generating two-dimensional cross-sectional images of the patient in much the same way that CT images are produced. The series of images or slices generated are displayed on a screen and recorded on film. As with CT, images are oriented as if the patient were supine and the observer at the patient's feet.

Tl weighted sagittal images of the brain were obtained. T2 weighted images with a TR of 2000 and TE of 20, 80 msec, were also obtained in the axial projection.

MRI has largely replaced conventional radiography for applications in which it provides superior discrimination among tissue densities. In the examination of the central nervous system (see ■ **Figure 18-8**), MRI

shows the plaques of demyelination characteristic of multiple sclerosis. Although CT is preferred for distinguishing between ischemic and hemorrhagic strokes and in identifying subarachnoid hemorrhage, MRI is a more sensitive indicator of early ischemia and infarction, and of lesions in the posterior cranial fossa (brain stem and cerebellum).

MRI is also valuable in determining the location, size, and shape of tumors, particularly in the brain and liver, and in the diagnosis of bone and joint disorders (internal derangements, ligamentous tears, spinal cord compression due to disk herniation or spinal stenosis).

Because the apparatus generates a strong magnetic field, jewelry, watches, and other metal objects must be removed before the examination. MRI is contraindicated for patients with ferrous metal prostheses or implanted cardiac pacemakers. For the duration of the examination, which may take more than an hour, the patient lies motionless on a narrow table within the cylindrical magnet. Some patients become claustrophobic in these circumstances or may find it difficult to remain still.

Contrast agents that are used in radiology are not effective in improving the clarity of MRI images; however, the metallic element **gadolinium** enhances the MRI signal of any tissue or area in which it accumulates by shortening the T1 of adjacent protons. Intravenously administered gadolinium is quickly distributed throughout the circulation, showing blood vessels, highly vascular tissues, and zones of hemorrhage with great clarity. MRI angiography with intravenous gadolinium is useful in rapid diagnosis of aortic aneurysm and renal artery stenosis.

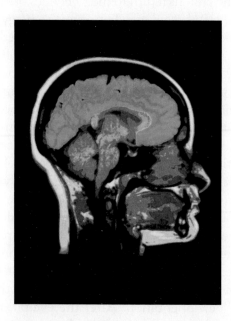

FIGURE 18-8. Color-enhanced MRI of the head at a lateral view (Source: Photo Researchers, Inc.)

Pause for Reflection

1. How does MRI differ from conventional radiography and ultrasonography?
2. Explain T1 and T2.
3. What are some indications for ordering an MRI?
4. What precautions must be taken when performing an MRI that do not need to be taken with other imaging procedures, and why?
5. What complaint are some patients likely to make when undergoing an MRI?
6. What element enhances the MRI signal, and what is its greatest benefit?

Nuclear Medicine

Nuclear medicine applies the principles of nuclear physics to both diagnosis and treatment. The basis of all nuclear diagnosis is the introduction into the body, by ingestion, injection, inhalation, or some other route, of a **radioactive tracer** (a substance that has been **tagged** or **labeled** by having a **radioactive isotope** incorporated into its chemical structure).

After an interval the distribution or concentration of the tracer is assessed or measured in some way. In nuclear imaging, that assessment results in a picture or graphic representation of the distribution of the tracer. The term **radiopharmaceutical** is sometimes applied to radioactive tracers used in diagnostic procedures, although strictly speaking it refers only to radioisotopes that are administered for therapeutic purposes, such as radioactive iodine used to suppress hyperactive thyroid tissue in Graves disease.

Unlike other imaging techniques, nuclear imaging appraises the **function of the structures** under study rather than their anatomy (size, shape, position). The significance of increased or decreased **uptake of a radiotracer** depends on the tissue under study and the biochemical nature of the substance into which the radioisotope has been incorporated. For example, radioiactive iodine is used to study the function of the thyroid gland, which normally extracts iodine from the circulation. If administration of radioactive iodine is followed after an interval by the finding of an even distribution of radioactivity throughout the thyroid gland, the conclusion is that the gland is functioning normally.

A **"hot" zone** (an area of increased uptake of radioisotope) corresponding to the position of a nodule in the thyroid gland suggests that the nodule consists of hyperactive thyroid tissue. A **"cold" nodule** is more likely to represent a malignant tumor, which is unable to concentrate iodine like normal thyroid tissue.

Standard scanning procedures have been devised for many tissues and organs, including the brain, heart, lungs, liver, and kidneys. For each of these examinations, the choice of radiotracer, the route of administration, the interval between administration and scanning, and the details of the scanning procedure depend on the metabolism of the organ or tissue in question and the type of information to be determined by the procedure. The amount of radiation absorbed by the patient in standard nuclear imaging studies is small and poses little threat to health. Nuclear studies are contraindicated, however, in pregnancy.

Radiation can be detected and measured in various ways. Like x-rays, radiation exposes photographic film that has been protected from light. A Geiger counter measures radiation by recording its ionizing effect on argon gas. A **scintillation counter** (from Latin *scintilla* 'spark') contains materials that fluoresce (emit light) when struck by radiation, similar to the coating on a television screen or computer monitor. This fluorescence can be used to expose photographic film or can be converted to an electrical signal.

As with radiography, the application of computer technology to nuclear imaging has greatly broadened its diagnostic potential and permitted the generation of two-dimensional (tomographic) and three-dimensional images. Most imaging studies today are performed with a gamma camera. This is a scintillation counter with many collimators and a complex electronic program that analyzes radiation from many sources at once and fuses the data into a two-dimensional image. This image can be displayed on a television monitor, recorded photographically, and stored digitally.

Cholescintigraphy is a nuclear medicine study of the gallbladder and biliary duct system after injection of an isotopically tagged substance that is rapidly concentrated by the liver and secreted in bile. Failure of radioactive material to appear in the gallbladder within four hours after injection suggests cholecystitis or cystic duct obstruction. This procedure is considered more sensitive than either contrast radiography or ultrasonography, but is much more expensive.

As in contrast studies, injection of **cholecystokinin (CCK)** promotes contraction of the gallbladder and permits estimation of an **ejection fraction**. Early cholescintigraphic procedures employed a technetium-tagged agent called **hepatobiliary iminodiacetic acid (HIDA)**. Although other substances are now preferred, the term "HIDA scan" remains in use as a synonym for cholescintigraphy.

In **multiple-gated acquisition (MUGA)** scanning, computer analysis of radionuclide emissions from the heart results in a composite scan assembled from a series of successive images, all taken at the same point in the cardiac cycle to eliminate blurring due to motion. Comparison of ventricular volumes at the end of diastole and at the end of systole permits calculation of the ejection fraction.

The radioactive tracer used in **positron emission tomography (PET)** (see ■ **Figure 18-9**) is a man-made isotope whose nuclear decay results in the release of subatomic particles called positrons. Scintillation data

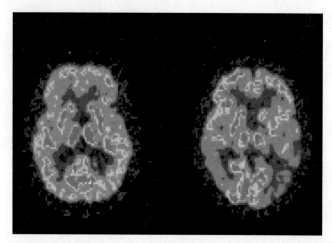

FIGURE 18-9. PET scan showing radioisotope-labeled chemicals to highlight areas of metabolic activity (Source: Getty Images, Inc.-Photodisc)

are collected simultaneously by a ring of counters surrounding the patient. In a manner analogous to computed tomography (CT), these data are then used to construct a two-dimensional image, color-coded to reflect concentration density.

PET scanning provides valuable information about brain function in Alzheimer and other dementias, parkinsonism, epilepsy, brain tumors, and stroke. This technique is also used to assess coronary blood flow and to study solitary pulmonary nodules and other masses.

Single-photon emission computed tomography (SPECT) is another form of nuclear imaging using computer software to generate two- and three-dimensional images. The incorporation of single-photon technology into nuclear imaging greatly improves the contrast and resolution of the images produced. SPECT has found particular application in providing information about regional blood flow, in assessing disorders of the heart and lungs, and in the evaluation of head injuries, seizure disorders, stroke, brain tumors, and dementia.

Ventilation-perfusion scintigraphy compares the integrity of the respiratory air passages with that of the pulmonary circulation. (This procedure is universally misnamed a **V/Q scan**, which is really something else.) Two scans are actually performed in succession with different radionuclides administered by different routes. First a ventilation scan with inhaled radioactive **xenon gas** is done to show which parts of the lungs are filled with inspired gas and which, if any, are not. After all of the xenon has been washed out of the respiratory tract with ordinary air, **technetium Tc 99m macroaggregated albumin** is administered intravenously. A second lung scan is then performed to assess the **perfusion** (circulatory distribution) of radionuclide through lung tissue.

A ventilation-perfusion scan is done when acute pulmonary embolism (blockage of a branch of the pulmonary artery by a clot that has traveled from elsewhere in the circulation) is suspected. Although such blockage may be evident on a simple perfusion scan, an abnormal scan can also result if a zone of lung tissue has poor circulation because of preexisting disease. Hence a ventilation scan is also done, so that any areas of lung tissue with chronic impairment of circulation can be identified. A **ventilation-perfusion mismatch** (an area with normal ventilation but blocked perfusion) probably represents a zone of acute pulmonary artery blockage due to embolism.

In a **bone scan**, an intravenously administered isotopic tracer binds to apatite, the crystalline calcium compound of which bone largely consists. The tracer is taken up in higher amounts by areas of bone in which there is heightened osteoblastic activity (new bone formation). This technique is useful in detecting osteomyelitis (infection of bone marrow), primary and **metastatic tumors of bone**, and subtle fractures missed by x-ray studies (including stress fractures, vertebral fractures due to sports injuries, and pathologic fractures due to osteoporosis or corticosteroid therapy). It may also be used to screen a child with unexplained evidence of trauma for abuse.

> ### Pause for Reflection
>
> 1. What is the basis of all nuclear diagnosis?
> 2. What is a radiopharmaceutical?
> 3. What is the significance of a "hot zone" or a "cold nodule" in a nuclear scan of the thyroid gland?
> 4. Define the following procedures: MUGA scan, PET scan, SPECT scan, HIDA scan.
> 5. Describe a ventilation-perfusion scan and its indications.
> 6. What are the indications for a nuclear bone scan?

Diagnostic Procedures

angiography (arteriography) The radiographic study of arteries into which radiopaque medium has been injected. Still pictures may be taken immediately after injection, or motion pictures may be made showing the flow of blood and contrast medium through vessels.

barium enema (BE) The standard radiographic examination of the large intestine by introduction of barium suspension into the rectum. Indications for barium enema are unexplained lower abdominal pain, change in bowel habits, hematochezia, detection of occult blood in stool, unexplained anemia or weight loss, and history of colonic polyps or cancer. (see ■ Figure 18-4).

chest x-ray (CXR) The standard PA chest film is the most frequently performed of all plain radiographic examinations. It provides diagnostic information on the respiratory passages and pulmonary aeration and vasculature; pleural and diaphragmatic margins; the configuration of the heart and great vessels; osseous structures; soft tissue contours; and abnormal infiltrates, masses, and accumulations of fluid.

computed tomography (CT) scan An application of computer technology to diagnostic imaging. Contrast medium may be injected into the circulation immediately before CT scanning. Intravenous contrast enhances the sensitivity of CT scanning of certain structures and body regions and improves the visibility of some tumors. Formerly called *computerized axial tomography (CAT) scan.*

full-column barium enema Barium enema examination in which the contrast medium is injected into the colon under full pressure, by elevation of the barium reservoir to the maximum safe height.

intravenous pyelogram (IVP) The delineation of the urinary tract (renal pelves, ureters, bladder, and urethra) by means of a contrast agent injected intravenously and then excreted by the kidneys (see ■ Figure 18-5). IVPs are performed for suspected urinary obstruction, bleeding from the urinary tract, or abdominal trauma, and can identify and localize renal calculi as well as tumors or cysts both within the urinary tract and adjacent to it. Also called *intravenous urogram (IVU), excretory urogram (XU).* Compare *retrograde pyelogram.*

kidneys, ureters, bladder (KUB) film. A plain film often done to screen for a radiopaque stone in the urinary tract.

magnetic resonance imaging (MRI) A method of obtaining cross-sectional "pictures" of the human body by computer manipulation of electronically acquired data.

mammography Radiologic evaluation of the female breast, primarily to search for or evaluate abnormal masses that may be malignant (see ■ Figure 18-3).

multiple-gated acquisition (MUGA) scan A study of cardiac shape and dynamics in which a radionuclide is introduced into the circulation and images of various points in the cardiac cycle are generated by computer manipulation of individual frames, called **gating**.

plain film A radiographic study performed without contrast medium.

portable film An x-ray picture taken with movable equipment at the bedside or in the emergency department or operating room when it is not feasible to move the patient to the radiology department.

positron emission tomography (PET) A nuclear imaging study that yields color-coded two-dimensional images to assess the metabolic activity and physiologic function of organs and tissues rather than their anatomic structure; particularly useful in diagnosis of subtle cerebral and cardiac lesions (see ■ Figure 18-9).

radionuclide scans The essence of any radioactive scan procedure is the introduction into the body of a radioactive substance (radionuclides, isotopes) whose distribution in tissues, vessels, or cavities can be detected and recorded by a device that senses radiation. In some cases the choice of material is governed by the tendency of certain organs or tissues to take up (absorb, concentrate) certain elements or compounds. Radionuclides may be swallowed, inhaled, or injected into a body cavity or into the circulation. Scanning may be performed immediately after the material is administered (as in studies of blood flow) or after an interval (as when absorption or concentration of a substance in an organ must occur first).

real-time examination Ultrasonographic examination performed by sweeping the ultrasound beam through the scan plane at a rapid rate, generating up to 30 images per second. The display of images at this frequency is in effect a motion picture, providing visualization of movement of internal structures as it actually occurs.

reconstruction study Generation of an image by computer processing of scan data.

retrograde pyelogram X-ray of one or both kidneys and ureters after retrograde injection of a contrast medium through a catheter into one or both ureters. Compare *intravenous pyelogram (IVP)*.

single-photon emission computed tomography (SPECT) A form of nuclear imaging that uses computer software to generate two- and three-dimensional images from data gathered after injection of a physiologically active substance bound to a gamma-emitting radionuclide. Used to evaluate regional blood flow, assess disorders of the heart and lungs, and evaluate head injuries, seizure disorders, stroke, brain tumors, and dementia.

stress cystogram A radiographic study of the bladder intended to demonstrate stress incontinence. Contrast medium is instilled into the bladder and films are taken while the patient coughs and bears down.

ultrasonography (US) A means of visualizing internal structures by observing the effects they have on a beam of sound waves (see ■ Figure 18-7).

upper gastrointestinal (GI) series Barium sulfate is given orally to outline the esophagus, stomach, and duodenum on x-ray film (see ■ Figure 18-10).

upper GI (UGI) series and small-bowel follow-through An upper GI series is done, and x-ray films are taken over a period of time to visualize the barium as it moves through the small bowel.

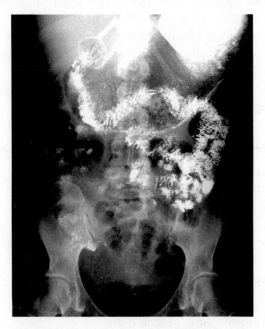

FIGURE 18-11. Upper GI series with barium

Imaging Techniques and Views

cine (for **cinematograph**) **view** A moving picture of events disclosed by an imaging technique and recorded in real time on film or tape.

coned-down view A radiographic study limited to a small area by the use of a cone that narrows and "focuses" the x-ray beam.

double-contrast technique A modification of the barium enema (BE) procedure. After the standard barium enema examination has been completed, the patient expels most of the barium, and the colon is then inflated with air. The coating of barium remaining on the surface may outline masses or defects not seen during the standard examination.

first-pass view An image or set of images obtained immediately after injection of radionuclide into the circulation, when its concentration in the blood pool is at its highest.

frogleg view An x-ray of one or both hip joints for which the patient lies supine with thighs maximally abducted and externally rotated and knees flexed so as to bring the soles of the feet together.

full-bladder technique An ultrasonographic examination of the pelvic region performed while the patient's bladder is distended with urine. This is done to improve the recognition of the bladder outline, which cannot be distinguished adequately when the bladder is empty.

gated view An image obtained by a technique synchronized with motions of the heart to eliminate blurring.

low-dose screen film technique A radiographic technique used in mammography to provide adequate imaging with less radiation than is used in conventional techniques.

multi-echo images On MRI, a series of spin-echo images obtained with various pulse sequences.

open-mouth odontoid view A view of the odontoid process of the second cervical vertebra, for which the x-ray beam is aimed through the patient's open mouth.

partial saturation technique A magnetic resonance technique in which single excitation pulses are delivered to tissue at intervals equal to or shorter than T1.

spin-echo technique An MRI technique by which T2 is determined indirectly, as a function of TE, the echo time.

sunrise view of the patella X-ray study of the knee region in which the patella is visualized above the distal femur and appears like a rising or setting sun.

swimmer's view An oblique view of the thoracic spine in which the arm nearer to the x-ray source hangs at the patient's side and the opposite arm is upraised.

T1-weighted image On MRI, a spin-echo image generated by a pulse sequence using a short TR (0.6 seconds or less).

T2-weighted image On MRI, a spin-echo image generated by a pulse sequence using a long TR (2.0 seconds or more).

washout phase Scintigraphic scanning of the lungs at the conclusion of the inhalation phase of a lung scan, after an interval during which all inhaled radionuclide would be expected to have been exhaled.

Pharmacology

contrast medium A substance that is introduced into or around a structure and, because of the difference in absorption of x-rays by the contrast medium and surrounding tissues, allows radiographic visualization of the structure.

gadolinium A nonradioactive metallic element that acts as a contrast agent in MRI studies by enhancing the signal of areas or tissues in which it is present. After intravenous injection it can show up narrowed areas or malformations in blood vessels, vascular tumors, and areas of hemorrhage. It can also be used to delineate joint spaces in arthrography.

iodinated contrast medium A contrast medium containing iodine rather than a metallic salt; used in angiography, intravenous pyelography, oral cholecystography, and other studies.

radioisotopes Radioisotopes are used as imaging agents in CT, MRI, PET, SPECT, and nuclear medicine studies. Transcribing them correctly can be a challenge. When typing nonproprietary (generic) isotope names, element symbols should be included with the name. It may appear to be redundant, but it is the correct form; therefore, we would type sodium pertechnetate Tc 99m, iodohippurate sodium I 131,

or sodium iodide I 125. Occasionally the physician may simply dictate isotopes such as Tc 99m, iodine 131 or I 131, or sodium iodide I 125, and unless a trademarked name is indicated, the element and number should be typed with a space, no hyphen, and no superscript (in healthcare documentation). Note that while the name of an element is written in lowercase (indium), the first letter of its symbol is in uppercase (In).

technetium (Tc) A synthetic radioisotope with wide applications in nuclear imaging. In a **HIDA (hepatobiliary iminodiacetic acid) scan**, an intravenously administered technetium compound outlines the biliary tract more precisely than is possible with conventional radiology or ultrasound. Other technetium compounds are used in scanning the scrotum to diagnose testicular torsion and in performing bone and other scans to identify local areas of inflammation such as abscesses or zones of osteomyelitis.

Common Imaging Agents

An imaging agent may also be called a contrast agent, a dye, a tracer, or a radiopharmaceutical. Many radiopharmaceutical imaging agents are identified by their abbreviations because the expansions are unwieldy. In healthcare documentation, radiopharmaceutical abbreviations can be transcribed as dictated; they need not be expanded unless instructed otherwise.

AdreView (iobenguane sulfate) Nuclear imaging agent for the detection of adrenal tumors, pheochromocytoma or neuroblastoma.

Ceretec (technetium Tc 99m exametazime injection preparation kit) Scintigraphy imaging agent (with or without methylene blue stabilization) is used as an adjunct in the detection of altered regional cerebral perfusion in stroke. Ceretec without methylene blue stabilization is indicated for leukocyte labeled scintigraphy as an adjunct in the localization of intraabdominal infection and inflammatory bowel disease.

Choletec (technetium Tc 99m mebrofenin) Hepatobiliary imaging agent used in cholescintigraphy.

DaTscan (ioflupane I 123 injection) Single photon emission computed tomography (SPECT) imaging agent for the evaluation of parkinsonian syndromes.

DMSA (technetium Tc 99m succimer injection preparation kit) **scan** Used to assess renal function.

FDDNP or **18F-FDDNP** PET scan imaging agent for diagnosis of beta-amyloid senile plaques and neurofibrillary tangles for early detection of Alzheimer disease.

FDG (fludeoxyglucose F 18) PET imaging agent for the detection of abnormal glucose metabolism with applications in oncology, cardiology, and neurology.

Gd-Tex (Now: MGd; motexafin gadolinium) Radio-sensitizing agent for the detection of brain metastases in patients with non-small cell lung cancer.

Indiclor (indium In 111 chloride) Used for radiolabeling of ProstaScint (capromab pendetide) in patients with prostate cancer and Zevalin (ibritumomab tiuxetan), used for radioimmunotherapy procedures. Indiclor is not to be administered directly.

multi-echo images On MRI, a series of spin-echo images obtained with various pulse sequences.

Myoview (technetium Tc 99m tetrofosmin) A cardiovascular imaging agent.

Omnipaque (iohexol) An iodinated radiopaque contrast medium administered by an intrathecal route for myelography (lumbar, thoracic, cervical, total columnar) and in contrast enhancement for computerized tomography (myelography, cisternography, ventriculography).

Omniscan (gadodiamide) An intravenous enhancing agent for MRI examinations.

ProstaScint (capromab pendetide, radiolabeled with indium In 111) A radiolabeled monoclonal antibody to prostate-specific membrane antigen, used to localize sites of soft tissue metastasis in prostate cancer patients.

TechneScan MDP (technetium Tc 99m medronate disodium) A bone imaging agent.

thallous chloride T1 201 injection Used in myocardial perfusion imaging with either planar or SPECT (Single Photon Emission Computed Tomography) techniques for the diagnosis and localization of myocardial infarction; with exercise stress testing as an adjunct to the diagnosis of ischemic heart disease (atherosclerotic coronary artery disease); in scintigraphic imaging of the myocardium to identify changes in perfusion induced by pharmacologic stress in patients with known or suspected coronary artery disease and who cannot exercise adequately; and localization of sites of parathyroid hyperactivity in patients with elevated serum calcium and parathyroid hormone levels.

Visipaque (iodixanol) Injected intra-arterially in digital subtraction angiography and indicated for angiocardiography (left ventriculography and selective coronary arteriography), peripheral arteriography, visceral arteriography, and cerebral arteriography. Administered by intravenous injection, it is used for contrast-enhanced computed tomography (CECT) imaging of the head and body, excretory urography, and peripheral venography.

Transcription Tips

1. Confusing terms related to imaging: Some of these terms sound alike; others are potential traps when researching. Memorize the terms and their meanings so that you can select the appropriate term for a correct transcript.

    bowel—the intestine
    bile—a fluid secreted by the liver
    bowl—a round container

    cistern—a closed reservoir for fluid
    system—an assemblage or arrangement of structures

    diffuse—spread out
    defuse—to make less dangerous, tense, or hostile

    discrete—distinct, separate
    discreet—circumspect, able to keep a secret

    effect (noun)—the result, outcome, a change (as in mass effect)
    affect—to influence (verb) or demeanor (noun)

    enterolithiasis—presence of calculi in the intestines
    anterolisthesis—slipped vertebra

    malalignment—displacement, out of line
    malignment—slanderous or disparaging remark

    plain—without contrast (when referring to x-rays)
    plane—a surface in which a straight line connecting any two points will be on the same surface

    spiculated—spiked, thorny
    speculated—considered or discussed, conjectured

    transverse (adj.)—at an angle across something
    traverse (verb)—to go across

2. Slang Terms. Expand these slang brief forms when encountered in dictation.

C spine	cervical spine
L spine	lumbar spine
LS spine	lumbosacral spine
T spine	thoracic spine
sono	sonogram
tib	tibia, tibial
fib	fibula, fibular
tib-fib	tibia and fibula, tibiofibular

3. Spelling. Memorize the spelling of these difficult-to-spell terms. Note silent letters, doubled letters, and unexpected pronunciation.

    dominant
    Doppler (always capitalized)
    dysraphism
    extraaxial (one word, no hyphen necessary)
    gallbladder (one word)
    hemorrhage
    heterogeneous
    homogeneous
    leukomalacia
    parenchyma
    sagittal (1 *g*, 2 *t*'s)
    silhouette (as in cardiac silhouette)
    sphenoid
    spondylolisthesis
    spondylolysis
    subtle (the *b* is silent)
    symphysis pubis
    uncinate process
    uncovertebral

    Use preferred spellings for the following terms unless instructed otherwise:

    anulus, *not* annulus
    distention, *not* distension
    disk, *not* disc

4. Watch out for spelling changes when forming derivatives.

bone	bony
caudal (adj.)	caudad (adv.)
	caudate (adj.)
cephalic (adj.)	cephalad (adv.)
foramen	foraminal
inflamed	inflammatory

    Directions can be expressed as adverbs by adding the suffix *ly*.

anterior	anteriorly
distal	distally
inferior	inferiorly
lateral	laterally
medial	medially
posterior	posteriorly

Transcription Tips

proximal   proximally
superior   superiorly

A combining vowel can be used to join directional and positional adjectives into a single word; the adjectives can also be combined using a hyphen. Notice the spelling changes in the combined forms. (*Note*: The choice is the dictator's, not the transcriptionist's. The term should be transcribed as dictated.)

anterior-posterior   anteroposterior
anterior-lateral   anterolateral
posterior-anterior   posteroanterior
posterior-lateral   posterolateral
superior-lateral   superolateral

5. Tricky Abbreviations. Some abbreviations are acronyms and pronounced as a word; others have soundalike letters; *B*, *D*, *P*, and *V* can all sound alike, as can *T* and *D*, *F* and *S*, *N* & *and*. Although some abbreviations do not need to be expanded, knowing what they mean is necessary in order to choose the correct abbreviation.

AP   anteroposterior
DVT   deep venous thrombosis
mCi   millicuries
mcCi   microcuries
         (Note: The abbreviation is actually
         µCi, but the *mu* symbol doesn't
         transfer well electronically.)
PA   posteroanterior
Tc   technetium

6. Dictation Challenges

X-ray can be used as a noun, referring to the image itself, or a verb, referring to the procedure. It is transcribed with a lowercase *x* except when it is the first word in a sentence.

An x-ray was taken of the abdomen.

The patient was x-rayed after admission.

The patient was re-x-rayed on the 2nd hospital day.

CAT (pronounced as a word) scan is an older term meaning *computerized axial tomography*. The more current term is *CT scan*, for *computerized tomography*. Occasionally, both terms may be used in the same report. It is acceptable to transcribe *CT* when *CAT* is dictated unless otherwise instructed.

The terms *cistern* and *system* can sound a lot alike (see #1), but noting context clues will ensure that you are transcribing the correct term. *Cisterns* occur only between the meningeal coverings of the central nervous system, and most of them are in the cranial cavity. The plural form might be preceded by the adjective *subarachnoid* (though all cisterns are subarachnoid). A reference to a specific cistern should be preceded by a distinguishing anatomic adjective (for example, *ambient, carotid, chiasmatic, cerebellomedullary, cerebellopontine, crural, interpeduncular, lumbar, pontine, superior, sylvian*). The phrase *ventricular cistern* is nonsense and would never be used; hence dictation that sounds like *ventricular cistern = ventricular system* always. Since *system* generally connotes an assemblage or array of structures, the plural form *systems* is less likely to be heard.

Like many other adjectives in medical terminology, the word *navicular*, meaning boat-shaped (from the Latin *navicula*, "little boat"), is often used without a noun, becoming in effect a noun itself. There are naviculars (navicular bones) in both the wrist and the ankle.

Prominent spurs were seen off the anterior surface of the talus and the navicular.

Students often transcribe words beginning with the prefixes *a* or *an*, such as *acute* and *asymmetric*, as two separate words. Remember when transcribing to concentrate on context—don't just transcribe what you hear—and you'll avoid these embarrassing types of mistakes.

Although *ensure* and *insure* can be synonyms, *ensure* is more commonly used in healthcare documentation to mean "to make certain" while *insure* is used in the same sense as *insurance*.

Becoming a Radiology Transcriptionist

by Ellen A. Drake

I started my transcription career in Radiology at St. Joseph's, a Catholic hospital in Tampa, Florida. I got married at 21 before graduating college, and one of us had to work. Never having had to seek a job before, I went through an employment agency. The "counselor" lied about my qualifications. She told them I could type the requisite 40 cwpm (corrected words per minute), but I had typed only 26 cpwm on the agency typing test. Incidentally, in high school typing class, I swore on a daily basis, "I will never make my living typing!" The employment agent literally pestered them about what a great "catch" I was until they hired me to keep her from calling them again.

The hospital didn't retest, but I lived in fear that this lie would be discovered. Fortunately, typing speed wasn't critical because all I did was fill in forms (insurance forms, the appointment calendar) all day. I was the receptionist, scheduler, insurance filer, phone answerer. A good portion of my first four to six checks went to that employment agency.

We had an open waiting room, and outpatients could hear everything that was said to other patients and over the phone. No fax, no Internet, no HIPAA in those days. I read the x-ray reports over the phone to the doctors' offices, and that's how I started picking up the terminology. With my English major background, I found learning the vocabulary easy and fascinating. During slow periods and breaks, I would browse the *Dorland's Medical* dictionary. When the transcriptionist would take ever-longer cigarette breaks, she would let me transcribe; when she returned, she would edit my work and show me my mistakes. My accuracy and speed improved as I transcribed more and more; eventually, she left and I got her job.

We had a "state-of-the-art" dictation system. It consisted of a continuous loop tape system, enough magnetic tape for hours and hours of dictation. The system had two heads, a recording head and a playback head. As a continuous loop, once the dictation was transcribed, the tape would go back through the dictation head. Sometimes, the tape would fall off one or the other of the heads and end up in a pile at the bottom of the box. This always meant loss of dictation because the tape could never be put back exactly at the same spot, and we could spend hours trying to find the point at which the dictation had been transcribed.

Untranscribed dictation was also lost when we had a stat report. We would have to scan ahead, using the fast forward, to find the stat report. When the doctors were "right on our heels," they could dictate over the untranscribed dictation that we had to scan through to get to the stat report. The doctors, nice as they were, did not like redictating!

The doctors were great at answering my questions, especially the chief radiologist. He would throw the film up on the light box with a resounding slap and show me all the abnormalities. On slow weekends, he also let me watch semi-invasive procedures that are probably no longer done in the radiology department. I watched a failed attempt at a venogram (I fainted), a fluoroscopy-guided lung biopsy (I got woozy), and a myelogram.

The chief radiologist was a perfectionist. For reports, we used four-part NCR packets; each part was a different color and we had little pieces of colored correction paper that we used to make corrections. We were allowed no more than two corrections per report. We strove for no errors because it was a pain to line up the copies and the colored correction tape on the typewriter platen.

If the chief radiologist received a letter that had his name misspelled or some other mistake on the envelope, he would toss it in the trash without opening it. It could have had a $10,000 check and he didn't care. His outgoing letters could have no mistakes and no corrections. He would hold the letter up to the light box, and if he saw a correction, no matter how carefully it had been made, the letter would have to be retyped. I remember coming to tears once when I had typed a letter about eight times, failing to obtain a perfect copy. His private secretary suggested I do something else for a while and come back to it later, and that worked. I finally typed a perfect letter. I learned about perfection on that job.

(continued)

Spotlight On Becoming a Radiology Transcriptionist (page 2)

Patients brought down from the floors were lined up in the corridor between the x-ray rooms on gurneys. As I walked back and forth to the record room, patients would reach out for comfort or to stop me and ask how much longer. Sometimes, I just stopped and held their hand and let them talk about their lives and their families to distract them. I remember going to one of the several restrooms inside the department, having to pass outpatient dressing rooms on the way. A patient sat on the bench in one of them, curtains open, hospital gown open in the front and not covering anything; I guess he was hot. I stammered an apology and backed out of the corridor as quickly as I could. He thought I was a nurse and didn't even react. After that I generally went to the restrooms outside the department.

The story about the venogram is an amusing vignette in itself. It was the first procedure I was allowed to watch. The radiologist asked if I had a problem with the sight of blood. I said, "Only if it's a relative." The patient was a stranger who had had eight children. She was just 28 years old. She was sitting on an examining table with her black legs over the side, feet resting on the radiologist's knees. He was sitting on a stool. I stood at the end of the table.

Both her legs were swollen, the skin was tight and shiny. I watched as he used a needle to find a vein in which to inject the dye in her foot/ankle area. He couldn't find one. He just kept poking the needle in and out, in and out. She didn't seem to feel a thing. The two of them were talking, cracking jokes, and laughing. I started to feel woozy. I knelt down on the floor, saying, "I think I need to get closer to the floor." He looked over and asked if I was okay. I nodded yes, and he kept poking at her foot with the needle. I never even saw any blood! They continued to carry on their animated conversation. Before long, I sat cross-legged on the floor. Again, he asked if I was okay. Again, I nodded yes. Almost instantly, the room was black and swirling around me, and I was lying on the floor. I could still hear him talking, but I couldn't see anything. I heard him ask the patient, "Are you related to her?" She just laughed loudly and said no.

Eventually, he gave up on the procedure and said they would try again on another day when her legs weren't so swollen. I stayed on the floor, but I had come around. After he sent the patient back to the room, he got me up, took me to his office, and gave me brandy.

The radiologist I worked for loved to challenge me. I'm sure he used words that he had never used when the previous transcriptionist had been there. One day, he dictated a barium enema for which the patient was poorly prepared. He said the colon was filled with "si-buh-lus" stool. We didn't have the research resources we have today; I had a *Dorland*'s dictionary and that was all. No Internet. No way to search phonetically or use a wild card search. I tried *si, se, so, su, sa,* and even *sy,* knowing that vowels can take on the sound of any other vowel, but I couldn't find the term. I went to him and verified the pronunciation and asked about the spelling. He just grinned and said, "keep trying." I knew that many words began with a silent *p,* so I tried *psi, pse, pso, psu, psa,* and *psy,* with no luck. Finally, in desperation, I went back to him, and he gave me the first three letters, *scy.* Of course, I found it instantly. Well, I found *scybala,* but I knew enough to substitute the adjective ending for *scybalous.*

Many years later, I told this story to my medical transcription students. One of them went to work for a local hospital transcription department. All the other transcriptionists were very experienced. She was the "newbie" and pretty much ignored unless she requested help. One day an MT was struggling to decipher a word. She asked every MT in the department except my former student to listen. None of them helped. Finally, as the MT was about to give up and leave a blank, the newbie asked, "May I listen?" Guess what she heard? Scybalous! She told the MT how to spell the word and what it meant and garnered a whole new level of respect from her coworkers. Less than a year and a half later, she was made supervisor of the MT department. Now, I'm sure that her promotion had more to do with her previous experience in another career, her maturity, her ability to work with people, and her organization skills, but I do think that the respect she gained from that incident helped make her promotion more acceptable to her more experienced MT coworkers.

Exercises

Medical Vocabulary Review

Instructions: Choose the best answer.

___ 1. The term *anterolisthesis* is most likely to appear in which type of radiology report?
A. X-ray of the spine.
B. X-ray of the skull.
C. X-ray of the pelvis.
D. X-ray of the hand.

___ 2. Which finding is likely on chest x-ray of a patient suspected of having a collapsed lung?
A. Extravasation.
B. An artifact.
C. Atelectasis.
D. Blurred costophrenic angle.

___ 3. Abnormal reduction in the amount of air in lung tissue is called ____
A. hypoinflation.
B. hypoaeration.
C. hyperaeration.
D. hyperinflation.

___ 4. Gliomas, astrocytomas, or metastatic disease are likely to be said to be _____ in the findings on a brain scan.
A. interstitial
B. intraaxial
C. ectopic
D. confluent

___ 5. A narrow connection between two larger bodies or parts is _____
A. an isthmus.
B. a pole.
C. a tail.
D. ectasia.

___ 6. _____ is a benign developmental abnormality consisting of a localized zone of increased density in a long bone.
A. An osteophyte
B. A filling defect
C. A bony island
D. Acoustical shadowing

___ 7. Abnormal reduction of mobility or motility; reduced contractile movement in one or both cardiac ventricles is referred to as

_____
A. akinesis.
B. dyskinesis.
C. hyperkinesis.
D. hypokinesis.

___ 8. A chest x-ray showing dilation or distention of the larger air passages of the lungs would be said to show _____
A. acoustical shadowing.
B. hyperinflation.
C. bronchiectasis.
D. peribronchial cuffing.

___ 9. On a chest x-ray, the angle at the junction of the ribs and diaphragmatic pleura is called the _____
A. echo pattern.
B. costophrenic angle.
C. collecting system.
D. air-fluid level.

___ 10. _____ is leakage of contrast medium from the structure into which it is injected through a perforation or other abnormal orifice.
A. Ectasia
B. Cuffing
C. Blunting
D. Extravasation

___ 11. Meningiomas, fluid, or hemorrhage on a brain scan are more likely to be _____ in location.
   A. extraaxial
   B. parietal
   C. anterior
   D. occipital

___ 12. Structures offering relatively little resistance to x-rays are said to be _____
   A. sonolucent.
   B. translucent.
   C. radiolucent.
   D. shadowy.

___ 13. _____ is a zone within a tubular structure that is not filled by injected contrast medium.
   A. Acoustical shadowing
   B. A gas density line
   C. A filling defect
   D. A peristaltic wave

___ 14. Structures resisting penetration by x-rays are said to be _____
   A. radiopaque.
   B. opacified.
   C. loculated.
   D. effaced.

___ 15. Tissue in the breast that is physiologically active, as opposed to fat and connective tissue is referred to as _____
   A. sonolucent.
   B. sacralization.
   C. tail of the breast.
   D. parenchyma.

___ 16. The proportion of blood left in the left ventricle of the heart at the end of diastole or the proportion of radiopaque bile left in the gallbladder after cholecystokinin stimulation is the _____
   A. air-fluid level.
   B. ejection fraction.
   C. summation artifact.
   D. filling defect.

___ 17. On chest x-ray, the normal radiographic appearance of the branches of the pulmonary arteries and veins about the hila of the lungs are referred to as _____
   A. air bronchogram.
   B. interstitial markings.
   C. pulmonary vascular markings.
   D. pulmonary vascular redistribution.

___ 18. _____ softening of the white matter of the brain.
   A. Demineralization
   B. Ectopia
   C. Ectasia
   D. Leukomalacia

___ 19. _____ is the displacement of a structure that is normally seen at or near the center of the body.
   A. Ectopia
   B. Midline shift
   C. Mass lesion
   D. Mass effect

___ 20. Maintenance of flow in an artery beyond an area of narrowing or obstruction by establishment of collateral circulation is _____
   A. reconstitution.
   B. loculated effusion.
   C. opacification.
   D. runoff.

Diagnostic and Surgical Procedures

Instructions: Match the following diagnostic and surgical procedures to their descriptions or definitions. Some answers may be used more than once or not at all.

____ 1. angiography

____ 2. barium enema

____ 3. intravenous pyelogram

____ 4. KUB x-ray

____ 5. magnetic resonance imaging

____ 6. mammography

____ 7. multiple-gated acquisition

____ 8. plain film

____ 9. positron emission tomography

____ 10. real-time examination

____ 11. retrograde pyelogram

____ 12. single-photon emission computed tomography

____ 13. stress cystogram

____ 14. ultrasonography

____ 15. upper gastrointestinal series

A. A contrast-enhanced radiologic examination of renal pelves, ureters, bladder, and urethra

B. Contrast-enhanced radiologic examination of large intestine

C. Contrast-enhanced study of the bladder for incontinence

D. Cross-sectional images obtained by computer manipulation of electronically acquired data

E. Form of nuclear imaging that uses computer software to generate two- and three-dimensional images from data gathered after injection of a physiologically active substance bound to a gamma-emitting radionuclide

F. Means of visualizing internal structures by observing the effects they have on a beam of sound waves

G. Nuclear imaging study that yields color-coded two-dimensional images to assess the metabolic activity and physiologic function of organs and tissues rather than their anatomic structure

H. Orally-administered contrast study to outline the esophagus, stomach, and duodenum on x-ray film

I. Plain film often done to screen for a radiopaque stone in the urinary tract

J. Radiologic evaluation of the female breast

K. Radionuclide-enhanced study of cardiac shape and dynamics in which images of various points in the cardiac cycle are generated by computer manipulation of individual frames

L. Still or motion pictures showing flow of blood and contrast medium

M. Ultrasound study performed by sweeping the ultrasound beam through the scan plane at a rapid rate, generating up to 30 images per second

N. X-ray of body part without contrast

O. X-ray of one or both kidneys and ureters after backward injection of a contrast medium via a catheter into one or both ureters

Imaging Techniques and Views

Instructions: Match the following imaging techniques and views to their descriptions or definitions. Some answers may be used more than once or not at all.

____ 1. cine view

____ 2. coned-down technique

____ 3. double contrast technique

____ 4. first pass view

____ 5. frogleg view

____ 6. gated view

____ 7. low-dose screen film technique

____ 8. multi-echo image technique

____ 9. partial saturation technique

____ 10. spin-echo technique

____ 11. sunrise view

____ 12. swimmer's view

____ 13. T1-weighted image

____ 14. T2-weighted image

____ 15. washout phase

A. Imaging technique recorded in real time on film or tape

B. A view that that narrows and "focuses" the x-ray beam down to a small area

C. Inflation of the colon with air after patient expels most of the barium as part of a barium enema

D. Images obtained immediately after injection of radionuclide into the circulation, when its concentration in the blood pool is at its highest.

E. Abduction and external rotation of thighs with knees flexed so as to bring the soles of the feet together for x-ray of hip joints

F. An image obtained by a technique synchronized with motions of the heart to eliminate blurring

G. Radiographic technique used in mammography to provide adequate imaging with less radiation

H. Series of spin-echo images obtained with various pulse sequences on MRI scanning.

I. Use of single excitation pulses delivered to tissue at intervals equal to or shorter than T1 on MRI scanning

J. Indirect determination of T2 as a function of TE, the echo time

K. Knee x-ray in which the patella is visualized above the distal femur

L. Oblique view of thoracic spine in which the arm nearer to the x-ray source hangs at the patient's side and the opposite arm is upraised

M. A spin-echo image generated by a pulse sequence using a short TR (0.6 seconds or less) on MRI

N. On MRI, a spin-echo image generated by a pulse sequence using a long TR (2.0 seconds or more)

O. Scintigraphic scanning of the lungs at the conclusion of the inhalation phase of a lung scan, after an interval during which all inhaled radionuclide would be expected to have been exhaled

Pharmacology

Instructions: Match the following pharmacology terms to their descriptions or definitions. Some answers may be used more than once, some not at all.

___ 1. contrast medium

___ 2. gadolinium

___ 3. iodinated contrast medium

___ 4. radioisotopes

___ 5. technetium Tc 99m

___ 6. Choletec

___ 7. DMSA

___ 8. FDDNP

___ 9. Gd-Tex

___ 10. Indiclor

___ 11. Myoview

___ 12. Omnipaque

___ 13. Omniscan

___ 14. ProstaScint

___ 15. Visipaque

A. A synthetic radioisotope with wide applications in nuclear imaging

B. Hepatobiliary imaging agent used in cholescintigraphy

C. Imaging agents in CT, MRI, PET, SPECT, and nuclear medicine studies

D. Iodinated radiopaque contrast medium administered intrathecally for myelography

E. Nonradioactive metallic element used in MRI that enhances the signal of areas or tissues in which it is present

F. Not administered directly used humans, used for radiolabeling of ProstaScint

G. PET scan imaging agent for detection of beta-amyloid senile plaques and neurofibrillary tangles for early detection of Alzheimer disease

H. Preparation of technetium Tc 99m tetrofosmin for cardiovascular imaging

I. Radiolabeled monoclonal antibody to prostate-specific membrane antigen, used to localize sites of soft tissue metastasis

J. Radiopaque contrast medium for thoracic, abdominal, pelvic, and retroperitoneal imaging and to enhance MRIs of the brain, spine, and other CNS tissues

K. Radiosensitizing agent for the detection of brain metastases in patients with non-small cell lung cancer

L. Substance that is introduced into or around a structure and that allows radiographic visualization of the structure

M. Technetium Tc 99m succimer preparation used to assess renal function

N. Used in angiography, intravenous pyelography, oral cholecystography, and other studies

O. Used in digital subtraction angiography, peripheral arteriography, visceral arteriography, and cerebral arteriography

Dissecting Medical Terms

Instructions: As you learned in your medical language course, words are formed from prefixes, combining forms (root word plus combining vowel), and suffixes. Combining vowels (usually **o** but not always) are used to connect two root words or a root and a suffix. By analyzing these word parts, you can often determine the definition of a term without even looking it up (if you know the definition of the parts, of course!).

Being able to divide and analyze the words you hear into their component parts will also improve your auditory deciphering ability and spelling and help you research those words that you cannot easily spell or define.

For the following terms, draw a slash (/) between the components and then write a short definition based on the meaning of the parts. Remember that to define a word based on its parts, you start at the end, usually with the suffix. If there's a prefix, that is defined next and finally the combining form is defined. The actual definition of medical words does not always equal the sum of their parts because of changes in meaning over time; when this is the case, adjust your final definition to fit today's use.

Example: intracranial

Divide & Analyze:
  intra/crani/al = pertaining to + inside + skull.
Define: Pertaining to inside the skull.

1. arthropathy _____
   Divide _____
   _____
   Define _____

2. atherosclerosis
   Divide _____
   _____
   Define _____

3. bronchiectasis
   Divide _____
   _____
   Define _____

4. craniocaudad
   Divide _____
   _____
   Define _____

5. costophrenic
   Divide _____
   _____
   Define _____

6. cystadenoma
   Divide _____
   _____
   Define _____

7. endobronchial
   Divide _____
   _____
   Define _____

8. extratesticular
   Divide _____
   _____
   Define _____

9. fibronodular
   Divide _____
   _____
   Define _____

10. gynecomastia
    Divide _____
    _____
    Define _____

11. hypervascular
    Divide _____
    _____
    Define _____

12. intravesicular
    Divide _____
    _____
    Define _____

13. leukomalacia
Divide _____

_____
Define _____

14. hyperinflation
Divide _____

_____
Define _____

15. lymphadenopathy
Divide _____

_____
Define _____

16. malalignment
Divide _____

_____
Define _____

17. multiloculated
Divide _____

_____
Define _____

18. neoplasm
Divide _____

_____
Define _____

19. osteopenia
Divide _____

_____
Define _____

20. paramedian
Divide _____

_____
Define _____

21. patellofemoral
Divide _____

_____
Define _____

22. periarticular
Divide _____

_____
Define _____

23. pnemothorax
Divide _____

_____
Define _____

24. thoracolumbar
Divide _____

_____
Define _____

25. uncovertebral
Divide _____

_____
Define _____

Spelling Exercise

Instructions: Review the adjective suffixes in your medical language textbook. Test your knowledge of adjectives by writing the adjectival form of the following pulmonary medicine words. Consult a medical dictionary to verify your spelling.

Noun	**Adjective**
1. abdomen	_____
2. asymmetry	_____
3. atelectasis	_____
4. bronchiectasis	_____
5. confluence	_____
6. foramen	_____
7. granuloma	_____
8. inflammation	_____
9. spondylolysis	_____
10. testicle	_____
11. ventricle	_____
12. vesical	_____

Combining Words

Instructions: Review the adjective suffixes in your medical language textbook. Test your knowledge of combined words by forming a single word from the following pairs. Consult a dictionary to verify your spelling and the definition.

Phrase	Answer
1. anterior and posterior	_____
2. anterior and lateral	_____
3. anterior and listhesis	_____
4. cranial and caudal	_____
5. inferior and lateral	_____
6. inferior and medial	_____
7. medial and lateral	_____
8. posterior and anterior	_____
9. posterior and lateral	_____
10. posterior and medial	_____
11. superior and lateral	_____
12. superior and posterior	_____

Abbreviations Exercise

Instructions: Expand the following common abbreviations and brief forms. Then memorize both abbreviations and definitions to increase your speed and accuracy in transcribing dictation

Abbreviation	Expansion
1. AP	_____
2. BE	_____
3. CABG	_____
4. CC (view)	_____
5. CCK	_____
6. COPD	_____
7. CT (scan)	_____

8. CTR	_____
9. CXR	_____
10. DEXA (scan)	_____
11. DPA	_____
12. DVT	_____
13. HIDA	_____
14. IV (contrast)	_____
15. IVC (filter)	_____
16. IVP	_____
17. L5-S1	_____
18. LM (projection	_____
19. mcCi	_____
20. mCi	_____
21. ML (projection)	_____
22. MLO (projection	_____
23. MRI	_____
24. MUGA	_____
25. Ob	_____
26. PA	_____
27. PET	_____
28. RV (of heart)	_____
29. SI (joint)	_____
30. SPA	_____
31. SPECT	_____
32. SXA	_____
33. T1 (on MRI)	_____
34. T2 (on MRI)	_____
35. Tc (radioisotope)	_____
36. TE (on MRI)	_____
37. TR (on MRI)	_____
38. UGI	_____
39. US (imaging)	_____
40. VCUG	_____

Transcript Forensics

Instructions: This section presents snippets of transcribed dictations from clinic notes; history and physical examinations and consultations; operative reports and procedure notes; and discharge summaries. Explain the passage so that a nonmedical person can understand it.

Example: Metastatic bone survey shows multiple **lytic skull lesions** with irregular margins involving the **occipital, parietal, and frontal bones**.

Explanation: This study is done to evaluate whether cancer has spread (metastasized) to the bones; specifically this portion of the study is related to the skull bones. There is evidence of uneven (irregular) bone destruction (lytic lesions) in the posterior (occipital), the upper side (parietal), and frontal bones of the skull.

1. PELVIC AND HIPS: **AP and frogleg views** of the left pelvis were obtained, and these show deformity to the right femoral head with a somewhat fragmented appearance to it.

   Explanation: _____
   _____
   _____
   _____
   _____

2. Hand x-ray: There is a **transverse fracture** of the **proximal** portion of the 1st digit **phalanx**. On the **oblique films** there appears to be a displaced fragment of bone between the 2nd and 3rd digits at the PIP.

   Explanation: _____
   _____
   _____
   _____
   _____

3. Mammogram: **Craniocaudal** and **mediolateral views** of each breast were done using low-dose film mammographic technique. Breasts are bilaterally **symmetric**, showing mostly fatty replacement of the glandular tissue with minimal **ductal ectasia** still present.

   Explanation: _____
   _____
   _____
   _____
   _____

4. **KUB** and **scout** tomographic studies prior to possible IVP reveal a considerable amount of **air and fecal material** in the colon, with moderate small-bowel contents partially obscuring the **renal structures** and lower abdomen and pelvis.

   Explanation: _____
   _____
   _____
   _____
   _____

5. CHEST X-RAY: An **alveolar consolidative process** in the left **basilar** region partially obscures the left diaphragmatic contour. **Strandy infiltrate** is also seen, but to a lesser degree, in the medial basal region of the right lung base. **Peribronchial cuffing** is present in both hilar regions. Vascularity appears normal. The **cardiac silhouette** is normal in size and configuration. The visualized bony thorax is normal.

   Explanation: _____
   _____
   _____
   _____
   _____
   _____

6. **UGI** series: Moderate-sized direct sliding-type **diaphragmatic hernia** with some gastric **reflux** and evidence of acute as well as chronic reflux esophagitis.

Explanation: _____
_____
_____
_____
_____
_____

7. SKULL: No **mass effect, midline shift**, or evidence of **subdural or epidural hemorrhage** is seen. Calcification is seen in the falx, the pineal, and the choroid plexus.

Explanation: _____
_____
_____
_____
_____
_____

8. LUMBAR SPINE, THREE VIEWS: Three views of the lumbar spine show mild degenerative change and **sacralization of transverse process** of L5 on the left. Loss of L5-S1 intervertebral disk space is present. IMPRESSION: Generalized **osteopenia**. Pedicles are preserved in appearance.

Explanation: _____
_____
_____
_____
_____
_____

9. CERVICAL SPINE X-RAY IMPRESSION: Diffuse **cervical spondylosis** consisting of **disk space narrowing** and marginal **osteophyte formation** both anteriorly and posteriorly at multiple levels, as described above. I see no obvious central **stenosis**, though there does appear to be compromise of the right C5-6 and left C4-5 and left C5-6 neural foramina.

Explanation: _____
_____
_____
_____
_____
_____
_____

10. **Tl-weighted sagittal images** of the brain were obtained. **T2-weighted images** with a **TR** of 2000 and **TE** of 20, 80 msec, were also obtained in the axial projection.

Explanation: _____
_____
_____
_____
_____
_____

Sample Reports

Sample diagnostic imaging reports appear on the following pages, illustrating a variety of reports. Fictional names are provided for illustration of proper format, and no resemblance to actual persons is intended. Sample transcripts were prepared according to *The Book of Style for Medical Transcription* (AHDI).

Diagnostic Imaging Report

MICHEL, THOMAS
#908397
10/19/[add year]

CHEST, PA AND LATERAL

The heart is normal in size. Trachea is at midline. Normal pulmonary vascular markings. Opaque sutures are seen in the projection of the right upper chest, and there are minimal fibrotic changes in the right lung. Lungs are expanded, and no active infiltrate is otherwise seen.

IMPRESSION
Presence of opaque sutures in the projection of the right upper chest and minimal fibrotic changes in the right lung. No active cardiopulmonary disease is otherwise demonstrated at this time.

DEREK NETHERWOOD, MD

DN:hpi

d&t: 10/19/[add year]

Diagnostic Imaging Report

RIBEIRO, LUCINDA
#837984
4/25/[add year]

Attending: Rachel Greenlee, MD

LOW-DOSE MAMMOGRAPHY

CLINICAL HISTORY
There is no family history of breast cancer. Patient had onset of menses at age 12 years, and her last menstrual period (LMP) was at age 50 years. Patient is a gravida 4, para 3, ab 1. Currently she is asymptomatic. There is no history of previous breast surgery. She is on intermittent estrogen therapy.

Bilateral mammographic examination reveals atrophic breasts with minimal fibrocystic residuals, predominantly fibrotic. There are no dominant mass lesions. No abnormal calcifications are detected. Small intramammary lymph nodes are noted in the tail of each breast. The skin and subcutaneous fat lines appear smooth. Vascularity is normal and symmetrical.

IMPRESSION
1. Atrophic breasts with minor fibrocystic residuals.
2. No evident malignant mass lesion.
3. Annual mammography is recommended in this age group.

JAMES VARGAS, MD

JV:hpi

D&T: 4/25/[add year]

Diagnostic Imaging Report

PIECZARKA, JON
#869391
August 27, [add year]
Attending: Erik Nutting, MD

LEFT LOWER EXTREMITY DOPPLER ULTRASOUND

CLINICAL INDICATIONS
Left leg pain and swelling. Left knee pain for 1 week.

FINDINGS
There is acute thrombus and deep vein thrombosis (DVT) noted over the distribution of the left trifurcation vessels. This is at the distal popliteal region. Proximal popliteal vein is normal and compresses normally and demonstrates normal respiratory variation.

No DVT identified within the left common femoral, superficial femoral vein. Both demonstrate normal compressibility, augmentation of flow and patency.

IMPRESSION
Acute deep venous thrombosis (DVT) at the trifurcation vessels distribution at the knee.

CHRISTINE BERTRAM, MD

CB:hpi

d&t: 8/27/[add year]

Diagnostic Imaging Report

ENGFER, JARED
#938589
July 19, [add year]
Attending: Charles Cheeseman, MD

KIDNEYS, URETERS, BLADDER (KUB)
The spinous processes, transverse processes, and pedicles of the lumbar vertebrae are fairly well maintained. A minimal amount of degenerative disease is seen within the hips. A large amount of gas and feces is noted throughout the colon. Some gas is noted within the small bowel. Calcified phleboliths are seen within the pelvis. There is also a large 2 x 4 cm mass of increased density in the midportion of the true pelvis.

IMPRESSION
Density within the midpelvis of undetermined etiology. In this first film on this patient, the possibilities include (1) a suppository, (2) residual barium from a previous study, (3) a foreign body.

INTRAVENOUS PYELOGRAM
The KUB study shows the 4 mm calcification in the lower midpole of the right kidney and is unchanged in the interval since our comparison study. The right kidney also appeared normal at that time. The left kidney showed exactly the same configuration on the outside study presented for review, with an irregular right upper pole and two small cystic changes lateral to the upper pole caliceal system, measuring 2 cm and 2.5 cm in diameter. The curvilinear displacement of the caliceal systems also suggests a larger cystic change in the parapelvic region, measuring approximately 5 cm in diameter. The compression of the renal pelvis and deviation of the left upper ureter are essentially the same as seen on the intravenous pyelogram. The bladder again appears normal with a minimal residual.

IMPRESSION
Right renal lithiasis and slight right nephroptosis on the upright study; otherwise normal-appearing right upper urinary tract and ureter. Deformity of the upper pole of the left kidney with some blunting of the caliceal system and the formation of cystic calices lateral to the main upper pole caliceal system suggests a pyelonephritis. Tuberculosis should be considered as an etiology. A larger parapelvic cyst is also noted, displacing the renal pelvis inferiorly and causing some deformity but no evident amputation of the middle or lower pole caliceal systems. The study is consistent with the same findings as on our recent intravenous pyelogram.

JOELLEN SLADEK, MD

JS:hpi

d&t: 7/19/[add year]

Diagnostic Imaging Report

DIETAL, ROLAND
#616670
June 17/[add year]
Attending: Jeffrey Busch, MD

MRI OF BRAIN WITH AND WITHOUT CONTRAST

Comparison is made to prior study. The prior study was performed without contrast.

Ventricles, cisterns, and sulci are symmetric. They are age-appropriate. They are unchanged from the prior study. Findings are consistent with atrophy. Patient shows confluent increased signal in the periventricular white matter with additional areas scattered in the white matter bilaterally. Overall pattern is unchanged. There are a few discrete lacunar infarctions, most notably along the left caudate head. All of these findings are stable. There is no new or significantly increased abnormality.

The postcontrast scan shows no abnormal enhancement in coronal or axial planes. As on the prior study, there is some limited sinus disease in the right sphenoid sinus. This is less prominent than it was previously but not completely resolved.

IMPRESSION
1. Pattern-stable atrophy, diffuse white matter disease, relatively prominent, and some discrete areas of lacunar infarction including left caudate head.
2. There is no new or increasing abnormality compared to the prior study.
3. Limited right sphenoid sinusitis, improved but not resolved.

ELDON DENAULT, MD

d&t: 6/17/[add year]

Comic Relief

Incorrect	Correct
The x-ray was frantically normal.	The x-ray was practically normal.
There were many radio loosened stones.	There were many radiolucent stones.
Excess study of the GI tract.	X-ray study of the GI tract.
The patient had an intrapenis pyelogram.	The patient had an intravenous pyelogram.
Mugger study.	MUGA study (for nuclear medicine).
X-rays of the vertebral column showed bunny fur formation.	X-rays of the vertebral column showed bony spur formation.

PEARSON
myhealthprofessionskit™

To access the online exercises and transcription practice, go to **www.myhealthprofessionskit.com**. Select "Medical Transcription," then click on the title of this book, ***Healthcare Documentation: Fundamentals & Practice***. Then click on the Diagnostic Imaging chapter.

Pathology

Learning Objectives

▶ Spell and define common pathology terms.

▶ Define gross description, microscopic description, biopsy, autopsy.

▶ Demonstrate knowledge of anatomical, medical, adjectival, and soundalike terms by accurately completing the exercises in this chapter.

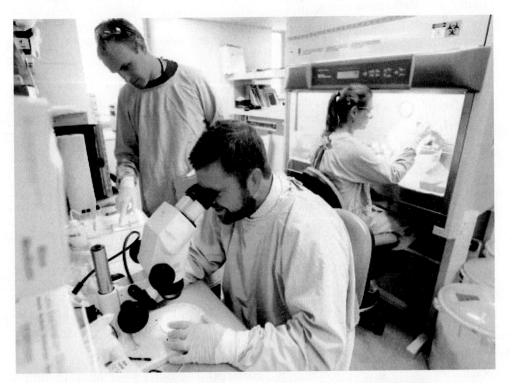

A typical pathology lab within a hospital. Source: Reuters, Corbis Images.

Transcribing Pathology Dictation

Introduction

Pathology is the branch of medicine that studies the structural and functional changes produced in the living body by injury or disease. The practice of pathology is divided into three principal branches. **Anatomic pathology** is concerned with the gross and microscopic changes brought about in living human tissues by disease. **Clinical pathology** refers to the laboratory examination of bodily fluids and waste products such as blood, spinal fluid, urine, and feces. **Forensic pathology** involves the application of knowledge comprised by the other two branches to certain issues in both civil and criminal law.

The standard pathology residency lasts four years, the training time being variously divided between anatomic and clinical pathology. Pathologists who serve as medical examiners, coroners, or forensic consultants usually have additional training in forensic pathology.

Much of the day-by-day work in clinical pathology is done by **medical technologists**. These are specially trained nonphysicians who, under the supervision of a pathologist, perform routine laboratory examinations of blood, urine, and other fluids, and prepare tissue specimens for microscopic examination by a pathologist.

This chapter is concerned chiefly with basic practices and dictation pertaining to anatomic pathology.

Vocabulary Review

acinus (pl., **acini**) A grape-shaped secretory unit in a gland or the saccular terminal dilatation of a pulmonary alveolus.

adenoma A benign tumor arising from glandular epithelium.

adipocere A waxy substance into which the soft tissues of a dead body are converted after prolonged immersion.

aggregate Clustered together (adjective). A cluster or the total amount (noun). To gather together, to amount to (verb).

alveolus (pl., **alveoli**) A hollow or cavity. *Dental alveolus*—tooth socket. *Pulmonary alveolus*—a pouchlike dilatation at the end of a bronchiole, the site of gas exchange between air and blood.

anthracotic pigmentation Gray or black discoloration of lung tissue caused by inhalation of carbon particles; observed in varying degrees in those who live in industrial or urban environments, cigarette smokers, and coal miners.

architecture In microscopic anatomy, the basic framework or structural pattern of an organ or tissue.

atypia Any abnormality in cellular form or type; it may be associated with cancer or a precancerous condition.

autolytic Pertaining to the breakdown or destruction of cells or tissues after death.

Barrett esophagus Peptic ulceration of the lower esophagus with metaplastic formation of columnar epithelium instead of the normal squamous epithelium. It can evolve into adenocarcinoma.

basement membrane A microscopic connective tissue layer underlying an epithelial surface and also investing certain kinds of cell.

benign Referring to a neoplasm or other disease process that poses no threat to life.

biliary dyskinesia Dysfunction of the sphincter of Oddi, which regulates the flow of bile and pancreatic juice into the duodenum.

calculous cholecystitis Cholecystitis associated with gallstones, the most common type.

carcinoma A malignant tumor arising from epithelial cells.

celiac sprue (or **disease**) A malabsorption syndrome precipitated by ingestion of gluten-containing foods and characterized by degeneration of intestinal villi.

centrilobular Affecting the central portions of lobules, as in the liver.

cholesterolosis The deposition of cholesterol in abnormal quantities in tissues.

collagenous colitis A type of inflammatory reaction in the colon characterized by deposits of collagen, the principal noncellular component of connective tissue, beneath the epithelium of the colon.

columnar epithelium Epithelium consisting of one or more layers of cells whose height is at least twice their width.

cortex (pl., **cortices**) The outer layer of an organ or other structure, usually referring to a zone of functioning tissue (parenchyma) rather than a connective tissue capsule.

cross-section A cut made perpendicular to the long axis of a structure (see ■ Figure 19-1) .

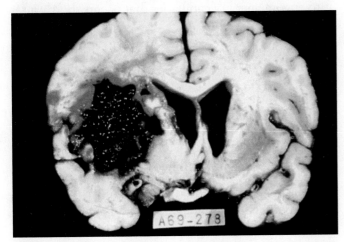

FIGURE 19-1. Cross-section of brain showing cerebrovascular accident. Source: Pearson Education, PH College.

crypt A blind pit or tube opening onto a free surface (skin or mucous membrane).

cytology The branch of biology concerned with the structure and function of living cells. In clinical pathology it refers to the diagnostic assessment of cells that have been detached from a surface for microscopic study, as in a Pap smear.

cytopathic effects Effects characterized by pathologic changes in cell structure.

cytoplasm The fluid medium within a cell in which the nucleus and other organelles are suspended.

diener (German, *servant*) A morgue attendant.

disseminated intravascular coagulation (DIC) A condition in which widespread clotting of blood in vessels consumes clotting factors and leads to hemorrhage.

dysplasia Cell abnormalities usually heralding eventual development of malignancy.

eosinophilic infiltrate The appearance of eosinophils (polymorphonuclear leukocytes with coarse granules appearing red with hematologic stains) in the interstitial tissues of a structure such as the lung, colon, or liver.

epidermal inclusion cyst A benign cutaneous lesion caused by the infolding of keratinizing squamous epithelium.

fibrinous exudate A semisolid film on a wound or ulcer consisting largely of the insoluble protein fibrin.

fixative A fluid used to arrest the process of decomposition in a biopsy or autopsy specimen, to kill bacteria and fungi in or on the specimen, and to begin hardening the tissue to facilitate preparation for microscopic study.

foamy histiocytes Histiocytes with a vacuolated appearance due to the presence of complex lipoids.

focus (pl., **foci**) The site or center of a morbid process.

friable Crumbly; fragmenting or bleeding easily on touch or manipulation; said usually of diseased tissue.

glandular epithelium Epithelium consisting of cells specialized to produce secretion.

glial reaction A process of scarring in inflamed or degenerating nervous tissue as a result of the action of microglia.

Glisson capsule The connective tissue sheath of the liver.

glomerulus (pl., **glomeruli**) One of numerous globular tangles of capillaries in the renal cortex, each surrounded by a Bowman capsule into which a filtrate of plasma is expressed as the first step in the formation of urine.

granulation tissue A layer of tissue on the surface of a healing wound or ulcer. Its granular appearance is due to the presence of numerous minute nodules of connective tissue, whose coalescence will eventually form a cicatrix (scar).

granuloma A small firm nodule consisting of tightly aggregated chronic inflammatory cells.

gross description The pathologist's narration of findings after examining a specimen with the naked eye.

H&E Hematoxylin and eosin, the most commonly used combination of stains in histology.

Helicobacter pylori A curved or spiral gram-negative bacillus, the causative agent of most peptic ulcers.

hepatocyte A cell of the liver parenchyma.

histiocyte Any of various macrophages found in connective tissue, including Kupffer cells in the liver, osteoclasts in bone, alveolar macrophages in the lungs, and giant cells of chronic inflammation.

histology The division of anatomy concerned with the microscopic study of tissues.

hyperchromatic and stratified nuclei Nuclei that are arranged in layers and stain more intensely than normal.

hyperplasia Abnormal increase in the number of cells.

hyperplastic polyposis syndrome An uncommon disorder characterized by the abnormal multiplication or increase in the number of normal cells in normal arrangement in tissue and occasionally associated with serrated adenomas or mixed polyps.

hypertrophy The enlargement or overgrowth of an organ or part due to an increase in the size of its constituent cells.

hypostatic Pertaining to, caused by, or associated with poor circulation of blood in a dependent body part or organ.

inked Marked for orientation purposes with black ink, referring to a pathology specimen (examples of use: inked black; inked, sectioned, and submitted).

in situ (Latin, *in position*) In its original or normal position; said of a malignancy that has not begun to extend or invade beyond its tissue of origin (e.g., carcinoma in situ).

in toto Totally or completely.

interstitial tissue Aggregation of similarly specialized cells which together perform certain special functions; e.g., adenoid tissue, lymphoid tissue.

livor mortis A purplish discoloration of the skin due to engorgement of capillaries that occurs shortly after death.

lobular Referring to tissue architecture characterized by division into circumscribed units (lobules).

lobulated Made up of or divided into lobules (small lobes).

malar Pertaining to or situated on the cheeks.

malignant Referring to a neoplasm or other disorder that poses a threat to life.

malpighian bodies Aggregations of B lymphocytes that occur at intervals along the periarteriolar lymphoid sheaths in the white pulp of the spleen.

metaplasia The presence of a type of mature cells that are not normal for the tissue in which they are found.

metastasis The spread of disease, especially malignant disease, to other sites in the body (see ■ Figure 19-2).

microscopic description The pathologist's narration of findings upon microscopic examination of a specimen.

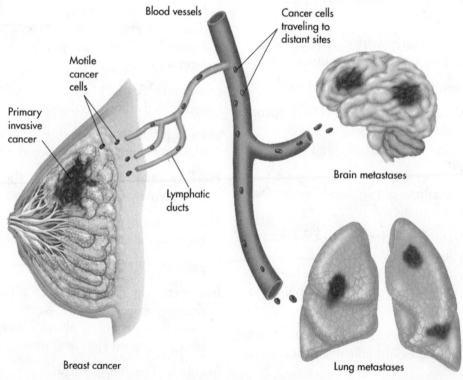

FIGURE 19-2. Invasion and metastasis by cancer cells

muscularis propria The muscular layer of a hollow or tubular organ, lying outside the submucosa.

neoplasm New or abnormal growth, tumor. May be benign or malignant. Malignant neoplasms show anaplasia (loss of differentiation of cells) and are invasive and metastatic.

neutrophilic cryptitis Microabscess formation in the crypts of Lieberkühn, a cardinal sign of ulcerative colitis.

normocephalic Denoting a head whose size, shape, and appearance are normal.

panlobular Affecting all parts of lobules with equal severity.

parenchyma The physiologically active tissue of an organ, as opposed to its connective tissue stroma.

patent Open, unobstructed, usually referring to a tubular structure or normal aperture.

paucicellular Containing relatively few cells, referring especially to highly anaplastic (undifferentiated) forms of certain malignant neoplasms

pigmented histiocytes Black-tinged or melanin-laden histiocytes (macrophages).

polypoid Relating to or resembling a polyp.

portal Pertaining to the hilum or porta of the liver, or to the portal vein, which enters there.

portal triad Hepatic triad, the grouping of tributaries of the hepatic artery, the hepatic vein, and the bile duct at the angles of the lobules of the liver.

post Short for *postmortem examination.*

preparation artifact An appearance or finding in a tissue specimen resulting from technical processing of the specimen rather than from disease or abnormality.

refractile Transmitting light rays in the manner of glass or water, with deviation of rays as they pass into the surrounding air.

rigor mortis Stiffening of the muscles that comes on within a few hours after death and passes off after another few hours.

serial sections Multiple slices of a specimen to provide a three-dimentional concept of a tissue or lesion.

serrate, serrated Having a sawlike edge.

sinus and conus A shortcut reference to the *coronary sinus,* a venous trunk that collects blood from the heart muscle and drains into the right atirum, and the *conus arteriosus,* a conical pouch in the right ventricle from which the pulmonary trunk arises.

sinusoid A thin-walled terminal capillary having little or no adventitia and often anastomosing with other sinusoids; found in the liver, adrenals, heart, parathyroid, parotid gland, spleen, and pancreas. As an adjective, sinusoid means resembling a sinus (a cavity, channel, or space).

smear and culture Study of specimen material by spreading it on a slide and staining for microscopic examination, and by culturing in one or more media suitable for the growth of pathogenic organisms.

stellate Star-shaped.

trabeculation Strands or bands of connective tissue extending from the capsule of an organ into its substance without dividing it into discrete lobes.

vacuole A clear space or cavity within the cytoplasm of a cell.

vacuolated Describing cells that contain vacuoles.

variant Something that differs in some characteristic from the class to which it belongs.

vascular proliferation Growth of new blood vessels as part of an inflammatory or neoplastic process.

Virchow-Robin space An extension of the subarachnoid space between the pia and arachnoid membranes surrounding a blood vessel for a short distance after it enters the brain.

villous adenoma See *adenoma.*

viscid Sticky, glutinous.

Medical Readings

Pathology Reports

by John H. Dirckx, MD

The pathology report. The pathology report usually consists of three parts: the **gross description**, the **microscopic description**, and the **diagnosis**.

In most settings, the pathologist dictates several cases consisting of only gross specimens. The **gross descriptions** are transcribed and the pathologist reviews them for accuracy. When the **microscopic descriptions** have been dictated, the transcriptionist carefully matches each document with the appropriate patient and specimen, transcribing each microscopic description on the page of the corresponding gross description.

The **tissue diagnosis** should be dictated at the same time as the microscopic description. Some specimens (teeth, for example) do not require a microscopic diagnosis, and the dictation will consist only of a gross description and diagnosis.

Although some pathologists prefer to dictate their findings after the examination has taken place, many dictate as they perform the exam. A microphone rigged to a headset or lapel is remotely attached to dictation equipment, and a pedal controls the dictation unit. This arrangement leaves the dictator's hands free to perform the exam while simultaneously operating the dictation equipment.

The autopsy report. A gross autopsy report will typically include an external examination, an internal examination, a summary of findings, and one or more provisional diagnoses. Some pathologists also include a clinical history.

The **external examination** includes a systematic description of the decedent by body system, noting the presence or absence of clothing; the condition of eyes, teeth, skin, and appendages; the degree of decompositional change; the presence or absence of scars, wounds, or obvious trauma; and palpation of the usual anatomic landmarks.

The **internal examination** includes a detailed gross examination of all body cavities. The body is usually opened through a Y-shaped incision (literally in the shape of the letter Y), and the findings are described categorically by body system. These findings include a description of the endocrine, respiratory, cardiovascular, gastrointestinal, urogenital, and central nervous systems in their unaltered state, as well as a description of specific organs that have been removed for measurement and closer examination, including the lungs, heart, liver, spleen, pancreas, kidneys, and brain.

The results of available **laboratory tests** (for example, screening tests for drugs and alcohol) are often reported at the conclusion of the autopsy report, as are the provisional (tentative) and/or clinical **diagnosis** and **cause of death**, if determined. Additionally, **tissue specimens** taken for microscopic examination may be listed.

The **microscopic autopsy** is similar to the microscopic description of a surgical specimen. Using a microscope, the pathologist examines representative tissue specimens taken during the gross autopsy examination. A final pathologic diagnosis is then rendered. Not included in student practice transcripts but encountered on the job is demographic information.

Autopsy reports also include the date and time (or estimated time) of death, as well as the date and time the autopsy was performed. The pathologist's name is entered at the bottom of each report.

Gross and Microscopic Examination of Tissue

by John H. Dirckx, MD

The materials examined by an anatomic pathologist fall into two major classes: specimens taken from living patients, and autopsy specimens. At autopsy it is feasible to remove vital organs such as the heart and the liver in their entirety and subject them to thorough, destructive dissection. Specimens from living patients are necessarily limited in type and volume. Such specimens are either tissues or organs removed during surgical operations (see ■ Figure 19-3) or samples of material (biopsy specimens) removed from the living body for the purpose of examination.

Whereas the pathologist obtains and selects autopsy material for examination, specimens from the living patient are generally obtained by other physicians and submitted for study to the pathologist. Virtually all tissue specimens, regardless of how and by whom they are obtained, are subjected to certain routine procedures.

As soon as possible after being removed from the body, the specimen is placed in a glass, plastic, fiberglass, or aluminum bottle, jar, or bucket containing a fluid called a **fixative**. The fixative has several purposes: to arrest the process of decomposition that begins

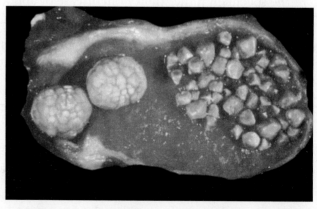

FIGURE 19-3. A gallbladder specimen with multiple gallstones
Source: Biophoto Associates, Photo Researchers, Inc.

almost at once in devitalized tissue, to kill bacteria and fungi in or on the specimen, and to begin hardening the tissue to facilitate preparation for microscopic study.

The most commonly used fixative is a 10% aqueous solution of **formalin**. Because formalin is made by bubbling formaldehyde gas through water, it is often called simply "formaldehyde." Formalin is inexpensive and highly suitable for most purposes. However, several other fixatives are available and may be preferred for special applications.

The pathologist's initial examination of a surgical or biopsy specimen is usually performed after the specimen has been placed in fixative. Although the fixative alters the color and consistency of the tissue to some extent, gross pathologic features can still generally be recognized. Occasionally specimens are brought directly from the operating room to the pathologist without being placed in preservative or fixative.

The pathologist performs the examination at a cutting board, which protects the top of the workbench from knife cuts and from the chemical action of fixatives. The specimens are handled with rubber gloves or with forceps. Excess fluid is soaked up with paper towels or other absorbent materials. Scalpels, razor blades, and scissors are used to open specimens for further examination and to trim them to the proper size for processing. One dimension, at least, of the trimmed specimen must be no more than 3–4 mm to allow penetration of processing chemicals. The trimmed pieces of tissue are placed in small flat round or oblong cassettes of perforated metal or plastic with lids of the same material, in which they will remain during the first stages of processing.

The pathologist dictates the findings during or immediately after the gross inspection and cutting of surgical specimens.

Identification of the specimen. The dictation always begins with basic identifying data: the patient's name as shown on the label of the container and on the laboratory requisition accompanying the specimen, and a general indication of what material has been submitted.

At every step in the handling of a specimen, care is taken to ensure that it is correctly identified. The container in which it is placed by the pathologist, surgeon, or operating room technician is labeled with the patient's name, the nature of the specimen, and often the date, the name of the person obtaining the specimen, and other information. Alternatively, a serial number or accession number may be assigned to the specimen container and the pertinent data kept in a register.

If only one specimen is taken during an operation, as in an appendectomy, it may be unnecessary to identify it other than by the patient's name. When anatomically indistinguishable specimens are submitted, such as abdominal lymph nodes taken from several areas and possibly containing metastatic malignancy, they must be kept carefully separated and distinguished as to their origins.

In removing a specimen, the surgeon may cut it to a certain shape to indicate its origin or its orientation in the patient's body. Orientation may also be indicated by placement of a suture (**surgical stitch**) at a certain place in the specimen, such as at the uppermost point of a tumor excised from the skin. In cutting autopsy specimens from paired organs such as the lungs and the kidneys, the pathologist may indicate by the shape of the specimen which side it came from—for example, triangular for left, square for right.

After identifying the specimen, the pathologist may include clinical information (patient's medical history) in dictation if this is available; often it is entered on the requisition.

Dimensions. The size of each specimen as submitted is usually determined and recorded in three planes in metric units (cm or mm). Solid organs or tumors may be weighed, if practicable, and the weight recorded in grams (g). The volume of any contained fluid (as in a cystic cavity) may be measured or (more often) estimated, and recorded in milliliters (mL) or cubic centimeters (cc).

Gross description. The pathologist then describes the physical features of the specimen, with particular attention to any abnormalities such as swelling, hemorrhage, scarring, or tumor. The description typically includes mention of the color, texture, and consistency of both the exterior and the cut surfaces of the specimen. Any well-defined abnormality (nodule, cyst, ulcer, perforation, scar, pigmentation) is measured as precisely as possible. Not only the exact size and location of any tumor, but also its relation to the margins of the surgical specimen, must be carefully determined to document the adequacy of removal.

Microscopic examination of certain kinds of surgical specimens is routinely omitted unless the pathologist's gross examination shows abnormalities needing further study. Surgically removed tissues that are not usually sectioned for microscopic study include hernia sacs, blood clots, varicose veins, healthy bone (e.g., a section of rib removed for access to thoracic organs), and teeth. If microscopic examination will not be done, the pathologist dictates a diagnostic impression at the conclusion of the report on gross findings.

Because the tissue specimens taken by the pathologist in the autopsy room are generally too large to be handed over directly to a histology technician for preparation of microscope slides, these specimens are subjected to further examination and selective cutting in the pathology laboratory, just as with surgical specimens. Ordinarily, however, the pathologist does not dictate a report after this second inspection and cutting of autopsy specimens, since gross findings are included in the report of the autopsy.

The histopathology laboratory and the microscopic examination of tissue. The preparation of microscope slides from a gross tissue specimen is a complex and exacting process consisting of many steps, some of which are performed by automatic machinery.

The process actually begins when the specimen is placed in fixative. The fixative arrests decomposition and hardens tissue. Before the tissue can be cut into transparent sections, it is necessary to make it still harder by replacing its water content with a rigid material such as paraffin or cellulose. (Bone, however, is too hard for sectioning. A specimen containing bone must be decalcified with either dilute acid, an ion exchange resin, or a chelating agent, or by electrolysis before it can be processed. The same is true of teeth and soft tissue specimens such as sclerotic arteries and scar tissue containing calcium.)

When the paraffin method is used, the tissue specimen is first dehydrated by immersion in a graded series of solutions of an organic solvent such as acetone, Cellosolve, ethyl alcohol, or isopropyl alcohol, which replaces the water. The dehydrated tissue is then immersed in a clearing agent such as xylene (xylol), benzene, cedarwood oil, or chloroform, which replaces the dehydrating agent and renders the tissue transparent. Certain agents (dioxane, tetrahydrofuran) can serve as both dehydrating and clearing agents. After clearing, the tissue is transferred to a bath of melted paraffin, which replaces the clearing agent and infiltrates the tissue spaces. When this infiltration is complete, a technician removes the specimen from the paraffin bath with warmed forceps and embeds it in a cube-shaped mold containing fresh melted paraffin.

When the mold has cooled, the result is a block of paraffin inside which the tissue is embedded with all its water replaced, and its empty spaces filled, by paraffin. This paraffin block is then trimmed to appropriate dimensions and cut on a microtome, a precision instru-

ment on the order of an electric meat slicer, which makes transparent slices that are only about 5 micrometers (0.005 mm) thick. For technical reasons, sections are usually made by cutting across the broadest flat surface of the tissue specimen, unless the pathologist has given special instructions for an edge cut or **cross section** (see ■ Figure 19-4). Usually only one or two sections from each paraffin block are chosen to be made into slides. Sometimes **serial sections** (for example, every tenth or twentieth slice) are taken so as to provide the pathologist with a three-dimensional concept of a tissue or lesion.

Immediately after cutting, the paraffin sections are floated on a bath of warm water, which helps to smooth out wrinkles and curled edges. Each section is affixed to a separate microscope slide (a thin strip of clear glass about 1 x 3 inches) by means of a film of albumin solution or other suitable adhesive. The slides are identified with labels bearing names or numbers matching those of the containers in which the gross specimens were submitted.

Substances other than paraffin are sometimes used to infiltrate and embed tissue for sectioning. With Carbowax, which is water-soluble, the dehydration and clearing steps can be omitted; however, obtaining satisfactory sections with Carbowax demands a high degree of technical skill. Celloidin is a suspension of a cellulose derivative in a volatile solvent. Because infiltration and embedding with celloidin do not require heat, there is less distortion of tissue than with the paraffin and Carbowax methods. Celloidin, however, takes much more time; as much as a month may elapse between fixation and sectioning. Commercially available embedding media besides Carbowax include Epon, Paraplast, and Parlodion.

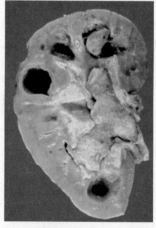

FIGURE 19-4. Photograph of sectioned kidney specimen with extensive renal calculi. Source: Dr E. Walker, Photo Researchers, Inc.

Microscopic examination of the slide at this stage would yield little information, because all of the tissue spaces are filled with the infiltrating medium. This must be removed and replaced with water or some other suitable fluid by a reversal of the procedures used in making the block. Once the infiltrating agent has been removed and the tissue section rehydrated, the slide is immersed in one or more coloring solutions called **stains**. These impart a more or less intense coloration to the tissues, which greatly facilitates microscopic examination (see ■ Figure 19-5).

Seldom is only a single color applied. Different stains have affinities for different components of tissue, depending on their chemical properties. Hence it is usual to apply at least two contrasting colors. The use of standard combinations of stains enables the pathologist to recognize normal and abnormal microscopic features of tissue consistently and confidently.

In practice, staining usually involves a number of steps besides immersion of the prepared slide in a coloring agent. First a **mordant** may be applied to render the tissue chemically more receptive to staining. Many fixatives have mordant properties. After the first stain has been applied, the slide is immersed in or washed with a **decolorizer**, which removes stain from all parts of the tissue to which it has not become chemically bound. The slide is then treated with a **counterstain** of a contrasting color, which is taken up by tissues decolorized in the preceding step. A **polychrome stain** is a mixture of two or more coloring agents in one solution. With a polychrome stain, differential staining of tissue components takes place even though the tissue is exposed to all of the coloring agents simultaneously. A **metachromatic stain** is one that changes color on becoming chemically bound to certain tissues.

By far the most commonly used combination of stains for routine histopathology work is **hematoxylin and eosin (H&E)**. Hematoxylin is a deep blue stain which imparts various shades of blue and purple to cell nuclei and other tissue components of slightly acidic nature. Eosin stains most of the other components pink to red. Many special stains and techniques are available to bring out certain features (nerve tissue, reticular fibers, lipid material, pathogenic microorganisms) that are not shown by routine stains. In submitting a tissue block to the histology technician, the pathologist may write instructions regarding the use of special stains. Some staining operations can be done by automatic machinery, but often part or all of the staining process is performed manually. Slides are placed vertically in

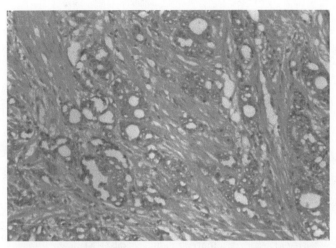

FIGURE 19-5. Microscopic photograph of prostate tissue showing cells that have become cancerous (the cancer cells line the white spaces). Source: CDC, Dr. Edwin P. Ewing, Jr.

tall narrow glass containers called Coplin jars, which are filled with stain or other solutions.

After staining and drying, the tissue section on the slide is ordinarily protected with a cover slip, a very thin sheet of glass about 7/8 of an inch square. A film of balsam or other mounting medium is first placed over the tissue section, and the cover slip is gently dropped into place. The balsam eventually hardens around the edges, but under the cover slip it remains fluid indefinitely, preserving the section in a clear, homogeneous, refractile medium. Mounting media in common use are Apathy medium, (Canada) balsam, Clarite, and Permount.

In most laboratories, slides are available for the pathologist's examination 24–72 hours after the tissue is removed from the body. Processing is speeded and simplified by the use of automated machinery that dehydrates, clears, and infiltrates tissue during the night. The preceding day's specimens are then embedded, sectioned, and stained on the following morning.

The pathologist examines or "reads" slides with a light microscope, using various magnifications as needed. The standard magnifications are scanning power (X35–50), low power (X100), and high power (X450–500). The greater the magnification, the more the detail that can be distinguished, but the smaller the zone of tissue that can be viewed without moving the slide. After reviewing the slides, the pathologist dictates the microscopic findings and then states one or more diagnoses or diagnostic impressions.

Since gross and microscopic reports are dictated on different days, they are seldom transcribed at the same session. Ordinarily the gross report is transcribed on the top half of a standard surgical pathology form. This transcription is made available to the pathologist when the slides of the tissue are examined. The dictation of microscopic findings and diagnosis is then transcribed on the bottom half of the form, and the form is returned to the pathologist for review and signature.

Pause for Reflection

1. Describe the major sections of a complete pathology report.
2. Describe the main parts of an autopsy report.
3. Describe the 2 major classes of materials examined by an anatomic pathologist.
4. What types of information are included in the gross description?
5. Briefly describe the "certain routine procedures" to which virtually all tissue specimens, regardless of how and by whom they are obtained, are subjected.
6. Define the following terms: mordant, decolorizer, counterstain, polychrome stain, metachromatic stain.
7. What is the most common stain used in preparing specimens for histologic examination?

Diagnostic, Surgical, and Laboratory Procedures

autopsy The examination of a body after death, consisting of detailed visual observations of external body tissues and internal organs, and microscopic analyses of the internal organs and structures following tissue dissection. Also called *postmortem examination*, *necropsy*, *"post."*

biopsy A sample of tissue removed from a living patient and submitted for pathologic examination.

curettage A surgical scraping.

electron microscopy The study of specimens with an electron microscope.

excisional biopsy The surgical removal of an entire tumor, lesion, or diseased organ from a living patient.

fine-needle aspiration A technique used to remove cells by suction from certain structures such as the prostate, subcutaneous lymph nodes and other neck masses, and breast masses.

frozen section Cutting of a flash-frozen surgical specimen for rapid staining and microscopic examination while the patient is still in the operating room, as a guide to further surgical decision-making.

incisional biopsy Refers to the surgical removal of part of a tumor, lesion, or diseased organ for pathologic study.

needle biopsy A needle is passed through the skin directly into the organ to be studied, and an inner cutting needle slices and removes a core of tissue.

permanent section Prepared, stained, and fixed specimen that is ready for microscopic examination.

punch biopsy A cylindrical instrument used to obtain a plug of tissue for examination.

shave biopsy A thin layer of skin consisting mostly or entirely of epidermis is removed with a blade held approximately parallel to the surface.

smear Material spread thinly over a microscopic slide.

Transcription Tips

1. Confusing terms related to Anatomic Pathology: Some of these terms sound alike; others are potential traps when researching. Memorize the terms and their meanings so that you can select the appropriate term for a correct transcript.

   discrete—distinct, separate
   discreet—prudent, able to keep a secret

   fascicle—a small bundle of nerve, muscle, or tendon fibers
   vesicle—blister

   fascicular—pertaining to nerve, muscle, or tendon fibers
   vesicular—pertaining to composed of blisters

   fibrinous—containing the insoluble protein fibrin
   fibrous—containing or composed of fibers

   liver—the large gland in the right upper abdomen that secretes bile and converts sugar into glycogen.
   livor—see *livor mortis* below

   pleural—pertaining to the membrane that lines the chest cavity and covers the lungs.
   plural—more than one.

   rigor mortis—the stiffening of muscles that comes on a few hours after death.
   livor mortis—the purplish discoloration of areas of the body closest to the ground after death.

   sheet—a thin, flat structure resembling a sheet or paper or a bed sheet.
   sheath—tubular structure enclosing or surrounding organs or other structures such as nerves and tendons.

   villous—hairy, shaggy, covered with villi (tiny hairlike structures).
   bilious—characterized by or consisting of bile.

   In addition, prefixes such as *hyper-* and *hypo-* or *peri-* and *para-* are easy to confuse. Context should help you determine which is correct, but if still uncertain, verify the term and its meaning in a medical dictionary.

   periductular fibrosis
   hyperorthokeratosis
   periglandular chronic inflammation

   Sections of specimen A show lymph nodes with paracortical and follicular **hyper***plasia ...*

   The squamous mucosa shows a mild degree of acanthosis and focal **para***keratosis.*

   Infiltrative nests of neoplastic urothelial cells extend into lamina propria of bladder mucosa, and into **peri***urethral prostatic stroma ...*

2. Slang Terms. Expand these slang brief forms when encountered in dictation.

ca	carcinoma
mets	metastasis
esoph	esophagus
micro	microscopic (expand when dictated as a heading)
tabby	therapeutic abortion

3. Spelling. Memorize the spelling of these difficult-to-spell terms. Note silent letters, doubled letters, and unexpected pronunciation.

   abundance (-*ance*, not -*ence*)
   aggregate (two *g*'s followed by one *g*)
   anulus (fibrosus)—*not* annulus or fibrosis
   columnar (the *n* can be lost in pronunciation)
   cystlike (no hyphen)
   disarray
   dyskinesia
   embalmed
   en bloc ("in block" or "ahn block")
   gallbladder (one word)
   gallstones (one word)
   in situ
   in toto
   leiomyoma
   malpighian (bodies)
   panlobular (one word)
   parenchyma
   paucicellular
   outpouching (one word)
   vacuoles (the *v* might sound like a *b*)
   viscid

Transcription Tips

4. Watch out for spelling changes when forming derivatives.

Combined forms
    fibrinopurulent
    glomangioma
    steatocystoma

Singular, Plural
    acinus, acini
    alveolus, alveoli
    cortex, cortices
    diverticulum, diverticula,
       not diverticuli or diverticulae
    foramen, foramina
    focus, foci ("foh-sigh")
    gyrus, gyri
    lacuna, lacunae
    lumen, lumina
    medulla, medullae
    pneumothorax, pneumothoraces
    sulcus, sulci

Adjectives
    calculus (noun) vs calculous (adjective)
    decidua (noun) vs decidual (adjective)
    mucus (noun) vs mucous (adjective)
    villus (noun, rarely used in the singular) vs
      villous (adjective)
    stroma (noun) vs stromal (adjective)

Note the proper forms of cross section (noun), cross-section (verb), and cross-sectional (adj.).

5. Dictation Challenges

"Little" words: A common problem in all types of medical transcription is confusing "little" words. However, these seemingly unimportant words can often have a significant meaning. Word pairs, like *in* and *on*, *to* and *through*, *toward* and *throughout*, *with* and *within*, as well as isolated words such as *not*, can have a contradictory or misleading impact on meaning if the wrong word is chosen. Listening carefully and paying attention to contextual clues is the best way to avoid making mistakes with these words.

left side of back, not left-sided back

Both are bisected and specimens submitted in toto, B (4) (*not* "bisecting specimens …")

This placental disk without cord or membranes is 326 g. (not "membrane is")

Specimen labels: Sometimes "quotation . . . end quotation" is dictated, sometimes it is not, but the label name should be put in quotation marks: Specimen labeled "plaque, left femoral artery." Tissue specimens are often referred to as "block #1," "block #2," and so on.

Do not confuse the terms for specimens with *en bloc* (pronounced "ahn block") which means "in a lump; as a whole." Example:

The specimen is submitted in its entirety as block #2.

The tumor was submitted en bloc, the superior margin tagged with a stitch.

Colors: The use of combination colors to describe tissues on gross examination is standard in pathology dictation. Two colors used together are hyphenated before and after the noun. Colors ending in *–ish* combined with another color preceding a noun are hyphenated but not when they follow the noun.

green-brown bile
tan-brown to tan-dark brown friable fragments
The specimen is tan-pink to brown.
The mucosal lining is red-brown.
greenish-black viscid bile
Bile is greenish black.

6. Confusion of word endings or confusing the end sound of one word with the sound of the next word: Listen carefully and observe context to determine the correct term. Note that *sinusoid* can be a noun, in which case it is often used in the plural form *sinusoids*, but it can also be an adjective.

consolidated vs consolidative
crypt distortion, *not* cryp distortion
flecked (the *–ed* may be difficult to hear)
infiltrative vs infiltrated
inked (the *–ed* may be difficult to hear)
patchy edema, *not* patchedema
representative vs represented
thickened, *not* thick and

Spotlight On

Hands-on Anatomy Lessons— My Pathology Experience

by Brenda J. Hurley

My first role in healthcare documentation was in the pathology department. We had two pathologists and two medical secretaries. We were called medical secretaries because the term *medical transcriptionist* was not used back in the early 1980s. Also, we had to perform other duties besides transcription, such as answer the phone for the department, send out correspondence, file reports, and a myriad of other tasks that were needed to have our department run smoothly for our pathologists and histologists.

In order to provide optimal departmental coverage, the medical secretaries staggered their working hours. I took the later shift of 9 a.m. to 5:30 p.m., while my colleague worked 7 a.m. to 3:30 p.m. Our histologists worked early in the morning in order to prepare the slides for gross, some started their shift at 5 a.m., with the last one on duty until 3:30 p.m. Because I worked the "late" shift in the department I was often asked to assist the pathologists with "gross" when surgical specimens arrived later in the afternoon.

Today, pathology departments have pathology assistants who handle much of the grossing duties so pathologists are not burdened with the dictation of the gross description and dissection of the surgical specimens received for tissue processing. But back in my day, it was the pathologist and me with gloves on working with the surgical tissue specimens. What an amazing experience this gave me to learn so much about disease processes and anatomy!

Briefly, my contribution to this process included verifying the specimen container label matched the pathology requisition card. Once verified, I would label tissue cassettes with the pathology accession number assigned to this case. Depending on the specimen received, there could be one tissue cassette or a dozen needed. The pathologist would determine how many were required. I got to know their preferences well and often would have

the correct number of cassettes ready by the time they were ready for that specimen.

The pathologist would take the specimen out of the container and then would dictate the estimated weight, the description of the specimen to include the color, texture, and its measurements. Then he would dissect the specimen according to standard protocol and take representative sections of the specimen, placing them in the assigned tissue cassette(s). Some smaller specimens, such as a skin biopsy, would be bisected and then the entire specimen would be placed in the tissue cassette(s). That would be identified as submitted "in toto." Specimens in a fragmented form, such as uterine curettings from a D&C, would be referred to as "in aggregate," meaning all the fragments were measured together such as in a cluster or mass. The pathologist would dictate all of these details in what would then be transcribed to become the microscopy section of the pathology report.

Granted this was not a job for anyone with a queasy stomach, as the formalin odor was strong and the surgical specimens that we examined could be pretty unpleasant to view (or smell), but I loved it! My pathologists enjoyed discussing what they were reviewing, so I asked plenty of questions. It is an entirely different lesson to actually see and hold a gallbladder rather than see a colored picture of it in a book. So when I transcribe that the gallbladder was packed full of stones, I have an instant replay in my head that takes me back to what I saw and held.

We had some tumors so large that they would be delivered from the surgical suite in a diaper pail—I am not kidding. At times when the case had the potential to be something unusual or mysterious, the pathologist would take pictures of the specimen for a permanent recording. One of the most interesting body structures, at least to me, is the uterus. It is smaller than the size of your fist and it is nearly impossible to imagine how it could expand large enough to hold a baby during a full-term pregnancy.

Some of our surgical pathology cases were tragic and difficult to get through, knowing the pain

Spotlight On Hands-on Anatomy Lessons *(page 2)*

and suffering the individual and their families would endure when the diagnosis was delivered. I remember one unusual day when we had four breast biopsies (from four different patients) that were all diagnosed as malignant. We all shared the pain when our pathologist had to deliver his findings to the waiting surgeons. Thank goodness there were a lot more happy days when the results delivered were in terms like benign, no abnormal findings, no atypical changes seen, and normal.

I usually did not assist with autopsies since those were scheduled to be done during the time when the histology technicians were available, but I would often help with specimen preparation when organs or portions of organs were removed for tissue processing at a later time. I remember a case when a middle-aged man fell on his side; unknowingly he had ruptured his spleen which caused internal hemorrhaging that resulted in his death. Autopsy did not reveal anything significant other than an enlarged spleen that had ruptured, but microscopically it was found that the man had an undiagnosed leukemia which was the reason for his splenomegaly that caused thinning of the splenic capsule.

Our role in pathology, at times, is providing answers. The answers we offer from an autopsy cannot always give comfort for the loss of a loved one but it can help with the understanding as to why when the cause was previously unknown.

A pathology department takes real teamwork to work efficiently and effectively. Interesting that I stepped in to help out the team when there was a need in the department, but found that each time I expanded my role to help the team, I learned something new. Take it from me, opportunities come in many different forms. Don't let yours slip away.

CODES IN PATHOLOGY REPORTS

The inclusion of codes in pathology reports for billing and research purposes is standard procedure. In some systems, such as PACS and other technologies where the dictation and transcription are integrated, the codes may be keyed in by the dictator or pulled from another source within the system. Sometimes, the dictator dictates the codes following the diagnoses. When dictated, codes are transcribed at the bottom of the report, below the signature block.

Pathology, as it is practiced today, captures data (information/reports) in several different ways:

Narrative reports

Structured reports

Coded data (ICD vs. SNOMED vs. Local Codes)

PACS

Many pathology departments use software known as PACS, a Picture Archiving and Communications Solution that allows them to integrate pathology imaging into the electronic patient record and enables surgeons and other specialists to view results and images remotely. Such systems help pathology departments improve workflow by tracking the specimen from the time it is ordered by the referring clinician, to its arrival in the lab, to staining, to the clinical work, transcription and report generation including all the corresponding ICD and CPT codes.

Thus, while the reports in this unit are straight transcription, you should be aware that on the job you may be working within a software system that incorporates templates and structured reports, embedded images, and captures coding data.

CANCER CLASSIFICATIONS, GRADING, AND STAGING

Classification of cancer refers to the site of origin, grading to cell analysis or histology, and staging to the extent of tumor.

Note: The terms *class*, *grade*, and *stage* are not capitalized in transcription unless they appear at the beginning of a sentence or follow a colon.

Common examples of **classification by site of origin** include the following:

Adenocarcinoma originates in glandular tissue.

Blastoma originates in embryonic tissue of organs.

Carcinoma originates in epithelial tissue lining organs and tubes.

Leukemia originates in tissues that form blood cells.

Lymphoma originates in lymphatic tissue.

Myeloma originates in bone marrow.

Grading is based on microscopic histological findings.

grade 1 is used for cells that are slightly abnormal and well differentiated.

grade 2 is used for cells that are more abnormal and moderately differentiated.

grade 3 is used for cells that are very abnormal and poorly differentiated.

grade 4 is used for cells that are immature and undifferentiated.

Dictation example: *Papillary urothelial carcinoma, grade 2-3/3* ("two to three over three").

Staging delineates the extent of the disease, and there are several methods. The **tumor, node, metastases (TNM) system** classifies cancer by tumor size (T), the degree of regional spread or node involvement (N), and distant metastasis (M). These three parameters are combined in one expression (T1 N0 M0).

Tumor (T)

T0 No evidence of tumor.

TX Primary tumor cannot be assessed.

Tis Carcinoma in situ (limited to surface cells).

T1- T4 Increasing tumor size, extent, or
involvement.

Node (N)

N0   No lymph node involvement.

NX   Regional lymph nodes cannot be assessed.

N1-N4 Increasing degrees of metastatic lymph node involvement; criteria vary for different anatomic sites.

Metastases (M)

M0   No evidence of distant metastases.

MX Extent of metastasis cannot be determined.

M1   Evidence of distant metastases.

Note: Parenthetic 3-letter abbreviations may be used to indicate site of metastasis, i.e., M1(HEP) for hepatic metastases. Other criteria or attributes of the tumor or stage may be indicated by lowercase prefixes: *a* for autopsy, *c* for clinical, *p* for pathologic, *r* for recurrent, *y* after multimodal treatment, e.g., pN0. Suffixes and numerals following the classification may further specify size, invasiveness, or extent of metastasis, e.g., pN0(i)(sn). See the *AMA Manual of Style* for further details.

The **extent of disease** may also be classified by a simple numerical method.

stage 0 Cancer in situ (limited to surface cells).

stage I   Cancer limited to the tissue of origin, evidence of tumor growth.

stage II   Limited local spread of cancerous cells.

stage III Extensive local and regional spread.

stage IV Distant metastasis.

Individual cancer stages may be subdivided as in the following examples:

stage 0a

stage 0is (is = in situ)

stage IB2

stage IIIE+S (E = extralymphatic spread; S = splenic involvement, as seen in Hodgkin disease)

stage IVA

Note: Cancer staging methods may be combined to define individual stages that differ among anatomic sites; e.g., pancreatic cancer, stage IIA: T3 N0 M0.

CANCER STAGING SYSTEMS

FIGO. The FIGO system is used for obstetric and gynecologic disorders. FIGO stages use Roman numerals, occasionally in combination with capital letters and Arabic numerals: 0, I, IA, IA1, IB, IB1, II, III, IV, IVA, IVB, etc.

Dukes. The Dukes staging system is used for colon and rectal tumors and is expressed as follows: Dukes A through Dukes D or Dukes stage A through Dukes stage D.

Bethesda system. The Bethesda system is used for reporting cervical cytology (Papanicolaou test results). Squamous intraepithelial lesions (SIL) are divided into low-grade and high-grade lesions in the Bethesda system for cytologic classification. ASC (atypical squamous cells), ASC-H (atypical squamous cells—cannot exclude high-grade SIL), ASC-US (atypical squamous cells of undetermined significance), CIN (cervical intraepithelial neoplasia), HGSIL (high-grade SIL), LSIL (low-grade SIL), T zone (transformation zone), and VAIN (vaginal intraepithelial neoplasia) are just a few of the abbreviations used in the Bethesda system. CIN 1 (mild dysplasia) and lesions showing clear-cut evidence of papillomavirus effect are classified as low-grade lesions. CIN 2 (moderate dysplasia) and CIN 3 (severe dysplasia and carcinoma in situ) are classified as high-grade lesions.

Note: Expand Bethesda system abbreviations on first use in a report and punctuate as shown above.

Low-grade squamous endoepithelial lesion (LGSIL, CIN 1) with features of human papillomavirus (HPV) infection, and focal high-grade squamous intraepithelial lesion (HGSIL) encompassing moderate squamous dysplasia (CIN 2) is represented.

Multiple endocrine neoplasia. Staging of multiple endocrine neoplasia incorporates Arabic numerals and letters as follows: MEN 1, MEN 2, MEN 2A, MEN 2B, MEN 3. Use a space between the abbreviation and the numeral to differentiate from similar genetic abbreviations in which the spaces are closed up.

Gleason score. The Gleason score or grade is used for classifying prostate carcinoma. Arabic numerals 1 through 5 are used. Generally, the pathologist will examine at least two specimens under the microscope to identify at least two architectural patterns, assigning a Gleason score for each one and reporting the combined score.

Gleason score 1 + 2 for a score of 3/10

AJCC staging. The American Joint Committee on Cancer (AJCC) prefers the TNM system for staging melanoma. AJCC stages are as follows:

Stage 0: Melanoma present only in the epidermis and has not spread.

Stage IA (T1a N0 M0): Melanoma localized and less than 0.75 mm thick, has spread to upper dermis.

Stage IB (T1b-2a N0 M0): Tumor between 0.75 mm and 1.5 mm thick, has penetrated further into dermis.

Stage IIA (T2b-3a N0 M0): Tumor between 1.5 and 4 mm deep, has reached lower dermis.

Stage IIB (T3b-4a N0 M0): Tumor more than 4 mm, still localized but has penetrated below dermis.

Stage III (T4 N1-4 M0): Melanoma has infiltrated lymph nodes, may occur at any thickness.

Stage IV (any T, any N, any M1): Melanoma metastasized to other organs or other areas of the skin, may occur at any thickness level, with or without lymph node involvement.

Clark scoring method. A less preferred method for classifying melanoma, the Clark scoring method measures how deeply the tumor has invaded the skin. Clark levels are roughly equivalent to AJCC stages as follows:

Clark level		AJCC stage
I	0	0
II	IA	IA
III	IB	IB
IV	IIA	IIA
V	IIB	IIB

Exercises

Medical Vocabulary Review

Instructions: Choose the best answer.

___ 1. A microscopic connective tissue layer underlying an epithelial surface and also investing certain kinds of cell is _____
A. the cortex.
B. the sheath.
C. columnar epithleium.
D. the basement membrane.

___ 2. Dysfunction of the sphincter of Oddi, which regulates the flow of bile and pancreatic juice into the duodenum, is _____
A. biliary dyskinesia.
B. Barrett esophagus.
C. calculous cholecystitis.
D. Virchow-Robin spaces.

___ 3. An entire specimen sample consisting of multiple smaller pieces of tissue is called _____
A. a foci.
B. cytology.
C. aggregate.
D. histology.

___ 4. The terms *portal* and *hepatic* both refer to the _____
A. lung.
B. liver.
C. pancreas.
D. gallbladder.

___ 5. Thin-walled terminal capillaries having little or no adventitia and found in the liver, adrenals, heart, parathyroid, parotid gland, spleen, and pancreas are called _____
A. acini.
B. crypts.
C. sinusoids.
D. sinus and conus.

___ 6. A benign tumor arising from glandular epithelium is _____
A. a carcinoma.
B. an adenoma.
C. a granuloma.
D. an adenocarcinoma.

___ 7. Highly anaplastic (undifferentiated) forms of certain malignant neoplasms containing relatively few cells might be said to be _____
A. serrated.
B. refractile.
C. hyperplastic.
D. paucicellular.

___ 8. Tissue that is crumbly; fragmenting or bleeding easily on touch or manipulation is said to be _____
A. frozen.
B. friable.
C. fibrinous.
D. collagenous.

___ 9. Grape-shaped secretory units in a gland are _____
A. acini.
B. villi.
C. crypts.
D. alveoli.

___ 10. The physiologically active tissue of an organ, as opposed to fat and connective tissue is the _____
A. cortex.
B. epithelium.
C. parenchyma.
D. interstitial tissue.

___ 11. _____ is another name for the connective tissue sheath of the liver.
A. Barrett esophagus
B. Glisson capsule
C. Malpighian bodies
D. Muscularis propria

___ 12. Black coloration of lung tissue of little or no pathologic significance caused by inhalation of tiny particles of carbon, seen in smokers and those who live in industrial or urban environments, might be referred to as _____
A. foamy histiocytes.
B. eosinophilic infiltrates.
C. pigmented histiocytes.
D. anthracotic pigmentation.

___ 13. A semisolid film on a wound or ulcer consisting largely of the insoluble protein fibrin is _____
A. fibrinous exudate.
B. columnar epithelium.
C. eosinophilic infiltrate.
D. glandular epithelium.

___ 14. Kidney capillaries that form the site of the filtration barrier between the blood and the kidney and projecting into the expanded end of the renal tubules are _____
A. hepatocytes.
B. glomeruli.
C. lobules.
D. portal triads

___ 15. An adenoma in the colon might be described as _____
A. autolytic.
B. polypoid.
C. malignant.
D. fibrinous.

___ 16. Cell abnormalities heralding eventual development of malignancy are evidence of _____
A. metaplasia.
B. anaplasia.
C. dysplasia.
D. hyperplasia.

___ 17. A malabsorption syndrome precipitated by ingestion of gluten-containing foods and characterized by degeneration of intestinal villi is called _____
A. celiac sprue.
B. cholesterolosis.
C. Barrett esophagus.
D. calculous cholecystitis.

___ 18. Small saclike structures in the lung or root sockets for the teeth are called _____
A. alveoli.
B. crypts.
C. nuclei.
D. sinusoids.

___ 19. Strands or bands of connective tissue sometimes extending from the capsule into the substance of an organ are called _____
A. portal triads.
B. trabeculation.
C. neutrophilic cryptitis.
D. vascular proliferation.

___ 20. Clear spaces or cavities within the cytoplasm of a cell are called _____
A. artifacts.
B. crypts.
C. variants.
D. vacuoles.

Diagnostic, Surgical, and Laboratory Procedures

Instructions: Match the following diagnostic, surgical, and laboratory procedures to their descriptions or definitions. Some answers may be used more than once or not at all.

____ 1. autopsy

____ 2. curettage

____ 3. excisional biopsy

____ 4. fine-needle aspiration

____ 5. incisional biopsy

____ 6. needle biopsy

____ 7. punch biopsy

____ 8. shave biopsy

____ 9. electron microscopy

____ 10. frozen section

____ 11. permanent section

____ 12. smear

A. Material spread thinly over a microscopic slide

B. Thin layer of skin consisting mostly or entirely of epidermis is removed with a blade held approximately parallel to the surface

C. Removal of a core of tissue from an organ using a special type of needle

D. Examination using a device that allows much greater magnification and resolution than a light microscopy

E. Surgical scraping

F. A specimen that is sent directly from surgery to pathology for immediate examination while the patient is still under anesthesia

G. Removal of cells by suction from certain structures such as the prostate, subcutaneous lymph nodes and other neck masses, and breast masses

H. Prepared, stained, and fixed specimen that is ready for microscopic examination

I. Surgical removal of part of a tumor, lesion, or diseased organ for pathologic study

J. Examination of a body after death

K. Surgical removal of an entire tumor, lesion, or diseased organ

L. Use of a cylindrical instrument to obtain a plug of tissue for examination

Dissecting Medical Terms

Instructions: As you learned in your medical language course, words are formed from prefixes, combining forms (root word plus combining vowel), and suffixes. Combining vowels (usually **o** but not always) are used to connect two root words or a root and a suffix. By analyzing these word parts, you can often determine the definition of a term without even looking it up (if you know the definition of the parts, of course!).

Being able to divide and analyze the words you hear into their component parts will also improve your auditory deciphering ability and spelling and help you research those words that you cannot easily spell or define.

For the following terms, draw a slash (/) between the components and then write a short definition based on the meaning of the parts. Remember that to define a word based on its parts, you start at the end, usually with the suffix. If there's a prefix, that is defined next, and finally the combining form is defined.

Example: collagenous

Divide & Analyze:
collagenous = collagen/ous = pertaining + collagen (the major component of connective tissue)
Define: pertaining to the major component of connective tissue

1. anthracotic
   Divide _____

   Define _____

2. autolytic
   Divide _____

   Define _____

3. bronchopneumonia
   Divide _____

   Define _____

4. cholesterolosis
   Divide _____

   Define _____

5. cytoplasmic
   Divide _____

   Define _____

6. dyskinesia
   Divide _____

   Define _____

7. dysplasia
   Divide _____

   Define _____

8. endocardium
   Divide _____

   Define _____

9. epithelial
   Divide _____

   Define _____

10. extrahepatic
    Divide _____

    Define _____

11. fibrinopurulent
    Divide _____

    Define _____

12. granuloma
    Divide _____

    Define _____

13. hyperchromatic
    Divide _____

    Define _____

14. hyperplastic
Divide _____
_____
Define _____

15. hypostatic
Divide _____
_____
Define _____

16. intraepithelial
Divide _____
_____
Define _____

17. lymphocytic
Divide _____
_____
Define _____

18. panlobular
Divide _____
_____
Define _____

19. paucicellular
Divide _____
_____
Define _____

20. tubulovillous
Divide _____
_____
Define _____

5. cytoplasm _____
6. eosinophil _____
7. epithelium _____
8. esophagus _____
9. fibrin _____
10. fiber _____
11. focus _____
12. gland _____
13. hyperplasia _____
14. column _____
15. lymphocyte _____
16. mesentery _____
17. metastasis _____
18. muscle _____
19. pericardium _____
20. polyp _____
21. porta (hepatis) _____
22. septum _____
23. sinus _____
24. trabecula _____
25. viscera _____

Forming Plurals

Instructions: Review the rules for forming plurals in your medical language textbook. Test your knowledge of plurals by writing the plural form of the following terms. Consult a medical dictionary to confirm your spelling.

Singular	Plural
1. acinus	_____
2. alveolus	_____
3. bronchus	_____
4. cortex	_____
5. calyx	_____
6. focus	_____
7. glomerulus	_____
8. medulla	_____
9. nucleus	_____
10. pelvis	_____

Spelling Exercise

Instructions: Review the adjective suffixes in your medical language textbook. Test your knowledge of adjectives by writing the adjectival form of the following pulmonary medicine words. Consult a medical dictionary to verify your spelling.

Noun	Adjective
1. alveolus	_____
2. calculus	_____
3. collagen	_____
4. column	

Transcript Forensics

Instructions: This section presents snippets of transcribed dictations from clinic notes; history and physical examinations and consultations; operative reports and procedure notes; and discharge summaries. Explain the passage so that a nonmedical person can understand it.

Example: The adipose tissue averages about 1 inch in thickness at the umbilical area. The ribs are incised and there are no pneumothoraces. The pleural cavities each contain approximately 50 mL of blood-tinged serosanguineous fluid.

Explanation: The fat tissue at the navel is about an inch in thickness. There is no air or gas in the area around the lungs but there is about 50 mL of fluid tinged with blood and serum.

1. The thyroid gland is enlarged and **nodular**. It has a red-brown **parenchyma**. There are no **discrete** tumors.

    Explanation: _____
    _____
    _____
    _____

2. There is only early **atherosclerosis** with 10% to 20% occlusion of the main coronary arteries and large branches. No **thrombi** are seen. The myocardium is flabby and pale. There are no large areas of **fibrosis**. There are no zones suggestive of recent **infarction**.

    Explanation: _____
    _____
    _____
    _____
    _____

3. The pleural surfaces are smooth and glistening. The pulmonary parenchyma is moderately **congested**. There is slight **edema**. There is equivocal nodularity of the lower lobes bilaterally. There is no **consolidation** or infarction. There are no **granulomas** or tumors.

    Explanation: _____
    _____
    _____
    _____
    _____

4. The stomach and duodenum show no **erosion** or **ulceration**. The small intestine is kinked due to numerous **fibrous adhesions**. The left colon contains soft green-brown fecal material. It is slightly dilated with gas. There are no gastrointestinal **neoplasms** or **diverticula**.

    Explanation: _____
    _____
    _____
    _____
    _____

5. The **hepatic parenchyma** shows a **micronodular fibrotic pattern**. There are no large tumors or nodules. The gallbladder is thin-walled. It contains greater than 100 dark green calculi, varying from 1 mm to 1.2 cm in greatest diameter. The **extrahepatic biliary ducts** are **patent** and undilated.

    Explanation: _____
    _____
    _____
    _____
    _____
    _____

6. On section there is minimal **atrophy** of the **renal parenchyma**. There is marked congestion of the renal tissue. The **calices** and **pelves** are patent and free of dilatation. The urinary bladder contains about 3 ounces of **turbid** yellow fluid. The mucosa of the bladder is slightly **trabeculated**.

Explanation: _____
_____
_____
_____
_____
_____

7. The scalp is **reflected**, revealing no hemorrhage in the temporal muscles, fatty tissues, or **periosteum**. The calvaria is removed, showing clear, colorless **CSF** and no **epidural**, **subdural**, or **subarachnoid hemorrhages**.

Explanation: _____
_____
_____
_____
_____
_____

8. Sections show fragments of antral and fundal-type gastric mucosa with patchy moderate chronic inflammation including some **eosinophils and neutrophils** that extends into the **glandular epithelium** in several areas associated with **neutrophilic pit abscesses**, foci of surface mucosal erosion, hemorrhage, and a few luminal neutrophil aggregates.

Explanation: _____
_____
_____
_____
_____
_____

9. Sections of the prostate gland show many foci of a well-differentiated adenocarcinoma in the **TURP** specimen. The tumor occurs mostly as well-differentiated glandular structures which have a very close, tight, back-to-back configuration. In a few areas the glandular structures are enlarged and somewhat irregular. Diagnosis: Well-differentiated adenocarcinoma of the prostate gland (**Gleason score 1 + 2 for a score of 3/10**).

Explanation: _____
_____
_____
_____
_____

10. Sections show gallbladder tissues with **necrosis** and/or absence of the **lining epithelium**, patchy moderate, acute and chronic inflammation, **fibrosis**, **vascular proliferation**, edema, and hemorrhage. Viable, intact lining epithelium is not seen. Tumor is not identified. An ascending infectious process should be considered.

DIAGNOSIS: Acute **gangrenous and chronic calculous cholecystitis**.

Explanation: _____
_____
_____
_____
_____

Sample Reports

Sample pathology reports appear on the following pages, illustrating a variety of reports. Fictional names are provided for illustration of proper format, and no resemblance to actual persons is intended. Sample transcripts were prepared according to *The Book of Style for Medical Transcription* (AHDI).

Pathology Report

HARVICK, DIANA
#706994
DATE: 11/20/[add year]

CLINICAL HISTORY
Thrombocytopenia.

MATERIAL SUBMITTED
Spleen.

GROSS DESCRIPTION
The specimen is labeled "spleen." Received in formalin is an 80 g spleen measuring 10.0 x 7.0 x 2.5 cm. The external capsule appears discretely lobulated and wrinkled purple-gray without evidence of lacerations or discolorations. A small amount of attached fatty tissue is present throughout the hilum. Upon sectioning the parenchyma appears glistening dark red, with pinpoint bulging follicles and unremarkable trabecular architecture. No areas suggestive of infarction or hemorrhage are grossly noted. Representative sections are submitted in four cassettes (A-D).

MICROSCOPIC EXAMINATION
Sections from the spleen reveal somewhat attenuated white pulp regions with only a rare small germinal center found. The sinuses are slightly congested with slight infiltration of neutrophils. Occasional plasma cells are also found. Small collections of 2 and 3 foamy histiocytes are found in some areas. A rare megakaryocyte is also present. There is no evidence of capsular fibrosis, granuloma formation, or malignancy in the tissue submitted.

DIAGNOSES
1. Spleen: Benign splenic tissue demonstrating mild sinus congestion together with small aggregates of foamy histiocytes.
2. No evidence of malignancy.

JOYCE LADINE, MD

JL:hpi
d&t: 11/21/[add year]

Surgical Specimen Cytology

NEEL, SUSAN ELLEN
#291863
Surgery: 8/21/[add year]

GROSS DESCRIPTION

Specimen #1 is received in the fresh state and consists of a nodular-shaped fragment of dark brown, firm, friable tissue. The received specimen measures 1.9 x 1.5 x 0.8 cm in greatest dimension. On sectioning there is noted an area that has a tannish-brown color and a firm, friable consistency. This area measures 1.2 cm in diameter. A frozen section is performed on the specimen and is submitted in entirety for histologic study and labeled "1A." Additional sections are submitted for histologic study and are labeled "1B."

Specimen #2 is received in the fresh state and consists of a segment of right colon with cecum and attached segment of terminal ileum. The segment of right colon measures 46 cm in length. The segment of terminal ileum measures 8.9 cm in length. The serosal adipose tissue is marked by irregular focal areas of surgical trauma. There is noted an obstructing napkin-ring-shaped lesion within the right colon. This lesion measures 3.9 cm in greatest dimension. It shows edges which are rolled. There is central ulceration in this lesion. This lesion is located 17.5 cm from the distal margin of resection and 30 cm from the ileocecal valve. The proximal and distal margins of resection are seen to be free of tumor. The segment of right colon, which is proximal to this obstructing lesion, is dilated. There is marked hyperemia to the mucosal surface. No polyps are seen. An irregular globular-shaped fragment of omental tissue is seen attached to the surface of the colon. The omental tissue shows focal areas of hemorrhage. There is not seen any gross area of metastatic tumor. Representative sections are submitted from the following areas for histologic study: A) primary lesion; B) proximal margin of resection; C) distal margin of resection; D) serosal surface over the lesion; E) mesenteric lymph nodes; F) omental tissue.

FROZEN TISSUE DIAGNOSIS

Biopsy of right hepatic nodule: Metastatic adenocarcinoma.

MICROSCOPIC EXAMINATION

Specimen #1 consists of multiple sections of biopsy of a right hepatic nodule. The sections demonstrate, within the parenchyma, a metastatic focus of hyperchromic nuclei with prominent nucleoli. Atypical mitoses are seen. The majority of the tumor shows distinct gland formation. Within the malignant glandular structures, the cells show loss of orientation and polarity. There is evidence of mucin production within the malignant glandular structures. The adjacent liver parenchyma shows no evidence of any hepatitis or granulomatous disease.

Specimen #2: Multiple sections from the primary lesion within the right colon show a moderately well differentiated adenocarcinoma arising from the mucosal surface. This is moderately well differentiated adenocarcinoma which extends into the lamina propria. There is extension into the muscularis. There is minimal extension into the adenocarcinoma. Proximal and distal margins of resection are free of adenocarcinoma. Several sections from the right colon show several distinct diverticula. Sections from 17 mesenteric lymph nodes are examined histologically. One of the 17 lymph nodes is positive for

(continued)

Surgical Specimen Cytology *(continued)*

NEEL, SUSAN ELLEN
#291863
SURGERY: 8/21/[add year]
Page 2

metastatic adenocarcinoma. A section from omental tissue shows edema and congestion to the omental tissues. The omental tissue shows no evidence of any metastatic adenocarcinoma.

PATHOLOGIC DIAGNOSES
1. Biopsy right hepatic dome nodule: Metastatic mucin-secreting adenocarcinoma. (56-8146, I)
2. Right colon (extended): Moderately well differentiated adenocarcinoma arising from the mucosal surface of the right colon. This is an obstructing napkin-ring-shaped, moderately well differentiated adenocarcinoma. The proximal and distal margins of resection are free of adenocarcinoma. Several diverticula are seen both proximal and distal to the adenocarcinoma. One of 17 mesenteric lymph nodes is positive for metastatic adenocarcinoma. The received omental tissue shows edema and congestion with no areas of metastatic adenocarcinoma. (67-8143, I)

CHARLES OHMAN, MD

CO:hpi
d&t: 8/21/[add year]

Autopsy, Gross and Microscopic

CAMPBELL, ALEXANDER
#736076
Expired: 10/14/[add year]

GROSS DESCRIPTION

EXTERNAL EXAMINATION
The body is that of a tall, somewhat obese Caucasian male who appears his stated age of 67 years. There is a white hypopigmented horizontal lesion located in the right mid abdomen, measuring up to 4 cm in maximal length. This may represent an old well-healed surgical scar. The patient has gray-brown hair in the normal distribution. The pupils are symmetric and measure 0.5 cm bilaterally. The face and neck are cyanotic. The chest appears symmetric. The abdomen is obese and distended. The extremities are symmetric and contain no obvious ulcerations.

INTERNAL EXAMINATION
A Y-shaped incision is made in the usual fashion, opening the thoracic and abdominal cavities. The pleural cavities and the pericardium contain no obvious adhesions or effusions. The abdominal cavity contains no ascites. There are no obvious abnormalities in the locations of the thoracic and abdominal organs.

Heart: The heart weighs 560 g. The epicardial surface is smooth and unremarkable. The coronary arteries show moderate atherosclerosis mainly involving the left anterior descending artery. Cross sections through the myocardium reveal no obvious focal scarring or recent infarct.

Gastrointestinal tract: The mucosal surfaces of the esophagus, stomach, small and large intestines are smooth and unremarkable.

Liver: The liver weighs 1500 g. The serosal surface contains one small white round discoloration on the superior surface of the right lobe measuring up to 0.3 cm in maximal dimension. Sectioning through the liver parenchyma reveals a somewhat nutmeg appearance. No obvious nodules or focal lesions are seen.

Spleen: The spleen weighs 380 g. The spleen parenchyma is markedly congested. However, no obvious nodules or focal lesions are seen.

Pancreas: The pancreas is of normal size and appearance. No obvious nodules or focal lesions are seen.

Kidneys: The right and left kidneys each weigh 210 g. The cortical surfaces of both kidneys are somewhat granular. Sectioning through the parenchyma reveals no obvious nodules or focal lesions.

Pelvic organs: The bladder mucosa is smooth and unremarkable. The prostate is somewhat nodular and irregular. Sectioning through the testes reveals no obvious nodules or focal lesions.

Vascular system: The distal aorta shows moderate atherosclerosis. No obvious thrombus formation is noted.

(continued)

Autopsy, Gross and Microscopic

CAMPBELL, ALEXANDER
#736076
Page 2

Bone marrow: The bone marrow is red and of normal consistency. No focal lesions are seen.

Nervous system: The formalin-fixed brain without dura mater weighs 1300 g (1220 g prior to fixation, 1289 g following draining of ventricular cerebrospinal fluid). The cerebellum weighs 138 g. The dura mater over the cerebral convexity is unremarkable. The superior sagittal sinus is patent and unremarkable. The cerebral hemispheres are symmetrical and show no edema or atrophy. No convolutional abnormality is recognized. The leptomeninx is thin and translucent.

The cranial nerves show no gross abnormality. The major cerebral arteries are well preserved and show moderate to marked atherosclerosis. The calvaria and dura are unremarkable. The cerebral hemispheres are symmetric and show no obvious edema or herniation.

GROSS IMPRESSION
Moderate to marked atherosclerosis of the cerebral arteries.

MICROSCOPIC DESCRIPTION

Heart: The anterior left ventricular wall and left main coronary artery show myocardial hypertrophy, focal myocardial scarring, and moderate atherosclerosis. The anterior left ventricular wall and left anterior descending artery show myocardial hypertrophy, increased interstitial and perivascular fibrosis, and marked atherosclerosis with 80% luminal occlusion. The anterolateral left ventricular wall and left circumflex arteries show myocardial hypertrophy, perivascular fibrosis, and moderate atherosclerosis with 60% luminal occlusion. The lateral left ventricular wall, posterolateral left ventricular wall, posterior left ventricular wall, and posterior interventricular wall show myocardial hypertrophy and perivascular fibrosis. The mid-interventricular septum shows myocardial hypertrophy. The anterior interventricular septum shows myocardial hypertrophy and perivascular fibrosis. The anterior right ventricular wall and right coronary artery demonstrate mild atherosclerosis. The posterior right ventricular wall shows no significant histopathology.

Lungs: The right lung periphery shows marked congestion and edema, as do the right lung hilum, left lung periphery, and left lung hilum.

Esophagus, stomach, small and large intestines: There is autolysis present.

Liver: The liver shows centrilobular congestion.

Spleen and pancreas: The spleen shows congestion. The pancreas demonstrates autolysis.

(continued)

Autopsy, Gross and Microscopic

CAMPBELL, ALEXANDER
#736076
Page 3

Kidneys and adrenals: There are autolysis and occasional totally sclerosed glomeruli of the right and left kidneys and adrenals.

Bladder, prostate, right and left testes: Benign prostatic hypertrophy is present.

Aorta and bone marrow: Mild to moderate atherosclerosis is demonstrated.

Brain: Serial coronal sections of the cerebral hemispheres show symmetrical lateral ventricles which are covered by a smooth ependymal lining. The cerebral cortex and white matter are unremarkable. The corpora striata, thalami, and hippocampi reveal no gross pathology. Serial horizontal sections of the brain stem demonstrate no gross lesions. Upon serial sagittal sections, the cerebellum is unremarkable.

MAJOR PATHOLOGIC DIAGNOSES
1. Moderate to marked atherosclerosis, coronary arteries and distal abdominal aorta.
2. Cardiomegaly (560 g).
3. Marked bilateral pulmonary congestion and edema.
4. Passive congestion of liver and spleen with splenomegaly (380 g).
5. Diabetes mellitus.

CAUSE OF DEATH
Atherosclerotic heart disease.

DAVID GALLARDO, MD

DG:hpi

d&t: 10/15/[add year]

Comic Relief

Incorrect	Correct
The tumor is attached to the mucosal surface by a broad pedestal and a tapering stock.	The tumor is attached to the mucosal surface by a broad pedicle and a tapering stalk.
Cause of death: Subarachnoid hemorrhoid due to trauma.	Cause of death: Subarachnoid hemorrhage due to trauma.
Vocal hemorrhages are grossly visible throughout both cerebral hemispheres.	Focal hemorrhages are grossly visible throughout both cerebral hemispheres.
Anasarca and widespread visceral edema indicate longstanding watery tension.	Anasarca and widespread visceral edema indicate longstanding water retention.
There is a zone of ecchymosis and crepitus overlying the left-off septal boss.	There is a zone of ecchymosis and crepitus overlying the left occipital boss.
Received informally is a mess of partially decomposed tissue with prominent vascular elephants.	Received in formalin is a mass of partially decomposed tissue with prominent vascular elements.

PEARSON
myhealthprofessionskit™

To access the online exercises and transcription practice, go to **www.myhealthprofessionskit.com**. Select "Medical Transcription," then click on the title of this book, ***Healthcare Documentation: Fundamentals & Practice***. Then click on the Pathology chapter.

Professional Issues

Learning Objectives

▶ Compare and contrast different work environments and options for medical transcriptionists.

▶ Evaluate questions and considerations that should be taken into account when choosing employment in healthcare documentation.

▶ Define and illustrate the components of a good cover letter and resumé.

▶ Describe and employ recommended strategies for searching for employment.

▶ List several strategies for obtaining opportunities to take employment tests even after being turned down for employment.

▶ Apply strategies for alleviating test anxiety and improving performance on employment tests.

▶ Differentiate among the different types of employment tests.

▶ List and describe various employment and networking resources.

▶ Describe and apply healthy ergonomic practices

Professional Issues:
Where to Work

Medical transcriptionists (MTs) work for hospitals, multispecialty clinics, physician practices, transcription companies, home offices, radiology clinics, pathology laboratories, tumor boards, law offices, and even veterinary hospitals. Some work as employees; others prefer the independence of being freelance MTs or independent contractors (ICs).

Qualified MTs may eventually become supervisors, managers, quality assurance specialists, proofreaders, speech recognition editors, and teachers, while others may establish their own transcription companies. In the not-too-distant future, some transcriptionists may become healthcare data integration analysts—ensuring the accuracy, completeness, and continuity of the patient's healthcare record.

Medical transcriptionists' earnings vary according to geographic area, skill level, place of employment, and method of compensation. MTs working for companies in large metropolitan areas generally earn more than those in smaller cities. Some facilities have incentive pay plans where transcriptionists are paid a bonus over and above the minimum production level and base pay for that facility; others pay on production alone. Production pay, contrary to some opinions, isn't always better than hourly, especially when how much you can produce per hour is impacted by so many things, like account mix, hardware, software, availability of support staff, and so on. The Bureau of Labor Statistics (**bls.gov**) Occupational Outlook Handbook provides up-to-date information on job outlook and median income for medical transcriptionists

Job opportunities exist all over the United States and Canada and in American hospitals in foreign countries. In addition to choice of work setting, transcriptionists can often find part-time or full-time employment with flexible scheduling. Furthermore, through the miracle of technology and high-speed Internet access, transcriptionists may live in the Deep South and work for a transcription service in the Pacific Northwest. A transcriptionist may move from the East Coast to the West Coast and never change employers.

Advances in technology have also made it possible for the blind or visually impaired and those confined to wheelchairs to become medical transcriptionists.

Hospitals and Medical Centers

Many hospitals have sent their transcriptionists home to work remotely or outsourced their transcription to a medical transcription service. However, MTs who perform specialty transcription, such as radiology or pathology, may work within or adjacent to those departments.

Hospitals may offer competitive salary and benefit packages, particularly larger hospitals in metropolitan areas. In addition, many offer some type of incentive pay plan that has the potential to increase income for productive MTs. In addition, some hospitals reimburse part or all of the tuition for advanced degrees or courses related to one's job.

Hospitals offer opportunities for advancement into supervisory positions for motivated employees. Hospital transcription provides a wide range of dictation types, covering all medical specialties and challenging areas of interest to transcriptionists. Facilities and equipment are often state of the art.

Even when working remotely, many hospital transcriptionists have access to the hospital's server, allowing them to check a patient's prescriptions for an unclear drug or dosage or the laboratory data for unintelligible lab results. Similar reports by a difficult physician may be consulted in order to fill in blanks caused by unclear dictation. Demographic data is usually imported into the document with the press of a single key or key combination.

Disadvantages of working in the hospital setting may include lack of autonomy, inflexible scheduling, a lackluster environment if on-site, supervisory personnel who are unfamiliar with or unsympathetic to the needs of transcriptionists, and the frustration of dealing with hospital bureaucracies. With the advent of managed care and its associated cost-cutting, more hospitals are outsourcing their medical transcription to transcription services.

A medical transcription student, almost without exception, is not prepared to move directly from the classroom to the hospital setting as a transcriptionist. It is virtually impossible to prepare most students to transcribe with the accuracy and efficiency required by inpatient transcription departments. Students may want to find positions transcribing for a solo physician, for a group practice, or for a transcription service. Once you have achieved enough experience to be productive and efficient, then the hospital setting is a realistic goal.

Physician Offices and Clinics

The small office environment can be decidedly more personal, often providing a family-like atmosphere. Employees in such environments may enjoy medical and retirement benefits and a predictable income, although with the decline in physician income due to managed care, some offices no longer offer benefits to their employees. Physician office or clinic hours may more readily accommodate the needs of MTs with school-age children, seldom requiring weekend work. In addition, transcriptionists may enjoy the direct contact with physicians, who may be more appreciative of their work, more accessible for questions, and more willing to take the time to teach and offer feedback—a real advantage to the new MT.

While the transcriptionist in a physician's office or clinic may become more proficient with practice, there are fewer opportunities for advancement in this environment, and the dictation will offer less of a challenge to the MT hoping to expand their knowledge and skills.

Transcription Services (MTSOs)

Employees of transcription companies usually enjoy competitive rates of pay. Because they transcribe a variety of dictation from different accounts (physician offices, clinics, hospitals), their skills are continually challenged. There may be greater flexibility of work schedules.

Disadvantages of working for a transcription service can include absence of immediate feedback concerning questions about dictation. The same resources an off-site employee of a hospital has access to are often not available to the employee of a service working on the same account. Client specifications and physician lists are often out-of-date or incomplete. Each client often has its own formats and specifications, and being switched from one client to another may adversely affect production.

Compensation may be based entirely on production, so that a day of poor-quality dictation, lack of dictation available for transcription, or personal illness can wreak havoc with the transcriptionist's income. Benefit packages may not be as comprehensive as those offered by a hospital, and health insurance is often unavailable. However, some transcription services are responding to the shortage of qualified transcriptionists by offering attractive benefit packages.

Freelance Transcription

Freelance transcriptionists function as independent contractors, most often working from home, although some prefer to maintain offices outside their homes. Because they are solo workers, few of them can individually handle the volume of a hospital account, but some transcribe hospital overflow (the excess of dictation that cannot be handled by a hospital's transcriptionists).

Advantages of freelancing include a sense of accomplishment and independence, high self-esteem, pride in entrepreneurship, and the opportunity to work flexible hours. For those who choose to work at home, the advantages also include decreased costs for transportation, including nonproductive commuting time, and office wardrobe.

For the freelance MT, disadvantages can include the burden of having to handle all areas of a business, including bookkeeping, arranging for pickup of dictation and delivery of finished work to each client's office, the cost of equipment and repair, and the need for finding other MTs to cover during times of overload, vacation, or sickness. The unpredictable level of income, difficulty with financial planning, lack of affordable medical benefits, and the necessity for complying with the IRS and other regulatory agencies are other disadvantages. Unless children are old enough to fend for themselves, childcare is still a necessity.

The transcriptionist working from home must be prepared to practice self-discipline and deal with distractions created by family members, neighbors, solicitors, and the telephone. Some at-home MTs complain that they are never able to "get away" from their work, household chores, or family concerns that demand their attention. Finally, there is often a sense of isolation, and the inability to ask questions or network with other transcriptionists and physicians can prove frustrating.

Other Employment Settings

Medical transcriptionists are often employed by insurance companies or government facilities. Others combine their transcription skills with clinical skills to function as medical assistants. Still others work in medical research facilities or tumor registries. In law offices that specialize in personal injury or medical malpractice cases, medical transcriptionists may be employed to analyze discrepancies in health records and translate medical language in a chart into lay language for attorneys.

Within all of these settings, MTs may perform transcription, or they may act as supervisors, managers, or quality assurance experts. MTs with strong technical skills have often transitioned to roles within the hospital's information technology department. In addition, many are called upon to teach medical transcription within hospitals, in community colleges, at vocational/technical schools, or in court-reporting schools. A few MTs have found alternative job pathways as researchers, editors, consultants, and authors in the areas of the publishing industry that service medical transcription.

Employment Options

by Judy Hinickle

The possibilities of employment in the transcription field today have increased in scope and variety. Many people are faced with decisions or options not open to them even 10 years ago.

Transcriptionists are paid in various employment settings by the hour, by production, by a combination of the two, or with the profits of self-employment. All sorts of personal needs are taken into consideration with each. Do you need the security of hourly wages or a salary? Or would you rather take risks that you will make more money when paid by production or through self-employment? Does a spotlight on production statistics cause you too much stress, or do you thrive on the challenge?

What about the other areas of compensation? Benefits are a major method of compensation, but perhaps we should consider whether a specific employer is the best choice for obtaining maximum benefits. Would you take a job because of the medical insurance, or the profit sharing, or the pension plan? Or would you rather make a better wage with a job having no benefits and make your own provisions for insurance, investment, and retirement?

When looking at these wage and benefit issues, MTs need to consider trade-offs. If your choice of employment gives you none of the benefits which traditionally equate to 25-33% of your wages, are you then getting that in cash and applying it to those benefits? As an independent contractor with no benefits, are you making that additional 25-33% after expenses so that you can pay your taxes and also purchase the insurance and a pension plan independently? If self-employed, do your wages and profit after expenses equal or exceed an equivalent wage and benefit package in a traditional setting?

There are, of course, lifestyle and personal benefits to be considered in alternate employment settings, but you must be careful not to shortchange your financial future with short-sightedness now.

Once you get past wage and investment issues, personal ability and satisfaction become important. What kind of work hours does your lifestyle require? How much responsibility do you want to accept? Do you like to supervise? Teach? Do you like to "plug in and tune out"? Would you rather not deal with people? Do you like taking risks? Do you think self-employment means there is no one to answer to? Do you want to work a certain number of hours per week and no more?

There are many things to consider in your employment decisions—certainly more than are described here. Within each opportunity you need to balance the wage and benefit issues with the personal fulfillment and family issues, and the spirit of independence with the risks of less security. Being aware of your own personal needs and giving them priority levels, while keeping a watchful eye on the future, will help ensure fruitful decisions.

> ### Pause for Reflection
>
> 1. Differentiate among the different work settings; what are the pros and cons of each setting?
> 2. Of the various options to be considered when seeking employment (compensation, benefits, schedule, environment), which are more important for you? Why?

Getting That First Job
Applying for Employment

by Ellen A. Drake

If you're like most students, you've been thinking about the job you want since your first days as a student, how much you're going to make, and how you're going to spend all that money. You probably have also been planning ahead and preparing your resumé, practicing for interviews, and learning all that you can so that you can make the best impression possible on a potential employer and live up to that impression.

There are many sources of information to help you in preparing a resumé, writing an application letter, and putting your best foot forward in an interview. Your school may have classes to help you. The counseling office or learning/tutoring center at your school may be able to help. The library has numerous references, and even some student dictionaries give advice in the appendix on preparing resumés. The Internet is also an excellent resource for this. It is common, today, to complete the entire application process online with cover letters and resumés being submitted via email and applications completed electronically.

Application letters. Application letters are written to accompany resumés, indicate the job you want, highlight your strengths, and state your availability for an interview. They should be only a page long, no more. If you are sending your resumé to the Human Resources Department of a large clinic or hospital, you may want to send a copy to the transcription supervisor as well, or at the very least, telephone to say that you have sent your resumé to the Human Resources Department. Be sure to proofread your letter and resumé carefully. In the area of transcription, quality is all-important, and many supervisors would look no further than the first error before discarding your application.

Resumés. The purpose of your resumé is to persuade an employer to interview you. It must look professional and present your qualifications in the best possible manner. It should be specific for the position for which you are applying. A resumé should be limited to one page if possible and should contain the following categories of information:

1. **Personal data**. Name, address, telephone number, email address. Age and marital status are not included.

2. **Educational background**. Include names of schools, degrees, areas of special training, certifications and credentials, and academic awards. You might also mention the medical specialties covered in your training program and that the dictation you transcribed was actual physician dictation (not reports read by actors or other readers).

3. **Work experience**. If work experience is unrelated to the position applied for, explain how the experience you've gained in the jobs you've held can be applied to the position you are seeking. Include any internship or practicum experience, and give dates.

4. **References**. Just list names and addresses; don't include actual letters at this point. Take the letters of recommendation to your interview. Be sure that you have contacted each of your references to be sure it is okay for you to list them. You do not want to list anyone who may give you a noncommittal or even negative recommendation.

5. **Professional affiliations**. Be sure to include professional association membership on the national, state/regional, and local level, any offices held, awards, and published works.

Testing. You should take as many on-line employment tests as you can; I have known many excellent students who surprised a potential employer by doing well on the screening tests. See Georgia Green's essay on Skills Testing for Employment in this chapter.

Although it may take longer and you may have to work harder to find a job due to your inexperience, it should not be impossible. Being inexperienced is an employment issue in almost every industry, not just medical transcription.

Job Searching Advice
by Sarah Barton

As a new MT graduate I found the job search to be pretty overwhelming. You rarely see transcription jobs advertised in the places we would find other jobs, such as a local paper or job bank, and it takes some time to find a mentor or employer willing to invest the significant time into getting a new transcriptionist up to quality and production goals.

Like many MT students I had chosen this path to further my education because I needed to be at home but also needed to bring in an income. I had education in sports medicine but had been a stay-at-home mother for nine years, lived in a small military town that didn't have an exciting job market, and I had four children, two of them not yet in school. I knew, like many of you did when you chose this path, that the cost of childcare would leave me with very little take-home pay. I very carefully selected what school to attend and felt I was on my way to have the best of both worlds—a career while staying at home with my children.

I waited until I graduated from my medical transcription program to begin applying for jobs, but I did start looking and familiarizing myself with the process a few weeks ahead of time. After reading countless discussions that had convinced me I might never find a job, just three weeks after graduation I had three offers to choose from and one was from my first choice company. A week after that I started. I was fortunate to find a position that paid hourly for six months while I got up to speed. I am not going to tell you those jobs are common or even easy to come by, but I know they do exist because I had one of them. I can't say I was top of the class in transcription school either but I was a very hard worker.

Finding a job probably feels pretty overwhelming to you too. While you might not want to start the search until you've actually completed your training, you can lay a foundation starting on the first day of school. I cannot encourage you enough to view your time as a student as a time of being a professional. Remember, today's graduate mentor could be tomorrow's MT recruiter. Here are some tips that I found helpful.

1. **Begin networking on your first day of school.** Make contacts and always present yourself as a professional. Don't share things you wouldn't want coworkers to know. Don't say inflammatory things on chat sites or MT groups because those same people could be hiring you one day. Get involved in the student alliance of your professional organization. Networking is powerful! Social networking sites have a number of open MT groups. Make sure your photograph on your profile is one you wouldn't mind a boss seeing, keep topics that commonly create conflict off your page, and act in a professional manner.

2. **Social networking** can be a great tool but it can also be your professional demise if you're not careful. Make sure you have nothing out there that could offend a recruiter or indicate that you're anything but someone who will be a great employee or independent contractor. If you feel a recruiter is rude, do not post that. Do not publicly trash a company. Recruiters do check Facebook, I promise.

3. If you have attended an MT training program that you know has an outstanding reputation and the name of your school alone could get you an interview, it is worth considering putting your **education** at the top of your resume instead of midway through. For me that meant putting education as the first section on my resume. I wanted the recruiter to see it at first glance. Believe me, that opened a lot of doors. My skills got me hired but the name of my school opened the door. If you have an RHDS or other professional credential, be sure to put the initials after your name right at the top of your resume. I have discussed this topic with an MT recruiter numerous times and she told me that 10-second rule really applies. Your resume needs to impress a recruiter in 10 seconds flat.

4. **Be careful what you put on a resume.** If you have a year of experience volunteering with an activity that involves a controversial issue, then you have to decide how that might be perceived. I am not telling you not to put this on your resume, but I am encouraging you to put some thought into every detail.

5. Have a second set of eyes **review your resume**. Your school may have someone available to do this. I sent mine to our student coordinator and she gave me a few tips. I had a rough start in MT school because I went into it thinking that with five-plus years of college behind me, it would be easy. As most of you know, it was far from easy. We were not assigned a GPA but I was often asked for my average score. Overall I had a 96% average, and in the MT world where only 98% and above is acceptable for accuracy, that might not be impressive. In the last module of the course I had pulled it together and had a 99% average. Our wonderful student coordinator advised me to focus on those scores. In the description of my education I wrote, "Attained 99% average level of accuracy in the advanced transcription module." I focused on the positive. Also remember you're applying for a job that requires attention to detail so it has to be perfect. You cannot have spelling or grammar errors on your resume.

6. Start making a list now of all the **MTSOs** and any medical facilities that hire MTs. I spent hours doing this before graduation but I would advise not getting distracted from your studies. There are lists on-line but there are far more than the lists have. The Internet is your friend.

7. With the lists you've made, you're going to want to **get organized**. Whom do you want to work for? If you know, as I did, apply to them after you've tested with other companies if possible. Work out your test-taking nerves before testing with your top choices. We all bombed our first tests! As you apply to those companies, write yourself a note on this list. As you receive e-mails back (and you won't get many), you should note if they rejected you, why, and anything else important. Make a note if you tested and also how you applied (application versus sending a resume).

8. You need **two versions of your resume**. You need a copy-and-paste version with no formatting, and you need one you can send as an attachment that does have formatting. Many applications will require you to paste a resume into a text box and the cut and paste version of your resume will be handy.

9. To make your life easier, start writing out **answers to application questions** in Word. You will encounter many applications that have questions with text boxes for your answer. If you have to fill out each and every one of them from scratch, it will be very time consuming. You can save these answers and next time you encounter a similar question just copy it into an application. They all tend to ask the same questions. After a while I caught on to this, and the process became

much easier after I had my document of answers ready to paste into the application. If you make applications a full-time job like I did, you will be very glad you took this bit of advice.

10. Have a **cover letter** ready. I had a nice one that I shared on my school board for others to use if they want. Perhaps someone has done the same at your school.

11. **Apply** no matter what the requirements are. Having gone to a reputable school, I knew that people often hired us because they knew we were ready to hit the ground running, so I applied no matter how much experience was required. If nothing else, applying gives you the experience of applying and possibly of testing. Testing is a very valuable experience. As I said earlier, you need to work your testing nerves out somewhere.

12. Get the **RHDS** (registered healthcare documentation specialist) **credential**. This shows a commitment to your professional advancement and a basic understanding of medical transcription.

13. **Follow up on applications**. I always gave it a week (this is why you have to stay organized and make notes) and then followed up with a very brief e-mail. You have to be careful to walk the line between being proactive and being annoying.

14. **Know what you're willing to do and be flexible**. If you will only work weekdays from nine to five, good luck finding a job. Acute care is going to need weekend work. MTSOs always need second and third shift and they pay a differential for it. If you are truly flexible, you will make yourself more marketable. If you know you cannot do weekends or odd hours, don't say you can. Be as flexible as you can be while being realistic. The more inflexible you are, the harder it is to find a job. Also know what you're willing to work for. I turned down offers that I felt were too low. This is a personal decision and many new MTs are willing to work for a less-than-ideal wage to get some experience.

15. Handle your **phone interviews** exactly as you would a face-to-face interview. You would not bring your children or your barking dog or your television to an interview in person so don't bring them to your phone interview either. Have a quiet environment and focus on your interview. It helped me to anticipate questions and have notes ready with answers. I anticipated behavioral interview questions like, "Tell me about a time you had to work with a difficult person." That made it so much easier and kept me from rambling too much. I was always asked about my computer so I wrote down my computer specifications (what version

of Windows, how much RAM, etc). Anything you can anticipate being discussed is helpful in preparing.

16. Lastly, grow a "thick skin" now and **be ready for rejection**. We were all rejected over and over and over again, and sometimes not so politely, before we got our first job. You are going to get canned e-mails telling you that you don't have enough experience. You may get e-mails back asking if you can comprehend English because the ad asked for experience. Most rejections will come in the form of no response at all. One day you'll get that e-mail you've been waiting for and this will all seem worth it. With dedication to your skill, perseverance in the job search, and marketing yourself well, you will become a working medical transcriptionist. Just hang in there and keep applying!

Skills Testing for Employment

by Georgia Green

So you've been spurned by a recruiter looking for experienced MTs to fill their vacancies. How do you turn a "no" into a "yes" and get a testing opportunity?

Start by doing your homework. How many workstations can this employer afford to devote to bringing a novice along and how are they currently staffed? How can you get this information? Is this the right job for you—does the available workload realistically match your skill set? If a workstation is potentially available in the near future, how can you ensure that you are considered for the job?

First, you need to show off your skills. There are several ways to get a testing opportunity:

1. Ask for it straight out.

2. Bond with your contact (on the phone or in person) and build sympathy for your cause. Bonding can be handled in the usual friendly way—get someone to laugh with you or find something in common. Ask for advice. Nothing warms up experienced MTs to your cause more than asking how they got started and who gave them their first opportunities.

3. If you hit a brick wall, try to go through someone else in the same office. If you always get the receptionist when you call and it is her job to "screen out newbies," you need to call at another time to get someone more sympathetic. Here is a tip: Managers work late! Call after the receptionist has gone home. But be careful not to come off as a pest or stalker. If you need to call a number of times to get someone else, don't give your name each time. If you are told to get lost, wait a reasonable time before trying again. If you are having trou-

ble relating to that idea, just think of a time you ever felt hounded by someone. It makes it hard to hear the message of the perceived hounder.

4. Go through someone else outside of the company—use your networking contacts to get someone to make an introduction and secure you a testing opportunity.

5. Ask your contact at this company to refer you to an associate in another company that can offer you a test.

6. Ask for a "mercy test": "I know you can't take me on, but can you just give me a test so I can see where I stand and what I should work on to prepare myself for a future opportunity with your company?" That will always work so long as you haven't annoyed anyone and you catch someone at the right time. As a supervisor or manager, I fell for it every single time if the message was presented in the right way.

7. Remember that there is more than one fish in the sea. If you can't get through one door, find another. I had an applicant I wanted to hire but his geographical location just didn't suit the needs of the office I was hiring for unless he could work full time. He couldn't do this, so there was nothing I could offer him. He needed to look elsewhere, but I don't think he ever got over his disappointment that I couldn't help him.

Overcoming Barriers to Success

• **Test anxiety** is the primary cause of failed tests. Tips for dealing with test anxiety include mastering the list of Do's and Don'ts that follow. Get adequate sleep and lay out everything in advance. If the test is given on-site, arrive early (practice the route you will drive to an on-site test), practice deep breathing and relaxation exercises. Imagine how you would handle a worst case scenario so that you can manage anything. Test for a job you know you don't want both for practice and for the joy of refusing a job opportunity (in case you get an offer!).

Lack of preparedness. Use the tips below to be prepared.

• **An unmatched skill set.** If your training did not include authentic dictation or enough practice hours, you are wasting your time applying for an acute care position or a multidictator environment. Look for a position that matches your existing skill set and then upgrade your skills. Some services do offer limited-dictator environment opportunities and will train you one dictator at a time. Use your networking skills to locate these opportunities.

• **Poor skills.** In spite of a lack of exposure to adequate authentic dictation, your grammar, spelling, and referencing skills can and should be top notch. If not, hit the books and bone up.

Do's and Don'ts

1. Do stay professional at all times even if you think you are alone. Applicants who display a "can do" attitude are given the benefit of the doubt in a borderline test.

This is what can happen. Recently someone I recommended for a position was not hired, and when I asked the employer the real reason for the nonhire (I knew the student had a good skill set), she said it was because her clerk had overheard the applicant swearing and grumbling under her breath at the testing station. She said she felt the applicant would be difficult to work with. I personally know this student to be a thoroughly professional individual who would make a great employee. She just goofed in this one area because she thought she was alone.

2. Never fabricate experience to get a test. By all means, build up the experiences you've had, but never lie to get a test because it will come back to haunt you.

3. Don't complain even if hit with the unexpected. Sometimes how you deal with the unexpected is actually part of the test. One employer used a ridiculously substandard workstation to "test the ingenuity and patience" of applicants. I don't agree with this technique, but it has been done.

4. Be prepared for every eventuality. Ask questions in advance of the employer and among your networking group so that you can anticipate as much as possible.

5. Dress right for the part. Even though you may wear your jammies when you work at home, wear business attire when applying for a job. This seems obvious, but you'd be surprised at how some people interpret "business attire." This is true even if you know for a fact that everyone in the office wears jeans and sweatshirts.

6. Keep your conversation professional. Never share details of your personal life, medical condition, and so on, even if you are baited into doing so. Resist this temptation, as it is likely to be held against you.

7. Keep your cool no matter what happens.

Strategies for Different Test Types

What is going to be on the test? Everyone tests differently, but here is an overview of what to prepare for. There is one primary screening instrument and one secondary, plus a whole host of other tests that may be administered. Let's go over each:

On-site transcription test. Ask in advance whether you will be allowed to use references and whether you can bring your own. If they provide references, find out which ones they use and become familiar with them. Ask what the test will cover. If it includes operative reports and you have little or no surgery transcription experience, own up to this prior to the test. Be prepared for every report type (i.e., find out what is unique about ops!). Ask about time limits and how much dictation you will be asked to do—and practice timing yourself. Remember it is always better to leave a blank than guess. Ask for instructions about blanks—do they want an underscore, a space, or a ("sounds like"). Don't rely on a spellchecker even if one is available. Most test sites won't care what format you use, but don't second-guess this—ask in advance.

Remote transcription test from your home office. Ask what references and resources you may use. Never assume a spellchecker is equivalent to looking something up—it isn't. The odds are that a better performance is expected with an off-site test since the testing situation cannot be monitored. If you are not told not to ask someone to proofread your work, plan to do so. In an uncontrolled testing environment, a valid test takes into account the fact that the applicant may have had some kind of outside help. If it is made clear to you that you are not to do so, follow the test instructions and let the employer know that your work is in fact your own.

Spelling test. Bone up on spelling, common abbreviations, and so on in advance. Take practice tests. Consult lists of frequently misspelled medical and English words. And if a spelling test or any written instrument is administered off-site, you can expect that only a 100% score is acceptable because it would be assumed that you had every possible reference available and possibly even asked for help from a friend (even if you did not).

Grammar test. Bone up on this as well. Take practice tests. There is no excuse for not doing well on a grammar test. Good grammar skills are a prerequisite for being an MT.

Written test of medical knowledge. Be comfortable with the multiple-choice format. Take practice tests.

Auditory discrimination—a dictated or written test of terms that sound alike or are similar in some way. You can find these kinds of test items in most transcription training materials, including *The Medical Transcription Workbook* by Health Professions Institute. Prepare for this, e.g., you should know there is an *ileum* and an *ilium* and which is which.

Editing skills. You may be given a proofreading test. This is also something you can practice in advance. Learn what errors are most egregious and which ones are most common.

Decision making/judgment. "What would you do if . . . ?" A test of this nature relies on common sense and your knowledge of confidentiality laws, ethics, and so on.

Reference book skills. You should know about all the common reference books found in the MT workplace, what they look like, and how to use them. You should be able to rattle off the names if asked. Get your hands on them even if you can't buy them (try bookstores and libraries) and read the preface material to help you know how they are organized.

Keyboarding. An inexpensive typing tutor program can be relied upon to bring your basic keyboarding up to 60-75 wpm in short order. Even though actual keyboarding speed has little relationship with transcription speed, a big deficit in keyboarding can impact your productivity. PLUS some human resource departments place way too much emphasis on this. Be prepared for something ridiculous like a copy-typing test.

Basic computer knowledge. You need to know how to use Windows and Microsoft Word. You need to know how to name and transfer files in each environment. You need to know about your own computer system in depth if you are working at home. You should know tons of stuff about the Internet, about FTP, wav files, and so on.

Essay test. Yes, a writing sample is legitimate. In fact, I personally recommend it to employers. If you can express yourself well in writing using good grammar, spelling, and organizational skills, you have the potential to be a good MT and a good employee who communicates well with others. This is also something you can be prepared for by practicing.

Personal Interview

As noted above, never discuss your personal life, illnesses, childcare problems, and so on, even if the employer seems to invite and encourage this discussion in a friendly way. It is a way employers try to get you to admit to being a problem employee from the start.

Steady eye contact and a firm handshake are also important. Have some reasonable questions prepared in case you are asked if you have questions. Even if you have unusual work requirements, don't tell an employer in advance how inflexible you intend to be on the job if you actually want to get hired. Think in terms of getting your foot in the door, showing how valuable you can be, and then earning the right to enjoy some flexibility.

Good questions to ask: What is most important to you in a new employee? Tell me more about how you got started with this company. Bad questions: When will I get a raise? When can I begin taking time off?

Watch for trap questions. You may be asked, What do you dislike or like most in a supervisor? Why did you leave your last job (never say anything negative, even if you worked for Attila the Hun). Good comments to make: I enjoy learning something new every day. I have a great deal of respect for experienced MTs and am privileged to work closely with you and your staff. It sounds sappy but it is tried and true. Bad comments: I'm looking forward to not having to pay a babysitter and to be able to work when I feel like it. I hate picky QA people.

Real-time chat and/or e-mail interview. Never send out an e-mail that is not grammatically correct and thoroughly spell-checked. Think of every e-mail to a potential employer as an extension of your resumé. Real-time chatting can be a bit more difficult. Pay attention to your text as you type it, and do correct your mistakes as you go, even if the employer tells you not to worry about it. S/he may be evaluating your basic grammar/spelling as you "chat."

Having a Plan B: What If I Don't Get Hired?

Securing a retest. So what if you get bad news or no news at all? Consider these factors: Did your test performance reflect your true skill set and abilities? If you honestly believe that something prevented your best performance, say so and ask politely for a retest. For example, ruffled nerves because you had a car accident on your way to the interview or a death in the family the previous day; an unexpected equipment failure during the test; a legitimate misunderstanding about the test instructions—any of which might be real reasons for a retest. Some companies require time to elapse before a retest. Ask for an exception to this rule and a different test and come to the retest better prepared.

Is this job the right match for your existing skills? If not, look for opportunities that do match and/or begin revising your skill set. Ask the employer for a referral to another company that might be able to use your skill set. Expand your network. Finding entry-level opportunities is about being in the right place at the right time. Sometimes you can achieve this randomly but you increase the odds by building a network in the industry—among your new MT grad peers, among your new more-experienced peers, and among employers. Keep a notebook with names, numbers, and contact dates. Follow up regularly with everyone from the day you enroll in school until you are gainfully employed in your dream job—and then keep your notebook just in case.

Skillbuilding. Expand your experience beyond a limited-dictator environment through additional training or stair-step jobs. If you can do acute care work but feel you cannot do operative reports or foreign accents, look for work opportunities that will broaden your exposure to areas where you feel weakest.

Never Burn Bridges

Estimates of the number of MTs in the U.S. vary from 250,000 to 500,000 or more. It is a tight-knit community and we all need to work together to build the profession. Be ever vigilant about the quality of your work and your professional reputation.

Pause for Reflection

1. Describe the purpose of a cover letter.
2. Describe the components of a resumé.
3. Briefly describe the tips Sarah Barton offers for job searching and getting that first job.
4. According to Georgia Green, what are some of the ways by which you can secure a testing opportunity?
5. How can you overcome barriers to being successful on a test when you do get the opportunity?
6. What tips for preparation does Green offer?
7. Realistically evaluate your own skill set. Looking at the different kinds of employment tests that you might encounter, which one(s) might pose an extra challenge for you and why?

Employment and Networking Resources

Professional Association

AHDI (Association for Healthcare Documentation Integrity)

The professional association for medical transcriptionists and healthcare documentation specialists is AHDI (**AHDIonline.org**), formerly AAMT (American Association for Medical Transcription). Join AHDI while you are still a student. It costs much less than being an active member; you can't beat the value.

You will be a student member for a year, even if you finish your program in the next month. While you won't technically be a student anymore, you won't be asked to renew your membership until your first year of membership ends. When your student membership expires, you will be able to join AHDI as a postgraduate for another year, still at a reduced membership fee although a little more than as a student. You will not have to pay the full member price until the third year of membership.

You will have two full years of membership under your belt before you have to pay the full cost of membership. AHDI does this in order to give new MTs a chance to get a job and be making some money before they need to pay the larger membership fee. This is a good deal!

The AHDI Career Connection site at **http://career-connection.ahdionline.org/search.cfm** provides:

- FREE and confidential resumé posting—Make your resumé available to employers in the industry, confidentially if you choose.

- Job search control—Find relevant industry job listings quickly and easily and sign up for automatic e-mail notification of new jobs that match your criteria.

- Easy job application—Apply online and create a password-protected account for managing your job search.

- Saved jobs capability—Save up to 100 jobs to a folder in your account so you can go back to apply when you are ready.

Get Connected

AHDI has a New Professionals Alliance. Join at no extra cost; it's listed under GetConnected/Volunteer-Central/ Alliances. You will also want to join a local chapter if there is one near you or the on-line association if you don't have a local chapter. See the GetConnected/Governance/Components section of the AHDI website. If there is no local chapter near you, join the Online Association; it is listed under state/regional under components.

You should also think about joining the New Professionals Alliance because networking is the way most MTs, experienced and inexperienced, find job openings. AHDI also has a presence on Facebook as do many formal and informal medical transcription groups, and that is a good place to network. Search Facebook for AHDI or medical transcription to find the groups. AHDI also has a jobs board.

Professional Credentials

Study for and sit for the RHDS (registered healthcare documentation specialist) credentialing exam. An RHDS credential will help open doors that might not otherwise be open to a recent graduate. An RHDS practice exam is part of this course. AHDI periodically has free webinars to explain credentialing and introduce you to the exams and the study materials that you can use to prepare for them. You can download the Candidate Guide from the AHDI website.

The RHDS exam is based on the level 1 AHDI Medical Transcriptionist Job Description and the competencies outlined in the AHDI Core Competencies and the AHDI Model Curriculum. The AHDI RHDS exam consists of both medical transcription-related knowledge items and transcription performance items. The medical transcription-related knowledge portion of the exam consists of multiple-choice questions in certain specified content areas and percentages.

The transcription performance portion of the RHDS exam consists of short items employing medical dictation and/or transcription that must be transcribed, proofread, and/or edited. It consists of dictation that is realistic and representative of that encountered under actual working conditions. Dictation is selected for its appropriate medical content. The practical portion of the exam is designed to test a candidate's knowledge, skills, and abilities to practice medical transcription effectively in today's healthcare environment. Emphasis in the practical portion of the exam is more on critical thinking skills rather than keyboarding, research, or other technical skills.

Usually, the Young Professionals Alliance, the Online Association, or one of the local chapters offers an on-line study group, and the Association offers printed preparatory materials for sale as well as an on-line practice exam. Health Professions Institute (**http://www.hpisum.com/**) has a free weekly newsletter. Each issue contains a self-assessment quiz that may be useful in preparing for the exam. Click on Subscribe from the home page to sign up for the newsletter.

AHDI's mastery-level CHDS (certified healthcare documentation specialist) examination was established to recognize individuals with specialized, advanced transcription competencies and is based on Level 2 competencies. Individuals interested in obtaining a CHDS should gain substantial transcription experience before taking this examination. It is not recommended for recent graduates who have completed a transcription certificate program and have no other transcription experience.

It is not acceptable to use the designation *MT* (medical transcriptionist) or *HDS* (healthcare documentation specialist) after one's name because doing so gives the impression that the appellation carries the weight of a professional certification designation. *RHDS* and *CHDS* are the recognized professional credentialing designations for medical transcriptionists, and they may be used only if authorized through the Association for Healthcare Documentation Integrity. The AHDI Credentialing Committee changed the names of these credentials to match the Association's name, at least for those who have taken the current versions of the two exams. The new names are Registered Healthcare Documentation Specialist to replace the RMT credential and Certified Healthcare Documentation Specialist to replace the CMT credential.

Web Resources

Search the Web for medical transcription services. **MedicalTranscription.com** has a "Find a Medical Transcription or EHR Vendor" database that you can use to find medical transcription service organizations (MTSOs) and contact information for many of them. Once you have an MTSO name, you can use a search engine to find its website, verify contact information and check to see if it has a careers or job openings link on its website.

Also, be sure to subscribe to *Advance for Health Information Professionals* and *For the Record* magazines. You can search for them on the Web; both magazines have electronic subscriptions and on-line content. Although most of their classifieds will be for HIM personnel or experienced MTs, you'll be able to keep up on the healthcare industry in general and important medical transcription news in particular.

Transcription Forums

MT Chat and several other of the medical transcription forums also list job opportunities. MT Chat has a jobs registry; you'll need to register there to access it. Beware of anyone offering to extend your training or provide externship opportunities for a fee. You can Google medical transcription forums but avoid sites that sound belligerent or negative. Some sites seem to attract negative or hateful people; just choose to stay away from them. When you register for MT Chat (and possibly other forums), you can set your preferences so that when there is a new posting to the specific forums you're interested in, like the jobs board, you will get an e-mail.

RSS Feeds

If a jobs board site has an RSS feed, use it. One of the easiest ways to do RSS is through Google Reader, but there are other ways. Your browser may have an RSS reader option (Mozilla Firefox does). You can also use e-mail notification; you should probably set up a separate e-mail address just for job applications with gmail, hotmail, yahoo, or your Internet service provider. Be sure to use a professional-sounding e-mail address. Recruiters are not impressed by **hotchick229@hotmail.com** or **studoncall@yahoo.com**.

RSS readers are better than e-mail notifications. They don't fill up your mailbox and you can choose when and how you want to read them. You can RSS almost anything you're interested in. Google will explain how to do all this in its Help pages.

Equipment

A good headset is essential for transcription, both for reasons of sound quality and confidentiality. Get one as soon as you can afford one. When buying a professional headset, you need to determine what kind you would prefer (ear-bud style, stethoscope style, noise-cancelling style). Some prefer the ear-bud style or stethoscope style headsets, but many use the sound-cancelling style. The sound quality is better, and distracting noise is minimized. Many headsets have volume controls built in. This is useful, even though your computer and the audio player software also have volume controls. Use an Internet search engine to search for medical transcription equipment or medical transcription headsets. Compare features and prices; don't make your decision on price alone.

If you work on-site, generally all your equipment except the headset will be provided for you. There could still be a few employers using analog tape which requires a tape player, but most use digital dictation systems. There are hand-held digital recorders where the dictation can be transferred to a computer using a USB port or by other means. There are a variety of formats for audio files besides MP3. Many systems use wav format and, unfortunately, many use a proprietary format for which you might need a proprietary player or software to convert it to a format that can be played by standard audio players.

To get around the larger file size of some of these formats, the dictations may be compressed or zipped (as may the transcribed documents) for transferring via the Internet. Encryption should also be used, especially to comply with HIPAA and the new HITECH act requirements for security and confidentiality.

If you work remotely or telecommute (let's start avoiding "at home" as it implies less than professional employment), whether you provide your own equipment depends on your status. If you are an employee, most likely your employer will provide equipment, but you will not be able to use that equipment for personal use. You also may be restricted from accessing the Internet for research or your Internet access may be limited in order to avoid viruses and other technical issues. Some MTs have two computers—their work computer and a personal computer with electronic references and Internet connection for research.

If you work as an independent contractor, then you must provide your own equipment (IRS rules), although you may have to meet certain requirements such as high-speed Internet access, security requirements, etc., set by your client or the MTSO with whom you subcontract.

It is not within the scope of this course to cover all the things you need to know to be an independent contractor or to run your own business. However, there are some good free digital player applications available online. Search for medical transcription audio player software. These programs usually have a paid version with additional features. You may want to try out the free download first and determine whether it is sufficient or whether the pro version would better suit your needs.

There are other software programs, such as EasyWMA, for converting proprietary audio formats to a format that your audio player can use. EasyWMA converts most audio formats to wavs or MP3s. If you end up working on your own, these software products may be all you need. Many small independent contractors depend on programs like this. On the other hand, as your business grows, you will almost certainly need more professional software and equipment. Do your homework before purchasing any software or hardware to make sure that it will meet your needs.

Variations on dictation and transcription platforms are widespread. Many platforms are what are known as **ASPs (application service providers)**, meaning that it's not just a means of transferring audio files and documents but also a digital player and word processor (an interface makes it possible to use your word processor). Some independent contractors and smaller companies subscribe to larger companies that operate ASPs. This is a way to keep overhead costs for equipment low and be able to provide some of the same services to clients that larger companies provide.

There is an immense amount of information available about Internet and computer security specific to medical transcription. When you are working, your employer will provide the means for keeping your data secure or information on how to secure it. All employers should require HIPAA/HITECH compliance courses for their employees. Should you become an independent contractor, you should take such a course to be sure you are in compliance with applicable laws for security and confidentiality.

You should not purchase new equipment, except possibly a headset, until you actually have employment and know what you will need. Generally speaking, you will want your PC to have as much RAM as you can afford, a good-sized hard drive, a backup external drive that backs up automatically. You'll be working with sound and word processing so you don't need video game-playing capabilities, but you'll want a good sound card (pretty standard these days). You'll want a system that is dedicated for work and not used by the family.

Computer Skills

If you work remotely, and especially if you become an independent contractor (IC), your computer skills must be exceptional. If you are feeling weak in this area, there are several things you can do. There are numerous online computer skills courses; most of them will not be MT-centric, but they don't need to be for you to learn to be comfortable with Windows and Microsoft Word. There are books written specifically for MTs on using Microsoft Word and on healthcare documentation technology; you may want to search for these.

You need to develop good habits now to avoid *viruses and malware*. Make a point of researching *computer security, computer hygiene,* and *Internet, e-mail,* and *listserv etiquette*.

Pause for Reflection

1. What is the name of the professional association for healthcare documentation specialists? What resources does it offer the new MT?
2. What on-line resources might be useful in networking and in seeking that first job?
3. What equipment considerations do you need to keep in mind as you enter the job market?
4. What is an ASP?

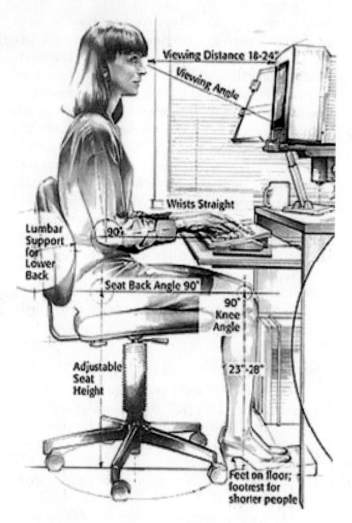

Ergonomic Tips

by Audrey Kirchner

Medical transcription doesn't seem as if it would be a physically taxing job but it is! One of the main pitfalls of medical transcription (or in fact any heavy use of computers) is **overuse syndrome**. There are ways to treat this, of course, but prevention by being well acquainted with ergonomics is preferable to treatment.

Ergonomics in the workplace is essential for the MT but just as essential for anyone working on a computer for more than 30 minutes per day. Let's examine some of the basic points of ergonomics for the medical transcriptionist.

Work Space

The computer monitor should be perpendicular to the window. Window coverings should be adjusted for sunlight as necessary. Keep references and other materials within easy and comfortable reach—arranged by impor-

tance and frequency of use. Avoid reaching and twisting to access anything. Avoid excess noise. Keep your work space clean and free of unnecessary items.

Your Body

Make sure that you quickly identify any symptoms (numbness, tingling, aching in arms, hands or wrists) of **carpal tunnel syndrome (CTS)** or overuse immediately. Take frequent breaks to help prevent overuse syndromes. Adjust your chair and keyboard to keep your wrists in a straight position—use a wrist leveler if needed. Do not rest your wrist on any hard surface or any sharp surface or put pressure on your wrists while typing. A light touch while typing is recommended to prevent muscle and tendon injuries.

Take care of your health in general. Smoking decreases circulation and can escalate overuse syndromes. Mouse and trackball should be located next to the keyboard. Support feet on a footrest or keep flat on the floor. Keep the lower back supported. Armrests can be used to support the arms though avoid pressure on elbows. Adjust your chair into different positions and settings throughout the day. Avoid doing repetitive tasks hour after hour.

Protect Your Sight

The monitor should be 18 to 30 inches from your eyes. Position desk light so that it does not shine on screen or in eyes. Reflective glare can be very fatiguing—watch out for shiny papers and posters. Adjust brightness and contrast controls on your computer monitor for maximum benefit. A clean screen helps you see better and with less effort. The top of the computer screen should be at eye level but lower if you wear bifocals. Reference materials should be placed at the same height as the monitor. Have your eyes checked regularly. Wear glasses if appropriate and make sure they are appropriate strength.

When it comes to medical transcription or any prolonged computer use, there are only so many firings of muscles that your body can take. Repetitive firing of muscles and tendons is what causes some of the worst overuse syndromes. Ensuring that your work environment is properly configured and that you make use of regular breaks will serve you well in medical transcription or with long-term computer use.

Make sure that your work space is properly configured to allow you the optimum benefit ergonomically. Invest in ergonomic furniture and equipment.

Future Roles for MTs

The electronic health record (EHR) and health information technology are opening up opportunities for transcriptionists who have honed their clinical knowledge and computer skills to grow and advance their careers. You should think of becoming a medical transcriptionist as the beginning of your adventure into healthcare, not the end.

The American Health Information Management Association notes that "as processes continue to evolve, additional training and fine-tuning of the core medical transcription knowledge set will be required to adequately prepare professionals" for new roles such as speech editor, documentation quality auditor, documentation assistant, medical scribe, data analyst, and ICD-10 coder. Speech editing is already a reality as a large portion of the MT workforce is involved in speech recognition editing,

At on an on-line meeting sponsored by AHDI, various EHR roles—including EHR analyst, EHR trainer, and scribe—that incorporate core knowledge and skills of the healthcare documentation specialist were evaluated. One of the future roles discussed was that of quality review in the outpatient EMR. Core competencies included in this role are terminology, formatting, ease of reading issues, validating the medical document through visit notes, and checking for signature deficiencies. There was also discussion about MTs moving to health IT certifications. These roles will work with planning, implementation, operation of the EHR for knowledge management, quality improvement, patient safety, and care coordination.

So you can see that through your training as a medical transcriptionist, you have an amazing foundation on which to build any number of related careers. Keep your eyes open for opportunities for continuing education and career advancement. You're already well on your way to an exciting new career; be ready to seize opportunities when they arise.

From Medical Transcriptionist to Data Abstractor

by Sarah Barton

After almost two years in medical transcription, I transitioned to clinical data abstraction work. My official title is newborn data systems operator, but the title doesn't really reflect what I do. I review charts in the electronic health record and look for specific information on the patients' diagnoses, treatment, and clinical outcomes. I review criteria for inclusion in our special diagnoses modules which includes information specific to necrotizing enterocolitis (NEC), hypothermia therapy, hypoxic ischemic encephalopathy (HIE), and a few other conditions that are specific to the neonatal period.

I have been in the neonatal intensive care unit (NICU, pronounced "nick-yoo") and seen the babies on various types of ventilators or on ECMO (extracorporeal membrane oxygenation) so I could learn more about these devices and what they do. For example, I have to look for details like the length of bowel a baby was left with after NEC was treated by bowel resection. Sometimes this means reviewing everything from autopsy reports to nutrition notes. Often, just like in paper charts, the information is not always in the same spot. The great thing about an electronic record is that I can use search features to narrow down where to look.

The decision to leave my home-based medical transcription position for an on-site position in an EHR environment was not easy. A big part of the reason was that my spouse is a veteran and became disabled; it took almost a year for his disability rating to be determined after he was discharged. That process did not go smoothly. During that time I had no choice but to become the breadwinner. It was very hard. Although my medical transcription career was never intended to support the family, I was doing well as a medical transcriptionist and was not in a low-paying job. I was fortunate to have a good job as an IC with a lot of flexibility. I was treated well and my contribution was valued. However, once I became the breadwinner I needed benefits including retirement, for my own peace of mind.

One night I was frustrated when transcribing a 48-minute consultation report from genetics, and my mind wandered to benefits and wanting to provide my children with healthcare insurance. I hadn't checked the job boards in probably a month. I saw a position on a popular job site for a data systems manager. As I later discovered, the real job title was newborn data systems operator. I read through the requirements and under "preferred skills" was medical transcription. I couldn't believe it! It was as if this position was written for me. It was in a NICU, and because I had been working for a children's hospital, I thought it might be perfect. I was stunned when the manager called me a few days later to schedule an interview.

During the interview I focused on the skills it takes to work at home. I talked about my ability to work well without supervision and stay motivated. I talked about my attention to detail and about my excellent knowledge of medical terminology. Just as with medical transcription phone interviews, I went in prepared with a list of questions I anticipated being asked and what my answers would be. I was able to glance at my list and stay focused and give clear answers. I knew the interview went well, and I left it feeling that I had done everything I could do to earn this job.

Fifteen minutes after I left the interview, the recruiter called and officially offered me the job and $2.50 per hour more than the advertised rate of pay because my medical transcription experience was counted as experience in this job. I was thrilled. I cried. I called my mother. I cried again. I knew this job would change my life. I wasn't getting rich doing it, but I also knew it was a starting point for greater things.

If I had gone only by the job title, I never would have found this job. It didn't sound like a job I would be qualified for. I had to click on the link and actually read the job details. For that reason, I always tell MTs who are seeking a transition to read job postings carefully. The most important thing you can do to transition into other healthcare documentation work is to recognize and value your skills. It might not be enough to say that you were a medical transcriptionist. Define what you did and highlight your skills.

Shortly after beginning this position I attended HIT Management Training that was sponsored by The Office of the National Coordinator for Health IT. I received a grant because I had experience in healthcare documentation as a medical transcriptionist. This qualifies me to take HIT Pro competency exams which are to become a credential in the future. Later that year my company started a scholarship fund for coders. I won a scholarship that paid my full tuition to attend a local university to become a medical coder.

If I implied that I'm doing a job that "any MT could do," perhaps I misled. I use my proofreading and research skills constantly and could not do my job without those skills. I have those impeccable research skills

because of MT school and 2 years of putting those skills to daily use. Pediatrics has been my niche in the MT world and specialized pediatrics terminology is critical to my particular position. Of course not all jobs are going to be in pediatrics hospitals so this is just something that is tremendously beneficial to my situation.

I also have to be able to communicate very effectively. I do not have a degree in IT, but my computer skills help tremendously. I've known a few MTs who have no knowledge of computers or technical skills, and those MTs could not do this job. If you're an MT who does not know how to e-mail an attachment or create a Microsoft Word document, you could not do my job and I'd dare say EHR training will be more challenging for you. As hard as it is for some of us to imagine, there are plenty of MTs out there who do not have these basic computer skills. If I were in those shoes, I would be remedying that right now.

For my job, and for most EHR jobs at the present time, you have to be able to go on-site. I also have to be able to work independently, but any successful MT is going to have that skill. In this position I need to work well with others and be a team player in a sometimes very stressful environment. If you're working from home to avoid human contact, that is something you would have to overcome to do my job.

What I am doing is not for everyone. We're all in medical transcription for different reasons and we all have different life circumstances. If I can pass anything on to you, it is to fully read a job description and don't let a title scare you away. Believe in yourself and don't let age or experience slow you down. Finally, realize that as an MT you have skills to contribute to other positions.

Things that are not requirements but certainly help are the graduate level technical writing courses under my belt and a few courses in HIPAA, health law, and health administration courses. None of these were required for the job but they help me on the job. If nothing else, I'm able to appear well informed. I could do my job without that training, but I don't think I would advance as quickly.

In the spirit of full disclosure, I have had 5+ years of college, but this was not a requirement for the job. I studied sports medicine and also took a number of health administration courses. I mentioned in my interview that I want to earn the RHIA certification in the next few years. That showed ambition and a plan for the future.

There are so many things I love about what I am doing, not the least of which is that if I get a really tough case I can spend hours working on it and make exactly the same income. My focus is 100% on quality in everything that I do. There is no production goal to make and my pay doesn't depend on how fast I go. I am treated well and I am respected. That feels so good! I go to work and can focus on work, not everything else going on in the house around me. When I'm home, work is over and I can focus on my family.

The last thing I want to share with you is that I love knowing that I am doing a good job. For some MTs, doing a good job means making more money. For me, doing a good job means being handed more responsibilities that are often fun and exciting and teach me new things. It means promotions and raises too. I also love seeing the patients. I love going in their room to update a chart and seeing these tiny little miracles that just a few years ago wouldn't have had a chance to survive, yet there they are right in front of me. This last week I've seen, or at least heard about, tragedies that made me go home and hug my kids extra tight, and I've seen miracles that amaze me. I haven't just listened to stories about it; I've seen it. I love being in the hospital.

The future is changing for medical transcription. You have a fantastic foundation as an MT, just as I did. Now is the time to consider how you want to build on that foundation. I would encourage you to look at every job posting even if it doesn't sound like you would qualify. Take a good look at your skills and knowledge and market yourself as the valuable professional you are.

Was it worth it? I no longer work as a medical transcriptionist so you might ask if it was worth it to become an MT. Yes, it was. My medical transcription skills gave me a foundation to be a very good clinical data abstractor. I learned to be thorough, to question everything, and the importance of the smallest details. I also did very well in coding school with my foundation in transcription, and I would like to think I will be a good coder sometime soon. I actually had a wonderful medical transcription job and a supervisor that was nothing but encouraging and helpful, but I needed benefits, wanted a retirement plan, and wanted to move up into management. Medical transcription served me well and I value the skills it taught me.

From Medical Transcriptionist to Scribe Manager

by Deborah R. Nolan

I wasn't really looking for a new job. But my husband spotted an ad on Craigslist and asked me, "What's a scribe?" I took a look at the ad; here's part of it:

Area Scribe Manager

• Lead scribe recruitment, hiring and on-boarding efforts by establishing relationships with local universities and pre-med societies in local market.

• Train scribes in the areas of medical terminology, anatomy, billing, coding, documentation, charting, and electronic medical records.

I was intrigued, and maybe a bit bored with my QA job. I read the ad description again and wondered if I could even be considered. I do have management and training experience, but they wanted an advanced degree, such as an RN. I was an LVN in a former life (pre-MT/QA, that is), but I let my license lapse when we moved to Oregon from California. At that point, I had been out of nursing school for 10 years, and I was burnt out. I moved on to medical transcription and was making decent money. Further education just didn't seem necessary.

In my killer cover letter and resumé I changed my title from medical transcriptionist to healthcare documentation specialist. I played up the fact that I had done some work with students and externs, was an expert in medical language, and was focused on quality. It didn't hurt that I had completed the ONC's program in EHR implementation and project management last year.

I got the job. The best part is that during my interview, after reading my resumé and talking with me, the CEO said, "You know, your background is just perfectly suited to this position. We never thought about hiring someone with your qualifications."

The scribes I train are typically college juniors or seniors, getting their pre-med prereqs in place. In no way do I expect that in six months, these young people will have the critical thinking skills necessary to replace an MT. The difference between MTs and scribes is huge because scribes are temporary workers at best who are paid minimum wage and should be grateful for the opportunity to even be in an ED, much less documenting the patient's health story in the EHR. Their acceptance rate to med school is an astounding 90% if they obtain this clinical experience before applying. I knew I had my work cut out for me.

The scary thing was that, beginning the next week, I would have to leave home a couple of days a week to drive to the hospital ED and manage the scribes and audit their work. Some days are spent training them at the office. Other days I still work at home. But I'll get to see the world from outside my home office window, and that's exciting. I'll also be enrolled in an RHIA program soon, so I'll be busy!

Here's how my first week as a scribe went:

Grab your COW (Computer On Wheels) and hope someone remembered to plug it in and clean off the keyboard. Fire it up and find out which physician you'll be running after for 8 hours. Look at the track board of patients waiting and be ready to hit the ground running (literally). "Chest pain in 2, let's go!" With one hand on the COW and one hand on the mouse, walking rapidly behind the doc, you find room 2 on the screen, assign that patient to yourself, open a new note/template, run into the patient's room, try to find a place to fit inside the room, and start typing the HPI (history of present illness) madly, interpreting the encounter like so:

Doc: Hi, Mrs. Jones. Where does it hurt?

Mrs. Jones: Oh, right here. (Points to area; you take your eyes off screen so you can see where the patient is pointing.)

Doc: Uh huh, and how long has this been going on?

Mrs. Jones: Just this morning. It kind of goes here, too. (Points again.)

You type: 72-year-old F c/o midline CP which radiates into her L shoulder.

Meanwhile, you are trying to listen and watch as you type the HPI. The doc then decides to do the ROS (review of systems), so you open that tab and start clicking boxes, but you can't find the correct boxes, so you open the "comment" icon and type it in. Then he goes back to examining the patient and doesn't dictate it, but he tells you earlier that if he doesn't dictate any pertinent positives, the exam is normal. Except didn't the patient just appear to exhibit some LLQ (left lower quadrant) guarding with palpation?

You leave the room and scoot back to the desk area. You remember to ask the doc about the abdominal exam. "Oh, yeah, she did have some LLQ tenderness." While popping in the patient's PMH (past medical history) and SH (social history), you remember to ask what his differential diagnoses might be. Good thing you have that medical background so you can figure them out yourself if he doesn't dictate them, right? Meanwhile, he's ordered a CT scan, UA (urinalysis), and CBC (complete blood count). You see that in the "orders" tab. You make note on your pad to check when those results come in so you can load them into the chart. You try to continue filling out your chart, which should be done in five minutes or less. "Hey, let's go see the knife wound in 15." Off you go, running again . . . My feet hurt.

The pace of the ED is maddening. I remember this from my nursing days, which is probably why I went into medical transcription. But transcription in real time? That's the tough part. As MTs, we think we have the greatest listening skills, but in this role it's crucial. There's no slowing down the audio or backspacing with your foot pedal. You could go back and ask the docs, but they have a ton of patients to see. You've got to be able to think on your feet and be incredibly organized because you can have 4 charts on 4 different tabs, and you don't want to place the wrong information on the wrong chart.

I've been sitting down for 20 years doing medical transcription and quality assurance. Being a scribe is completely different. Last week I was present for two codes, one an MI, one a drowning victim. There is nothing like being there in the room with a team of 20 nurses, medics, techs, and docs, all trying to save this person's life—while you trying to type and stay out of the way.

Normally, it takes a couple of months for scribes to be up to speed. As noted before, these are people still in college, hopefully moving on to medical or nursing school. Getting scribe experience gives them valuable clinical experience which gives them a better chance of making it into school. It's great for the scribes. It's great for the doctors. A couple of the providers told me that before scribes, they were spending an additional 2-3 hours after their shift was over, just inserting data into the electronic medical record (EMR). Having an EMR ends up costing you more money after all. What a surprise! With scribes, the charts are complete at the end of the doctors' shifts. There's no dictating, no waiting for reports to come back in 24 hours; it's practically instantaneous.

Of course, there are issues. The scribes generally have no medical terminology experience. They are expected to take a free on-line course. They are also encouraged to look up unfamiliar terms or ask the doctors while they are working. The scribes I manage are mostly part time due to their college schedules, and because they are planning to move on to medical school, they are temporary workers (1-2 years at best).

The doctors I've spoken with feel frustrated that they have so many different part-time scribes, and there's no consistency. They would like to have a few great scribes to count on. Although they recognize the importance of the scribes getting this clinical experience, the doctors are paying a premium for this service that allows them more time to do their jobs.

So I asked my boss, why don't we hire some full-time MTs to work on-site? After all, they hired me not just for my nursing background but also for my medical language expertise. The scribes were mostly working nights and weekends. If we had a handful of MTs working full-time days at the hospital, the docs could count on them. The MTs could become "lead scribes" who train and mentor the new scribes. They are already medical language specialists. While it takes new scribes a couple of months to get up to speed, it took me a week. I already had the background, had the computer savvy to learn Epic (the EHR system) quickly due to working on multiple platforms throughout my career, and had the organizational skills needed to keep the work flowing. And so do my fellow MTs. Last week my boss allowed me to place two ads for local MTs to work as scribes, and I have had a wonderful response.

I see so many possibilities here. The EHR is here to stay. While there are point-and-click boxes, there's a lot of narrative that is important and that the doctors want in these records. You simply cannot tell a patient health story with checkboxes. Even the checkboxes have narrative comment boxes, and I use these a lot. I think there is really an unmet need for good MTs who want to keep doing what they are doing.

The downside is that we have to leave our cozy home offices and get out into the real world. That was tough for me. The upside is the ability to continue to utilize our extensive knowledge and skills in the rapidly changing healthcare arena without having to switch professions altogether. Without giving away any confidential information about my company, I can tell you that scribes are paid better than minimum wage, and that I've been given approval to pay the full-time hourly MTs much better, with full benefits.

Personally, I love my job. I cannot even fathom going back to sitting at a desk doing QA for 8 hours at a time. Although I miss being home every day, I do get to work out of my home office two or three days a week. The rest of the time I am either training scribes or working on their quality evaluations. I've developed higher quality standards as well. While I am at home, I perform lots of administrative duties. I've also started to assist with other accounts as well, most of which will require implementation, or "go-lives," and will require me to travel every couple of months.

I truly enjoy working with the scribes. These are college graduates with heavy emphasis on the sciences including A&P and organic chemistry. Yes, they mostly require training in medical terminology, and sometimes this is their first job. They are eager to learn, and they have energy and enthusiasm to spare.

Research this field because your skills as MTs are needed to lead this new workforce. You'll need EHR skills and experience in utilizing multiple MT platforms. We need to be creative and sell our skills and knowledge. There is a place for healthcare documentation specialists as permanent, well-paid experts to assist providers in telling an accurate health story for their patients.

WE TAKE OURSELVES WITH US

My friend Judy tells the story of her six-year-old daughter who talked all the time in class instead of doing her work. She asked the teacher if her daughter could move to another seat where she would not be as likely to talk so much. The teacher observed, "Wherever Ann Marie goes, she takes herself with her."

Perhaps that is why some of us have the same difficulties wherever we go—we take ourselves with us. Most of us blame everything and everybody but ourselves for our failures. "I lost that job because . . . " "I lost that account because . . . " "That relationship failed because . . . " We aren't happy in our jobs so we change jobs, thinking the job is the problem. Then we have the same or similar problems in the next job, and think another job is the answer. Or we can't get along with a client, so we dump that one, and sign up another. Or one consulting job after another is unsatisfactory, and we always blame the client. We think if we just change jobs, or change cities, or change clients, or change friends or family, things will work out.

If our personal insight enabled us to recognize that "wherever we go, we take ourselves with us," then perhaps we could better see who or what needs to be changed. Without self-awareness of our strengths and weaknesses, and using that knowledge to our advantage, we can't successfully control our speed, or strategies for moving forward, on the racetrack of life or business.

Sally C. Pitman

Spotlight On

Criticism

by Marcy Diehl

Criticism first became a subject for conversation in my life many years ago when I went to work for a prominent thoracic and cardiovascular surgeon. During the course of the interview, he asked me if I was able to take criticism gracefully. Well, I was stumped. No one had ever asked before; they had just handed it out, and I really didn't know how gracefully I had accepted what I had had so far. It depended on who was dishing it out, I guess.

I thought about my response, worrying that my prospective job somehow hinged on what I had to say one way or the other. I felt he would have liked for me to say something like "Oh, I love criticism" or even "I never need it!" Evidently I gave the right answer, however (he did hire me), when I replied, "Well, I guess we'll have to find out, won't we?" This answer implied to him that he would hire me and that we would both see how his criticism and my acceptance of it went along.

But I was now on the alert. I was forewarned that criticism was, in fact, a big possibility, and I worked very hard against the day when "we" would find out how gracefully I could accept it. I really didn't know where it would come from. There were a lot of possibilities; the day seemed fraught with them.

That was just the first day.

By the second day, I found out. That was the day my first transcripts were returned. Large permanent blue-black ink circles covered the many carefully prepared documents. It was hard to be graceful when I looked at the ruination of a half-day's labors (actually, half a night, too, as I had spent long hours at home researching unfamiliar words).

We had weeks of that, and I was getting discouraged; still graceful, I presume, but discouraged. The errors were becoming fewer and fewer, but that didn't seem to help much, since I wanted them to disappear. It was harder and harder to face up to them somehow, now that I was feeling more secure in the job. Grace was wearing thin. He never said anything. I never said anything. I just retyped. A lot.

Then two things happened. The surgeon's wife came into the office on Saturday morning when he proofread and busily marked up my work. She watched, appalled. Monday morning shortly after I arrived for work, she called "to see how you're taking it." "Fine," I said. She was relieved, and reported that she had talked to him about it, feeling that he had been too harsh. "Well," he said, "she won't learn if I don't teach her, and she's worth teaching."

I learned about grace that day. He took his precious time to teach and to help me. He had a B.S. in journalism and knew his Greek and Latin roots to a fine degree as well. I was pretty much humbled by his constant criticism, his love of perfection, and his belief in my potential for growth.

All of our lives we are both subjected to and the dispensers of criticism. If we can remember to accept it with the spirit in which it is given, realizing it took some time to critique our performance and that it was done because of our ultimate potential, we then must accept it not only with grace but with thanks.

Secondly, we must try to remember to give our criticism only with graciousness, knowing that we can help someone in whom we see the potential for personal or professional betterment, and not criticize to showcase our own skills. If we cannot criticize fairly, with love and in private, then we need to withhold it.

This is a lifelong relationship—us and criticism. We never should feel we have outgrown the need. If we protect ourselves by not doing anything new anymore, sticking to only what we do perfectly, then we will no longer grow in grace and wisdom.

Exercises

Chapter Review

1. With your instructor's guidance, locate and interview a supervisor and a transcriptionist or speech recognition editor in each of the major employment settings: hospital, MTSO, and freelance or independent contractor. Questions you might ask include:

    How did you get into this field? What degrees or credentials do you have? What do you like best about your job? What do you like least? What goals do you have for the future? What advice would you give to a beginner?

2. Using the many questions in the essay "Employment Options," write a brief summary of your desires or expectations regarding work setting, compensation, work schedule, and benefits. Do you think your expectations are realistic?

3. Using any or all of the resources mentioned in this chapter, find one or more opportunities for employment as a medical transcriptionist or speech recognition editor. List the name of the company, contact information, and job description and requirements.

4. Prepare a cover letter and a resumé (remember, two versions, one with and one without formatting) for one or more of the jobs you found. If your school or program does not provide help preparing cover letters and resumés, find sites on the Internet that provide guidelines.

5. With your instructor, school or program job counselor, or a classmate or relative, practice phone and person-to-person interviews. For the person-to-person interview, be sure to dress and conduct yourself as you would for a real interview.

Online Exercises

These exercises are located at **www.myhealthprofessionskit.com**. To access the exercises, select the discipline "Medical Transcription," then click on the title of this book, *Healthcare Documentation: Fundamentals & Practice*, and the chapter title. When you have completed each exercise, follow your teacher's instructions for submitting the assignment for grading or obtaining access to the answer key to check your own work.

RHDS Practice Test

Click on the title of this practice test for the registered healthcare documentation specialist (RHDS) credential. It consists of 100 multiple-choice questions and 50 audio clips. Follow the instructions at the beginning of the test. It will be scored immediately upon completion. Make notes about the questions you miss so that you can review those knowledge areas.

PEARSON
myhealthprofessionskit™

To access the online exercises, go to **www.myhealthprofessionskit.com**. Select "Medical Transcription" click on the title of this book, ***Healthcare Documentation: Fundamentals & Practice***. Then click on the Professional Issues chapter.

Comic Relief

The Gourmet Medical Transcriptionist

by Renee M. Priest

No matter what kind of dictation we transcribe—acute care or chart notes—the words we listen to daily, in all their graphic detail, have a profound and direct impact on the food we plan to eat. Let's face it, transcribing bowel resections and the odd proctoscopy or two does not make that hunk of liver, thoughtlessly tossed in the sink to thaw, look appetizing at all. In fact, the sight of it will undoubtedly quell any desire to come near the kitchen for a very long time.

It is important to realize that there is an art to this, a subtle matching of words and ingredients. While I cannot be considered an expert, I have had considerable experience in making those critical dinner menu decisions. Sometimes the determining factor is a dictator's accent, some tiny little thing in the patient history, and sometimes just a background noise. I have to admit that acute-care dictation, with its wide variety of accents, dictators, and different reports, is a virtual cornucopia of fertile food for thought.

For instance, the proctoscopy . . . every now and then I get a French physician who makes a proctoscopy sound positively romantic. The sound of those sibilant syllables can lead me directly to mental visions of mussels gently steamed in white wine, crusty French bread, real butter, and little green cornichon pickles for tartness.

A certain Asian dictator had me considering stir fry one day until I remembered there was no shrimp in the freezer. I continued transcribing until I heard the sound of a radiologist from Pakistan and remembered I had some cans of white beans on hand, pita bread, and eggplant in the garden. A Southern physician is sure to trigger a frenzy of black-eyed peas, cornbread, ham slices, or maybe buttermilk biscuits, collards, fried chicken, and sliced tomatoes from the garden with a tiny sprinkling of olive oil.

One of my favorites (I keep these ingredients on hand because I have this dictator frequently) is a surgeon from Jamaica. Just the way those vowels roll around, the cadence of his spoken words, you can bet we are having jerk chicken done on the grill.

Patient names can do it as well. A woman from Hungary created quite a dilemma for me as I had no paprika in the spice rack. A desperate phone call to a friend finally solved that problem. You simply cannot make a proper goulash without paprika!

No matter how you look at it, this matching up stuff is not easy. The consequences of a mismatch are immediately obvious. A little forethought and planning are essential ingredients in the process. Just because you hear island music in the background of a dictation does not mean the family is going to be particularly enthusiastic about recreating an official version of a Hawaiian cooking pit in the front yard. The desire to create authenticity is most certainly going to suffer a setback if someone has to put on rubber boots and slog through the Florida swamp searching for the right palm tree to cut down in order to produce a genuine hearts of palm salad.

Asian dictators bring out my creative side. I have discovered that it is possible to use up practically anything lurking in the refrigerator just by plopping it in a wok. So it was indeed disheartening when the family simply sat in silence when I presented them with a truly inspired dish of baby corn, shiitaki mushrooms, and fried softshell crab.

I still cannot figure out why those blue corn tortillas, lovingly created one night because one of my dictators happened to examine a native American Indian, remained untouched. It is true that they were slightly more gray than blue, with a texture reminiscent of fried washing machine lint, but that is no excuse.

While I cannot exactly blame that 90-year-old Polish patient (he kept singing Polish ditties during his neurological exam), it is certainly true that Southern smoked sausage does not blend with sauerkraut and caraway seeds as well as kielbasa would have. I did discover that chicken gizzards make a suitable substitution for sweetbreads in a dish from Provence. But someone forgot to mention that when making a cassoulet, it is essential to use a really DEEP dish because, if you , those beans and juices just ooze to the bottom of the oven, making a stink you would not believe.

I am constantly amazed when I read threads on Internet message boards on how boring medical transcription can be, typing the same thing day after day, same procedures, same words. I never seem to have that problem. After all, there is always that evening meal to plan ahead for, and who knows what might spark the creative juices!

Appendix A: Resources

Alder, Cynthia C., BSHSA, RHIT, CMT. "Healthcare Documentation Specialists," 18

Barton, Sarah. "From Medical Transcriptionist to Data Abstractor," 709-711

Barton, Sarah. "Job Searching Advice," 699-701.

Bogdanovich, Jody. "My Husband's Journey," 607-608

Campbell, Linda C. "A Caregiver's Perspective: My Last Two Years with Marion," 256-258

Campbell, Linda C. "Patient Confidentiality," 16-18

Campbell, Linda C. "War Souvenirs," 157-158

Diehl, Marcy. "Criticism," 714

Dirckx, John H., MD. "Adventures in Thought Transference," 78-82

Dirckx, John H., MD. "Arterial Blood Gases," 310-312

Dirckx, John H., MD. "Assessment of Pulmonary Function," 308-310

Dirckx, John H., MD. "Depression," 144-145

Dirckx, John H., MD. "Diagnostic Radiology," 626-640

Dirckx, John H., MD. "Drug Dependency," 146-147

Dirckx, John H., MD. "Gross and Microscopic Examination of Tissue," 670-674

Dirckx, John H., MD. "Hyperbaric Oxygen Therapy," 179-180

Dirckx, John H., MD. "Insomnia," 145-146

Dirckx, John H., MD. "Laboratory Examination of Urine," 427-430

Dirckx, John H., MD. "Mechanical Ventilation," 312-313

Dirckx, John H., MD. "Negative Pressure Wound Therapy," 177-179

Dirckx, John H., MD. Numerous excerpts from *H&P: A Nonphysician's Guide to the Medical History and Physical Examination*, 4th ed. (HPI, 2009)

Dirckx, John H., MD. Numerous excerpts from *Human Diseases*, 3rd ed. (HPI, 2009)

Dirckx, John H., MD. Numerous excerpts from *Laboratory Tests & Diagnostic Procedures in Medicine* (HPI, 2004)

Dirckx, John H., MD. "Ocular Imaging," 349-350

Dirckx, John H., MD. "Pathology Reports," 670

Dirckx, John H., MD. "Perspectives on Dermatology," 174-177

Dirckx, John H., MD. "Vision Testing," 348-349

D'Onofrio, Mary Ann and Elizabeth. "Curve Balls," 139

Drake, Ellen, CMT. "A Flock of Floaters," 363-364

Drake, Ellen, CMT. "Applying for Employment," 698-699.

Drake, Ellen, CMT. "Basic Research Skills," 82-85

Drake, Ellen, CMT. "Becoming a Radiology Transcriptionist," 647-648

Drake, Ellen, CMT. "Making the Most of Your Studies," 103-104

Drake, Ellen, CMT. "Mishears," 80

Drake, Ellen, CMT. "Proofreading Skills," 89-90

Drake, Ellen, CMT. "Traditional Editing," 90-93

Drake, Ellen, CMT. "What Is Vulgar?," 193

Drake, Ellen, CMT. "What MTs Do That Speech Recognition Cannot," 97-100

Drake, Ellen, CMT, and Georgia Green, CMT. "Searching the 'Wild, Wild Web'," 85-89

Drake, Ellen and Randy. "Orphan Drugs," 41

Green, Georgia, CMT. "Abbreviation Expansion Software," 69-70

Green, Georgia, CMT. "A View from the HIM Director's Chair," 28-31

Green, Georgia, CMT. "Feeling the Need for Speed," 100-103.

Green, Georgia, CMT. "How the HDS Fits into Healthcare Documentation," 8-12

Green, Georgia, CMT. "Skills Testing for Employment," 701-704

Guyer, Diane. "Absurdity Recognition," 108

Hinickle, Judy. "Employment Options," 698

Hurley, Brenda J., CMT. "Evolution of the Medical Transcription Role," 5

Hurley, Brenda J., CMT. "Hands-on Anatomy Lessons —My Pathology Experience," 677-678

Hurley, Brenda J., CMT. "HIPAA—What Is It?," 12-16

Hurley, Brenda J., CMT. "Listening to Your Body," 495-496

Hurley, Brenda J., CMT. "Our Health Story—Being a Patient Advocate," 45

Hurley, Brenda J., CMT. "Technology, Security, and Beyond for the Remote Workforce," 65-69

Kirchner, Audrey, CMT. "Ergonomic Tips," 708-709

Kirchner, Audrey, CMT. "Speech Recognition Editing," 93-96.

Lederer, Richard, PhD. "Jest for the Health of It," 58

Lederer, Richard, PhD. "A Little Bit of Comma Sense," 132

Marshall, Judith. "Check Mates," 287

Marshall, Judith. "Confessions of an Addict," 326-327

Marshall, Judith. "Totally Hip," 570-571

Martin, April L., MSL, RHIA, CMT. "Evolution of the Healthcare Documentation Specialist," 7

National Institute on Drug Abuse. "Commonly Abused Drugs," 155

Nolan, Deborah R. "From Medical Transcriptionist to Scribe Manager," 711-713

O'Donnell, Michael J., MD. "A Cardiovascular Surgeon's View," 383-386

Pitman, Sally C. "We Take Ourselves with Us," 713

Priest, Renee M., CMT. "Ergonomics: It's All in the Tushie," 72-73

Priest, Renee M., CMT. "Editing on the Fly," 105

Priest, Renee M., CMT. "The Gourmet Medical Transcriptionist," 716

Pyle, Vera. "The Mind Behind the Machine," 2

Roth, Sherry, PA-C, CMT. "Tips on Dictating and Transcribing Speech Recognition Reports," 96

Starkey, John. "Surviving Bladder Cancer," 444

Taylor, Bron. "How I Became a Medical Transcriptionist," 19-20

Taylor, Bron. "Transcribing Gastroenterology Dictation," 534

Turley, Susan M. "Needle Classification," *Understanding Pharmacology for Health Professionals*, 43

Turley, Susan M. "Who Nose?," 232

Woods, Kathleen Mors. "Transcribing Cardiology Dictation," 401

Web Sites

http://www.hpisum.com/

Health Professions Institute: Free articles for students and teachers. Click on Downloads or e-Perspectives links. Check out the Useful Websites article with more extensive lift of resources than this one.

http://www.ahdionline.org/

Association for Healthcare Documentation Integrity (AHDI): Information on the RHDS and CHDS credentials, networking, position papers, and other industry resources. Click on tabs under banner for detailed menus.

http://grammar.ccc.commnet.edu/grammar/

Capital Community College: Comprehensive grammar site and quizzes. Click on drop-down menus for detailed menus.

http://www.ismp.org/

Institute for Safe Medication Practices: Click on Tools tab and scroll down for Error-prone Abbreviations list.

http://www.jointcommission.org/

The Joint Commission: Use search box for official Do Not Use List of Abbreviations.

http://emedicine.medscape.com/

eMedicine: Register free. Free information on diagnoses, diseases, and treatments, with illustrations.

http://meded.ucsd.edu/clinicalmed/introduction.htm

Practical Guide to Clinical Medicine: Very useful in understanding the history and physical examination.

http://www.fpnotebook.com/index.htm

Family Practice Notebook: This site is organized by specialties, each specialty by chapters. There's an examination section for each specialty or condition which can prove very helpful.

http://www.labcorp.com/datasets/labcorp/html/chapter/

Search for tests by name, number, CPT code or keyword, or click on the first letter of the test you're looking for and browse. Also search by specialty.

http://www.arupconsult.com/index.html

Physician's Guide to Laboratory Test Selection and Interpretation: You can use the search box to search for specific laboratory tests or the topic list (by letter or category) to find a disease or condition. Contains a lot of information both about the disease and the diagnostic tests used to diagnose the disease.

http://www.ncbi.nlm.nih.gov/sites/entrez?db=pubmed&TabCmd=Limits

National Library of Medicine: The best place to search for specific information about medical topics with over 16 million abstracts. Abstracts are synopses of articles. Click the Limits tab and then the Human and English language box to restrict your searches. Register and set preferences, save searches, etc. Set it so that it remembers you and you never have to log in again. This site has good tutorials and Help tools which are strongly recommended.

http://www.ncbi.nlm.nih.gov/sites/entrez?db=PMC

PubMed Central: Same thing as above except that citations have access to the full text article.

http://cdc.gov/

Centers for Disease Control and Prevention: Use the index or search for infectious and communicable diseases and information about vaccinations, pests, parasites, toxins, poisons, etc. The CDC also exposes disease- and health-related hoaxes.

http://www.onelook.com/

Good online dictionary, wild card searches, and reverse lookup (using the definition instead of the word). OneLook will find medical and nonmedical words. Use options to set preferences.

Appendix B: Glossary

A&P (anterior and posterior) repair A combination of anterior and posterior colporrhaphy for the repair of cystocele, rectocele, and uterine prolapse.

ABGs (arterial blood gases) Unlike most blood tests where blood is drawn from a vein, this test requires that blood be drawn from an artery. It measures the pH and the levels of oxygen (O_2) and carbon dioxide (CO_2) in the blood from an artery. It is a measure of lung function (how well your lungs move oxygen into and carbon dioxide out of the blood). Values include partial pressure of oxygen (PaO_2), partial pressure of carbon dioxide ($PaCO_2$), pH (normal values are between 7.35 and 7.45), bicarbonate (HCO_3), oxygen (O_2) content and saturation.

ablation Total removal of a part, normal or abnormal, by surgical or chemical means.

ABO incompatibility A hemolytic disease in which a mother makes antibodies against her baby's blood when her blood type is different from the baby's. The antibodies can cross the placenta and cause hemolytic disease of the newborn or erythroblastosis fetalis, resulting in jaundice and anemia. This condition can also be caused by Rh incompatibility between the mother and baby.

ABR (auditory brainstem response) A hearing test done on newborns or infants. It measures activity in the brainstem in response to sounds. Three small sensors are placed on the baby's head and neck and headphones on the ears. Clicking sounds are played and the brain's response is recorded by a computer. Also, *BAER (brainstem auditory-evoked response)*.

abscess A collection of pus in any part of the body that, in most cases, causes swelling and inflammation around it. Pus forms in a tissue space walled off from surrounding tissues by fibrin, coagulated tissue fluids, and eventually fibrous tissue.

absence ("absáhnce") **seizure** (petit mal) Brief loss of attention and perception.

absorption tests Based on determination of blood or stool levels of substances that have been ingested in measured amounts.

acanthosis nigricans A diffuse hyperplasia and darkening of the skin in areas such as the axilla or groin. One form accompanies internal carcinomas and is called malignant acanthosis nigricans. A benign nevoid form in adults may accompany endocrine diseases. A benign form in children is called pseudoacanthosis nigricans.

accessory muscles of respiration Neck and upper chest muscles not needed for normal breathing.

acid phosphatase Enzyme whose level in the serum is often increased in prostatic carcinoma.

acid-fast stain A staining procedure in which sputum, tissue, or other material is exposed to fluorochrome dye and then washed with acid-alcohol. Organisms of the genus Mycobacterium and some others retain the dye and are said to be acid-fast.

acinus (pl., **acini**) A grape-shaped secretory unit in a gland or the saccular terminal dilatation of a pulmonary alveolus.

acoustical shadowing The inability of ultrasound to reach and delineate structures located in the "shadow" of an organ or tissue that reflects a large amount of ultrasound.

acromegaly Abnormal growth of the body, especially facial features and extremities due to excess of pituitary growth hormone.

acute tubular necrosis A generalized failure of the renal tubules to perform their excretory functions. Also referred to as *renal shutdown* or *shock kidney*.

ad lib. According to pleasure (Latin *ad libitum*).

adipocere A waxy substance into which the soft tissues of a dead body are converted after prolonged immersion.

adjustment disorder A persistent state of emotional or physical distress triggered by a major life event or situation, such as the death of a loved one, interpersonal conflict, divorce, financial problems, or loss of employment.

ADLs (activities of daily living).

adnexa (plural only; takes a plural verb) Organs adjacent to the uterus—ovaries, tubes, broad ligaments, round ligaments, and associated blood vessels.

AdreView (iobenguane sulfate) Nuclear imaging agent for the detection of adrenal tumors, pheochromocytoma or neuroblastoma.

ADT (admission, discharge, transfer) **information** Demographic data about the patient that includes name, patient number, and dates of admission and discharge or transfer and can include age, sex, and other information. This data is electronic and can often be incorporated directly into a medical report.

adynamic ileus Bowel obstruction caused by decreased bowel motility, often secondary to peritonitis.

AF (atrial fibrillation, atrial flutter) Abnormal heartbeat in which the heart rhythm is fast and irregular.

affect One's prevailing mood or emotional state, pleasant or unpleasant, particularly as perceived by the examiner: basic emotional state, and emotional content of responses to examiner (apathetic, blunted, depressed, elated, euphoric, flat, inappropriate, labile).

AFI (amniotic fluid index) An ultrasound procedure used to assess the amount of amniotic fluid that surrounds the fetus.

AFP (alpha fetoprotein) A test performed on maternal serum, usually around 16-18 weeks' gestation. Maternal AFP may be abnormally low when the fetus has Down syndrome and abnormally elevated when the fetus has a neural tube defect. AFP is also a marker for certain cancers. This test is included in a triple screen or quadruple screen.

agglutinins, cold Antibodies formed by persons with mycoplasmal pneumonia, which cause red blood cells to clump when chilled but not at room or body temperature.

agglutinins, febrile A group of antibody tests, each for a specific febrile (fever-causing) infectious disease, used as a screening procedure in patients with fever of unknown origin (FUO).

aggregate Clustered together (adjective). A cluster or the total amount (noun). To gather together, to amount to (verb).

air bronchogram A radiographic shadow of an air-filled bronchus passing through an airless segment of lung.

air-fluid level A line representing the level of a collection of fluid seen in profile, with air or gas above it.

air-space disease As seen on chest x-ray, disease or abnormality of lung tissue that encroaches on space normally filled by air.

AK amputation Above-the-knee amputation.

ALT (alanine aminotransferase) An enzyme whose level in the serum is elevated in hepatitis, cirrhosis, and other liver diseases.

altered level of consciousness Varying from slight drowsiness or inattentiveness, to confusion and disorientation, to deep coma from which the subject cannot be aroused by any stimulus.

alveolus (pl., **alveoli**) A hollow or cavity. Dental alveolus—tooth socket. Pulmonary alveolus—a pouchlike dilatation at the end of a bronchiole, the site of gas exchange between air and blood.

amenorrhea Absence of menstruation.

amorphous sediment Unformed and generally insignificant debris seen in a urine specimen under microscopic examination.

ampulla of Vater Also known as the *hepatopancreatic ampulla*. Formed by the union of the pancreatic duct and the common bile duct.

Amsler grid A tool used in visual field testing.

amylase, serum An enzyme whose level is increased in pancreatitis and mumps.

ANA (antinuclear antibody) An antibody detected by immunofluorescence in patients with rheumatoid arthritis, lupus erythematosus, and other autoimmune diseases.

anal verge The distal end of the anal canal, forming a transitional zone between the skin of the anal canal and the perianal skin.

anastomosis Surgical joining of two organs or vessels.

ankyloglossia Tongue tie.

ankylosis Immobility and consolidation of a joint due to disease, injury, or surgical procedure.

anovulation Failure of ovulation to occur at the expected times.

antepartum Before childbirth.

anterior colporrhaphy Plication of the vaginal muscularis fascia overlying the bladder (pubocervical fascia) to repair a cystocele. A midline incision is made in the vaginal mucosa and the vagina dissected sharply away from the pubocervical fascia lateral to the inferior pubic ramus. Absorbable mattress sutures are placed in layers on the pubocervical fascia, excess vaginal mucosa trimmed away, and remaining mucosa closed with running or interrupted sutures.

anterior drawer test With the patient supine, the injured knee is bent to 90 degrees. The physician then grasps the upper end of the tibia and pulls it anteriorly. Excessive movement means the anterior cruciate ligament (ACL) within the knee joint is damaged or torn.

anterolisthesis Spondylolisthesis, a forward displacement of one vertebra over another resulting from congenital deformity of or damage to vertebral articular processes.

anthracotic pigmentation Gray or black discoloration of lung tissue caused by inhalation of carbon particles; observed in varying degrees in those who live in industrial or urban environments, cigarette smokers, and coal miners.

anuria Total cessation of urinary output.

AOE (automated otoacoustic emission) **testing** A hearing test done usually on newborns. A small earpiece is placed into a baby's outer ear which sends out gentle clicking sounds. If a baby has a functioning middle and inner ear, an echo response will be generated that can be measured by a computer.

A1c See *hemoglobin A1c*.

aphakia (adj., **aphakic**) Absence of the lens of the eye; it may be congenital, traumatic, or as a result of cataract extraction.

aphasia Impairment of the ability to communicate through spoken or written language, or to understand spoken or written language, or both.

apnea Cessation of breathing.

arrhythmia Irregular rhythm of the heartbeat, with or without an abnormally slow or fast rate.

arthrocentesis Insertion of a needle into the joint cavity in order to remove or aspirate fluid. May be done to remove excess fluid from a joint or to obtain fluid for examination.

artifact Something present in an image which isn't natural to the structure or tissue. An aliasing artifact in ultrasonography is due to a sampling error. In MRI, an aliasing artifact is due to the appearance of a structure outside the field of view within the image. A summation artifact in mammography is the appearance of harmless shadows photographically superimposed to resemble cancerous lesions that disappear when the breast is viewed from another angle.

ASO (antistreptolysin O) **titer** A blood test to measure antibodies against streptolysin O, a substance produced by group A streptococcus bacteria. The value is measured in Todd units.

AST (aspartate aminotransferase) An enzyme whose level in the serum is elevated in myocardial infarction, liver disease, and other conditions.

ataxia Impairment of complex movements due to loss of proprioceptive impulses from the muscles of the trunk or limbs.

atelectasis Collapse of lung tissue.

atelectatic otitis media See *tympanic membrane atelectasis*.

athetosis Slow, writhing, involuntary movements of the face or limbs.

atypia Any abnormality in cellular form or type; it may be associated with cancer or a precancerous condition.

auricle The protruding flap of the external ear, also known as the pinna.

AV (atrioventricular) **block** Impairment of the conduction between the atria and ventricles of the heart.

AV (arteriovenous) **nicking** Tapering of a venule where an arteriole crosses it.

avascular necrosis Death of bone tissue with destruction of adjacent joint due to obstruction of blood supply as a result of trauma; long-term systemic treatment with corticosteroids in patients with lupus, rheumatoid arthritis, or vasculitis; chronic alcohol abuse; blood disorders; and other diseases.

aversion therapy A form of behavior therapy that associates an objectionable or undesirable pattern of behavior with an unpleasant experience or consequence, so as to reduce or extinguish the behavior.

avulsion The ripping or tearing away of a part.

azotemia See *uremia*.

Babinski reflex Consists of dorsiflexion of the great toe and flaring of the other toes in response to stroking the sole of the foot toward the toes; an indication of disease or injury affecting a corticospinal tract. A normal reflex is downgoing, except in newborns and infants, in which the normal Babinski reflex is upgoing.

bacteriuria The presence of bacteria in the urine.

BAL (bronchoalveolar lavage) Obtaining of material from lung tissue by washing.

balloon angioplasty Stretching or breaking up atherosclerotic plaques in a coronary artery. See also *PTCA*.

band forms, bands Immature neutrophils whose nuclei appear as bands, in contrast to mature neutrophils whose nuclei are segmented or lobed.

barium enema (BE) The standard radiographic examination of the large intestine by introduction of barium suspension into the rectum.

barrel chest In pulmonary emphysema the anteroposterior diameter of the chest is often increased so that the rib cage approaches a cylindrical shape (like a barrel).

Barrett esophagus Peptic ulceration of the lower esophagus with metaplastic formation of columnar epithelium instead of the normal squamous epithelium. It can evolve into adenocarcinoma.

Bartholin glands A pair of glands located on either side of the vaginal orifice that secrete mucus for lubrication during intercourse.

basal body temperature Daily determination of oral temperature on arising is useful in confirming and dating ovulation. Daily graphing of basal body temperature will show a rise of 0.75 to 1.0ºF (0.2 to 0.5ºC) approximately one day after ovulation.

basement membrane A microscopic connective tissue layer underlying an epithelial surface and also investing certain kinds of cell.

basilar Pertaining to the bases (lowermost parts) of the lungs.

basos An acceptable brief form for *basophils*.

Battle sign Postauricular mastoid ecchymosis, a sign seen in basilar skull fractures. Named for William Henry Battle.

beta HCG See *HCG*.

biliary colic Pain in the gallbladder region due to passage of gallstones along the bile duct.

biliary dyskinesia Dysfunction of the sphincter of Oddi, which regulates the flow of bile and pancreatic juice into the duodenum.

BiliBlanket A portable phototherapy device for the treatment of neonatal jaundice (hyperbilirubinemia). It uses fiberoptics and represents advanced technology in phototherapy treatment given in the hospital or at home. See also *phototherapy*.

bilirubinemia The presence of bilirubin in the blood. Hyperbilirubinemia is an excessive amount of bilirubin in the blood, evidenced by jaundice (yellowing of the skin and mucous membranes).

bilirubinuria The presence of bilirubin in the urine resulting from liver disease or biliary duct obstruction.

bimalleolar fracture Fracture of the medial and lateral malleoli, the bony prominences on the sides of the ankle.

BK amputation Below-knee amputation.

blast forms, blasts Very immature cells, particularly leukocytes, not normally found in peripheral blood but present in acute leukemia.

bleeding time The number of minutes it takes for a small incision in the skin, made with a lancet, to stop bleeding. Either the Duke method (puncture of the earlobe) or the Ivy method (puncture of the forearm) may be used.

blepharitis Inflammation of one or both eyelids.

blepharochalasis Drooping eyelid skin.

blepharoplasty Surgery on the eyelids to remove skin and fat and reinforce surrounding muscles and tendons to improve vision impaired by sagging eyelids.

blepharospasm Spasm of the eyelids, usually due to local irritation, photophobia, or both.

bloating An overly full, distended feeling, usually from excessive intestinal gas.

blood pool The circulating blood, into which radionuclides are injected for various types of circulatory scans.

blood type A genetically determined and permanent characteristic of a person's red blood cells based on the presence of certain antigens. Two blood type systems of clinical importance are the ABO (comprising types A, B, AB, and O) and the Rh (comprising Rh-positive and Rh-negative).

blunted costophrenic angle On chest x-ray, a costophrenic angle that is flattened or distorted by scarring or pleural fluid.

BMD (bone mineral density) test Measures the amount of calcium in regions of the bones.

BMI (body mass index) A measure of the proportion of fat to lean body mass.

BMP (basic metabolic panel) A panel of 7 or 8 chemical blood tests used as a screening tool or to assess and monitor fluid and electrolyte status, kidney function, blood sugar levels, and response to therapy. It includes sodium, potassium, chloride, and bicarbonate, or CO_2 (the electrolytes), plus BUN, creatinine (measures of kidney function), and glucose (blood sugar). Calcium may be included although not technically part of a BMP. May be referred to as a chem-7, or chem-8 if calcium is included. Cf. *BNP*.

BNP (brain natriuretic peptide; B-type natriuretic peptide) A blood test used to detect, diagnose, and evaluate the severity of congestive heart failure; rising levels may also indicate worsening acute coronary syndrome. BNP is made by the heart and normally only a low amount of BNP is found in the blood. Not to be confused with *BMP*; the context of the report and the values given determine which test is meant

boggy uterus More spongy or elastic than expected.

bone wax Gel-like material that is exactly like wax used in the kitchen. It has the ability to seal little pores in the bone that are exuding blood.

bony crepitus The crackling sound produced by the rubbing together of fragments of fractured bone.

bony island Benign developmental abnormality consisting of a localized zone of increased density in a long bone.

bony process A component of bone, not bone itself. The greater and lesser trochanters are processes of the femur (thigh) bone.

borborygmus (pl., **borborygmi**) Audible rumbling and gurgling sounds i n the digestive tract.

both-bone fracture Fracture of two adjacent bones in a limb, either radius and ulna (forearm) or tibia and fibula (leg).

bowel gas pattern On abdominal film, the normal radiographic appearance of gas in the intestine.

Bowman layer (or **membrane**) Anterior limiting lamina, a thin layer of the cornea beneath the outer layer of stratified epithelium.

BPH (benign prostatic hyperplasia) An overgrowth of androgen-sensitive glandular tissue that normally accompanies aging and causing varying degrees of urinary obstruction. It does not evolve into cancer.

brachytherapy A form of cancer treatment in which radioactive material is inserted into the body close to the tissues to be treated.

bradyarrhythmia A pulse that is both irregular and abnormally slow.

brawny Thickened or hardened as a result of severe inflammatory response. Examples: brawny edema, brawny erythema.

Braxton Hicks contractions Weak and irregular contractions of the uterus occurring during mid to late pregnancy.

breech birth The delivery of a newborn buttocks first.

bridging Formation of a bridge from one bone to another by abnormal calcium deposition, as in osteoarthritis.

bridging osteophytes Osteophytes (bony outgrowths) on adjacent vertebrae that meet and fuse, forming a "bridge" across the joint space.

bronchiectasis Abnormal, irreversible dilatation of bronchi, related to chronic infection.

bronchoscopy Inspection of the interior of the trachea and main bronchi with a fiberoptic instrument. Specimens and biopsies can be taken through the instrument.

bruit A rough vascular sound, synchronous with the heartbeat, heard with a stethoscope on auscultation over a narrowing in an artery.

BSI (Brief Symptom Inventory) A brief questionnaire-based survey used to screen psychiatric patients and monitor their progress during treatment. Analysis of patient-reported data helps to identify anxiety, depression, hostility, somatization, and other mental conditions, to estimate the severity of the patient's distress, and to provide a basis for treatment.

BSS (balanced saline solution) An irrigating solution commonly used during eye surgeries.

bucket-handle fracture Microfractures through the immature part of the bone edge of the metaphysis in infants, caused by shearing, often seen in rapid acceleration and deceleration forces to the extremity.

buckle fracture A type of impaction fracture that generally occurs at the transition from diaphysis to metaphysis.

bulla (pl., bullae) A blister or bleb; a fluid-filled epidermal sac larger than a vesicle.

BUN (blood urea nitrogen) The serum level of urea nitrogen, a waste product of protein metabolism. Elevation indicates an impairment of kidney function.

burr cell An abnormal red blood cell with a jagged contour.

BUS Bartholin glands, urethra, and Skene glands.

butterfly fracture A long-bone fracture in which the central fragment is triangular-shaped.

bx Abbreviation for *biopsy*.

CABG (coronary artery bypass graft) Surgical procedure done to bypass one or more occluded coronary arteries by using a vein graft (often from the leg).

cachexia General appearance of debility and malnutrition.

calculous cholecystitis Cholecystitis associated with gallstones, the most common type.

calculus (pl., calculi) Stone; abnormal concretion, usually of mineral salts. May be found in the kidneys (renal calculi), bladder, and ureters. Can usually be successfully crushed in situ and the fragments flushed out by means of a cystoscope, but ESWL or an open procedure (generally laparoscopic) may sometimes be appropriate.

callus formation An unorganized meshwork of woven bone, which is formed following fracture of a bone and is normally replaced by hard adult bone.

canaliculus (pl., canaliculi) An extremely narrow tubular passage or duct; in ophthalmology, the lacrimal duct.

C&S (culture and sensitivity) Laboratory test that grows a colony of bacteria removed from an infected area in order to identify the specific infecting bacteria and then determine their sensitivity to a variety of antibiotics. Do not confuse with CNS (central nervous system).

CAP (community-acquired pneumonia) Pneumonia not acquired in a hospital or a long-term care facility.

capsulorrhexis In cataract extraction surgery, a continuous circular tear in the anterior lens capsule to allow expression or phacoemulsification of the lens nucleus. Also, *capsulorhexis*.

carbuncle A spreading lesion made up of furuncles communicating by subcutaneous passages.

cardia The first of five portions of the stomach adjacent to and surrounding the cardiac opening where the esophagus connects to the stomach; it is not anatomically divided but used for reference.

carotid endarterectomy Removal of hardened plaque from an obstructed carotid artery.

cast Application of a solid material to immobilize an extremity or position of the body in the treatment of a fracture, dislocation, or severe injury. It may be made of plaster of Paris or fiberglass.

casts Plugs of material formed in renal tubules, detected on urinalysis. Casts are always abnormal.

causalgia Burning or stinging due to irritation or inflammation of nerves.

cavitation A pathological hollow space or place in tissues or organs such as occurs in the lungs in pulmonary tuberculosis.

CBC (complete blood count) A group of blood tests, including hemoglobin (hgb), hematocrit (hct), white blood count (WBC), WBC differential, red blood count (RBC), and platelets.

CEA (carcinoembryonic antigen) A glycoprotein occurring in the normal embryo and also detectable in the serum of some adults with cancer of the colon.

celiac sprue (or disease) A malabsorption syndrome precipitated by ingestion of gluten-containing foods and characterized by degeneration of intestinal villi.

cellulitis A type of infection occurring in soft tissues, including the skin, whose cardinal features are diffuse and spreading tissue swelling, redness, pain, and fever; often caused by streptococci.

centrilobular Affecting the central portions of lobules, as in the liver.

cephalgia, cephalalgia Headache. Local or generalized, intermittent or constant; can result from infection, neoplasm, or hemorrhage within the cranium, obstruction to the flow of cerebrospinal fluid, trauma, or migraine.

Ceretec (technetium Tc 99m exametazime injection preparation kit) Scintigraphy imaging agent (with or without methylene blue stabilization) is used as an adjunct in the detection of altered regional cerebral perfusion in stroke.

ceruloplasmin A copper-carrying protein in blood plasma that is absent in Wilson disease.

cervical cerclage A surgical treatment for cervical incompetence in which a ring of strong suture of special tape is placed around the cervix and tightened to prevent the cervix from thinning and stretching so as to avoid premature delivery.

cervical incompetence A medical condition in which a pregnant woman's cervix begins to dilate (widen) and efface (thin) before her pregnancy has reached term. It may cause miscarriage or preterm birth during the second and third trimesters.

cesarean delivery (cesarean section, C-section) Removal of the fetus (usually term or near-term) surgically through an incision in the abdomen and uterus.

Chaddock reflex Extension of the great toe elicited by tapping the ankle behind the lateral malleolus, a sign of disease or injury of a corticospinal tract.

Chadwick sign Purplish discoloration of the cervix and vagina in early pregnancy.

chem-7 panel A blood test for sodium, potassium, chloride, bicarbonate, BUN, creatinine, and glucose.

chem-8 panel Chem-7 panel plus calcium.

chem-20 A comprehensive panel of blood chemistry tests that includes the tests included in a BMP plus liver function tests (ALT, AST, alkaline phosphatase, total protein and albumin, and bilirubin) and cholesterol (HDL, LDL, triglycerides, and total cholesterol), and LDH. The more common name is CMP (comprehensive metabolic panel). May also be referred to as a *chemistry panel.*

chemotherapy protocol A program according to which cancer drugs are administered to a given patient; specifies choice of agents, routes of administration, dosages, intervals, and duration of treatment.

Cheyne-Stokes respirations Cyclic alternations between periods of apnea or hypopnea and periods of tachypnea.

chocolate agar A culture medium containing blood which, when autoclaved, turns chocolate brown. It is used to culture *Neisseria gonorrhoeae* and *Haemophilus influenzae.*

cholesteatoma A benign but locally invasive growth of the tympanic membrane caused by prolonged negative pressure (partial vacuum) in the middle ear. It contains cholesterol, hence the name.

cholesterol, serum A lipid (fatty) material formed in the liver and transported in the blood, which serves as a building block for various hormones and other substances. Elevation of serum cholesterol, which is usually due to an inherited disturbance of lipid metabolism, is associated with increased risk of atherosclerosis. See *HDL, LDL, VLDL.*

cholesterolosis The deposition of cholesterol in abnormal quantities in tissues.

Choletec (technetium Tc 99m mebrofenin) Hepatobiliary imaging agent used in cholescintigraphy.

chorea Rapid, jerky, purposeless involuntary movements of one or several muscle groups.

choriocarcinoma A malignant tumor that can develop from either the chorion of a normal pregnancy or a hydatidiform mole. It grows rapidly and metastasizes early, often before an abnormal pregnancy is suspected. Quantitative assay of hCG plays a role in the detection and management of both of these placental neoplasms.

chorionic villus sampling Removal of a biopsy specimen from the chorion, which carries a significant risk of causing miscarriage, for the purpose of genetic testing to see if the patient is at risk for having a baby with Down syndrome or other genetic defect.

Chvostek sign Twitching of the face after percussion over the facial nerve in front of the ear, a sign of latent tetany due to hypocalcemia.

cicatrix (scar) A zone of fibrous tissue occurring at the site of a healed injury or inflammatory or destructive lesion extending into the dermis.

CIN (cervical intraepithelial neoplasia) Dysplasia that is seen on a biopsy of the cervix and classified as follows: CIN I—mild dysplasia; CIN II—moderate to marked dysplasia; CIN III—severe dysplasia to carcinoma in situ.

cine (for **cinematograph**) **view** A moving picture of events disclosed by an imaging technique and recorded in real time on film or tape.

CK (creatine kinase) A serum enzyme that can be chemically distinguished into three isoenzymes or fractions: the BB (CK-BB) isoenzyme is elevated in cerebral infarction, the MM (CK-MM) in muscular dystrophy and muscle crush injury, and MB (CK-MB) in myocardial infarction. When separated in the laboratory by electrophoresis, these isoenzymes appear as distinct bands in a visual display. Hence the expression MB band is roughly synonymous with MB isoenzyme. Do not confuse *creatine* with *creatinine.* CPK (creatine phosphokinase) is an outdated abbreviation for CK.

clean-voided specimen (**clean catch**) Obtained after cleansing of the area around the urethral meatus to prevent contamination of the specimen with material from outside the urinary tract.

client The recipient of psychotherapy; a term preferred to "patient" when the therapist is not a physician.

client-centered therapy A form of psychotherapy in which the client is encouraged, with a minimum of direction by the therapist, to discover the sources of distressing mental symptoms and means of resolving them.

clinical correlation (**advised** or **recommended**) Interpreting an imaging study in light of the patient's medical history and objective findings on physical examination and laboratory testing.

clinicians Healthcare professionals who treat patients or provide direct patient care of any type. These include physicians, nurses, and allied health professionals (technologists and therapists).

CLO (Campylobacter-like organism) **test** To detect *H. pylori* in acid peptic disease. Also *rapid urease test*.

closed fracture Fracture with no open skin wound. Also called a *simple fracture*.

closed reduction of fracture Correcting a fracture by realigning the bone fragments by manipulation without entering the body.

clotting time The time needed for a clot to form in a tube of freshly drawn blood under standard conditions. The Lee-White method is the one most often used.

clubbing Club-shaped deformity of fingertips, seen in chronic pulmonary disease.

CMP (comprehensive metabolic profile) A group of 14 specific blood tests including glucose, calcium, albumin, total protein, sodium, potassium, carbon dioxide or bicarbonate, chloride, BUN, creatinine, ALP, ALT, AST, and bilirubin.

CMV (cytomegalovirus) A herpesvirus that is often not symptomatic but can cause infections, and particularly virulent in persons with AIDS, resulting in CMV retinitis. It is used as a broad screening tool to evaluate organ function and check for conditions such as diabetes, liver disease, and kidney disease, and to monitor known conditions such as hypertension.

coags Slang term for *coagulation studies*.

coagulation panel Platelet count, bleeding time, clotting time, prothrombin time, partial thromboplastin time, and clot retraction. In addition, plasma assay for specific coagulation factors is possible.

cognitive therapy A form of psychotherapy based on promoting the client's rational understanding of the source of distressing emotions, thought patterns, and undesirable behaviors, and correction of these by adoption of more mature, balanced, and realistic attitudes.

collagenous colitis A type of inflammatory reaction in the colon characterized by deposits of collagen, the principal noncellular component of connective tissue, beneath the epithelium of the colon.

collar button (ventilation) **tubes** Surgical placement of tiny tubes in the eardrum to prevent chronic ear infections. See *myringotomy tubes*.

collateral vessels Vascular channels newly formed from existing ones to maintain the circulation of a tissue or organ whose normal blood supply has been impaired by disease or injury.

Colles fracture Fracture of the distal radius with dorsal displacement, with or without involvement of the ulna.

coloboma (iridis) A congenital defect in the iris, in which a wedge-shaped segment is absent, giving a keyhole appearance to the pupil; similar defects are created by certain types of ocular surgery.

colostomy A surgically created opening from the colon to the abdominal wall, through which feces are passed rather than by the rectum; may be temporary or permanent.

colposcopy Examination of the cervix with an illuminated low-power microscope, which facilitates identification of suspicious cervical lesions requiring biopsy.

columnar epithelium Epithelium consisting of one or more layers of cells whose height is at least twice their width.

comminuted fracture Fracture in which the bone is shattered, splintered, or crushed into many small pieces or fragments.

commissurotomy Surgical enlargement of the aperture of a stenotic heart valve, particularly the mitral, by stretching or cutting.

complex seizure Impaired alertness or unconsciousness; sometimes with psychic symptoms or automatisms.

conchal bowl (or **concha**) The cartilage that is situated right near the ear canal and looks like a bowl.

condyle A rounded projection on a bone. It usually serves as an articulation site at which two anatomical structures meet.

condyloma (pl., **condylomata**) Genital wart.

coned-down view A radiographic study limited to a small area by the use of a cone that narrows and "focuses" the x-ray beam.

confabulation Invention of stories about one's past, often bizarre and complex, to fill in gaps left by amnesia; a typical feature of Korsakoff syndrome in chronic alcoholics.

confluent Merged, not discrete or distinct.

conization of the cervix Removal of a cone of tissue from the cervix for microscopic examination.

consolidative process An abnormal process that increases the density of a tissue or region. Also, *consolidation*.

contiguous images A series of scans without intervals of unexamined tissue between them.

Coombs test, direct A test to determine whether the patient's red blood cells have become coated with an antiglobulin. The test is positive in newborns with hemolytic disease due to Rh incompatibility and in other patients with acquired hemolytic disease.

Coombs test, indirect A test to determine whether the patient's serum contains antiglobulin to red blood cells. This test is positive in the mother of an infant with hemolytic disease due to Rh incompatibility and in other patients with acquired hemolytic disease.

cor pulmonale Dilatation, hypertrophy, or failure of the right ventricle due to acute or chronic pulmonary disease.

corpectomy Excision of all or part of a vertebral body for decompression of the spinal cord with the removed bone being replaced by a graft.

cortex (pl., **cortices**) The outer layer of an organ or other structure, usually referring to a zone of functioning tissue (parenchyma) rather than a connective tissue capsule.

cortical bone Compact bone which is dense and hard on the bone surface, like the bark of a tree.

corticosteroid Cortisol or aldosterone (hormones of the adrenal cortex), or any synthetic drug having similar effects.

costophrenic angle The angle at the junction of the ribs and diaphragmatic pleura.

cough May be variously described as brassy, bubbling, croupy, hacking, harsh, hollow, loose, metallic, nonproductive, productive, rasping, rattling, or wracking.

CPAP (continuous positive airway pressure) A method of positive pressure ventilation to keep the airways open at the end of exhalation, increase oxygenation, and improve breathing. Often prescribed for patients with obstructive sleep apnea.

CPD (cephalopelvic disproportion) The fetal head is too large to pass through the maternal pelvis.

CPR (cardiopulmonary resuscitation) The use of external compression of the heart coupled with breathing techniques to revive a victim whose heart and respirations have stopped.

CPT (*Physicians' Current Procedural Terminology*) A formal classification of diagnostic and therapeutic procedures published by the American Medical Association and revised annually, in which each procedure is assigned a five-digit code. CPT codes are universally used in billing third-party payers for medical services.

crackles Rales.

craniectomy Surgical removal of part of the bone of the skull.

craniotomy Surgical incision into the cranium, which necessitates drilling or sawing through the bone of the skull.

creatinine clearance A measure of kidney function, calculated from the serum creatinine level and the amount of creatinine excreted in the urine in 24 hours.

crepitant rale A fine crackling rale.

crepitus See *bony crepitus* and *joint crepitus*.

cross-section A cut made perpendicular to the long axis of a structure.

crossed (or **contralateral**) **straight leg raising** With the patient supine, the unaffected leg is held straight and flexed at the hip. If sciatica is present, the patient will experience pain in the opposite, affected side.

CRP (C-reactive protein) A test used to detect rheumatoid arthritis.

crust A hard, friable, irregular layer of dried blood, serum, pus, tissue debris, or any combination of these adherent to the surface of injured or inflamed skin; a scab.

cryopexy Surgical treatment of retinal detachment consisting of localized freezing of the surface of the sclera to fix the retina to the choroid.

cryoprobe A cryosurgical instrument containing a circulating refrigerant, which can be rapidly chilled so as to deliver subfreezing temperature to tissues.

cryosurgery The application of liquid nitrogen (at a temperature of -196°C) to destroy superficial skin lesions.

cryotherapy Local treatment of neoplasms or other lesions by freezing.

crypt A blind pit or tube opening onto a free surface (skin or mucous membrane).

cryptorchidism Failure of one or both of the testes to descend into the scrotum; also cryptorchism and undescended testicle.

crystalline lens The natural lens of the eye.

crystals, urinary Detected on urinalysis.

CSF (cerebrospinal fluid) The fluid medium of the central nervous system (brain and spinal cord), which can be sampled by lumbar puncture (spinal tap) for chemical testing, cell counts, and culture.

CT (computed tomography) **scan** An application of computer technology to diagnostic imaging. Contrast medium may be injected into the circulation immediately before CT scanning to enhance the imaging of certain structures and body regions and improve the visibility of some tumors. Formerly *computerized axial tomography* (CAT) *scan*.

C3F8 (perfluoropropane) **gas** An intraocular gas used to tamponade the retina in retinal detachment surgery or to replace intravitreal fluid that may have leaked out during other surgeries such as trabeculectomy. Other gases used for similar purposes are sulfur hexafluoride (SF6), perfluoroethane (C2F6).

cubital tunnel syndrome A type of entrapment neuropathy with a complex of symptoms resulting from injury or compression of the ulnar nerve at the elbow,

cuffing, peribronchial Thickening of bronchial walls as seen on chest x-ray.

culdoscopy Endoscopic inspection of the cul-de-sac (pouch of Douglas), the lowermost part of the peritoneal cavity, which lies between the uterus and the rectum. The instrument is introduced vaginally under anesthesia.

cupping of the disc The normal optic nerve head has a slight central depression (physiologic cupping). Increase in the depth of the cup occurs with increased intraocular pressure (glaucoma) or atrophy of the optic nerve.

curettage A surgical scraping.

Cushing syndrome Truncal obesity, moon facies, hypertension, impairment of glucose tolerance, osteoporosis, and other metabolic abnormalities caused by an excess of adrenocortical steroid, either from a tumor or hyperactivity of the adrenal gland or as a result of prolonged therapeutic administration of hormone.

cut A CT section or image; a scan.

CXR (chest x-ray) The standard *PA chest* film is the most frequently performed of all plain radiographic examinations. A PA film shows the lungs as the x-rays pass from the back of the body to the front. It provides diagnostic information on the respiratory passages and pulmonary aeration and vasculature; pleural and diaphragmatic margins; the configuration of the heart and great vessels; osseous structures; soft tissue contours; and abnormal infiltrates, masses, and accumulations of fluid. Other routine views are *AP* (anteroposterior) and *lateral*. An AP film shows the lungs as the x-rays pass from the front of the body (anterior) to the back (posterior). In the lateral view, the x rays pass from side to side. Other views that may be referenced are *oblique* (the patient is positioned at a 45-degree angle to the film) and *lateral decubitus* (the patient is lying on either side). Images obtained as the patient takes a deep breath and holds it are called *inspiratory* x-rays; images taken after exhalation and before inspiration are called *expiratory* x-rays.

cyanosis Bluish color of skin, particularly lips and nail beds, due to presence of excess unoxygenated blood in the circulation.

cyclothymia Abnormal lability of mood, which varies between excitement and depression without becoming severe enough to be called bipolar disorder.

cystocele Bulging of the urinary bladder through the anterior vaginal wall.

cystolitholapaxy An endoscopic procedure in which bladder stones are crushed with a lithotrite and the resulting fragments are flushed out by irrigation.

cystourethrocele Prolapse of the urethra and bladder into the vagina.

cystourethroscopy A combination procedure consisting of urethroscopy and cystoscopy.

cytology The branch of biology concerned with the structure and function of living cells. In clinical pathology it refers to the diagnostic assessment of cells that have been detached from a surface for microscopic study, as in a Pap smear.

cytopathic effects Effects characterized by pathologic changes in cell structure.

cytoplasm The fluid medium within a cell in which the nucleus and other organelles are suspended.

dacryorhinocystotomy A variation on dacryocystorhinotomy, passage of a probe through the lacrimal sac into the nasal cavity.

D&C (dilatation and curettage) Scraping of the endometrium, after stretching of the cervix with graded dilators, to obtain specimen material for the diagnosis of endometrial disease. This procedure, performed under anesthesia (general, spinal, or intravenous), is also used therapeutically for various endometrial disorders.

dark-field microscopy A microscopic technique using special lighting that makes it easier to identify *Treponema pallidum*, the organism that causes syphilis.

DaTscan (ioflupane I 123 injection) Single photon emission computed tomography (SPECT) imaging agent for the evaluation of parkinsonian syndromes.

debridement Successive scraping away of dead skin down to viable tissue that bleeds from a wound or burn to prevent infection and promote healing.

decompensation Failure to maintain a stable status of diseases or symptoms.

decubitus ulcer An erosion of the skin and subcutaneous tissues due to prolonged pressure, occurring chiefly in immobile persons confined to bed. Also known as a *bedsore* or *pressure ulcer*. The word *ulcer* is often omitted in dictation.

delusion A false belief or wrong interpretation of observed facts, sometimes associated with hallucinations. May be categorized as delusions of grandeur (believing that one is a monarch or other celebrity), reference (a false perception that the words or actions of others refer to oneself), or persecution (thinking one is the target of official surveillance or a hostile plot).

dementia Deterioration of mental function.

demineralization Reduction in the amount of calcium present in bone, due to disease or immobilization.

dependent edema Swelling of the lower extremities, aggravated by the downward hanging position.

dermatographism The property of abnormally sensitive skin by which strokes or writing with a pointed object are reproduced on the skin surface as raised red lines. Also *dermographism*.

dermatome 1) An instrument used to obtain thin slices of skin for grafting. 2) An area of skin that is mainly supplied by a single spinal nerve (dermatome distribution).

Descemet membrane Posterior limiting lamina, a thin hyaline membrane between the substantia propria and the endothelial layer of the cornea.

DEXA (dual-energy x-ray absorptiometry) Enhanced form of x-ray technology that is used to measure bone loss. Stationary devices usually check the spine and hips. Portable devices, some utilizing ultrasound as well, are used on wrists and hands.

diaphoresis Sweating.

diarrhea Abnormal frequency, urgency, and looseness of stools.

diascopy Inspection of red or purplish lesions through a transparent plastic or glass plate, which compresses the skin. If the color is due to dilated blood vessels, it blanches (fades) with compression; color due to deposition of pigment, including blood pigment, in tissues is not altered by surface pressure.

diastasis Dislocation of two bones normally attached to each other.

DIC (disseminated intravascular coagulation) A condition in which widespread clotting of blood in vessels consumes clotting factors and leads to hemorrhage.

differential white blood cell count A determination of the relative numbers of the six types of white blood cells normally found in peripheral blood. When the count is performed visually, a technician observes 100 white blood cells in a stained smear of whole blood and reports the number of each cell type found as a percent. The differential count can also be done electronically. The six types of white blood cells are segmented neutrophils (PMNs or segs), band neutrophils (bands, representing the immature form), eosinophils (eos), basophils (basos), lymphocytes (lymphs), and monocytes (monos).

digital subtraction angiography X-ray images of the head with and without contrast medium are processed by a computer, which deletes all shadows common to both films (skull bones, soft tissue profiles and interfaces), leaving only the vascular system visible.

dilatation and curettage (D&C) Scraping of the endometrium, after stretching of the cervix with graded dilators, to obtain specimen material for the diagnosis of endometrial disease. This procedure, performed under anesthesia (general, spinal, or intravenous), is also used therapeutically for various endometrial disorders.

diopter (D) A unit of refractive power of lenses. For example, reading glasses may be rated as 2.25 diopters; intraocular lenses may be rated 19.0 diopters.

dipstick A commercially produced strip of plastic or paper bearing a series of dots or squares of reagent, each designed to assess a specific chemical property of urine; often used to refer to the test itself.

discoid Consisting of small, flat plaques.

diskectomy Excision of an intervertebral disk.

diuresis An increase in the production of urine by the kidneys as a result of renal or systemic disease, toxic substances, or drugs administered to reduce body water, sodium, or both.

diverticulum (pl., **diverticula**) An abnormal outpouching of a hollow organ such as the colon.

DMSA (technetium Tc 99m succimer injection preparation kit) **scan** Used to assess renal function.

dorsiflexion Bending upward of the hand or foot.

double-contrast technique A modification of the barium enema procedure. After the standard barium enema examination has been completed, the patient expels most of the barium, and the colon is then inflated with air. The coating of barium remaining on the surface may outline masses or defects not seen during the standard examination.

double-J stent A ureteral stent of flexible material with a J-shaped curl at each end, one to anchor the stent in the renal pelvis and the other to anchor it in the bladder.

DRE (digital rectal examination) Examination of the interior of the rectum and adjacent structures, especially the prostate gland, with a finger inserted through the anus.

DRG codes Diagnosis-related group codes that determine the amount of reimbursement the hospital will receive.

dribbling Uncontrollable passage of drops of urine, particularly just after voiding.

DSM (*Diagnostic and Statistical Manual of Mental Disorders*) A description and classification of mental disorders based on objective criteria. Recognized as a diagnostic standard and widely used for reporting, coding, and statistical purposes, DSM is published by the American Psychiatric Association. The current (fifth) edition (DSM-V) appeared in 2013.

DTRs (deep tendon reflexes) Occur in response to sudden stretching of a muscle, usually induced by tapping a tendon with a rubber-headed reflex hammer. Tendon reflexes are tested in several muscles of the upper and lower extremities, with comparison of the two sides.

dual photon densitometry A quantitative assessment of a patient's bone density, and comparison with normal ranges for persons of the same age and sex.

Duke bleeding time The number of minutes it takes for a small incision in the earlobe, made with a lancet, to stop bleeding. The Ivy method (puncture of the forearm) is another method for assessing bleeding time.

dullness to percussion Muffling on percussion due to consolidation of lung tissue by infection or neoplasm, or to fluid in the pleural space.

DXA scan (dual x-ray absorptiometry) The preferred technique for measuring bone mineral density. Formerly called *DEXA* (dual-energy x-ray absorptiometry). The DXA scan is typically used to diagnose and follow osteoporosis. It is not to be confused with the nuclear bone scan, which is sensitive to certain metabolic diseases in which bones are attempting to heal from infections, fractures, or tumors.

dysequilibrium Loss of balance sense; tendency to fall without support.

dyslipidemia Any of various disorders characterized by abnormally high levels of lipids (cholesterol, triglycerides) in the blood.

dysmenorrhea Pain occurring with menstruation and often severe. The lay term for dysmenorrhea is "menstrual cramps."

dyspareunia Pain in the vulva, vagina, or pelvis with sexual intercourse.

dysphagia Difficulty swallowing.

dysphoria A general feeling of mental or emotional discomfort.

dysplasia Alteration in size, shape, and organization of adult cells usually heralding eventual development of malignancy.

dyspnea Shortness of breath.

dysthymia A depressed mood, usually chronic or recurrent, that is not severe enough to be called major depression.

dystocia Abnormal slowing or arrest of the progress of labor.

dysuria Pain in the urethra or vulva with urination.

eardrum Strictly speaking, the middle ear. In everyday usage, both lay and professional, the term refers only to the tympanic membrane, a thin, tough layer of tissue at the inner end of the ear canal that receives sound waves and transmits them to the inner ear by the chain of ossicles in the middle ear.

eburnation Increased density of articular ends of bone.

ECCE (extracapsular cataract extraction) Surgical removal of the clouded lens of the eye leaving the capsule intact for implantation of an intraocular lens.

ECG, EKG (electrocardiogram) A tracing of the electrical activity of the heart.

echocardiography A noninvasive diagnostic procedure in which an ultrasonic beam is directed at the heart and the returning echoes are recorded and analyzed; valuable for the measurement of cardiac chambers (wall thickness and cavity volume), assessment of ventricular function, and identification of valvular malfunction.

echo characteristics The frequency, intensity, and distribution of echoes produced by a structure or region on ultrasound examination.

echo pattern The ultrasonographic appearance of a structure as seen on a visual display.

E. (Escherichia) coli Gram-negative bacterium normally found in the intestine and responsible for many urinary tract infections.

ectasia (-ectasis) Dilatation or distention of a tubular structure, as in the bronchi or intestines.

ectopic pregnancy Pregnancy in which implantation has occurred somewhere other than the endometrium—in the uterine tube, on the pelvic peritoneum, or even on an ovary.

ectopy, ectopia The appearance of a structure or organ outside its normal location.

ectropion Eversion (turning outward) and drooping of the lower eyelid, exposing the conjunctival surface and allowing overflow of tears.

eczema Superficial dermatitis of unknown cause accompanied by redness, vesicles, itching, and crusting.

EDC (estimated date of confinement). Calculated by going back 3 months and then forward 7 days from the first day of the last menstrual period. May also be called *EDD* (estimated date of delivery).

edema Swelling due to the presence of fluid in tissue spaces.

EEG (electroencephalography) Measurement and recording of electrical activity in the brain from several sites simultaneously. Electrodes are attached with fine needles to standard sites on the scalp, and the record is made on a strip of moving paper. Tracings are usually made after administration of a short-acting sedative (with the subject asleep, if possible). The effects of hyperventilation and of photic stimulation (exposure to a flashing light) are recorded also. The EEG is particularly useful in identifying and classifying seizure disorders.

effacement Abnormal flattening of the contour of a structure; in obstetrics, the flattening of the cervix from a tubular structure to a ring during labor.

effusion An abnormal accumulation of fluid in a body cavity, such as the pericardium.

EGD (esophagogastroduodenoscopy) Endoscopic procedure to view the esophagus, stomach, and duodenum.

EG (esophagogastric) **junction** The transition site from the stratified squamous epithelium of the esophagus to the simple columnar epithelium of the cardia of the stomach. Also, *cardioesophageal* or *gastroesophageal* (GE) *junction*.

egress Escape or come out of.

electroconvulsive (electroshock) **therapy** Delivery of controlled electric shocks to the brain to alter electrochemical function, primarily in depression. The treatment, administered only by a physician, causes convulsions and loss of consciousness; the patient awakens in a state of disorientation. Several treatment sessions may be necessary before improvement is noted.

electrodesiccation See *fulguration*.

electrolytes The electrolytes are sodium (Na), potassium (K), chloride (Cl), and bicarbonate (HCO_3) which is sometimes reported as total carbon dioxide (CO_2). They are used to monitor acid-base balance, kidney function, hypertension, response to diuretics, and potassium supplementation. Reference ranges: potassium 3.5–5.2 mEq/L; sodium 135–147 mEq/L; chloride 95–107 mEq/L; bicarbonate 19–25 mEq/L. Numerical values are sometimes dictated, in the order shown here, without mention of the electrolytes by name. One can determine which electrolyte goes with which value by knowing the normal reference ranges.

electrolytes, sweat Sodium and chloride ions in the sweat, increased in persons with cystic fibrosis.

electrolytes, urinary Sodium, potassium, and chloride ions in the urine. Abnormal concentrations could indicate kidney disease.

electrophysiologic studies Measurement of electrical activity in nerves and muscles. See *EMG* and *NCV*.

embolism Obstruction of a blood vessel by a detached blood clot, air, fat, or injected material. An embolus is the material that causes the obstruction.

EMG (electromyogram) Test to determine the response pattern of muscles when stimulated by an electrical impulse from a needle electrode inserted into the muscle.

encephalopathy Any organic disease or damage of the brain, particularly the cerebral cortex, that causes impairment of mental or physical functioning; often due to degenerative diseases (Alzheimer disease, Creutzfeldt-Jakob disease) or chemical intoxications (alcohol, lead).

endodiathermy A procedure using a probe for cauterizing bleeding retinal vessels such as in diabetic retinopathy or before large and more central retinectomies. Another indication is to mark a break in retinal detachment surgery or in preparation for a retinotomy.

endolymph The fluid medium contained in the inner ear.

endometrial ablation Surgical destruction (ablation) of the endometrium (uterine lining) for dysfunctional uterine bleeding. A variety of ablating modalities including laser, radiofrequency, thermal balloon (ThermaChoice), electricity, cryosurgery (freezing), and microwave may be used. The procedure may be done under local or spinal anesthesia. A hysteroscope may be used for visualization.

endometrial stripe On an ultrasound, refers to the thickness of the endometrium; an endometrial stripe of more than 4 or 5 mm is an indication for an endometrial biopsy in a postmenopausal woman.

enterocolitis Inflammatory disease of both the small and large intestines.

entropion Inward turning of the margin of the lower eyelid, often so that the lower lashes touch the eyeball.

enuresis Urinary incontinence. Do not confuse with anuresis (inability to urinate). See *anuria*.

eos Brief form for *eosinophils*.

eosinophilic infiltrate The appearance of eosinophils (polymorphonuclear leukocytes with coarse granules appearing red with hematologic stains) in the interstitial tissues of a structure such as the lung, colon, or liver.

epidermal inclusion cyst A benign cutaneous lesion caused by the infolding of keratinizing squamous epithelium.

epiphora Chronic overflow of tears from the lower eyelid onto the cheek; may be due to blockage of the nasolacrimal duct or to deformity of the lower lid (ectropion).

epiphysis The expanded articular end of a long bone.

episiotomy An incision in the posterior midline to enlarge the vulvar opening during childbirth.

ERG (electroretinography) Instrumental determination of changes in electrical potential of the retina in response to light stimuli; identifies visual abnormalities due to retinal disease.

erosive gastritis Inflammatory condition characterized by multiple erosions of the mucous membrane lining the stomach.

eschar The crust that forms on a burn.

ESR (erythrocyte sedimentation rate) The rate at which red blood cells settle to the bottom of a specimen of whole blood that has been treated with anticoagulant. The rate is expressed in millimeters per hour (mm/h), as measured in a standard glass column. Elevation of the sedimentation rate occurs in various inflammatory and malignant diseases but is diagnostic of none. An acceptable brief form is *sed rate*.

ESWL (extracorporeal shock wave lithotripsy) A method of shattering stones in the urinary tract (also in the biliary tract) by means of ultrasound waves generated outside the body. This noninvasive procedure can break up more than 90% of urinary tract stones in adults, permitting passage of the fragments in the urine.

ethmoidectomy A surgical procedure to remove the partitions between the ethmoid sinuses in order to create larger sinus cavities.

euthyroid Normal thyroid.

exacerbation Worsening in severity of symptoms.

excoriation Abrasion of the epidermal surface by scratching.

extraarticular Affecting or pertaining to structures other than joints.

extraaxial Outside the brain or external to the pia mater, the meningeal membrane that covers the brain, spinal cord, and the proximal portions of the nerve root. Extraaxial masses are more likely to be meningiomas, fluid, or hemorrhage. Compare *intraaxial*.

extravasation of contrast Leakage of contrast medium from the structure into which it is injected through a perforation or other abnormal orifice.

exudate Protein-rich fluid, inflammatory cells, and tissue debris deposited in or on tissues as a result of inflammation or degeneration.

facies Distinctive facial expressions associated with specific medical conditions.

failure of descent, failure to descend A delay in the progression of labor in which the baby fails to descend into the birth canal.

Falope ring sterilization A small silastic band is placed around a loop of the uterine (fallopian) tube to close it off to prevent pregnancy. Although intended to be permanent, some women choose this method because it is sometimes reversible.

FBS (fasting blood sugar) A measure of the concentration of glucose in the plasma after a 12-hour fast.

FDG (fludeoxyglucose F 18) PET imaging agent for the detection of abnormal glucose metabolism with applications in oncology, cardiology, and neurology.

FDDNP or **^{18}F-FDDNP** PET scan imaging agent for diagnosis of beta-amyloid senile plaques and neurofibrillary tangles for early detection of Alzheimer disease.

FDG (fludeoxyglucose F 18) PET imaging agent for the detection of abnormal glucose metabolism with applications in oncology, cardiology, and neurology.

FEF$_{25-75}$ (forced expiratory flow 25%-75%): the average flow rate during the midportion of a forced expiration, measured in liters per second (L/sec).

femoral neck fracture Fracture through the neck of the femur, proximal to the greater and lesser trochanter.

femoral-popliteal bypass Implantation of a vessel graft (real or artificial) into the femoral and popliteal arteries to bypass one or more blockages.

fetal macrosomia Excessive body size and weight.

fetal pyelectasis Dilatation of a renal pelvis observed in a fetus.

FEV$_1$ (forced expiratory volume in 1 second): the volume of air that is exhaled during the first second of forceful exhalation, in liters.

FEV$_1$/FVC: the ratio of FEV$_1$ to FVC, expressed as a percent.

fibrinous exudate A semisolid film on a wound or ulcer consisting largely of the insoluble protein fibrin.

fibrosis Excess fibrous connective tissue in an organ or tissue formed as a reparative or reactive process, as opposed to formation of fibrous tissue as a normal constituent of an organ or tissue.

filling defect A zone within a tubular structure that is not filled by injected contrast medium (usually a tumor or abnormal mass).

fine-needle aspiration A technique used to remove cells by suction from certain structures such as the prostate, subcutaneous lymph nodes and other neck masses, and breast masses.

fine-needle biopsy Sampling of a gland or organ tissue via insertion of a fine-bore needle and collecting a specimen for pathologic diagnosis.

finger-to-nose test The patient extends the arms outward laterally, closes the eyes, and tries to touch the finger to the nose. Tests coordination.

first-pass view An image or set of images obtained immediately after injection of radionuclide into the circulation, when its concentration in the blood pool is at its highest.

first-voided specimen The first urine passed after arising in the morning.

fissure A linear defect or crack in the continuity of the epidermis.

fistulotomy A fistulotomy is surgery to open a fistula to allow it to heal.

5'-nucleotidase (pronounced "five prime nucleotidase") A serum enzyme whose level increases in biliary obstruction. Testing for this enzyme helps to distinguish liver disease from bone disease as possible causes of elevated serum alkaline phosphatase.

fixation Procedure to stabilize a fractured bone while it heals. External fixation includes casts, splints, and pins inserted through the skin. Internal fixation includes pins, plates, rods, screws, and wires that are applied during an open reduction.

fixation device A plate, pin, nail, or screw used to hold fracture fragments in place.

fixative A fluid used to arrest the process of decomposition in a biopsy or autopsy specimen, to kill bacteria and fungi in or on the specimen, and to begin hardening the tissue to facilitate preparation for microscopic study.

flaccidity Absence of muscle tone and absence of reflexes.

flare and cells Diminished clarity of the aqueous humor due to protein leakage from the iris and swirls of inflammatory cells in the anterior chamber due to inflammation.

flash pulmonary edema Rapid onset of pulmonary edema (accumulation of fluid in the pulmonary tissues and air spaces) brought on by decompensated congestive heart failure, acute myocardial infarction, or mitral regurgitation.

flatulence, flatus Excessive intestinal gas.

flexure A bend. The hepatic flexure and splenic flexure are bends in the large bowel where it bends first to the left and then downward respectively.

fluorescein staining Fluorescein dye is applied to the cornea and conjunctiva, and the surface of the eye examined with a cobalt blue light, to detect injuries, ulcerations, or foreign bodies. See also retinal arteriography.

foamy histiocytes Histiocytes with a vacuolated appearance due to the presence of complex lipoids.

focus (pl., **foci**) The site or center of a morbid process.

fornix An archlike structure or the vaultlike space created by such a structure. The inferior fornix of the conjunctiva is the inferior line of reflection of the conjunctiva from the eyelid to the eyeball; the superior fornix is the superior line of reflection of the conjunctiva from the eyelid to the eyeball, which receives the openings of the lacrimal duct.

fornix-based peritomy A conjunctival incision starting at the base of the fornix. Also *fornix-based conjunctival flap*.

fourchette A fold of skin crossing the posterior commissure of the labia minora. Episiotomy may be performed during delivery to avoid irregular tearing of the fourchette.

FRC (functional residual capacity) The volume of air remaining in the lungs after normal expiration.

free air Air or gas in a body cavity where it does not belong, usually after escape from the GI tract.

free T$_4$ test A measure of the plasma concentration of thyroxine (T$_4$) that is free (not bound to protein).

frenuloplasty Surgical repositioning of an abnormally attached lingual frenum, the restraining structure under the tongue. Also called *frenoplasty*. Used to correct *tongue tie*.

friable Crumbly; fragmenting or bleeding easily on touch or manipulation; said usually of diseased tissue.

frogleg view An x-ray of one or both hip joints for which the patient lies supine with thighs maximally abducted and externally rotated and knees flexed so as to bring the soles of the feet together.

frozen section Cutting of a flash-frozen surgical specimen for rapid staining and microscopic examination while the patient is still in the operating room, as a guide to further surgical decision-making.

FSH (follicle-stimulating hormone) A hormone secreted by the anterior pituitary gland that stimulates ovulation in women and spermatogenesis in men. Measurement of serum FSH is part of the evaluation of a patient for infertility or gonadal dysfunction.

FTA (fluorescent treponemal antibody) **test** An indirect immunofluorescence test, highly specific for syphilis.

FTA-ABS Fluorescent treponemal antibody absorption test, to detect syphilis.

fulguration The application of an electrical current to destroy superficial skin lesions.

full-bladder technique An ultrasonographic examination of the pelvic region performed while the patient's bladder is distended with urine. This is done to improve the recognition of the bladder outline, which cannot be distinguished adequately when the bladder is empty.

full-column barium enema Barium enema examination in which the contrast medium is injected into the colon under full pressure, by elevation of the barium reservoir to the maximum safe height.

fundus The rear of the interior of the eye, consisting of the retina, its blood vessels, and the optic nerve head.

funduscopic examination Inspection of the fundus (the rear of the interior of the eye, consisting of the retina, its blood vessels, and the optic nerve head). The examination is performed with an ophthalmoscope. Also called *ophthalmoscopy*.

funic souffle (rhymes with "truffle") A whistling sound due to the flow of blood in the umbilical cord, heard on auscultation of the pregnant abdomen.

furuncle A deep, solitary abscess; a boil.

FVC (forced vital capacity) The maximum volume of air that can be forcefully exhaled after a maximal inspiration, in liters.

gadolinium A nonradioactive metallic element that acts as a contrast agent in MRI studies by enhancing the signal of areas or tissues in which it is present. After intravenous injection it can show up narrowed areas or malformations in blood vessels, vascular tumors, and areas of hemorrhage. It can also be used to delineate joint spaces in arthrography.

GAF (Global Assessment of Functioning) A subjective rating by a mental health professional, on a scale of 0-100, of the social, occupational, and psychological functioning of an adult subject. The scale is published in DSM.

gallop rhythm A cardiac rhythm that simulates the sound of a galloping horse on auscultation, usually due to the presence of a third or fourth heart sound, or both.

Gamma Knife stereotactic radiosurgery A form of radiation therapy using specialized equipment that focuses hundreds of tiny beams of radiation on a tumor in the brain delivering a strong dose of gamma radiation to the site where the beams meet but having little effect on the brain tissue as the individual beams pass through. Gamma Knife is a trademarked device.

gas density line A linear band of maximal radiolucency, representing or appearing to represent a narrow zone of air or gas.

gastrostomy button, balloon-tipped A small skin level gastrostomy tube made of silicone. It has an inflatable balloon at one end (inside the body) and an external base (outside the body) at the other.

gated view An image obtained by a technique synchronized with motions of the heart to eliminate blurring.

Gd-Tex (MGd; motexafin gadolinium) Radiosensitizing agent for the detection of brain metastases in patients with non-small cell lung cancer.

gestational diabetes Carbohydrate intolerance first occurring or first noted during pregnancy. This is a risk factor for polyhydramnios (excessive volume of amniotic fluid) and fetal macrosomia.

Glasgow coma scale Used to assess a patient's level of consciousness after a head injury. Verbal, motor, and sensory responses to stimuli are graded on a scale of 1 through 5. The values for each are added together for a total score. A score of 7 or less indicates coma; a score of 3 or less indicates brain death.

glaucoma Any of several related disorders in which sustained elevation of increased intraocular pressure can lead to irreversible impairment of vision.

Gleason score A numerical indicator of the malignant potential of prostatic carcinoma, determined by adding the grades of the two least differentiated biopsy specimens. Example: Gleason score 1+2 for a score of 3/10.

glial reaction A process of scarring in inflamed or degenerating nervous tissue as a result of the action of microglia.

Glisson capsule The connective tissue sheath of the liver.

glomerulus (pl., **glomeruli**) One of numerous globular tangles of capillaries in the renal cortex, each surrounded by a Bowman capsule into which a filtrate of plasma is expressed as the first step in the formation of urine.

glottic Pertaining to the larynx. Glottal or glottic spasm is laryngospasm.

glycated hemoglobin, glycosylated hemoglobin See *hemoglobin A1c*.

glycosuria The abnormal presence of glucose in the urine.

goiter Enlarged thyroid gland.

grand mal seizure See *tonic-clonic*.

graphesthesia The ability to recognize letters or numbers traced on the skin.

gravid Pregnant.

gravida Pregnant woman.

great vessels The major vascular trunks entering and leaving the heart: the superior and inferior venae cavae, the pulmonary arteries and veins, and the aorta.

greenstick fracture Fracture in which there is an incomplete break; one side of bone is broken and the other side is bent. This type of fracture is commonly found in children due to their softer and more pliable bone structure.

growth plate The area of growing tissue near the ends of the long bones in children and adolescents. Also known as the *epiphyseal plate*.

hallucination A sensory perception for which no basis exists in fact. Hallucinations may affect any one or more of the five senses (visual, auditory, tactile, olfactory, or gustatory); a typical feature of schizophrenia, delirium tremens, and some seizure disorders.

H&E Hematoxylin and eosin, the most commonly used combination of stains in histology.

H&H Slang abbreviation for *hemoglobin* and *hematocrit*. The hemoglobin level is usually dictated first.

HCG, hCG (human chorionic gonadotropin) A hormone produced by the placenta and detected in various blood and urine tests for pregnancy. A more specific test detects only the beta subunit of this hormone, hence the term beta-HCG.

Hct, HCT Abbreviation for *hematocrit*.

HDL (high-density lipoproteins) Lipid-carrying serum proteins associated with a relatively low risk of cholesterol deposition in arteries.

heartburn Burning pain in the epigastrium or chest due to digestive disorders. Also called *pyrosis*.

heel-to-shin test With the patient standing straight, the heel of one foot is placed against the shin of the opposing leg. Tests coordination.

HEENT Abbreviation for *head, eyes, ears, nose, and throat*. If dictated, does not need to be expanded.

Hegar sign Softening of the cervix in early pregnancy, as palpated on pelvic examination.

Helicobacter pylori (*H. pylori*) A curved or spiral gram-negative bacillus, the causative agent of most peptic ulcers.

hematemesis Vomiting blood.

hematochezia Passage of blood from the rectum.

hemicolectomy Surgical excision of approximately half the colon.

hemilaminectomy Excision of part of a vertebral lamina.

Hemoccult test For occult blood in the stool.

hemoglobin A1c (Hgb A1c, HbA1c, glycated hemoglobin) Hemoglobin in red blood cells that has united chemically with plasma glucose. The concentration of hemoglobin A1c reflects plasma glucose levels during the preceding several weeks and so serves as a measure of long-term glucose control in diabetes mellitus.

hemoptysis Coughing up blood from respiratory passages.

hemorrhoidectomy Surgical excision of hemorrhoids (anal varicose veins).

hepatocyte A cell of the liver parenchyma.

hepatojugular reflux Bulging of jugular veins when the liver is compressed because of increased pressure in the venous system. Note: *Not* reflex.

hepatorrhaphy Suturing a ruptured or lacerated liver.

herniorrhaphy Surgical repair of a hernia (protrusion of organ or tissue through an abnormal opening).

hertz Abbreviated *Hz*, a measure of the frequency of a vibration, particularly one producing sound; equivalent to one cycle (or double vibration) per second. The normal human ear can detect sounds ranging in pitch from 20 to 20,000 Hz.

hesitancy Difficulty initiating the urinary flow.

Hgb, HGB Abbreviation for *hemoglobin*, the oxygen-carrying complex of iron and protein in red blood cells. The hemoglobin level is reduced in anemia.

histiocyte Any of various macrophages found in connective tissue, including Kupffer cells in the liver, osteoclasts in bone, alveolar macrophages in the lungs, and giant cells of chronic inflammation.

histrionic Referring to a style of speech and behavior in which the subject acts in an excessively dramatic fashion, as if performing on stage.

HLA (human leukocyte antigen) Patients with HLA-B27 antigen are genetically predisposed to acute anterior uveitis. HLA-A29 antigen is associated with posterior uveitis conditions such as birdshot retinochoroidopathy.

Holter monitoring A continuously recorded EKG as monitored by a portable EKG machine worn by the patient. This procedure is done on an outpatient basis for 24 hours to detect arrhythmias.

Homans sign Pain on passive dorsiflexion of the foot indicative of deep venous thrombosis.

hospitalist A physician who oversees the care of patients admitted to the hospital, works exclusively in a hospital, and does not have a private practice.

hyaloid membrane The vitreous membrane, a delicate boundary layer enveloping the vitreous body of the eye.

hydrocele A circumscribed collection of fluid, especially a collection of fluid in the serous membrane covering the front and sides of the testis and epididymis (tunica vaginalis testis) or along the spermatic cord.

hydrocelectomy Excision of a hydrocele.

hydrocephalus An increase in the volume of cerebrospinal fluid in the ventricular system of the brain, usually accompanied by an increase of pressure and eventually by reduction of brain substance.

hydronephrosis Distention of the renal pelvis due to filling of the ureters and renal pelves with urine under pressure.

hydroureter Distention of the renal pelvis due to filling of the ureters and renal pelves with urine under pressure.

hyperbilirubinemia High concentrations of bilirubin in the blood causing yellowing of the skin and mucous membranes (jaundice).

hyperchromatic and stratified nuclei Nuclei that are arranged in layers and stain more intensely than normal.

hyperemia Redness due to dilatation of superficial blood vessels.

hyperglycemia Elevated blood glucose.

hyperkalemia Elevation of serum potassium.

hyperplasia Abnormal increase in the number of cells in a tissue or organ.

hyperplastic polyposis syndrome An uncommon disorder characterized by the abnormal multiplication or increase in the number of normal cells in normal arrangement in tissue and occasionally associated with serrated adenomas or mixed polyps.

hyperresonance Accentuated breath sounds on auscultation due to a cavity within lung tissue or air in the pleural space.

hypesthesia Partial loss of sensation on one or more parts of the body surface.

hyphema Presence of blood in the anterior chamber.

hypoglycemia Low level of blood glucose.

hypokinesis Abnormal reduction of mobility or motility; reduced contractile movement in one or both cardiac ventricles.

hypopnea Very shallow breathing.

hypostatic Pertaining to, caused by, or associated with poor circulation of blood in a dependent body part or organ.

hypovolemia A significantly decreased volume of circulating blood, usually due to excessive blood loss.

hypoxemia Reduction of oxygen tension.

hysterosalpingogram A test to assess infertility in which radiopaque dye is injected into the uterus and fallopian tubes, and x-rays are taken to show if the tubes are patent (clear) or obstructed.

I&D (incision and drainage) A procedure used to open and drain an abscess that has not been responsive to conservative measures.

I&D (irrigation and debridement) A procedure in which an open wound or burn is bathed with a solution to achieve wound hydration, remove deep debris, and aid visual examination. Cellular debris and surface pathogens contained in wound exudates or residue are irrigated away. Dead, devitalized, or contaminated tissue can then be scraped away down to viable tissue to prevent infection and promote healing.

ICD codes International Classification of Diseases codes assigned to diagnoses and surgical procedures for purposes of reimbursement and other uses.

ileus Intestinal obstruction. See *adynamic ileus*.

impacted fracture Fracture commonly seen in children in which the broken ends of the bone are driven into each other. May also be called a *buckle fracture*.

impaction Plugging of an orifice with a dense mass of some material, as cerumen (earwax) in the external auditory meatus.

impingement Contact or pressure, generally abnormal, between two structures.

IMV (intermittent mandatory ventilation) The patient is allowed to breathe on their own but assisted by a ventilator; the ventilator takes over (this is the mandatory part) when patient effort is not sensed. Usually followed by a number, e.g., IMV of 5, which refers to the ventilator setting.

in situ (Latin, "in position") In its original or normal position; said of a malignancy that has not begun to extend or invade beyond its tissue of origin; e.g., carcinoma in situ.

in toto Totally or completely.

incontinence Involuntary passage of urine or stool.

incoordination Jerkiness and awkwardness in activities requiring smooth coordination of several muscles.

Indiclor (indium In 111 chloride) Used for radiolabeling of ProstaScint (capromab pendetide) in patients with prostate cancer.

infarction Death of tissue due to interruption of its blood supply.

infiltrate Diffusion of inflammatory fluid or exudate into air cavities of the lung, or their walls, producing cloudiness of lung tissue on chest x-ray.

injection (or injected) When pertaining to the eyes, injection refers to congestion or dilation of the visible vessels with blood. See also *hyperemia*.

inked Marked for orientation purposes with black ink, referring to a pathology specimen (examples of use: inked black; inked, sectioned, and submitted).

INR (international normalized ratio) A modification of the prothrombin time test in which the test result is multiplied by a constant established for the batch of thromboplastin reagent used.

intention tremor Tremor occurring only during voluntary movement.

intercondylar fracture Fracture of the humerus between its two condyles, the rounded prominences at the end of the humerus, in the shape of a T, also *T-shaped fracture*.

intercostal retractions Sucking in of muscles between ribs on inspiration.

IOL (intraocular lens) An artificial lens used to replace the native lens after cataract extraction.

internal fixation device Any appliance placed surgically in or on a bone to stabilize a fracture during healing.

interstitial markings The radiographic appearance of lung tissue, as opposed to the appearance of air contained in the lung.

interstitial tissue Aggregation of similarly specialized cells which together perform certain special functions; e.g., adenoid tissue, lymphoid tissue.

intertrochanteric fracture Fracture between the greater and lesser trochanters of the hip.

interval change Change in the radiographic appearance of a structure or lesion in the interval between two examinations.

intervals On EKGs, AH or A-H, PA or P-A, PR or P-R, ST or S-T, and QT or Q-T when coupled with interval are all acceptable. By convention, QRS interval is transcribed without hyphens, and AV (atrioventricular) interval is not hyphenated.

intima (tunica intima) The innermost layer or lining of an artery.

intraaxial Inside the brain. Intraaxial tumors are more likely to be gliomas, astrocytomas, or metastatic disease. Compare extraaxial.

intracorporeal lithotripsy The application of a shattering force directly to a stone by means of a device inserted endoscopically into the urinary tract. Electrohydraulic and pneumatic lithotripters function exactly like miniature jackhammers.

intradermal test The injection into the dermis of a chemical or other type of substance known to produce an allergic reaction in sensitive individuals. This creates a wheal which is outlined with a pen and/or measured. The area is examined again in 30 minutes. A reddened, enlarged area at the site of the injection indicates a positive allergic reaction to that chemical or allergen.

intravesical immunotherapy Instillation of an immunologic agent, often BCG, into the bladder for the treatment of superficial transitional cell carcinoma.

introitus The vestibule of the vagina, at the level of the labia minora, urethral meatus, and Bartholin glands.

intussusception Prolapse of one part of the intestine into another.

iodinated contrast medium A contrast medium containing iodine rather than a metallic salt; used in angiography, intravenous pyelography, oral cholecystography, and other studies.

IOL (intraocular lens) An artificial lens used to replace the native lens after cataract extraction.

irregularly irregular pulse An arrhythmia associated with atrial fibrillation; the pulse rate is irregular and the pulse amplitude varies.

ischemia Inadequate blood supply.

isoenzyme Any of a group of enzymes having similar chemical effects but differing in structure and often arising from different sources in the body. See CK, LDH.

isorhythmic dissociation A type of atrioventricular dissociation characterized by atria and ventricles beating at similar rates, although independently.

isthmus A narrow connection between two larger bodies or parts.

IUD (intrauterine device) A device placed in the uterus to prevent conception. Two types available in the U.S. are the copper Paragard and the hormonal Mirena.

IUP (intrauterine pregnancy) A normal pregnancy that develops within the uterus.

IVP (intravenous pyelogram) The delineation of the urinary tract (renal pelves, ureters, bladder, and urethra) by means of a contrast agent injected intravenously and then excreted by the kidneys. IVPs are performed for suspected urinary obstruction, bleeding from the urinary tract, or abdominal trauma, and can identify and localize renal calculi as well as tumors or cysts both within the urinary tract and adjacent to it. Also called *intravenous urogram* (IVU), *excretory urogram* (XU). Cf. *retrograde pyelogram.*

jaundice Discoloration of skin and sclerae by excessive bile pigment.

joint crepitus A grating sensation caused by the rubbing together of the dry synovial surfaces of joints.

joule (J) SI unit of electric power.

keloid A firm, nodular, irregular, often pigmented mass of fibrous tissue representing a hypertrophic scar.

KUB A plain radiograph of the kidneys, ureters, and urinary bladder. It need not be expanded.

kyphosis Forward hunching of the upper spine.

label To render a substance radioactive by incorporating a radionuclide in it; also, to cause a tissue or organ to take up radioactive material.

Lachman test Similar to the anterior drawer test, but performed with the patient's knee flexed only to 15-20°. Also used to evaluate anterior cruciate ligament stability.

lacrimal punctum (pl., **puncta**) A minute aperture in either eyelid at the inner canthus, through which tears pass into a nasolacrimal duct.

lacrimation Tearing.

lamina of vertebral arch Either of the pair of broad plates of bone flaring out from the pedicles of the vertebral arches and fusing together at the midline to complete the dorsal part of the arch and provide a base for the spinous process. L., *lamina arcus vertebrae.*

laminectomy Surgical cutting through the posterior arch of one or more vertebrae and removal of herniated disk material.

laminotomy Division of the lamina of a vertebra.

laparoscopy Inspection of abdominal cavity through an endoscope inserted through an incision in the abdominal wall. Minor surgical procedures can be performed through the instrument.

larynx The voice box, containing the vocal cords and situated between the laryngopharynx (the lowermost part of the throat) and the trachea (windpipe).

LDH Abbreviation for *lactic dehydrogenase*, an isoenzyme. LDH1 is found in heart muscle; levels are increased after myocardial infarction. LDH2 is normally found in higher amounts in the serum than is LDH1. When the level of LDH1 surpasses that of LDH2, this is called a "flipped LDH." *LDH* need not be translated in reports.

LDL (low-density lipoproteins) Lipid-carrying serum proteins associated with a relatively high risk of cholesterol deposition in arteries.

LE cell prep Lupus erythematosus cell test.

LEEP (loop electrosurgical excision procedure) Use of a thin low-voltage wire loop to remove cervical tissue for histological analysis as part of a colposcopy; it may be performed in a doctor's office or as an outpatient surgical procedure in a hospital or clinic.

left shift See *shift to the left.*

leukocytes White blood cells (WBCs), including neutrophils, eosinophils, basophils, lymphocytes, and monocytes.

leukomalacia Softening of the white matter of the brain.

LFTs (liver function tests).

LH (luteinizing hormone) A hormone produced by the anterior pituitary gland. In women it stimulates ovulation and formation of the corpus luteum, and in men it stimulates production of androgens in the testicle. Measurement of LH is part of the evaluation of a patient for infertility or gonadal dysfunction.

lid lag Slowness of upper eyelids to move with eye movements, noted in exophthalmos.

lipid Fat.

lipid profile A measure of the plasma concentrations of total cholesterol, high density lipoprotein cholesterol (HDL-C), low density lipoprotein cholesterol (LDL-C), and triglycerides.

lipoproteins, serum Serum proteins that bind and transport lipid materials including cholesterol.

livor mortis A purplish discoloration of the skin due to engorgement of capillaries that occurs shortly after death.

LMP (last menstrual period) Used in calculating EDC in pregnancy and also pertinent in menstrual disorders.

lobectomy Surgical removal of a lobe of the thyroid gland.

lobular Referring to tissue architecture characterized by division into circumscribed units (lobules).

lobulated Made up of or divided into lobules (small lobes).

loculated effusion A collection of fluid in a body cavity whose distribution is limited by adjacent normal or abnormal structures.

longitudinal lie The relation of the long axis of the fetus to that of the mother. In the longitudinal lie the fetal axis is parallel to mother's.

lues ("loo-eez") Syphilis.

Lugol solution An iodine-based staining solution. During a colposcopy, Lugol's is applied to the vagina and cervix. Normal tissue will stain, but tissue suspicious for cancer will not. Also called a *Schiller test*, so Schiller-positive indicates that the tissue did not stain, a seeming paradox.

lumbar Pertaining to the mid back.

lumen The hollow interior of a vessel or other tubular structure.

lumpectomy Surgical removal of a tumor from the breast rather than removing the entire breast.

lung biopsy Removal of tissue from the lung for microscopic examination and diagnosis. The technique may be percutaneous (needle biopsy), by transbronchial lavage (washing) through a fiberoptic bronchoscope, transthoracic (via needle or open procedure), or aspiration (through a needle). See *pleural biopsy*.

lytic (osteolytic) **lesion** A disease or abnormality resulting from or consisting of focal breakdown of bone, with reduction in density.

macule A flat patch or mark differing in color from surrounding skin.

malaise A vague sense of being unwell.

malar Pertaining to or situated on the cheeks.

marsupialization Surgical technique of cutting a slit into a cyst and suturing the edges of the slit to form a continuous surface from the exterior surface to the interior of the cyst. Sutured in this fashion, the cyst remains open and can drain freely. This technique is used to treat a cyst when a single draining would not be effective, and complete removal of the surrounding structure would not be desirable.

mass effect The radiographic appearance created by an abnormal mass in or adjacent to the area of study.

mass lesion Anything that occupies space within the body and is not normal tissue.

MB bands See **CK** (creatine kinase).

MCH (mean corpuscular hemoglobin) The average weight of hemoglobin per red blood cell, calculated from the hemoglobin level and the red blood cell count.

MCHC (mean corpuscular hemoglobin concentration) The average concentration of hemoglobin in red blood cells, calculated from the hemoglobin level and the hematocrit.

McMurray test or **sign** Extension of the knee from full flexion with the leg and foot externally rotated causes an audible or palpable snap in medial meniscus tear; extension with the leg and foot internally rotated causes a snap in lateral meniscus tear.

MCV (mean corpuscular volume) The average volume of a red blood cell, calculated from the hematocrit and the red blood cell count.

meconium Stool formed in the fetal intestine before birth.

melena Black stools (often due to the presence of blood).

menarche The onset of the first menstrual period.

menometrorrhagia Excessive menstrual bleeding occurring both during menses and at irregular intervals.

menopause The cessation of regular menstrual periods.

menorrhagia Regularly occurring menstrual flow that is excessive in volume and lasts longer than a normal menstrual period.

mesentery The fan-shaped membrane on the posterior (back) wall of the abdominal cavity that supports the ileum and jejunum.

metaplasia The presence of a type of mature cells that are not normal for the tissue in which they are found.

metastasis The spread of disease, especially malignant disease, to other sites in the body.

microdiskectomy Debulking of a herniated nucleus pulposus using an operating microscope or loupe for magnification. This procedure may be performed as a minimally invasive procedure using an arthroscope to access the site of herniation.

midline shift Displacement of a structure that is normally seen at or near the midline of the body, such as the pineal gland or the trachea.

miosis Sustained constriction of the pupil, which may be due to ocular or nervous system disease or to the effect of drugs (pilocarpine, morphine).

miscarriage Spontaneous abortion.

monos Brief form for *monocytes*.

MRI (magnetic resonance imaging) A method of obtaining cross-sectional "pictures" of the human body by computer manipulation of electronically acquired data. MRI is contraindicated when the patient has a medical device, such as a cardiac pacemaker. In such cases, a CT scan may be performed.

mucopus Mucus mixed with pus.

MUGA (multiple gated acquisition) **scan** Radiologic procedure in which a radioactive isotope is injected into the arteries with a subsequent scan showing uptake of the isotope by the heart. These radioactive emissions are electronically collected and analyzed by computer, resulting in a series of successive images all taken at the same point in the cardiac cycle. This test is used to assess heart size, shape, and function.

multi-echo images On MRI, a series of spin-echo images obtained with various pulse sequences.

multigravida A woman who has been pregnant more than once.

multipara A woman who has given birth more than once.

muscularis propria The muscular layer of a hollow or tubular organ, lying outside the submucosa.

mydriasis Sustained dilatation of the pupil, which may be due to ocular or nervous system disease or to the effect of drugs (atropine, cyclopentolate).

myelography Visualization of the spinal canal (the tubular enclosure of the spinal cord formed collectively by the vertebrae) with real-time fluoroscopy with contrast medium introduced into the subarachnoid space by lumbar puncture. The procedure may be followed by a CT scan to better define the anatomy and any abnormalities.

myoclonic seizures Repeated shocklike, often violent contractions in one or more muscle groups.

Myoview (technetium Tc 99m tetrofosmin) A cardiovascular imaging agent.

myringotomy A surgical procedure in which a tiny incision is created in the eardrum to relieve pressure caused by excessive build-up of fluid, or to drain pus from the middle ear.

myringotomy tubes (often called *ear tubes*) Small tubes that are surgically placed into a child's eardrum by an ear, nose, and throat surgeon. The tubes may be made of plastic, metal, or Teflon and are placed to help drain the fluid out of the middle ear in order to reduce the risk of ear infections.

nasal smear Examination of a stained smear of scrapings from the nasal mucosa for evidence of infection (neutrophilic leukocytes) or allergy (eosinophilic leukocytes).

nebulizer Any of various devices used to convert water, usually containing dissolved medicine (bronchodilator, surfactant), into a fine mist that can be inhaled into the respiratory tract through a mouthpiece.

needle biopsy A needle is passed through the skin directly into the organ to be studied, and an inner cutting needle slices and removes a core of tissue.

neoplasia The progressive multiplication of cells that results in the formation and growth of a tumor.

neoplasm New or abnormal growth, tumor. May be benign or malignant. Malignant neoplasms show anaplasia (loss of differentiation of cells) and are invasive and metastatic.

nephron The anatomic and functional unit formed by a glomerulus and its renal tubule.

nephroscopy A ureteroscope that is of sufficient length and maneuverability to reach the renal pelvis is called a nephroscope. Direct examination of the renal pelvis can provide information about hematuria, calculous disease, tumors, and other disorders of the kidney.

nerve conduction velocity (NCV) Measured by timing the passage of nerve impulses between a stimulating and a recording electrode, which are a precisely measured distance apart.

neutrophil, segmented A mature neutrophil with a segmented or lobulated nucleus. Also called *polymorphonuclear leukocytes* or *polys*.

neutrophilic cryptitis Microabscess formation in the crypts of Lieberkühn, a cardinal sign of ulcerative colitis.

nevus (1) A pigmented lesion of the skin. (2) A skin lesion present since birth (birthmark).

non-Hodgkin lymphoma Cancer of the lymphatic tissues other than Hodgkin's lymphoma.

nondisplaced fracture Fracture in which the break is partial or complete, but the alignment is maintained.

nonunion fracture Fracture in which the realigned bone fragments have failed to heal.

normocephalic Denoting a head whose size, shape, and appearance are normal. .

normochromic MCHC is in the normal range.

normocytic anemia Erythrocytes normal in size but decreased in number.

NST (nonstress test) A noninvasive (thus, nonstress) test to monitor the fetal heart rate during fetal movement and during contractions in labor by means of an external monitor placed around the mother's belly.

nuchal cord Occurs when the umbilical cord becomes wrapped around the fetal neck 360 degrees. Half of nuchal cords resolve before delivery.

nuchal rigidity Marked stiffness of the neck, a cardinal finding in meningitis.

nystagmus A rhythmic back-and-forth movement of the eyes usually due to congenital abnormality or central nervous system disease.

O&P (stool for ova and parasites) Examination of stool for parasites or their ova (eggs).

oblique fracture Fracture that is curved or slanting, neither transverse nor at an acute angle, caused by a rotational force.

obstipation Total inability to pass stool.

obstructive uropathy Disease or pathology of the urinary tract caused by obstruction.

oligohydramnios Less than the normal amount of amniotic fluid, defined as 500 mL or less at term and smaller amounts at earlier gestational ages. Too little amniotic fluid can cause severe fetal abnormalities, and the mortality rate is high.

Omnipaque (iohexol) An iodinated radiopaque contrast medium administered by an intrathecal route for myelography (lumbar, thoracic, cervical, total columnar) and in contrast enhancement for computerized tomography (myelography, cisternography, ventriculography).

Omniscan (gadodiamide) An intravenous enhancing agent for MRI examinations.

oophorectomy Surgical removal of an ovary.

open fracture Fracture in which the broken end of a bone pierces through the skin. It may recede back and be hidden, but leaves an open wound. This type of fracture is particularly ominous because of the risk of a deep bone infection. Also called *compound fracture*.

odontoid fracture Fracture of the odontoid process of the second cervical vertebra.

odontoid process A small, toothlike, upward projection from the second cervical vertebra around which the first vertebra rotates.

ophthalmoscopy See *funduscopic examination*.

OraQuick In-Home HIV test The first over-the-counter in-home HIV test kit approved by the FDA that does not need to be sent to a laboratory for analysis. An oral fluid sample is taken by swabbing the upper and lower gums and placed into a developer vial, and results are obtained within 20 to 40 minutes.

orchiectomy Removal of a testicle.

oriented in all spheres A standard phrase indicating that the subject is aware of time (date, day of week, season), person (identity of self and others), place (state, city, address), and situation (at home, at a relative's home, in a hospital).

ORIF (open reduction, internal fixation) A surgical procedure to correct a fracture that requires alignment and fixation with a plate, pin, or screw.

orthopnea Shortness of breath (dyspnea) relieved by assuming an upright position. Two-pillow orthopnea means the patient's shortness of breath is relieved when the upper body is supported on two pillows.

orthostatic hypotension Low blood pressure brought on by a sudden change in body position, most often when shifting from lying down to standing.

ossicles The small bones of the middle ear—the malleus (hammer), incus (anvil), and stapes (stirrup).

osteophytes, osteophyte formation Outgrowths of bone from the surface.

Oswestry Disability Index An assessment of functional impairment by chronic low back pain based on a self-administered questionnaire.

palliative Providing relief but not curative, for example, giving morphine to terminal cancer patients in doses necessary to relieve pain.

palpitation(s) Various abnormal sensations accompanying heartbeat: unduly rapid heartbeat; noticeably irregular beat; a feeling that some or all heartbeats are unusually strong; a sense of missed beats; or intermittent flip-flop sensations in the heart. Do not confuse with *palpation*.

panendoscopy Cystoscopy performed with an instrument that permits wide-angle viewing of the urinary bladder and urethra.

panlobular Affecting all parts of lobules with equal severity.

panretinal photocoagulation Use of a laser to destroy almost the entire retina to treat neovascularization, such as in diabetic retinopathy.

Pap (Papanicolaou) smear A vaginal speculum is inserted and cells detached from the vaginal walls, the squamo-columnar junction, and the endocervical canal by gentle scraping. Smears are stained by the Papanicolaou technique and screened, usually with computer assistance, for signs of cellular dysplasia or other abnormalities. Results are reported according to the Bethesda system.

papilledema Swelling of the optic disk, as observed with an ophthalmoscope; usually due to increased intracranial pressure ("choked disc") (caused by intracranial hemorrhage, neoplasm, or disturbance of cerebrospinal fluid circulation) or intrinsic eye disease (optic neuritis). The disk appears edematous and perhaps injected, and the retinal vessels as they emerge from the swollen disc appear to be kinked ("stepping" of vessels).

papule A small elevated zone of skin.

para Live birth.

paralysis Complete loss of muscular function.

paranoia (adj., **paranoid**) An abnormal mental state characterized by delusions, especially delusions of persecution.

parenchyma The physiologically active tissue of an organ, as opposed to its connective tissue stroma.

paresis Muscle weakness.

paresthesia A sense of tingling or prickling ("pins and needles") on a part of the body surface. The lay term "numbness" is applied indiscriminately to hypesthesia, anesthesia, and paresthesia.

paroxysmal Occurring in sudden attacks or seizures (paroxysms).

partial saturation technique A magnetic resonance technique in which single excitation pulses are delivered to tissue at intervals equal to or shorter than T1.

partial seizure Seizure in which only part of one cerebral cortex is involved.

patch test The application to the skin of a piece of filter paper containing a chemical or other type of substance known to produce an allergic reaction in sensitive individuals. Many patches are taped to the skin and labeled. After 24–48 hours the skin underneath is examined. A reddened, raised area of skin indicates sensitivity to the substance applied.

patent ("PAY-tent") (1) Open, unobstructed, usually referring to a tubular structure or normal opening, hole, or gap. (2) Apparent, evident.

pathologic reflexes Present only in neurological disorders, such as Babinski reflex or Chaddock reflex.

pathological fracture Fracture of a bone weakened due to disease such as osteomyelitis or other disease, not due to injury.

paucicellular Containing relatively few cells, referring especially to highly anaplastic (undifferentiated) forms of certain malignant neoplasms

PCP Abbreviation for *Pneumocystis pneumonia*, due to *Pneumocystis jiroveci* (formerly *P. carinii*).

PCP (primary care provider) The physician, usually a family practice or internal medicine specialist, who takes care of a patient's healthcare on a routine basis. The PCP may be an admitting or attending physician who has privileges at a hospital or other healthcare facility.

PEF (peak expiratory flow): the highest flow rate attained during forced expiration, measured in liters per second (L/sec).

pelvic relaxation Weakening of the pelvic floor muscles and ligaments, often a result of childbirth or aging and resulting in prolapse of the uterus or bladder.

peribronchial cuffing Thickening of bronchial walls by edema or fibrosis, as seen in asthma, emphysema, cardiac failure, and other acute and chronic respiratory and circulatory disorders.

pericarditis Inflammation of the pericardium, the membranous sac surrounding the heart.

perimetry A means of assessing peripheral vision by testing the subject's ability to discern moving objects or flashing lights at the extreme periphery of the visual fields.

perineal area The region between the thighs and containing the roots of the external genitalia; in males, it is the area between the scrotum and anus, in the female the area between the vulva and anus.

peripheral edema Swelling of the extremities due to fluid retention in the subcutaneous tissues.

peripheral iridotomy Puncture of the iris without the removal of iris tissue to decrease intraocular pressure in patients with angle-closure glaucoma. Standard surgical instruments or a laser may be used to make the puncture, allowing the aqueous to pass directly from the posterior chamber into the anterior chamber, bypassing the pupil. A laser peripheral iridotomy (LPI) uses a laser beam to selectively burn a hole through the iris near its base. Either an argon laser or Nd:YAG laser may be used.

peripheral neuropathy Damage to the nerves in the lower legs and hands as a result of diabetes mellitus. Symptoms include either extreme sensitivity or numbness and tingling.

peritomy An incision made completely around the periphery of the conjunctiva in surgical repair of a retinal detachment.

PET (positron emission tomography) **scan** A nuclear imaging study that yields color-coded two-dimensional images to assess the metabolic activity and physiologic function of organs and tissues rather than their anatomic structure; particularly useful in diagnosis of subtle cerebral and cardiac lesions. PET scanning of the brain with stereotactic surface projection has yielded 90% accuracy in the diagnosis and differentiation of Alzheimer and frontotemporal dementias. It has also proved useful in assessing parkinsonism, Huntington disease, epilepsy, neoplasms, and acute stroke.

petechia (pl., **petechiae**) A very small spot of hemorrhage under the surface of skin or mucous membrane, usually multiple, due to a local or systemic disorder.

PFTs (pulmonary function tests) To measure the rate and volume of gas exchange in the respiratory system by means of finely calibrated instruments.

pH A measure of alkalinity or acidity.

phacoemulsification Fragmentation of the lens of the eye with ultrasound.

phototherapy Light treatment is the process of using light to eliminate bilirubin in the blood of newborns. These light waves are absorbed by the baby's skin and blood and change bilirubin into products which can pass through their system. See also biliblanket.

pigmented histiocytes Black-tinged or melanin-laden histiocytes (macrophages).

pilonidal cyst, sinus, abscess A cyst that develops along the tailbone (coccyx) near the cleft of the buttocks, approximately 5 cm from the anus. These cysts usually contain hair and skin debris.

pit A small depression in the skin resulting from local atrophy or scarring after trauma or inflammation.

pitting edema Edema that retains the mark of the examiner's fingers after release of pressure.

pivot shift test With the patient supine, the foot is held in the physician's hand. The physician then turns the foot inward while pushing on the outside of the knee with the opposite hand, at the same time flexing and extending the patient's leg. This test is also used to evaluate anterior cruciate ligament stability.

plain film A radiographic study performed without contrast medium.

plantar (not planter) Pertaining to the sole of the foot.

plantar flexion Bending downward of the hand or foot.

platelets Noncellular formed elements in circulating blood, produced in bone marrow and active in blood coagulation. Also called *thrombocytes*.

pleura A delicate serous membrane protecting the lungs.

pleural biopsy A procedure to remove a sample of the tissue lining the lungs and the inside of the chest wall for microscopic examination and diagnosis. It may be done percutaneously (needle through the skin and chest wall) or by open technique. See *lung biopsy*.

pleural effusion An abnormal accumulation of fluid in the pleural cavity. Types of effusion include chylothorax (fluid from the intestine), hemothorax (blood), hydrothorax (serous fluid), and pyothorax or empyema (pus).

pleural friction rub A creaking, grating, or rubbing sound caused by friction between inflamed pleural surfaces during breathing.

pleuritic pain Sharply localized stabbing pain in the chest that is aggravated by taking a deep breath, and virtually abolished by breathholding. It typically results from irritation of the pleura due to pleurisy, pneumonia, pulmonary infarction, or chest wall injury.

PMI (point of maximal intensity) The point on the chest wall where the impulse of the beating heart is most distinctly felt by the examiner's fingers.

pneumatic retinopexy Fixation of the retina in its proper position with the injection of a bubble of gas into the interior of the eye in the vitreous cavity. With proper postoperative positioning, the retina can be pushed back into proper position and then the gas will spontaneously disappear in a few weeks. Gases used in this procedure may be either perfluoropropane (C3F8), sulfur hexafluoride (SF6), or perfluoroethane (C2F6).

pole of kidney The upper or lower extremity of a kidney.

polypectomy The surgical removal of outgrowths (polyps).

polys Brief form for *polymorphonuclear leukocytes*.

Pomeroy technique Used in tubal ligation.

portable film An x-ray picture taken with movable equipment at the bedside or in the emergency department or operating room when it is not feasible to move the patient to the radiology department.

portal Pertaining to the hilum or porta of the liver, or to the portal vein, which enters there.

portal triad Hepatic triad, the grouping of tributaries of the hepatic artery, the hepatic vein, and the bile duct at the angles of the lobules of the liver.

post Short for *postmortem examination*.

postcoital Occurring after sexual intercourse.

posterior colporrhaphy Repair of a posterior vaginal defect (rectocele). Typically, a transvaginal approach is used and incorporates a posterior colpoperineorrhaphy with plication of the levator ani muscle. The rectovaginal fascia is plicated in the midline and excess vaginal mucosa excised and repaired with absorbable sutures.

posterior drawer sign A test designed to detect instability of the posterior cruciate ligament.

posterior sulcus The groove formed by the intersection of the diaphragm and the posterior thoracic wall, as seen in a lateral chest x-ray.

postpartum Following childbirth.

postvoiding residual Urine remaining in the bladder, as detected by catheterization after the patient has voided.

PPD (purified protein derivative) A tuberculin skin test for tuberculosis. The abbreviation does not need to be expanded in medical reports. Also, Mantoux test, tine test.

precordial In front of the heart.

preeclampsia Abnormal development of high blood pressure that may be accompanied by proteinuria and edema, all due to toxemia during pregnancy.

presenting part The part of the fetus that is nearest to, or has entered, the birth canal. With a longitudinal lie this is either the head or the breech (buttocks).

probe Ultrasound transducer.

propofol A rapidly acting hypnotic used in the induction of general anesthesia and as procedural sedation for ophthalmic surgery.

proprioception Position sense.

ProstaScint (capromab pendetide, radiolabeled with indium In 111) A radiolabeled monoclonal antibody to prostate-specific membrane antigen, used to localize sites of soft tissue metastasis in prostate cancer patients.

prostatectomy Removal of the entire prostate gland.

proteinuria The abnormal presence of protein in the urine.

pruritus, pruritic Itching.

PSA (prostate specific antigen) A screening test that measures the amount of prostate specific antigen in the blood. High levels of PSA may indicate the presence of prostate cancer.

psyche A vague term roughly equivalent to "mind." Pronounced "SY-kee." Do not confuse with the slang term psych (psychiatry or psychology).

psychodrama A type of group therapy in which clients resolve conflicts and distressing emotional states by acting out their fantasies and fears in the setting of a dramatic performance before an audience of fellow clients.

psychosis A mental disorder in which, in addition to emotional distress, the patient experiences a break with reality, manifested by delusions, hallucinations, and grossly bizarre or socially inappropriate behavior.

PTCA (percutaneous transluminal coronary angioplasty) Procedure used to dilate an occluded artery, usually a coronary artery, by passing a catheter (with a deflated balloon section) to the site of the occlusion and inflating the balloon to compress the obstruction and enlarge the lumen of the vessel.

PT, pro time (prothrombin time) The time required for a clot to form in blood treated with certain reagents. The result, reported in seconds, is converted to an international normalized ratio (INR) by application of a factor established for the batch of thromboplastin used in the test. The prothrombin time is prolonged in deficiency of certain coagulation factors and after treatment with heparin or coumarin anticoagulants.

PT/PTT Prothrombin time and partial thromboplastin time.

PTT (partial thromboplastin time) The time required for a clot to form in blood treated with certain reagents. Abnormal prolongation of this time occurs in deficiency of various coagulation factors and after treatment with heparin.

ptosis (1) Drooping of an upper eyelid that cannot be fully corrected by voluntary effort. (2) Sagging of an organ or other structure, such as the breasts.

pulmonary vascular markings As seen on chest x-ray, the normal radiographic appearance of the branches of the pulmonary arteries and veins about the hila of the lungs.

pulmonary vascular redistribution Increased prominence of upper pulmonary vessels and reduced prominence of lower pulmonary vessels at the lung hila in left ventricular failure and other disturbances of circulatory dynamics.

pulse The heartbeat, and by extension the rate of heartbeat, as measured at the wrist (radial pulse), the cardiac apex (apical pulse), or elsewhere.

punch biopsy A cylindrical instrument used to obtain a plug of tissue for examination.

purulent Containing or consisting of pus.

pyuria The presence of pus or pus cells (neutrophils) in voided urine.

quadriceps exercises Repeatedly bringing the knee into full extension, with tensing of the muscles of the front of the thigh.

RA test Rheumatoid arthritis test.

radical In surgery, directed to the cause; directed to the root or source of a morbid process; it usually means removal of an entire organ or body part along with surrounding structures and sometimes lymph nodes.

radical mastectomy Removal of the entire breast as well as surrounding and underlying tissues and axillary lymph nodes as appropriate with certain types and stages of cancer.

radiculopathy A general term for disease of the nerve roots.

radioisotopes Radioisotopes are used as imaging agents in CT, MRI, PET, SPECT, and nuclear medicine stud-

ies. Transcribing them correctly can be a challenge. When typing nonproprietary (generic) isotope names, element symbols should be included with the name. It may appear to be redundant, but it is the correct form. Therefore, we would type sodium pertechnetate Tc 99m, iodohippurate sodium I 131, or sodium iodide I 125. Occasionally the physician may simply dictate isotopes such as Tc 99m, iodine 131 or I 131, or sodium iodide I 125, and unless a trademarked name is indicated, the element and number should be typed with a space, no hyphen, and no superscript (in healthcare documentation). Note that while the name of an element is written in lowercase (indium), the first letter of its symbol is in uppercase (In).

radiolucent Offering relatively little resistance to x-rays (by analogy with translucent).

radionuclide scans The essence of any radioactive scan procedure is the introduction into the body of a radioactive substance (radionuclides, isotopes) whose distribution in tissues, vessels, or cavities can be detected and recorded by a device that senses radiation. In some cases the choice of material is governed by the tendency of certain organs or tissues to take up (absorb, concentrate) certain elements or compounds. Radionuclides may be swallowed, inhaled, or injected into a body cavity or into the circulation. Scanning may be performed immediately after the material is administered (as in studies of blood flow) or after an interval (as when absorption or concentration of a substance in an organ must occur first).

radiopaque Resisting penetration by x-rays.

rale An irregular discontinuous sound, like bubbling fluid, crackling paper, or popping corn. Rales are heard on auscultation of the lungs and are due to passage of air through fluid—mucus, pus, edema fluid, or blood—or to the sudden expansion of small air passages that have been plugged or sealed by mucus.

rapid strep test (RST) The most rapid in-office test done by a clinician to test for streptococcal pharyngitis (strep throat), a group A streptococcal infection of the pharynx.

rasp, raspatory A surgical file.

RBCs (red blood cells) The most numerous cells of the blood, which carry oxygen from the lungs to the tissues, and carbon dioxide from the tissues to the lungs.

real-time examination Ultrasonographic examination performed by sweeping the ultrasound beam through the scan plane at a rapid rate, generating up to 30 images per second. The display of images at this frequency is in effect a motion picture, providing visualization of movement of internal structures as it actually occurs.

rebound tenderness Additional stab of pain when pressure on abdomen is released, often indicating peritoneal irritation.

recalcitrant (1) Stubborn, not responding as desired (said of an illness). (2) Defiant of authority or guidance (said of a child).

rectocele Bulging of the rectum through the posterior vaginal wall.

red blood cell count The number of red blood cells per cubic millimeter of blood, as counted by a technician using a microscope or by an electronic cell counter. The count may be reported either as a simple numeral (e.g., 5,300,000/mcL [microliter]) or as the product of a number less than ten and 10^6 (e.g., 5.3×10^6). The count may be dictated simply as 5.3 and may be so transcribed or may be expanded to 5,300,000.

red blood cell indices Measures of the volume and hemoglobin content of red blood cells, derived by calculating from the hemoglobin, hematocrit, and red blood cell count. The red cell indices are the MCV, MCH, and MCHC.

red reflex A luminous red appearance seen when a beam of light is projected into the eye onto the surface of the retina.

reflex A muscular contraction occurring in response to a sensory stimulus.

reflux The backward flow of urine within any part of the urinary tract.

refractile Transmitting light rays in the manner of glass or water, with deviation of rays as they pass into the surrounding air.

refractory Resistant to treatment; not responding to stimulus.

renal failure A severe decline in kidney function, with retention of urea, creatinine, potassium, and other substances normally excreted. Acute renal failure refers to abrupt onset.

renal hypertension The type of high blood pressure resulting directly from compromise of the circulation in at least one kidney.

resection Surgical removal.

respiratory distress Indicated by increased effort to breathe, pursing of lips, and use of accessory muscles of respiration.

resting tremor Tremor occurring only when the affected muscles are not being used for purposeful activity.

retinal detachment A separation of the retina from its supporting layers. Surgical treatment includes laser repair of tears or holes in the retina before detachment occurs, pneumatic retinopexy, scleral buckle, or vitrectomy.

retinitis Inflammation of the retina, the light-sensitive membrane at the back of the eyeball.

retrobulbar block A type of regional anesthetic nerve block in which a local anesthetic is injected into the area located behind the globe of the eye (the retrobulbar space) providing akinesia of the extraocular muscles and preventing movement of the globe. Sensory anesthesia of the cornea, uvea, and conjunctiva is also achieved by blocking the ciliary nerves.

retrograde pyelography, retrograde pyelogram Radiography of the kidneys, ureters, and bladder following the injection of a contrast medium backward through a urinary catheter into the ureters and the calyces of the pelves of the kidneys. Useful in locating urinary stones and obstructions.

rhabdomyolysis Rapid destruction of skeletal muscle tissue, associated with excretion of myoglobin in the urine. Myoglobin is harmful to the kidney and often causes kidney damage. Causes include excessive exercise, dehydration, severe burns, electrolyte imbalance, and medications.

RHDS (registered healthcare documentation specialist).

rhegmatogenous Arising from or caused by a tear, as in rhegmatogenous retinal detachment.

rheumatoid arthritis Chronic inflammatory disease of joints and synovial membranes leading to muscle atrophy and rarefaction of the bones and late-stage deformity and ankylosis, of unknown cause but thought to be autoimmune in origin.

rhinitis Inflammation of the nasal mucous membrane.

rotator cuff tear repair Re-attaching the tendon to the head of humerus (upper arm bone). A partial tear may need only a trimming or smoothing procedure called a debridement. A complete tear within the thickest part of the tendon is repaired by stitching the two sides back together.

RPR (rapid plasma reagin) Test for antibody to *Treponema pallidum*. Used in the diagnosis of syphilis.

RV (right ventricle).

salpingectomy Surgical removal of a uterine (fallopian) tube.

Salter-Harris fracture Fracture of the epiphyseal plate in children.

scab See *crust*.

scale A flake of epidermis shed from the skin surface.

scar See *cicatrix*.

scleral buckle procedure The most common procedure to treat a retinal detachment. A piece of silicone sponge, rubber, or semi-hard plastic is sewn onto the sclera of the eye, either over the area of detachment or encircling the eyeball like a ring, pushing the sclera toward the middle of the eye and relieving traction on the retina. Other procedures may be performed in conjunction with a scleral buckle to scar the retina and hold it in place until a seal forms between the retina and the choroid to keep the retina detachment from recurring.

sclerostomy Treatment of glaucoma by means of the surgical creation of an opening through the sclera.

sclerotomy Incision into the sclera.

scoliosis Lateral curvature of the spine.

sed rate See *erythrocyte sedimentation rate*.

segs An acceptable brief form for *segmented neutrophils*.

seizures Sudden, transitory impairment of central nervous system function, with or without loss of consciousness, and with or without local or generalized tonic and clonic contractions of voluntary muscles.

septoplasty A corrective surgical procedure to straighten the nasal septum, the partition between the two nasal cavities. Ideally, the septum should run down the center of the nose. When it deviates into one of the cavities, it narrows that cavity and impedes airflow. Often the inferior turbinate on the opposite side enlarges, which is termed compensatory hypertrophy. Deviations of the septum can lead to nasal obstruction.

septorhinoplasty A procedure similar to rhinoplasty, but it not only improves the appearance of the nose but removes any internal obstructions that may be blocking nasal breathing.

serial scans A series of scans made at regular intervals along one dimension of a body region.

serial sections Multiple slices of a specimen to provide a three-dimensional concept of a tissue or lesion.

serology Blood tests used to measure serum antibody titers in infectious disease and to detect antigens. Example: Serology was negative for syphilis, HBsAg, chlamydia, gonorrhea, and HIV. Also, *serologic test*.

serous cystadenoma A benign cystic tumor of the ovary.

serous effusion Noninfected fluid in the middle ear space; fluid behind the eardrum.

serous gland One producing a thin, watery secretion, not containing mucus.

serrate, serrated Having a sawlike edge.

sessile polyp A relatively flattened growth that is usually benign but can transform into a malignant growth.

seton A silk string or a rubber band used to help a fistula to drain.

shave biopsy A thin layer of skin consisting mostly or entirely of epidermis is removed with a blade held approximately parallel to the surface.

shift to the left An increase in the relative number of immature neutrophils, as detected in a differential white blood count. The various types of cells were formerly recorded on forms arranged in columns, the more immature neutrophils being recorded at the extreme left of the form. Sometimes dictated as *left shift*.

shock (precordial) An abnormally strong thrust applied to the chest wall by the beating heart, as detected by the examiner's fingers.

shortness of breath Feeling out of breath; breathlessness; difficulty catching one's breath.

sickle cell (sickling) An abnormal red blood cell found in persons with sickle cell anemia; the cell assumes a sickle or crescent shape at reduced oxygen levels.

signal intensity The strength of the signal or stream of radiofrequency energy emitted by tissue after an MRI excitation pulse.

simple seizure No unconsciousness; local twitching or jerking; perception of flashing lights or other abnormal sensory phenomena.

sinus and conus A shortcut reference to the coronary sinus, a venous trunk that collects blood from the heart muscle and drains into the right atrium, and the conus arteriosus, a conical pouch in the right ventricle from which the pulmonary trunk arises.

sinusoid A thin-walled terminal capillary having little or no adventitia and often anastomosing with other sinusoids; found in the liver, adrenals, heart, parathyroid, parotid gland, spleen, and pancreas. As an adjective, *sinusoid* means resembling a sinus (a cavity, channel, or space).

situs solitus The normal position of organs.

skin graft, full-thickness A skin graft consisting of the epidermis and the full depth of the dermis.

skin graft, split-thickness A skin graft consisting of the epidermis and a portion of dermis, or a mucosal graft consisting of only a partial thickness of mucosa.

small bowel transit time The time required for swallowed contrast medium to pass through the small bowel and appear in the colon.

smear Material spread thinly over a microscopic slide.

smear and culture Microbiologic study of secretions or other materials from the cervix, vagina, urethra, rectum, or from superficial lesions, to identify causes of infection.

somatosensory evoked potential Waves recorded from the spinal cord or cerebral hemisphere after electrical stimulation or physiological activation of peripheral sensory fibers; analysis of deviations in latency or amplitude can detect or characterize lesions of the peripheral or sensory conduction pathways.

somatostatin A hormone that inhibits production and release of growth hormone.

sonogram See *ultrasound*.

sounds Clicking, popping, rubbing, grating.

spasm Sustained contraction, usually painful, of a muscle.

spasmodic torticollis Twisting of the neck and unnatural position of the head caused by spasms of neck muscles, particularly the sternocleidomastoid and trapezius muscles.

specific gravity The weight of a substance per unit of volume compared to pure water, which by definition has a specific gravity of 1.000. The specific gravity of urine (normally 1.001 to 1.030) is a rough measure of the amount of material dissolved in it.

SPECT (single-photon emission computed tomography) A form of nuclear imaging that uses computer software to generate two- and three-dimensional images from data gathered after injection of a physiologically active substance bound to a gamma-emitting radionuclide. Used to evaluate regional blood flow, assess disorders of the heart and lungs, and evaluate head injuries, seizure disorders, stroke, brain tumors, and dementia.

speculum An instrument for inspecting a body cavity or orifice, often equipped with a light source, a magnifying lens, or both.

spermatocele An abnormal sac (cyst) filled with milky or clear fluid that may contain sperm that develops in the epididymis. Generally painless and noncancerous but if a spermatocele grows large enough to cause discomfort, surgery can be performed.

sphincter A muscular ring that constricts passage or closes an orifice, e.g., the lower esophageal sphincter (cardiac sphincter), the pyloric or prepyloric sphincter, cricopharyngeal sphincter, and anal sphincter.

spiculated Spiked, thorny.

spinal tap See *LP* (*lumbar puncture*).

spiral fracture Also called a torsion fracture in which the bones have been twisted apart by a rotational force. Often seen in cases of physical abuse.

spirometry The measurement of lung volumes and inspiratory and expiratory flow rates with a spirometer according to a standard testing protocol.

splint Flat nail that is placed across a fracture or osteotomy to hold it in place.

splitting Separation of the first or second heart sound, or both, into two distinctly audible components.

spondylolisthesis Forward displacement of one vertebra over another.

spondylosis (1) Ankylosis—immobility and consolidation of a joint due to disease, injury, or surgical procedure, or (2) degenerative spinal changes of the vertebrae, intervertebral disks, and surrounding ligaments and connective tissue due to osteoarthritis, sometimes accompanied by pain and paresthesias.

spontaneous abortion Miscarriage.

spontaneous ventilation Unaided natural ventilation or breathing, as opposed to mechanical or artificial ventilation.

spurring Formation of one or more jagged osteophytes, as in osteoarthritis.

sputum Phlegm from the respiratory passages. May be variously described as blood-streaked, bloody, clear, foul-tasting, frothy, gelatinous, green, purulent, putrid, ropy, rusty, viscid, viscous, watery, or yellow.

sputum smear and culture Microscopic examination of respiratory secretions for pathogenic organisms, neoplastic cells, or other abnormal findings.

station The position of the fetal presenting part with respect to the maternal ischial spines as labor progresses. Station minus two means that the presenting part lies 2 cm above the spines.

STD screen Sexually transmitted disease screen.

stellate Star-shaped.

stenosis An abnormal narrowing in a blood vessel or other tubular organ or structure. The term *coarctation* is synonymous, but is commonly used only in the context of aortic coarctation.

strabismus A general term for any condition in which the direction of gaze is different in the two eyes, as noted by an observer.

straight leg raising With the patient supine, the leg is elevated with the knee straight to the point where pain is experienced in the back or leg itself, or dorsiflexion of the foot causes an increase in pain. This test is done to determine if nerve root irritation such as sciatic nerve root compression is present. Also known as *Lasègue sign* or *test*.

strep screen Faster than a culture, but detecting only beta-hemolytic streptococci. *Strep* is an acceptable brief form for *streptococcus*.

stress fracture A crack in the cortex of a bone caused by repetitive stress, as in running, rather than by a single violent event.

stress incontinence Loss of urine when mechanical stress is placed on the bladder, as by coughing, laughing, sneezing, straining, or change in position.

STS (serologic test for syphilis) A general term referring to any test used to identify syphilis by a serologic method.

ST-T wave changes A customary abridgment of the phrase "ST segment and T-wave changes." The ST segment is the part of the EKG tracing extending from the S wave to the T wave. There is no "ST wave."

subcutaneous emphysema Air or gas in subcutaneous tissue.

submucous resection of inferior turbinates A surgical procedure in which the bone expanding the turbinates on the inside is shaved down, allowing for significant long-term reduction in the size of the turbinates. This procedure is often performed in conjunction with septoplasty when there is a deviated septum and nasal obstruction is significant.

suboptimal Not as good as might have been expected; usually referring to technical factors in an x-ray study, such as positioning, film quality, and patient cooperation.

suicidal ideation Thoughts of committing suicide as a relief from mental distress, without actual attempts at suicide.

superficial reflexes Muscle contractions in response to stroking the skin; those of the abdominal wall are tested as part of a complete neurologic examination.

syncope (fainting) Sudden loss of consciousness, usually transitory, due to circulatory or neurologic abnormality, including central nervous system intoxication or injury, but frequently the result of strong emotion in the absence of organic disease.

syndactyly Webbing of the fingers or toes, the most common congenital anomaly of the hands and feet.

tachyarrhythmia A pulse that is both irregular and abnormally rapid.

tachycardia Rapid heart rate (over 100/min).

tag Same as *label*.

TAH-BSO Total abdominal hysterectomy and bilateral salpingo-oophorectomy.

tail of breast A wedge-shaped mass of normal breast tissue extending toward the axilla.

takeoff of a vessel The origin of a branch from a larger vessel, as demonstrated radiographically with injected contrast medium.

tamponade Surgical compression by placement of a pack, a pad or plug made of cotton, sponge, or other material.

T&A (tonsillectomy and adenoidectomy) Surgical removal of the palatine tonsils and adenoids in the throat due to recurrent episodes of infection and chronic hypertrophy. Also called *adenotonsillectomy*.

tarsus A plate of connective tissue forming the framework of the eyelid. Also, *tarsal plate*.

TE (echo time) The interval between the first pulse in a spin echo examination and the appearance of the resulting echo.

TechneScan MDP (technetium Tc 99m medronate disodium) A bone imaging agent.

technetium (Tc 99m) A synthetic radioisotope with wide applications in nuclear imaging. In a HIDA (hepatobiliary iminodiacetic acid) scan, an intravenously administered technetium compound outlines the biliary tract more precisely than is possible with conventional radiology or ultrasound. Other technetium compounds are used in scanning the scrotum to diagnose testicular torsion and in performing bone and other scans to identify local areas of inflammation such as abscesses or zones of osteomyelitis.

tenesmus Straining at stool, usually without result and often painful.

Tenon capsule, membrane The sheath of the eyeball.

tension pneumothorax Accumulation of air or gas in the pleural space so that the pressure within the pleural space is greater than atmospheric pressure. This can result when the patient is on positive pressure ventilation or when the tissues around an open chest wound act as valves, allowing air to enter but not to escape. The resultant positive pressure in the cavity displaces the mediastinum to the opposite side, with consequent interference with respiration.

tenting of hemidiaphragm On PA chest x-ray, a distortion of the diaphragm by scarring, in which an up-pointing angular configuration (like a tent) replaces all or part of the normal curved contour of a hemidiaphragm.

thallous chloride T1 201 injection Used in myocardial perfusion imaging with either planar or SPECT techniques for the diagnosis and localization of myocardial infarction; with exercise stress testing as an adjunct to the diagnosis of ischemic heart disease (atherosclerotic coronary artery disease); in scintigraphic imaging of the myocardium to identify changes in perfusion induced by pharmacologic stress in patients with known or suspected coronary artery disease and who cannot exercise adequately; and localization of sites of parathyroid hyperactivity in patients with elevated serum calcium and parathyroid hormone levels.

third-party payer An insurance company, Medicare, Medicaid, etc., that will pay all or a portion of a patient's covered medical expenses.

thoracic Pertaining to the chest.

thoracoscopic wedge excision Resection of a small piece of lung that contains a suspicious nodule or known cancer with a margin of healthy tissue around it through a special videoscope. The procedure is usually done on patients whose lung function is such that a more invasive or extensive surgery would be contraindicated.

thrill An abnormal sensation felt by the examiner over the heart when blood jets through an anomalous or narrowed orifice.

thyroid function test (TFT) Blood test to measure the levels of thyroxine, triiodothyronine, and thyroid-stimulating hormone in the bloodstream to determine thyroid function.

thyroidectomy Surgical removal of the thyroid gland.

thyromegaly Enlarged thyroid gland.

tibial plateau The flattened surface at the upper end of the anterior aspect of the tibia.

tic A rapid involuntary muscle twitch, typically recurrent and stereotyped, affecting one or several body areas.

TIMI score (Thrombolysis In Myocardial Infarction) A risk-scoring system developed to categorize a patient's risk of death and ischemic events and provide a basis for therapeutic decision making. The lower the number (from 0 to 3), the more serious the flow limitation.

Tinel sign Shocklike pain when the volar aspect of the wrist is tapped; indicative of carpal tunnel syndrome.

titrate To adjust the dosage of a drug up or down to maintain maximum effectiveness or to reduce side effects.

TNTC (too numerous to count). This usually refers to a very large number of red blood cells or white blood cells seen on microscopic examination of urine. Because any number higher than 15–20 cells per high-power field indicates significant hematuria or pyuria, an exact count of 50 or more cells would provide no additional useful information. Doctors frequently dictate simply *TNTC*.

T1-weighted image On MRI, a spin-echo image generated by a pulse sequence using a short TR (0.6 seconds or less).

tongue tie (ankyloglossia) A condition in which the bottom of the tongue is attached to the floor of the mouth. This restricts a patient's ability to freely move the tip of the tongue. The surgical correction of the condition is called frenuloplasty.

tonic-clonic seizure In the tonic phase the victim becomes rigid, often cries out, loses consciousness, falls, stops breathing. In the clonic phase there is generalized muscular jerking; may bite tongue or lips, may be incontinent of urine or stool.

tonometry Determination of the pressure of the aqueous humor (intraocular pressure), to detect glaucoma. Tonometers of various types are used; one of the more common ones is the Schiøtz tonometer.

toxicology screen A panel of blood tests for toxic substances and drugs of abuse including alcohol, amphetamines, barbiturates, benzodiazepines, cannabinoids, cocaine, opiates, and others. Urine tests for some of these substances are also available. Screening may identify the cause of some cases of coma, delirium, or dementia.

TR (repetition time) On MRI, the interval between one spin echo pulse sequence and the next.

trabeculation Strands or bands of connective tissue sometimes extending from the capsule into the substance of an organ. Trabeculation of the bladder may be a secondary result of a bladder outlet obstruction due to hypertrophy and hyperplasia of the bladder muscle and the infiltration of the connective tissue.

trabeculectomy Surgical removal of a portion of the trabecular meshwork to create a fistula between the anterior chamber of the eye and the subconjunctival space to facilitate drainage of the aqueous humor in glaucoma.

transrectal Said of a diagnostic or surgical procedure that is performed through the rectum.

transrectal ultrasound (TRUS) An ultrasound procedure to examine the prostate gland for tumors that cannot be felt by a digital rectal exam, and to estimate the size of the prostate gland. In a prostate needle biopsy, it is used to guide the needle to the right part of the prostate gland.

transthoracic needle biopsy Excision of tissue for microscopic examination and diagnosis using a needle inserted through the skin and chest wall.

transurethral resection of bladder tumor (TURB, TURBT) A resectoscope is inserted through the urethra into the bladder, and tumors are resected by means of an electrical loop; usually performed in conjunction with a cystoscopy.

transurethral resection of the prostate (TUR, TURP) A resectoscope is inserted through the urethra and advanced to the level of the hyperplastic prostate. The surgeon then shaves away surplus prostatic tissue encroaching on the lumen of the urethra by means of an electrical loop, which also seals severed blood vessels. The instrument is equipped with an irrigating system that flushes away blood and tissue.

transverse fracture of the radius Complete fracture that is straight across the bone at right angles to the long axis of the bone.

treadmill stress test See *exercise stress test*.

Treitz, ligament of A fibromuscular band extending from the diaphragm to the small intestine at the site of transition from duodenum to jejunum.

tremor(s) Shaking of parts of the body supplied by voluntary muscles, principally the arms, forearms, and hands.

triglycerides, serum The level of fat in the serum, usually measured in the fasting state.

trimalleolar fracture Fracture of the medial and lateral malleoli and the posterior process of the tibia.

triple screen A panel of tests that includes AFP (alpha-fetoprotein), hCG (human chorionic gonadotropin), and uE3 (unconjugated estriol) obtained during the second trimester to evaluate for certain fetal abnormalities such as trisomy 21 (Down syndrome), trisomy 18 (Edwards syndrome), neural tube defect, spina bifida, or anencephaly. May be dictated as "tri screen."

troponins Troponins are the preferred tests for a suspected heart attack; they also help in evaluating the extent of heart injury and in distinguishing noncardiac chest pain. Troponin I and T are cardiac-specific whereas other tests such as the CK-MB or myoglobin are not.

Reference ranges: troponin I 0-0.1 ng/mL (onset: 4–6 hrs, peak: 12–24 hrs, return to normal: 4–7 days); troponin T 0–0.2 ng/mL (onset: 3–4 hrs, peak: 10–24 hrs, return to normal: 10–14 days).

TRUS (transrectal ultrasound) Examination to assess the size and configuration of the prostate gland.

T2-weighted image On MRI, a spin-echo image generated by a pulse sequence using a long TR (2.0 seconds or more).

tubal ligation Surgical division of the uterine (fallopian) tubes to obtain sterility.

tubo-ovarian abscess An abscess formed between a uterine tube (fallopian tube) and its adjacent ovary.

TUIP (transurethral incision of the prostate) Longitudinal incisions are made in the prostatic urethra without removal of any tissue.

TULIP (transurethral ultrasound-guided laser incision of the prostate) Resembles TUIP, but the incisions are made with a laser.

TUR Transurethral resection.

TURB, TURBT (transurethral resection of bladder tumor) A resectoscope is inserted through the urethra into the bladder, and tumors are resected by means of an electrical loop; usually performed in conjunction with a cystoscopy.

TURP (transurethral resection of the prostate) A resectoscope is inserted through the urethra and advanced to the level of the hyperplastic prostate. The surgeon then shaves away surplus prostatic tissue encroaching on the lumen of the urethra by means of an electrical loop, which also seals severed blood vessels. The instrument is equipped with an irrigating system that flushes away blood and tissue.

Tv (Vt) (tidal volume) The volume of air inhaled and exhaled during normal breathing, measured in liters (L).

tympanic membrane Same as *eardrum*.

tympanic membrane atelectasis A complication of chronic serous otitis media in which the middle ear contains a viscous fluid and the tympanic membrane (eardrum) has become thin, atrophic, retracted, and adherent to middle ear structures; there is usually conductive hearing loss.

tympanostomy Incision of the tympanic membrane with insertion of a tube for drainage.

tympanotomy Incision of the tympanic membrane. See *myringotomy*.

upper GI (UGI) series and **small-bowel follow-through** An upper GI series is done, and x-ray films are taken over a period of time to visualize the barium as it moves through the small bowel.

UPJ (ureteropelvic junction) The origin of the ureter from the renal pelvis.

uptake Absorption or concentration of a radionuclide by an organ or tissue.

ureteral stent A flexible tube placed within a ureter to maintain its patency .

urethroscopy A rigid urethroscope is a short tubular instrument designed to provide a view of the interior of the urethra. Used principally in examining the male urethra for prostatic enlargement or infection, urethral stricture (local narrowing due to scarring), varices, infectious lesions, and foreign bodies.

uric acid, serum A breakdown product of purine metabolism, increased in gout and other disorders.

urinalysis (UA) A group of standard laboratory examinations of the urine, including determination of pH and specific gravity, chemical testing for sugar, albumin, occult blood, leukocyte esterase, nitrite, acetone, and bilirubin, and microscopic examination for red and white blood cells, bacteria, casts, crystals, and other formed elements.

uterine descensus Prolapse of the uterus. Also called *descensus uteri*. In first-degree descensus, the cervix of the uterus is within the vaginal orifice; second-degree, the cervix is outside the orifice; and third-degree, the entire uterus is outside the orifice.

uterine sound A long flexible instrument with graduated measurements used for exploring the length and direction of the cervix and uterus. May be used as a verb, as in "The uterus was sounded to a depth of 8 cm."

UTI (urinary tract infection) Infection of the bladder or of one or both ureters or kidneys.

UVJ (ureterovesical junction) The point at which a ureter enters the urinary bladder.

vacuolated Describing cells that contain vacuoles.

vacuole A clear space or cavity within the cytoplasm of a cell.

variant Something that differs in some characteristic from the class to which it belongs.

vascular proliferation Growth of new blood vessels as part of an inflammatory or neoplastic process.

vasculitis Inflammation of blood vessels.

vasectomy Surgical division of the vas deferens in the male to effect sterility.

VDRL Venereal Disease Research Laboratory test for syphilis. Abbreviation does not need to be expanded.

vein stripping Surgical removal of (usually) the saphenous leg vein and its branches to treat varicose veins.

venipuncture Insertion of a needle into a vein for the purpose of removing blood for testing, or to inject fluids, medicines, or diagnostic materials.

venous stasis (ulcer, discoloration) Cessation or impairment of venous flow, initially causing skin discoloration but may lead to a skin ulcer.

ventricular ectopy Ventricular ectopic beats (VEB) are also called premature ventricular contractions (PVCs) as they may occur just before the normal beat of the ventricle. VEBs are easily seen on an electrocardiogram.

ventricular ejection fraction That portion of the total volume of blood in a ventricle that is ejected during ventricular contraction (systole); usually expressed as a percent rather than a fraction.

vertigo A subjective sense of spinning. Dysequilibrium and vertigo sometimes occur together, and both are indiscriminately referred to as dizziness by the laity.

vesicle A small thin-walled sac containing clear fluid. Do not confuse with *vesical*, meaning pertaining to the bladder.

villous adenoma See *adenoma*.

Virchow-Robin space An extension of the subarachnoid space between the pia and arachnoid membranes surrounding a blood vessel for a short distance after it enters the brain.

viscid Sticky, glutinous.

Visipaque (iodixanol) Injected intraarterially in digital subtraction angiography and indicated for angiocardiography (left ventriculography and selective coronary arteriography), peripheral arteriography, visceral arteriography, and cerebral arteriography. Administered by intravenous injection, it is used for contrast-enhanced computed tomography (CECT) imaging of the head and body, excretory urography, and peripheral venography.

visual field defect See *visual field testing*.

visual field testing Use of a black felt sheet or screen mounted on a wall to map areas of impaired or absent vision. An Amsler grid consists of a network of lines, usually white on black, around a central point at which the subject is instructed to gaze while the examiner moves a small object through various parts of the visual field to detect defects.

vitrectomy Surgical extraction of the contents of the vitreous chamber (vitreous humor, vitreous gel) of the eye. An anterior vitrectomy removes only a small amount of aqueous fluid from the front of the eye. A posterior or pars plana vitrectomy removes some or all of the fluid from the deeper portions of the eye.

VLDL Abbreviation for *very low-density lipoproteins*.

vulva The group of structures that make up the female external genitalia (labia majora, labia minora, clitoris, the vaginal orifice, and the urinary meatus).

WAIS (Wechsler Adult Intelligence Scale) A testing instrument designed to assess intellectual functioning in specific cognitive domains, including verbal comprehension and reasoning ability, and to provide a measure of general intellectual capacity. The current edition is WAIS-IV.

washout phase Scintigraphic scanning of the lungs at the conclusion of the inhalation phase of a lung scan, after an interval during which all inhaled radionuclide would be expected to have been exhaled.

water brash Heartburn with regurgitation into the mouth of fluid that may be sour or almost tasteless.

WBCs (white blood cells) See *leukocytes*.

wean To gradually discontinue or deprive, as in to wean off ventilation.

wet-field cautery Irrigation of the surgical field while applying cautery to achieve hemostasis. The Wet-Field coagulator is a trademarked device "designed to provide precise episcleral, intrascleral, and intraocular hemostasis with reduced peripheral tissue trauma" but wet-field is generally used in a generic sense.

wheezing Whistling sound made in breathing.

white blood cell count (white count, white cell count) The number of white blood cells per cubic millimeter of blood, as counted by a technician using a microscope or by an electronic cell counter. The count may be reported as either a simple numeral (e.g., $7,200/mm^3$ or mcL) or as the product of a small number and 10^3 (e.g., 7.2×10^3). In the latter case, the report may be dictated simply as 7.2 and may be so transcribed or may be expanded to 7,200.

x-ray To identify foreign bodies, masses, or abnormalities of the airway due to injury or disease.

Appendix C: Normal Laboratory Test Values

Tests Grouped by Panel or Profile	Normal Range (Metric)	
CBC (Complete Blood Count)		
hemoglobin (Hgb)	13.2–16.2 g/dL (Male)	12.0–15.2 g/dL (Female)
hematocrit (Hct)	40–52% (Male)	37–46% (Female)
RBC (red blood cell count)	4.3–6.2x10^6/mcL (Male)	3.8–5.5x10^6/mcL (Female)
WBC (white blood cell count)	4.1–10.9x10^3/mcL	
WBC differential		
polys (polymorphonuclear cells)	35-80%	
bands (immature polys)	0-10%	
lymphs (lymphocytes)	20-50%	
monos (monocyte)	2-12%	
eos (eosinophils)	0-7%	
basos (basophils)	0-2%	
platelet count	140-450x10^3/mcL	
RDW (red cell distribution width)		
coefficient of variation	11.5-14.5%; standard deviation 35-47 fL	
MCV (RBC mean cell volume)	82-102 fL (Male) 78-101 fL (Female)	
MCHC (mean cell Hgb concentration)	31-35 g/dL	
reticulocyte	0.5-1.5% (Adult)	
CMP (Complete Metabolic Profile)		
albumin	3.5-5.0 g/dL	
alkaline phosphatase	20-120 U/L	
ALT (alanine aminotransferase)	8-45 U/L	
AST (aspartate aminotransferase)	<35 U/L	
bilirubin, total	1.7-8.5 mcmol/L	
BUN (blood urea nitrogen)	5-20 mg/dL	
calcium	8.2-10.2 mg/dL	
carbon dioxide (CO_2)/bicarbonate	24-30 mEq/L	
chloride	100-106 mEq/L	
creatinine	0.6-1.2 mg/dL	
glucose	60-115 mg/dL	
potassium	3.5-5.0 mEq/L	
protein	6.0-8.3 g/dL	
sodium	136-145 mEq/L	
BMP (Basic Metabolic Profile; Electrolytes)		
calcium	8.2-10.2 mg/dL	
carbon dioxide (CO_2)/bicarbonate	24-30 mEq/L	
chloride	100-106 mEq/L	
creatinine	0.6-1.2 mg/dL	
glucose	60-115 mg/dL	
potassium	3.5-5.0 mEq/L	
sodium	136-145 mEq/L	
BUN (blood urea nitrogen)	5-20 mg/dL	

Tests Grouped by Panel or Profile Normal Range (Metric)

Renal (Kidney) Function Panel

albumin	3.5-5.0 g/dL
calcium	8.2-10.2 mg/dL
carbon dioxide (CO_2)/bicarbonate	24-30 mEq/L
chloride	100-106 mEq/L
creatinine	0.6-1.2 mg/dL
glucose	60-115 mg/dL
phosphorus	2.5-4.5 mg/dL
potassium	3.5-5.0 mEq/L
sodium	136-145 mEq/L
BUN (blood urea nitrogen)	5-20 mg/dL

Hepatic (Liver) Function Panel

albumin	3.5-5.0 g/dL
alkaline phosphatase	20-120 U/L
ALT (alanine aminotransferase)	8-45 U/L
AST (aspartate aminotransferase)	<35 U/L
bilirubin, direct	0.1–0.4 mg/dL
bilirubin, total	1.7-8.5 mg/dL
protein	6.0-8.3 g/dL

Lipid Panel

cholesterol, total	< 200 mg/dL
HDL (high-density lipoprotein) cholesterol	35–80 mg/dL
LDL (low-density lipoprotein) cholesterol, calculated	40–130 mg/dL
triglycerides	< 160 mg/dL

Thyroid Function Tests

T_3, total	60-181 ng/mL
T_4, free	0.8-1.5 ng/dL
T_4, total	5.5-12.3 ng/mL
TBG (thyroid binding globulin)	12-30 mg/L
thyroid stimulating hormone (TSH)	0.4-4.5 mcU/mL

Cardiac Panel

total CK	38-120 ng/mL	
CK-MB	0-3 ng/mL	
CK-index	0-3	
troponin	<0.4 ng/mL	
C-reactive protein	0-1.0 mg/dL	less than 10 mg/L (SI units)

Acute Hepatitis Panel

hepatitis A, IgM antibody	negative
hepatitis B core, IgM antibody	negative
hepatitis B surface antigen	negative
hepatitis C antibody	negative

Tests Grouped by Panel or Profile   Normal Range (Metric)

Coagulation Panel

prothrombin time (PT)	12-14 seconds
partial thromboplastin time (PTT)	18-28 seconds
fibrinogen	170-420 mg/dL

Iron Studies

total serum iron (TSI)	76-198 mcg/dL (Male) 26-170 mcg/dL (Female)
total iron-binding capacity (TIBC)	262-474 mcg/dL
transferrin	204-360 mg/dL
ferritin	18-250 ng/mL (Male) 12-160 ng/mL (Female)

Urinalysis

specific gravity	1.002-1.030
pH	5-7
protein	negative-trace
glucose	negative
ketone	negative
bilirubin	negative
blood	negative
nitrite	negative
leukocyte esterase	negative
urobilinogen	0.2-1.0 ehr u/dL
microscopic	
RBCs	0-2/hpf
WBCs	0-2/hpf
RBC casts	0/hpf

Arterial Blood Gases

pH	7.34-7.44
pCO_2	35-45 mmHg
pO_2	75-100 mmHg
HCO_3	22-26 mEq/L

CSF (Cerebrospinal Fluid)

glucose	50-80 mg/dL
protein	15-45 mg/dL
RBCs	0/mcL
WBCs	0-3/mcL

Stool

fat	< 5 g/day in patients on a 100 g fat diet
nitrogen	< 2 g/day
urobilinogen	40–280 mg/24 h 68–473 mg/24 h
weight	< 200 g/day

Tests Performed on Whole Blood, Plasma, or Serum

Note: Test results depend on methods used. Normal ranges and other interpretive data given in this book are intended solely for purposes of orientation and should not be applied to actual test results.

Analyte or Procedure	Normal Range (Metric)	Normal Range (SI)
acid phosphatase	< 0.6 U/L	< 0.6 U/L
ACTH (adrenocorticotropic hormone)	10–50 pg/mL	2.2–11.1 pmol/L
A/G (albumin/globulin) ratio	1.5–3.0	1.5–3.0
albumin	3.5–5.0 g/dL	35–50 g/L
aldolase	2.5 U/L	2.5 U/L
aldosterone, recumbent	3–16 ng/dL	0.08–0.44 nmol/L
upright	7–30 ng/dL	0.19–0.83 nmol/L
alkaline phosphatase (slang "alk phos")	20–120 U/L	20–120 U/L
alpha$_1$-antitrypsin (AAT)	100–300 mg/mL	20–60 mmol/L
alpha–fetoprotein (AFP)	< 15 ng/mL	< 15 mcg/L
ALT (alanine aminotransferase)	8–45 U/L	8–45 U/L
ammonia, serum	15–45 mcg/dL	11–32 mcmol/L
amylase	< 125 U/L	< 125 U/L
anion gap	12–20 mEq/L	12–20 mmol/L
AST (aspartate aminotransferase)	< 35 U/L	< 35 U/L
bands (banded neutrophils)	4–8%	4–8%
basophils (basos)	0–1%	0–1%
B cells	5–15%	5–15%
bicarbonate	24–30 mEq/L	24–30 mmol/L
bilirubin, direct	0.1–0.4 mg/dL	0.1–0.5 mg/dL
bilirubin, indirect	0.1–0.9 mg/dL	1.7–6.8 mcmol/L
bilirubin, total	1.7–8.5 mcmol/L	1.7–15.3 mcmol/L
bleeding time	< 4 minutes	< 4 minutes
BNP (brain natriuretic peptide)	< 50 pg/mL	< 50 ng/L
BUN (blood urea nitrogen)	5–20 mg/dL	1.8–7.1 mcmol/L
calcitonin, male	0–15 pg/mL	0–4.20 pmol/L
calcium	8.2–10.2 mg/dL	2–2.5 mmol/L
CD4 cell count	500–1500 cells/mm^3	0.5–1.5 x 10^9 cells/L
CEA (carcinoembryonic antigen)	< 2.5 ng/mL	< 2.5 mcg/L
chloride	100–106 mEq/L	100–106 mmol/L
cholesterol	< 200 mg/dL	< 520 mmol/L
cholinesterase (pseudocholinesterase)	8–18 U/L	8–18 U/L
clotting time, Lee–White	6–17 minutes	6–17 minutes
copper	0.7–1.5 mcg/mL	11–24 mmol/L
cortisol, 8 a.m.	5–23 mcg/dL	138–635 nmol/L
4 p.m.	3–16 mcg/dL	83–441 nmol/L
creatinine	0.6–1.2 mg/dL	50–100 mcmol/L
electrolytes: see individual values for sodium, potassium, chloride, and bicarbonate		
eosinophils (eos)	2–4%	2–4%
EPO (erythropoietin)	5–30 mcU/mL	5–30 U/L
erythrocyte sedimentation rate, Westergren	0–20 mm/hr	0–20 mm/hr
Wintrobe	0–15 mm/hr	0–15 mm/hr
estradiol	24–149 pg/m	90–550 pmol/L

Analyte or Procedure	Normal Range (Metric)	Normal Range (SI)
ferritin	20–200 ng/mL	20–200 mcg/L
fibrin degradation products (fibrin split products)	< 3 mcg/mL	< 3 mg/L
5-nucleotidase	< 12.5 U/L	< 12.5 U/L
free fatty acids (FFA)	8–20 mg/dL	0.2–0.7 mmol/L
free T_4 index	0.9–2.1 ng/dL	12–27 pmol/L
FSH (follicle-stimulating hormone), female	1.1–24 ng/mL	5.0–108 U/L
male	0.5–4.5 ng/mL	2.2–20.0 U/L
FSP (fibrin split products)	< 3 mcg/mL	< 3 mg/L
gastrin	21–125 pg/mL	10–59.3 pmol/L
GFR (glomerular filtration rate)	90–135 mL/min/1.73 m²	0.86–1.3 mL/sec/m²
GGT (gamma–glutamyl transpeptidase)	< 65 U/L	< 65 U/L
globulin, total	1.5–3.0 g/dL	15–30 g/L
glucagon	50–200 pg/mL	14–57 pmol/L
glucose	60–115 mg/dL	3.3–64 mmol/L
HDL (high density lipoprotein) cholesterol	35–80 mg/dL	1–2 mmol/L
hematocrit (Hct)	40–48%	40–48%
hemoglobin (Hgb)	12–16 g/dL	7.5–10 mmol/L
hemoglobin A_{1C} (glycosylated hemoglobin), normal	4–7%	4–7%
acceptable diabetic control	< 8%	< 8%
hexosaminidase A	2.5–9 U/L	2.5–9 U/L
homocysteine	< 1.6 mg/L	< 12 mcmol/L
insulin	5–25 mcU/mL	34–172 pmol/L
iron, males	50–160 mcg/dL	9.0–28.8 mcmol/L
females	45–144 mcg/dL	8.1–26 mcmol/L
iron–binding capacity	250–350 mcg/dL	45–63 mcmol/L
lactic acid	4.5–19.8 mg/dL	0.5–2.2 mmol/L
LDH (lactate dehydrogenase)	< 110 U/L	< 110 U/L
LDL (low density lipoprotein) cholesterol	40–130 mg/dL	1–3 mmol/L
leucine aminopeptidase, serum (SLAP)	< 40 U/L	< 40 U/L
LH (luteinizing hormone), females	0.5–2.7 mcg/mL	4.5–24.3 U/L
males	0.4–1.9 mcg/mL	3.6–17.1 U/L
lipase	< 1.5 U/L	< 1.5 U/L
lymphocytes (lymphs)	25–40%	25–40%
magnesium	1.5–2.3 mg/dL	0.6–1.0 mmol/L
MCH (mean corpuscular hemoglobin)	27–31 pg/cell	27–31 pg/cell
MCHC (mean corpuscular hemoglobin concentration)	32–36 g/dL	320–360 g/L
MCV (mean corpuscular volume)	82–92 mcm³	82–92 fL
melatonin, 8 a.m.	0.8–7.7 pg/mL	3.5–33 pmol/L
midnight	3.7–23.3 pg/mL	16–100 pmol/L
methemoglobin	< 3%	< 3%
monocytes (monos)	4–6%	4–6%
myeloid/erythroid ratio	2.0–4.0	2.0–4.0
myoglobin	14–51 mcg/L	0.8–2.9 mol/L
osmolality, serum	280–295 mOsm/kg	280–295 mOsm/kg
oxygen saturation (slang "O_2 sat")	95–100%	95–100%

Analyte or Procedure	Normal Range (Metric)	Normal Range (SI)
parathyroid hormone	11–54 pg/mL	1.2–56 pmol/L
pCO_2 (partial pressure of carbon dioxide)	35–45 torr	35–45 torr
pepsinogen	124–142 ng/mL	124–142 mcg/L
pH	7.35–7.45	7.35–7.45
phenylalanine	2–4 mg/dL	121–242 mcmol/L
phosphorus	2.5–4.5 mg/dL	0.8-1.5 mmol/L
platelets	150 000–400 000/mm³	150–400 x 10⁹/L
pO_2 (partial pressure of oxygen)	75–100 torr	75–100 torr
potassium	3.5–5.0 mEq/L	3.5–5.0 mmol/L
progesterone	0.1–28 ng/mL	0.3–89 nmol/L
prolactin (nonpregnant)	2.5–19 ng/mL	1.1–8.6 nmol/L
PSA (prostate specific antigen)	< 4 ng/mL	< 4 mcg/L
pseudocholinesterase (cholinesterase)	8–18 U/L	8–18 U/L
red blood cells (RBCs)	4,800,000–5,600,000/mm³	4.8–5.6 x 10¹²/L
red cell distribution width (RDW)	< 15%	< 15%
renin, reclining	0.2–2.3 ng/mL	1.6–4.3 ng/mL
upright	4.7–54.5 pmol/L	38–102 pmol/L
reticulocytes	0.5–1.5%	0.5–1.5%
sedimentation rate (sed rate)		
Westergren, male	0–15 mm/h	0–15 mm/h
Westergren, female	0–20 mm/h	0–20 mm/h
Wintrobe, male	< 10 mm/h	0–10 mm/h
Wintrobe, female	< 20 mm/h	< 20 mm/h
segmented neutrophils (segs)	40–70%	40–70%
SLAP (serum leucine aminopeptidase)	< 40 U/L	< 40 U/L
sodium	136–145 mEq/L	136–145 mmol/L
somatotropin, child	5–10 ng/mL	5–10 ng/mL
adult	232–465 pmol/L	232–465 pmol/L
T cells	55–65%	55–65%
testosterone, male	300–1200 ng/d	10.5–42 nmol/L
thyroxine (T_4 or T4)	4.5–12.0 mcg/dL	58–154 nmol/L
transferrin	250–430 mg/dL	2.5–4.3 g/L
triglycerides	< 160 mg/dL	< 1.80 mmol/L
TSH (thyroid stimulating hormone)	0.4–4.2 mcU/mL	0.4–4.2 mU/L
T_3 or T3	70–190 ng/dL	1.1–2.9 nmol/L
T_3 uptake	25–38%	0.25–0.38
2-hour postprandial glucose	< 140 mg/dL	< 7.7 mmol/L
uric acid	3.4–7 mg/dL	202–416 mcmol/L
vasopressin	2-12 pg/mL	1.85–11.1 pmol/L
white blood cells (WBCs)	5-10 x 10⁹/L	5000–10 000/mm³
zinc	0.75–1.4 mcg/mL	11.5–21.6 mcmol/L

Index

Note: Terms with *f* indicate figures.